The metric system is employed throughout this text, and the physician is strongly urged to use these measures exclusively for writing prescriptions. The following tables are included because on occasion they may prove useful. It is essential to ensure that there is no confusion between grams (ggm, Gm or G) and grains (gr).

Approximate Metric and Apothecaries' Equivalents of Household Measures

Household measure	Metric	Apothecaries'
1 drop	0.06–0.1 milliliter	1–1.5 minims
1 teaspoonful	5 milliliters	1 fluid dram
1 dessertspoonful	8 milliliters	2 fluid drams
1 tablespoonful	15 milliliters	0.5 fluid ounce
1 water glass	250 milliliters	8 fluid ounces

Approximate Metric and Apothecaries' Equivalents

Metric	Apothecaries'
1 milligram	1/60 grain
1 gram	15 grains
1 kilogram	2.20 pounds (avoirdupois)
1 milliliter	15 minims
1 liter	1 quart
1 liter	34 fluid ounces
1 grain	60 milligrams
1 dram	4 grams
1 ounce	30 grams
1 minim	0.06 milliliter
1 fluid dram	4 milliliters
1 fluid ounce	30 milliliters
1 pint	500 milliliters
1 quart	1000 milliliters

Apothecaries' System of Equivalent Weights and Measures

Weights

20 grains	1 scruple
60 grains	1 dram
480 grains (8 drams)	1 ounce troy
5760 grains (12 ounces)	1 pound troy

Measures

60 minims	1 fluid dram
480 minims (8 fluid drams)	1 fluid ounce
7680 minims (16 fluid ounces)	1 pint
32 fluid ounces	1 quart

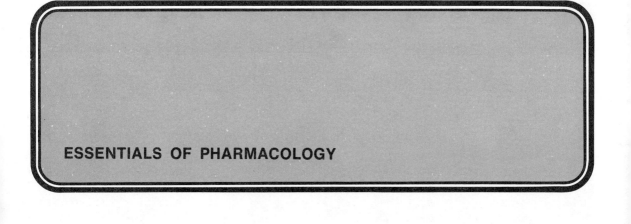

ESSENTIALS OF PHARMACOLOGY

EDITED BY

JOHN A. BEVAN B. SC., M.B., B.S

WITH 32 CONTRIBUTORS

ESSENTIALS OF PHARMACOLOGY

INTRODUCTION TO THE PRINCIPLES OF DRUG ACTION

SECOND EDITION

MEDICAL DEPARTMENT
HARPER & ROW, PUBLISHERS
HAGERSTOWN, MARYLAND
NEW YORK, SAN FRANCISCO, LONDON

The authors and publisher have exerted every effort to insure that drug selection and dosage set forth in this text are in accord with current recommendations and practice at the time of publication. However, in view of ongoing research, changes in government regulations, and the constant flow of information relating to drug therapy and drug reactions, the reader is urged to check the package insert for each drug for any change in indications and dosage and for added warnings and precautions. This is particularly important when the recommended agent is a new and/or infrequently employed drug.

Cover and text designed by Maria S. Karkucinski

Composed in Helvetica, linofilm by Progressive Typographers, York, Pa.
Printed by Quinn & Boden Company, Inc. Rahway, NJ

76 77 78 79 80 81   10 9 8 7 6 5 4 3 2 1

Essentials of Pharmacology: Introduction to the Principles of Drug Action,
Second Edition. Copyright © 1976 by Harper & Row,
Publishers, Inc. All rights reserved. No part of this book may be
used or reproduced in any manner whatsoever without written permission
except in the case of brief quotations embodied in critical articles
and reviews. Printed in the United States of America. For information
address Medical Department, Harper & Row, Publishers, Inc., 2350
Virginia Avenue, Hagerstown, Maryland 21740

Library of Congress Cataloging in Publication Data
Main entry under title:

Essentials of pharmacology.

Includes bibliographical references and index.
1. Pharmacology. I. Bevan, John A., 1930-
[DNLM: 1. Pharmacology. QV4 E78]
RM300.E84 1976   615'.1   75-40101
ISBN 0-06-140464-0

CONTENTS

I. GENERAL PHARMACOLOGY

II. SYSTEMATIC PHARMACOLOGY

DRUGS ACTING ON THE PERIPHERAL NERVOUS SYSTEM

DRUGS ACTING ON THE CENTRAL NERVOUS SYSTEM

DRUGS ACTING ON THE CARDIOVASCULAR SYSTEM

DRUGS ACTING ON THE GASTROINTESTINAL, RENAL, AND HEMATO-POIETIC SYSTEMS

HORMONES AND DRUGS MODIFYING ENDOCRINE ACTIVITY: AUTOCOIDS

CHEMOTHERAPY OF INFECTIONS AND NEOPLASIA

III   MISCELLANEOUS TOPICS AND REFERENCE MATERIAL

CONTRIBUTORS

ROBERT D. ANSEL, M.D.
Clinical Instructor, Department of Neurology, University of California, Los Angeles, School of
Medicine, Los Angeles, California
Chapter 31

JAY M. ARENA, B.S., M.D.
Director, Poison Control Center; Professor, Department of Pediatrics, Duke University School of
Medicine, Durham, North Carolina
Chapter 13

JOSEPH H. BECKERMAN, M.Sc., Pharm.D.
Lecturer, Department of Pharmacology, University of California, Los Angeles, School of Medicine,
Los Angeles, California
Chapters 12, 68, 78, 79

JOHN A. BEVAN, B.Sc., M.B., B.S.
Professor, Department of Pharmacology, University of California, Los Angeles, School of Medicine,
Los Angeles, California
Chapters 1, 14, 18, 19, 20, 32, 33, 35, 70, 71, 72, 80

MARGARET C. BOADLE-BIBER, B.Sc., D.Phil.
Assistant Professor, Department of Pharmacology, Yale University School of Medicine, New Haven,
Connecticut
Chapter 24

BENJAMIN S. BUNNEY, B.A., M.D.
Assistant Professor, Departments of Psychiatry and Pharmacology, Yale University School of
Medicine, New Haven, Connecticut
Chapter 25

ARTHUR K. CHO, Ph.D.
Professor, Department of Pharmacology, University of California, Los Angeles, School of
Medicine, Los Angeles, California
Chapters 2, 3

MARTIN J. CLINE, M.D.
Bowyer Professor of Medical Oncology, Department of Medicine, University of California, Los
Angeles, School of Medicine, Los Angeles, California
Chapter 67

WILLIAM L. DEWEY, B.S., M.S., Ph.D.
Associate Professor, Department of Pharmacology, Medical College of Virginia, Virginia
Commonwealth University, Richmond, Virginia
Chapter 29

MARK A. GOLDBERG, Ph.D., M.D.
Associate Professor, Departments of Neurology and Pharmacology, University of California, Los Angeles; Chief, Department of Neurology, Harbor General Hospital, Torrance, California
Chapter 30

LOUIS S. HARRIS, Ph.D.
Professor and Chairman, Department of Pharmacology, Medical College of Virginia, Virginia Commonwealth University, Richmond, Virginia
Chapter 29

CHARLES M. HASKELL, B.A., M.D.
Assistant Professor, Departments of Medicine and Surgery, University of California, Los Angeles, School of Medicine, Los Angeles, California
Chapter 67

LEO E. HOLLISTER, M.D.
Professor, Departments of Medicine and Psychiatry, Stanford University School of Medicine, Palo Alto, California
Chapter 9

DONALD J. JENDEN, M.B., B.S.
Professor and Chairman, Department of Pharmacology, University of California, Los Angeles, School of Medicine, Los Angeles, California
Chapter 5

JOHN E. JONES, A.A., B.S., M.D.
Dean and Professor of Medicine, West Virginia University School of Medicine, Morgantown, West Virginia
Chapters 41, 42, 43, 44, 45, 46, 47, 48

BENJAMIN M. KAGAN, M.D., F.A.A.P., F.A.C.P.
Director, Department of Pediatrics, Cedars-Sinai Medical Center; Professor and Vice Chairman, Department of Pediatrics, University of California, Los Angeles, School of Medicine, Los Angeles, California
Chapter 11

HAROLD KALANT, M.D., Ph.D.
Professor, Department of Pharmacology, University of Toronto Faculty of Medicine; Associate Research Director, Biological Studies Department, Addiction Research Foundation, Toronto, Ontario, Canada
Chapter 10

JOHN P. KANE, M.D., Ph.D.
Assistant Professor, Department of Medicine, Cardiovascular Research Institute, University of California, San Francisco, School of Medicine, San Francisco, California
Chapter 36

RONALD L. KATZ, M.D.
Professor and Chairman, Department of Anesthesiology, University of California, Los Angeles, School of Medicine, Los Angeles, California
Chapter 27

BERTRAM G. KATZUNG, M.D., Ph.D.
Professor, Department of Pharmacology, University of California, San Francisco, School of Medicine, San Francisco, California
Chapter 34

BERT N. LA DU, JR., M.D., Ph.D.
Professor and Chairman, Department of Pharmacology, University of Michigan Medical School, Ann Arbor, Michigan
Chapter 8

PETER LOMAX, M.D. D.Sc.

Professor, Department of Pharmacology, University of California, Los Angeles, School of Medicine, Los Angeles, California
Chapters 22, 38, 39, 40, 62, 69

CHARLES H. MARKHAM, M.D.

Professor, Department of Neurology, University of California, Los Angeles, School of Medicine, Los Angeles, California
Chapter 31

JORDAN D. MILLER, M.D.

Assistant Professor, Department of Anesthesiology, University of California, Los Angeles, School of Medicine, Los Angeles, California
Chapter 27

HAROLD E. PAULUS, M.D.

Associate Professor, Department of Medicine, University of California, Los Angeles, School of Medicine, Los Angeles, California
Chapters 6, 28

ROBERT H. ROTH, B.S., Ph.D.

Associate Professor, Departments of Pharmacology and Psychiatry, Yale University School of Medicine, New Haven, Connecticut
Chapters 23, 24, 25, 26

CHE SU, Ph.D.

Associate Professor, Department of Pharmacology, University of California, Los Angeles, School of Medicine, Los Angeles, California
Chapter 51

DERMOT B. TAYLOR, M.A., M.D.

Professor, Department of Pharmacology, University of California, Los Angeles, School of Medicine, Los Angeles, California
Chapter 21

JOHN A. THOMAS, B.S., M.A., Ph.D.

Assistant Dean and Professor, Department of Pharmacology, West Virginia University School of Medicine, Morgantown, West Virginia
Chapters 41, 42, 43, 44, 45, 46, 47, 48

JEREMY H. THOMPSON, M.D., F.R.C.P.I.

Professor, Department of Pharmacology, University of California, Los Angeles, School of Medicine, Los Angeles, California
Chapters 4, 7, 37, 49, 50, 52, 53, 54, 55, 56, 57, 58, 59, 60, 61, 63, 64, 65, 66, 73, 74, 75, 76, 77

JUDITH R. WALTERS, Ph.D.

Assistant Professor, Department of Psychiatry, Yale University School of Medicine, New Haven, Connecticut
Chapter 26

THOMAS C. WESTFALL, Ph.D.

Professor, Department of Pharmacology, University of Virginia School of Medicine, Charlottesville, Virginia
Chapters 15, 16, 17

PREFACE TO SECOND EDITION

For a perfect sight of the old medicine, let me conduct you to the bedside of Charles II: With a cry he fell. Dr. King, who, fortunately, happened to be present, bled him with a pocket knife. Fourteen physicians were quickly in attendance. They bled him more thoroughly; they scarified and cupped him; they shaved and blistered his head; they gave him an emetic, a clyster, and two pills. During the next eight days they "threw in" fifty-seven separate drugs; and towards the end, a cordial containing forty more. This availing nothing, they tried Goa stone, which was a calculus obtained from a species of Indian goat; and as a final remedy, the distillate of human skull.

Sir Andrew MacPhail
The Source of Modern Medicine, 1933

There is no doubt that the "new medicine" is different. Part of the progress is due to the adoption of a rational drug therapy based upon knowledge of the useful as well as the adverse effects of pharmacologic agents.

Many changes have been made in the second edition of this text. A number of new and distinguished authors have been added to the roster of contributors. The whole text has been revised, brought up to date and expanded, particularly into general pharmacology, the pharmacology of the peripheral and central nervous system and the endocrine glands, and anticancer agents. Completely new chapters have been added, including those on pharmacogenetics, drugs of abuse, poisons, alcohol, pediatric pharmacology and drugs used in the treatment of the hyperlipidemias. I would like to thank all those who made suggestions and gave advice on the reshaping of the contents.

As before, the text is designed primarily for medical and dental students although it would be of considerable value to those in the ancillary sciences of medicine, particularly pharmacy and optometry. Despite its modest increase in length it still remains a relatively short text, a distillate of essential pharmacologic knowledge, a sufficient core of knowledge upon which to base drug therapeutics of the new medicine. An understanding of its contents would be sufficient preparation for the National Boards in Pharmacology.

It is a pleasure to thank those to whom I am greatly indebted for their help in the preparation of this edition. The constructive critical review of various chapters by the following members of the Clinical Staff of the Center for Health Sciences, University of California, Los Angeles, is deeply appreciated: Victor D. Newcomer, M.D., Gary S. Rachelefsky, M.D., Ronald M. Reisner, M.D., Arthur D. Schwabe, M.D., Jerrold A. Turner, M.D., and Lowell S. Young, M.D. Dr. Jeremy H. Thompson has been a continual source of invaluable support, comment, and encouragement. Barbara Friedman has carefully drawn the new figures and helped remedy deficiences in existing ones: Nell Crewe has assisted with typing. The staff of the Medical Department of Harper & Row have redesigned the layout of the text. Partial support for compiling the index was obtained from Roerig Division of Pfizer Pharmaceuticals. Finally, my sincere thanks go to Elizabeth Ainley without whose constant, meticulous help and management of the whole revisionary process this edition would not have been possible.

Los Angeles, California   *J.A.B.*

PREFACE TO FIRST EDITION

This textbook is based upon the course in pharmacology for medical and dental students given by the staff of the Department of Pharmacology, The Center for the Health Sciences, University of California at Los Angeles. These students have completed their preclinical studies and are commencing their clinical work. The aim is to present an essential core of pharmacologic knowledge sufficient for those proceeding to clinical clerkships, specific enough to guide others during internship, and yet provide a grounding in basic principles for both that will be valuable during the balance of professional life.

The text has been written within the constraints imposed by a recently adopted shorter curriculum. It has been recognized that although all students should understand the principles of the various basic sciences, and for professional reasons must assimilate and retain an essential compendium of facts, much that has been committed to memory in the past need not have been. Often detailed factual knowledge of a subject has been acquired at the sacrifice of a thorough understanding of its principles. Only the latter will prepare the student to understand and make new claims, developments, and advances. The authors of this book have attempted to effect a compromise between an understanding of the principles of drug action and the pragmatic requirements of practice.

Events of the past few years have drawn the attention of both professional and layman to the price we seem to have to pay for our increasingly bountiful therapeutic cornucopia. New drugs can control and cure disease and make our lives longer and more pleasant. Unfortunately, they cause undesirable adverse reactions, interfere with important laboratory testing procedures, and by their very number, often make the choice of the best drug in any particular instance difficult or impossible. For these reasons the adverse effects of drugs have been given unusual emphasis throughout the book. Until agents with new actions or safer substitutes for those commonly used are found, we must learn to use those we have more circumspectly.

Since this book is designed as a teaching text for students, it is not claimed to be a complete exposition of the discipline, nor to be an *infallible* guide to the clinical indications, uses, limitations, adverse effects, and dosage of drugs. The practicing physician is urged to check the drug package insert and other sources before administration especially if the drug is fairly new or used infrequently.

Los Angeles, California   *J.A.B.*

FOREWORD TO FIRST EDITION

George Bernard Shaw sighed hopelessly but fondly for a world in which "the young *knew* and the old *could*." Similar difficulties beset the teacher and the student, the writer and the reader, and nowhere more poignantly than in pharmacology. Relatively few can keep abreast of this explosive field, and only they really know what there is for the student to learn. But it is difficult for these scholars to appreciate how vast and bewildering the territory to be covered appears to the student, and especially to the student who aspires to be a physician or a dentist rather than a pharmacologist. This great separation between the pharmacologist and the many students who depend upon him for guidance can be bridged best by teachers whose understanding of their students is no less than their comprehension of the subject. Understanding of this kind is developed most helpfully as a continuing cooperative effort, and this textbook is the result of such an effort at the UCLA School of Medicine.

Not all of pharmacology is included, for if it were, the result would be not a book but a library. Rather, the needs of medical and dental students have been sympathetically and carefully learned by the teachers, the better to enable them to condense, to select, and to organize the total material in such a way that it is a textbook for undergraduate students.

But the basic medical sciences are continually changing, and those of us who try to be students of pharmacology for a longer time will find this concise book a useful means of keeping abreast of new drugs and new knowledge of their mechanisms of action.

Sherman M. Mellinkoff, M.D.
Dean, School of Medicine,
The Center for the Health Sciences,
University of California, Los Angeles

PART I

GENERAL PHARMACOLOGY

JOHN A. BEVAN

1. INTRODUCTION AND GENERAL PRINCIPLES

SELECTIVE ACTIVITY

Pharmacology may be defined as the study of the **selective biologic activity** of chemical substances on living matter. A substance has biologic **activity** when in small doses, it initiates cellular and subcellular changes; it is **selective** when the response occurs in some cells and not others. Pharmacology is concerned with the nature of these selective changes, the systematization of the responses and the chemicals that cause them and the mechanism whereby these changes are brought about.

Many chemicals possess selective activity of value in the treatment of disease. Strictly speaking these are **drugs,** and their use is part of **therapeutics.** Historically, interest in drugs and their effects has been closely associated with medicine. Today, the need for new compounds with selective activity useful in combating disease is still the strongest and most compelling incentive to further investigative research. Although modern pharmacology is still closely associated with medicine, it depends heavily upon the basic physical, chemical and biologic sciences for theory and technique.

Selectivity of action may be manifest at different levels of biologic organization. For example, antibiotics act on one species but not another; general anesthetics act on one organ system but not another; morphine acts on one part of an organ but not another. Most commonly used drugs, with the major exception of antibiotics, are classified according to the organ system on which they exert their chief selective action. Provided the selective activity of a compound is of therapeutic value, the greater the degree of selectivity, the more valuable the drug.

DRUG–RECEPTOR INTERACTION

Since drugs, or selectively active substances, act on some cells and not on others, they must exert their effect at some specific site or system which is unique to or uniquely associated with the response. This component of the responsive cell is called a **receptor** and may be loosely defined as the site of attachment of a drug from which it exerts its selective action.

DRUG–RECEPTOR BINDING

The forces that govern the interaction between atoms and between molecules underlie the interactions between drugs and their receptors. Four types of bonds have been described. These are discussed below in order of their increasing strength, decreasing incidence in drug–receptor interaction and probably decreasing importance in determining selective biologic activity. It is assumed that the receptor is comparatively stable in form and that only the alteration of drug structure will affect pharmacologic selectivity and potency.

VAN DER WAALS' FORCES. These are weak binding forces which are ubiquitous. They operate between *any* atoms brought into close proximity. The force of attraction of these bonds is inversely proportional to the seventh power of the distance of separation of the atoms or molecules. When the drug and its receptor can come into close contact, these forces become highly significant. The larger and more specific the molecule, the greater is the contribution of these forces. They are the main reason why drugs react or bind at one site and not another.

HYDROGEN BONDS. Many hydrogen atoms on the surface of molecules possess a partial positive charge and can form bonds with negatively charged oxygen and nitrogen atoms. Since these act over greater distances than van der Waals' forces, close approach is not so important for their effect. These bonds together with van der Waals' forces represent the basis of most drug–receptor interaction.

IONIC BONDS. Such bonds form between ions of opposite charge, e.g., acetylcholine$^+$ and chloride$^-$. The importance can be clearly seen with such neuromuscular blocking agents as *d*-tubocurarine (Ch. 21). They act at very high velocity.

These three types of bonds dissociate reversibly at body temperature.

COVALENT BONDS. These bonds are formed when the same pair of electrons is shared by adjacent atoms and they are responsible for the cohesion of organic molecules. They are uncommon in pharmacology. Because of their strength and the difficulty of reversal or cleavage, drugs acting in this manner cause a prolonged effect. Chloroquine (Ch. 63), dibenzyline (Ch. 19) and the organophosphorus anticholinesterases (Ch. 16) form such bonds. Such compounds tend to be extremely toxic.

RECEPTORS AND ACCEPTORS

Certain biologic molecules, presumably because of their peculiar steric and physicochemical characteristics, bind with specific drugs. As a result of their location and cellular role, the perturbation that results from such binding leads to changes in cellular activity. These molecules are *receptors.* The relative strength of binding, the presence or absence of these molecules in the cell and the relative importance and role of these molecules in the special function of the cell forms to a great extent the basis of selective biologic action. A study of these factors, one of extreme difficulty and complexity, represents one of the most fundamental in pharmacology.

Receptors should be contrasted with the so-called **acceptors,** which are functionally silent sites of drug attachment in the body. Binding presumably takes place in a manner similar to that at receptors, but no selective biologic activity is initiated. Hence, the alternative names for acceptors—"silent receptors" and "sites of loss."

Some drugs react with receptors which are not distributed uniformly over the cell surface but are aggregated in discrete areas of the cell membrane. Perhaps the best example is *d*-tubo-curarine (Ch. 21), which exerts its effects at the synaptic junction between the motor nerves and voluntary muscle by reacting with receptors limited to the end–plate region of the muscle cell. This region represents 0.01–1.0% of the surface area of the cell. If the amount of drug effective at the end plate were evenly distributed one molecule thick over this specialized area, it would cover only 1% of its surface. Thus, *d*-tubocurarine paralyzes voluntary muscle by its reaction with receptors restricted to 0.0001–0.01% of the cell surface. Only a very small fraction of the *d*-tubocurarine injected into an animal is actually responsible for its selective biologic action. Much of the drug remains in the body fluids, and a considerable proportion reacts with the plasma proteins and acceptors in connective and other tissues. It follows, therefore, that sites of drug binding are not necessarily sites of pharmacologic action.

STRUCTURE–ACTIVITY RELATIONS

Drugs that exert the same or similar specific biologic activity usually exhibit similar chemical or physicochemical properties. A study of sympathomimetic amines (Ch. 18), voluntary muscle relaxants (Ch. 21) and muscarinic agents (Ch. 15) clearly illustrates this principle. However, very small changes of chemical structure can sometimes result in a dramatic loss or reduction of specific activity. For example, *l*-norepinephrine and *d*-norepinephrine are identical except that one is the mirror image of the other. Yet the *l*-form is 50 times more active than its isomer.

Such considerations led to the conclusion that the common denominators for selective activity among a given group of drugs are dictated by the chemical and physical characteristics of the receptor.

The term **affinity** is used to describe the propensity of a drug to bind at a given receptor site, and **intrinsic activity** describes its ability to initiate biologic activity as a result of that binding. Presumably because of the complexity of the binding process, a drug may possess affinity, i.e., be bound at a receptor site and yet not initiate specific activity, i.e., possess no intrinsic activity. This is not the same as binding at an acceptor, since other drugs may have affinity for the receptor and be intrinsically active, and still be inactive at an acceptor. A study of the relation between drug structure and selective activity will go a long way to reveal the nature and characteristics of the receptor site.

Our knowledge of receptors is entirely inferential, and in most instances, their location and nature are largely unknown. Currently a very considerable research effort is being made to isolate receptors. The receptors for the anticholinesterases (Ch. 16) and monoamine oxidase inhibitors (Ch. 24) are located on or are enzymes. Many drugs act on the same receptors as those via which physiologically important substances such as the neurotransmitters exert their effects. However, many other drugs seem to bear little resemblance to known cellular constituents, and the existence of receptors for these drugs must be assumed fortuitous.

Biochemical research has elaborated many of the cyclic and sequential series of chemical reactions which proceed to some final cellular event, whether it be a metabolic change, the shortening of contractile proteins or mitosis. In a number of instances, the precise site of influence of a drug on such reaction chains is known, as with penicillin (Ch. 55).

DRUG ANTAGONISM

The selective activity of many drugs may be specifically blocked or antagonized by other agents. For example, a drug such as *d*-tubocurarine that antagonizes the effect of acetylcholine at the end plate of the skeletal muscle cell (Ch. 21) does not antagonize at the same dose the other effects of acetylcholine nor those of histamine, serotonin or epinephrine. Frequently, the antagonism between a drug (agonist) and its selective or specific blocking agent (antagonist) occurs at the same receptor. Such an interaction is known as **pharmacologic antagonism.** Such specific blocking agents can be considered to have a high affinity for the receptor but have little or no intrinsic activity. Not infrequently they share some of the same required structural common denominators as their agonists. Many blocking molecules are more bulky than the molecules of the drugs they antagonize. We can but assume that they react with the receptors by virtue of the affinity characteristics they share with their agonists, but because of their more bulky form prevent access of agonist molecules to the receptor. Quantitative studies have demonstrated that agonist and antagonist molecules, which seem to have no direct influence on each other, when they compete for the same receptor obey physicochemical laws as we know them.

DOSE AND POTENCY

Individuals vary in their response to drugs even when an attempt is made to select as homogenous a group as possible. When an unselected group of individuals is studied, as is the case in most medical practice, the variation in drug effects is considerably greater. Thus the dose for one is not an appropriate dose for another.

It is reasonable to conclude that the factors governing the affinity and intrinsic activity of an agonist for the same type of receptor in any one individual show a variation of properties. Some receptors are more readily bound to the selectively active molecule than others and therefore react with the agonist at a lower concentration. If this is true, the greater the dose given, the greater the concentration of the drug in the region of the receptors, the greater the number of drug-receptor interactions and the greater the pharmacologic effect. A dose- or concentration-related effect is an attribute of drug action invariably seen in clinical practice except in those uncommon situations when a dose of a drug producing a maximum effect is administered.

Two chemically similar drugs that initiate the same selective activity probably do so by acting on the same population of receptors. If one is effective at a lower molar concentration than the other, it is said to be more *potent* than the other. If all other factors that influence the concentration of the drug in the region of the receptor (e.g., absorption, distribution, penetration, binding and metabolism) do not account for this difference in potency, it must be related to the relative affinity of two drugs for the same group of receptors.

The term potency is often used to express other ideas. For example, if one drug produces a greater maximum effect than another, irrespective of the dose used, it is often said to be more potent. It might be more correct to say that one drug can cause a greater particular effect. Alternatively, drugs are sometimes considered to be of similar potency if, when used in recommended doses, they cause similar effects. It might be best to consider the doses therapeutically equivalent in these circumstances.

Drugs of high potency are not necessarily the most valuable therapeutically. The best criterion of the relative value of drugs causing the same effect is selectivity. Obviously a drug of low potency and high selectivity is more desirable than one of high potency and low selective activity. This concept of selectivity is often fairly easy to measure objectively in the experimental animal (Ch. 5), but difficult in man. It depends upon measuring the ratio of the dose producing the desired effect to the dose causing significant adverse effects. The means used in man to measure this varies with each class of drug and is one of the important problems of the clinical pharmacologist. It is often referred to as the **therapeutic ratio.** This ratio varies very considerably from one drug to another. It is extremely high in the case of the antibiotic penicillin, usually considered to be a safe drug in patients who are not hypersensitive to it, and low with digitalis, an indispensable drug in the treatment of heart disease, but one that must be used with care.

ACCESSIBILITY

Selective activity may result from the accessibility to a given drug of some receptors, but not others. This is often the result of a diffusion barrier. For example, certain antibiotics used to sterilize the gastrointestinal tract appear to be specific in this effect, because when taken by mouth they are not absorbed. The same drugs administered systemically do not exhibit such specificity. Other drugs that have dramatic effects on the peripheral, but not the central, nervous system are denied access to the latter by the blood–brain barrier. Under certain experimental circumstances when the same drugs are tested in the absence of this barrier, their effect on the CNS becomes clearly apparent. Many barriers, such as the plasmalemma and lysosomal and mitochondrial membranes, can exist between the extracellular space and the sites of pharmacologic receptors. Such molecular characteristics as lipid solubility, molecular size, ionization constant, molecular shape and biologic stability influence the ability of a drug to reach its ultimate pharmacologic destination (Ch. 2). Access to some cells or parts of cells is sometimes made possible by special molecular transport systems.

QUANTITATIVE ASPECTS OF DRUG ACTION

The relationship between drug dose and effect is one of the most fundamental in pharmacology. In the whole animal, although the relationship between dose and effect often appears simple, this may well be fortuitous as the final drug induced change is influenced by a multitude of factors. For example, when epinephrine is injected intravenously (Ch. 18), the resultant changes in arterial pressure are the consequence of the effect of the drug on a variety of tissues, including the heart and blood vessels, some of which lead to a rise and others to a fall in arterial pressure. The measured effect is influenced by the drug distribution among various body compartments, its temporary storage in some sites, its metabolism and excretion and by the activity of homeostatic reflexes. Thus any experimentally determined relationship in the whole animal is unlikely to have fundamental significance.

Pharmacologists frequently employ simple, isolated preparations of tissues in vitro to determine basic drug effects. Such tissues, although isolated from the body, can be maintained in reasonably satisfactory condition for some time. Under these circumstances, the relationship between dose and effect is likely to be more meaningful, although there are many complicating factors. In Figure 1–1, a typical drug dose–response curve is shown. When response is plotted against dose or log dose, the curve is typically nearly symmetrical and S-shaped. Several features of this curve are important. A **threshold** dose can be recognized. Although difficult to define, since ability to measure threshold change varies with circumstances and, possibly, the observer, it is common experience that a certain amount of drug must be given before its effects are apparent. The magnitude of a drug's effect does not increase indefinitely. There is a dose, the **maximum** dose, which just elicits a

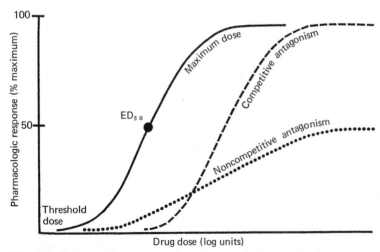

FIG. 1–1. Relationship between drug dose and pharmacologic response for an agonist drug and the effect on this relationship of a competitive and noncompetitive antagonist.

maximum response. Here again, the precision with which this dose can be determined is not very great. In contrast, the drug dose to produce a half maximum response or effect can usually be determined experimentally with some accuracy. This is the **effective dose**$_{50}$ (**ED**$_{50}$) and is a measure of drug potency. Finally, the slope of the dose–response curve provides an indication of the rate at which a drug's effect will change with dose.

The shape of a dose–response curve is similar to that obtained when the percentage of a large group of animals showing a particular drug effect is plotted against the dose of drug required to produce that effect (Ch. 5). In this latter case, the change is quantal (all or none), and thus the shape of the curve reflects the variation in sensitivity of the population of animals. It might be argued by analogy that the dose–response curve obtained from experiments on isolated tissues reflects the variation in sensitivity of individual cells that respond in an all or none fashion to the drug. This population of cells has a Gaussian distribution of sensitivity.

Various explanations have been advanced for the general shape of the drug dose–response curve. It is usually assumed that one drug molecule reacts with one receptor molecule and that the size of the response is related to the number of drug–receptor combinations. If the distribution of sensitivity of the receptors to a drug is normal or log normal, i.e., Gaussian, then the dose–response curve can be considered to be an integrated normal Gaussian curve. This is a symmetric S-shaped curve. Certainly many experimentally derived relationships can be adequately represented by such a relationship.

A. J. Clarke (1885–1941) was the first to apply laws of chemical mass action to the drug dose–response relationship. If a drug D combines with a receptor site R, the response would be proportional to the number of DR complexes

$$[D] + [R] \underset{K_2}{\overset{K_1}{\rightleftharpoons}} [DR] \overset{K_3}{\longrightarrow} \text{Response}$$

produced where K_1, K_2 and K_3 are rate constants.

The expected relationship derived from this function is a hyperbolic curve, which also adequately represents much experimentally derived biologic data. It is only at its extremes that this curve differs significantly from the integrated Gaussian curve, and it is here that pharmacologic measurement is inaccurate. This relationship is similar to that seen in classic Michaelis–Menten kinetics that describes the velocity of an enzyme reaction in relation to the concentration of substrate.

COMPETITIVE ANTAGONISM. A pharmacologic antagonist can have a variety of effects on the dose–response curve. If the antagonist reacts reversibly with the same receptors as the agonist, they will compete for occupation of the same receptor. Their relative effectiveness would depend on their relative affinity for the receptor and their concentration. A pharmacologic antagonist that acts in this manner would displace the dose–response curve to the right, without changing its shape, slope or maximum response (Fig. 1–1). Such an antagonism or blockade is said to be **competitive** or **surmountable** although the response to a particular dose of agonist is reduced or blocked by an antagonist, a higher dose of agonist could surmount this blocking action and be effective.

NONCOMPETITIVE ANTAGONISM. If an antagonist formed a more stable bond with its receptor, which was not displaced by a high concentration of agonist acting on the same receptor, the dose–response curve would be displaced to the right and its maximum and slope decreased (Fig. 1–1). Such a blockade is considered **non-competitive** or **unsurmountable.**

Should an antagonist cause this pattern of change in the dose–response curve, it does not necessarily imply that it is acting on the same receptor as the agonist. For example, it might act at some point between receptor activation and the final event responsible for effector response. With most drug effects, there are a series of chain reactions between receptor activation and response. These represent many possible sites of drug effect. Whether an agonist and antagonist react with the same receptor must be determined in a different type of experiment.

FURTHER READING

Albert A (1973): Selective Toxicity. (5th ed) New York, Halsted Press

Goldstein A et al. (1974): Principles of Drug Action. (2nd ed) New York, Wiley

ARTHUR K. CHO

2. DRUG ABSORPTION, DISTRIBUTION AND EXCRETION

The nonpharmacologic events that occur after drug administration are described in this chapter. A drug is absorbed into the blood stream, distributed throughout the body and then eliminated either by conversion to another compound or by excretion. These events are important in relation to the pharmacologic action of a drug because they determine the quantity of drug that reaches the site of action and length of time that it is available to exert pharmacologic action.

PROPERTIES OF ORGANIC MOLECULES

The movement of a drug throughout the body is determined by its **polarity** and **ionic** characteristics. The ionization of most drugs is the result of acid–base reactions of organic compounds. An organic acid is a weak electrolyte that can ionize to give a hydrogen ion and the conjugate base:

$$CH_3-COOH \rightleftharpoons CH_3-COO^{\ominus} + H^{\oplus}$$

Analogously, an organic base is a weak electrolyte that ionizes by accepting a proton:

$$CH_3-NH_2 + H_2O \rightleftharpoons CH_3NH_2^{\oplus} + OH^{\ominus}$$

When organic compounds are ionized, they are more soluble in aqueous solutions, and for this reason many drugs are administered as their ionized salt forms. For example, (Fig. 2–1), acetylsalicylic acid is usually administered as its sodium salt (I) and diphenhydramine, an organic base, is administered as its hydrochloride salt (II). In their neutral or unionized forms, these organic acids and bases are more soluble in lipid-like or fatty material, i.e., they are **lipophilic.**

The **polarity** of an organic molecule is a measure of its ability to dissolve in water and is determined by the number of polar groups (e.g., OH, NH$_2$, COOH) it contains. A compound like inositol (III) would be much more polar than cyclohexanol (IV). The polarity of a molecule also determines its partition between two immiscible solvents. Thus, the equilibrium concentration ratio (C) of compound III in a two-phase system consisting of an organic solvent and water would be much smaller than the corresponding ratio of compound IV, i.e.,

$$C = \frac{C_{III\,org}}{C_{III\,Aq}} \ll \frac{C_{IV\,org}}{C_{IV\,Aq}}$$

The polarity of a weak electrolyte is much greater in the ionized state, and this is the basis for its increased solubility in aqueous systems and reduced solubility in most organic solvents and lipids. The transfer of weak electrolytes from aqueous systems to lipid material, on the other hand is maximal when the electrolyte is in its neutral form.

THE PENETRATION OF MEMBRANES

The movement of a drug molecule throughout the body is dependent on its ability to pass through the membranes that separate the different tissue compartments. There are several mechanisms by which this is accomplished and the most common one is **passive diffusion.** In

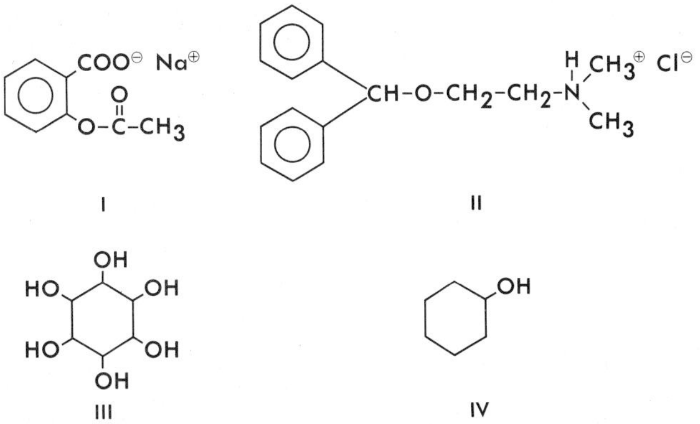

FIG. 2–1. Chemical structures.

diffusion the drug passes through the membrane by dissolving in it and moving across at a rate proportional to the concentration gradient along the direction of diffusion. In order to dissolve in the membrane which is lipid in character, the drug must be lipid soluble. Therefore, compounds that are neutral and nonpolar, e.g., the volatile anesthetics, diffuse through membranes much more readily than charged polar compounds, such as decamethonium.

Polar compounds, such as sugar and amino acids, that are physiological substrates penetrate membranes by a **carrier mediated process** in which the compound combines with a specific site at the outer surface of the cell membrane to form a complex which crosses the membrane. The complex is unstable on the inside of the membrane, so that the material transported is released and the carrier moves back across the membrane to bind another molecule which in turn is transported. There are different types of carrier mediated transport based on the energetics involved. In some cases the transport is by **facilitated diffusion,** where the movement driving force is the concentration gradient across the cell membrane. In other processes, the movement is in opposition to a thermodynamic gradient and energy is needed to maintain transport. This second process is called **active transport.** Drugs that enter cells by carrier mechanisms are usually similar in chemical structure to the normal carrier substrate so that they bind to the carrier.

Other polar, low molecular weight substances, i.e., water, ethyl alcohol and urea, are thought to penetrate membranes through pores or breaks in the bimolecular lipid layer. The entry of high molecular weight compounds, such as proteins and molecular aggregates, into cells is achieved by **pinocytosis,** in which the entire cell engulfs the material.

ABSORPTION, DISTRIBUTION AND EXCRETION OF DRUGS

Drugs are usually introduced into an organism at locations remote from their site of action, and unless the drug is given intravenously, it must enter the circulation. This total process is called **absorption.** Two key factors affecting the rate of absorption are the pH at the site of absorption and the route chosen for its administration.

EFFECT OF pH

When there is a substantial pH difference between the site of absorption and the blood such as exists between the stomach and the blood, the rate of absorption of weak electrolytes is altered markedly. For example, the gastric contents are usually quite acidic (ph ~ 1) so that the state of ionization of acids and bases in the stomach will be markedly different from that in the plasma (pH 7.4). If a weak electrolyte is introduced into either side of the membrane, it will diffuse across the membrane as the neutral nonpolar form and approach equilibrium (Fig. 2–2). The rate at which it will attain equilibrium or the rate at which the drug will move from one compartment to the other will depend on the concentration of the diffusable form. Thus conditions that favor the neutral form of the drug will enhance absorption and vice versa.

Using as an example an acid of pK_a − 5.0, the relationship at equilibrium is illustrated in Figure 2–2. The stomach and plasma can be regarded as two compartments separated by a membrane which can be penetrated only by the neutral, nonpolar form of the drug. At equilibrium the concentration of freely permeable or neutral form of the acid will be equal, but since the charged form of the acid cannot penetrate the membrane, two separate equilibria will be established on either side of the membrane. In the plasma compartment the relative concentration

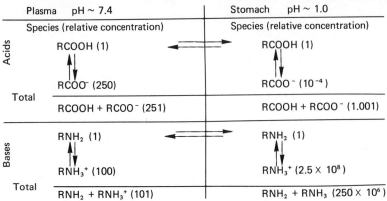

FIG. 2–2. The partition of weak electrolytes between plasma and stomach. The plasma and stomach compartments are separated by a barrier representing a membrane or a series of membranes. Only the neutral, nonpolar form of weak electrolytes can penetrate the barrier so that the equilibria indicated are established with only the neutral form at equal concentrations across the membrane barrier. The total drug in each compartment is given by the sum of neutral and ionized species.

of neutral to ionized form calculated from the Henderson Hasselbach equation is:

$$\text{Log } \frac{[A^-]}{[HA]} = pH - pK_a = 7.4 - 5 = 2.4$$

$$\frac{[A^-]}{[HA]} = \frac{250}{1}$$

The concentration of carboxylate anion is 250 times that of the free acid. In the high acidity of the stomach, the neutral form predominates and a concentration ratio of 1/10,000 results. The ratio of plasma to stomach concentration will be given by the ratio of the total amount of acid in each compartment which is 251:1.001 in favor of the plasma compartment. The analogous calculation for an organic base is also shown in Figure 2–2: the ratio of plasma/stomach concentration is $1:2.5 \times 10^6$. Thus basic compounds are extensively concentrated in the stomach because of its high acidity.

Because of the dynamic state of these compartments, the equilibrium described above and in Figure 2–2 is rarely attained. The important feature of this description is the role of ionization in the rate of absorption. When a drug such as salicylic acid is introduced into the stomach compartment, its rate of absorption is proportional to the concentration of the unionized form of the drug, which in this case is 99.999% of the total amount present in the stomach (Fig. 2–2). Essentially all of the drug is present as the diffusable form. In contrast, only 0.00000148% of a base such as amphetamine with a pK_a of 9.83 will be present in the stomach in the neutral, diffusable form. It follows that if the same quantity of the two drugs were introduced into the stomach, the rate of absorption of the weak acid would be substantially greater. The intestinal pH is estimated to be about 5.3 and in this environment, the rate of amphetamine absorption would be increased several hundred-fold.

ROUTES OF DRUG ADMINISTRATION

A drug can be introduced into an organism as a gas, in solution, as a suspension or as a solid. In the latter two states the rate at which the drug is dissolved or extracted into **biologic fluids** is a significant factor in the rate of absorption. Some drugs, e.g., the hormones are given as oil suspensions to decrease their rate of absorption. The role of the rate of dissolution of solid drugs in their absorption has been explained to us with nauseating frequency by the mass media. In some slow release forms (Ch. 77), the drug is incorporated into a bead of slowly dissolving material. The rate of absorption becomes dependent on the rate of solution of the bead matrix, usually a wax-like material.

The vascularity of the site of administration and the area of absorbing surface also influence the absorption rate. Drugs are absorbed much more rapidly from highly vascular areas, e.g., the lungs, than from subcutaneous sites.

The routes of drug administration used for systemic drug effects can be divided into two major groups, **enteral** (into the gastrointestinal tract) or **parenteral,** when the gastrointestinal tract is bypassed by injection or by introduction into the lungs. The oral route of administration is the most common in clinical practice as it is the most suitable for self-administration.

The mucous membranes of the oral cavity have a thin epithelium and are richly vascular. This is conducive to rapid absorption, and drugs can be prescribed for sublingual or buccal administration. One advantage of this route of administration is that once absorbed, the drug enters the general circulation without first passing through the liver. When absorbed from the stomach or intestines, the drug must pass through the hepatic portal system before entering the general circulation. Since the liver is the major site of drug metabolism (Ch. 3), a substantial amount of drug can be metabolized. Neutral and acidic drugs are readily absorbed from the stomach (see above). The gastric mucosa has an extensive blood supply and, as a consequence of its many folds, a large surface area. The low pH prevents significant absorption of basic drugs; they are absorbed more effectively from the oral cavity (pH $\sim$ 6.0) or the intestine (pH $\sim$ 5.0).

The physiologic role of the intestine is to absorb end products of food digestion. The large surface area, rich vascularity, near-neutral pH and the length of time spent in the intestine all promote the absorption. Drugs can also be introduced into the distal end of the gastrointestinal tract rectally.

When a drug is administered parentally it can be introduced directly into the circulation intraarterially or IV, into subcutaneous sites or into muscles (IM). Intravenous administration has the distinct advantages of speed, precision and complete absorption. However, IV injections can cause adverse cardiovascular effects such as hypotension and cardiac irregularities, and for this reason are usually made very slowly. Additional problems that result from intravascular injection and the high plasma concentration of drug that results, include anaphylactoid reactions, which are usually more severe because of the rapid and intense antigen-antibody reaction, and CNS effects, e.g., stimulation after procaine (Ch. 22).

The absorption of drugs from subcutaneous and IM sites is dependent upon local tissue vascularity and the ability of the drug to penetrate capillary membranes. This route of administration is especially important for drugs such as insulin and some penicillins that decompose in the gastrointestinal tract. Absorption from IM and subcutaneous sites is usually quite rapid. Modifications of the physical state of the drug have been used to decrease the rate of absorption from these sites. For example, steroid-containing pellets have been implanted subcutaneously, and drugs in an oily vehicle have been given by deep IM injection to form a depot. A more pharmacologic approach is to inject the drug with a small amount of epinephrine, a vasoconstrictor that reduces local blood flow at the site of administration (Ch. 18).

OTHER TECHNIQUES USED TO OBTAIN LOCAL DRUG EFFECTS. Direct intraarterial infusion is used to administer antineoplastic agents locally to a diseased area (Ch. 67). These compounds have a low therapeutic index and cannot be given systemically in doses that will selectively affect the malignant tissue. Local effects of antihistamines, antibiotics and antiinflammatory agents are obtained by direct administration to the desired area. A summary of the routes of drug administration is given in Table 2–1.

DISTRIBUTION

When a drug is absorbed into the circulation, it is distributed into all organs including those which are not relevant to its pharmacologic or therapeutic action. The relationship between these various "depots" of the drug and the free drug in plasma is shown in Figure 2–3. The drug can be reversibly associated with its site of action, with plasma proteins and with tissues not involved in its primary action. The two pathways of drug loss, excretion and metabolism will be considered later.

There are three major factors that control the entry of a drug into an organ and its retention: blood flow or perfusion rate, the ease of penetration of the organ and special cellular mechanisms for retention of the drug by the tissue. The wide range of perfusion rates for different organs are shown in Table 2–2, with kidney and lung as the most highly perfused tissues. Tissues that are highly perfused will tend to accumulate more drugs because they have a greater opportunity to equilibrate with plasma.

The ease of penetration of a drug into a given organ varies with the organ as well as with the drug. Certain tissues are less permeable than others. For example, the brain is separated from the general circulation by the **blood-brain barrier,** and an analogous barrier separates the fetal from the maternal circulation. In general lipophilic, neutral compounds will readily penetrate these tissue barriers and polar, charged compounds will not.

Many drugs accumulate within cells, i.e., their intracellular concentration becomes higher than their concentration in plasma or extracellular water. One of the reasons for this accumulation is the pH difference between the inside and outside of the cell. Most cells have intracellular pH values that are lower than 7.4, so that basic drugs would be expected to accumulate within

TABLE 2–1. Routes of Drug Administration

For local effects	For systemic effects
Topical (skin, mucous membranes)	IV
	IM
Oral	Subcutaneous
(of compounds active in the G.I. tract)	Intradermal
	Oral
Direct injection techniques	Rectal
(into specific tissues or into arteries supplying a specific tissue)	Inhalation

the cell. This has been demonstrated by a number of investigators. The stomach is a good example of an organ with this pH difference, and many basic drugs are concentrated in the acid stomach relative to the plasma after parenteral administration.

Alternatively, some drugs are localized in tissues by carrier systems. These drugs are frequently closely related to a physiologically occurring substrate and act as competitive substrates for the carrier. For example, the sympathomimetic amines, metaraminol and tyramine, are transported into the presynaptic adrenergic nerve ending by the carrier normally involved in the reuptake of *l*-norepinephrine. They are retained in this tissue in opposition to a concentration gradient that would predict much lower tissue levels.

The distribution of selected drugs is shown in Table 2–3. The data are expressed as tissue to plasma ratios, reflecting the extent to which the tissue accumulates the drug relative to plasma. Chlorpromazine, a highly lipophilic substance can be contrasted with methylatropine, a highly polar hydrophilic, quaternary amine. Meperidine, a narcotic analgesic, is intermediate in polarity.

Note that the highly perfused organs have higher tissue levels. Chlorpromazine is extensively concentrated in tissues, while antipyrine is distributed throughout body water, i.e., is not localized at all. The ionic compound, methylatropine, does not enter the brain, although it is accumulated in peripheral tissues in approximately the same tissue to plasma ratios as meperdine. The 0.2 tissue to plasma ratio of methylatropine for brain reflects the amount of material in cerebral vascular bed. This low level is a consequence of the blood–brain barrier.

THE BLOOD-BRAIN BARRIER

The endothelial cells of capillaries in muscle are separated by gap junctions that are 50–100 Å wide. These openings allow the passage of molecules into the extracellular space that are unable to diffuse through the membranes of the endothelial cell. In contrast, the endothelial cells of cerebral capillaries have much tighter junctions and indeed form an essentially continuous layer. This is the morphologic basis of the blood-brain barrier.

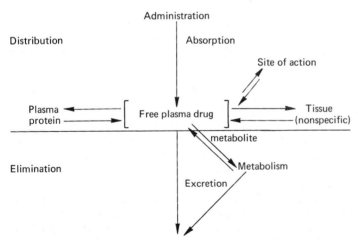

FIG. 2–3. Pathways of drug movement. After absorption drug in the plasma moves reversibly into the different compartments indicated. The two unidirectional processes are metabolism, where the drug is converted to another compound, and excretion, where the drug is removed from the body.

TABLE 2-2. Blood Perfusion Rates in Adult Humans

Organ	% of cardiac output	% of body weight	Perfusion rate (ml $\cdot$ min^{-1} $\cdot$ 100 g tissue^{-1})
Lungs	100	1.5	400
Kidney	20	0.5	350
Liver	24	2.8	85
Heart	4	0.5	84
Brain	12	2.0	55
Muscle	23	40.0	5
Skin	6	10.0	5
Adipose tissue	10	19.0	3

This barrier prevents or restricts the entry and exit of polar molecules so that permanently charged molecules like methylatropine do not readily enter the brain (Table 2-3), while lipid soluble compounds like meperidine and chlorpromazine are found at brain to plasma ratios approximating those of the lungs. For this reason most drugs that have effects on the CNS are nonpolar lipophilic compounds, while those whose action is primarily peripheral are generally polar or charged. For example, methylatropine is used as a peripheral anticholinergic, while its nonquaternary analog has been used to treat Parkinson's disease because it can enter the brain and exert central anticholinergic actions (Ch. 31).

The blood-brain barrier also prevents the passive entry of polar physiologic substrates such as sugars and amino acids. These substances must enter the brain by carrier mediated transport systems. One of these transport systems is utilized in the treatment of Parkinsonism. This disease can be ameliorated by increasing the brain concentration of dihydroxyphenylethylamine (dopamine). However, dopamine does not penetrate the blood-brain barrier so that its administration will have no effect on brain dopamine levels. The therapeutic solution is to administer L-dihydroxyphenylalanine (L-Dopa), an amino acid that can enter the brain by an existing carrier mechanism where it is converted to dopamine by a decarboxylase present in the brain.

THE PLACENTAL BARRIER

In the pregnant female, the maternal circulation is separated from the fetal circulation by several layers of fetal tissues in the placenta, resulting in a barrier that restricts the passive diffusion of compounds between the maternal and the fetal circulation. The substances that penetrate the placental barrier, like those that enter the CNS, are lipophilic nonpolar compounds. Thus it might be expected that obstetric anesthetics would also enter the fetus. Fortunately, however, there is a significant time delay in the equilibration between the two circulatory systems so that the high initial levels of CNS depressants found in the maternal blood are not immediately achieved in the fetus, and vigorous infants are delivered by mothers under anesthesia. However, if the anesthesia is prolonged 1 hr or more, and longer acting drugs such as meperidine have an opportunity to equilibrate, depression of the neonate can occur. The practical significance of these findings is that the protection afforded the fetus from drugs given to the mother is temporary, dependent on the rate of equilibration between the two circulatory systems. This rate of equilibration is, of course, dependent on the physical properties of the drug; e.g., highly lipophilic compounds such as thiopental (Ch. 26) can reach pharmacologically effective levels in fetal plasma within 7 min after administration to the mother.

TABLE 2-3. Localization of Drugs in Various Organs

Organ	Chlorpromazine*	Merperidine†	Antipyrine**	Methylatropine††
		(Concentrations relative to plasma)		
Brain	68.0	5.5	0.95	0.2
Heart	6.7	4.2	0.98	2.1
Lung	52.0	5.6	0.91	3.3
Liver	15.5	3.9	0.98	1.2
Kidney	23.0	4.9	1.04	0.6
Muscle	4.7	1.8	0.98	—
Plasma	1.0	1.0	1.0	1.0

*Salzman NP, and Brodie BB (1956): J Pharmacol Exp Ther 118:46
†Burns JJ et al. (1955): J Pharmacol Exp Ther 114:289
**Brodie BB et al. (1949): J Biol Chem 179:31
††Albanus L et al. (1969): Acta Pharmacol Toxicol 27:97

PLASMA PROTEIN BINDING

The plasma proteins affect the distribution of some drugs by forming a reversible drug protein complex. The complexed drug behaves like a macromolecule and as such does not equilibrate with other tissues nor interact with its site of action. The complex is not filtered through the glomerulus nor taken up by the liver so that the rate of removal of a drug is also reduced. Albumin is the plasma protein most frequently involved in this interaction, but globulins can also participate.

The binding of drugs and other small molecules by plasma proteins is a reversible process which in some cases has an extremely high affinity. The protein drug complex acts as a body depot, and, as free drug is eliminated from the plasma, an equivalent amount of bound drug dissociates. Certain hormones such as cortisone and thyroxin (Ch. 41) also bind with specific globulins in plasma so that low free plasma levels of the hormones are maintained with a readily available store. The drugs that bind with plasma proteins (Table 4–1, Ch. 4) are generally lipid soluble compounds of moderate molecular weight. Many of them bind to albumin at the same site. When more than one such drug is introduced into the plasma, a competition for binding sites occurs and the total amount of free drug increases. When this occurs, an increase in the pharmacologic response to each drug results. Perhaps the most often quoted example is the interaction between bilirubin, a toxic heme metabolite, and the sulfonamides (Ch. 11).

ADIPOSE TISSUE

Although adipose tissue has a high affinity for lipophilic drugs, it is poorly perfused so that the rate at which it equilibrates with plasma drug is slow. Once accumulated in the fat, however, this tissue acts as a reservior from which the drug is slowly released back into the circulation. The chlorinated insecticides, such as DDT, are highly lipophilic compounds to which individuals are exposed for long periods of time. The compound is slowly accumulated in the fat, and tissue to plasma ratios of 306:1 have been found in autopsy specimens.

VOLUME OF DISTRIBUTION

A quantitative estimate of the tissue localization of a drug may be obtained from its volume of distribution. The volume of distribution (V_d) of a drug is the volume in which it would have to be dissolved in order to give the plasma concentration obtained if no elimination occurred. It is thus a hypothetical number and is calculated from the total dose given (Q) and the extrapolated initial plasma concentration (C_o):

$$V_d(ml/kg) = \frac{Q(mg/kg)}{C_o(mg/l)}$$

The extrapolated initial plasma concentration is obtained experimentally from plots of plasma concentration versus time. When the plasma level of the drug decays with first order kinetics [log (C) versus time is a straight line], (Fig. 2–4), (C_o) can readily be extrapolated. It is obvious from the above equation that the lower the plasma concentration the larger the volume of distribution.

In Table 2–4, the volumes of distribution of some drugs and other compounds that are used to measure different body compartments are shown. The theoretic plasma concentration attained immediately after administration of 10 mg/kg of drug is also given. A difference of three orders of magnitude in the volume of distribution is observed. Highly lipid soluble compounds like meperidine and chlorpromazine have a large volume of distribution, while the polar, permanently charged molecules such as decamethonium have a much smaller V_d. Like methylatropine (Table 2–3), they do not penetrate tissues easily.

The volumes of distribution of reference compounds are given for comparison. Labeled albumin is retained in the plasma volume, whereas mannitol enters only extracellular space. The volume of distribution of labeled water is a measure of total body water. The volumes of distribution of the drugs shown can be compared to those of the reference compounds. Thus decamethonium is restricted to extracellular space, while chlorpromazine is highly localized in different tissues

TABLE 2–4. Volumes of Distribution of Various Drugs and Reference Compounds

	Volume of distribution (ml/kg body weight)	Theoretic plasma level after 10 mg/kg dose (μg/ml)
Reference compounds		
[131]I Albumin (plasma volume)	40	
Mannitol (extracellular volume)	200	
[3]H$_2$O (total body water)	600	
Drugs		
Decamethonium	180	55.0
Antipyrine	515	19.5
Clonidine	12,500	0.8
Meperidine	20,000	0.05
Chlorpromazine	100,000	0.01

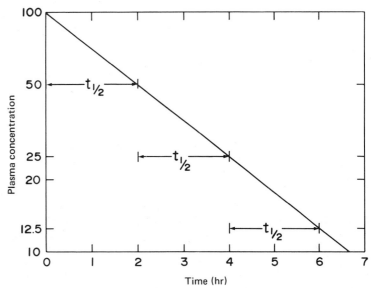

FIG. 2–4. First order decay. Graphic representation of a first order decay process. Note that the ordinate is a logarithmic scale. When plotted this way the time necessary for the plasma concentration to decrease by a half is constant.

so that a low plasma concentration results (Table 2–2).

The volume of distribution of a drug varies between individuals as well as with pathologic states, so that a given dose can give widely varying plasma concentrations in different patients. These differences should result in a wide range of responses to a given dose. In studies with the tricyclic antidepressent, nortriptyline, investigators found a tenfold difference in plasma level of the drug in a group of 25 patients given the same dosage where presumably the disease did not alter the volume of distribution. The therapeutic results were also variable but correlated with plasma levels; low levels were without effect and the high levels were sufficient to cause side effects. Other causes of individual differences in response to drugs are described in Chapter 8. Pathologic states can also alter the volume of distribution. When the pharmacokinetics of lidocaine, an antiarrhythmic agent, were examined in patients with heart failure, a significant decrease in volume of distribution was noted in comparison to patients with other cardiovascular problems. The result of this lower volume of distribution would be a raised plasma concentration which could account for the higher incidence of side effects from lidocaine in patients with heart failure. This change in volume of distribution is thought to be due to the decrease in perfusion rate resulting from the failing heart.

EXCRETION

RENAL EXCRETION

The most important route of drug excretion is through the kidney in the urine. Urine is formed from the plasma by the processes of glomerular filtration, absorption and secretion that are carried out in the nephron. Filtration is a physical process in which the blood is fractionated according to the molecular size of its components. Most drugs have molecular weights less than 500 and so are readily filtered unless bound to plasma proteins. The glomerular filtrate is acted upon by mechanisms in the proximal and distal tubules which involve removal from the filtrate of physiologically useful material such as inorganic ions, sugars, amino acids and water. In the proximal tubule glucose, amino acids and sodium ions are removed by carrier transport systems. Chloride ion is passively reabsorbed to maintain electrical neutrality, and water is absorbed to maintain the isotonicity of the urine. The proximal tubule wall also secretes substances into the ultrafiltrate from the peritubular capillaries. These include organic anions, e.g., salicylates and penicillins, and cations, such as the quaternary ammonium anticholinergics. The blood in the peritubular capillaries has ample opportunity to equilibrate with the glomerular filtrate so that nonpolar compounds can freely move back and forth.

As the ultrafiltrate or urine proceeds through Henle's loop, water and sodium ions are removed so that the contents become more concentrated in those components that are not removed by transport systems. The removal of water is 99% of that filtered so that the concentration of drug in the urine increases substantially as it proceeds through the nephron. This results in a concentration gradient of drug between plasma and urine in favor of the urine. If the drug can readily penetrate the membranes separating the two fluids, the drug will diffuse back into plasma along its concentration gradient. Lipophilic compounds are extensively reabsorbed by this mechanism.

When the drug is a weak electrolyte, its reabsorption is affected by the pH of the urine in the same way that pH differences control concentration gradients between stomach and plasma. The excretion of a basic drug will therefore be favored in acidic urine, whereas the excretion of an acidic drug will be favored by an alkaline urine. The pH of the urine can be acidic or alkaline depending on diet and drug treatment. For example, high doses of ascorbic acid decrease urine pH, while bicarbonate ingestion increases it. This effect is utilized in treatment of barbiturate overdose. The removal of barbiturates, being weak acids with pK_a values about 7.0, is facilitated by administering sodium bicarbonate to alkalinize the urine.

BILIARY EXCRETION

The liver secretes 0.5–1.0 liter of bile daily. Significant levels of organic compounds are present in this fluid. Many of the substances present in the bile are reabsorbed from the small intestine, but certain highly polar compounds are not and are excreted through the feces. There are three classes of materials present in bile: inorganic ions and sucrose present in concentrations equal to those in the plasma, proteins and phospholipids present in levels below those in plasma and organic compounds, molecular weight about 400, that are present in bile in concentrations 10–1000 times that of plasma. Most of the drugs excreted through the bile are in this latter category. These drugs usually contain large hydrocarbon radicals with a polar functional group and frequently are conjugates of drugs or their metabolites (Ch. 3).

The compounds of the third group are concentrated in the bile by transport processes; separate carriers for anions, cations and glycosides appear to exist in the liver. These systems are responsible for the biliary excretion of such drugs as the barbiturates (Ch. 26), the quaternary antimuscarinics (Ch. 17) and the cardiac glycosides (Ch. 33). Conjugates of other drugs such as the phenothiazines, morphine and steroids, are also excreted in significant amounts in the bile as these polar compounds are not readily reabsorbed through the intestines.

Other excretion routes of lesser importance include the breath, saliva, sweat and milk. The excretion of drugs into the fluids is largely dependent on passive diffusion and, for weak electrolytes, the pH difference between plasma and the secretion. The excretion of drugs in the milk becomes an important consideration in nursing mothers since the breast fed infant can receive the drugs taken by the mother (Ch. 75). Volatile anesthesics and other low molecular weight compounds that arise by degradation of drugs can be eliminated through the lungs.

PHARMACOKINETICS

The level of drug in any tissue is in a constant state of flux. As the drug moves from one compartment to another via the plasma and is being removed simultaneously from the body by metabolism or excretion. The quantitative interrelationships between these processes, the pharmacokinetics of a given drug, determine its dosage and control its duration of action. In the case of drugs acting reversibly, the concentration of a drug at its site of action is proportional to its free plasma concentration. As the free plasma level declines, the drug response should also decline. While there are a number of irreversibly acting drugs, most act reversibly, and a proportionality between plasma level and concentration at the site of action is assumed. Typical tissue level versus time curves for an IV administered drug are shown in Figure 2–5. The curve is biphasic with an initial steep and then a more gradual slope. In essence, the curve reflects two processes, distribution and elimination, that occur simultaneously after introduction of the drug into the circulation. The process of absorption in this case has been excluded by the route of administration. The initial decline in plasma level reflects the rapid distribution to and entry into tissues and a relatively constant rate of elimination. Once the plasma and most of the tissues have achieved a steady state, then the rate of decline decreases. The slope reflects mostly elimination by excretion and/or by metabolism to another compound. When the drug is administered orally, the rate of absorption becomes a significant rate limiting process, and a slow rise in plasma level is seen together with a slower decline. The peak plasma level is also lower. These

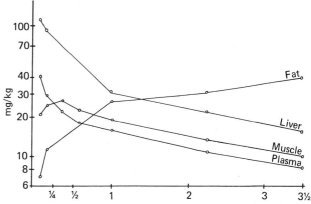

FIG. 2–5. Tissue levels of thiopental. Tissue concentrations of thiopental after an IV dose of 25 mg/kg to a dog. The ordinate is a logarithmic scale demonstrating the first order decline of the drug in liver, plasma and muscle 1 hr after injection. The level of the drug in fat tissue increases slowly because of the poor perfusion of the tissue and its high affinity for this lipophillic compound. The slower rise in muscle level also reflects poor perfusion compared to the liver. (Brodie BB et al. (1952): The role of body fat in limiting the duration of action of thiopental. J Pharmacol Exp Ther 105:422.)

curves can be used to obtain the volume of distribution and other relevant pharmacokinetic constants by computer techniques, but such manipulations are beyond the scope of this book (Wagner, 1971).

Even without sophisticated analysis, data on plasma levels versus time are useful in understanding the pharmacokinetics of drugs, and approximate values for some parameters can be obtained. For example, the initial distribution phase can be ignored approximately 1 hr after IV administration. After that time the plasma decay curve should reflect elimination and approximate a first order process. This means that the plasma decay curve in which log C plasma versus time are plotted should be a straight line (Fig. 2–4 and 2–5). Extrapolation of this line back to zero time gives a plasma concentration value from which an apparent volume of distribution can be calculated (see above).

Another pharmacokinetic parameter obtainable from this graph is the plasma half-life, the time necessary for the plasma concentration to decrease by half. The half-life is a constant for all first order processes such that it can be used in pharmacokinetics to predict the duration of action of a drug and determine the optimal dosing sequence necessary to maintain therapeutic drug levels.

The role of distribution and elimination in controlling the efficacy of a multiple dosage regimen is shown in Figure 2–6 in which a family of plasma decay curves is plotted and therapeutic range indicated. The object of the regimen is to maintain the level of drug within the therapeutic range. When one of parameters that affect this curve is altered however, plasma levels can change markedly. If, e.g., the rate of elimination is decreased from 50% by renal impairment or inhibition of metabolism, the plasma levels increase into the toxic range. Furthermore, since the plasma levels are also a function of the volume of distribution, a change in this parameter will also alter plasma levels (see Fig. 2–6). Drugs are usually used in a therapeutic regimen lasting several days. The object of this plan of administration is to obtain a steady state plasma level of drug that is neither toxic nor pharmacologically ineffective.

Pharmacokinetic parameters can be used to calculate the steady state plasma level (C) after prolonged administration utilizing the equation:

$$\overline{C} = \frac{F\,D}{V_d K T}$$

where D = dose, F = fraction of dose absorbed, V_d = volume of distribution, K = rate constant for elimination $\left(= \dfrac{0.693}{\text{half-life}} \right)$ and T is the dosage interval.

A drug given at a total dose of 50 mg three times a day, when $F = 1$, $V_d = 50$, $k = 0.11$ days and $T = 0.333$ days will have a steady state plasma concentration of

$$C = \frac{50}{50 \times 0.11 \times 0.33} = 27.6 \text{ mg/liter.}$$

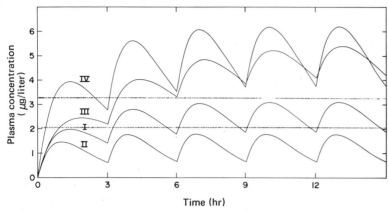

FIG. 2–6. Plasma levels during a dosage regimen. The curves represent plasma levels during a dosage regimen of 5 mg/kg drug every 6 hr. The horizontal lines enclose the therapeutically effective range with the upper line representing the toxic level. The effects of changes in volume of distribution and rate of elimination are shown. The $t_{1/2}$ values are the half-life for elimination[1].

Curve	Dose (mg · kg⁻¹)	Volume of distribution (liter · kg⁻¹)	Rate constant absorption (hr⁻¹)	Rate constant[1] elimination (hr⁻¹)	(t^{1/2})
I	5	1.3	2.0	1.0	(0.64hr)
II	5	1.3	2.0	2.0	(0.32hr)
III	5	1.3	2.0	0.5	(1.28hr)
IV	5	0.65	2.0	1.0	(0.64hr)

This equation implies that the steady state concentration of a drug being administered repeatedly is dependent on its absorption, the size of the individual as reflected in the volume of distribution and its half-life which could reflect individual differences in metabolism. Thus administration of a drug using the same dosage regimen to different people should result in widely differing steady state plasma levels. It is not surprising that under these circumstances the drug is ineffective in some patients and toxic in others. This problem is recognized in the administration of gentamycin (Ch. 56) and digitoxin (Ch. 33), since these drugs have a narrow therapeutic range. The usual technique is to administer an initial "loading" or high dose(s) to rapidly attain the desired effect. The subsequent maintenance doses depend upon how closely this objective is attained but are usually much smaller. They should be given at such intervals that the maximal and minimal plasma levels are not above the toxic and not below the effective levels.

While much of this last section may be self-evident, the use of these pharmacokinetic principles to determine dosage regimen is an exception rather than a rule. The usual dosage regimen as indicated by the drug manufacturer in the package is followed regardless of size, pathologic state or additional therapy.

FURTHER READING

Brodie BB, Gillette JR (1971): Concepts in Biochemical Pharmacology, Vol 28 of Handbook of Experimental Pharmacology. Berlin, Springer-Verlag

Goldstein A, Aronow L, Kalman SM (1974): Principles of drug action. The Basis of Pharmacology, (2nd ed) New York, Harper and Row

LaDu BN, Mandel HG, Way EL (1971): Fundamentals of Drug Metabolism and Drug Disposition. Baltimore, Williams and Wilkins

Levine RR (1973): Pharmacology–Drug Actions and Reactions. Boston, Little Brown

Wagner JG (1971): Biopharmaceutics and Relevant Pharmacokinetics. Hamilton, Hamilton Press

ARTHUR K. CHO

3. DRUG METABOLISM

Drug metabolism refers to the processes by which administered drugs are modified by the organism. The metabolites that result are chemically distinct from the parent drug and are usually more polar. This increased polarity means that the metabolites diffuse through cellular membranes less readily than the original drug. Such substances also tend to persist less in the body, as their renal tubular reabsorption is reduced, i.e., their excretion is increased. The restricted distribution and more rapid excretion will limit pharmacologic activity so that metabolism usually converts a drug to a less active metabolite. However, this is not always the case, and pharmacologically active or even toxic metabolites are known. Thus, drug metabolism and the enzymes responsible for these processes are important considerations in the evaluation of drug actions.

The subject of drug metabolism will be presented in terms of individual reactions. However, it should be remembered that, like other biochemical reactions, drug metabolism can occur as a series of interdependent reactions, with the product of one reaction becoming the substrate for another. Metabolic reactions can be classified under four headings: 1) oxidation—involving the addition of oxygen, OH or the removal of hydrogen; 2) reduction—the addition of hydrogen which is not as important as oxidation; 3) conjugation—this pathway includes several reactions which involve the condensation between the drug or its metabolite and an endogenous compound and, 4) hydrolysis—in which a molecule is generally cleaved with the addition of the elements of water.

OXIDATION

Oxidation is a common process in drug biotransformation. It is catalyzed by several different enzymes, the most prominent one being the mixed function oxidase of the liver endoplasmic reticulum.

LIVER MIXED FUNCTION OXIDASE

This enzyme system is also called the liver microsomal drug metabolizing enzyme because of its presence in an artifact of subcellular fractionation, the microsomes. This microsomal fraction, obtained by differential centrifugation procedures, consists mostly of fragments of the endoplasmic reticulum, a network of membranous structures present in most cells. The close association of these enzymes with membrane lipids requires that substrates for this system be lipo-

philic. The enzyme system catalyzes the general reaction:

$$R\text{—}H + O_2 + NADP\bullet H \xrightarrow{\text{Microsomes}}$$

$$ROH + H_2O + NADP$$

and is called a mixed function oxidase because it requires oxygen as well as a reduced cofactor, in this case nicotinamide adenine dinucleotide phosphate (NADP $\bullet$ H). Similar enzyme systems. are also found in kidney, lung and adrenal tissue, but the most important tissue from the point of view of drug metabolism is the liver.

The mixed function oxidase is remarkable in its nonspecificity. The only requirement appears to be lipid solubility. The chemical nature of the reaction product formed is dependent on the structure of the substrate, and a summary of the different products is shown on Fig. 3–1. All of the reactions can be rationalized in terms of an initial hydroxylation of carbon or other atoms which may be followed by hydrolysis. Two different mixed function oxidases have been demonstrated in microsomes on the basis of their sensitivity to carbon monoxide. One oxidase oxygenates the nitrogen of amines to the hydroxylamine or to the amine oxide. This enzyme system has a flavin containing protein as its terminal oxidase and is not affected by carbon monoxide. The second enzyme system has a heme protein as the terminal oxidase and is inhibited by carbon monoxide. This carbon monoxide sensitive oxidase appears to be more general in the reactions it catalyzes and is usually considered to be the primary drug metabolizing enzyme system.

The heme dependent oxidase has three major components: a phospholipid, probably phosphatidyl choline, a NADP•H-dependent cytochrome reductase, which is a flavin containing protein, and the heme protein called cytochrome P_{450}. Cytochrome P_{450} is responsible for the transfer of electrons from NADP•H to the oxygen and transfer of OH to the substrate. The term P_{450} originated in studies of the interaction of this heme with carbon monoxide, and 450 refers to the wave length, in nanometers, of maximal absorption of the reduced heme carbon monoxide complex. More recently, other heme proteins have been demonstrated in this enzyme system with slightly different absorption maxima so that there appears to be a family of such proteins.

The activity of the P_{450} oxidase is modified by other drugs and foreign compounds. The repeated administration of compounds, such as the barbiturates, oral antidiabetics, phenytoin and halogenated hydrocarbons, causes an increased synthesis or induction of the enzyme system, while other drugs, such as chloramphenicol, inhibit this system. One class of inhibitor used commercially is the so-called insecticide synergists, such as piperonyl butoxide. This compound inhibits the oxidase in all species including insects and is included in the formulation of certain insecticide sprays. Piperonyl butoxide prolongs the action of the insecticide by inhibiting its metabolism. A more common clinical basis for inhibition is by a competitive substrate. Thus, the metabolism of one drug can be inhibited by the simultaneous administration of another drug that is also a substrate for the mixed function oxidase. For example, the rate of metabolism of the antidiabetic agent tolbutamide is decreased when bishydroxycoumarin, an anticoagulant, is administered at the same time. Some of the drugs that affect the liver mixed function oxidase are listed in Tables 4–2 and 4–3 (Ch. 4). These changes in activity of the oxidase can alter the duration of action of drugs whose half-life is dependent on metabolism and constitute one category of drug interactions (Ch. 4).

MONOAMINE OXIDASE

Monoamine oxidase is another mixed function oxidase but with a more physiological role than the liver mixed function oxidase. It is responsible for the metabolic oxidation of a variety of endogenous amines including norepinephrine, epinephrine and 5-hydroxytryptamine. The enzyme is present in nervous tissue (Ch. 14,24), but it is also found in the liver and bowel mucosa where it can effect the metabolic oxidation of ingested amines. Ingestion of the sympathomimetic amine tyramine by a patient receiving a monoamine oxidase inhibitor can result in a serious adverse reaction (Ch. 24).

DOPAMINE β-HYDROXYLASE

Dopamine β-hydroxylase is an enzyme found in adrenergic nervous tissue that converts dopamine to norepinephrine. It is also capable of oxidizing compounds related to dopamine to form compounds that can be retained and subsequently released by adrenergic nerves. These compounds are called false transmitters and have been implicated in the action of several antihypertensive agents (Ch. 20).

DEHYDROGENASES

Oxidation of organic compounds can result from the removal of hydrogen. There are a variety of dehydrogenases present in the body. Alcohol dehydrogenase is a liver enzyme that catalyzes the following reaction:

$$NAD + CH_3CH_2-OH \xrightarrow{\text{Alcohol dehydrogenase}}$$

$$CH_3-CHO + 2NAD•H$$

The cofactor for this enzyme is nicotinamide adenine dinucleotide (NAD) which is reduced. There is also an aldehyde dehydrogenase which converts the acetaldehyde to acetic acid. Because of the high doses of alcohol that are usually taken, its kinetics of metabolism are different from most other foreign compounds. Alcohol dehydrogenase becomes saturated with

(I) Oxidative and Degradative Reactions.

PATHWAY	ENZYME (SOURCE)	SUBSTRATE	METABOLITE	OTHER DRUGS
Aromatic C hydroxylation	Mixed function oxidase (liver)	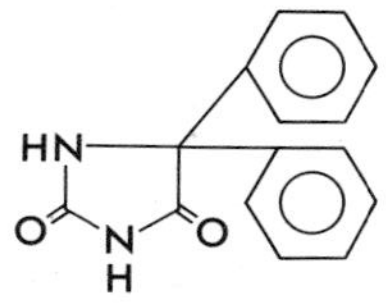 DIPHENYLHYDANTOIN	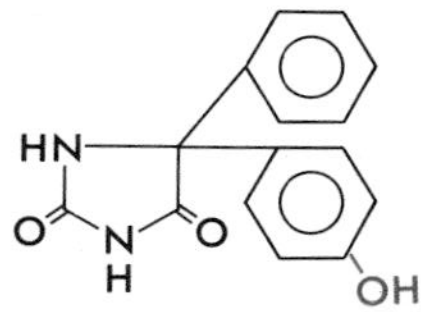	Amphetamine phenobarbital, phenylbutazone, propanolol
Aliphatic C hydroxylation	Mixed function oxidase (liver)	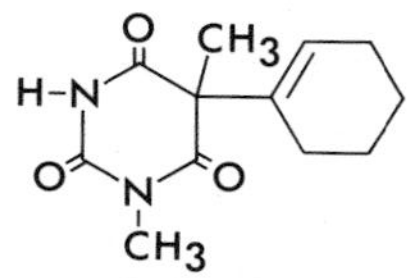 HEXOBARBITAL	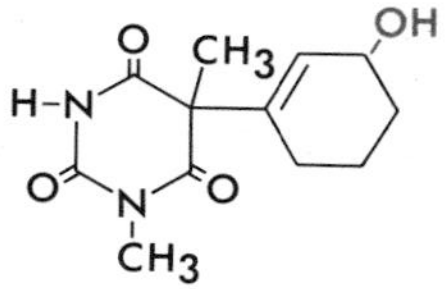	Pentobarbital, tolbutamide
N demethylation	Mixed function oxidase (liver)	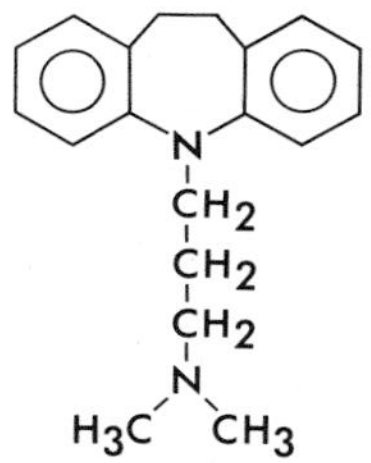 IMIPRAMINE	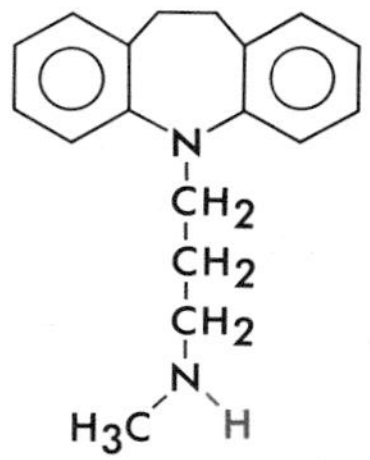 DESIPRAMINE*	Morphine, chlorpromazine, protriptyline
O dealkylation	Mixed function oxidase (liver)	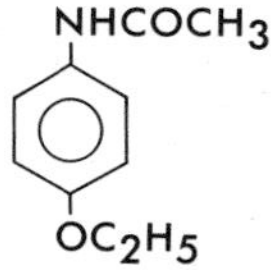 ACETOPHENETIDINE	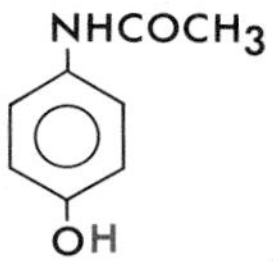 ACETAMINOPHEN*	Indomethacin
N hydroxylation	Mixed function oxidase (liver)	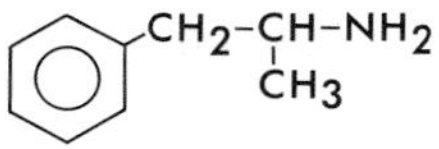 AMPHETAMINE	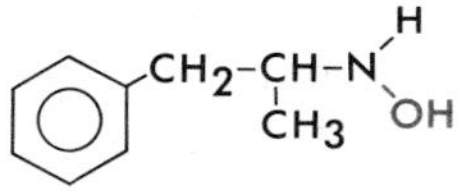	Carinogenic aromatic amines, chlorpromazine

FIG. 3–1. Chemical structures of selected drugs and their metabolites. The changes in structure that result from metabolism are shown in red. * Pharmacologically active metabolites that are also administered directly.

PATHWAY	ENZYME (SOURCE)	SUBSTRATE	METABOLITE	OTHER DRUGS
N Acetylation	Acetyltransferase	ISONIAZID (INH) — pyridine ring, $CONHNH_2$	pyridine ring, $CONHNH\,COCH_3$	p Aminosalicylic acid, sulfanilamide
Glucuronylation	Glucuronyltransferase	4-OH-DIPHENYLHYDANTOIN (METABOLITE)	glucuronide conjugate (COOH, OH, HO, HO)	Morphine
Sulfonation	Sulfokinase (liver, kidney)	ACETAMINOPHEN — $NHCOCH_3$, OH	$NHCOCH_3$, $O\text{-}SO_3H$	Steroids
Amino acid conjugation	Transacetylase	SALICYLIC ACID — COOH, OH	$CONHCH_2COOH$, OH	Benzoic acid
Mercapturic acid	Aryltransferase (liver, kidney)	BENZENE	$NHCOCH_3$ / $SCH_2\text{-}CH\text{-}COOH$	Aromatic hydrocarbons and halocarbons
Dehydrogenation	Alcohol dehydrogenase (brain, liver, etc)	ETHANOL CH_3CH_2OH	$CH_3\overset{H}{C}=O$	

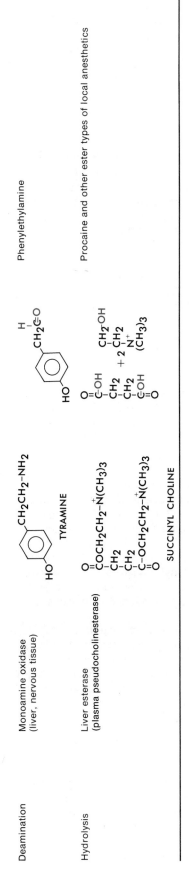

| Deamination | Monoamine oxidase (liver, nervous tissue) | HO—⟨benzene⟩—CH₂CH₂–NH₂
TYRAMINE | HO—⟨benzene⟩—CH₂CHO
Phenylethylamine |
| Hydrolysis | Liver esterase (plasma pseudocholinesterase) | O=C–OCH₂CH₂–N⁺(CH₃)₃
CH₂
CH₂
C–OCH₂CH₂–N⁺(CH₃)₃
O
SUCCINYL CHOLINE | O=C–OH   CH₂–OH
CH₂ + 2 CH₂
CH₂   N⁺
C–OH   (CH₃)₃
O
Procaine and other ester types of local anesthetics |

$$\text{HO}-\bigcirc-\text{CH}_2\text{CH}_2-\text{NH}_2 \quad \text{(TYRAMINE)}$$

$$\text{HO}-\bigcirc-\text{CH}_2\text{C}(\text{H})=\text{O} \quad \text{(Phenylethylamine)}$$

$$\begin{array}{l} O=\overset{}{C}-OCH_2CH_2-\overset{+}{N}(CH_3)_3 \\ CH_2 \\ CH_2 \\ \overset{}{C}-OCH_2CH_2-\overset{+}{N}(CH_3)_3 \\ \parallel \\ O \end{array} \quad \text{SUCCINYL CHOLINE}$$

$$\begin{array}{l} O=\overset{}{C}-OH \\ CH_2 \\ CH_2 \\ \overset{}{C}-OH \\ \parallel \\ O \end{array} + 2 \begin{array}{l} CH_2-OH \\ CH_2 \\ \overset{+}{N} \\ (CH_3)_3 \end{array}$$

respect to alcohol, and thus the rate becomes dependent only on the availability of NAD. This means that the rate at which alcohol is metabolized is independent of the quantity of ethanol ingested (Ch. 10). For example, if metabolism will take 1 hr to lower body alcohol 200–100 mg/kg, it will take 3 hr to reduce it 400–100 mg/kg. In contrast, if the metabolism of alcohol followed first-order kinetics (Ch. 2) with a half-life of 1 hr, body alcohol elimination by metabolism 400–100 mg/kg would take only 2 "half-lives" or 2 hr (i.e., 1 hr for reduction 400–200 and 1 hr further for reduction 200–100). The oxidation of acetaldehyde to acetic acid can be inhibited by disulfuram, a drug used to treat alcoholism (Ch. 10).

REDUCTION REACTIONS

Compounds containing sites of unsaturation, such as carbonyl, azo and nitro groups, are reduced by enzymes that oxidize other substrates. For example, liver alcohol dehydrogenase can reduce aldehydes and aliphatic ketones to the corresponding alcohols in the presence of NAD • H. Aromatic ketones are reduced by an NADP • H dependent enzyme, aromatic aldehyde reductase. Both of these enzymes are present in the cytoplasm of the liver cell. The conversion of carbonyl groups to alcohols does not increase the polarity of the compound very much, but the alcohol function can be readily converted to a highly polar conjugate (see below) which is rapidly excreted.

Azo and nitro functions are reduced by the liver mixed function oxidase under certain conditions. Nitro compounds, such as chloramphenicol, are reduced to the corresponding amines in the presence of NADP • H under anaerobic conditions. Nitro reductase activity is inhibited by carbon monoxide in vitro and is induced by phenobarbital, supporting the view that the P_{450} dependent mixed function oxidase is involved. Prontosil is an azo compound that is reduced by the liver to form sulfanilamide:

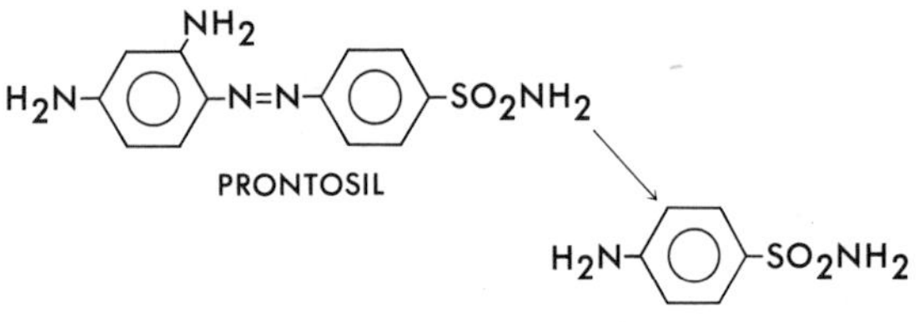

This reaction is an example of the metabolic activation of a drug. The azo group is also present in food dyes, many of which are metabolized by this route.

CONJUGATION REACTIONS

There are a number of different conjugative reactions in which the foreign compound or its metabolite is coupled to an endogenous compound. The most important conjugative enzymes for drugs are found in the liver, emphasizing once again the importance of this organ in drug metabolism. Figure 3–1 summarizes the common conjugative reactions. The conjugated product is considerably more polar than the parent drug, since the endogenous compound coupled is highly polar and usually charged. The most common conjugative reaction is glucuronide formation, occurring with a variety of different functional groups. Several endogenous compounds, such as steroids, thyroxin and bilirubin, the degradation product of heme, are eliminated as glucuronides. The formation of glucuronide is very important for bilirubin excretion, and in newborn infants, where levels of glucuronyl transferase are marginal, toxicity due to bilirubin can occur (Ch. 11). In Figure 3–1 a phenolic hydroxyl is shown as the functional group participating in this reaction, but aliphatic hydroxyl, hydroxylamine, amine, carboxyl and thiol groups are also substrates. Glucuronyl transferase, the enzyme catalyzing this reaction, is present in the endoplasmic reticulum and is induced with drugs such as phenobarbital.

N-Acetylation is an important pathway for the metabolism of isoniazid, and differences in isoniazid half-lives have been attributed to genetic differences in acetyl transferase activity. Although the acetyl derivative is the only conjugate listed in Figure 3–1 that is not charged, it is a polar compound and is readily excreted.

HYDROLYSIS

Plasma contains a hydrolytic enzyme called "pseudocholinesterase," which is capable of hydrolyzing a variety of choline or aminoethanol esters (Ch. 16). The drugs succinylcholine and procaine are substrates for this enzyme, and the duration of their pharmacologic activity is dependent on enzymatic hydrolysis. Both of these compounds have very short half-lives, and succinylcholine, a neuromuscular blocking drug (Ch. 21), must be continuously infused to maintain effective plasma levels. When infusion stops, the effects rapidly disappear, so that the drug is well

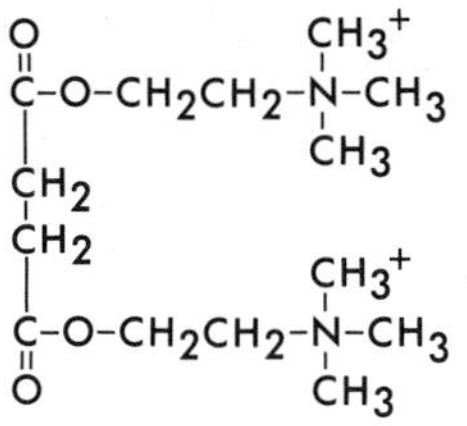

SUCCINYLCHOLINE

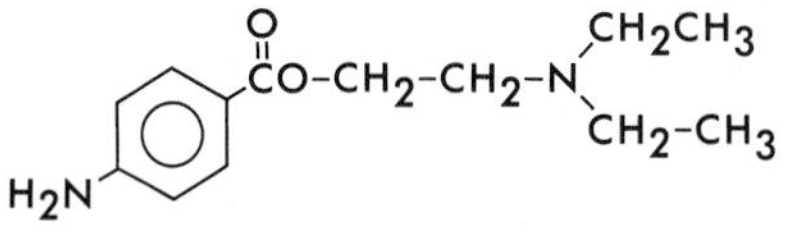

PROCAINE

suited for use as a muscle relaxant in surgical procedures.

Procaine is a local anesthetic with an appropriately short half-life. It also has antiarrhythmic properties (Ch. 34). For use as an antiarrhythmic, a longer duration of action was desirable, and the corresponding amide (procainamide) was synthesized. This compound is hydrolyzed much more slowly than the ester and consequently has a longer half-life. There are individual differences in the activities of the esterase. Genotypes with deficiencies in plasma pseudocholinesterase were discovered when groups of people were found to slowly recover from the effects of succinylcholine (Ch. 8). In addition to pseudocholinesterase, there is also a carboxyesterase present in the liver that catalyzes the hydrolysis of exogenous esters such as procaine. Amides such as procainamide are hydrolyzed by this enzyme but much more slowly.

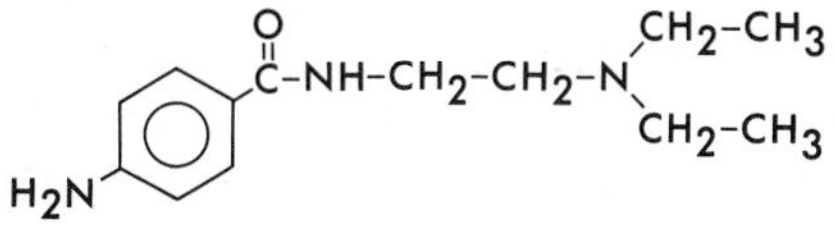

OVERVIEW

Drugs are frequently metabolized in a sequence of reactions. For example, as shown in Figure 3–2, amphetamine (I) can be metabolized by

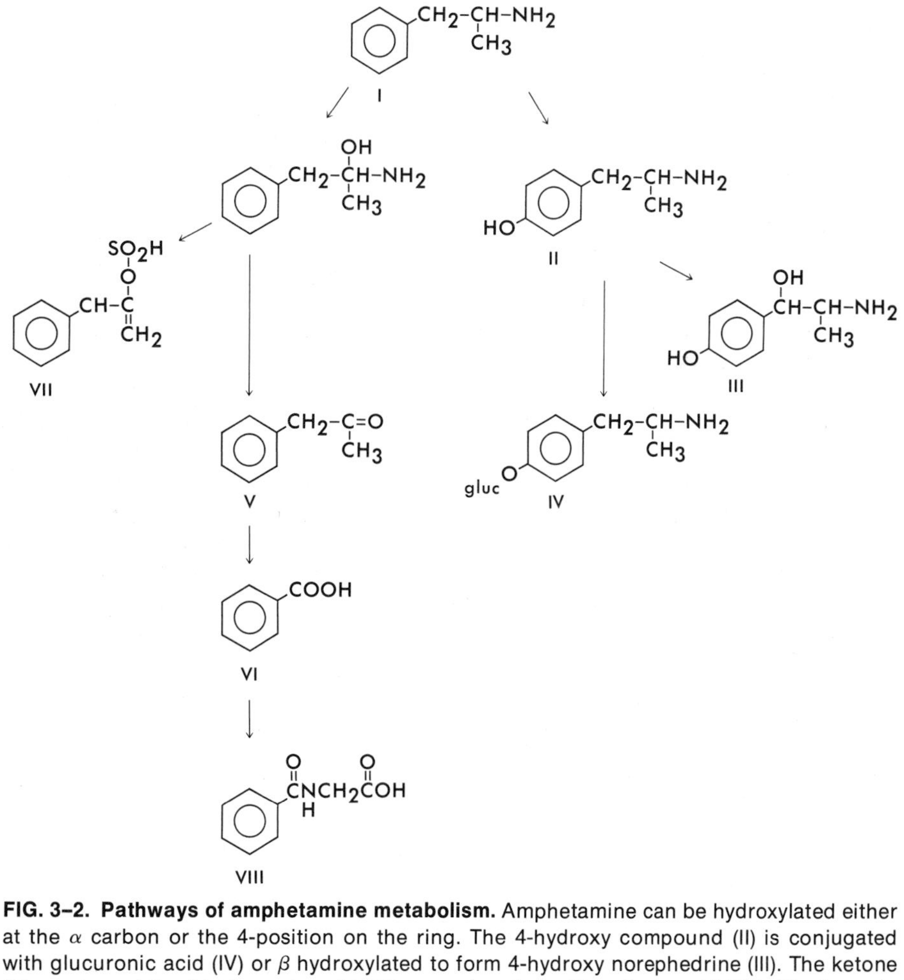

FIG. 3–2. **Pathways of amphetamine metabolism.** Amphetamine can be hydroxylated either at the α carbon or the 4-position on the ring. The 4-hydroxy compound (II) is conjugated with glucuronic acid (IV) or β hydroxylated to form 4-hydroxy norephedrine (III). The ketone (V) can be oxidized to benzoic acid (VI) or conjugated with sulfuric acid (VII). The benzoic acid can be conjugated with glycine (VIII).

the mixed function oxidase to p-hydroxyamphetamine (II) which in turn can be hydroxylated by dopamine β-hydroxylase to form p-hydroxynorphedrine (III). p-Hydroxyamphetamine can be conjugated with glucuronic acid to form the glucuronide (IV) which is rapidly excreted. Compounds II and III are pharmacologically active and can contribute to the actions of the parent drug. Amphetamine can also be oxidized at the carbon attached to the nitrogen with subsequent hydrolysis resulting in the corresponding ketone (V). The ketone in turn can be oxidized to benzoic acid (VI) or conjugated with sulfuric acid (VII). The benzoic acid formed can be conjugated with glycine (VIII). All of the metabolites have been identified in urine and plasma of animals given amphetamine, but the predominate metabolite varies with the species. The major metabolite in man is the deaminated product whereas in rats it is the p-hydroxy compound.

Species differences in drug metabolism make it difficult to predict metabolic pathways of a drug in one species from data obtained in another. This difference is very important with respect to drugs that have metabolites that are pharmacologically active. The species differences that have been observed probably reflect quantitative rather than qualitative differences in drug metabolizing enzymes.

Developmental differences in drug metabolism have also been observed (Ch. 11). Drug metabolizing enzymes of the endoplasmic reticulum continue to develop after birth, so that infants have low drug metabolizing capability. For this reason new born infants are more sensitive to drugs such as chloramphenicol whose duration of action is dependent on metabolism. They are also more sensitive to bilirubin which is removed by conjugation. An increase in the free bilirubin concentration in plasma resulting from the introduction of a drug that displaces bilirubin from albumin can result in neonatal jaundice (Ch. 11).

JEREMY H. THOMPSON

4. DRUG INTERACTIONS

A *drug interaction* occurs whenever the *prophylactic, therapeutic* or *diagnostic* action of a drug is altered in or on the body by a second chemical. The second substance (interactant) may be another drug, or a dietary or environmental chemical. As the number of "drugs" used together increases, the *potential* for drug interactions increases *geometrically.*

As a result of interacting, the action of either or both interactants may be *increased, decreased, altered,* or *show no change.* Thus, a patient may experience a therapeutic failure, an adverse drug reaction or a potentiated therapeutic effect; rarely does the interaction result in *no obvious alteration* in the expected therapeutic effect of the individual agents.

The clinical significance of individual drug interactions is difficult to assess. Almost certainly only a fraction of the more dramatic instances are recognized, since, with most therapeutic agents, there is no readily measured end point of drug effect, and there is wide variation between blood levels and therapeutic response following standard dosage regimens. Furthermore, prediction of patient response to multiple drug therapy is frequently difficult, since drugs may act at more than one site, or by more than one mechanism. Additionally, species variation in mechanisms of drug interactions makes animal data unreliable for predicting human response. For example, clofibrate enhances coumarin activity in the dog by inhibiting its metabolism, whereas in man, clofibrate enhances coumarin activity by displacing the anticoagulant from plasma protein binding sites.

DRUG INTERACTIONS: CLASSIFICATION AND CATEGORIES

Drugs are usually administered to influence a specific target tissue (e.g., a microorganism, heart muscle, the medullary chemotrigger zone, etc.). To do so, the agent must be absorbed, transported throughout the body and metabolized and excreted. Thus there are numerous sites at which drugs may interact to alter the level of free drug or active metabolite at the receptor site or to modify response.

The mechanisms of drug interactions may be quite varied and complex, and in some cases more than one mechanism may be involved. Thus, any classification tends to oversimplify the problem. In general, drugs may interact before administration (when mixed in IV bottles, syringes, etc.); during absorption, distribution, receptor or acceptor binding; on the processes of effector response; at sites of metabolic processes or during metabolism or excretion (Fig. 2–2).

Several important categories of drug interactions are not covered in this chapter; in vitro interference with, or direct in vivo drug induced alterations in clinical laboratory determinations (Ch. 74); and chemical and physical interactions which may develop during drug formulation, and which influence bioavailability (Ch. 7). Chemical and physical interactions that are covered however, are those which may develop in the patient or in the infusion bottles or syringes when drugs are mixed.

Knowledge of mechanisms of drug interactions enables the physician to minimize toxicity, to treat toxicity more adequately with minimum interference with therapy and often to engender beneficial interactions. Drug interactions *per se* may or may not be dangerous. However, *ignorance, or failure to recognize interactions, may be dangerous.*

Mechanisms of drug interactions and some

pertinent examples are cited here. Numerous other interactions are described throughout the book and in Chapter 74.

DRUG INTERACTIONS BEFORE ADMINISTRATION TO THE PATIENT

Our acceptance of drugs as therapeutic agents rather than as chemicals has blunted appreciation that they may interact chemically and physically when mixed prior to administration. Interactions in these areas are discussed elsewhere (Ch. 74).

DRUG INTERACTIONS DURING ABSORPTION

Drug interactions may develop following administration by any route, but those associated with oral, topical and parenteral administration are the most important.

Oral Administration

DRUG INTERACTIONS DUE TO ALTERATION IN FUNCTION. Drugs that **alter the rate of gastric emptying or bowel motility** may produce significant drug interactions. Atropine and other anticholinergic drugs, or fatty drugs (e.g., castor oil), delay gastric emptying, increasing or decreasing absorption of the second drug depending upon whether or not it is absorbed in the stomach or small intestine, respectively; parasympathomimetic agents will have the opposite effect. Similarly, anticholinergic agents or constipating drugs (opiates, ganglion blocking agents) will slow tablet disintegration and dissolution, and the second drug may not be brought into optimum contact with the mucosa. Additionally, by delaying drug passage, excessive toxicity may be seen, e.g., clindamycin induced enterocolitis in patients taking antidiarrheal drugs (Ch. 59).

Increased peristalsis produced by laxatives and other drugs may reduce the time for dissolution or absorption of enteric coated or "slow release" tablets. Additionally, cathartic abuse leading to potassium loss will potentiate digitalis toxicity.

By altering the **rate or level of mucosal blood flow,** drugs may affect the absorption of other agents. This can be seen in the treatment of congestive heart failure.

Modification or elimination of the host microflora can substantially alter the susceptibility of patients to drugs. For example, broad spectrum antibiotics by destroying vitamin K synthesizing flora will potentiate oral anticoagulants (Ch. 40). Similarly, methotrexate, which undergoes an enterohepatic circulation, is markedly more toxic if the microflora is depressed, since the drug is normally metabolized by intestinal organisms to a nontoxic metabolite (Ch. 65).

DRUG INTERACTIONS PRODUCING ALTERATIONS IN THE PHYSIOCHEMICAL PROPERTIES OF THE LUMENAL CONTENTS. The wide range in gastrointestinal pH favors direct (e.g., antacid) or indirect (e.g., anticholinergic) drug induced alterations in acid/base gradients which may modify drug **ionization, solubility** or **stability.**

Since many drugs are weak electrolytes (Ch. 2), lowering or raising the pH will profoundly influence the rate and extent of absorption by influencing the degree of ionization. For example, the absorption of nalidixic acid, salicylates, oral anticoagulants, nitrofurantoin, probenecid and phenylbutazone (all weakly acidic drugs) is depressed with elevation of pH. Similarily, the absorption of amphetamines, quinine and ephedrine (all basic drugs) is depressed with lowering of pH.

The stability or solubility of many drugs is dependant upon pH; e.g., the acid labile penicillins are variably destroyed in an acid environment (Ch. 55), whereas an acid medium is optimal for iron absorption. Alterations in gastric or duodenal pH profoundly influence gastric emptying (see above).

Various components of foods or drugs may actively **chelate** or **adsorb** drugs intraluminally, reducing their adsorption. For example, calcium, barium, magnesium, aluminum and iron salts form chelates with tetracycline antibiotics, and charcoal or cholestyramine adsorb and chelate many acidic drugs such as warfarin and thyroxine.

Other physiochemical interactions can be of therapeutic importance. **Osmotically active agents** (e.g., saline cathartics) may alter absorption of other drugs: **salts** may be formed which are more or less stable, soluble or absorbable than the original agents; fat soluble agents (e.g., vitamins A,D,E and K) will be **sequestered** in fatty drugs, such as castor oil or mineral oil; surface active agents (e.g., dioctyl sodium sulfosuccinate) may increase the absorption of poorly absorbed drugs by lowering surface tension or by facilitating intralumenal mixing and drug/mucosa contact.

DRUG INTERACTIONS ASSOCIATED WITH ALTERATIONS IN THE MUCOSA. Some drugs (e.g., neomycin, PAS, phenolphthalein) may produce varying degrees of villus atrophy leading to a generalized malabsorption. In contrast, excessively rapid drug absorption may be seen if the intestinal villi have been partially destroyed by toxic agents such as tannic acid.

DRUG INTERACTIONS AND TRANSPORT MECHANISMS. Drug induced alteration of gastrointestinal active and passive transport mechanisms may strongly influence drug absorption: pH effects on passive diffusion have been discussed above. Primary phenolic amino acids compete for the same transport mechanism as that absorbing α-methyl dopa, and naturally occurring purine and pyrimidines can interfere with the absorption of purine and pyrimidine antimetabolites. Additionally, barbiturates, diphenylhydantoin, nitrofurantoin, glutethimide and oral contraceptives prevent ileal mucosal folate conjugase from splitting off monoglutamate from polyglutamates, and tyramine in food will not be destroyed on absorption in patients taking monoamine oxidase inhibitors, possibly producing a hypertensive crisis (Ch. 20).

Parenteral Administration

Epinephrine is frequently used to retard the absorption of local anesthetics (Ch. 22). Conversely, hyaluronidase injected subcutaneously with a primary drug can increase the rate of its absorption. Interactions developing on IV administration are covered in Chapter 74.

Topical Administration

Systemically and topically administered drugs may interact. Thus systemic glucocorticosteroids may modify intradermal skin test antigens, and topically administered cholinesterase inhibitors in the eye (e.g., echothiopate) may be sufficiently absorbed to potentiate systemically administered muscle relaxants.

Many drugs applied topically interact with one another; e.g., soaps can depress the antibacterial properties of polymyxin B.

DRUG INTERACTIONS ALTERING DISTRIBUTION

Important drug interactions may alter drug distribution by affecting **drug plasma binding, blood flow** or **drug transport** across membranes.

Plasma Binding

Plasma proteins and plasma cellular elements (particularly the red blood cells) are common carriers of a variety of endogenous (hormones) and exogenous (drugs) substances. Binding depends upon the number of binding sites available and the affinity of the drug for the binding site. The bound drug is usually inactive but is in reversible equilibrium with the free active fraction (Ch. 2). Binding to plasma albumen has been

TABLE 4–1. Some Drugs That Displace Other Drugs from Plasma Protein-Binding Sites

Acetaminophen	Mefenamic acid
p-Aminobenzoic acid (PABA)	Methotrexate
	Nalidixic acid
Barbiturates	Oxyphenbutazone
*Chloral hydrate	Phenylbutazone
Clofibrate	Salicylates
Cyclosphosphamide	Sulfinpyrazone
Diazoxide	Sulfonamides
Diphenylhydantoin	Tolbutamide
Ethacrynic acid	Tranquilizers
Ethyl biscoumacetate	Triiodothyronine
Indomethacin	Warfarin

*A metabolite of chloral hydrate, trichloroacetic acid is the actual displacer.

studied more frequently than binding to plasma globulin or cellular elements.

Since there are only a limited number of available attachment sites on proteins, one drug may displace another drug if the affinity of the displacing agent for the attachment site is greater than that of the bound agent. If a drug is displaced, the increase in the free active fraction of that drug will be associated with an immediate **increase in therapeutic response** and, paradoxically, with **an accelerated half-life,** since the free drug is susceptible to metabolism and excretion. Eventually a new equilibrium between bound and free drug develops with restabilization of drug response. Obviously, a 2% displacement of a drug bound 98% is of far greater clinical importance than a similar displacement of a drug bound 20%.

It is usually highly acidic drugs that bind to plasma proteins and displace other drugs (Table 4–1). For example, warfarin is about 98% bound. If the patient ingests another acidic agent and the bound fraction of warfarin falls to 96%, this small change is actually associated with a **doubling** of the free active fraction, provided that the volume of distribution does not change. This is equivalent (for a short while) to **doubling** the dose of warfarin (Ch. 40). Numerous deaths due to hemorrhage were reported prior to recognition of this interaction. Similarly, sulfonamides and aspirin may displace tolbutamide, producing fatal hypoglycemia, and a variety of acidic drugs may displace methotrexate, dramatically increasing its toxicity (Ch. 67). The antiinflammatory activity of phenylbutazone and aspirin may be due in part to their displacement of glucocorticosteroids from plasma binding sites.

Blood Flow

Epinephrine/local anesthetic interaction has been mentioned above under absorption. Since most nonpolar drugs are metabolized in the liver, concomitantly administered drugs which influence hepatic blood flow may alter the response of agents such as propranolol that are measureably cleared by single passage through the liver bed. Similarly, cardiovascular agents, by altering blood pressure and plasma volume, may have a profound effect on the distribution of a second agent.

Transport Across Membranes

Most drugs after absorption have to cross a variety of membrane barriers to reach their receptor (Ch. 2); other drugs may alter such passage. For example, the antihypertensive agent guanethidine is taken up into the adrenergic nerve terminal by the norepinephrine pump (Ch. 20). Tricyclic antidepressants, phenothiazines and some antihistamines by blocking the norepinephrine pump can reverse the action of guanethidine.

DRUG INTERACTIONS AT RECEPTOR AND ACCEPTOR SITES

Receptors are sites of drug action. They may range from enzymes in the wall of *Staph. aureus,* to the neuroeffector junction in muscles or glands. Drug interactions at the level of receptors are invariably complex and are the **basis of the mode of action of many drugs.** The following mechanisms can be identified: 1) **alteration in the release of an endogenously stored compound** (tyramine and amphetamine potentiate each other in the release of epinephrine): 2) **alteration in the concentration of endogenous compound at the receptor** (desmethylimipramine and cocaine block the uptake of norepinephrine): 3) **alteration in the sensitivity** of a receptor for a drug (thyroxine increases the sensitivity of receptors to coumarins). Finally, drugs can **interact at the same receptors:** the actions of particular agonists can be antagonized by specific antagonists. Many examples occur among the drugs that act on the autonomic nervous system (Chs. 1,14).

Drug interactions at acceptor sites (other than plasma binding sites) are difficult to quantitate. However, quinacrine may displace the 8-aminoquinolines, thus potentiating their toxicity (Ch. 63).

DRUG INTERACTIONS ASSOCIATED WITH METABOLISM

The intensity and duration of the pharmacologic effect of many drugs depends upon their rate of metabolism. Through actions on tissue microsomal enzymes, particularly those of the liver, the kidney and the gastrointestinal mucosa, drugs or drug metabolites may **accelerate** (enzyme induction) or **reduce** (enzyme inhibition) the rate of metabolism of themselves or other related or unrelated drugs. There is no simple chemical relationship between inducers and inhibitors and the drugs that are affected in either category. Furthermore, some drugs may have a biphasic effect. Since the metabolite(s) may be relatively more or less pharmacologically active or toxic than the parent drug, the end result and clinical response are often complex. Thus, when two inducers, both of which produce sedation (e.g., a barbiturate and an antihistamine) are given together, it is impossible to predict the clinical outcome with regard to the net effect of *potentiation* versus *induction.* In general, the microsomal enzymes involved in induction and inhibition are those mediating dealkylation, aromatic hydroxylation, side chain oxidation, deamination, sulfoxidation, azolink reduction and glucuronidation.

Enzyme induction and inhibition usually take about 1–3 weeks to revert to normal after the offending agent has been discontinued. However, with agents such as the chlorinated insecticides, which are lipid soluble, profound effects may persist for months after cessation of exposure due to slow release of the inducer from adipose tissue.

Enzyme Induction

An increase in the quantity of drug metabolizing enzymes usually arises through **augmented synthesis** of microsomal protein: **reduced catabolism** of enzyme protein may rarely be involved. In the liver, enzyme induction is associated with an increase in liver weight, an increase in production of cytochrome P_{450} and changes in the smooth membrane of the endoplasmic reticulum; enzyme induction is prevented by inhibitors of RNA synthesis, such as actinomycin D.

Several hundred drugs are known to produce enzyme induction in laboratory animals, but only a few have been proven to do so in man (Table 4–2). As a general rule, a compound is likely to cause enzyme induction if it is lipid soluble at physiologic pH, not rapidly metabolized and moderately bound to plasma proteins. Phenobarbital appears to be a universal inducer, since it increases the metabolism of more than 60 different agents, including diphenylhydantoin, griseofulvin, digitalis, cortisol and the oral anticoagulants.

The interaction between phenobarbital and bishydroxycoumarin has been well studied and will serve to illustrate the clinical importance of enzyme induction. If a patient's prothrombin time is well controlled on a daily dosage of bishydroxycoumarin, the introduction of phenobarbital

TABLE 4—2. Some Drug Metabolizing Enzyme Inducers

Alcohol (ethanol)	Chlorcyclizine	Heptachlorepoxide	Phenacetin
Aldrin	Chlorobutanol	Hexachlorocyclohexane	Phenaglycodol
Aminopyrine*	Chlordane	Hexobarbital*	Phenobarbital*
Amobarbital*	Chlordiazepoxide	Imipramine*	Phenylbutazone*
Androstenedione	Chlorinated hydrocarbons	Insecticides, halogenated	Prednisolone
Antihistamines	Chlorinated insecticides	Lindane	Prednisone*
Barbiturates*	Chlorpromazine*	Meprobamate*	Probenecid*
Bemegride	Cortisone	Methoxyflurane*	Promazine
Benzene*	Cotinine	Methylphenylethylhydantoin	Pyridione
3,4-Benzpyrene (charcoal broiled meats, cigarette smoke, etc.)*	o,p -DDD	Methyprylon	Secobarbital*
	Dieldrin	Nicotine (tobacco smoking)	Stilbestrol*
Butabarbital	Diphenhydramine	Nikethamide	Testosterone and its derivatives
Carbromal	Diphenylhydantoin*	Nitrous oxide	
Carbutamide	Ethchlorvynol	Norethynodrel	Tolbutamide*
Carcinogens (polycyclic aromatic hydrocarbons)	Glutethimide*	Orphenadrine*	Trifluperidol
	Griseofulvin	Paramethadione	Triflupromazine
Chloral betaine	Haloperidol	Pentobarbital*	Urethane
Chloral hydrate	Heptabarbital	Pesticides	

*These drugs stimulate their own metabolism either in test animals or in man during chronic administration.

TABLE 4—3. Some Drug Metabolizing Enzyme Inhibitors

Acetohexamide	Chlorpropamide	Methylphenidate	Procarbazine
Allopurinol	Clofibrate	Metronidazole	Prochlorperazine
p-Aminosalicylic acid	Coumarins	Mushrooms (*Coprinus atramentarius*)	Quinacrine
Anabolic steroids	Disulfiram		SKF-525A
Androgens	Estrogens	Nialamide	Sulfonylureas
Anticholinesterases	Furazolidone	Nitrofurantoin	Sulfaphenazole
Bishydroxycoumarin	Insecticides	Norethandrolone	D-Thyroxine
Calcium carbimide	Iproniazid	Oral contraceptives	Tolbutamide
Carbon disulfide	Isocarboxazid	Pargyline	Tranylcypromine
Chloramphenicol	Isoniazid	Phenelzine	Triparanol
Chlordiazepoxide	MAO inhibitors	Phenyramidol	Warfarin
Chlorpromazine	Methandrostenolone	Prednisolone	

(which increases the rate of metabolism of the anticoagulant) will be associated with the risk of **thrombosis.** On the other hand, if the patient is concomitantly taking phenobarbital while the dose of bishydroxycoumarin is being adjusted, fatal hemorrhage may develop 2–3 weeks after the phenobarbital is discontinued if the dose of bishydroxycoumarin is not adjusted downwards.

Enzyme induction may be responsible for the development of **tolerance** to such drugs as barbiturates, glutethimide and meprobamate, since these drugs stimulate their own metabolism. The ability of drugs to increase the rate of metabolism of themselves or other drugs often confuses the results of new drug studies.

The phenomenon of enzyme induction may also be used in the treatment of disease. For example, phenobarbital, phenytoin, o,p' DDD, diphenylhydantoin and phenylbutazone enhance hepatic hydroxylase activity and are associated with an accelerated metabolism of cortisol to the inactive 6-β-hydroxycortisol; this therapeutic approach has been used in the treatment of certain patients with **Cushing's syndrome.** Similarly, inducers have been used to treat **hyperbilirubinemia** in neonates and in patients with **familial unconjugated hyperbilirubinemia.**

Enzyme induction is not rapid enough to be of value in the treatment of overdosage with drugs such as phenobarbital. Enzyme induction may alter the results of clinical laboratory test values (phenobarbital and phenytoin increase the metabolism of cortisol, estrogens, progestagens and androgens) and be responsible for disease (griseofulvin, by inducing α-amino levulinic acid synthetase may precipitate acute intermittent porphyria).

Enzyme Inhibition

Many drugs or drug metabolites (Table 4–3) inhibit **microsomal enzymes** by either *competitive inhibition,* or by *inducing functional impairment* (direct toxicity or depletion of glycogen stores) of organ function. In general, the effects produced are opposite to those seen with enzyme induction (see above). For example, bishydroxycoumarin, phenyramidol, phenylbutazone and some sulfonamides inhibit the metabolism of tolbutamide to carboxymethyl and hydroxymethyltolbutamide, thus potentiating the hypoglycemic effect of the sulfonylurea (Ch. 45). Phenylbutazone and the sulfonamides have an additional potentiating effect in that they displace tolbutamide from plasma protein binding sites. Phenindione is a useful anticoagulant to use in diabetics since it does not alter drug metabolism.

Enzyme inhibition may be associated with either therapeutic failure, or with an adverse drug response. For example, PAS, isoniazid, bishydroxycoumarin, disulfiram, methylphenidate, phenylbutazone, phenyramidol and sulfonamides depress the hepatic metabolism of diphenylhydantoin. Thus, if a patient is stabilized (with respect to control of seizure activity) on diphenylhydantoin, and if an inhibitor is introduced, anticonvulsant toxicity may rapidly develop (Ch. 30). On the other hand, if the patient is initially stabilized on diphenylhydantoin and an inhibitor, seizure activity may rapidly develop if the inhibitor is discontinued.

Inhibition of **nonmicrosomal** enzymes by drugs is common. Azathioprine and 6-mercaptopurine are metabolized to less toxic compounds by xanthine oxidase. If allopurinol, a xanthine oxidase inhibitor, is given concomitantly, severe toxicity to the antimetabolites will appear (Ch. 67).

Interactions associated with the monoamine oxidase inhibitors are classical. Concomitant use with sympathomimetic amines, therapeutically administered or ingested, will be associated with symptoms of catecholamine excess (Ch. 18).

Enzyme inhibition can also be associated with altering the results of clinical laboratory tests. For example, glutethimide inhibits the biosynthesis of cortisol by depressing the 2α-hydroxylation of cholesterol.

DRUG INTERACTIONS DURING EXCRETION

There are numerous routes of drug excretion (Ch. 2), but drug interactions involving the urinary tract are the only ones of clinical importance.

Drug interactions may alter the urinary excretion of other drugs by **increasing** or **decreasing glomerular filtration, tubular secretion** or **active or passive tubular reabsorption.** The most important mechanisms involved in these interactions are alterations in glomerular blood flow, changes in osmotic or pH gradients within the tubules or competition for tubular transport systems. Examples of two of these mechanisms will be discussed briefly.

pH Effects

These are primarily of clinical importance if the pK_a of the "affected" drug or active metabolite is in the range of 3.0–7.5 for acids and 7.5–10.0 for bases, and if a significant proportion of the drug or metabolite is normally excreted unchanged in the urine. Thus, urinary alkalinizers (thiazide diuretics, acetazolamide, potassium citrate, sodium bicarbonate, citrate or lactate) will favor the ionization of acidic drugs augmenting their excretion but will favor nonionization of basic drugs augmenting their absorption. Urinary acidifiers (ammonium chloride) will have the opposite effect. Control of urinary pH is of great importance in treating overdosage of drugs, such as the barbiturates, aspirin, amphetamines, etc. (Ch. 13).

The urinary solubility of many drugs is critically dependant upon pH; e.g., sulfonamides readily precipitate out in acid urine (Ch. 60).

Tubular Mechanisms

Many acidic drugs, such as aspirin, sulfonamides, sulfonylureas, methotrexate, acetazolamide, thiazide diuretics, probenecid, phenylbutazone, indomethacin and the penicillins, are actively secreted by the renal tubules. Drug interactions may arise through competition for their sites of transport. Probenecid, for example, blocks the secretion of penicillins, some cephalosporins (Ch. 55) and indomethacin, and the hypoglycemic effect of acetohexamide is enhanced by phenylbutazone which inhibits the tubular secretion of hydroxyhexamide, an active metabolite. Additionally, aspirin, by blocking the secretion of methotrexate, can rapidly produce serious toxicity (Ch. 67).

FURTHER READING

Hansten PD (1973): Drug Interactions. (2nd ed) Philadelphia, Lea & Febiger

Hussar DA (1973): Drug interactions. AM J Hosp Pharm 145:65–116

Martin EW (1971): Hazards of Medication. Philadelphia and London, J. B. Lippincott

Morselli PL, Garattini S, and Cohen SN (1974): Drug Interactions. New York, Raven Press

Prescott LF (1969): Pharmacokinetic drug interactions. Lancet 2:1239–1243

Raisfeld IH (1973): Clinical pharmacology of drug interactions. Annu Rev Med 24:385–418

DONALD J. JENDEN

5. BIOLOGIC VARIATION AND THE PRINCIPLES OF BIOASSAY

Most drugs are pure chemical compounds of known structure, and quantities suitable for therapeutic use may be dispensed by weighing or by chemical estimation. Many agents commonly used in therapeutics, particularly extracts of plants or animal tissues, are not pure, and the chemical structure of the active principles is not always known. In these cases it is necessary to determine the quantity to be used by observing the biologic responses to the drug. The estimation of drug potency by the reactions of living organisms or their components is known as **bioassay.** The principles of bioassay are important not only because some of the most valuable drugs presently in use must be subjected to bioassay to determine the activity of each batch, but also because the same basic principles are applicable to all comparisons of drug effectiveness, including clinical trials of new drugs and their continuing practical evaluation.

Whereas physical or chemical properties such as weight and optical density may be measured with great precision (0.001–1%), the errors involved in measurement of biologic properties are much greater (5–50%), and it is necessary to design and analyze a bioassay in such a way as to minimize the effects of biologic variation.

NATURE AND SOURCES OF BIOLOGIC VARIATION

The net effect produced by a drug is the result of a number of interacting factors. In addition to the basic propensity of a compound to react with and alter a normal physiologic or biochemical function, the observed response depends on the rate at which the drug is absorbed and excreted; its ability to bind with, and hence be removed by, nonspecific tissue acceptors; reversible binding to plasma proteins; (Ch. 2) its rate of metabolism in the organism as a whole and sometimes in the tissues which it affects; its distribution throughout the body and the efficiency of normal compensatory and adaptive mechanisms of the organism. All these factors not only vary from animal to animal but change in a single animal in response to alterations in the internal and external environment. It is not surprising that the quantity of drug required to produce a given effect may vary widely in different experiments. The principal objective of bioassay design is to minimize this inherent variability.

DOSE-RESPONSE CURVES

A graphic picture of biologic variation may be obtained by plotting the percentage of a large group of animals responding to a drug in a specific way against the dose of the drug (Fig. 5–1). A sigmoid curve is generally obtained, the steepest part of which is roughly in the middle of the curve. Because a given change in dose corresponds to the greatest change in response where the curve is steepest, the dose required to produce a given effect can be most accurately estimated at the 50% point. It is conventional to refer to this dose as the ED_{50} (effective dose for 50%) or median effective dose. If the "effect" is a lethal response, the dose is called the LD_{50} or median lethal dose. The ratio of the LD_{50} to the ED_{50} is a measure of the safety margin of a drug and is sometimes known as the therapeutic index (Ch. 1). The term therapeutic index is sometimes used more generally to refer to the ratio of ED_{50} for a toxic and desired therapeutic effect. It

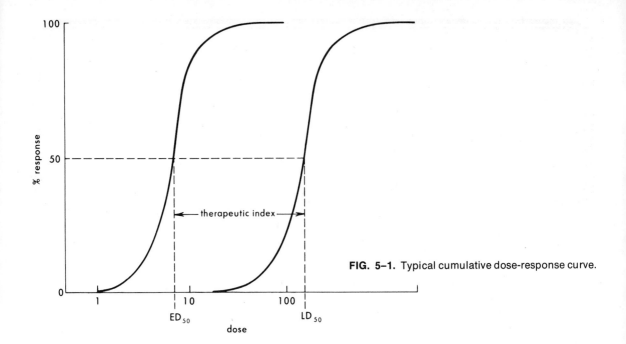

FIG. 5–1. Typical cumulative dose-response curve.

should be noted that a symmetric curve like that in Figure 5–1 is usually not obtained unless the dose is plotted logarithmically on the abscissa. Partly because of the greater ease with which a symmetric curve can be analyzed, bioassay data are usually collected with logarithmically spaced doses.

A curve of similar shape is usually obtained if a continuous measure of mean drug response is plotted on the ordinate instead of the percentage showing a specific threshold response, but in this case the ordinate usually has no intrinsic limit and a different type of statistical analysis must be employed. When two different drugs are being compared in this way, it is often found that they differ not only in their potency (the dose required to produce 50% of their maximum effect) but also in the maximum effect they are capable of exerting. Figure 5–2 illustrates schematically an example of this in which the analgesic effects of morphine and codeine are compared. The curves for morphine and codeine differ in two respects. First, the entire morphine curve is located to the left of the codeine line, indicating that morphine is more potent than codeine regardless of the response level at which they are compared. Second, the codeine curve shows a ceiling, indicating that the drug is in-

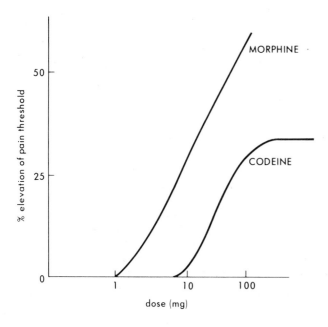

FIG. 5–2. Schematic representation of dose-response curves for analgesic action of morphine and codeine. Morphine is more potent in the sense that the required dose is lower and it is capable of producing more profound analgesia than any dose of codeine.

capable of producing more than a certain degree of analgesia whatever the dose. In contrast, morphine produces an increasing analgesic effect over the entire practical dose range. Note that the relative potency of these two drugs is not a fixed number but a function of the degree of analgesia (i.e., response) at which it is measured. A nonparallel shift in the dose-response curve is also produced by a noncompetitive antagonist (Ch. 1), in contrast to a competitive antagonist, which causes a shift to the right of the dose-response curve of an agonist without changing the slope.

Because of the greater ease with which straight lines may be fitted to data both visually and statistically, an empirical or semiempirical transformation is usually applied to the response measurement so that a straight line relation is obtained. There are both theoretical and empirical reasons to believe that many quantal responses like that represented in Figure 5–1 follow a normal, or gaussian, probability distribution. In this case the cumulative dose-response curve can be transformed into a straight line if the number of standard deviations above the mean is plotted as the ordinate instead of the percentage corresponding to it. This is the basic procedure employed in probit analysis. Because of the exaggeration of random error at extreme values of the ordinate, an iterative weighted regression procedure must be used for statistical analysis of the results and not a simple linear regression.

DESIGN OF BIOASSAYS

THE REFERENCE STANDARD

At one time the biologic activity of some drugs was expressed directly in terms of a simple pharmacologic response. For example, the quantity of digitalis extract required to kill a frog was defined as a "frog unit." Since frogs differ greatly in their sensitivity, depending on season, species, weight and many other factors, this kind of definition does not provide a sufficiently stable measure to permit the confident prescription of clinical dosage. These units have been replaced by absolute reference standards, therefore the role of the biologic test is to compare the effect of the standard with that of the unknown preparation rather than to provide a direct unit of drug activity. A reference standard is a stable sample of the drug maintained in the United States by the Board of Trustees of the United States Pharmacopeial Convention and other agencies and distributed to pharmaceutical manufacturers for standardization of their products. A specific quantity of the standard is defined as possessing one unit of activity, and pharmaceuticals requiring biologic standardization must be labeled according to the number of units of activity per gram or milliliter. The use of reference standards in pharmaceutical standardization is analogous to the internationally accepted definitions of length and weight and has been the most important single factor in establishing confidence in and reliability of bioassay. In clinical drug evaluation or trial it is equally important to include one or more established drugs to serve as standards with which a new agent may be compared.

MINIMIZATION OF BIOLOGIC VARIATION

In order to minimize the effects of biologic variation, the responses to the standard and unknown samples should be observed in animals which are as similar as possible in every respect. Factors such as age, sex, genetic strain, weight and environment can exert a major influence on the sensitivity to drugs, and unless they are carefully controlled, the precision of the assay will be reduced and the result may be biased. Individual animals should then be assigned to receive standard or unknown preparations on an objectively random basis, such as the throwing of dice or the use of a table of random numbers. Ideally, a crossover design should be employed in which the assay is repeated with the standard and unknown preparations administered to the opposite group of subjects, so that an independent comparison of standard and unknown is made in each animal. When more than two drugs are being compared or more than one dose level of each is being tested, a more complicated type of balanced experimental design such as a Latin Square should be employed, in which the same principle is observed. This is not always possible because observation of the response may involve sacrifice of the animal. Some of the most accurate bioassays are made on a single piece of isolated tissue such as a strip of rat uterus or guinea pig ileum, thus eliminating most of the factors contributing to variability of response between animals. Whatever the experimental format, it is imperative that both the selection of animals and the procedure itself be rigorously controlled and precisely reproduced (see Appendix at end of this chapter).

OBJECTIVE EVALUATION

Wherever possible, the biologic response should be objectively measured. Sometimes, particularly in clinical trials, no relevant objective criterion of response is available, and assessment of efficacy depends primarily on subjective evaluation by the patient and/or the physician. In this case, subjective bias should be minimized by use of a double-blind system in which neither the patient nor the observing physician knows to which group the patient is assigned. Unfortunately, it is not always possible to keep a study double-blind, because both the patient and the physician can sometimes easily recognize either the therapeutic or adverse effects of a drug and thus distinguish it from a placebo.

CLASSIFICATION OF BIOASSAYS

Bioassays may be classified in various ways depending on the quantal or continuous nature of the response, the empirical relation between dose and response, the system used for assignment of subjects to different groups and many other considerations. The most important distinction is between assays employing a single predetermined end point (direct assays) and those which establish a dose-response relation (indirect assays).

DIRECT ASSAY

The *United States Pharmacopeia (U.S.P.)* assay for *d*-tubocurarine is an example of a direct assay. The end-point response is head drop in rabbits, which results from neuromuscular paralysis. A sample of the drug is injected intravenously in small aliquots at constant time intervals until head drop is observed, and this is repeated with a series of 12–16 animals, half of which receive the reference standard and the other half the unknown. From the relative mean amounts of standard and unknown required to produce head drop, the relative activity may be estimated. The reliability of the assay is estimated from the variability of the results by standard statistical procedures and is expressed in terms of 95% confidence limits for the activity of the unknown preparation.

INDIRECT ASSAY

Direct assay is the simplest type of bioassay, in which an end-point response is predetermined, and the dose required to produce it is measured. Such an end point cannot always be established, and an indirect assay must be carried out. Here, two or more fixed doses of both standard and unknown are used, and the responses to each are measured. From the results, log dose-response curves are constructed (Fig. 5–3), and the potency of the unknown sample relative to the reference standard is estimated by fitting parallel lines to the data statistically and by calculating the horizontal distance between the two lines. This gives the logarithm of the relative potency.

The statistical calculations required to determine this ratio and its confidence limits are more complex than those for a direct assay. However, they yield an additional piece of information which may be important when the sample contains a mixture of pharmacologically active components, namely, an assessment of whether the log dose-response curves are parallel. When only a single active substance is present, the standard and the unknown differ only in dilution, and this difference should be the same no matter how it is measured. If more than one active component is present in the preparation, the standard and the unknown may differ in their dose-response curves, and the relative activity of the standard and the unknown may depend upon the response level chosen for the comparison, i.e., the log dose-response curves may not be parallel (Fig. 5–4). A direct assay uses only one end-point response and cannot detect this lack of parallelism. Since nonparallelism indicates that the potency ratio is not constant, the active components are probably not present in the same proportions in the standard and the unknown preparations, and projection of the results to clinical use may involve serious errors. A statistical test for parallelism is therefore included in the routine analysis and may lead to rejection of the assay or of the drug preparation. Complete instructions prescribed by the *U.S.P.* for the indi-

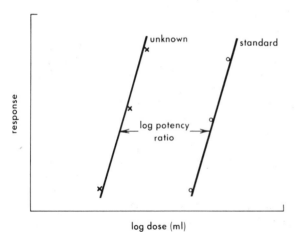

FIG. 5–3. Typical indirect bioassay in which the log dose-response curves are parallel. The unknown preparation is less active than the reference standard by a factor given by the antilogarithm of the horizontal distance between the lines. Confidence limits can be calculated from the scatter of the experimental points about the fitted parallel lines.

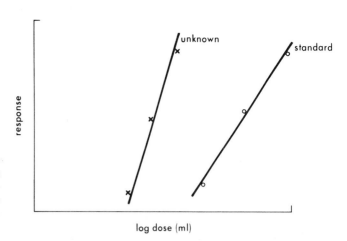

FIG. 5–4. Schematic representation of an indirect assay in which the log dose-response curves are not parallel. The activity of the unknown increases relative to the standard as the response level chosen for comparison increases.

rect assay of insulin are given in the Appendix at the end of this chapter to illustrate the precise control of both design and analysis required in the standardization of a drug for clinical use.

RELATIVE ADVANTAGES OF CHEMICAL AND BIOLOGIC ASSAY

Because of the much greater accuracy and simplicity of most chemical assays, these are always to be preferred when the results are in agreement with bioassay, as they generally are when the agent is available in pure form and its chemical composition is precisely known. If the results of bioassay conflict with those of chemical assay, the former must be relied upon. In at least two other situations bioassay may be preferable and chemical procedures inadequate or impossible: 1) in the early stages of experimental investigation of a new agent, when the material is not available in pure form and its exact nature is not known and 2) when chemical methods are insufficiently specific to distinguish between an active compound and active congeners, inactive impurities or degradation products.

CLINICAL TRIALS

A clinical trial is basically a bioassay in which the response to a drug is assessed in human subjects. Ethical considerations place significant limitations on the design of the assay.

The principles underlying a clinical trial are the same as those governing any other type of assay, but they are more difficult to implement. A new drug should not be assessed alone but must always be compared with a placebo and one or more accepted agents (analogous to the reference standard). Each drug should be tested using at least two dose levels in order to establish meaningful estimates of relative potency. The patients involved in the trial should be divided into groups which are balanced to every possible extent. Obviously, although animals of inbred strains can be grouped rather simply, the number of variables in a clinical trial is much greater: sex, race, weight and age can easily be balanced if the groups are sufficiently large, but when pathologic states are superimposed, it may be possible to equate the groups only approximately.

Whereas in a conventional bioassay a single simple objective measurement generally provides the information from which drug potency is estimated, there is usually no such simple measurement to be made clinically. Judgment of efficacy in disease states is usually based not only on several objective tests but also on subjective evaluation by both the patient and the physician. Clearly, objective measurements are preferable to subjective judgments, but a relevant subjective judgment is better than the most precise measurement of a variable which gives no direct information about the drug effect sought. The format and basis of the evaluation must be completely determined before the trial, and, in order to avoid bias, both the physician and the patient should be ignorant of which drug any individual is receiving (double-blind format).

FURTHER READING

Design and analysis of biological samples (1970): US Pharmacopeia XVIII, pp 867–882

Finney DJ (1952): Statistical Method in Biological Assay. New York, Hafner

Gaddum JH (1953): Bioassays and mathematics. Pharmacol Rev 5:87

Hill AB (1963): Medical ethics and controlled trials. Brit Med J 1:1043–1049

May CD (1961): Selling drugs by "educating" physicians. J Med Educ 36:1

Talalay P (1964): Drugs in Our Society. Baltimore, Johns Hopkins Press

APPENDIX: *U.S.P* INSTRUCTIONS FOR INDIRECT ASSAY OF INSULIN*

Standard solution. Dissolve a suitable quantity of U.S.P. Zinc-Insulin Crystals Reference Standard, accurately weighed, in sufficient water, containing 0.1 to 0.25 per cent (w/v) of either phenol or cresol, 1.4 to 1.8 per cent (w/v) of glycerin, and sufficient hydrochloric acid to make a *Standard solution* containing 40 U.S.P. Insulin Units in each ml. and having a pH between 2.5 and 3.5. Store in a cold place, protected from freezing, and use within 6 months.

Standard dilutions. Dilute portions of the *Standard solution* to make two solutions, one to contain 1.0 U.S.P. Insulin Unit in each ml. (*Standard dilution 1*), and the other to contain 2.0 U.S.P. Insulin Units in each ml. (*Standard dilution 2*). Use as a diluent a solution containing 0.1 to 0.25 per cent (w/v) of either cresol or phenol, 1.4 to 1.8 per cent (w/v) of glycerin, and sufficient hydrochloric acid to produce a pH between 2.5 and 3.5.

Sample dilutions. Employing the same diluent used in preparing the *Standard dilutions,* make two dilutions of the preparation to be assayed, one of which may be expected, on the basis of the assumed potency, to contain 1.0 U.S.P. Insulin Unit in each ml. (*Sample dilution 1*), and the other to contain 2.0 U.S.P. Insulin Units in each ml. (*Sample dilution 2*).

Doses of the dilutions to be injected. Select on the basis of trial or experience the dose of the dilutions to be injected, the volume of which usually will be between 0.30 and 0.50 ml. For each animal the volume of the *Standard dilution* shall be the same as that of the *Sample dilution.*

The animals. Select suitable, healthy rabbits each weighing not less than 1.8 Kg. Keep the rabbits in the laboratory for at least 1 week before use in the assay, maintaining them on an adequate uniform diet, with water available at all times except during the assay.

Procedure. Divide the rabbits into four equal groups of preferably not less than six rabbits each. On the preceding day, approximately 20 hours before the assay, provide each rabbit with an amount of food that will be consumed within 6 hours. Follow the same feeding schedule before each test day. During the assay, withhold all food and water until after the final blood sample is taken. Handle the rabbits with care in order to avoid undue excitement, and inject subcutaneously the doses indicated in the following design, the Second Injection being made on the day after the First Injection or not more than 1 week later.

At 1 hour and 2½ hours after time of injection obtain from each rabbit a suitable blood sample from a marginal ear vein. Determine the blood-sugar concentration in each sample as directed under *Blood-sugar Determination.*

Calculation. Calculate the response of each rabbit to each injection from the sum of the two blood-sugar values, and subtract its response to *Dilution 1* from that to *Dilution 2,* disregarding the chronological order in which the responses were observed, to obtain the individual differences, y, shown below. When the data for one or more rabbits are missing in an assay, allow for differences in the sizes of the groups by suitable means.

Group	Differences	Individual response (y)	Total response (T)
1	Standard 2— Sample 1	y_1	T_1
2	Sample 2— Standard 1	y_2	T_2
3	Sample 2— Standard 1	y_3	T_3
4	Standard 2— Sample 1	y_4	T_4

When the number of rabbits, f, carried through the assay is the same in each group, total the y's in each group and compute $T_\alpha = -T_1 + T_2 + T_3 - T_4$ and $T_\beta = T_1 + T_2 + T_3 + T_4$. The logarithm of the relative potency of the test dilutions is $M' = 0.301 T_\alpha/T_\beta$. The potency of the Injection in U.S.P. Units per ml. equals the antilog (log $R + M'$), where $R = v_s/v_u$, in which v_s is the number of U.S.P. Units per ml. of the Standard dilution and v_u is the number of ml. of Injection per ml. of the Sample dilution. Determine the confidence interval of the log-relative potency M'. If the confidence interval is more than 0.1212, which corresponds at $P = 0.95$ to confidence limits of 87 and 115 per cent of the computed potency, repeat the assay until the combined data of the two or more assays, redetermined as described under *Combination of Independent Assays,* meet this acceptable limit.

* Reproduced from *The United States Pharmacopeia,* ed. XVII, official September 1, 1965, by permission of the Board of Trustees of the United States Pharmacopeial Convention. The board is not responsible for any inaccuracies in the text thus reproduced.

HAROLD E. PAULUS

6. DEVELOPMENT OF NEW DRUGS*

Perhaps the single most significant occurrence in the Twentieth Century has been the remarkable increase in the average life expectancy of human populations; substantial changes in the organization and goals of society are occurring in response to the increased number and longevity of its members. Although improvements in public health engineering, sanitation, insect control and agricultural productivity have been vital prerequisites to this increased life expectancy, the development and dissemination of new drugs and vaccines have contributed substantially to the elimination of many scourges that previously held human populations in check. The development of new methods of birth control soon may provide a more acceptable method of population limitation. The rate of introduction of drugs with significant new actions has accelerated greatly, and, to a considerable extent, the methodology involved in the development of new drugs has become codified and organized into the pharmaceutical industry and is regulated by governmental agencies. The goal of this collaboration between government, industry, academicians and practicing physicians is the safe and orderly evaluation and introduction of new drugs in such a way that the risk: benefit ratio is favorable at all stages of the process.

FINDING A POTENTIAL NEW DRUG

New drug candidates may be found in a number of ways:

SERENDIPITY. The astute appreciation and exploitation of an unanticipated effect has been responsible for the introduction of many important classes of drugs. It originated with the prehistoric tribal medicine man who observed a reduction in fever when he chewed on (salicylate containing) willow bark, or relief of pain upon ingesting the sap of the opium poppy. Other important drugs in this category include colchicine (autumn crocus), digitalis (foxglove), atropine (belladonna plant), quinine (cinchona tree bark) and penicillin (*penicillium* mold).

NEW USES FOR OLD DRUGS. This method of finding new drugs is a derivative of serendipity. An unanticipated drug effect may be noted and exploited when a drug is used for a known indication, or when a drug is given for a nonstandard indication. These new applications tend to be developed by the physicians using the drugs rather than by the scientists producing them, e.g., the use of the local anesthetic lidocaine and the anticonvulsive diphenyl-hydantoin to control cardiac arrhythmias, the amphetamines to control hyperkinetic behavior in children, the anticancer agent methotrexate to control severe psoriasis and the anticancer drugs cyclophosphamide and azathioprine as immunosuppressive agents to prevent rejection of kidney transplants and to treat autoimmune diseases.

EXTRACTION OF A NATURAL REGULATOR from an animal product. Examples include the extraction of insulin from the pancreas, heparin from mast cells, adrenocorticotropin from the pituitary, thyroid extract from the thyroid and estrogens from the urine of pregnant mares. These drugs are usually obtained as a byproduct of the processing of domesticated meat producing animals such as hogs and cattle. The deliberate hyperimmunization of animals to certain antigens has used the animal as a factory to produce drugs (antisera) effective against a variety of bacteria and toxins, e.g., tetanus and,

* The author gratefully acknowledges the support of the U.S. Public Health Service (GM 15759).

diphtheria antitoxin, type specific pneumococcal and rabies antisera.

EMPIRICAL SCREENING of chemicals for a desired effect. This time honored method, perfected by the pharmaceutical industry, requires a relatively easy and inexpensive method for detecting the desired effect. In vitro examples include the use of bacterial cultures to detect the antibacterial effects of antibiotics and the use of tissue cultures of tumor cell lines to detect the effects of potential antitumor agents. Small animals may be used to screen for hypnotic, sedative and anesthetic effects, while the injection of irritating substances into small animals may be used to screen for antiinflammatory activity. When a reproducible routine test system has been standardized, there is no limit to the number of chemicals that can be processed. The rapid proliferation of antibiotic compounds is a tribute to the effective application of this approach.

DELIBERATE CHEMICAL MODIFICATION OF A KNOWN ACTIVE AGENT to enhance an effect (or a side effect). Having found and characterized the effects and side effects of a drug, pharmaceutical chemists can synthesize a myriad of cogeners of its basic chemical structure. By careful correlation of the changes in drug effect that occur with changes in structure, it is sometimes possible to develop rational structure-effect relationships in order to maximize the desired effects and minimize the undesired effects of a particular family of chemicals. Examples are modification of antihistamines to produce the phenothiazine tranquilizers, of the steroid molecule to enhance the potency of corticosteroids and of the basic structure of sulfa compounds to enhance hypoglycemic or diuretic effects.

LOGICAL FORMULATION OF A NEW CHEMICAL to produce a desired effect. Based on a detailed knowledge of physiological chemistry in the normal and diseased state, it should be possible to specifically formulate new drugs to correct a defect or modify an undesired manifestation of disease. Detailed structural characterization of a physiologic mediator may permit the development of an analog to block its effects. An example is allopurinol, an analog of xanthine, which blocks the enzyme xanthine oxidase, thus preventing the production of uric acid; use of this drug results in decreased concentrations of uric acid in the blood and benefits patients with gout. Although few currently available drugs were discovered in this way, the increasing knowledge of molecular biology should make this an important source of new drugs.

PRECLINICAL EVALUATION OF A CANDIDATE COMPOUND

The purposes of preclinical drug evaluation are to reasonably document that the drug may be tested safely in humans and to obtain some indication that it may be effective in certain human disease states. Thus the two major areas of preclinical evaluation are *efficacy evaluation* and *toxicity screening.* The major effort in these areas is expended by the pharmaceutical industry and is conducted by the experimental pharmacologist. Specialization may limit the role of an individual pharmacologist to the evaluation of a particular class of drug actions or to toxicology. At this stage there are many candidate drugs, but the investment in each is relatively small. Since the cost of drug development increases exponentially as the drug progresses through preclinical and clinical evaluation, the emphasis at this stage is the elimination of compounds that may later prove to be unacceptable.

SCREENING FOR EFFICACY

Several approaches may be taken. Many compounds may be screened for a specific effect, and those with the desired effect may then be more extensively evaluated for the presence of other (side) effects. Another approach is to screen all new compounds in a standard set of test systems to evaluate efficacy in a variety of organ systems. In vitro assays are used when appropriate, particularly when searching for antibacterial properties or for effects on cell metabolism that can be elicited in tissue culture systems. Sometimes drug effects can be studied in an isolated organ system; examples include the evaluation of ion transport across the excised toad bladder, the transmission of nerve impulses through the squid axon and the effects of various substances on the contractility of isolated segments of guinea pig intestine, rat uterus or other muscle preparations. More frequently, however, drug effects are evaluated in intact animals. Cardiorespiratory, renal, endocrine and CNS effects may be studied in normal animals. A useful technique for evaluation of drug effects on gastric acid secretion and transport across the gastric mucosa is the preparation of an isolated gastric pouch that permits one to quantitate these factors in a normal unanesthetized animal.

In general, drug actions that are intended to modify normal physiologic response patterns can be studied in normal animals. For the evaluation of drug activity against specific disease processes, diseases or models of disease may be induced in the animal, or inbred animal strains may be selected for the natural occurrence of certain diseases. The NZB mouse and certain inbred dog strains that develop an autoimmune illness similar to systemic lupus erythematosus can be used to evaluate immunosuppressive therapy. Antitumor drugs may be studied in strains of mice that either develop specific tumors or accept transplanted tumors. Specific infections or hypertension may be induced and treated with candidate compounds. Drug effects on hyperuricemia and gouty nephropathy may be evaluated in rodents who are fed oxonic acid (an inhibitor of uricase) and uric acid. Mice, rats, guinea pigs and dogs are the most frequently used experimental animals, but various monkey species are also used for some studies.

Activity of a drug in preclinical tests of efficacy does not necessarily mean that the drug will be active or useful in human disease states. The reliability with which in vitro and animal models can select drugs that will be effective in human diseases is constantly being reevaluated against the performance of new compounds. Results tend to be better when the pathophysiology of the human disease process is clearly understood.

METABOLIC STUDIES. If a compound appears to be promising, its absorption and metabolism are generally studied in several species of animals, usually rats, dogs and sometimes monkeys. These metabolic studies should establish the relative bioavailability of the compound when administered orally and parenterally, should determine the rate at which it is metabolized and excreted and should characterize its metabolic products. Usually the administration of radioisotope tagged compounds is followed by timed collections of serum, urine, stool and sometimes bile for quantitative analysis. In addition, relative drug concentrations in various tissues and organs may be determined following acute or chronic administration of the drug. The metabolites themselves should be evaluated for efficacy because active compounds frequently have pharmacologically active metabolic products. The rate of excretion can be expressed as a **half-life,** i.e., the time required for one-half of the drug to be excreted (Ch. 2). This information is useful in estimating optimal dosage intervals, but information obtained in animals can be applied to humans in only a very general way.

EVALUATION FOR DRUG TOXICITY

If given in sufficient dosage, all pharmacologically active drugs produce toxic effects. Those candidate compounds that, on the basis of their preclinical efficacy are considered worthy of evaluation in humans are subjected to rigorous preclinical toxcity evaluation. Preclinical toxicity screening has been substantially standardized and in the United States is regulated by the Food and Drug Administration (FDA). Its purpose is to characterize the toxic effects and to determine the relative margin of safety, i.e., the difference between the median lethal dose (LD_{50}) and the median effective dose (ED_{50}) (Ch. 5). This margin of safety, or **therapeutic index,** cannot be precisely defined for a compound because it may vary with the conditions of administration and the drug effect being observed.

Initially, a wide range of single doses are given to mice or rats to determine the minimum lethal dose and to estimate the biologic activity of the drug. Based on the results of the acute toxicity studies, the range of doses and routes of administration are determined for subsequent subacute toxicity studies. The drug is evaluated in several species of animals by repeated administration at a number of dose levels ranging from median effective levels to levels that are lethal after only a few doses. Chronic toxicity studies require continued drug administration for up to 2 years in several dosage ranges, at least one of which must be high enough to produce substantial toxicity. Generally three species of animals are studied, frequently the rat, the dog and the monkey. Additional studies are done to determine the effects of the compound on fertility and pregnancy. Decreased fertility, increased fetal wastage and fetal malformations are sought.

At the end of the preclinical evaluations, one should be confident that the candidate compound is safe for initial introduction into human subjects, and there should be reasonable indication that it may be therapeutically effective. Only a small percentage of the originally synthesized candidate compounds are selected for clinical evaluation. At this point the sponsor is required to submit the results of the preclinical investigations to the FDA, along with proposals for initial clinical evaluations. If the FDA is satisfied that the compound is reasonably safe, permission is given to begin initial clinical trials.

CLINICAL EVALUATION OF THE NEW DRUG

Having survived the rigors of preclinical efficacy and toxicity evaluation, the candidate compound, which may now be called a new drug, must be evaluated in the human subjects for whom it is intended. The purpose of clinical evaluation is to determine whether a new drug is effective for its projected therapeutic indications and to characterize its toxicity in order to define the conditions under which it may be ultimately prescribed for general use. The standards and conditions for clinical evaluation of new drugs are specifically regulated by the FDA, and drugs cannot be dispensed in the United States without its approval. In 1938, the FDA was made legally responsible for determining the safety of new drugs before their release. Until 1962, however, it was not necessary to prove that a new drug was therapeutically effective. Stimulated by the thalidomide tragedy in 1962 (Ch. 7), the FDA was directed to require proof of effectiveness as well as safety. This new requirement substantially increased the complexity of the clinical evaluation of new drugs and slowed the flood of new preparations into the pharmacy. In order to carry out its responsibility, the FDA requires complete information about the methods and quality controls used for the synthesis and manufacture of the compound, in addition to complete records of all preclinical studies. For each clinical study, both the protocol and the clinical investigators must be approved by the FDA; upon its completion, detailed case reports of each subject must be submitted, in addition to general summaries of the conclusions drawn from the trials.

THE CONTROLLED CLINICAL TRIAL

The crucial element in the clinical evaluation of a new drug is the controlled clinical trial, which in essence is the application of the scientific method to clinical investigation. It is used to prove or disprove a prestated hypothesis. Controlled clinical trials compare a treated group with an untreated, or control group. This comparison is necessary because of the complexity of human subjects and the multitude of uncontrollable or unknown variables that may affect the results of the trial. A prerequisite of any clinical trial is the **informed consent** of its participants. Each subject must understand the general structure of the trial, what therapeutic agents he may be exposed to and all of the possible risks of the trial, whether from treatment, lack of treatment or diagnostic maneuver. Alternative treatment methods must be explained, and the patient's privacy must be protected. Frequently, an institutional review committee is required to determine that proposed trials are safe and that the methods used to obtain informed consent are satisfactory. The time used to carefully explain a proposed clinical trial to its subjects is amply repaid because the subjects then become active, cooperating participants in the trial rather than merely passive subjects upon whom observations are made.

The *elements of a controlled clinical trial* collectively may be referred to as the design of the trial:

1. A clearly defined therapeutic objective (hypothesis)
2. A quantitative scale of accomplishment (to indicate attainment of the objective)
3. Representative subjects
4. Unbiased subject assignment to treatment or control groups
5. Control of bias (of investigator and subject)
6. Equal distribution of uncontrollable environmental and genetic factors
7. Statistical methodology to determine the significance of differences between study groups

The therapeutic objective, or hypothesis, must be clearly stated and must be answerable. The methods by which attainment of the objective will be recognized must be defined and should be quantitated by an appropriate scale. The scale may be based on the patient's report, e.g., severe, moderate, mild or none with respect to pain, or on a laboratory observation, e.g., blood sugar or serum drug concentration. The study subjects must be representative of the population to whom the hypothesis is to be applied. The results of a study of normal subjects cannot be indiscriminately applied to patients with a disease, and the findings of a study of subjects with minimal disease manifestations may not be applicable to those with severe disease manifestations.

The subjects must be assigned to the treatment or control group in an unbiased manner. This is generally done by *random assignment*, using a list of randomly generated numbers to determine the sequence in which subjects are assigned to the study groups. In the case of a *crossover trial*, each subject receives both the investigative and the control treatment, but the order in which they are given is randomly predetermined. The crossover trial has an additional advantage in that uncontrollable environmental and genetic factors tend to remain more or less constant within the individual subject, who acts as his own control. However, either spontaneous or treatment induced changes in the subject during the course of the study, and carryover effects of one drug upon the subsequent treatment may confound the investigator. These problems are avoided in a *parallel study* design in which each subject receives only one treatment, but larger numbers of subjects must be studied in order to equally distribute uncontrollable factors by randomization. The unavoidable bias of both the investigator and the subjects is frequently controlled by using a *double-blind* study design; here neither the investigator nor the subject knows which of the possible therapies is being given. Blindness is insured by preparing the various treatments in identical dosage forms, i.e., identical capsules, tablets, injections, etc. A code indicating the patient's actual treatment is readily available if this information should be needed. During a double-blind trial, the investigator or the subject frequently feels that he can recognize the treatment by its characteristic side effects or in some other way, but his lack of insight is usually evident when the code is broken at the end of the study. As long as some element of uncertainty is present, the double-blind design has attained its objective. At the conclusion of the clinical trial the treatment codes are broken, the data is tabulated and then subjected to *statistical analysis* to determine the significance of observed differences between the study groups. A variety of statistical methods may be applied, but these should be preselected in order to avoid bias. Mathematically massaging the data until the desired result is obtained is not a legitimate application of statistical methods to controlled clinical trials.

Placebos are frequently used as the control therapy in double-blind trials. A *placebo* is a substance, e.g., lactose capsules or saline injections, that is thought to be pharmacologically inert. The use of placebos is particularly helpful in controlled trials because it helps quantitate the degree to which subject responses are due to the study situation, the mere ingestion of capsules or other incontrollable variables. Subject response to the administration of a placebo is called *placebo effect* and, when specifically studied, has been seen in about one-third of subjects. Placebo effects are more likely to be seen when the pertinent effect is subjectively reported by the patient rather than when it is objectively measured by the investigator or by his laboratory. To some extent, the placebo effect is due to the suggestibility of the subject. It may be either positive or negative and applies not only to therapeutic effects but also to side effects of the treatment.

PHASES OF CLINICAL EVALUATION

Evaluation of a new drug in humans follows a logical pattern and is usually subdivided into distinct stages referred to as phases. Phase I is the initial exploratory introduction of the drug to human subjects. Its purpose it to determine that the drug is not generally toxic and to accumulate information that will be helpful in establishing dosage and dosage intervals for subsequent studies. A single tiny dose is usually given to the first subject. If it is well tolerated, single doses of increasing size are then given to a series of subjects until a dose in the anticipated therapeutic range is reached, or until some side effects are

observed. Clinical laboratory evaluations are done in all subjects to detect possible adverse effects on the blood, liver, kidneys or gastrointestinal tract, and the subjects are carefully observed for subjective or objective evidence of drug effects. The choice of the initial dose and the maximum dose to be used in a phase I trial is difficult to decide upon; the doses chosen depend to a greater extent on the "gut reaction" of the clinical pharmacologist conducting the trial than on any scientific formula. As part of the single dose trials, a metabolic study is usually done to determine that the drug can be found in the plasma (is bioavailable) and to determine the rate at which it disappears from the plasma. In addition, the rate and character of urinary excretion products may also be determined. The rate at which a drug disappears from plasma, or its half-life, is important in estimating the frequency with which doses should be administered in subsequent multiple dose trials. A drug that is metabolized rapidly must be given frequently to maintain plasma concentrations, while a slowly metabolized drug must be given less frequently to avoid accumulation. If no problems develop during single dose studies, multiple dose trials are begun. Again, a small number of subjects are given small doses of the drug in trials of 4–6 weeks duration. If no problems are encountered, other subjects are given larger doses, and thus the dose and duration of treatment are gradually increased, always with the knowledge that the previous dosage level was safe. Metabolic studies should be done during the multiple dose studies to ascertain the plateau concentrations developing during clinical therapy. Phase I studies are usually carried out in healthy normal volunteer subjects, although sometimes patients for whom the drug might reasonably be used as treatment are permitted to volunteer for Phase I studies. In either case, the subjects must understand that there is no likelihood that they will benefit personally from phase I drug administration. If the drug has an action that can be measured in normal subjects, this can be studied during phase I; e.g., the effects of a diuretic or an antihypertensive agent could be evaluated. However, evaluation of safety is the prime concern. Phase I studies are almost always undertaken by experienced clinical pharmacologists. Double-blind, placebo controlled studies are not always necessary, but this design is useful because it establishes a reference group against which incidental or minimal abnormalities can be judged.

Phase II is divided into early and late stages and consists of the initial introduction of the drug into patients who have the disease or condition that the drug is intended to treat. Early phase II studies should establish that the drug is as safe in patients as it was in the normal volunteers studied in phase I. Small numbers of patients are intensively studied to assess the potential usefulness and dosage range of the drug. Increasing doses of the drug may be given in an open or blind fashion by an experienced investigator. In addition to routine monitoring of safety, there is an intensive evaluation of the beneficial effects. If the new drug shows promise of being useful therapeutically and has not shown excessive toxicity, extensive and expensive clinical and preclinical studies are initiated. These consist of long term chronic toxicity studies and evaluations of drug effects on reproduction and fertility in animals and the entire spectrum of clinical studies leading to eventual approval of the drug for general distribution. Because the investment in these subsequent studies is so great, a drug that has modest toxicity or uncertain efficacy is very likely to be dropped at the end of the early phase II studies.

Assuming that the drug appears safe, and that therapeutic effects were shown at some dosage level in the early phase II studies, late phase II studies are begun. Late phase II studies represent a substantial commitment to the drug and are intended to provide statistical proof that the drug is therapeutically beneficial in the dosage to be ultimately recommended. Larger numbers of patients are studied in tightly controlled double-blind trials in which the drug is compared to placebo and to standard forms of therapy. At the end of phase II, one should be convinced that the drug is therapeutically useful and that it is generally safe for its proposed indication, and one should know the therapeutic dose range. Late phase II studies tend to merge into phase III studies in which the role of the drug in clinical practice is ascertained. A large number of patients are studied by a variety of investigators, and the drug is given in situations similar to those of actual clinical practice. The duration of administration should approach that anticipated in subsequent clinical practice. A sufficient number of subjects should be studied to uncover the possibility of rare but serious toxicity. Special aspects of safety and metabolism are evaluated, e.g., drug dosage in patients with hepatic or renal insufficiency, interactions with other drugs, drug concentrations in milk and transmission across the placental barrier. If it is anticipated that the drug may be used during pregnancy or in children, studies in these subjects are done late in phase III. Although many phase III studies are more valid if they are carried out in a double-blind controlled manner, unblinded administration of the drug in a clinical setting is also useful, if drug effect and side effects are carefully documented.

At the end of phase III, both the sponsor and the FDA must be satisfied that the drug is both safe and effective for its proposed uses, even when prescribed by busy physicians to sometimes forgetful patients. At this time, the "package insert" is written by the sponsor under the watchful eye of the FDA. This important document, which is inserted in every package of the drug and is quoted in the Physician's Desk Reference (PDR), summarizes everything that is known about the drug and specifies the conditions under which it should be used, dosage information, possible side effects, precautions and any other significant factors known about the drug. Whenever one uses an unfamiliar drug, the package insert should be carefully and completley read rather than being hastily discarded, for it contains the most authoritative current statement available about that drug.

The evaluation of a new drug does not stop when it has been released for general prescription. Drug evaluation is then referred to as phase IV and consists of continued surveillance during general clinical use. Unusual types of toxic reactions are often noted during phase IV, sometimes many years after the drug was originally introduced to medicine. Examples include bone marrow suppression by chloramphenicol and by phenylbutazone, hepatitis induced by isoniazide, hepatic fibrosis induced by methotrexate and the drug induced lupus syndrome caused by a variety of agents. An aspirin induced hepatitis was only recently recognized, even though this ubiquitous drug has been used for more than 75 years. Thus, phase IV evaluation continues as long as the drug is used. In addition to observations regarding toxicity, further refinement of dosage schedules, metabolism, interactions with other drugs, effects of various disease states on the drug and its metabolism and additional clinical indications for use of the drug frequently develop during phase IV.

SCIENTIFIC PERSONNEL INVOLVED IN NEW DRUG DEVELOPMENT

In addition to the individuals needed for the commercial aspects of the pharmaceutical industry, a number of distinct scientific roles are involved in new drug development. The *pharmaceutical chemist* must be well versed in both synthetic biochemistry and pharmacology in order to synthesize the compounds that may become new drugs. He must be able to isolate, identify and then synthesize the active principle of a naturally occurring herb or other product with medicinal properties. The *experimental pharmacologist* searches for evidence of drug activity in experimental animal and in vitro models of physiologic processes or diseases. Although he may evaluate the whole spectrum of drug activity, an individual may limit his work to a specific organ system or type of drug action. *Toxicologists* are experimental pharmacologists who specialize in the preclinical assessment of drug toxicity and are generally distinct from the individuals who evaluate the drugs for preclinical efficacy. Sometimes *veterinarians* are employed to supervise the care of the large variety of experimental animals used in preclinical studies; their knowledge of the naturally occurring incidence of certain abnormalities or diseases in these animal populations is particularly important. Early human studies are usually undertaken by *clinical pharmacologists,* i.e., physicians, especially trained in the design, conduct and evaluation of studies of drug effects in humans. Later trials in patients are conducted by *clinical investigators,* who are individuals with experience and expertise in the treatment of patients with diseases for which the drug is indicated. These studies are monitored by other physicians who attempt to assure that the study protocol is properly adhered to and finally are evaluated by physicians or pharmacologists employed by the FDA. Of great importance in the evaluation of both preclinical and clinical studies in the *biostatistician,* who is frequently assisted by specialists in computerized data storage retrieval and processing.

Thus the development of a new drug requires the diligent application of skills drawn from a number of disciplines. The long and torturous path involved in the development of a successful new drug is frustrating because so few candidate drugs complete it, but the satisfactions gained from the introduction of a substantial therapeutic advance make the effort worthwhile.

FURTHER READING

Melmon KL, Morrelli HF (eds) (1972): Clinical Pharmacology. Basic principles in therapeutics. New York, Macmillan

Feinstein AR (1967): Clinical Judgement. Baltimore, Williams & Wilkins

JEREMY H. THOMPSON

7. ADVERSE DRUG REACTIONS

"The remedy often times proves worse than the disease,"
William Penn, 1693.

Two types of actions may or may not be seen following drug administration: **desired drug actions,** those clinically desirable and beneficial effects sought by the physician, and/or **undesired drug actions,** which are additional drug effects not primarily sought. Undesired drug actions may be harmful or harmless; if harmful they are called **adverse drug reactions.**

Adverse drug reactions are consequently one facet of **iatrogenic disease** which encompasses the entire spectrum of adverse effects produced unintentionally by physicians while caring for their patients. Iatrogenic disease includes not only the direct injuries which may result from drugs or from diagnostic or therapeutic procedures, but also the disease states which may arise from personality conflicts between the physician and the patient. This chapter is concerned only with adverse effects produced by drugs.

A classification of drug effects into those desired and those not desired is unsatisfactory, since the same drug effect may fall into either group, depending upon the clinical situation. Sedation, e.g., with the antihistamine drugs may be undesirable when it occurs in a taxi or bus driver being treated for allergic rhinitis, but it may also be desirable when the drug is used primarily as an hypnotic (Ch. 49), or to treat a severe pruritic drug reaction where sedation is an additional "beneficial" effect. Thus, "adverse" is one of many qualifying adjectives applied to drug effects. In the past there has been a tendency to classify all unwanted drug effects as adverse, a practice which has led to some confusion.

Although the laity expect drugs to cure most disease and suffering without danger or undesirable effects, the use of any drug inevitably entails some risk. Both the patient and the doctor should recognize and accept this. The physician should not become a therapeutic nihilist for fear of adverse drug reactions, nor should he prescribe indiscriminately. Before administering a drug, he should carefully consider its possible adverse effects versus the potential therapeutic benefit.

Ideally, the right drug, in the right patient, in the right dosage (form, amount, interval), by the right route, at the right time and for the right disease will not yield an adverse effect(s). However, *this situation is rarely attained,* since no drug is so specific that it produces only desired drug effects in all patients. *No clinically useful drug (not even a placebo) is entirely devoid of toxicity.* Adverse drug reactions may also develop following the administration of the wrong drug(s), to the wrong patient, in the wrong dosage, by the wrong route, at the wrong time or for the wrong disease.

The terminology of adverse drug reactions is not standardized, and the distinctions, if any, among *drug side effects, drug toxicity, drug allergies, drug intolerance, drug idiosyncrasies and drug induced diseases* have not yet been clearly established. Because of this confusion, the comprehensive term "adverse drug reaction" will be used to *summarize the ways in which the use of drugs may cause harm to the patient.*

FREQUENCY OF OCCURRENCE AND CONSEQUENCES OF ADVERSE DRUG REACTIONS

Because of the difficulties outlined above and below, data concerning the frequency of occurrence of adverse drug reactions tend to minimize the problem and should be interpreted carefully.

Adverse drug reactions have accounted for 3–20% of hospital admissions, and 5–40% of patients in hospitals experience an adverse drug reaction. Also, 30% of patients admitted for a drug reaction have a further reaction while in the hospital, and the average length of hospital stay is doubled for patients who experience a reaction.

The "incidence" of adverse drug reactions has increased in recent years mainly because more people are taking more drugs, often for longer periods of time; more drugs are being used together without a parallel increase in our knowledge of their pharmacokinetics and of the diseases for which they are being given; the pattern of diseases being treated is changing, i.e., a greater percentage of older patients, or those on chronic immunosuppressive therapy, etc., are involved; and there is greater exposure to environmental agents which may alter the response to drugs.

PROBLEMS IN ASSESSING THE INCIDENCE OF DRUG REACTIONS

The "incidence" of adverse drug reactions is highly variable, as is the "incidence" of reactions to specific agents. True incidence values depend upon many factors, some of which are discussed below.

IMPRECISE DEFINITION. The definition of an adverse drug reaction is often imprecise. For example, to some physicians dryness of the mouth following atropine (Ch. 17) is an adverse reaction, whereas to others this is merely a useful indicator in determining the correct dose. Similar problems occur with other drugs such as antihistamine induced sedation (see above).

Reaction rates differ widely depending upon whether they were obtained prospectively or retrospectively, or upon how the reaction was defined, i.e., by clinical impression, biochemical or immunological test, drug rechallenge, etc.

IMPRECISE PRESCRIPTION FIGURES. It has been reliably estimated that physicians write prescriptions for about 80% of their patients, and that about two billion prescriptions are written each year in the United States. However, except under rare circumstances, e.g., with a new drug under trial, or with agents such as the narcotics, no accurate records are available on the *use* of prescription or nonprescription (over-the-coun-

ter) drugs. If figures on the use of individual drugs are not known, no true incidence rates on adverse reactions can be calculated, and *it is virtually impossible to assess the benefit:risk ratio of any agent for any patient.*

Acquisition of precise prescription figures is complicated in turn by numerous problems, particularly the question of nursing errors (see below) and patient noncompliance (see below).

LACK OF AN APPARENT CAUSE/EFFECT RELATIONSHIP. Some of the adverse effects of x-irradiation, teratogens and anticancer drugs may not be apparent for years after the subject has been placed "at risk." Similarly, adverse effects may not appear until after prolonged exposure to the drug (chloroquine retinopathy, Fig. 7–1, Ch. 63), or else they may continue long after the offending agent has been discontinued (kidney and bone marrow toxicity from gold salts).

FAILURE TO REPORT REACTIONS. In this law-suit conscious age, many physicians fail to report adverse reactions for fear of legal reprisals.

ERRORS IN DRUG ADMINISTRATION. These are surprisingly common (see below), and their occurrence clouds incidence rates. It is essential to establish if a patient suspected of suffering an adverse drug reaction has or has not received the drug in question.

CONFUSED THINKING. There is often failure to recognize that a new "symptom" developing under therapy is in fact a drug reaction rather than some manifestation of the underlying disease process. The physician must cultivate a high index of suspicion.

DEVELOPMENT OF "ADVERSE" NONDRUG REACTIONS. Symptoms often listed as adverse effects of drugs are common. A survey of 414 healthy university students and hospital staff *who were not taking medications* indicated that 81% of the subjects experienced in the preceding 72 hr a variety of symptoms (Table 7–1). The median number of symptoms experienced was two per person, and 10% of the subjects experienced six or more.

MULTIPLE DRUG EXPOSURE. It is the rare patient who receives only a single drug. Thus, if a "drug" reaction develops during multiple drug administration, it may be impossible to decide which agent, if any, was responsible.

PREDISPOSING FACTORS TO ADVERSE DRUG REACTIONS

Even though it is impossible to derive any accurate figures on the occurrence of adverse drug

reactions, many of the variables that influence their incidence are known (Table 7–2). *It must be*

TABLE 7—1. Percentage of Subjects Reporting Each Symptom

Symptom	Medical group	Nonmedical group
Skin rash	8	3
Urticaria	5	1
Bad dreams	8	3
Excessive sleepiness	23	23
Fatigue	41	37
Inability to concentrate	25	27
Irritability	20	17
Insomnia	7	10
Loss of appetite	3	6
Dry mouth	5	3
Nausea	3	2
Vomiting	0	0
Diarrhea	5	2
Constipation	4	3
Palpitations	3	3
Giddiness or weakness	2	3
Faintness or dizziness on first standing up	5	5
Headaches	15	13
Fever	3	1
Pain in joints	9	5
Pain in muscles	10	11
Nasal congestion	31	13
Bleeding or bruising	3	3
Bleeding from gums after brushing teeth	21	20
Excessive bleeding from gums after brushing teeth	1	1

Reidenberg MM, Lowenthal DT (1968): Adverse, non-drug reactions. N. Engl J Med, 279: 678–679

stressed, however, that it is still impossible for the most part to predict which patients are most likely to suffer adverse reactions to drugs.

PREDISPOSING DRUG FACTORS

Chemical Characteristics

Various chemical characteristics are associated with certain types of adverse drug reactions.

DEGREE OF POLARITY. Highly polar (water soluble) drugs (Ch. 2) (e.g., thiazide diuretics), being slowly absorbed from the gastrointestinal tract, and primarily excreted by the kidney unchanged, are likely to accumulate in patients with renal insufficiency. Conversely, nonpolar (fat soluble) drugs (Ch. 2) (e.g., phenothiazines, barbiturates) are rapidly absorbed from the gastrointestinal tract but poorly eliminated by the kidney, and additionally tend to be highly protein bound and to depend upon hepatic enzyme systems for their metabolism. Frequently they are associated with enzyme induction. Thus knowledge of the chemical characteristics that determine polarity and the pK_a and pH of a drug (see below) may facilitate prediction of adverse drug reactions in patients with disease of excretory organs and prediction of drug interactions at the level of plasma protein binding and hepatic metabolism (Ch. 4).

ACIDIC AND BASIC PROPERTIES. Weak acids (sulfonamides, aspirin, phenobarbital, etc.) are poorly excreted in acid urine but well excreted in an alkaline urine. Conversely, weak bases (amphetamines, antihistamines, etc.) are well excreted in acid urine but poorly excreted in alkaline urine. Consideration of urinary pH and its control will enable safer use of drugs with regard to controlling drug excretion (e.g., barbiturate overdosage, Ch. 13) and in preventing drug interactions (Ch. 4).

ABSORPTION OF ULTRAVIOLET LIGHT. Nearly all drugs capable of causing photoallergy (Table 75–8) absorb ultraviolet light, suggesting some common chemical characteristic(s). (See "Allergic Diathesis.")

CHEMICAL SIMILARITIES. Certain chemical groupings predictably yield adverse reactions, although they may occur in drugs with totally different pharmacologic actions. For example, hepatic damage induced by one "hydrazine" will almost invariably develop with another agent containing that grouping, and there is a range of aniline-like drugs which may produce hemolysis in subjects with glucose-6-phosphate dehydrogenase deficiency (Table 75–23).

Similarly, in individuals hypersensitive to certain chemical groups, related drugs usually produce symptoms of allergy. For example, a patient hypersensitive to the sulfonamides will usually

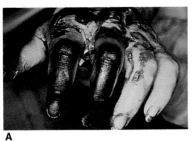 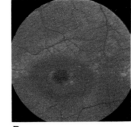 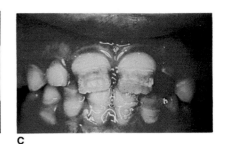

A

B

C

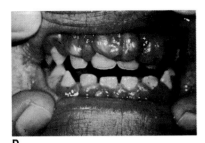

D

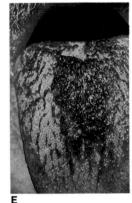

E

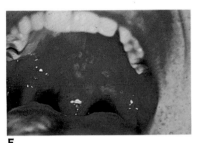

F

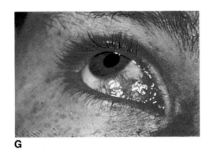

G

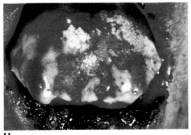

H

FIG. 7-1. Some representative drug reactions.

A. Necrosis of fingers due to accidental intraarterial injection of thiopental.

B. Retinopathy from chronic Chloroquine administration.

C. Tetracycline-induced staining and enamel hypoplasia of secondary dentition.

D. Diphenylhydantoin-induced gum hyperplasia.

E. Tetracycline-induced "black hairy tongue."

F. Sulfonamide-induced agranulocytosis.

G. Lesions of Stevens-Johnson syndrome in conjunctiva due to Sulfonamide.

H. Lesions of Stevens-Johnson syndrome in mouth due to Sulfonamide.

(continued)

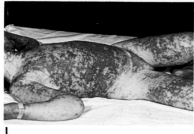

I

FIG. 7-1. Some representative drug reactions. *(continued)*

I. Toxic epidermal necrolysis due to Penicillin.
J. Exfoliative phototoxic reaction to a Tetracycline.
K. Lesions of erythema multiforme on wrist due to a Sulfonamide.
L. Penicillin-induced angioedema.
M. Bullous skin eruption due to Griseofulvin.
N. Phenolphthalein-induced skin pigmentation.
O. Glucocorticosteroid-induced "acne."
P. Bromoderma.

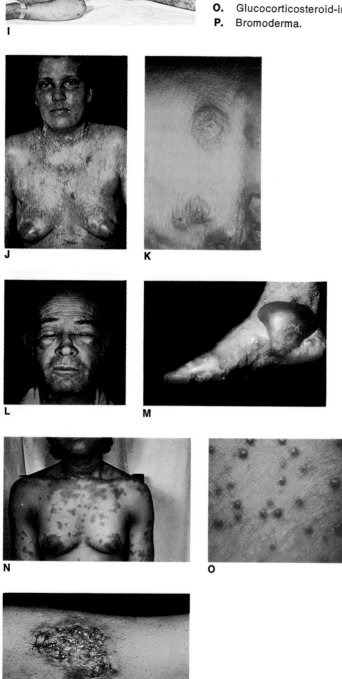

J

K

L

M

N

O

P

TABLE 7-2. Predisposing Factors to Adverse Drug Reactions

Drug factors

Chemical characteristics
Route of drug administration
Number of drugs administered
Drug dosage and duration of treatment
Addition of pharmacologic effects
Combination with adjuvants
Drug cost

Host factors

Age: pediatric; geriatric
Weight and body composition
Sex
Blood group
Race and heredity (pharmacogenetics)
Temperament
Skin color
Environment and diet
"Allergic" diathesis
Concomitant disease
Pregnancy
Lactation
Patient errors
Physiologic variations
Status of host microflora

Physician and nurse factors

Physician factors
Nurse factors

product against decomposition under normal storage conditions. If a drug degrades, three main problems may be associated with its use: the patient is deprived of active ingredient, the degraded product may produce toxicity (e.g., the Fanconi-like syndrome with tetracyclines Ch. 57), and if either of these occurs, the physician is open to litigation.

Nonexpired drugs (due to adverse storage conditions) may degrade prematurely; out of date drugs are not necessarily degraded, but they should not be used.

THERAPEUTIC INEQUIVALENCY. Samples of the same "drug" from different manufacturers, although containing equal quantities of chemically derived active ingredients, may differ dramatically in therapeutic effect due to altered bioavailability. Important properties influencing drug bioavailability are indicated in Table 7-3. Although the degree of bioavailability is important for most therapeutic agents, it is of critical importance to patients stabilized on long term therapy with antiepileptic drugs, antibiotics, anticoagulants, digitalis and endocrine agents. For example, switching to the same antiepileptic chemical supplied by a second manufacturer may lead, if the bioavailability of the new formulation does not equal that of the initial preparation, to redevelopment of seizure activity.

cross react with all other sulfonamides and with the chemically related drugs the sulfonylureas, the thiazide diuretics and acetazolamide.

DRUG DEGRADATION. Unstable drugs are supplied with an expiration date which indicates the period of time a manufacturer guarantees his

DRUG PURITY. The average tablet or capsule is anything but a simple preparation of "pure drug." Additional items are present for specific pharmaceutical formulation reasons, and some

TABLE 7-3. Some of the Factors Contributing to Therapeutic Inequivalency*

Formulation and manufactoring factors

Additives (adjuncts)	Excipients agents	Preservatives
Adjuvants	Flavors	Pressure of tablet punches
Binders	Formulation	Purity
Buffers	Friability	Solubility (of adjuncts)
Chelators	Granulators	Solubility (of drug)
Coating composition	Hardness	Solvation
Coating thickness	Hydration, degree of	Stereoisomeric stability
Coloring agents	Impurities	Stereoisomerism
Compactness of fill	Incompatabilities	Surface activity
Complexation	Lubricants	Surface area
Crystal structure	Packaging materials	Surfactants
Deaggregation rate	Particle size	Suspending agents
Diluents	pH	Uniformity of composition
Disintegrators	Porosity	Vehicles
Dissolution rate	Potency	Wettability
Emulsifying agents		

Distribution Factors

Age of drug product	Moisture, atmospheric	Stability of ingredients
Deterioration	Oxidation	Stereoisomeric shifts
Epimerization	Packaging	Storage conditions
Humidity	Radiation	Temperature of environment
Inertness of atmosphere	Reduction	Transportation stress

*Modified from Martin (See "Further Reading")

of these assume importance when evaluating drug bioavailability and the problems created by "generic inequivalency" (see above).

It is rare that the active (drug) ingredients of any preparation are not what the manufacturers state they are, but several mistakes have been discovered. In the United States, e.g., some early preparations of digitalis glycosides contained estrogens that caused puzzling gynecomastia in several patients, and a minor epidemic of precocious puberty in young girls taking isoniazid was traced to contamination of the drug by female sex hormones in an improperly cleaned tablet making machine. Impure drugs rarely reach the United States market today. However, the tourist or alien may bring in a drug purchased abroad which, because of less stringent controls in its country of manufacture, contains contaminants.

It is more common that questions arise concerning the safety or dangers of nondrug components of drug preparations. For example, the sodium content of antacids may pose a significant hazard to patients with compromised cardiovascular function, and many drug solutions are contaminated by bacteria. In recent years considerable publicity has been directed towards the potential dangers of particulate matter (fibers) in solutions for IV administration.

Route of Drug Administration

Generally speaking, serious adverse reactions are more common following parenteral administration, particularly by the IV route, compared to oral or topical administration. However, the topical administration of some drugs, e.g., the penicillins or the sulfonamides, is more frequently followed by sensitivity reactions than is parenteral or oral administration, respectively. "Nonabsorbable" drugs given for an effect in the bowel lumen, e.g., group 4 sulfonamides (Ch. 60), magnesium and aluminum antacids (Ch. 37) and neomycin (Ch. 56), are absorbed to a slight degree. Under normal circumstances such absorption is harmless, but in the face of hypersensitivity to the compound or in the presence of compromised excretory organ function, toxicity may readily develop. Localized toxicity is also common when specific routes of drug administration are used, e.g., thrombophlebitis from too concentrated a drug solution infused IV, or chemical meningitis, and neuropathies, etc., following poorly controlled intrathecal drug administration.

Number of Drugs Administered

In one detailed epidemiological study of medical patients, adverse drug reactions increased ex-

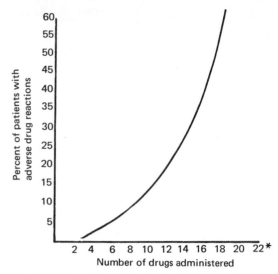

FIG. 7–2. The relationship of rate of adverse drug reactions to number of drugs administered. (Smith JW, Seidl LG, Cluff LE (1966): Studies on the epidemiology of adverse drug reactions V. Clinical factors influencing susceptibility. Ann Intern Med 65:629–640)

ponentially with the number of drugs given (Fig. 7–2). The types of medication given to patients receiving many drugs and fewer drugs were similar. Furthermore, although patients who received more drugs had a higher mortality rate and a longer hospital stay than those who received fewer drugs, the types of illnesses in the two groups were not different. Considerable sophistication is required to evaluate the multipotential for drug interactions when many drugs are given together (Ch. 4). The **"benefit:risk" ratio for each drug decreases when multiple drugs are given.**

Drug Dosage and Duration of Treatment

In general, the longer the duration of treatment and the higher the dosage, the greater the chance of development of adverse drug reactions. Repeated short courses of some drugs, however, can be just as dangerous, e.g., as the antibiotics (Ch. 53).

Most responses to drugs are dose dependent, but drugs may have more than one effect each with a different dose response, e.g., sedation and antihistaminic actions with the antihistamines (Ch. 47). However, only minute quantities of a drug can generate severe anaphylactic shock in subjects hypersensitive to that agent.

Addition of Pharmacologic Effects

If the pharmacologic effects of two drugs are additive, adverse drug reactions may develop. A patient taking PAS, e.g., may develop salicylism on taking small doses of aspirin (Ch. 28). Similarly, atropinism may readily develop if an antihistamine and phenothiazine are combined, since both drugs possess some parasympatholytic activity (Ch. 49).

Combination of Drugs with Adjuvants

Adjuvants combined with drugs for parenteral administration sometimes increase their sensitizing potential. Examples are the inclusion of procaine or benzathine in penicillin preparations (Ch. 55) or the use of heparin in oil.

Drug Cost

The high cost of some drugs may increase the rate of patient noncompliance (see below).

PREDISPOSING PATIENT (HOST) FACTORS

Several patient variables may alter the pharmacology or pharmacokinetics of drugs, producing adverse effects. Computer based data gathering programs, e.g., the Boston Collaborative Drug Surveillance Programme (Ch. 79), will doubtless identify numerous other important factors.

Age

At the extremes of life, the functions of absorption, metabolism and excretion may be imperfectly developed, as in the newborn (particularly the premature infant), or diminished, as in the elderly subject. Furthermore, the responsiveness of certain tissues and homeostatic mechanisms may be different from the adult, and the ability of the body to oppose drug effects may be altered. Thus, therapy based on pharmacokinetic data derived from the adult may lead to unexpected toxicity.

PEDIATRIC AGE GROUP. Compared to adults, children have a more rapid gastrointestinal transit time, a higher body water content (70–75% compared to 60%), a relatively greater body surface area, differences in tissue distribution of drugs (e.g., the relative permeability of the blood brain barrier), a relatively low glomerular filtration rate and renal plasma flow, plasma proteins that do not bind drugs as well and difficulty (and therefore unreliability) with oral therapy. All these factors influence the development of adverse drug reactions. For a discussion of specific aspects of drug therapy in the pediatric age group see Chapter 11.

GERIATRIC AGE GROUP. In 60–70 year-olds the risk of an adverse drug reaction is about double that of the young adult. This results from a diminution in function of the organs of absorption, metabolism and excretion due to age or associated disease. For example, symptom free patients of 65 years of age may have lost as much as 50% of their renal glomerular and tubular functions. Diminished renal function is accentuated by dehydration, congestive heart failure, urinary retention, electrolyte abnormalities, etc. Thus, drugs excreted by the kidney, e.g., digoxin and phenylbutazone, may rapidly achieve high plasma levels in the geriatric patient if dosage is not adjusted downwards.

Geriatric patients can exhibit reduced sensitivity (responsiveness) to some drugs compared to adults. Thus a gradual loss in sensitivity of autonomic reflexes in the CVS may influence the response of patients to drugs such as guanethidine (Ch. 20). Similarly, phenothiazines are more prone to produce Parkinson's disease in the elderly. Emotional problems and cerebral arteriosclerosis can contribute to unintentional drug abuse or imperfect compliance (see below).

Weight and Body Composition

Body weight, composition (fat) and degree of physical fitness can influence the development of adverse drug reactions. Pentobarbital (e.g., a nonpolar drug) rapidly accumulates in adipose tissue from where it is slowly released to act on the CNS (Chs. 2,26,27). Thus the pattern and deviation of pharmacologic effect may vary with the amount of body fat.

Sex

Although various sex differences in drug distribution, response and metabolism have been described in animals, these are not (excluding those associated with pregnancy and lactation, see below) of major importance in man. Oral contraceptive steroids retard the metabolism of certain drugs (Ch. 4). Furthermore, epidemiologic studies have shown that the incidence of adverse drug reactions is higher in women compared to men, e.g., the incidence of blood dyscrasias with phenylbutazone, aminopyrine and chloramphenicol has an unexplained 3:1 preponderance in women.

Sex differences influence the severity of some diseases in man, e.g., essential hypertension. Since hypertension is associated with greater end organ damage in men compared to women, more potent drugs tend to be used in men. Thus the sex of a patient is often an important factor in planning therapy and indirectly in the development of adverse drug reactions.

Blood Group

Associations between blood group and secretor status and various disease states, although unexplained, have been recognized for many years. It has recently been found, e.g., that women of blood group A are nearly three times more likely to develop thromboembolism while on oral contraceptive steroids than are women of blood group O.

Race and Heredity (Pharmacogenetics)

The study of the genetic control of drug metabolism is part of pharmacogenetics (Ch. 8), and genetic polymorphisms of drug metabolism can be responsible for the production of adverse drug reactions.

Temperament

The patients temperament may influence the development of adverse drug reactions. Emotional, sensitive, frail, asthenic, high strung, hypochondriacal subjects report more adverse drug reactions and tend to be greater placebo responders than more stable, stoic individuals. Geriatric patients may exhibit wide swings of mood due to cerebral arteriosclerosis and other factors, and thus suffer more "subjective" drug reactions.

Skin Color

The presence of melanin in the skin protects against injury by external agents, e.g., radiant energy. Thus photodermatitis (see below) is very rare in the Black subject but common in the Caucasian, and particularly in the albino of any race.

Environment and Diet

The phenotype of each organism is the result of the interplay between its genetic makeup and environmental influences. Genetic influences are discussed in Chapter 8.

Foods or drugs may depress the absorption of therapeutic agents (Ch. 4). In patients taking monoamine oxidase inhibitors, foods containing tyramine (cheese, pickled herrings, beer, wine, etc.) may prove fatal (Ch. 18). The precise influence of tobacco smoking is not clear. Smoking does increase the activity of some enzymes, notably benzpyrene reductase and hepatic oxidases, and heavy cigarette smokers are less likely than nonsmokers to suffer reactions from benzodiazepines. Exposure to DDT and other insecticides is unavoidable for almost everybody in the United States, and some foodstuffs contain up to 5 ppm of DDT, a concentration which produces enzyme induction in animals. Many other common substances produce enzyme induction (Table 4–2), and various industrial solvents can produce hepatic or renal damage. Extremes of heat or cold are associated with hypovolemia or hypervolemia, respectively, with the concomitant development of pH and electrolyte changes in tissue fluids. Hypoxia (living at high altitude) is a stimulus to enzyme induction. Picas, e.g., clay or starch eating can be associated with drug interactions. Undoubtedly many environmental and dietary factors are unknown.

Allergic Diathesis

Patients with an "allergic diathesis" (eczema, hay fever, asthma, urticaria, angioedema, etc.) are more likely to develop drug allergy than nonhypersensitive individuals. Patients with ulcerative gastrointestinal disease may be more likely to develop drug allergy to orally administered drugs than are other patients. A patient known to have suffered an allergic drug reaction should not be exposed again to this or to related agents *without full consideration of the risk of inducing fatal anaphylaxis.* In one study, barbiturates, the penicillins, meprobamate, codeine and the thiazide diuretics, were responsible for 70% of the allergic reactions encountered. Allergy to the penicillins is covered more fully in Chapter 55; little is known about allergies to other drugs.

Concomitant Disease

Disease states may predispose to adverse drug reactions in one of five main ways.

DISEASES NECESSITATING MULTIPLE DRUG THERAPY. In some diseases (e.g., infections, hypertension, congestive heart failure), multiple drug therapy is required, a situation predisposing to adverse drug reactions (see above).

DISEASES AFFECTING THE ORGANS OF ABSORPTION, METABOLISM AND EXCRETION. Diseases of the gastrointestinal tract, diarrhea, obstruction, ulcerative lesions, malabsorptive states, pernicious anemia, etc., are frequently associated with altered drug absorption leading to adverse drug reactions. Similarly, congenital or acquired liver or renal disease can alter the metabolism or excretion of drugs or drug metabolites. In alcoholism the rate of hepatic microsomal oxidase activity is increased, whereas in advanced cirrhosis it may be reduced. Similarly, in renal disease, drugs which are not readily excreted can produce severe toxicity, e.g., the aminoglycoside antibiotics (Ch. 56).

Little is known about the way disease states may alter drug handling or tissue sensitivity. Many diseases are associated with hypo or hyperproteinemia, but whether or not plasma protein binding of drugs is measurably altered in all these situations is not known. Certainly low serum albumin levels have been associated with increased diphenylhydantoin and prednisone toxicity; reduced protein binding of many drugs, e.g., the sulfonamides, occurs in uremia.

EXAGGERATION OF OVERT OR LATENT DISEASE. Drugs may exaggerate overt disease, or they may precipitate latent disease. A few examples will be mentioned.

Therapeutic agents may produce hyperuricemia either directly (ethionamide, pyrazinamide, thiazide diuretics, etc.) or indirectly (methotrexate) precipitating gout. Glucocorticosteroids can induce diabetes mellitus through gluconeogenesis and possible other mechanisms. Barbiturates, by depressing the synthesis of δ amino levulic acid, may precipitate an acute attack of porphyria. Neuromuscular blockade in patients with myasthenia gravis is accentuated by aminoglycoside antibiotics and various antimalarial agents. In patients with the Crigler-Najjar syndrome, jaundice can be produced by drugs which are cleared via glucuronidation, since glucuronyl transferase is poorly developed in such patients, and the drugs compete successfully with bilirubin for the enzyme.

ADVERSE REACTIONS IN PATIENTS WITH INFECTIONS. Drug reactions are more likely to develop in patients with infections. The reason is unclear, but under experimental situations the CNS toxicity of some drugs is increased in the presence of fever.

Pregnancy

Major alterations in body function develop during pregnancy. It has been suggested, e.g., that the increased demand for protein anabolism makes the liver more susceptible to drugs such as the tetracyclines which depress this function (Ch. 57). Additionally, during pregnancy the metabolism of some drugs is delayed, e.g., succinylcholine, and there is a depression of transport processes which clear drugs (e.g., bromsulphalein) through the liver cell. Changes in hemodynamics and renal function can alter drug clearance and response. The fetus may suffer adverse drug reactions (see below).

Lactation

Many drugs are excreted in the milk (Table 75–26), and thus can produce adverse effects in the infant.

Patient Errors

Patient errors influencing adverse drug reactions can be *failure to take medicine as prescribed* and/or *self-medication,* which may interfere with the prescribed medication through drug interactions (Ch. 4).

FAILURE TO TAKE MEDICINE AS PRESCRIBED. Patients may take either more or less than the prescribed dose; both usually result in suboptimal therapy. The usual and fallacious rationale for taking more than the prescribed dose is "if three of these pills a day are making me better, six of them a day will make me better twice as quickly." However, irregular medication (patient noncompliance) is far more common than overmedication.

PATIENT NONCOMPLIANCE. A careful study of 40 outpatients receiving a total of 143 different drugs in a medical clinic indicated that *only 10% were taking their drugs as prescribed.* Noncompliance rates of 20–80% were reported in studies involving antibiotics, antacids, antidepressants and antimalarials. Noncompliance may be serious. In a study of patients with congestive heart failure, 92% continued to take their digitalis as prescribed, whereas 83% persisted with their thiazide diuretic; only 60% continued to take potassium supplements.

Noncompliance is more difficult to predict than to detect, since the causes are poorly understood. Correlations between noncompliance and old age, low income, socioeconomic status, marital status (widowed, separated or divorced) and type of, or duration of disease have been made, but with inconstant results.

Two points are clear: the error rate increases with increasing dose (increasing number of tablets) and the number of different drugs prescribed, and in many instances, failure to comply results from failure of the physician to fully inform the patient about the drug, the purpose of using it and it's dose schedule.

CONSEQUENCES OF NONCOMPLIANCE. The consequences of noncompliance are either adverse drug reactions or apparent therapeutic failure. For example, failure to take antibiotics regularly often leads to relapse of the original infection, emergence of resistant organisms or superinfection (Ch. 52). On occasion, however, no real disadvantage can be observed. For example in a study of antacid therapy in the treatment of peptic ulcer disease, noncompliance was not associated with increased morbidity, suggesting that antacids may have a minimal role, if any, in therapy!

Since noncompliance rates are high, it should be suspected in every patient. Many techniques have been tried to measure the degree of compliance, but they are rarely foolproof. Direct tests for the drug or drug metabolite in urine or feces, or for the presence of an inert marker (e.g., riboflavin produced fluoresence), are more satisfactory than pill counting, special drug dispensers or quantitation of a measurable side effect (e.g., dry mouth with atropine). Tests which can directly measure drug effect (prothrombin time) are more valuable.

The best treatment for noncompliance is prophylaxis. Physicians should thoroughly explain the drug to the patient, outlining its name, why it is being given and how it should be taken. In addition, prescription drugs, over-the-counter drugs, or foods which could possibly interfere with the agent should be identified, in so far as they are known.

SELF-MEDICATION. Self-medication with drugs left over from previous prescriptions, or with over-the-counter preparations (tonics, vitamins, aspirin, iron tablets, laxatives, etc.), is not unusual, and may lead to drug interactions (Ch. 4). Similarly, care must be taken with regard to other drugs the patient may be taking concomitantly under prescription from another physician. One of the most important parts of history taking is a thorough inquiry into the nature and dosage of all "drugs" taken in the immediate past.

Physiologic Variations

Many physiologic changes occur in the body during the day, and these functions alter if a patient is placed on complete bed rest. Additionally, prolonged bed rest is associated with a reduced plasma volume and depressed cardiovascular function. Stresses of heat, exercise and fluid deprivation alter the rate of drug metabolism, and circadian effects with regard to drug absorption, metabolism and excretion are only now being identified. Fluctuations in urinary pH develop, particularly in relationship to meals, and this may alter drug effects.

Status of Host Microflora

The normal human organism is populated by 60 or more different microorganisms, particularly in the gastrointestinal tract. That these microflora are important in drug metabolism is only just being realized. Patients stabilized on anticoagulants, e.g., usually need their dose adjusted downwards if broad spectrum antibiotics are added to the drug regimen (Ch. 57). Additionally, colonic microflora metabolize chenodeoxycholic acid to lithocholic acid, a potential hepatotoxin (Ch. 37).

PHYSICIAN AND NURSE FACTORS

Physician and nurse factors have been partially covered above under host factors, but bear elaboration here.

PHYSICIAN FACTORS. Physicians may be tempted to use drugs when little or no clinical benefit can be expected, e.g., the unwise prophylactic use of antibiotics (Table 52–4), or the use of digitalis glycosides in subjects with aortic stenosis or mitral insufficiency, where clinical benefits are minimal. Under such circumstances, digitalis may be "pushed" to toxic levels in an attempt to produce some clinical improvement.

NURSE FACTORS. Some degree of error is inevitable in all human performance, but studies have indicated that in some hospitals, where the quality of drug therapy should be at the highest level, between 20–30% of all doses of medication were either incorrect or harmful. A careful study of nine nurses in a teaching hospital indicated that for every six drug doses ordered, there was one error. Statistically, 40% were omission of a dose, 20% were the administration of a drug not ordered and 40% were drugs administered at the wrong time, in the wrong dosage form, in an extra dose or in under or overdosage. Medication errors increase logarithmically with the number of drugs prescribed.

CLASSIFICATION OF ADVERSE DRUG REACTIONS

Adverse drug reactions are difficult to classify because of the many variables or "risk" factors which may influence their development, and because the definition of an adverse drug reaction is not clear cut (see above). A simple classification is given here which, although by no means comprehensive, will hopefully clarify this heterogenous and complex subject; many of the categories overlap each other. Specific reactions, and the drugs which may cause them, are tabulated in Chapter 75.

Reactions Associated with the Therapeutic Effect of Drugs

Many adverse reactions are produced through an extension of the drugs therapeutic effect.

Overdosage is seen when too large a dose of an agent is given, e.g., respiratory depression and coma with the barbiturates, or hemorrhage with the anticoagulants. Overdosage may also be seen with "standard" therapeutic doses due to failure of drug metabolism and/or excretion, e.g., antibiotic toxicity in the presence of renal failure (Table 52–1), the Grey Baby Syndrome with chloramphenicol (Ch. 57), or succinylcholine sensitivity (Ch. 8).

A therapeutically useful action of a drug may be harmful when it involves a tissue **other than the target organ,** e.g., with autonomic or anticancer agents (Chs. 15,17,67).

Depression of host "resistance" is a direct extension of the mode of action of many drugs which interfere with leucocyte function, lysosomal activity and immune mechanisms. Examples occur with glucocorticosteroids (Ch. 46; Table 52–1), immunosuppressants (Table 52–1), anticancer drugs (Ch. 67; Table 52–1) and oral contraceptives (Ch. 48; Table 52–1).

Depression of the inflammatory and repair processes is the basis of the use of the glucocorticosteroids and immunosuppressive agents in autoimmune and some chronic inflammatory diseases, and to suppress graft versus host reactions. However, in some quiescent infections (e.g., peptic ulcer disease, postoperative wound healing), such effects may be dangerous.

Interference with the normal body flora may lead to superinfections (Ch. 52), and often poses a therapeutic problem. For example, antibiotic suppression of the normal bowel bacterial flora may lead to symptoms of vitamin B deficiency (Ch. 57) or to an altered responsiveness to anticoagulants.

Reactions Associated with the Nontherapeutic Effect of Drugs

Direct pharmacologic effects are very common. Drowsiness from the antihistamines or morphine induced constipation are two typical examples. Reactions associated with the **intensification of concurrent disease** are an exceedingly important category. Thus, a patient with peptic ulcer may have a relapse if treated with corticosteroids, reserpine, aspirin or anticoagulants. Similarly, hepatic coma may follow administration of morphine, ammonium chloride or thiazide diuretics in those with cirrhosis of the liver.

Many drugs cause local **tissue irritation.** Upper gastrointestinal symptoms (nausea, vomiting, dyspepsia, heartburn) are common after oral administration of antibiotics, iron preparations, aspirin, etc. These are mild adverse effects, and slight reduction in dosage or proper spacing of the drug in relation to meals reduces symptoms. Similarly, hypertonic or hypotonic parenteral injections may cause considerable local edema or pain. Occasionally a sterile abscess develops following a large parenteral injection or following repeated injections to the same muscle of, e.g., an iron–dextran complex. Tetracycline antibiotics are notoriously prone to produce thrombophlebitis (due to endothelial irritation) following IV administration.

Tissue deposition of drug crystals may develop in the urinary tract, for example, sulfonamide crystalluria (Ch. 60). Some drugs have the capacity to produce **blockade of nutrient absorption.** For example, several agents produce malabsorption (Table 75–27). Similarly, barbiturates and diphenylhydantoin may block the utilization of folic acid and vitamin B_{12}, resulting in megaloblastic anemia (Table 75–24).

Delayed adverse effects may be seen following the use of **radioactive drugs.** Thorium dioxide (Thorotrast), e.g., used for many years as a radiopaque dye in arteriography, is stored in the reticuloendothelial system and has been incriminated, after a latency of up to 20 years, in producing generalized atrophy, fibrosis and malignant degeneration. Similarly, the use of radioactive iodine (^{131}I) in the treatment of hyperthyroidism has been linked with the subsequent development of thyroid carcinoma and leukemia.

Effects due to **drug degradation** have been discussed above.

Reactions Associated with Allergy

Hypersensitivity (allergic) reactions represent the largest single group of adverse drug reactions. While most drugs are capable of producing an allergic response, penicillin, streptomycin, the sulfonamides and quinidine are notorious offenders. To give rise to an allergic reaction, the drug or drug metabolite(s) (haptene) must combine strongly with a tissue or plasma protein. This complex is processed by the reticuloendothelial system, with ultimately the production of antibody. Antibodies can react with both the complex and the haptene, but our knowledge of their production is far from clear. Antibodies against the offending drug or its metabolites cannot be demonstrated in every case of suspected drug allergy, and reexposure of the patient to the original drug may not elicit an allergic reaction.

Allergic reactions to drugs are either *immediate, accelerated* or *delayed.* Immediate reactions usually are combinations of atopy, angioneurotic edema and serum sickness. In severe cases death may occur from anaphylactic shock. (See Chapter 55 for a discussion of penicillin allergy.)

REACTIONS ASSOCIATED WITH SUNLIGHT.

By far the most important precipitating exogenous factor is sunlight, and reactions are either **phototoxic** or **photoallergic** (Table 7–4). In addition, drug photosensitivity has been documented in at least three diseases, porphyria, lupus erythematosus and pellagra. Phototoxic reactions occur when a nontoxic substance changes into a toxic one in the patient's skin by the absorption of photoenergy. Photoallergic reactions occur when the absorption of radiation energy by a chemical changes it into a metabolite which may then sensitize the patient. Photosensitization may also arise following topical exposure of various compounds, particularly antiseptics and antibiotics in soaps, hair rinses, shampoos, perfumes and antiseptic creams (Table 75–8). Drugs that produced photoallergies, absorb light in the ultraviolet and near ultraviolet range. Thus blue discoloration after exposure to ultraviolet light occurs only in those phenothiazine derivatives which are able to induce photoallergy, not in other representatives of this class. Similar changes have been noted with the tetracyclines and the sulfonamides. Photoallergic rashes may persist for long periods of time after termination of drug exposure. Frequently, the patient remains permanently sensitized to the offending drug, even in the absence of sunlight.

PREGNANCY AND FETAL DEVELOPMENT

Effects on Reproduction

Parasympatholytic drugs (Ch. 18) may produce impotence. Thorazine and related psychopharmacologic agents have been shown to interfere with ejaculation without affecting orgasm. Monoamine oxidase inhibitors are reported to increase and progestational agents to decrease female fertility.

Effects During Intrauterine Development

Adverse drug effects are nowhere more dramatically evident than in the fetus and neonate. Most drugs with a molecular weight of 1000 or less can easily cross the placental barrier (Table 75–25). The effects of rubella virus (German measles) during the first trimester of pregnancy are well known. Of more importance and not generally recognized is that many drugs can cause similar effects. The effect of a drug given

TABLE 7–4. Characteristics of Drug Induced Photosensitivity

Reaction	Phototoxic	Photoallergic
Reaction possible on first exposure	Yes	No
Incubation period necessary after first exposure	No	Yes
Chemical alteration of photosensitizer	No	Yes
Covalent binding with carrier	No	Yes
Clinical changes	Usually like sunburn	Varied morphology
"Flares" at distant previously involved sites possible	No	Yes
Can persistent light reaction develop	No	Yes
Cross-reactions to structurally related agents	Infrequent	Frequent
Broadening of cross-reactions following repeated photo-patch testing	No	Possible
Concentration of drug necessary for reaction	High	Low
Incidence	Usually relatively high (theoretically 100%)	Usually very low (but theoretically could reach 100%)
Action spectrum	Usually similar to absorption spectrum	Usually higher wavelength than absorption spectrum
Passive transfer	No	Possible
Lymphocyte stimulation test	No	Possible
Macrophage migration inhibition test	No	Possible

Baer RL, Harber LC (1971): Reactions to Light, Heat, and Trauma. Immunologic Diseases. Vol. II, Swater M (ed) Boston, Little Brown

early in pregnancy may be fetal death. During organogenesis, in the first trimester, malformations may be produced. Later in pregnancy or during labor, drugs may cause fetal morbidity or death. Morbidity in the perinatal period is more common in premature infants.

Drug exposure during pregnancy is unfortunately commonplace. Studies reported that 82–92% of women were given at least one drug during pregnancy, and four was the average number of drugs prescribed; 4% of patients were given ten drugs or more.

TERATOGENESIS. The thalidomide disaster focused attention on the potential danger of administering drugs during pregnancy. Although thalidomide is no longer available, a brief discussion of the incident is instructive.

A German pharmaceutical firm developed in the late 1950s, thalidomide, a drug which induced sleep without residual hangover. Subsequently, because of its apparently minimal side effects, thalidomide was manufactured and sold in many countries, often combined with analgesics, hypnotics and antiinflammatory drugs. Some 90 different brand names under which thalidomide was sold have been identified. The first cases of phocomelia, or seal limbs (Figs. 7–3 and 7–4), were detected in Germany in September 1960, and since then, according to the German minister of health, approximately 6000 cases have been reported in that country alone. Of these, about half have died. Besides phocomelia, malformations of the gastrointestinal tract, ears and heart were seen. Facial hemangiomas were fairly common, but the babies were usually normal mentally. Parenthetically, it should be stressed that the only notable adverse effect in the adult taking thalidomide is peripheral neuritis.

It is usually considered that there is a critical time during organogenesis for an individual tissue to be affected by teratogenic agents. This time coincides with the greatest mitotic activity in that organ. For example, the limb buds exhibit maximal susceptibility between 18–28 days of gestation, or, in other words, 38–48 days after the first day of the last menstrual period. This indicates the importance of not exposing women of childbearing age to unnecessary medication, as *teratogenic effects may be produced before pregnancy is diagnosed or even suspected.*

Many experiments have been undertaken in animals in an attempt to demonstrate thalidomide teratogenicity. Most have been unsuccessful. This poses the question of how accurate and useful are animal experiments in predicting the potential toxicity of new drugs to human beings (Ch. 6).

Several other potent pharmacologic agents, anticancer drugs, sulfonylurea compounds and corticosteroids are suspected of producing teratogenic effects during pregnancy.

MASCULINIZATION OF THE FEMALE FETUS. Before embryonic sexual structures differentiate, they are susceptible to the influence of exogenous endocrine agents. Female pseudohermaphroditism, e.g., has been produced by testosterone (given for hyperemesis gravidarum) and by a variety of synthetic progestational agents commonly used in the treatment of habitual or threatened abortion.

Perinatal Effects

Drugs given to the mother before or during labor may cross the placenta, and the baby may be born still under their influence (Table 75–25). In most instances, the drug is an anesthetic, analgesic, tranquilizer, antidiabetogenic agent, antibiotic or antihypertensive. Side effects of simple overdosage tend to be produced, similar to those seen in the adult. Paralytic ileus from antihypertensive drugs and ventilatory depression following reserpine, hypnotics and narcotics are not unusual. Occasionally, barbiturates induce hemorrhagic disease of the newborn due to depression of the Stuart-Power factor.

Neonatal Effects

The neonate is not just a miniature young adult. This point is discussed above under Age Factors and in Chapter 11.

MISCELLANEOUS REACTIONS

Effects Following Use of Placebos

The basic emotional pattern of a patient may influence his response to drugs. This is particularly true of drugs affecting the central nervous system and of placebos (Ch. 6). Many physicians have observed mild adverse reactions to placebos, such as depression, sleepiness, sleeplessness, anorexia, nausea, tremulousness, dizziness, palpitations and lassitude. Some puzzling severe reactions to placebos have been reported, such as fixed drug eruptions, anaphylactic shock and even death.

A placebo is by definition innocuous. It is a pharmacologically inert agent, or a food substance (iron capsule, bread pill, sugar pill, vitamin C tablet). No substance should be used as a placebo if there is even remote danger of a harmful effect. Thus aspirin should not be used, especially in children. Similarly, the ever present danger of serum hepatitis makes it impossible to guarantee the harmlessness of parenteral injections of normal saline, a common placebo. On the other hand, there is the danger of failing to recognize the need for precise treatment and substituting a placebo for necessary drug (or psychiatric) therapy.

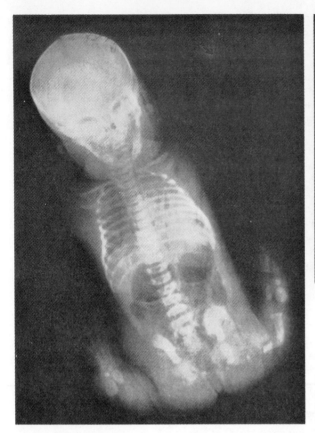

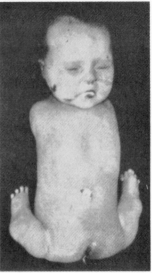

FIG. 7–3. Female infant who died 24 hours after birth. (Ward, Shirley P (1962): Brit Med J Sept. 8 p. 646. Reprinted from the *British Medical Journal* by permission of the author, editor, and publishers, B.M.A. House, Tavistock Square, London, W.C. 1)

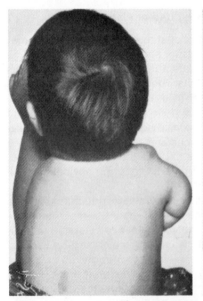 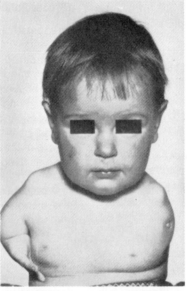

FIG. 7–4. Boy, aged 18 months, whose mother had taken thalidomide during early pregnancy. Note saddle nose and hemangioma situated on the right cheek. The left upper limb is absent; on the right side, there is a rudimentary humerus, no radius, and two rudimentary digits. (Gillis L (1962): Brit Med J Sept. 8. Reprinted from the *British Medical Journal* by permission of the author, editor, and publishers, B.M.A. House, Tavistock Square, London, W.C. 1)

Drug Interactions

Adverse drug reactions may develop through drug interactions (Ch. 4).

Effects on Laboratory and Diagnostic Procedures

It is now recognized that many commonly prescribed drugs can invalidate diagnostic tests (Ch. 76). Furthermore, drugs may produce pathologic changes in tissue; for example, a megaloblastic bone marrow may be associated with ingestion of barbiturates, and lymph node changes suggestive of sarcoidosis or lymphoma may attend diphenylhydantoin administration.

Effects Due to Failure to Institute Correct Therapy

Frequently drugs are prescribed because the patient expects a pill. In these instances (by giving a potentially harmful agent without a true indication for its use), the physician can be criticized justifiably. For example, the administration of antibiotics to patients with uncomplicated coryza is therapeutically unsound. On the other hand, indirect harm can be caused by postponing correct therapy.

A related topic of particular importance in the United States is the long time lag in FDA approval of new drugs developed overseas.

FURTHER READING

D'Arcy PF, Griffin JP (1972): Iatrogenic Disease. England, Oxford University Press

Forfar JO, Nelson MM (1974): Epidemiology of drugs taken by pregnant women: drugs that may affect the fetus adversely. Clin Pharmacol Ther 14:632–642

Harber LC, Baer RL (1972): Pathogenic mechanisms of drug-induced photosensitivity. J Invest Dermatol 58:327–342

Martin EW (1971): Hazards of Medication. Philadelphia, Lippincott

Smithells RW (1966): Drugs and human malformations. Adv Teratol 1:251

Zbinden G (1963): Experimental and clinical aspects of drug toxicity. Adv Pharmacol 2:1

BERT N. LA DU, Jr.

8. PHARMACOGENETICS

Although it has been recognized for many years that genetic differences in people can modify their response to drugs, it has been only during the past 20 years that systematic studies have been conducted to evaluate the importance of genetic traits in drug effectiveness and adverse drug reactions. The scientific study of genetically determined individual variability in drug metabolism and unusual drug reactions is called *pharmacogenetics.* This relatively new field of pharmacologic investigation seeks answers to some important questions: how do genetic differences in people account for individual variability in the transformation, detoxification and excretion of drugs? Do genetic factors explain clinical observations that some patients, given the recommended amounts of appropriate drugs, develop unexpected or adverse drug reactions? Certain human genetic traits are associated with unusual drug effects, and definite relationships exist between genetic factors and drug disposition and metabolism.

DETECTION AND ANALYSIS OF PHARMACOGENETIC CONDITIONS

The observation that a patient has shown an exaggerated drug response or developed an unexpected drug reaction has been the starting point for many pharmacogenetic studies. Careful investigation of an individual patient's symptoms, however, is not enough to decide whether genetic or environmental factors are responsible, and a genetic approach, or a **genetic analysis** of the condition is required. It must be determined whether the unusual drug response is familial (runs in certain families) and, if this is so, whether it occurs among selected members of the family pedigree in a pattern that agrees with expectation for an inherited trait. For example, a recessively inherited trait should occur, on the average, in one-fourth of the sibs (brothers and sisters) of the index patients. Other patterns of drug sensitive family members would, of course, be expected for dominant traits, or for sex linked hereditary conditions. If the unusual drug reaction is closely associated with a specific biochemical "marker," such as the deficiency of a particular enzyme, or the presence of an abnormal drug metabolite in the urine or blood, more conclusive genetic evidence can be obtained. These biochemical and genetic steps are rather easily followed for pharmacogenetic conditions that are inherited as simple Mendelian dominant or recessive traits. The investigation becomes much more complicated, however, if several different genes are involved, and a particular combination of these genes must be inherited for patients to show the unusual drug reaction.

One general method that has been employed in pharmacogenetics is to measure the relative contributions of genetic and environmental influences using identical and fraternal twins. This method has the advantage that important information about the relative genetic contribution can be obtained from only a few test subjects, even though it does not indicate how many genes are involved or how the genetic factors operate. Basically, the twin study method is a comparison of variability of some pharmacologic measurement between pairs of identical (monozygotic) twins and pairs of fraternal (dizygotic) twins. Since monozygotic twins have the same genetic constitution, their variability is much less than the intrapair variability of fraternal twins for genetically determined traits.

A comparison of the percent of a test dose of isoniazid excreted as acetylisoniazid in 24 hr (Table 8–1) by identical and fraternal twins shows this metabolic (conjugation) pathway for iso-

TABLE 8–1. Excretion of Isoniazid by Identical and Fraternal Twins*

	Identical twins			Fraternal twins	
Twin pair number	Sex	Isoniazid excreted in 24 hr (% of dose)	Twin pair number	Sex	Isoniazid excreted in 24 hr (% of dose)
1	M	8.8	6	F	12.1
	M	8.3		F	13.7
2	F	26.0	7	F	10.9
	F	25.2		F	4.6
3	M	11.8	8	M	11.0
	M	12.4		M	8.5
4	F	12.2	9	F	3.9
	F	11.5		F	15.2
5	F	4.1	10	M	10.5
	F	4.4		M	15.6

*Bonicke R, Lisboa BP (1957): Uber die Erbbedingtheit der intraindividnellen Konstanz der Isoniazidausscheidung beim Menschen. Naturwissenschaften. 44:314

niazid to be determined primarily by genetic factors. Twin studies with several other drugs (phenylbutazone, antipyrine, bishydroxycoumarin and ethanol) led to similar results. The latter drugs are all handled mainly by biotransformation rather than by excretion into the urine as unchanged drug, and the rate of decline of the drug concentration in plasma was used as a measure of the rate of elimination. Close agreement in biological half-times was found within identical twin pairs; much wider variation occurred in pairs of fraternal twins. From all of these results, it is concluded that genetic factors, primarily, determine the rate of metabolism of most drugs and chemicals in man.

Pharmacogenetic conditions can also be investigated through population surveys by making some pharmacologic measurement in many people to see if the collected responses follow a unimodal, bimodal or multimodal distribution. Bimodality suggests that there may be two distinct subpopulations, but it does not prove that there must be a genetic basis for the two groups. Tests can be made, on that premise, to find out if a genetic hypothesis is supported, e.g., blood concentrations of isoniazid 6 hr after an oral dose of the drug show bimodality (Fig. 8–1). Further work has established that the rate of disappearance of the drug (rapid or slow) depends upon the rate of isoniazid acetylation, and the latter is proportional to the level of an enzyme, N-acetyl transferase, in the liver. Slow acetylators of isoniazid have appreciably less N-acetyl transferase in their liver than rapid acetylators. Family studies and other genetic tests have led to the conclusion that two allelic genes (R = rapid acetylation, r = slow acetylation) at one locus control the rate of isoniazid metabolism. Thus, there are three possible genotypic combinations (RR, Rr and rr) and two phenotypes: **rapid** (RR or Rr) and **slow** (rr). Slow acetylators are homozygous for a recessive gene, but since about one-half of

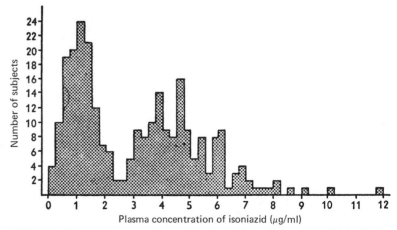

FIG. 8–1. Plasma concentrations of isoniazid 6 hr after oral administration to 267 members of 53 families. (Evans DA, Manley KA, McKusick VA, (1960): Genetic control of isoniazid metabolism in man Br Med J 2:485)

the United States population are slow, the recessive gene is far from rare. The respective gene frequencies are r = 0.723 and R = 0.277. The relative gene frequencies differ in other geographic areas according to the particular ethnic groups and their genetic history. Asiatic groups are generally much higher in rapid acetylators, and Middle Eastern groups are higher in slow acetylators than European and American populations.

OBJECTIVES OF PHARMACOGENETIC STUDIES

Whatever approaches are used in pharmacogenetic investigations, the objectives are the same: 1) evaluate how genetics contributes to the condition, 2) determine the inheritance pattern (dominant, recessive; sex linked or autosomal), 3) measure the frequency of the genes involved in the general population and different ethnic groups, 4) find the biochemical basis for the variation and 5) establish the clinical importance of the condition.

VARIATIONS IN DRUG METABOLISM

SERUM CHOLINESTERASE VARIANTS AND SUCCINYLCHOLINE SENSITIVITY

Several genetic variants of serum cholinesterase have been detected that are less effective in hydrolyzing the muscle relaxant drug, succinylcholine, than the common form of the esterase most people have in their blood. Succinylcholine, a dicholine ester of succinic acid, is inactivated by cleavage of one of the ester groups. After succinylcholine is given, an appreciable portion of the drug is hydrolyzed as it circulates through the blood and distributes to the tissues. Part of the drug reaches the tissues and binds to the myoneural junction sites. The enzyme is probably less important in destruction of the drug at this point than it is while the drug is being distributed through the blood and tissues. People with deficient serum cholinesterase have an exaggerated response to a standard dose of the drug because more drug escapes hydrolysis and reaches the tissues. They develop muscular paralysis, including the respiratory muscles, which may last for several hours. Artificial respiration must be given during this period until the drug effects disappear, but patients properly oxygenated and cared for should completely recover. One might suppose that many other esterases in the body could also act on succinylcholine and compensate for a deficiency of serum cholinesterase, but clinical experience shows this not to be so. Serum cholinesterase is the principal enzyme responsible for succinylcholine hydrolysis in man.

After succinylcholine was introduced into general use in the 1950s, occasional patients with prolonged and exaggerated response were noted, and it was suspected that they had a deficiency (reduced amount) of serum cholinesterase. However, it was found that the serum esterase from sensitive patients was not reduced in quantity but modified, probably in its structure, to give it different **qualitative** properties. The **atypical** cholinesterase from these patients had a lower affinity for choline ester substrates, and it was a less efficient catalyst by far than the usual esterase from succinylcholine hydrolysis. It was also less susceptible to dibucaine inhibition and a variety of other inhibitors. A simple inhibition test with dibucaine was developed to measure cholinesterase activity (with and without the inhibitor) to classify the type of esterase present. The inhibition by dibucaine or *dibucaine number,* for the usual cholinesterase cholinesterase is about 80%; atypical cholinesterase has a dibucaine number of about 20%, and heterozygous carriers with serum cholinesterase of mixed or intermediate quality have dibucaine numbers of about 60%. The dibucaine inhibition test is useful in family studies, since both homozygous atypical (AA) individuals and heterozygous (UA) can be distinguished from homozygous usual (UU) people by analyzing serum samples; drug administration is not necessary to determine each individual's genotype. Family pedigree studies established that the subjects with atypical cholinesterase inherited a rare gene (A) from both parents and that all people with atypical esterase would be sensitive to succinylcholine if they were ever given the drug. In the general Canadian population, and probably in the United States, about 3.8% are heterozygous carriers of the atypical gene and 1:2820 are homozygous for the atypical gene (AA). Unless serum cholinesterase activity is greatly reduced, heterozygous carriers of the atypical gene (AU) are not unusually sensitive to succinylcholine. Clinically, then, sensitivity to succinylcholine is inherited as an autosomal, Mendelian recessive trait.

Finding one genetic variant of an enzyme often leads to the discovery of others. Further variants of cholinesterase are known which also affect the response to succinylcholine. A **fluoride resistant** variant, detected by its greater resistance to fluoride inhibition than the usual cholinesterase, also has a lower affinity for choline ester substrates. Fluoride inhibition tests give "fluoride numbers" which can be used to distinguish whether individuals have inherited a single or a double dose of the fluoride resistant cholinesterase gene. Family studies in selected families carrying both the atypical (dibucaine resistant) and fluoride resistant genes showed that these genes segregate as allelic genes at the same genetic locus, rather than as genes determined at different loci.

This evidence, and the fact that genes (A and F) produce active esterases with reduced affinities for substrates and inhibitors, suggest they are both structural gene mutations in which the cholinesterases differ very slightly, perhaps only by single amino acids, from the amino acid sequence in the usual serum cholinesterase.

Another rare serum cholinesterase variant of interest is determined by the "silent" gene. Individuals homozygous for this gene have essentially no detectable cholinesterase activity. They show no signs or symptoms from this enzymatic deficiency and no disturbance in their normal intermediary metabolic reactions; the only expression of the hereditary enzymatic defect is an exaggerated response to succinylcholine if they should receive the drug.

There are additional rare variants of serum cholinesterase which could be mentioned, but those given above illustrate some general pharmacogenetic principles worth noting again. The enzyme affecting succinylcholine hydrolysis does not participate in the metabolism of endogenous or dietary esters, and the enzymatic deficiency is apparent only when succinylcholine is given. The unusual drug reaction can be clearly associated with the altered quantity or quality of the specific enzyme protein. Susceptible patients can be detected and predicted by a simple blood test and the same test can be used in families and sample populations to determine the frequency of the rare genes concerned with the drug reaction.

OTHER EXAMPLES OF HEREDITARY VARIATIONS IN DRUG METABOLISM

ISONIAZID. Slow acetylators of isoniazid are more likely to accumulate the drug with repeated doses and to develop a peripheral neuritis. This complication can be prevented by pyridoxine, and the vitamin does not interfere with the antitubercular activity of isoniazid.

DIPHENYLHYDANTOIN. Families are known with members who metabolize (p-hydroxylation) diphenylhydantoin much more slowly than expected. They are likely to develop overdose toxicity symptoms, nystagmus, ataxia and drowsiness if given the usual doses of the drug.

ACETOPHENETIDIN. Rarely, patients have been reported to develop red cell hemolysis and methemoglobinemia after small doses of acetophenetidin. It is believed that they have an inherited inability to metabolize the drug by the usual pathway (O-dealkylation and sulfate or glucuronide conjugation) and transform the drug *via* deacetylation and p-phenetidin to hydroxyphenetidin derivatives, which are toxic metabolites.

HEREDITARY METABOLIC DISORDERS OF PHARMACOGENETIC INTEREST

RED CELL DEFICIENCIES

Some inherited traits not directly concerned with drug metabolism can change the cellular environment in such a way as to make cells vulnerable to adverse drug effects. For example, there are a number of inherited enzymatic deficiencies of red blood cells that will result in hemolysis if primaquine and certain other drugs are taken. Best known are the deficiencies of glucose-6-phosphate dehydrogenase (G6PD). At least 80 distinct variants of the enzyme have been identified, but not all of these are associated with drug induced hemolysis. Generally, those variants with activity reduced to less than 30% of the normal are regularly associated with hemolytic reactions. It is not known exactly why a reduction in G6PD activity leads to hemolysis. G6PD is recognized as an important means of supplying NADPH, the cofactor for glutathione reductase, and glutathione appears to be essential for maintaining red cell membrane functions. This explanation may not be entirely correct, but it is clear that the glutathione concentration falls in erythrocytes deficient in G6PD if they are incubated with acetylphenylhydrazine. This simple in vitro test has been used to identify individuals who would be susceptible to drug induced hemolysis.

Since the gene determining the characteristics of G6PD is carried on the X chromosome, G6PD deficiencies are inherited as sex linked traits. Males are more likely to show drug related hemolysis than females. A survey of American Negroes (Table 8–2) indicated that 15% of the males and 1.6% of the females were classified as "reactors" by the glutathione stability test. Although the test does not discriminate well between intermediate and normal responses, the figures obtained establish the inheritance to be sex linked, without dominance. Females are classified as reactors, intermediate or normal, depending upon whether

TABLE 8–2. Glutathione Stability in Erythrocytes from American Negroes

	Genotype*	Expected frequency†	Observed frequency**
Females (184 subjects)			
Normal	AA	0.742	0.935
Intermediate	Aa	0.239	0.049
Reactor	aa	0.019	0.016
Males (144 subjects)			
Normal	AY	0.864	0.833
Intermediate	—	0	0.021
Reactor	aY	0.136	0.146

*A, normal X chromosome; a, X chromosome with gene causing primaquine sensitivity.
†Calculated on the assumption of sex linked inheritance without dominance, frequency of 0.136 for the reactor gene and a frequency of 0.864 for the normal gene (after Childs B et al [1958] : A genetic study of a defect in glutathione metabolism of the erythrocyte. Bull Johns Hopkins Hosp 102:21.
**The glutathione stability test does not discriminate well between normals and intermediates.

both, one or neither of the X chromosomes carry the defective gene; males, having one X chromosome, are either reactors or normal.

In addition to red blood cell enzymatic defects, there are abnormal forms of hemoglobin that predispose the patient to hemolysis when sulfonamides and antimalarial drugs are given. Hemoglobin H and hemoglobin Zurich are hemoglobins of this type.

CONJUGATION DEFECTS

Several inherited deficiencies in glucuronide conjugation are known which are characterized by hyperbilirubinemia and jaundice. Not only is the conjugation of bilirubin affected, but there may also be reduced glucuronide formation of such drugs and foreign chemicals as salicylates, menthol and tetrahydrocortisone. Since these inherited disorders vary considerably in severity and in the specific molecular deficiency from family to family, the degree of drug conjugation impairment will also be variable.

VITAMIN RESPONSIVE CONDITIONS

Some individuals have greatly increased requirements over the average for particular vitamins and may show symptoms of a vitamin deficiency unless the vitamin intake is increased manyfold over the usual daily requirement. Specific examples are known of defective conversion of B_{12} to cofactor forms of the vitamin. Some respond to very high B_{12} administration. The therapeutic use of vitamins to treat hereditary disorders of this type illustrates the need to individualize therapy for each patient's particular genetic constitution.

INHERITED RESISTANCE TO COUMARIN ANTICOAGULANT DRUGS

It is unusual to find a true difference in responsiveness to drugs at the tissue level; most of the genetic differences in "response" can be explained by alterations in drug dynamics of drug distribution and drug metabolism, changing how much reaches the tissue sites. The local dose-response relationships rarely change. One exception is the hereditary resistance to coumarin anticoagulants. Such patients require nearly 20 times as much drug to produce the expected increase in prothrombin time, an amount that would cause a fatal hemorrhage in the usual patient. Discovery of the condition was unusual, since the first patient happened to be an identical twin, and his brother also required anticoagulant treatment and showed the same remarkable resistance to coumarin drugs. Their entire family, and one other large pedigree, have been tested for this genetic trait. Coumarin resistance is inherited as an autosomal dominant trait. The resistant individuals show another unusual feature: they are about 20 times more sensitive than usual to the antidotal effects of vitamin K. Since metabolism of the anticoagulant drugs is not unusual in these people, the most reasonable explanation for their resistance is a genetically altered tissue protein which regulates the synthesis of the blood clotting factors II, VII, IX and X in the liver.

Surprisingly, there seems to be a natural animal model for this human pharmacogenetic condition. Warfarin is used as a rat poison, but natural resistance to this agent has been noted in rat populations with repeated use. Studies on some of the resistant rats indicated that rare genes for resistance have been selected out, and the rats had the same mechanism of resistance as found in human variants.

MISCELLANEOUS HEREDITARY CONDITIONS WHICH MODIFY DRUG EFFECTS

Drugs may produce undesirable effects in certain other patients with hereditary conditions or traits. A few will be briefly noted (Table 8–3).

Malignant hyperthermia with muscular rigidity is a rare but very serious complication associated with anesthesia. The condition is familial and appears to be inherited as an autosomal dominant trait. Since hyperthermia may occur with or without muscle rigidity, it is probable that more than one genetic disorder is represented. Patients are often young, healthy individuals who unexpectedly develop these symptoms during surgery using halothane and succinylcholine. It can occur with other anesthetic agents. Succinylcholine is not specifically associated with

TABLE 8–3. Some Hereditary Conditions Which Modify Drug Effects

Conditions	Drugs	Pharmacologic effects
Malignant hyperthermia	General anesthetics	Hyperthermia and rigidity
Angle closure glaucoma	Atropine	Intraocular pressure increased
Chronic, simple glaucoma	Dexamethasone	Intraocular pressure increased
Porphyria (hepatic)	Barbiturates	Porphyrin synthesis increased
Idiopathic hypertrophic subaortic stenosis	Digitalis	May not increase cardiac output
Mongolism	Atropine	Response increased
Familial dysautonomia	Norepinephrine	Increased pressor response

hyperthermia, but this combination is most frequently noted in the cases reported to date. Approximately one-half of the patients who develop hyperthermia and rigidity do not survive. Muscle biopsies from survivors respond abnormally to caffeine, and it has been suggested that the intracellular distribution of calcium is disturbed. However, the exact cause of this hereditary disorder is still unknown.

It is intentional to close with an example of a pharmacogenetic condition whose investigation is still in progress and unsolved, as there are many such problems awaiting study and solution today.

Aside from making use of the specific examples of pharmacogenetic conditions mentioned above, it is hoped that those using drugs will appreciate that genetic differences must be considered in selecting the best drugs and the doses most appropriate for each individual patient. Furthermore, when unexpected drug reactions do occur, the possibility of an inherited drug anomaly ought to be considered, and at least a family history should be taken. Even in experimental pharmacology, more use should be made of genetics, and unusual drug responses in animals should not be ignored. Studies over the years on hereditary metabolic diseases in man have given us valuable insight into normal metabolism and the role of specific proteins; the same rewards can be expected if animal pharmacogenetic models are properly utilized.

FURTHER READING

Kalow W (1962): Pharmacogenetics, Heredity and the Response to Drugs. Philadelphia, W. B. Saunders

La Du BN, Kalow W (eds) (1968): Pharmacogenetics. Ann NY Acad Sci 151:691

La Du BN (1972): Pharmacogenetics: defective enzymes in relation to reactions to drugs. Annu Rev Med 23:453

Vesell ES (1973): Advances in Pharmacogenetics. Steinberg AG, Bearn AG (eds) Progr Med Genet IX:291

Stanbury JB, Wyngaarden JB, Fredrickson DS (1972): Metabolic Basis of Inherited Disease. New York, McGraw Hill

LEO E. HOLLISTER

9. DRUGS OF ABUSE

One person's social drug is another's drug of abuse. One person's treatment may be another's treat. When we speak of "drug of abuse," we make a judgment. On the other hand, "drug dependence" refers to a biologic phenomenon. The one term is socially defined, according to local custom; the other term is universal. Perhaps it would be better to speak of "drugs used for non-medical purposes" or "drugs of social use," but these terms are less familiar. In any case, the term "drug of abuse" creates a paradox by including marihuana and excluding alcohol. In this discussion, we shall deal with opiates, sedatives, stimulants, hallucinogens and marihuana—those drugs most widely "abused" at present.

HIERARCHIES OF DRUG USE AND ABUSE

Each culture, including our own, has its special drugs. In the United States, the three national drugs are caffeine, nicotine and alcohol. Habituation to each is widespread, some citizens having the dubious distinction of taking all three drugs simultaneously. Yet few of us even think of these as drugs.

PERMISSIVE DRUGS. Our attitude to these drugs is almost completely permissive. Caffeine is available to children in the form of cola containing beverages and to adults as these, plus the ubiquitous coffee and tea. Because caffeine is a mild stimulant, its action is not likely to be discernible during the working day; rather, it may become more apparent in the form of a sleepless night following a dinner finished with too many cups of coffee. Caffeine is not considered to be much of a drug as we customarily take it.

Nicotine is available in a number of different forms of tobacco smoking, not to mention recently revived intranasal and buccal forms. While a strong campaign is currently being waged to discourage the use of cigarettes, with little success to date, the objection is not to the drug effect, but to the inhalation of noxious matter accompanying the combustion of tobacco. Although large acute doses (say, 60 mg) of nicotine could kill a human being, the constant doses taken by smokers, and the tolerance which develops, allow that much or more to be taken daily with relatively few physiologic effects. While smoking is associated with an increased number of deaths from coronary artery disease, it is questionable whether the pharmacologic effects of nicotine in cigarettes contribute directly to this harmful effect. Thus, this drug also is considered to be rather innocuous as usually taken.

By far the most dangerous of our national drugs is ethyl alcohol, which is available in a great variety of potable forms (Ch. 10). This drug is addicting in every sense of the word. Apparently our society values the beneficial aspects of the use of alcoholic beverages more than it fears the evil consequences, for they are readily available to all adults in unlimited quantities.

Alcohol is primarily a CNS depressant. It produces enough "disinhibition" to produce the desired social facility, although this is attended by impairment of function. Much could be said for and against the use of alcoholic beverages, but the plain fact is that we accept their use and their presumed benefits, as well as the dangers of abuse. No serious attempt has been made to prohibit use of alcoholic beverages since the universally disregarded Eighteenth Amendment to the United States Constitution was repealed in 1933.

PRESCRIPTIVE DRUGS. Under this category would be classified those used therapeutically for their central effects. As such, they are readily available when prescribed by physicians. Drugs of this type constitute some of the most widely prescribed and used drugs in our country.

The opiate analgesics are among the most valuable drugs in medical practice; no physician would think of attempting to practice without them (Ch. 29). Although a great variety of natural derivatives have been extracted from crude opium and many synthetic analogs manufactured, it is really doubtful whether overall any is superior to morphine. Codeine is virtually irreplaceable.

Barbiturates have been used for over 60 years, their annual consumption in the United States being measured in tons. These drugs are enormously useful in clinical practice, having sedative, hypnotic, muscle relaxant, anticonvulsant and anesthetic effects in different forms or varying doses (Ch. 26). Currently, diazepam and chlordiazepoxide, two new sedatives of the benzodiazepine class, are the first and third most prescribed drugs, respectively (Ch. 25).

Amphetamines have been used as stimulants for over 30 years and as appetite suppressants for nearly as long (Ch. 18). These drugs are potent stimulants, as compared with caffeine, with strong sympathomimetic effects. In recent medical practice they have been more often used as appetite suppressants. A number of amphetamine analogs have been produced for this specific purpose: diethylproprion, phenmetrazine and others.

PROSCRIPTIVE DRUGS. This group of drugs includes those which have been placed under special controls because of a great amount of illicit or illegal use. The situation at present is rapidly changing, owing to recent laws which expand the list of controlled drugs.

Proscriptive drugs would include many that are used medically, such as opiates, sedatives and stimulants, whenever they are used for nonmedical purposes and have usually been obtained from some illicit source. They would also include drugs such as marihuana and the hallucinogens, for which no medical uses have been established and whose only sources of supply, under prevailing laws, are illicit.

CONCEPTS OF TOLERANCE AND DEPENDENCE

Tolerance to and dependence on drugs are closely linked. Without tolerance to a drug, physical dependence is most unlikely.

TOLERANCE. Several possible mechanisms of tolerance to a drug may be distinguished. First, "behavioral" tolerance may develop. This type is best exemplified by chronic alcoholics who even with high plasma levels of ethanol may appear to be functioning normally. Second, "metabolic" tolerance may ensue. With continued exposure to the drug, enzymes may be induced that enhance its biotransformation to inactive metabolites. Meprobamate is an example of such a drug; its rate of hydroxylation is doubled after a week of use. When such drugs are clinically used over long periods of time, patients either experience a loss of the initial sedative effects or a need to increase the dose to maintain them. If the difference between the therapeutic dose of a drug and that which may result in physical dependence is small (with meprobamate this may be as low as a factor of 2–3), this type of tolerance may rapidly place the patient in danger of becoming physically dependent. Third, "immune" tolerance may develop from the formation of antibodies to the drug. Most drugs are of low molecular weight substances not ordinarily antigenic, but when bound to protein they may act as haptens. Antibodies to many have now been demonstrated, although their role in development of tolerance is not entirely clear. Finally, tolerance may be "pharmacodynamic," that is, be based on a lessened degree of drug effect due to homeostatic or compensatory mechanisms elicited by its initial effects. As this type of tolerance is conceptually linked with physical dependence, it will be discussed further below.

DEPENDENCE. Two types are recognized, psychologic and physiologic, although the boundaries between the two are sometimes difficult to define. Psychologic dependence is manifested by a strong craving for the drug, but not necessarily with the appearance of physical signs of withdrawal when it is stopped abruptly. Physical dependence is defined as the appearance of psychologic and physical symptoms of withdrawal, as exemplified by the well-known withdrawal reactions that occur in heavy users of alcohol, barbiturates or opiates. Psychologic dependence is seen in all who develop physical dependence, although the converse is not true.

The social drugs, caffeine and nicotine, or "abused" drugs, such as marihuana, hallucinogens or amphetamines in small doses, produce largely psychologic dependence. The consequence of stopping these drugs is the loss of comfort they may provide. Physical symptoms

TABLE 9–1. Scheme of Possible Sequence Tolerance-Withdrawal-Dependence

Assume	a) drug x to be a CNS depressant
	b) a neurohumor c to be a CNS excitant
Initially	x blocks c, producing SEDATION
Block of	c derepresses enzyme e synthesis
Increased	e compensates for block of c
Increased	c restores equilibrium, TOLERANCE
Increased	x must be taken to obtain desired effect of sedation; repeated through several cycles yielding marked increases of e and c
WITH-DRAWAL	of x in presence of increased e and c produces marked EXCITEMENT unmasking PHYSICAL DEPENDENCE

are minimal or nonspecific. Physical dependence to opiates has long been recognized, manifested by the withdrawal syndrome: sneezing, sweating, runny nose, shivering, gooseflesh, muscle aching, abdominal cramps and diarrhea. Proof that delirium tremens is due solely to physical dependence on ethanol was only firmly established in the past quarter century. A short time later, similar physical dependence was shown to follow barbiturate use. Both syndromes were manifested by apprehension, sweating, tachycardia, tremors, mental confusion, hallucinations and occasionally convulsions.

A scheme that explains how tolerance and later physical dependence develops is shown in Table 9–1. Homeostatic mechanisms in the body produce first tolerance and later on physical dependence and withdrawal signs.

SPECIFIC TYPES OF DRUGS OF ABUSE

HEROIN AND OTHER OPIATES

Although heroin is the most notorious of all abused opiates, other drugs which share many of its pharmacologic properties may also be subject to abuse (Ch. 29). Hundreds of thousands of doses of morphine and codeine are administered daily for medical purposes with little consequent abuse. Synthetic drugs resembling opiates, the opioids, are represented primarily by meperidine, pentazocine, methadone and dextropropoxyphene.

For reasons to be mentioned later, heroin is the preferred drug for street use. Although morphine seems to be in the most respects its full equivalent, a mystique about heroin makes it preferable. Codeine is not a widely abused drug, as large doses cause too many unpleasant side effects, such as itching from release of histamine.

Most opioids were introduced as narcotics less prone to cause addiction. This belief was rapidly dissipated in the case of meperidine, although its abuse has been largely restricted to those with easy access to it, such as physicians, nurses and other health personnel. Pentazocine represents the present culmination of a long search for drugs with mixed agonist–antagonist actions and less potential for abuse. To some extent this hope has been realized, large doses tending to produce unpleasant reactions of a hallucinogenic type; the few cases of dependence to pentazocine have been mild. Methadone is a potent narcotic quite useful as a substitute for morphine when patients are intolerant of the latter drug. It is highly addicting. D-Propoxyphene most resembles methadone chemically. Despite an undeservedly wide clinical use, instances of abuse are rare, undoubtedly due to its extreme lack of potency.

HISTORY. References are made to an opium-like drink in Greek mythology. Until comparatively recently, it was most widely used in the Orient and the Near East. For many years, China was the leading user of opium, although from all reports available, its use on the Chinese mainland had declined to the vanishing point under the present political regime. Not only has Indochina been one of the leading areas of opium production, but for many years Saigon was a leading opium port. Therefore, the great exposure to opium of United States troops in Vietnam should not have been unexpected.

The widespread use of opium for treating wounds during the United States Civil War led to the first of several "epidemics" of opiate use. It was estimated that 4% of Americans used opiates during the post Civil War period. Just prior to World War I, the estimate had dropped to 1 in 400 adults, but the rate of use was considered to be so alarming as to merit the passage of the Harrison Narcotic Act. From the end of World War II until 1964, the prevalence of heroin use was relatively constant, but a new epidemic followed the wake of increased nonmedical use of many drugs. By 1972, heroin was being used by an estimated 700,000 persons in the United States.

CHEMISTRY. Morphine was first isolated from opium early in the 19th century; a little less than a century ago it was found that a diacetyl derivative (heroin) could be produced by exposing it to acetic anhydride. Heroin was actually a Bayer trade name, just like aspirin, but both are now definitely generic. After opium has been harvested in growing areas such as Turkey or Lebanon, it was converted to morphine at one of the nearest transhipment points such as Beirut.

Most conversion of morphine to heroin occurs in France, particularly in Marseilles. A yield of 1 kg of 90–98% pure heroin might be expected from conversion of 12 kg of high grade opium. Scarcely ever does such pure material reach the consumer; usually it is first diluted considerably either with inert materials, such as lactose or talc, or with other drugs, such as quinine or barbiturates.

PHARMACOLOGIC CONSIDERATIONS. Heroin is about three times as potent as morphine, so it can be easily smuggled and is therefore a more acceptable illicit drug. It is also more water soluble, affording a more rapid onset of action by IV injection. Monoacetylmorphine, as well as morphine itself, is an active metabolite, readily passing into the brain and possibly accounting for its increased potency. The drug is excreted as conjugated or unconjugated morphine, which is the substance actually measured by urine tests. As with most drugs, duration of action depends somewhat on dose, with most street doses lasting for 3–5 hr. Thus, the addicted person is never very far removed from withdrawal symptoms.

Tolerance to opiates is well known. Many of the symptoms of the opiate withdrawal syndrome resemble those of increased cholinergic activity. Although withdrawal may be quite uncomfortable, it is rarely life threatening. The need for ever increasing amounts of drug to maintain the expected euphoriant effects, as well as the discomfort of withdrawal, have the expected consequence of strongly reinforcing the addiction once it is started. The prevalent belief is that both immediate reward (in the form of relief of physical or psychic pain) and the act of self-administration are strongly reinforcing factors in opiate addiction.

TOXICITY. Death from inadvertent overdose (an omnipresent possibility when injecting an IV dose of an unknown material) is probably due to acute respiratory depression accompanied by pulmonary edema with a highly viscid proteinaceous fluid. Such deaths rank high in the age group 15–25 years in cities such as New York. This syndrome is treated by prompt administration of a morphine antagonist (naloxone), endotracheal intubation, intermittent positive pressure oxygen and antibiotics for any complicating pneumonitis. Many other medical complications are associated with the use of heroin, principally due to lack of aseptic techniques in its administration. These include hepatitis B infection (the majority of chronic users) and a multitude of infections, most notably bacterial endocarditis.

ETIOLOGIC AND EPIDEMIOLOGIC CONSIDERATIONS. The notion of drug "fiends," that persisted until fairly recently, has been largely supplanted by the illness model of drug addiction. Use of drugs is construed as an attempt by certain individuals to attain pharmacologic relief from anxieties and depressions. One wonders whether the drug addict might not best be considered an "exploitee," preyed upon by those who exploit human folly. In any case, addiction to heroin and other drugs is a complex interplay between many factors, personal, environmental and pharmacologic.

Since the end of World War II, two rather stable patterns of opiate addiction have existed in the United States. The larger group was confined to the ghettos of northern cities and affected primarily persons who for one reason or another had not been assimilated fully into society: Blacks and Puerto Ricans in Harlem, blacks in Detroit or Chicago or Chicanos in Los Angeles. A much smaller group was found in the rural south, with addiction to opiate-containing cough syrups. Estimates of the total number of addicts in the country ranged between 75,000–200,000 until a few years ago.

The situation changed drastically in the 1960s so that by 1972 an estimated 700,000 persons were heroin users. By 1974, the estimate was reduced to 400,000, of whom about 160,000 were undergoing some kind of treatment. About 80,000 were in methadone maintenance programs, another 70,000 were in some drug free treatment and about 10,000 in detoxification. All estimates of the extent of drug use are suspect, but the latest heroin epidemic shows some signs of abating.

TREATMENT. Two contrasting styles of treatment have been used for opiate dependent individuals. The most widely used approach is methadone maintenance. The main idea behind this treatment is that methadone, which given once daily by mouth is both more active orally and longer lasting than most other opiates. The person's dependent need for drug is sustained without interfering with his activities. He does not "nod," nor is he obliged to sustain his dependence with criminal activity. Drug treatment is never given alone but is accompanied by sustained efforts at social and vocational rehabilitation. The cost of such treatment for each patient is usually not more than a few hundred dollars per year. Problems have arisen with diversion of methadone with "take home doses" and with difficulty in maintaining frequent clinic attendance once rehabilitation has been accomplished. Moralistic objections concern the desirability of maintaining drug dependence, yet methadone treatment is generally preferable to maintenance of heroin dependence. A methadone-like drug with a much longer duration of action, methadyl acetate (L-acetyl-α-methadol, LAAM) may obviate some of the difficulties mentioned above.

Drug free programs are variations on the theme of therapeutic communities, as pioneered for opiate users by Synanon. They are based on the general assumption that drug use is symptomatic of some emotional disturbance or inability to cope adequately with life. The most common technique uses peer group pressures, emphasizing confrontation. Other techniques include variations on group or individual psychotherapy, didactic approaches, alternative life styles through work or communal living and a variety of meditative techniques such as transcendental meditation, Zen or hypnosis. Treatment may last for months or years with costs depending on the degree to which professional staff is used.

As each treatment approach has a self-selected clientele, it is difficult to compare results. One has the general impression that more chronic users of opiates prefer methadone maintenance, whereas those with shorter histories of drug use are more amenable to the drug free approach. Unfortunately, proponents of each treatment have become markedly polarized.

Additional treatments under investigation include the use of narcotic antagonists or immunologic techniques to render opiate use unrewarding. Long acting depot forms for administration of methadone or a narcotic antagonist are also being sought.

BARBITURATES AND OTHER SEDATIVES

HISTORY. Barbiturates have been used medically for most of the present century, being one of the most widely prescribed classes of drugs. Their indications are many, including the relief of anxiety, the production of sleep, the control of epilepsy and either an adjunctive use in the control of pain or a direct use as an anesthetic. The experimental demonstration of physical dependence to barbiturates in the early 1950s led to a decline in their use, especially following the development of new barbiturate surrogates (often only technically "nonbarbiturates") or new chemicals with sedative properties labeled "tranquilizers" or "antianxiety drugs." Thus, newer drugs, such as glutethimide (a barbiturate surrogate more dangerous than its analog, phenobarbital), meprobamate, chlordiazepoxide and its congeners, and more recently methaqualone,

have to some extent replaced the barbiturates in clinical practice.

PHARMACOLOGY. Phenobarbital, amobarbital, pentobarbital, secobarbital and thiopental are the barbiturates most often used medically (Ch. 26). Phenobarbital is a very long acting drug. The very short acting thiopental is used exclusively as an IV anesthetic. Other members of the group with an intermediate length of action are most often employed as hypnotics. Meprobamate is a relatively weak sedative, with a span of action similar to that of secobarbital. Methaqualone and glutethimide are also weak drugs with relatively short durations of action. Chlordiazepoxide, diazepam and other drugs of the benzodiazepine series are more potent and much longer acting.

Those who abuse sedatives do so in order to obtain a rapid but fairly brief state of intoxication, not too unlike that caused by alcohol. It would be expected, therefore, that the drugs most likely to be abused would be those that are rapidly absorbed and have a short span of action. These requirements are well met by secobarbital, pentobarbital or amobarbital among the barbiturates, and by meprobamate, methaqualone or glutethimide among other classes. Drugs that are longer lasting, such as phenobarbital or the benzodiazepines, do not lend themselves so well to repeated bouts of intoxication. Thus, the biological half-life of the drug seems to have an important bearing on its potential for abuse. For a variety of reasons, including easier availability and cheaper price, secobarbital sodium is the preferred street drug.

Most abuse of these drugs is by oral ingestion, and the effects from secobarbital appear rather quickly. These are primarily a drunken state akin to alcohol intoxication, with relief of tension, euphoria and later sleepiness. By titrating the dose, users can maintain a constantly intoxicated state during the day but sleep it off at night. Tolerance rapidly develops so that the dose must be constantly raised to attain the same effects. Such tolerant individuals can take with impunity normally lethal doses up to 1–2 g daily. When such levels of dose are reached, severe withdrawal reactions resembling delirium tremens may occur. Like delirium tremens, these withdrawal reactions are life threatening if not treated appropriately. The principles of treatment are the same as with most other types of withdrawal from drugs: substitution of a pharmacologically equivalent drug (usually sodium pentobarbital), gradual withdrawal of the substituted drug and supportive treatment.

TOXICITY. Chronic intoxication of animals with barbiturates has been said to produce abnormal histologic changes in the brain, but such changes are not established in humans. Withdrawal reactions or inadvertent overdosage are the major hazards of sedative abuse. As these drugs are commonly used by alcoholics, the combination having synergistic depressant effects, unwitting suicides have occurred. Their concurrent use with heroin seems to be a major factor in "overdose" deaths attributed to the latter.

EPIDEMIOLOGY.

Instances of iatrogenic abuse have been reported periodically for many years. Recently, most sedative abuse has been by youngsters who obtain their supplies on the illicit market and only occasionally from the family medicine chest. More recent stringent controls on barbiturates may force a shift in the pattern of sedative abuse to other drugs. It is not clear why some users may prefer drugs of this type, commonly called downers, to stimulants (uppers). Many use either, depending on the availability, or may use one to counter the effects of the other. Sedatives may also be used in a pattern of multiple drug use involving other sedative drugs such as alcohol, marihuana or heroin.

TREATMENT OF SEDATIVE ABUSE.

The same treatment model might be applied to sedatives as to alcohol abuse, considering their pharmacologic similarities. The social context of use, including sedatives in a pattern of polydrug use, is somewhat different, so that it is by no means certain that similar treatment would be equally effective.

AMPHETAMINES AND STIMULANTS

HISTORY.

The stimulant effects derived from chewing coca leaves were discovered by folk pharmacologists in the Andes centuries ago. The active component cocaine, discovered in 1860, is a local anesthetic (Ch. 22). Although cocaine has little chemical resemblance to the amphetamines and other more modern stimulants, its pharmacologic actions are quite similar.

Chemical analogs of epinephrine and norepinephrine were known even before the identity of either hormone was established. Medical use of amphetamine dates from 1935, and in very short order most of the common indications were discovered (Ch. 18). Racemic amphetamine was quickly replaced by dextroamphetamine, and other homologs such as methamphetamine were developed. Newer homologs include drugs such as methylphenidate, phenmetrazine, diethylpropion and pipradol.

CHEMISTRY AND PHARMACOLOGY.

Amphetamines are indirect sympathomimetic amines. Thus the usual central effects are alertness, tremor and increased deep tendon reflexes. The mechanism for appetite suppression, which is only temporary, is not clear.

Methamphetamine is the most widely abused preparation, possibly because it is more easily made in the illicit market. It is usually sold as the raw chemical (slang term "crystal"). Most D-amphetamine reaching the illicit market is diverted from marginal pharmaceutical houses.

The familiar clinical effects of mild oral doses, such as an increased sense of well-being and perhaps a slight degree of nervousness, are quite different from those obtained from the massive doses taken IV by confirmed users. These doses may range 50–4000 mg daily. Such doses would be fatal in intolerant subjects, who have died from as little as 120 mg IV. Following IV injection, users report an immediate "rush" characterized by general sensations of tingling (said to be something like an orgasm). Great alertness and feelings of confidence and power soon follow. Users develop repetitive writhing movements of the extremities or masticatory movements of the mouth. As effects subside over a few hours, a new dose may be taken. Such repetitive doses (a "run") may last a week or more, during which time sleeping and eating are minimal. Exhaustion at the end of a run is followed by withdrawal characterized by marked depression and restlessness. Often "coming down" or "crashing" is so painful that the user seeks relief by taking downers, such as barbiturates or heroin. The latter drug is so effective that many heroin addicts are first initiated into its use as a treatment for a crash reaction from shooting amphetamines.

TOXICITY.

Abusers of this drug frequently develop paranoid thinking during its use. These symptoms may appear rapidly after a rather small total dose. In its full blown state, the paranoid psychosis from amphetamine resembles naturally occurring schizophrenia more closely than any other drug induced state. Recent studies suggest persistence of abnormal brain function and sleep disturbances lasting for months after termination of a run.

A recently recognized adverse effect of amphetamine abuse is necrotizing arteritis, resembling periarteritis nodosa. Once established, this complication is irreversible. It is often fatal, providing some credence to the popular slogan "speed kills." As amphetamines are often taken IV with unsterile apparatus, users of this drug are exposed to the same infectious complications as heroin users.

EPIDEMIOLOGY. The exact extent to which drugs of this class are abused is not really known. Two patterns of abuse exist, oral and IV. The former often stems from initial use of the drug either self-administered to enhance performance or prescribed by physicians to assist weight reduction. The consequences of this pattern of abuse are seldom great. A larger number of users quite early administer the drug IV, the desired effect being the "rush." Although some pure "speed freaks" exist, often this pattern of amphetamine use is associated with multiple drug abuse.

Tighter controls over manufacture and strong persuasion against its medical use have reduced its prescription. However, the reduction in amphetamine abuse has not been proportionate to the decreased medical use. More likely, reduced use stems from a better appreciation of its disastrous effects.

The encouraging decline in amphetamine abuse has been paralleled by an ominous increase in abuse of cocaine. The latter drug has attained a certain cachet among middle and upper class circles as well as among those who find it a ready substitute for street amphetamine. The drug has a low margin for safety, so that mucosal absorption through the nose ("sniffing") is preferred to oral or IV administration.

TREATMENT. No specific pharmacologic or psychologic treatment programs have been devised. Patients using amphetamines to treat a prevailing depression may be best treated with conventional antidepressant drugs. Some who have experienced the psychotic reaction evoked by the drug may have been destined to become schizophrenic, especially if the psychosis is long lived. Antipsychotic drugs would then be the treatment of choice. Psychologic approaches to treatment would be similar to those described for addiction to opiates.

HALLUCINOGENS

HISTORY. Almost every society, however primitive, has found some bark, skin, leaf, vine, berry or weed which contains "hallucinogenic" materials. Although the fortuitous discovery of the amazing properties of lysergic acid diethylamide (LSD) occurred in a chemical laboratory three decades ago, it was a case of art imitating nature. Similar compounds were known in morning glory seeds, and drugs such as mescaline and psilocybin had long been used by North and Central American Indians in the form of cactus buttons or magical mushrooms. Deliriants, such as the materials in belladonna (Datura stramonium), were also known to ancient man.

Drugs termed "hallucinogens" do not often produce hallucinations. Other terms have been proposed, such as "psychedelic" or "psychotomimetic," but these are equally inappropriate. Drugs of this type are taken for many reasons. According to those most widely given, the hallucinogenic drugs provide new ways of looking at the world and new insights into personal problems. The former action implies varying degrees of perceptual distortion; whereas the latter implies changes in mood and increased introspection. At times, it seems as though drug users will use any drug which alters thinking or mood, including deliriants such as the synthetic central anticholinergic drug, Ditran or organic solvents taken by inhalation. The prototypic hallucinogenic drug is LSD because of the extent of its use, because it represents a family of drugs that are similar and because it has been most carefully studied.

CHEMICAL AND PHARMACOLOGIC CONSIDERATIONS. LSD is based on the lysergic acid nucleus, within which one can discern resemblances both to the phenethylamine structure of mescaline and the indolethylamine structure of psilocybin. It is also readily apparent that both structures occur in brain biogenic amides, such as norepinephrine and dopamine in the case of phenethylamines, and 5-hydroxytryptamine (serotonin) in the case of the indolethylamines. Whether these chemical resemblances account for the similarity of action of the three types of drugs or for a mechanism of action mediated by effects on brain biogenic amines is still not certain.

The effects of LSD, mescaline and psilocybin are so similar that most persons regard them as a specific group of hallucinogens. The ratio of dose between LSD and psilocybin is approximately 1 : 250, whereas with mescaline it may be 1 : 4000. LSD may be one of the most potent pharmacologic materials known. The usual doses in man are 1–2 μg/kg. The drug is equally effective when taken orally or by injection, so the former route is preferred.

Like marihuana, hallucinogens of the LSD type are of very low acute toxicity, and deaths from overdose are rare. The mode of action of these drugs is uncertain, despite much experimental study. At the neurophysiologic level they induce a state of hyperarousal of the CNS. Pharmacologically, they block the central neurotransmitter, serotonin.

Usual doses of LSD in man produce a series of somatic, perceptual and psychic effects which overlap each other. Dizziness, weakness, tremors, nausea and paresthesias are prominent somatic symptoms. Blurring of vision, distortions of perspective, organized visual illusions or "hallucinations" and less discriminant hearing are common perceptual abnormalities, as well as the hallmark of hallucinogenic activity, a change in time sense.

Many of the psychic effects are similar to those observed with marihuana, but they are usually much more intense. Physiologically, the drug produces signs of overactivity of the sympathetic nervous system and central stimulation, in contrast to marihuana which has marked sedative action. The onset of effects is fairly rapid, usually within 30 min of ingestion, the duration varying with the dose. As with most drugs of this type, the phenomena experienced may vary considerably owing to such factors as the personality of the drug taker, the expectations of the experimenters or the circumstances under which the drug is taken. Waxing and waning of effects are typical.

The deliriant hallucinogens, exemplified by scopolamine or a series of synthetic anticholinergic drugs with strong CNS activity, produce a different clinical syndrome. The degree of mental disorganization is marked; usually the experience is terrifying and not fully remembered and residual confusion may last for days. Stramonium containing cigarettes, or proprietary remedies containing scopolamine or atropine, or the Datura plant itself, have been used by those who prefer, for whatever curious reason, to use drugs of this type.

A series of amphetamine analogs with varying alphabetical chemical designations (DOM, also called "STP," MDA, MMDA) are also hallucinogenic. In most respects they fit into the LSD group of drugs, although they are more potent than mescaline, which they resemble chemically. A synthetic dissociative anesthetic, phencyclidine, produces a sense of detachment of the mind from the body which evokes variable types of hallucinogenic effects. The form of phencyclidine (Sernylan) most widely abused is a product for veterinary anesthesia, which has been given the epithet "hog." Ketamine, a related compound, is used as an anesthetic for brief operations in children and occasionally produces adverse mental effects.

TOXICITY. A number of adverse psychologic consequences of the use of hallucinogenic drugs have been reported. Most common is a panic reaction associated with a "bad trip." These are often best managed by simple sedation with a barbiturate or with a benzodiazepine rather than a phenothiazine; simple "talking down" often suffices, if one has the time. Acute psychotic or depressive reactions may be evoked by use of these drugs, but these are generally in patients strongly predisposed. Errors of judgment may

lead to reckless acts which may threaten life; everyone on these drugs should be monitored by someone who is not.

EPIDEMIOLOGY. In the late 1950s, most of these drugs were regarded as laboratory curiosities, but under the spell of Huxley, Leary and the lay press, their alleged benefits for opening minds created an explosive increase in their use. This epidemic pattern seems to be over, although there is still extensive residual use of these agents. LSD has fallen from favor because it is synthetic, while mescaline is fashionable because it is organic. Almost without exception what is sold as mescaline is really LSD.

TREATMENT. Except for treating complications from the use of these drugs, no systematic program of treatment has been defined specifically for this class of drugs. The most successful way to have people stop using them is to separate them from the drug culture, but this is not feasible unless it is voluntarily accepted.

MARIHUANA

HISTORY. Marihuana is one of the oldest of all socially used drugs, its use being recorded several millennia ago. It may also be the most frequently used drug; current estimates vary between 200–300 million users throughout the world. During the past decade, a remarkable increase in the social use of this drug has occurred in western society, so that at the moment, an estimated 20 million people in the United States, mostly youth, have used the drug, but only a small proportion on a regular basis. This recent trend has stimulated renewed interest in its pharmacologic effects, especially as these may relate to socially undesirable consequences.

CHEMICAL AND PHARMACOLOGIC CONSIDERATIONS. Of the three principal cannabinoids in marihuana; cannabidiol, tetrahydrocannabinol (THC) and cannabinol, only THC has been definitely proven to be active. Two isomers of THC exist in marihuana; the Δ-1 isomer accounts for about 99% of the total THC, while the Δ-6 isomer often cannot be clearly identified in chemical analyses. A number of other THC isomers and analogs have been synthesized and have varying degrees of activity.

The availability of synthetic Δ-1-THC, as well as chemical techniques for quantifying its content in marihuana, has made possible for the first time pharmacologic studies which provide some but not complete precision in dose. When the material is smoked, a still uncertain and perhaps variable fraction of THC is either lost by smoke escaping into the air or exhaled incompletely absorbed from the respiratory dead space. Relatively little is lost by pyrolysis. The efficiency of delivery of a dose by smoking has been estimated from 20–80%, but with most experienced smokers it should approximate 50%. Synthetic Δ-1-THC and marihuana extracts are also taken orally, but doses equivalent in effect to those from smoking are severalfold larger.

When it is smoked, absorption of THC is rapid and effects appear within minutes. If marihuana is of low potency, effects may be subtle and brief. Seldom do they last longer than 2–3 hr after a single cigarette, although users prolong effects by repeated smoking. Oral doses delay the onset of symptoms for 15 min to 2 hr; the total time course is much longer than from smoking. Because synthetic THC, as well as marihuana extracts, requires nonpolar solvents, even the administration of accurate doses for animal pharmacologic studies has been a problem, despite the greater latitude of animal experimentation.

Clinically, the drug has a biphasic effect with initial symptoms of "stimulation" and euphoria followed later by sleepiness and dream-like states. These effects are highly dose dependent, ranging from a brief and mild high with minimal sleepiness to a prolonged intoxication with many features similar to psychotomimetic drugs.

The major physiologic effects of the drug are reddening of the conjunctivae, an increase in pulse rate, muscle weakness and some incoordination. Perceptual and psychic changes predominate and may include uncontrollable laughter, difficulty in concentration or thinking, depersonalization, dream-like states, slowing of the sense of time, visual distortions or illusions and less discriminant hearing. Almost all psychologic tests show impairment if the dose is high enough; if the task is difficult enough, even small doses induce impairment.

So far as the entire profile of pharmacologic actions is concerned, marihuana is unique. Attempts to fit it into some existing category of drugs, such as hallucinogens, sedatives, stimulants or anticholinergics, are therefore useless. It most resembles the combined effects of hallucinogens and alcohol—and this may explain its great popularity.

TOXICITY. Lethal doses of THC in animals are almost astronomic in size. No lethalities have been proven from use of marihuana in man. Thus the drug must certainly rank as one of the safest of intoxicants. Adverse mental effects may parallel those for hallucinogens, but they are far less common. It is still not certain that use of marihuana leads to an "amotivational syndrome;" it might very well be that its use is a consequence rather than a cause of some change in one's life style. A variety of adverse physical effects from marihuana use have been described, but few have been definitely proven. Respiratory tract irritation from smoking is definite and may have consequences similar to that of smoking cigarettes.

EPIDEMIOLOGY. The dramatic increase in marihuana use closely followed the increased use of hallucinogenic drugs. So far as one can tell, the same general influences obtained, supplemented by the symbolic value of marihuana as a sign of revolt by the young. Marihuana is preferred to hallucinogenic drugs by many, who describe its effects as "mellow," presumably signifying a milder and more pleasant type of reaction.

The number of users seems to have stabilized, but patterns of use vary as greatly as those for alcohol. Many people use marihuana only on social occasions. Others may avoid it during the work week but indulge on weekends, although not in a typical "binge" pattern. Still others may use the drug daily, but only at the end of the work day. The percentage of true "potheads," those who use the drug several times a day and who remain in a permanent state of intoxication, is unknown, but it is probably no more than that of users of alcohol who become alcoholics.

It appears that marihuana will remain as a social drug, although acceptance by society is still far from complete. Efforts at reducing the criminal penalties for possession and use have had partial success, but attempts at full legalization seem to be entirely fruitless.

TREATMENT. Few users seek treatment, although many who have stopped using the drug have been pleasantly surprised at the increased clarity of thinking. Although marihuana has been alleged to be a substitute for alcohol, it is more commonly used along with alcohol; alcoholism complicating marihuana use is rare. Marihuana may also be used in a pattern of multiple drug use, in which case treatment may be required for the more serious drugs being taken.

FURTHER READING

Brecher EM and the editors of Consumers Reports (1972): Licit and illicit drugs. The Consumers Union Report on Narcotics, Stimulants, Depressants, Inhalants, Hallucinogens and Marijuana—including Caffeine, Nicotine and Alchol. Mt. Vernon, New York, Consumers Union

Lewin L (1931): Phantastica. Narcotic and stimulating drugs. Their use and abuse. New York, E. P. Dutton p 335.

Mule SJ, Brill H (ed) (1972): Chemical and biological aspects of drug dependence. Cleveland, The Chemical Rubber Company Press p 561

Wald P, Hutt PB et al. (1972): Dealing with Drug Abuse. A Report to the Ford Foundation. New York, Praeger Publishers p 396

HAROLD KALANT

10. ALCOHOLS AND DISULFIRAM

THE ALCOHOLS

ETHANOL

History and Uses

Ethanol (grain alcohol) has been known in almost all parts of the world since prehistoric times. It is formed naturally by yeast fermentation of starch or sugar in fruits, grains, potatoes or sugar cane, and in many countries the law permits only naturally formed alcohol to be used for human consumption. Ethanol for industrial use is produced mainly by organic synthesis from ethylene.

Though brandy and whiskey were, in earlier times, considered "stimulants," alcohol is really a hypnotic and anesthetic drug. It is used very little in modern medicine, except as a solvent for some drugs given in liquid form. The great bulk of alcohol consumption by humans is for nonmedical purposes: with meals, in social gatherings, for relaxation or as "problem drinking."

Chemistry

The aliphatic alcohols form a homologous series beginning with methanol (wood alcohol):

$$CH_3OH$$
METHANOL

$$CH_3—CH_2OH$$
ETHANOL

$$CH_3—CH_2—CH_2OH$$
N-PROPANOL

$$CH_3—\underset{\underset{CH_3}{|}}{\overset{\overset{OH}{|}}{CH}}—CH_3$$
ISOPROPANOL   etc.

The first three are completely soluble in water, in all proportions, but as the carbon chain length increases, water solubility decreases, and octanol (eight carbons) is almost insoluble. These higher alcohols, together with methanol, are used mainly in industry.

ALCOHOLIC BEVERAGES. Only ethanol is used for human consumption, although trace amounts of methanol, higher alcohols, aldehydes and esters are present as the "congeners" which give different alcoholic beverages their distinctive tastes and aromas. Fermentation stops when the alcohol concentration becomes high enough to inhibit the yeast; beers contain only 3–6% alcohol by weight and table wines about 12–15%.

Distillation can increase the alcohol concentration greatly, and in most countries the law sets limits on the content which may be sold. In the United States, proof spirit is 50% alcohol by volume; in Britain and Canada it is about 57%. An American whiskey is usually 90% proof (10 under proof) and therefore contains 45% alcohol by volume, or about 36 g of ethanol/100 ml. Canadian whiskey is usually about 40% ethanol by volume, or 32 g/100 ml. Roughly speaking, one bottle of beer, 1½ oz of whiskey or gin and 4 oz of table wine all contain about the same amount of ethanol.

ABSORPTION, DISTRIBUTION AND ELIMINATION

Alcohol is absorbed by simple diffusion across any mucosal surface. This occurs in the stomach but is faster across the thinner mucosa of the small intestine, so that anything which delays gastric emptying (e.g., food, exercise and anticholinergic drugs) will retard absorption of ethanol. Reduction of visceral blood flow, excessive dilution of the ingested alcohol or anything else which reduces the ethanol concentration gradient across the mucosa will also slow the absorption. Fastest absorption occurs with an intragastric concentration of 20–30%; less than this reduces the diffusion rate, while higher concentrations may delay gastric emptying by causing irritation and pylorospasm.

Ethanol diffuses rapidly from the blood across all capillary walls and cell membranes and equilibrates with the *total* body water including the CSF and urine. Ethanol dilution methods can therefore be used for measuring body water. The vapor pressure of ethanol in the alveolar air is in equilibrium with that in the plasma; this is the basis of the Breathalyzer test. However, the amount of ethanol eliminated in breath, sweat and urine is usually less than 5% of the ingested dose. The rest is metabolized chiefly in the liver.

Metabolism

The first step in alcohol metabolism takes place very largely in the liver and consists of NAD–dependent oxidation, first to acetaldehyde and then to acetate:

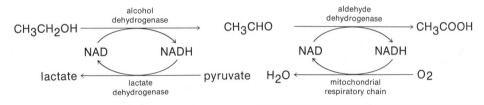

The NADH can be reoxidized to NAD either by the mitochondrial respiratory chain or by cytoplasmic redox reactions such as conversion of pyruvate to lactate. Ethanol oxidation therefore results in output of small amounts of acetaldehyde and large amounts of acetate and lactate from the liver into the peripheral circulation. Conversely, infusion of pyruvate or fructose can speed up alcohol oxidation by reoxidizing NADH to NAD. Ethanol can be oxidized in vitro, but probably not in vivo, by a peroxidative reaction in liver microsomes (MEOS). Minute amounts of ethanol are conjugated with sulfate or glucuronate or esterified with fatty acids.

BLOOD ALCOHOL CURVE. Liver alcohol dehydrogenase shows zero-order (saturation) kinetics at blood alcohol levels (BAL) above 25 mg/100 ml. There are differences between individuals, and in the same person at different times, but on the average, a 70 kg man can oxidize about 10 g ethanol per hour. Therefore, after a single dose, the BAL usually rises to a peak level in 30–90 min, depending on the dose, falls steadily at a rate of 15–20 mg/100 ml/hr until it reaches 20–25 mg/100 ml, then falls off exponentially (Fig. 10–1).

INTERACTION WITH OTHER DRUGS. As chloral hydrate (trichloracetaldehyde) competes with ethanol and acetaldehyde for their respective dehydrogenases, chloral and alcohol potentiate each other. Large doses of thyroxine, chlorpromazine and various other drugs can impair the oxidation of ethanol by inhibiting alcohol dehydrogenase.

ACTIONS

Three types of pharmacologic effects of ethanol can be distinguished: those caused by a direct action of ethanol on cell membranes, disturbances resulting from ethanol metabolism and stress reactions secondary to severe intoxication.

DIRECT EFFECTS ON CELL MEMBRANES. Like hypnotic, sedative and general anesthetic agents, ethanol dissolves in the lipids of the cell membrane, making it more dense and mechanically stable. This interferes with a number of processes which require the membrane to undergo rapid reversible changes in structure: 1) Rapid changes in Na^+ and K^+ flux, the basis of the action potential, are impaired. Nerve impulse conduction and muscle contraction (smooth, skeletal and cardiac) are therefore depressed at fairly high alcohol concentrations. The smaller the nerve fiber diameter, the greater is the effect at a given alcohol concentration. 2) Active transport of Na^+, K^+ and amino acids is decreased by inhibition of the membrane ATPase. This also reduces Na^+-linked processes such as reuptake of norepinephrine into sympathetic nerve endings (Ch. 14).

In the CNS, these changes lead to decreased neuronal activity, reflected in lower turnover of acetylcholine, lower ATP utilization and lower oxygen consumption. Effects are more marked in polysynaptic than monosynaptic pathways. Thus spinal reflexes, primary afferent sensory input and basic motor pathways are affected only at very high alcohol levels, while modulatory systems such as the reticular activating system, limbic system, extrapyramidal motor pathways and hypothalamus are sensitive to much lower levels.

Typically, small doses of alcohol (1–2 drinks) cause relaxation and mild **sedation,** together with centrally mediated **autonomic changes:** cu-

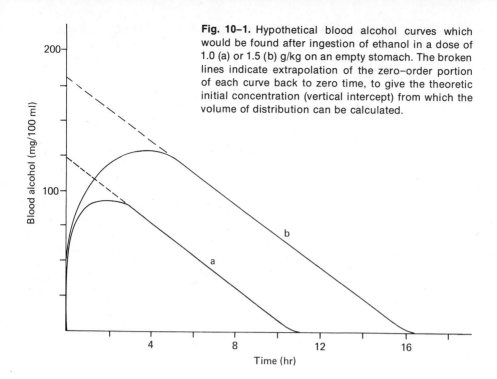

Fig. 10–1. Hypothetical blood alcohol curves which would be found after ingestion of ethanol in a dose of 1.0 (a) or 1.5 (b) g/kg on an empty stomach. The broken lines indicate extrapolation of the zero–order portion of each curve back to zero time, to give the theoretic initial concentration (vertical intercept) from which the volume of distribution can be calculated.

taneous vasodilatation, tachycardia and increased gastric acid secretion and motility. The sedation is usually accompanied by reduced conscious control over **emotional expression,** so that the person may become talkative, jovial, aggressive or morose, according to his underlying mood. Small doses do not hinder higher **intellectual processes** if there is no time limit and may even improve them by reducing nervous tension. However, **complex reactions** involving rapid decisions are impaired even by small doses. Other early changes include **positional nystagmus** and positive **Romberg sign** when the eyes are closed.

With higher doses, when the blood alcohol level is 100 mg/100 ml or higher, secretion of **vasopressin** is inhibited, causing diuresis of variable intensity. Oxytocin secretion is also inhibited; ethanol infusion has been used clinically to stop premature labor. Motor **incoordination** becomes marked, with slurred speech, motor ataxia and loss of balance. **Analgesia** occurs, and the intoxicated person may burn himself with a cigarette without noticing. Tendon **reflexes** are sometimes increased at first by loss of descending inhibitory control at the spinal synapses, but at high blood alcohol levels the reflexes disappear. Mental processes are progressively slowed; attention span is reduced. Finally, sleep progresses to **coma** at levels of 250 mg/100 ml or higher.

DISTURBANCES DUE TO ALCOHOL METABOLISM. NADH, formed during ethanol oxidation, modifies other NAD-linked enzyme reactions in the liver cytoplasm and mitochondria. Oxidation of fatty acids is inhibited, and phosphoglyceraldehyde is reduced to glycerolphosphate that is esterified with the fatty acids to form triglycerides, giving rise to **hyperlipemia** and **fatty liver.** Conversion of pyruvate to lactate interferes with gluconeogenesis, and the fasting subject may show **hypoglycemia.** The excess lactate passes into the blood contributing to metabolic acidosis. It also inhibits renal tubular clearance of urate, and thus can precipitate attacks of **gout.**

SECONDARY EFFECTS DUE TO STRESS. Loss of emotional control during intoxication may cause **excitement,** anger, fighting and other stressful behavior. With deeper intoxication, including coma, respiratory depression and fall in effective blood volume (due to peripheral vasodilatation), **hypoxia** may result. In both cases, stress induced catecholamine release may cause hepatic glycogenolysis, mobilization of free fatty acids from adipose tissue and reduced visceral blood flow. The latter may help explain why large doses of alcohol reduce drug metabolism in the liver.

Toxicity

Death from acute ethanol poisoning is usually due to respiratory depression at a blood alcohol level of 500 mg/100 ml or higher. If respiration is maintained artificially, death can result from direct inhibition of myocardial contractility at a BAL of about 1 g/100 ml.

These effects can occur at considerably lower levels in people who are also using other depressant drugs. Barbiturates and other sedatives, major and minor tranquilizers, antihistamines, cannabis and tricyclic antidepressants may be additive or synergistic with ethanol, due mainly to interaction in the nervous system.

TREATMENT OF TOXICITY. Since even the most severe acute toxic effects of ethanol are reversible, treatment consists essentially of maintaining respiration, blood pressure and body temperature until the ethanol has been removed by metabolism or by hemodialysis. Stimulants have very little place in therapy.

OTHER ALCOHOLS

Methanol

Methanol (wood alcohol, CH_3OH) has very similar pharmacologic actions to ethanol but is only about half as potent. Its special toxicity arises from its oxidation by alcohol dehydrogenase to yield **formaldehyde,** which in turn is oxidized to

formic acid. These metabolites are toxic to the retina and optic nerve and may cause permanent blindness. The formate also gives rise to metabolic acidosis which is sometimes fatal.

Treatment requires rapid correction of the acidosis by IV $NaHCO_3$ solution and elimination of the remaining unoxidized methanol by hemodialysis. An alternative method is to give small doses of ethanol which competitively inhibits oxidation of the methanol. The latter is then gradually lost in the urine.

Higher Alcohols

Small amounts of propanols, butanols, pentanols and their corresponding aldehydes and esters are found in alcoholic beverages, making up the so-called "congeners" or "fusel oil." There is some evidence that they may enhance ethanol toxicity. When the higher alcohols are drunk in place of ethanol, either alone or mixed with gasoline, benzene and other organic solvents, the treatment is basically the same as for ethanol or methanol poisoning.

ALCOHOLISM

Nature of the Problem

Though alcoholism is now widely considered a disease, it is perhaps best viewed as a form of *conditioned behavior.* If alcohol is used repeatedly and in large amounts to obtain relief from problems that the person does not know how to solve in other ways, drinking becomes a firmly established and automatic behavioral response to all sorts of other difficulties. Unfortunately, alcohol seldom solves the original problems and usually gives rise to many new ones.

As a form of acquired behavior, alcoholism should not be expected to have a single cause. Recent evidence suggests that there may be a hereditary predisposing factor. Parental and prevailing social attitudes toward drinking and drunkenness, personal emotional conflicts, availability and relative cost of alcohol and the drinking practices of one's friends have a great deal to do with the amount of alcohol use by society as a whole and by any particular individual within it. In the United States and Canada, about 85% of all adults drink alcohol; about 6% of these drink enough to be considered alcoholics.

Complications

The consequences of alcoholism include high rates of automobile and other accidents, loss of work productivity and earnings, family and social conflict and high incidence of various kinds of

disease. There are three main pharmacologic problems: 1) Oxidation of ethanol yields 7 kcal/g. Because it is possible to derive well over half the daily caloric requirement from alcohol, the rest of the alcoholic's diet tends to be reduced. Deficiency of protein and vitamins is common and may lead to peripheral neuritis, Wernicke's disease, Korsakoff's psychosis and pellagra. 2) The direct effects of alcohol on cell membrane functions in the liver, gastrointestinal tract and other organs are probably related to the production of liver cirrhosis, folate deficiency anemia, alcoholic cardiomyopathy and other diseases. 3) Chronic exposure of the brain to high concentrations of alcohol gives rise to adaptive changes which result in tolerance and physical dependence.

Tolerance and Dependence

Chronic heavy users of alcohol show a shift to the right of the dose-response curve. Larger doses are needed to produce the same effect. This reflects both **metabolic tolerance** produced by faster oxidation in the liver and **functional tolerance** in the nervous system. The depressant effects of ethanol provoke an adaptive hyperexcitability in the affected neurons. Thus the nervous system functions relatively normally in the continued presence of the drug, and the subject is said to be tolerant.

When the ethanol is withdrawn, the changes in

the nervous system are left unbalanced, and the hyperexcitability is revealed. This constitutes an alcohol **withdrawal reaction,** which can be relieved by taking more alcohol; the person is therefore said to be **physically dependent** on alcohol (Ch. 9).

WITHDRAWAL REACTIONS. The withdrawal reaction can range from mild to the very severe. After a single episode of intoxication, signs of mild hyperexcitability are found for a few hours, coinciding with the "hangover." After prolonged intoxication for days or weeks, withdrawal symptoms usually include sleeplessness, tremor, increased reflexes, sweating and loss of appetite. In more severe reactions there may be hallucina-

tions and convulsions. The most severe type (*delirium tremens*) includes, in addition, fever, delirium, intense hyperactivity and tachycardia which may end in cardiovascular collapse and death. Treatment usually includes sedation, fluid replacement and avoidance of environmental disturbance. Diphenylhydantoin (Ch. 30) is not always effective against convulsions in these patients; phenothiazines (Ch. 25) may make matters worse. Diazepam is perhaps the most widely favored drug because it has both sedative and anticonvulsant effects (Ch. 26). Propranolol (Ch. 19) and lithium (Ch. 24) are both being investigated at present for possible therapeutic value against tremor and other milder withdrawal symptoms.

DISULFIRAM

Chemistry and Metabolism

Disulfiram, or tetraethylthiuram disulfide, consists of two molecules of diethyl-dithiocarbamate (DDC), probably the pharmacologically active material, joined through a disulfide bond. It is split in the body to give DDC, and this in turn is broken down to yield carbon disulfide, which appears in the breath.

Actions and Use

Disulfiram is a vulcanizing agent, and rubber workers using it found that they became violently ill if they drank alcohol. This proved to be due to inhibition of acetaldehyde dehydrogenase, so that oxidation of ethanol led to an accumulation of acetaldehyde in the blood, causing intense flushing, tachycardia, nausea, vomiting and circulatory collapse. If an alcoholic treated with disulfiram knows that such consequences are likely to follow drinking, it usually aids his resolve to avoid alcohol. Disulfiram is absorbed from the gastrointestinal tract, begins to act in 2–4 hr and reaches maximum effect in 12–24 hr. Some patients, after starting on disulfiram, lose their will to take it; to prevent this, clinical trials

of a long acting parenteral form of disulfiram are under way.

Toxicity

Disulfiram inhibits other enzymes and may interfere with the metabolism of other drugs by the liver. It inhibits dopamine β-hydroxylase (Ch. 14), thus interfering with catecholamine synthesis. This may account for such symptoms as weakness, dizziness and cardiac arrhythmias seen in some patients. Skin allergies and toxic psychosis occasionally occur. Many patients complain of headache, sexual impotence and tiredness, but it is not really clear whether these are due to the disulfiram or to the strain of learning to live without alcohol.

Related Drugs

A number of other drugs cause disulfiram-like reactions to alcohol. **Citrated calcium carbimide** has a similar, more rapid and shorter action. It is also less severe, probably because dopamine β-hydroxylase is not affected. Animal charcoal and tolbutamide (Ch. 45) may also provoke similar reactions to alcohol, and physicians should warn patients who are given these drugs.

FURTHER READING

Hawkins RD, Kalant H (1972): The metabolism of ethanol and its metabolic effects. Pharmacol Rev 24:67–157

Israel Y, Mardones J (eds) (1971): Biological Basis of Alcoholism. New York, Wiley-Interscience

Kalant H, LeBlanc AE, Gibbins RJ (1971): Tolerance to, and dependence on, some nonopiate psychotropic drugs. Pharmacol Rev 23:135–191

Kalant H, Kalant OJ (1971): Drugs, Society and Personal Choice. Toronto, General Publishing

Kissin B, Begleiter H (eds) (1971, 1972 & 1974): The Biology of Alcoholism, Vol 1 (Biochemistry), Vol 2 (Physiology & Behavior) and Vol 3 (Clinical Pathology). New York, Plenum Press

Seeman P (1972): The membrane actions of anesthetics and tranquilizers. Pharmacol Rev 24:583–655

Wallgren H, Barry H, III (1970): Actions of Alcohol. Amsterdam, Elsevier

BENJAMIN M. KAGAN

11. PEDIATRIC PHARMACOLOGY

DIFFERENCES BETWEEN PEDIATRIC AND ADULT PHARMACOLOGY

An important difference between the pediatric individual and the adult is size. In addition, the growth and development of the infant and child are continually changing. In contrast, in the normal adult a relative plateau of maturation has been achieved, after which change proceeds in the opposite direction of aging and deterioration. The rate of change of different organ systems varies throughout life. It follows, therefore, that there is considerable variation in the phar-macology of different drugs at different stages of life, particularly during the actively growing and developing period of infancy and childhood. In this chapter, pharmacology from the time of birth, whether premature, full term or post mature through adolescence (set arbitrarily through the sixteenth year of life) will be considered. A related and important subject, that of the effect of maternal drugs on the fetus, and consequently upon the infant, will also be discussed.

VEHICLES AND ROUTES

For the older child who can swallow a pill or capsule, vehicles are generally not a serious problem. However, for the younger ones the palatability of a suspension or a solution may make the difference between their receiving or not receiving the drug. An extreme example is the odor of the indanyl ester of carbenicillin in suspension which makes it impossible to administer. On the other hand, candy-like chewable medications are a hazard as toddlers may eat them like candy. Jam, jelly, honey, applesauce or sauce can be used to make some oral preparations more palatable.

Some drug forms, for example those in solution and suspension, are less stable than others and have a shorter "shelf life." This must be borne in mind in order to avoid the use of preparations which may be either ineffective or worse yet, toxic. For example, outdated tetracycline with its shorter half-life in suspension can produce renal tubular dysfunction.

In general, from the standpoint of safety, the oral route is preferred. This route tends to minimize "psychic" trauma and to preserve rapport for future visits to the physician's office or hospi-tal. However, the tendency to vomit and the potential for aspiration when a child or infant is forced to take medication may create obvious problems. Aspiration of oily or chemically irritating substances may lead to a lipoid or chemical pneumonia.

When the oral route is not practical, some drugs can be given by rectum. Others, however, are not absorbed by this route, and diarrhea (sometimes even that resulting from this procedure) may make this route impractical. Drugs can be suspended in 1 or 2 oz of water or in a starch solution and introduced rectally via a catheter or bulb syringe. The buttocks should be held or taped together to prevent loss. In general, the oral dose is given by rectum, but the evidence that this rule holds generally is not available.

When necessary, the IV, IM, intrathecal or even intraventricular route is used. Each drug must be considered separately. It cannot be assumed that because any one of these routes is safe and effective, the other will also be so. For example, chloramphenicol can be given IV but not IM to attain predictable blood levels.

ABSORPTION

Because some intestinal transport mechanisms are underdeveloped in the neonate, some drugs, although eventually completely absorbed, are absorbed very slowly. Under such circumstances, these drugs must be administered less frequently than in the adult. Riboflavin is a good example of such a substance. In the older infant and adult, it is absorbed in as little as 3–4 hr, whereas in the newborn its absorption is only complete after 16 hr, as it is absorbed almost exclusively by passive diffusion over a long segment of the intestinal tract.

Some orally administered antibacterial agents, such as triple sulfonamides, chloramphenicol, erythromycin and the tetracyclines, are absorbed much more slowly in prematurely born than in full term infants.

METABOLISM

Distribution of a drug depends in part upon whether it is water or fat soluble. The process of growing older is a process of drying out. The egg has the highest percentage of water; as the fetus, the infant and the child grow, the percentage of water decreases. The newborn, e.g., may be 70% water, the premature as much as 80%. The extracellular water volume in the newborn is much greater than that in the adult. On the other hand, the fat content of the prematurely born may be only 1%, whereas the normal full term infant has an average of 16%.

Distribution is also dependent upon binding. Thus, diphenylhydantoin (CH_{30}), when given to a mother about to deliver, is found in unbound form in twice the concentration in the cord blood of the infant as it is in the mothers's blood. If hyperbilirubinemia develops, the unbound fraction may be three times that in the mother. It is this unbound fraction which crosses the cell membrane and reaches receptor sites.

During the period of infancy and childhood, marked differences in detoxification mechanisms are seen. An example is the relative inability of the neonate liver to inactivate or to conjugate such drugs as the sulfonamides or chloramphenicol. Giving several drugs at the same time may modify the problem by affecting enzyme sites, as is the case with the barbiturates that induce liver enzyme activity. Barbiturates have been shown to increase liver weight and also the size of the microsomal portion. Because of this effect, administration of phenobarbital to newborns significantly reduces blood bilirubin levels. This effect is of interest as an example of such activity, but is not used clinically because it takes too long to achieve maximum effect and because there are other methods of achieving reduction of serum bilirubin levels without the possible undesirable effects of the barbiturates in these infants.

EXCRETION

The ability of the liver and the kidney to excrete some drugs is incompletely developed in the full term infant and even more so in the prematurely born. Some antibacterial agents, e.g., such as penicillin G, are excreted primarily via the kidney without prior metabolism. The renal excretion rate is, therefore, a most important consideration in determining dosage and the time interval between doses.

Many drugs are metabolically transformed prior to excretion. The liver microsomal enzymes are primarily involved in these transformations. In general, these systems function less well in the neonate than in older individuals and reach a mature status at varying periods of time after birth.

Individuals vary greatly in their ability to conjugate via the glucuronide pathway. The normal adult excretes 40–50% of an oral dose of salicylamide as the glucuronide. However, glucuronide excretion by 14 full term infants in the 5th day of life was found to vary 8–45%. If this small sample is representative, there would be considerable variation in response to drugs detoxified via this pathway. On the other hand, some excretory pathways such as sulfation appear to be as active in the neonate as in the adult.

The kidneys are the most important route for excretion of most drugs. However, glomerular filtration rates and renal plasma flows in the newborn are only 30–40% of that in the adult. Excretion of hydrogen ion depends largely upon tubular function, and the infant cannot excrete as much hydrogen ion as an older child.

Ampicillin is almost entirely excreted by the kidney. The serum half-life of ampicillin is quite long during the first 2 weeks of life and declines over the next 2–3 weeks to a mature rate at about 1 month of age. The situation is similar for kanamycin, neomycin, streptomycin and other penicillins such as carbenicillin. However, there is no rule which can be applied to all antibacterial agents. For example, the half-life of colistin is not prolonged in the neonate.

The pediatric patient is subject to the same drug idiosyncrasies or allergic reactions as the adult. These are, usually, drug dependent rather than dose dependent. The incidence may vary from that in the adult. With benemid, there are more reactions in children than in adults. With others, such as the penicillins, the reverse is the case.

The process of development itself may be responsible for some untoward results. For example, tetracycline causes change in tooth texture and brown discoloration of the teeth (Ch. 7). The primary teeth may be affected when exposure through the mother occurs from about 4–6 months of gestation and until the infant is 12 months old. If no more tetracycline is given, the secondary teeth are not likely to be discolored. Tetracycline given between 12 months and 6 years of age may discolor the developing second teeth.

Some drugs have greater toxicity in the newborn than at other ages. When chloramphenicol was widely used, the mortality rate among newborns actually rose. The "gray syndrome" which was responsible in large part for this increase in mortality rate (Ch. 7) developed as a result of high blood levels of this drug. These in turn are a consequence of poor glucuronide conjugation, competition for the carrier by serum albumin or other compounds such as bilirubin, and relatively poor renal excretion.

Both infants and young children tend to have problems with drugs which disturb acid base balance. Thus overdosage with salicylates leads rather easily to metabolic acidosis, which is rarely seen in adults even with the same blood levels of salicylate. Likewise, when diuretics are given, serious depletion of sodium or potassium is more likely to occur in children than in adults.

The CNS of a developing fetus is peculiarly susceptible to toxicity. For example, when given to a neonate, a dose of morphine equivalent (based upon surface area) to that given to the adult may produce severe depression. Yet the same is not true of meperidine. It is not uncommon in children for doses of salicylate, antihistaminics, amphetamines, aminophyllin or atropine to produce delirium or convulsions, whereas equivalent amounts tend not to do so in the adult. On the other hand, while premature infants may have a diminished tolerance to digitalis, full term and older infants and children are more resistant to the therapeutic effects of digitalis and related glycosides than are adults.

It has long been known that small infants develop methemoglobinemia when exposed to well water containing high concentrations of nitrates or when their skin comes in contact with aniline dye from freshly stamped diapers or clothes or even from some compounds formerly used in laundries. This may also result from the use of bismuth subnitrate, some local anesthetic ointments or suppositories, sulfonamides or phenacetin.

At any period of growth, the use of cortisone or related compounds may result in slowing of growth or osseous development. Usually there is "catch up growth" when these are discontinued. On the other hand, androgens, such as testosterone, stimulate the rate of growth but also the rate of closure of epiphyses so that ultimate height is reduced.

SELECTION

The selection of drugs in infants and children is based upon similar basic principles as that for adults. However, the etiology of disease and clinical symptoms and signs tend to be very different. Delays in starting therapy can in general be more devastating than similar delays with adults. Therefore, early clinical diagnosis with a keen awareness of etiologic possibilities as well as a good knowledge of pediatric pharmacologic principles becomes paramount for the best care of pediatric patients.

DOSAGE

Relating the dose given to infants and children to a percentage of that given to an adult has been found to be unreliable, at times ineffective and sometimes dangerous. Too much of the metabolic effect and the difference in binding, absorption and excretion, etc., depends upon the state of growth and development of the particular organ system involved. The development of the various systems does not correspond uniformly to differences in weight, surface area, age or other simple parameter. In general, each drug must be considered on its own. Many "rules" have been promoted to relate adult dosage to pediatric use. These rules or methods have been known under the names of Gaubius, Brunton, Cowling, Dilling, Starkenstein, Young, Fried, Clark, Augsburger, Cullis, and there are others. However, none of these have been shown to be scientifically sound, for reasons that must be obvious from reading this chapter. Clearly there is a relationship between surface area and many physiologic functions, such as heat production, extracellular body water, plasma volume, cardiac output, glomerular filtration rate, organ size, oxygen consumption and also nitrogren, caloric, water and electrolyte requirements. Thus body surface measurements relate fairly well to dosage, but they are still imperfect since they do not take into account important variations such as those related to gestational age, age itself, variations in drugs unrelated to variations in body surface, individual variations between patients of the same surface area and differential development of different organ systems. In the absence of better guidelines, however, the surface area relationships may be used as a preliminary estimate of drug dosage (Table 11–1). For some drugs in pediatrics, such as morphine, pentobarbital, atropine and scopolomine, this must be considered as especially crude.

While body surface is the most reliable single guide to dosage, no method provides for individual variations in response or for the need of careful consideration of many factors in each individual patient as well as of each individual drug and route of administration. Since there is so much to be considered which can make for large differences in the safe and effective use of drugs in pediatrics, frequent reference to the

TABLE 11–1. Determination of Children's Doses from Adult Doses on the Basis of Body Surface Area

	Weight (kg.)	(lb.)	Surface area* (sq. M.)	Fraction of adult dose†
	2.0	4.4	0.15	0.09
Birth	3.4	7.4	0.21	0.12
3 wk	4.0	8.8	0.25	0.14
3 mo	5.7	12.5	0.29	0.17
6 mo	7.4	16	0.36	0.21
9 mo	9.1	20	0.44	0.25
1 yr	10	22	0.46	0.27
1-1/2 yr	11	25	0.50	0.29
2 yr	12	27	0.54	0.31
3 yr	14	31	0.60	0.35
4 yr	16	36	0.68	0.39
5 yr	19	41	0.73	0.42
6 yr	21	47	0.82	0.47
7 yr	24	53	0.90	0.52
8 yr	27	59	0.97	0.56
9 yr	29	65	1.05	0.61
10 yr	32	71	1.12	0.65
11 yr	36	78	1.20	0.70
12 yr	39	86	1.26	0.74

*Approximate average for age
†Based on adult surface area of 1.73 sq. M.

"package insert" is recommended, especially when drugs are being used with which the physician is not very familiar.

MATERNAL DRUGS, EFFECT ON FETUS AND CONSEQUENTLY UPON THE INFANT

Few women go through pregnancy without taking some drugs. During the period of embryogenesis, that is, especially during the first 3 months of pregnancy, the effects of drugs on the fetus can be significant and even devastating, causing disorganization of the developing process or even death of the fetus. Some severe malformations are clearly related to drugs taken by the mother in the first trimester. In the second trimester, or even the third, the result may be a malfunction of specific organ systems. Toxic effects tend to be more acute and serious the more rapid the rate of growth and development. Even during labor, drugs may change placental perfusion and thus affect transfer of drug to fetus. For example, drugs during labor may lead to hypotension and consequently poor perfusion of the placenta, to respiratory depression, to changes in the Apgar score of the newborn, alterations of the electroencephalogram or of neurologic signs. A good example are the sulfonamides; when one is given to the mother at a time close to delivery, it is transferred to the infant and thus potentiates the danger of hyperbilirubinemia and kernicterus. Sulfonamide competes with bilirubin for the limited glucuronide pathway for conjugation in the liver after which it

is readily excreted by the kidney. The sulfonamide also competes with bilirubin for albumin binding, resulting in more "free" bilirubin. Because of these factors, higher blood levels of free bilirubin develop, and the bilirubin enters and permanently damages brain tissue which results in kernicterus. This process is further aggravated by the fact that the normal newborn, especially the prematurely born infant, has less circulating albumin available for binding than do older infants or adults.

In addition to the sulfonamides, the following drugs have been found to displace bilirubin from protein binding: novobiocin, caffeine and sodium benzoate, salicylates and probably also indomethacin, lanatoside C, menadiol, lobelin, strophanthin, tolbutamide, polymyxin, sodium glucuronide, acetazolamide, epinephrine, penicillin, erythromycin, prednisolone and the phenothiazines.

Other drugs increase the potential for kernicterus by increasing the rate of hemolysis of red cells. These include the sulfonamides, the nitrofurans, naphthyl and quinone derivatives, some antimalarials, perhaps some antibiotics and large doses of vitamin K analogs. Because of the latter, care is taken to limit the dosage of vitamin K in the newborn to a parenteral dose of 0.5–1.0 mg or an oral dose of 1–2 mg.

Nursing mothers may also pass drugs to their infants via their own breast milk in concentrations sufficient to have an effect upon the suckling infant (Ch. 43).

In summary, the infant and the child are by no means merely small editions of the adult. The choice of pharmacologic agents, the doses and the routes for their administration must take into account the very important role of growth and development. Growth and development affect applied pharmacology through their influence upon the manifestations and the etiology of various diseases, and also upon the absorption, metabolism, excretion and tolerance of drugs. Finally, drugs given to the mother may affect the fetus and newly born via the placenta and the infant via the breast milk.

FURTHER READING

Done AK, Jung AL (1970): Neonatal pharmacology. Gellis SS and Kagan BM (eds) Current Pediatric Therapy. Philadelphia, Saunders, pp 995

Gellis SS, Kagan BM (1976): Current Pediatric Therapy. (7th ed) Philadelphia, Saunders

Kagan BM (ed) (1974): Antimicrobial Therapy. (2nd ed) Philadelphia, Saunders

Klein JO (1969): Consideration of gentamicin for therapy of neonatal sepsis. J Infect Dis 119:457–459

Klingberg MA, Abramovici A, Chemke J (eds) (1974): Drugs and fetal development. Vol 27 Advances in Experimental Medicine and Biology. New York, Plenum

Leach RH, Wood BSB (1967): Drug dosage for children. Lancet 2:1350

Wilson JT (1972): Developmental pharmacology: a review of its application to clinical and basic science. Annu Rev Pharmacol 12:423–450

Yaffe SF (1973): Pharmacokinetics in the fetus and newborn infant. Rev Can Biol 32:125–132

JOSEPH H. BECKERMAN

12. PRESCRIPTION WRITING

History records that prescription writing antedates the pyramids by a thousand years. One of the most important medical writings of Egyptian civilization, the Ebers Papyrus, contains many prescriptions. The symbol Rx is an indication that prescriptions are connected with the ancient past. It probably represents the sign of Jupiter (♃), the father of the gods whose help the prescriber wished to invoke to make his prescription effective.

The term prescription is associated with the order of specific medication for a certain person at a particular time. The medication is to be prepared by a pharmacist upon the direction of a licensed physician, dentist, veterinarian or other medical practitioner who has been given this legal responsibility. A prescription may be written or oral. The prescriber must sign his name to the forms. The pharmacist must immediately reduce to writing and file all oral requests.

The practitioner who writes a prescription should realize that it is a legal document for which he and the dispensing pharmacist are equally responsible. Of more importance, the prescriber should also remember that this document reflects his ability to apply his knowledge of medicine or dentistry to the treatment of disease. It is that vital link in which the patient actively participates.

Prescriptions should never be hastily conceived or incompletely written. They should be well composed, concise and legible. Incomplete or hard to read prescriptions may lead to medication errors, delays in administration of drugs to patients and breakdowns in interprofessional communication. Prescription writing cannot and should not be assigned to nurses, secretaries or other personnel.

The language of today's prescription is English. However, a considerable number of Latin phrases and words or their abbreviations are still commonly used. Unless these are correct, this practice can lead to confusion and error. Table 12–1 presents a current list of the Latin words and abbreviations.

Many prescribers prefer to write their prescriptions on small printed forms, usually 4 by 5 in. in size. Printed at the top of the blank are the name, address and telephone number of the practitioner. Space is provided for the name and address of the patient and the date. At the bottom of the form there is a line for the prescriber's signature. Today's forms also make provision for the prescriber to indicate the number of refills his patient may have and include a box to be checked following the word "label." Should the prescriber wish the dispensing pharmacist to place the name of the drug and its strength on the label of the patient's container, he checks this box. The use of prescription forms imprinted with the name of a specific pharmacy is in poor taste and unethical.

LAWS REGULATING PRESCRIBING AND DISPENSING OF DRUGS

Many regulations affect the prescriber and the dispenser of medications. In addition to federal laws, a number of rulings have been promulgated by the state boards of pharmacy which are in effect laws binding on the prescriber. It is essential that the prescriber familiarize himself with the legal requirements of the state in which he practices.

The first Federal Food and Drugs Act went into effect on June 30, 1906; after several amendments, it was completely rewritten and reenacted by Congress in 1939. Primarily, the Act regulates

TABLE 12–1. Latin Words and Phrases Used in Prescription Writing

Abbreviation	Latin	English meaning
aa	ana	of each
a.c.	ante cibum	before meals
ad	ad	to, up to
ad lib.	ad libitum	at pleasure (as desired)
aur.	auris	ear
b.i.d.	bis in die	twice a day
bis	bis	twice
c	cum	with
caps.	capsula	capsule
d.	dexter	right
d.	dies	day
disp.	dispensa	dispense
d.t.d.	dentur tales doses	give such doses
f., ft.	fac, fiat	make
gm., Gm., g.	gramma	gram
gr.	grana	grain
gtt.	gutta	drop
h.	hora	hour
h.s.	hora somni	at bedtime
m.	misce	mix
mixt.	mixtura	mixture
no.	numerus	number
non rep.	non repetatur	do not repeat
o.d.	oculus dexter	right eye
o.h.	omni hora	every hour
o.s.	oculus sinister	left eye
o.u.	oculus uterque	each eye
p.c.	post cibum	after meals
p.r.n.	pro re nata	as needed
pulv.	pulvis	powder
q.	quaque	each, every
q.h.	quaque hora	every hour
q.i.d.	quater in die	four times a day
-s	sine	without
sig.	signa	label
sol.	solutio	solution
s.s.	semi	one-half
stat.	statim	at once
syr.	syrupus	syrup
tab.	tabella	tablet
t.i.d.	ter in die	three times a day
tinct., tr.	tinctura	tincture
ung.	unguentum	ointment
ut dict.	ut dictum	as directed

the quality and movement of drugs and devices in interstate commerce. The Act was further amended to require FDA certification of insulin, penicillin, streptomycin, bacitracin, chlortetracycline, chloramphenicol and any derivatives of these compounds. "Dangerous" drugs, such as atropine, hyoscine, digitalis and thyroid, were restricted to sale only on prescription.

Because of the lack of specificity in the Food, Drug and Cosmetic Act, the original rulings concerning restricted drugs were clarified by the Durham-Humphrey Amendment of 1952. Under this amendment, drugs are divided into two general classes: 1) prescription legend drugs (those drugs bearing on the label the statement "Caution: Federal law prohibits dispensing without a prescription"), a prescription for which can be refilled only on specific authorization by the prescriber; and 2) those drugs which can be legally sold over the counter without a prescription (the patented or proprietary medicines).

The recent enactment of Public Law 91–513 (Controlled Substances Act), replaced or amended numerous federal laws relating to the control of drugs and other substances of abuse. The new law subjects every person who legitimately handles controlled substances to regulation by the Drug Enforcement Administration (DEA), an agency of the United States Department of Justice.

There are established five schedules on controlled substances to be known as schedules I, II, III, IV and V, defined as follows:

Schedule I
   A. The drug has a high potential for abuse.
   B. There is **no currently accepted medical use** for the drug in the United States.
   C. There is a lack of accepted safety for the use of the drug under medical supervision.
   Examples: Heroin, LSD, marihuana, mescaline and psilocybin

Schedule II
   A. The drug has a high potential for abuse.
   B. There is a currently accepted medical use in treatment in the United States.
   C. Abuse of this substance may lead to severe psychologic or physical dependence.
   Examples: Amobarbital, amphetamine, cocaine, codeine, dihydromorphinone, meperidine, methadone, methaqualone, methylphenidate, morphine, pentobarbital and secobarbital

Schedule III
   A. The drug has a potential for abuse less than those in Schedules I and II.
   B. There is a currently accepted medical use in the United States.
   C. Abuse of this substance may lead to moderate or low physical dependence or high psychologic dependence.
   Examples: Benzphetamine, codeine combined with nonnarcotic ingredients, glutethimide, methyprylon and paregoric

Schedule IV
   A. The drug has a low potential for abuse relative to the other schedules.
   B. There is a currently accepted medical use in the United States.
   C. Abuse of this substance may lead to limited physical or psychologic dependence relative to drugs in Schedule III.
   Examples: Barbital, chloral hydrate, diethylpropion, fenfluramine, meprobamate, paraldehyde and phenobarbital

Schedule V

A. The drug has a low potential for abuse relative to substances in Schedule IV.

B. The drug has a currently accepted medical use in the United States.

C. Abuse of this substance may lead to less physical dependence or psychologic dependence relative to drugs in Schedule IV.

Examples: This schedule contains drugs which were formerly treated as "exempt" narcotics. They are generally narcotic substances containing one or more nonnarcotics. Cough mixtures such as Elixir Terpin Hydrate and Codeine, Brown Mixture and Phenergan Expectorant with Codeine. Also included is Lomotil

The prescriber should remember that a state law regulating controlled substances can be and often is more stringent than federal regulations. California, e.g., requires the use of an official triplicate narcotic form for prescribing narcotics. These forms are consecutively numbered, are not transferable and should be kept under secure conditions.

COMPOSITION OF THE PRESCRIPTION

The prescription form has six basic components (Fig. 12–1): 1) the patient's name and address, the date and where necessary the age of the patient; 2) the superscription; 3) the inscription; 4) the subscription; 5) the signatura; and 6) the prescriber's name.

The **name** of the patient, including initials or first name, is essential to prevent errors. The **address** of the patient is needed for legal purposes. In addition to the patient's name and address, many prescribers note the patient's age on the prescription form. This practice provides an additional safeguard, since the pharmacist can then check the prescribed dosage for accuracy.

The **superscription** is the familiar symbol Rx, an abbreviation of the Latin word *recipe* (take thou). A prescriber may write a valid prescription on a blank slip of paper, in which event he should identify the document by writing the symbol Rx at the top of the slip.

The **inscription** constitutes the principal part of the prescription. This portion contains the names, concentrations and quantities of the prescribed ingredients. Because of the nature of today's therapeutic agents, considerable thought should be given to completing this section. To avoid serious errors, the prescriber should be familiar with the correct spelling of the name of the medication. The individual dose of the drug should be correctly given and clearly stated. The metric system should be used and the position of the decimal point correctly determined. On some printed prescription blanks, the decimal is replaced by a vertical line.

The **subscription** contains directions from the prescriber to the pharmacist for compounding the prescription. Because many of today's medications are commercially prepared, this portion of the prescription is rapidly becoming obsolete. In most prescriptions, the subscription serves merely to designate the dosage form desired and the number of doses to be dispensed to the patient.

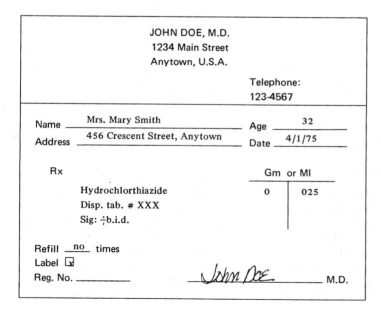

Fig. 12–1. Examples of prescriptions.

JOHN DOE, M.D.
1234 Main Street
Anytown, U.S.A.

Telephone:
123-4567

Name _____ Mrs. Mary Smith _____ Age _____ 32 _____

Address _____ 456 Crescent Street, Anytown _____ Date _____ 4/1/75 _____

Rx   Gm or Ml

Hydrochlorthiazide   0 | 025
Disp. tab. # XXX
Sig: ÷b.i.d.

Refill __no__ times
Label ☒
Reg. No. _____   ~John Doe~ _____ M.D.

```
                          JOHN DOE, M.D.
                          1234 Main Street
                          Anytown, U.S.A.
                                            Telephone:
                                            123-4567

    Name _____ John Smith _____     Age _____ 35 _____

    Address __ 456 Crescent Street, Anytown __  Date  4/1/75 ____

       Rx                                  Gm  or Ml

                Tab. Aspirin Compound
                     with Codeine Phosphate    0  |  032
                Disp. # XXX
                Sig. ÷ q. 4h. p.r.n. pain
                                                  |

    Refill __no__ times
    Label ☒
    Reg. No. _AD1234567_      _John Doe_____ M.D.
```

The **signatura** (also known as the signa, abbreviated as sig.) comprises the instructions for the patient's use. Because the effectiveness of the prescribed medication depends on the patient's adherence to the prescriber's dosage schedule, it is absolutely necessary that these instructions be both clear and concise. The use of the phrase "as directed" should be avoided. If the directions are complex and require considerable explanation, they should be written on a separate blank and given directly to the patient. Since the space on the prescription label is limited, the directions on the label must be concise and clearly understandable.

The **signature of the prescriber** should appear on every prescription. Federal law requires that the prescriber's address and registry number appear on every narcotic prescription and that such prescriptions be signed with ink or indelible pencil.

In general, the physician is advised against prescribing a mixture of several active drugs dispensed together in the same tablet or capsule. Although this practice has the advantage of ease for the doctor, is readily accepted by the patient and ensures, when this is important, that both drugs and never one alone is taken, it also has some disadvantages. First, patients vary in their response to drugs, and it is unlikely that their response to two drugs will vary in parallel. Consequently, if the dose of one drug in a two-drug combination is suited to the patient's needs, it is unlikely that the dose of the other will always be appropriate or optimal. There is no flexibility of dosage. Second, it is sometimes more expensive to prescribe drugs together than separately. Third, if adverse effects appear, it may be difficult to tell which drug is responsible, and all medication must be discontinued, at least temporarily. If the drugs are given separately, the ill effects can more easily be traced to their cause.

JAY M. ARENA

13. GENERAL PRINCIPLES OF TREATMENT OF POISONS AND THEIR AVAILABLE ANTIDOTES

INTRODUCTION

The causes of poisoning are many: accidental and deliberate, civilian and industrial. In pediatric patients, the chief etiologic factors are poor or faulty child supervision and parental unawareness of the problem. Each year more than one million incidents of poisoning occur in the United States, with over 3000 deaths, including those from gases and vapors. About half of these deaths are accidental, and one-third occur in children under 5 years of age. In fact, poisoning is the most common medical emergency among young children. These are somber statistics for a mechanism of injury and death that is largely preventable.

The above figures are undoubtedly much too low. Many more children succumb each year to the accidental ingestion of, or exposure to, toxic chemicals in household agents or drugs, but the correct diagnosis is never made because incriminating evidence is not detected or recognized. The natural curiosity of children to learn by exploration, questioning, sampling and trial and error leads them to investigate more than a quarter of a million household products and a myriad of drugs which are now available. With the increasing number of potentially toxic household agents and family drugs in our homes, this problem, enormous now, promises to be even more serious in the next decade.

When an acutely ill individual (particularly a child) with a bizarre chain of signs and symptoms is seen and presents an obscure and uncertain diagnosis, ingestion of a drug or exposure to a toxic chemical compound should always be considered. In patients who have not been observed to ingest or to have contact with a poison, the problem of an accurate diagnosis can be a most difficult one. Many symptoms and signs are tabulated as a quick aid in diagnosis in Table 13–1.

Treatment for acute poisoning, whether drug or chemical, is mainly symptomatic and supportive. Overtreatment of the poisoned patient with large doses of stimulants, sedatives and other therapeutic agents often does far more harm and damage than the poison itself. A calm and collected attitude with the judicious use of drugs, electrolytes and the maintenance of an adequate airway is for more effective than heroic measures, which usually are unnecessary. As a matter of fact, it is impossible at times to determine whether recovery occurred because of, or in spite of, the treatment used.

SPECIFIC THERAPEUTIC MEASURES

Vomiting

When poisons have been taken orally, empty the stomach quickly. This is the most important treatment that one could possibly use and there should be no procrastination here. Most poisons are in themselves emetics, but if vomiting does not occur spontaneously, it should be induced if possible if it is not contraindicated. (Contraindications include ingestion of corrosives, strychnine, or petroleum distillates and coma.) In children, when syrup of ipecac is not available, vomiting is best induced by having them drink a glass of water or milk, then gagging them with a finger (with precautions to prevent biting) or by stroking the posterior pharynx with a blunt object. To prevent aspiration in small children, the body should be inverted with the head down but supported and the feet elevated. Syrup of ipecac (not the fluid extract), if available, can be given in doses of 10–15 ml and repeated once in 15–30 min if emesis did not occur. Fluids (1–2 glasses) should be given several minutes before the ipecac is swallowed, since emesis may not occur if the stomach is empty. Use of ipecac, if ineffective, makes gastric lavage doubly imperative because when left in the stomach it is an irritant, and when absorbed it is a specific cardiotoxin capable of producing disturbances of conduction, atrial fibrillation or fatal myocarditis. The contraindications for using ipecac are the same as those for gastric lavage. If more than an hour has elapsed since an antiemetic drug was ingested, ipecac should not be used. Salt water as an emetic can be dangerous (hypernatremia) in children, and mustard is impractical.

The injection of apomorphine, 0.03 mg/lb subcutaneously, for prompt emesis followed by naloxone HCl, 0.01 mg/kg IV, IM, or SC, to terminate both the emetic and narcotic effects of apomorphine (the use of this narcotic antagonist can be omitted in most instances) is gaining widespread acceptance and is being used at many poison control centers. For best results, water (1–2 glasses) should be given beforehand (also true for the use of syrup of ipecac), since emesis does not occur readily if the stomach is empty. This therapy has three very distinct advantages: 1) rapid vomiting (within 3–5 min) with emptying of all gastric contents, 2) no obstruction of lavage tubes which may produce delays and incomplete emptying and 3) reflux of contents (enteric coated tablets, etc.) from the upper intestinal tract into the stomach. This treatment, however, should not be used if the patient is greatly depressed or comatose, or if the solution is green, which indicates decomposition of the tablet.

GASTRIC LAVAGE

If vomiting cannot be induced or is contraindicated, gastric lavage should be instituted at once. It is clearly indicated within 3 hr after ingestion of a poison and even later (up to 8 hr) if large amounts of milk or cream have been given or if enteric coated drugs have been taken. However, there are certain contraindications. These include: 1) ingestion of strong corrosive agents like alkali (concentrated ammonia, lye, etc.) or mineral acids (lavage probably can be safely carried out within 1 hr of ingestion); 2) ingestion of strychnine (a convulsion may be induced if much time has elapsed); 3) ingestion of petroleum distillates (kerosene, mineral seal oil, etc.) and 4) presence of coma with depression of cough reflex (aspiration pneumonia may occur).

In children, the only equipment needed is a common urethral catheter (8–12 French) and a syringe (20 or 50 ml). Davol plastic duodenal tubes are preferable because of their durability, flexibility and ease of passage with lubrication. For adults, a tube with a diameter between $5/_{16}$ and ½ in. (about 1 cm), 24F or greater, is usually satisfactory. The larger the tube that can be passed, the more rapidly the lavage can be completed.

In older children and adults the nasal route is preferred. However, oral passage is easier and less traumatic for infants and young children. The distance from the bridge of the nose to the tip of the xiphoid process should be marked on the lavage tube with adhesive tape prior to passage. Passage will be facilitated by immersing the tube in cold water or a water miscible jelly (avoid oils). Dentures and other foreign objects should be removed from the mouth. Restraints will be required for most children. In centers where anesthesiologists are readily available, patients can be lightly anesthetized, given succinylcholine and lavaged, after inserting into the trachea an endotracheal tube with an inflatable cuff. (In most community hospitals and in physicians' offices this method, although ideal, would be impractical.)

The patient should be placed on his left side with his head hanging over the edge of the examining table and with his face down. If possible, the foot of the bed or table should be elevated. This position is particularly important if the patient is drowsy, since the chances of aspiration are thus minimized. The tube should be passed gently, since no great force is necessary. If the patient will cooperate, have him swallow frequently; this permits the tube to move easily and rapidly. If the catheter enters the larynx instead of the esophagus, dyspnea and severe coughing are produced, but this may be absent if the patient is deeply narcotized. If this occurs, the tube should be partially withdrawn before proceeding. If in doubt as to the placement of the tube, the free end should be dipped in a glass of water; continuous bubbling on expiration implies placement in the trachea, whereas gas from the stomach is usually expelled in two or three bursts. In every instance, aspiration should be performed before instilling the lavage solution or antidote. When the tube has reached the stomach, the glass syringe is then attached and the stomach contents aspirated.

The fluid ordinarily used for lavage is tap water containing an antidote if one is available. However, the substitution of isotonic or one-half isotonic saline solution is far safer, particularly for children who have a limited tolerance for electrolyte depletion. A 5% increase in body fluid volume with electrolyte free water is sufficient to initiate the cardinal symptoms of water intoxication,

TABLE 13—1. Signs and Symptoms of Poisoning

Sign or symptom	Poison
EYE	
Dilatation of pupil (mydriasis)	Belladonna group, meperidine, alcohols, ether, chloroform, papaverine, sympathomimetics, parasympatholytics, antihistamines, gelsemium, cocaine, camphor, aconitine, benzene, barium, thallium, botulinus toxin, cyanide, carbon monoxide, carbon dioxide
Constriction of pupil (miosis)	Opium, morphine group, sympatholytics (ergot), parasympathomimetics, dibenamine, barbiturates, cholinesterase inhibitors, chloral hydrate, picrotoxin, nicotine, caffeine
Purple-yellow vision	Marihuana, digitalis, carbon monoxide, santonin
Blurred vision	Belladonna group (atropine), methyl alcohol, ethyl alcohol, ergot, carbon tetrachloride, irreversible cholinesterase inhibitors (DFP, TEPP, HETP), vesicant war gases (mustard gas), camphor
Partial or total blindness	Methyl alcohol
Photophobia, lacrimation, pain	Vesicant war gases (mustard gas), Mace, tear gases (bromacetone, etc)
FACE AND SCALP	
Dull and mask-like expression	Barbiturates, bromides, gelsemine, manganese, thallium
Facial twitchings	Lead, mercury
Alopecia	Thallium, arsenic, ergot, hypervitaminosis A, gold, lead, boric acid, thiocyanates
SKIN AND MUCOUS MEMBRANES	
Pale	Aniline derivatives, colchicine, sympathomimetics (epinephrine), insulin, pilocarpine
Livid, ashy pale	Dinitrocresol, dinitrophenol, ergot, lead, phenacetin
Cyanotic, brown-bluish (in absence of respiratory depression and shock)	Nitrobenzene, chlorates, acetanilids, carbon dioxide, methane, nitrous oxide, aniline derivatives, nitrites, morphine, sulfides, ergot, amyl nitrite, and well over 100 other drugs and chemicals
Pink	Carbon monoxide, cyanides
Yellow	Atabrine; jaundice from hepatic injury (chlorinated compounds, arsenic and other heavy metals, chromates, mushrooms, and many drugs); jaundice from hemolytic anemias (aniline, nitrobenzene, quinine derivatives, arsine, fava beans, and many drugs)
Sweating	Pilocarpine, nicotine, physostigmine, picrotoxin
Dry, hot skin	Belladonna group (atropine), botulinus toxin
Blue-gray	Silver salts
LOCAL COLORING OF THE SKIN	
Brown, black	Iodine, silver nitrate
Deep brown	Bromine
Yellow	Nitric acid, picric acid
White	Phenol derivatives
Gray	Meruric chloride
NERVOUS SYSTEM	
Coma	Morphine derivatives and analogues, all hypnotics, sedatives and general anesthetics, barbiturates, chloral hydrate, sulfonal, trional, paraldehyde, chloroform, ethers, bromides, alcohols, lead, cyanide, carbon monoxide, carbon dioxide, nicotine, benzene, atropine, phenols, scopolamine, xylene, irreversible cholinesterase inhibitors, (DFP, TEPP, HETP, parathion), insulin, aniline derivatives, mushrooms, salicylates, copper salts
Delirium, mental disturbances	Belladonna group (atropine, hyoscine), cocaine, alcohol, lead, marihuana, arsenic, ergot, amphetamine and derivatives, antihistamines, camphor, benzene, barbiturates, DDT, aniline derivatives, physostigmine, veratrine, nerve gases (DFP, TEPP)

(continued)

TABLE 13–1. (continued)

Convulsions	Strychnine, picrotoxin, camphor, santonin, cocaine, belladonna group (atropine), veratrine, aconite, irreversible cholinesterase inhibitors (DFP, TEPP, HETP, parathion), pentylenetetrazol, amphetamine and derivatives, ergot, nicotine, lead, antipyrine, barium, sodium fluoroacetate, mushrooms, caffeine, carbon monoxide, cyanides, salicylates, copper salts
Headache	Carbon monoxide, phenol, benzene, nitrobenzene, nitrates, nitrites, aniline, lead, indomethacin (Indocin)
Muscle spasms	Atropine, cadmium, strychnine, copper salts, bites of black widow spider, scorpion, and sting ray
General or partial paralysis	Carbon monoxide, carbon dioxide, botulinus toxin, alcohols, physostigmine, curare group, DDT, aconite, nicotine, barium, cyanide, mercury, arsenic, lead

GASTROINTESTINAL TRACT

Nausea, vomiting, diarrhea, dehydration, abdominal pain	Heavy metal salts, corrosive acids and alkalies, halogens, cathartics (croton oil, castor oil), ergot, nicotine, aconitine, cantharides, solanine, acetanilid and derivatives, phosphorus, phenols, cresol, methyl alcohol muscarine, cardioactive glycosides (digitalis), fluorides, morphine and analogues, DDT, irreversible cholinesterase inhibitors (DFP, TEPP, HETP, OMPA, parathion), pilocarpine, veratrine, colchicine botulinus toxin, mushrooms, boric acid and sodium borate, cocaine, procaine and local anesthetics, salicylates
"Burning" throat and stomach	Camphor, picrotoxin, iodine, arsenicals, antimony compounds

ABNORMAL COLOR OF FECES:

Pink to red to black (resulting from internal bleeding)	Salicylates, anticoagulants
Orange-red	Phenazopyridine (Pyridium)
Whitish	Antacids, such as aluminum hydroxide preparations
Blue	Dithiazinine (Delvex)
Red	Pyrvinium pamoate (Povan)
Black	Bismuth sodium triglycollamate (Bristrimate), bismuth glycolylarsanilate (Milibis), bismuth subsalicylate (Pepto-Bismol), iron preparations
Brownish staining of rectal mucosa	1,8-Dihydroxyanthraquinone (Dorbane, Doxan)

ODOR OF VOMITUS, BREATH OR BODY FLUIDS

Phenolic	Phenols, cresol
Etheric, ethereal sweet	Ether
Sweet	Chloroform, acetone
Bitter almond-like	Cyanides
Stale tobacco-like	Nicotine
Pear-like	Chloral hydrate
Alcoholic	Alcohols
Garlic-like	Phosphorus, tellurium, arsenic, malathion
Shoe polish-like	Nitrobenzene
Violets	Turpentine

COLORED MATERIAL AND GASTRIC LAVAGE OR VOMITUS

Pink or purple	Potassium permanganate
Blue, green	Copper salts, chemical dyes added to fluorides or mercury bichloride
Green	Nickel salts
Pink	Cobalt salts
Yellow	Picric acid, nitric acid
Bright red	Mercurochrome, nitric acid
Black, coffee-like grounds	Sulfuric acid, oxalic acid, nitric acid
Brown	Hydrochloric acid
Luminescent in dark	Yellow phosphorus
Discolored, bloody	Alkalis

(continued)

TABLE 13—1. (continued)

MOUTH

Excess salivation — Ammonia, cantharides, pilocarpine, arecoline, physostigmine, muscarine, nicotine, mercury, irreversible cholinesterase inhibitors (DFP, HETP, TEPP), salicylates

Dry mouth — Belladonna group (atropine), botulinus toxin, barium, diphenhydramine, ephedrine

EARS

Impaired hearing ("roaring") — Salicylates, quinine, streptomycin

"Buzzing" — Camphor, tabacco, ergot, methyl alcohol, quinidine

GENITOURINARY SYSTEM

Uterine cramps, uterine bleeding, abortion — Phosphorus, lead, pilocarpine, physostigmine, nicotine, ergot, quinine, mustard, cantharides, apiol, cathartics (croton oil, castor oil)

ABNORMAL COLOR OF URINE:

Blue — Methylene blue

Brown to black — Aniline dyes, cascara, chlorinated hydrocarbons, hydroxyquinone, melanin, methocarbamol (Robaxin), naphthalene, naphthol, nitrites, nitrofurans—furazolidone (Furoxone), nitrofurazone (Furacin)—phenol, phenyl salicylate (salol), pyrogallol, quinine, resorcinol (resorcin), rhubarb, santonin, senna, thymol

Green (blue plus yellow) — Anthraquinone, arbutin, bile pigments, eosins, methocarbamol (Robaxin), methylene blue, resorcinol (resorcin), tetrahydronaphthalene, thymol

Magenta to purple — Fuchsin, phenolphthalein

Orange — Indandione derivatives in alkaline urine: anisindione (Miradon), diphenadione (Dipaxin), phenindione (Danilone, Eridione, Hedulin)

Orange to orange-red — Phenylazopyridine (Pyridium)

Orange to red-brown — Combinations of phenylazopyridine (Pyridium) and other drugs used as urinary antiseptics; many of the trade names begin with Azo-; also santonin

Pink and red to red-brown — Aminopyrine, dipyrone, anthraquinone and its dyes, antipyrine (Pyrazoline), beets, chrysarobin (alkaline urine), cinchophen, danthron (Dorbane) (pink to violet in alkaline urine), deferoxamine (Desferal) (with elevated serum iron), diphenylhydantoin (Dilantin), emodin (alkaline urine), eosins (red with green fluorescence), hematuria producers (mercuric salts, irritants, etc.), hemolysis producers, phenindione (Danilone, Hedulin), phenolic metabolites (glucuronides), phenolphthalein (alkaline urine), phensuximide (Milontin), porphyrins, prochlorperazine (Compazine), rhodamine B (a food dye), santonin (alkaline urine), thiazolsulfone (Promizole), urates (especially in newborn infants and during tumor lysis)

Rust — Chlorzoxazone (Paraflex)

Yellowish or brownish — Danthron (Dionone, Dorbane, Istizin) (acid urine), heavy metals (bismuth, mercury), liver poisons (jaundice)—alcohol, arsenicals, carbon tetrachloride, chloral hydrate, chlorinated hydrocarbons, chlorobutanol (chlorbutol, Chloretone), chloroform, cinchophen—naphthalene, neocinchophen, nitrofurantoins, pamaquine (Aminoquin), Beprochine, Gamefar, Plasmoquine, Praequine, Quipenyl, sulfonamides, tribromomethanol with amylene hydrate (Avertin)

Yellow or green — Carotene containing foods, methylene blue, riboflavin, vitamin B complex, yeast concentrate

RESPIRATORY SYSTEM

Slow respiration — Opium, morphine derivatives and analogs, chloral hydrate, alcohols, picrotoxin, fluorides, cyanides

Rapid or deep respiration, or both — Belladonna group (atropine), cocaine, amphetamine and derivatives, strychnine, carbon dioxide, lobeline, salicylates, nikethamide, camphor

(continued)

TABLE 13–1. (continued)

Dyspnea	Cyanides, carbon monoxide, volatile organic solvents (benzene), snake venoms, suffocating war gases (phosgene), carbon dioxide
Respiratory paralysis	Morphine derivatives and analogues, general anesthesia, hypnotics and sedatives (barbiturates), alcohols, snake venoms, carbon monoxide
Edema (pulmonary)	Chlorine, bromine, phosgene, methyl perchloroformate
Burning pain in chest and throat	Tear gases
Sneezing	Adamsite, Clarc I, Clarc II
Restlessness	Caffeine
Laryngitis, coughing	Vesicant war gases (mustard gas, Lewisite, etc.), nerve gases (DFP, TEPP)
Difficult breathing	Alkalis
CARDIOVASCULAR SYSTEM	
Slow pulse (bradycardia)	Barium, aconite, cardioactive glycosides (digitalis), muscarine, physostigmine, pilocarpine, quinine, quinidine, veratrine, picrotoxin, lead, phenylephrine
Fast pulse (tachycardia)	Amphetamine and derivatives, atropine, cocaine, sympathomimetics (ephedrine), epinephrine, caffeine, alkalis
Angina pectoris-type pain	Nicotine
Pain in heart area	Sternutators (Adamsite, Clarc I, Clarc II)
Hypotension	Chloral hydrate, alkalies, nitrites, nitrates, quinine, volatile oils, iron salts, chlorpromazine (Thorazine)
Hypertension	Epinephrine or substitute, veratrum, ergot, cortisone, vanadium, lead, nicotine, amphetamines
Vascular collapse	Lead, acids, alkalis

*Material taken largely from Arena JM (1974): Poisoning: Toxicology, Symptoms, Treatment. 3rd ed., Springfield, Ill, Charles C Thomas

which are tonic and clonic seizures with coma. These may start without prodromes.

Only small amounts of fluids should be instilled at one time so that the passage of the poison into the upper intestinal tract will not be promoted. Lavage should be repeated 10–12 times or until the returns are clear. All washings should be saved, with the first separated from the others, for any analyses that might be indicated. As soon as the lavage is completed, an antidote if indicated should be instilled through the tube and allowed to remain in the stomach. Before the catheter is withdrawn, it should be either pinched off or suction maintained in order to prevent aspiration.

Recently, a device consisting of a double lumen tube designed to deliver and aspirate simultaneously (or separately) allows the entire procedure of gastric lavage to be done in as little as 5 min.

Lavaging Fluids

The following substances are useful in gastric lavage:

1. *Tannic acid* is mildly acidic (for neutralizing strong alkalis, diluted acetic acid is more effective) and precipitates a large number of organic and inorganic compounds, including alkaloids, metals and some glucosides. The tannates formed often redissolve and hydrolyze later and, therefore, should not be allowed to remain in the stomach. Approximately 30–50 g of tannic acid in 1000 ml of water is an effective concentration. Among the compounds rapidly precipitated by tannic acid are apomorphine, hydrastine, strychnine, veratrine, cinchona alkaloids, as well as salts of aluminum, lead and silver. Because of its hepatotoxic properties, tannic acid should be used with care and only in the recommended dilutions.

2. *Potassium permanganate* is an oxidizing agent that reacts well with organic substances. It effectively neutralizes such compounds as strychnine, nicotine, physostigmine and quinine. Because potassium permanganate is itself a strong irritant, caution must be taken to use it well diluted (1:10,000 approximately and not stronger than 1:5000) and to be sure that no undissolved particles come in contact with the stomach or other tissues. It is recommended that a thoroughly dissolved 5% solution be kept on hand to be diluted to the needed strength. A 1:10,000 solution may be prepared by dissolving 0.1 g in 1 liter of water or 1 g may be dissolved in 100 ml of water

and 10 ml of this solution added to 1000 ml of water to make a 1:10,000 solution.

3. *Dairy or evaporated milk* may be used. The latter may be diluted with equal parts of water or used without dilution particularly when the demulcent action is desired—e.g., with copper sulfate, croton oil, chlorates and thioglycollic acid.

4. *Sodium bicarbonate* in a 5% solution is advised for gastric lavage in cases of ferrous sulfate posioning, since it forms the less corrosive and more insoluble ferrous carbonate. The bicarbonate, although an effective alkaline solution, is usually not recommended for neutralizing acids because the liberated CO_2 might cause increased gastric distension and thus predispose the patient to perforation if the stomach wall has been partly corroded by the acid.

5. *Calcium salts* are helpful in fluoride and oxalate poisoning and in preventing tetany from hypocalcemia in certain types of poisoning. Lavage with a dilute solution of calcium lactate is recommended for many of these toxic substances. Approximately 15–30 g of calcium lactate (or gluconate) in 1000 ml of water may be used. Calcium chloride, 4 g in 1000 ml of water, is an alternate treatment.

6. *Magnesium oxide* (or hydroxide) is used primarily as a neutralizing agent for acidic substances, including aspirin, sulfuric and other mineral acids and oxalic acid. It does not release CO_2 to distend the stomach, and if too much is not allowed to remain in the stomach, the depressant effect of magnesium on the central nervous system is negligible. Approximately 25 g of magnesium

TABLE 13–2. Approximate Amount of Substance Adsorbed by 1 g of Charcoal

Adsorbendum	Maximum adsorption (mg)
Mercuric chloride	1800
Sulfanilamide	1000
Strychnine nitrate	950
Morphine hydrochloride	800
Atropine sulfate	700
Nicotine	700
Barbital (Veronal)	700
Barbital sodium (Medinal)	150
Phenobarbital sodium (Luminal) Alurate sodium Dial sodium (Dial) Evipal sodium Phanodorn calcium	300–350
Salicylic acid	550
Phenol	400
Alcohol	300
Potassium cyanide	35

TABLE 13–3. Some Substances Effectively Adsorbed by Activated Charcoal

Organic compounds		Inorganic compounds*
Aconite	Muscarine	Antimony
Alcohol	Nicotine	Arsenic
Antipyrine	Opium	Iodine
Atropine	Oxalates	Lead (to limited extent)
Barbiturates	Parathion	Mercuric chloride
Camphor	Penicillin	Phosphorus
Cantharides	Phenol	Potassium permanganate
Cocaine	Phenolphthalein	Silver
Delphinium	Quinine	Tin
Digitalis	Salicylates	Titanium
Elaterin	Stramonium	
Hemlock	Strychnine	
Ipecac	Sulfonamides	
Methylene blue	Veratrum	
Morphine		

*Cyanide is a known exception; it poisons the charcoal

oxide in 1000 ml of water is the concentration recommended.

7. *A starch solution* is considered particularly efficacious in neutralizing iodine. About 75–80 g of starch in 1000 ml of water is used and the lavage continued until the return fluid is no longer blue.

8. *Ammonium acetate* or dilute ammonia water, approximately 4 ml in 500 ml of water, combines with formaldehyde to form relatively harmless methenamine.

9. *Normal saline solution* (0.8% or approximately 1 tsp of salt in 1 pt of water) is an effective gastric lavage solution for silver nitrate since it reacts with it to form a relatively insoluble and noncorrosive silver chloride.

10. *Activated charcoal* is the residue from destructive distillation of various organic materials, treated to increase its absorptive powers; vegetable charcoals made from wood pulp, which has a low ash content, are of particular value. This is a potent adsorbent that rapidly inactivates many poisons, if it is given early before much of the poison has been absorbed (Table 13–2). It is effective for virtually all chemicals (except cyanide) whether they be organic, inorganic, large or small molecule compounds (Table 13–3). The potency of adsorption is not reduced by the acidity or alkalinity of the poison or by a wide range of pH in the gastrointestinal tract. Adsorbed material is retained tenaciously throughout passage in the gut.

Activated charcoal is one of the best, least expensive and most practical emergency antidote available. One to two tbsp in an 8 oz glass of water or a mixture of soupy consistency would be a suitable concentration for oral use or lavaging. Bone chars are not effective because of their high mineral content, and the mineral charcoals are relatively little used.

We have had favorable experience with four commercial activated charcoals on the American market. They are Norit A (American Norit Co., Jacksonville, Fla.), Darco G 60 (Atlas Powder Co., Wilmington, Del.), Nuchar C (West Virginia Pulp and Paper Co., 230 Park Ave., New York City) and Requa's (Requa Manufacturing Co., Inc., 1193 Atlantic Ave., Brooklyn 16, N.Y.). Undoubtedly many good ones other than these are available.

A minor drawback to activated charcoal is that it is black. Many children will refuse to drink it, and, if spewed, it spots uniforms, clothes, wall and personnel. An effective, palatable, easier to administer suspension preparation, hopefully, will soon be on the market.

Activated charcoal should not be used simultaneously with syrup of ipecac, since it is capable of adsorbing the emetic principle and inactivating it. It should be administered only after emesis has been induced successfully.

ANTIDOTES (See Table 13-6, page 101)

Effective and useful specific antidotes for poisoning are limited in number, and often their overuse may complicate the initial injury by producing other forms of poisoning. The sensible selection and use of drugs and therapeutic measures for the general and supportive treatment of poisoning are more likely to save lives than ill-considered and heroically applied specific antidotes. The most useful and practical antidotes now available to the physician for emergency use are outlined in Table 13–4. Because of its frequency of occurrence, the treatment of barbiturate intoxication is summarized in Table 13–5, and these, combined with the symptomatic and supportive drugs and measures on hand, are all that are usually necessary.

ANTIBIOTICS

Antibiotics are often of considerable value in such inflammatory conditions as pneumonitis, mediastinitis, peritonitis, etc., which often follow the ingestion of certain toxic substances—petroleum distillates, turpentine, cedar oil, lye, acids and other corrosives.

The selection of a specific antibiotic should be determined on an individual basis, depending on the severity and nature of the poison. In the hope of forestalling infection, some physicians advise that these antibiotics be administered even prior to the onset of signs and symptoms of infection when it is certain that substantial amounts of the particularly dangerous substances have been swallowed or aspirated in the lungs. Others feel that skilled and discriminating use of antibiotics would exclude their prophylactic use, except in already infected individuals, if aspiration occurs or if an indwelling catheter is necessary.

Increasing the Excretion of Poisons
Dialysis

HEMODIALYSIS (ARTIFICIAL KIDNEY). Dialysis can be used in cases of severe posioning from dialyzable substances as well as for non-dialyzable nephrotoxic compounds which produce acute tubular damage and renal failure. In general, poisons circulating in the blood or reversibly bound to tissue or colloids in equilibrium with the unbound poison can be removed by dialysis, while those irreversibly bound cannot. Dialyzable poisons include barbiturates, borates, bromates, bromides, ethylene glycol, glutethimide, methanol, salicylates, salt, thiocyanates and many others. Nephrotoxic compounds are not dialyzable.

Contraindications to this procedure are: inexperience of the operator and inadequate knowledge of the problem to which the apparatus is to be applied; bleeding, particularly from the gastrointestinal tract and destruction of platelets and white blood cells by the cellophane membrane during the course of hemodialysis.

Lipid Dialysis

Lipid dialysis is a new technique in the treatment of poisonings by glutethimide, pentobarbital, secobarbital, phenothiazines, camphor and other lipid soluble substances that cannot be effectively removed by hemodialysis employing an aqueous dialysate. Lipid dialysis is similar to aqueous hemodialysis, except that oil is circulated on the dialysate side of the membrane. An inexpensive and readily available effective, safe, nontoxic and nonpyrogenic dialysate is soybean oil. The oil does not cross the cellophane membrane and will absorb large quantities of lipid soluble substances.

A Klung or Kiil membrane can be easily used for lipid dialysis with only a few modifications. Two gallons of soybean oil will absorb a large quantity of the drug and compounds, and only a slow flow of the oil past the membrane is necessary for complete removal of lipid soluble substance in each circulation of the blood through the membrane. Glutethimide is highly soluble in alcohols and lipids, but it is very poorly soluble in water.

PERITONEAL DIALYSIS. Peritoneal dialysis is much more efficient than the natural kidney (but less efficient than the artifical kidney) for ridding

TABLE 13—4. Treatment of Convulsions Due to Poisoning*

Drug	Method of administration and dosage	Advantages	Disadvantages
Ether	Open drop	Dosage easily determined; good minute-to-minute control; no sterile precautions	Difficult to give in presence of convulsion; requires constant supervision by physician
Thiopental sodium (Pentothal sodium)	Give 2.5% sterile solution IV until convulsions are controlled; maximum dose: 0.5 ml/kg	Good minute-to-minute control; can be given easily during convulsion	Doses larger than recommended may cause persistent respiratory depression; requires sterile equipment and administration
Pentobarbital sodium (Nembutal sodium)	Give 5 mg/kg gastric tube, rectally, or IV as sterile 2.5% solution at a rate not to exceed 1 ml/min until convulsions are controlled	Good control of initial dose	No control of effects after drug has been given; requires sterile precautions; may produce severe respiratory depression
Phenobarbital sodium	Give 1—2 mg/kg IM or gastric tube and repeat as necessary at 30 min intervals up to a maximum of 5 mg/kg	Effect lasts 12—14 hr	Causes severe persistent respiratory depression in overdoses
Succinylcholine chloride	Give 10—50 mg IV slowly and give artificial respiration during period of apnea; repeat as necessary	Will control colvulsions of any type; effect lasts only 1—5 min; circulation not ordinarily affected	Artificial respiration must be maintained during use; no antidote is available; apnea may persist for several hours in some cases
Trimethadione (Tridione)	Give 1 g IV slowly; maximum dose: 5 g	Little depression of respiration	Not effective in all types of convulsions
Tribromoethanol (Avertin)	Only by rectal instillation; 50—60 mg/kg causes drowsiness, amnesia; 70—80 mg/kg produces light unconsciousness and analgesia	Ease of administration and pleasant induction without mental distress and respiratory irritation	A nonvolatile anesthetic given by a route which prevents adequate control once it is administered; contraindicated when renal or hepatic injury exists
Amobarbital sodium (Amytal)	Give 2% sterile solution; dose range 0.4—0.8 g	Immediate action and lasts 3—6 hr	Inhibits cardiac action of vagus; may produce severe respiratory depression
Diphenylhydantoin sodium ,(Dilantin)	Give IV slowly 150—250 mg from steri-vial and repeat 30 min later with 100—150 mg if necessary	Lack of marked hypnotic and narcotic activity	Solution is highly alkaline and perivenous infiltration may cause sloughing; not always effective and other anticonvulsants frequently must be used; cardiac arrest has been reported after IV therapy
Paraldehyde	Give 5—15 ml gastric tube, rectally or IM	Little depression of respiration, effects last 12 hr	Harmful in presence of hepatic disease; old and loosely stoppered solutions can break down to acetic acid and produce serious intoxication
Diazepam (Valium)	Give 2—5 mg IV or IM; repeat 2 hr later if necessary	Good muscle relaxant for skeletal muscle spasm	Hypotension; respiratory depression or muscular weakness may occur if used with barbiturates

*Convulsions can occur with almost any compound in a toxic dose

TABLE 13—5. Management of Barbiturate Poisoning

Condition	Treatment	Guides
Respiratory insufficiency	Airway, suction; endotracheal intubation, cuffed tube, lavage; humidified oxygen; mechanical ventilation, pressure or volume controlled ventilator	Arterial P_{O_2}, O_2 saturation, P_{CO_2}, pH, minute ventilation; x-ray film of chest; airway pressure
Hypovolemia	Albumin, 5% solution, 1 liter, then dextrose, 10% in sodium chloride 0.9 solution; potassium chloride supplement, 40—120 mEq	Central venous pressure, arterial pressure, urine output and osmolality
Low urinary output	Fluid infusion furosemide, 40 mg IV or ethacrynic acid, 25 mg IV	Urinary output and osmolality
Heart failure	Digoxin, 0.5 mg IV, followed by 1—4 doses of 0.25 mg digoxin at 1—2 hr intervals	Central venous pressure, ECG
Pneumonia	Ampicillin sodium, 1 g every 4 hr IV; methicillin sodium, 1 g every 6 hr IV; chloramphenicol sodium succinate, 500 mg every 6 hr IV; gentamicin sulfate, 0.75 mg/kg every 6 hr IM	Sputum and blood culture, with antibiotic sensitivity; chloramphenicol after aspiration of gastric contents, gentamicin for gram-negative bacteria resistant to other antibiotics
Dialysis	Peritoneal Lipid Hemodialysis (preferred)	Barbiturate levels of 3.5 mg/100 ml for short acting drugs and 8—10 mg/100 ml for long acting agents; impaired hepatic and renal function

the body of overdoses of many exogenous poisons. The artificial kidney is always preferable for dialysis, but one is not always available. Peritoneal dialysis, therefore, because of its availability and simplicity, is used much more frequently for dialysis. The development and use of simple disposable equipment with accompanying solutions for those with or without edema have brought this type of therapy within the reach of every physician and hospital, regardless of size. Contraindications are *absolute:* infection of the peritoneal cavity, and *relative:* recent or extensive abdominal surgery.

Exchange Transfusion

Blood transfusion is particularly efficacious when the toxic products of the poison tend to remain in the circulating bloodstream rather than become fixed or deposited in the viscera, bones or other tissues—in particular, the various types of drugs causing methemoglobinemia; e.g., the aniline dyes and their derivatives, such as acetanilid and phenacetin, nitrites, nitrates, bromates, chlorates, sulfanilamide, Pyridium (phenazopyridine), nitrobenzene and related nitro compounds. The object is to supply normal hemoglobin capable of transporting oxygen. In more severe instances, exchange or exsanguination transfusions may be life saving, if facilities and blood are available. This procedure offers certain advantages over other methods, such as hemodialysis, in that it is familiar to most physicians, requires little specialized equipment and does not necessitate exceptional experience as does the safe use of hemodialysis. It has obvious limitations in other than very small children, is technically difficult and presents the hazard of blood transfusion reaction, since it may be necessary to use blood from several sources. It is used with best results in infants under one year of age, poisoned from salicylates, barbiturates or other dialyzable drugs.

Forced Diuresis

Forced osmotic diuresis and alkalinization of the urine with large quantities of parenteral fluids are now being used effectively in the treatment of barbiturate and other intoxications.

GENERAL THERAPEUTIC MEASURES

1. Establish adequate airway by inserting an oropharyngeal or endotracheal tube. Often, however, extension of the head and forward displacement of the mandible are sufficient. The situation may require mouth-to-mouth breathing or mechanical respiratory equipment. Physiologic improvement of the patient's condition is often notable when tissues receive adequate oxygen.

2. Generally, legs and head are elevated to the level of the right atrium to allow venous drainage of the lower extremities and to promote circulatory pooling in the head and thorax. Cardiac failure may necessitate alterations in position.

3. Elastic bandaging of the legs prevents venous stasis. Passive leg exercises are advisable if depression is extreme. The patient is turned

from side to side every 2 hr to promote pulmonary drainage and reduce atelectasis.

4. Homeostasis is maintained by parenteral fluid according to blood electrolyte concentrations and urine output. An indwelling urethral catheter is placed in the bladder to permit accurate hourly measurement of output. When the kidney is not damaged, fluid therapy is aided by hourly measurement of urine specific gravity.

5. If oliguria is associated, electrocardiographic examination and frequent measurement of serum potassium are required.

6. Vital signs are recorded every 15 min or more frequently if values are labile or vasopressors are administered.

7. CNS stimulants should not be used to improve respiration. These drugs impart a false sense of security, and harmful reactions such as rebound depression or convulsions may occur. If the myocardium is hypoxic, epinephrine may induce fatal ventricular fibrillation.

8. IV vasopressors such as phenylephrine, methoxamine or other adrenergic drugs may be required if the patient has tachycardia above 110 pulse beats per minute, prolonged capillary filling time, pallor or diaphoresis. Moderate hypotension as low as 80 mm. Hg does not necessitate vigorous therapy with vasopressors unless urinary output is depressed. Extremely potent agents, such as levarterenol bitartrate, are used for severe shock, but vasoconstrictors may significantly depress urinary output.

9. Convulsions can occur with almost any compound in a toxic dose. Table 13–4 gives the various types of treatment available for convulsions.

TREATMENT OF NON-ORAL POISONING

ABSORBED DERMAL POISONS. There are any number of poisonous compounds that are capable of producing intoxication of various degrees through transcutaneous absorption as well as local dermatitis of many kinds. These compounds include the chlorinated and organic phosphate insecticides, the halogenated hydrocarbons, the caustics and corrosives and many others. The contaminated skin should be thoroughly washed with water from a hose or shower or even poured from a bucket. Clothing should be removed while a continuous stream of water is played on the skin. A 24 hr continuous shower has not been found effective for chemical burns. Chemical antidotes should increase the extent of injury. Corroded and burned areas should be treated as any burn.

INHALED POISONS. In cases of gas poisoning, the first act should be to move the victim from the presence of the gas and apply artificial respiration, if necessary.

INJECTED POISONS. If an injection of a poison has occurred, application of tourniquets central to the point of injection may slow absorption. Quantities of unabsorbed poison may be removed by means of surgery and suction similar to that commonly advised for the treatment of snake bite. Cryotherapy is also beneficial in delaying absorption.

CHEMICAL EYE BURNS. A chemical burn of the eye results from local contact with a chemical—solid, liquid, dust, mist or vapor—of such a degree as to alter the structure of the cornea and conjunctiva. Some alterations not visualized readily may be demonstrated by staining with a 2% solution of fluorescein, after a local anesthetic. The basic treatment of all types of chemical eye injuries is the quick, thorough irrigation of the eye with water at the nearest source of supply for 5 min. An ophthalmologist should be consulted for degree of damage and specific therapy.

FURTHER READING

Arena JM (1974): Poisoning: toxicology, symptoms, treatments 3rd ed. Springfield, Ill, Charles C Thomas

Berry FA, Lambdin MA (1963): Apomorphine and levallorphan tartrate in acute poisonings. Am J Dis Child 105:160

Lasagna L (1954): (N-allylnormorphine): practical and theoretical considerations. Arch Intern Med 94:532

Robertson WO (1962): Syrup of ipecac—a slow or fast emetic? AM J Dis Child 103:136

TABLE 13–6. Antidotes

Antidote	Dose	Poison	Reaction (antidote) and comments

Acids, weak
  Acetic acid, 1%
  Vinegar, 5% acetic acid
    (diluted 1:4 with water)
  Hydrochloric acid, 0.5%
	100–200 ml	Alkali, caustic	

Activated charcoal
  Darco G (Atlas Chem)
  Nuchar C (W Va Pulp & Paper)
  Norit A (Amer Norit Co)
	1–2 tbs to glass water or a mixture of soupy consistency	Effective for virtually all poisons (except cyanide), organic and inorganic compounds of large and small molecules	Broad spectrum of activity
			No reaction except staining

Alcohol, ethyl	IV as 5% solution in bicarbonate or saline solution PO as 3–4 oz of whiskey (45%) every 4 hr for 1–3 days	Methyl alcohol Ethylene and other glycols	Metabolizes methyl alcohol and prevents formation of toxic formic acid and formates; glycols into oxalates

Alkali, weak
  Magnesium oxide (preferred)*
  Sodium bicarbonate
	2.5% solution (25 g/liter)
	
	5% solution (50 g/liter)
		Acid, corrosive	Gastric distension from liberated CO_2 (from use of $NaHCO_3$)

Ammonium acetate Ammonium hydroxide	5 ml in 500 ml water 0.2% solution Both are for gastric lavage	Formaldehyde (formalin)	Forms relatively harmless methenamine
Atropine sulfate	1–2 mg IM and repeat in 30 min	Organic phosphate esters and other cholinesterase inhibitors	Atropinization
Barbiturate antidotes			See Table 13–5
Bromobenzene	Adult: 1 g Child: 0.25 g (in lavage solution)	Selenium	
Calcium EDTA or Versene (ethylenediamine tetra-acetate) [DTPA: (diethylenetriamine penta-acetic acid), more promising analogue]	25 to 50 mg/kg, 2% solution 2 times a day for 5 days 50 mg/kg, 20% solution (0.5% procaine) IM daily for 5–7 days Repeat these courses after 2-day rest period	Cadmium Cobalt Copper Nickel, and other metals Iron Lead (combined therapy with BAL for encephalitis)	Nephrotoxic Increases urinary potassium excretion Oral EDTA should not be used until all lead has been removed or absorbed from the gastrointestinal tract
Calcium lactate	10% solution (in lavage solution	Chlorinated hydrocarbons Fluoride Oxalates	
Calcium gluconate	10% solution, 5–10 ml IM or IV, may be repeated in 8–12 hr	Black widow spider and other insect bites	Muscle relaxant Bradycardia Flushing Local necrosis from perivenous infiltration (methocarbamol, etc., also effective)
Chlorpromazine**	1–2 mg/kg IM	Amphetamine	Drowsiness Hypotension Neuromuscular (Parkinsonian)

(continued)

TABLE 13–6. (continued)

Copper sulfate	0.25–3.0 g in glass of water	Phosphorus	Forms insoluble copper phosphide
Cyanide poison kit (Eli Lilly stock M76)		Cyanide	Hypotension
Amyl nitrite pearls	0.2 ml (inhalation)		
Sodium nitrite	follow with 3.0% solution (10 ml) in 2–4 min and		
Sodium thiosulfate	25% solution (50 ml) in 10 min through same needle and vein. (repeat with ½ doses if necessary)	Iodine	Sodium thiosulfate used alone for iodine; forms harmless sodium iodide
Deferoxamine B Desferal isolated from streptomyces pilosus	1–2 g IM or IV (adults), repeat if necessary every 4–12 hr; also 5–10 g via nasogastric tube after gastric lavage	Iron Hemochromatosis	Diarrhea Hypotension
Dimercaprol (BAL)	Severe intoxication Day 1: 3.0 mg/kg every 4 hr (6 inj) Day 2: same Day 3: 3.0 mg/kg every 6 hr (4 inj) Days 4–13 (or until recovery): 3.0 mg/kg every 12 hr (2 inj) Mild intoxication Day 1: 2.5 mg/kg every 4 hr (6 inj) Day 2: same Day 3: 2.5 mg/kg every 12 hr Days 4–13 (or until recovery): 2.5 mg/kg daily (1 inj.)	Antimony Arsenic Bismuth Gold Mercury (acrodynia) Nickel Lead (combined therapy with EDTA for encephalitis) Contraindicated for iron	Flushing Myalgia Nausea and vomiting Nephrotoxic Hypotension Pulmonary edema Salivation and lacrimation Fever (children)
Diphenhydramine hydrochloride	10–50 mg IV or IM	Phenothiazine tranquilizers (for extrapyramidal neuromuscular manifestations)	Atropine-like effect Drowsiness
Dithizon	10 mg/kg twice a day orally with 100 ml 10% glucose solution for 5 days	Thallium	Diabetogenic Not available for therapeutic use; may be obtained through a chemical supply company
Household antidotes Milk		Arsenic Mercury and other heavy metals	These are useful and readily available antidotes that can be used in an emergency; all have demulcent properties
Raw eggs Flour Starches Hydrogen peroxide	3% solution (10 ml in 100 ml water as lavage solution)	Iodine Potassium permanganate Oxidizing agent for many other compounds	Irritation of mucous membranes Distension of abdomen from release of gas
Iodine, tincture	15 drops in 120 ml water	Precipitant for: Lead Mercury Quinine Silver Strychnine	Precipitants must be thoroughly removed by gastric lavage

(continued)

TABLE 13–6. (continued)

Magnesium sulfate
Sodium sulfate
	2–5% solution for
	  lavage
	10% solution IM and
	  repeat in 30 min;
	  also as catharsis for
	  rapid elimination of
	  toxic agent from
	  gastrointestinal
	  tract
		Precipitant for:
		  Barium
		  Lead
		  Hypervitaminosis D
		  Hypercalcemia (glucocorticoid
		    therapy preferable)	

Methylene blue	IV: 1% solution given
	  slowly (2 mg/kg) and
	  repeat in 1 hr if
	  necessary
	Orally: 3–5 mg/kg
	  (action much slower)
		Methemoglobinemia
		  produced by:
		  Acetanilid
		  Aniline derivatives
		  Chlorates
		  Dinitrophenol
		  Nitrites
		  Pyridium
		  Over 100 other
		    chemicals and
		    drugs
			Perivenous infiltration
			  can produce severe
			  necrosis
			Hypertension
			Hemolysis

Monoacetin (glyceryl
  monoacetate)
	0.5 ml/kg IM or in saline
	  solution IV; repeat as
	  necessary
		Sodium fluoroacetate "1080"	Not available commercially; if
			  parenteral therapy not
			  feasible, can give 100 ml of
			  monoacetin in water

Nalorphine	Adult: 5–10 mg IM or IV
	  and repeat in ½ hr
	Child: 0.1–0.2 mg/kg IM
	  or IV and repeat in ½ hr
		Codeine
		Demerol
		Dionin
		Heroin
			Withdrawal symptoms
			Depressant effects in other
			  than narcotic compounds

Levallorphan
  and
	Adult: 0.5–1.0 mg IM or IV
	Child: 0.01–0.02 mg/kg IM
	  or IV
		Methadone
		Morphine
		Pantopon	

Naloxone	0.01 mg/kg IV, IM or SC	(For respiratory and
		  cardiovascular depression)
			Naloxone produces no
			  respiratory depression,
			  psychotomimetic effects,
			  circulatory changes or
			  miosis and is preferable

Petrolatum, liquid
  (mineral oil)
		Stomach concretion
		  (castor oil preferred)
			Solvent
			Demulcent

Pralidoxime iodine (2-PAM iodine)	Adult: 1–2 g	Organic phosphate esters	Diplopia

Pralidoxime chloride
  (2-PAM chloride)
	Child: 25–50 mg/kg IM or
	  IV as 5% solution
		Cholinesterase inhibition
		  by any agent: chemical,
		  drug, etc
			Dizziness
			Headache

Penicillamine and its
  derivatives
	1–5 g orally	Mercury and other heavy
		  metals
		Lead (investigational drug
		  permit necessary)
			Fever
			Stupor
			Nausea and vomiting
			Myalgia
			Leukopenia, thrombocytopenia
			Nephrosis, reversible
			Optic axial neuritis,
			  reversible
			Ineffective when severe
			  vomiting is prominent

Physostigmine	1–2 mg IV	Anticholinergic compounds
		  (peripheral and central
		  effects)
			Only cholinergic drug that
			  crosses the blood-brain
			  barrier

Pilocarpine (available
  only as a powder—
  Wyeth Lab)
	Orally: 2–4 mg	Atropine and related
		  alkaloids
			Antagonizes the
			  parasympathetic (mydriasis
			  and dry mouth), not
			  central, effects of
			  atropine

Potassium permanganate	1:5,000 and 1:10,000
	  solution for gastric
	  lavage
		Nicotine
		Physostigmine
		Quinine
		Strychnine
		Oxidizing agent for many
		  alkaloids and organic
		  poisons
			Severe irritant and should
			  not be used in stronger
			  dilutions or with any
			  residual particles

(continued)

TABLE 13—6. (continued)

Protamine sulfate	1% solution IV slowly (mg/mg) to that of heparin	Heparin	Sensitivity effects
Sodium chloride	1 tsp salt to 1 pt water (approximately normal saline solution) 6—12 g orally in divided doses or in isotonic saline IV	Silver nitrate Bromides	Forms noncorrosive silver chloride Hypernatremia
Sodium formaldehyde sulfoxalate	5% in lavage solution (preferably combined with 5% sodium bicarbonate)	Mercury salts	BAL therapy should follow gastric lavage
Sodium thiosulfate	Orally: 2—3 g or IM: 10 or 25% solution Repeat in 3—4 hr	Iodine Cyanide	
Starch	80 g/1000 ml water	Iodine	
Tannic acid	4% in lavage solution; never use in greater concentrations	Precipitates alkaloids, certain glucosides, and many metals	Hepatotoxic Tannates formed should not be allowed to remain in the stomach Because of its hepatotoxicity, should be used cautiously and in no greater than 4% solution
Universal antidote (activated charcoal alone preferable)	Two parts pulverized charcoal (burned toast); One part magnesium oxide (milk of magnesia); One part tannic acid (strong tea solution)		Over rated and ineffective; may actually be harmful in that it can give false sense of security to those who use it; mentioned here only to negate its popularity in lay journals and books
Vitamin K_1	25—150 mg IV Rate not to exceed 10 mg/min	Coumarin derivatives: Coumarin Marcoumar Warfarin, etc.	Bleeding Focal hemorrhages

* Paradoxical as it may seem, magnesium oxide should be used for (alkali) hypochlorite (bleaches) ingestion, to prevent the formation of irritating hypochlorous acid

** Recent reports have indicated that haloperidol is more effective in much smaller doses than chlorpromazine for the treatment of amphetamine intoxication

PART II

SYSTEMATIC PHARMACOLOGY

DRUGS ACTING ON THE PERIPHERAL NERVOUS SYSTEM

JOHN A. BEVAN

14. INTRODUCTION

The peripheral nervous system is composed of the afferent and efferent neurons of the autonomic and somatic nervous system. All drugs of clinical importance that act on the peripheral nervous system, with the exception of local anesthetics (Ch. 22) and the veratrum alkaloids (Ch. 20), do so by modifying the transmission of excitation between two serial neurons or between the junction of neurons with gland or muscle (effector cells. The region of close contact between two nerve cells or between a nerve and effector cell utilized for the transference of excitation or inhibition is termed a **synapse.** The synapse between a motor neuron and an effector cell is also known as a **neuroeffector junction.**

It is generally assumed that the peripheral junctional sites are models of synapses in the central nervous system. Consequently, the mode of action of drugs on the brain is frequently inferred from a study of their peripheral effects.

A knowledge of the anatomy, physiology and biochemistry of the peripheral nervous system, particularly its junctional sites, is an essential prerequisite to an understanding of its pharmacology. The pharmacology of those drugs that modify the neuroeffector mechanism at the synapse between motor nerves and voluntary muscle, the *neuromuscular junction* is discussed in Chapter 21.

ANATOMY OF THE AUTONOMIC NERVOUS SYSTEM

The autonomic (visceral, vegetative, automatic) nervous system innervates almost all the tissues of the body; the notable exception is voluntary muscle.

Visceral afferent, or sensory fibers are more numerous than autonomic motor fibers. (Fig. 14–1). They pass via either somatic nerves or the various ramifications of the autonomic nervous system into the cerebrospinal axis. Such fibers carry general visceral sensation and also information from the specialized reflexogenic areas of the cardiovascular, ventilatory, and other system (Chs. 16, 25).

Integration of autonomic activity occurs at all levels of the cerebrospinal axis. A study of patients with high spinal cord lesions shows that a number of reflex changes are mediated at the spinal or segmental level. The medulla and pons contain the so-called "vital" centers, important in the control of the ventilatory and cardiovascular systems. The principal site of organization and coordination of the autonomic nervous system is the hypothalamus. Sympathetic functions are controlled by the posterior, and parasympathetic by the middle and some anterior, nuclei. The supraoptic nuclei are anatomically and functionally associated with the posterior lobe of the pituitary. Integration of autonomic with somatic motor and sensory function, as for example in fainting at the sight of blood, must occur in higher centers.

Although the pharmacology of these integrative centers will not be systemically described, many drugs owe some of their important effects to actions upon them; examples are reserpine (Ch. 20), barbiturates (Ch. 26), morphine (Ch. 29), and digitalis (Ch. 33).

Visceral efferent fibers are divided among the two divisions of the autonomic nervous system. These divisions are distinguished anatomically (Fig. 14–2) and functionally. The fibers of the **sympathetic division** emerge from the thoracolumbar levels of the spinal cord and those of the **parasympathetic division** from the sacral part of the spinal cord and in association with certain cranial nerves. Both divisions can be represented

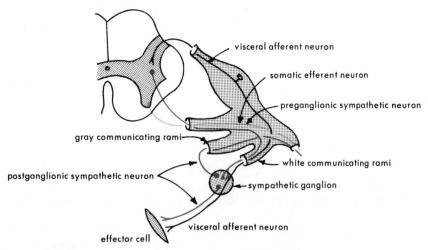

FIG. 14-1. Neuronal arrangement of the afferent and efferent neurons of the perpheral autonomic nervous system.

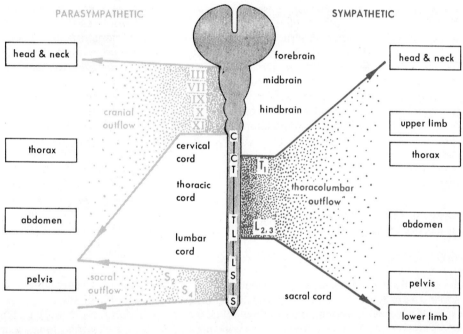

FIG. 14-2. Autonomic efferent outflow.

schematically as two serial neurons (Figs. 14-1 and 14-4). The proximal (preganglionic) neurons originate in the parasympathetic components of the nuclei of some cranial nerves and from the interomediolateral gray column of the spinal cord and synapse with distal (postganglionic) neurons in **ganglia.**

The sympathetic, or thoracolumbar division arises from segmental levels T_1 to L_2 or L_3 of the spinal cord (Fig. 14-2). Fibers pass via white communicating rami (myelinated fibers) and by nerves to ganglia most of which are found in the sympathetic chains and the paravertebral ganglia (Figs. 14-1 and 14-2). Postganglionic fibers are distributed to visceral structures via terminal plexuses and by specific autonomic nerves and to somatic tissues via the gray communicating rami (nonmyelinated fibers) and the spinal nerves. The cells of the adrenal medulla are homologous to sympathetic postganglionic neurons, and are innervated by preganglionic fibers, that pass in the splanchnic nerves. They form an integral part of the sympathetic autonomic division.

Sympathetic postganglionic fibers are subdivided into "long" fibers which innervate the heart, blood vessels, smooth muscle, glands and intramural ganglia and "short" fibers to the vas deferens, uterus and urinary bladder. The neuronal organization of the long fibers of the sympathetic nervous system is designed to ensure a generalized influence on the innervated viscera. One preganglionic fiber influences a large number of postganglionic neurons, and any one ganglion contains neurons which are distributed to a number of organs. Furthermore, the adrenal medulla, an integral part of this division, upon activating releases epinephrine and norepinephrine into the circulation to act on all tissues.

The parasympathetic, or craniosacral division emerges in association with cranial nerves III, VII, IX, X and XI and at segmental levels S_2 to S_4 of the spinal cord (Fig. 14–2). The cranial outflow of this division carries fibers to most structures in the head, neck, thorax and abdomen. The left half of the transverse colon, the descending colon and the pelvic viscera are supplied by the sacral outflow (pelvic nerve). Parasympathetic ganglia are small and are situated either close to, or buried within, innervated structures.

In contrast to the sympathetic division, the neural arrangement of the parasympathetic efferent limb is consistent with discrete, limited, localized effect. A typical parasympathetic preganglionic neuron synapses with only a few postganglionic neurons. Juxtaposition of parasympathetic ganglia to the viscera ensures a limited distribution of postganglionic fibers. The main exception to this generalization is Auerbach's plexus.

PHYSIOLOGY OF THE AUTONOMIC NERVOUS SYSTEM

Many tissues are innervated by both divisions of the autonomic nervous system. Although the actions of the two divisions are supplementary in some tissues (e.g., the salivary gland), in general (as in the bladder, bronchi, gastrointestinal tract, heart and pupil) activities of the two divisions produce opposite effects. In vivo, however, the two divisions act synergistically and tend to be complementary. Denervation studies show that many autonomically innervated structures possess intrinsic activity which is modified by autonomic activity. A few tissues, including most blood vessels, sweat glands and the spleen, are innervated by only one division.

The autonomic nervous system acts to regulate and maintain the constancy of the internal environment of the body despite many influences that threaten to alter it, such as temperature change, alteration in posture, exercise, food ingestion and anger. In Table 14–1 the responses of the various organs to autonomic activity and, where known, the dominant regulating division are summarized. If it is remembered that the sympathetic system discharges diffusely in response to fear or anger causing the physiologic changes appropriate to fight of flight, the seemingly unrelated effects listed in Table 14–1 appear to have more cohesion and are more readily understood and remembered. They are similar to the effects of epinephrine described in Chapter 18.

Sympathetic activity causes an elevation of cardiac output due to an increase in heart rate and stroke volume and an increase in total peripheral resistance. There is generalized venous constriction. These changes, together with the contraction of the spleen that occurs in some species are responsible for the rise in arterial pressure. The cardiac output is redistributed among the various regions of the body. As a result of active vasoconstriction it is shifted away from the skin, gastrointestinal tract, glands and, to a less extent the kidney to organs of more immediate biologic importance, the heart, voluntary muscle, brain and lungs. Glandular secretions dry up, sphincters of the gastrointestinal tract and urinary system contract, peristalsis is inhibited, and the tone in the wall of these organs is reduced. Pupils and bronchi dilate. Erector pili and sweat glands are activated. Glycogenolysis is stimulated. Blood levels of free fatty acids rise. There is transient elevation and depression respectively of potassium and inorganic phosphate.

In contrast, the parasympathetic nervous system is designed for conservative and discrete action. It can effect changes in a single organ; for example, vagal bradycardia can occur without concomitant salivary secretion or a change in gastric tone. It only of the two divisions is essential for life.

NEUROHUMORAL TRANSMISSION

It is generally accepted that transmission of excitation across junctional regions of the peripheral nervous system in mammals occurs through the mediation of liberated chemical substances. Of the many experimental studies that led to the establishment of this theory, those of Otto Loewi, in 1921, are the most simple and convincing. Loewi perfused two frog hearts (Fig. 14–3). He stimulated the vagus of one **(A)** and then transferred the fluid present in this heart to the second **(B)**. The second heart slowed. When the sympathetic supply was stimulated the transferred fluid accelerated the second heart. Loewi argued that the autonomic nervous activity influenced the

TABLE 14–1. Effector Responses to Autonomic Nervous Activity

Effector system	Predominant division*	Response	Receptor type	Response to other division	Receptor type
IRIS					
Dilator pupillae	Symp.	Contraction (mydriasis)	α	————	————
Sphincter pupillae	Parasymp.	Contraction (miosis)	Chol.	————	————
CILIARY MUSCLE	Parasymp.	Contraction (near vision)	Chol.	Opposite (weak)	β
BRONCHI BRONCHIOLES	Parasymp.	Contraction	Chol.	Relaxation	β
HEART	See Ch. 33				
Atria	Parasymp.	Increased conduction velocity, decreased contractility	Chol.	Mixed; increased conduction velocity; increased contractility	β
AV node and bundle	Parasymp.	Decreased conduction velocity; lengthened refractory period	Chol.	Opposite	β
SA node	Parasymp.	Slowing	Chol.	Opposite	β
Ventricles	Symp.	Increased conduction velocity; increased contractility; increased automaticity	β	————	————
BLOOD VESSELS					
Abdominal viscera	Symp.	Constriction	α	————	————
Coronary	Symp.	Dilation	β	?Same	Chol.
Glands	Parasymp.	Dilation	Chol.	Opposite	α
Pulmonary	Symp.	Constriction	α	?Opposite	Chol.
Skeletal muscle	Symp.	Complex dilation	β, Chol.	————	————
Skin, mucosa	Symp.	Constriction	α	————	————
GASTROINTESTINAL TRACT					
Liver	Symp.	Glycogenolysis, lipolysis, etc.	————	————	————
Muscle wall	Parasymp.	Increased tone and motility	Chol.	Opposite	α, β
Sphincters	Parasymp.	Relaxation	Chol.	Opposite	α
GLANDS					
Gastrointestinal	Parasymp.	Secretion	Chol.	————	————
Lacrimal	Parasymp.	Secretion	Chol.	————	————
Nasopharyngeal	Parasymp.	Secretion	Chol.	————	————
Respiratory	Parasymp.	Secretion	Chol.	————	————
Salivary	Parasymp.	Thin secretion	Chol.	Same, thick secretion	α
SKIN					
Pilomotor	Symp.	Piloerection	α	————	————
Sweat glands	Symp.	Secretion	Chol.	Symp. similar in special areas	α
URINARY BLADDER					
Detrusor	Parasymp.	Contraction	Chol.	Opposite	β
Sphincter and trigone	Parasymp.	Relaxation	Chol.	Opposite	α
SEX ORGANS	Parasymp.	Erection	Chol.	Ejaculation	?α

Parasymp., parasympathetic   Symp., sympathetic   Chol., cholinergic α, alpha adrenergic receptor
β, beta adrenergic receptor
* During rest and normal physiologic function

myocardium through the liberation of a specific chemical substance. Such a substance was contained in the fluid transferred from heart A to heart B.

The supporting evidence for the theory of neurohumoral transmission is overwhelming. The minimum criteria necessary to establish a substance as a neurohumoral transmitter are as follows: 1) demonstration of liberation of the active substance from junctional sites during presynaptic nervous activity; 2) identification by chemical or biologic methods of the liberated substance; 3) identity of the response to nerve stimulation and local injection of liberated substance; 4) similar modification of responses to nerve stimulation and the local injection of transmitter substance by drugs and other procedures; 5) demonstration of synthetic and destructive mechanisms for the proposed transmitter in the region of the junction.

It has been established that acetylcholine mediates transmission between the pre and postganglionic neurons of both parasympathetic and sympathetic divisions (ganglionic transmission). The same substance, acetylcholine, is the chemical transmitter between postganglionic parasympathetic neurons and their effector cells, and between the motor nerves of the somatic nervous system and voluntary muscle. The transmitter released at the postganglionic sympa-

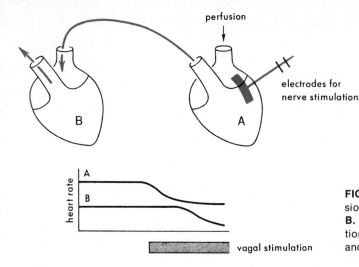

perfusion

electrodes for
nerve stimulation

B

A

heart rate

A

B

vagal stimulation

FIG. 14–3. Loewi's experiment. The perfusion fluid flows from frog heart **A** to heart **B**. Stimulation of the autonomic innervation of heart **A** causes changes first in **A** and then in **B**.

FIG. 14–4. Anatomic, physiologic, and pharmacologic classification of efferent neurons and junctional sites of the peripheral nervous system. **Ach,** acetylcholine; **Norepi,** norepinephrine; **Epi,** epinephrine.

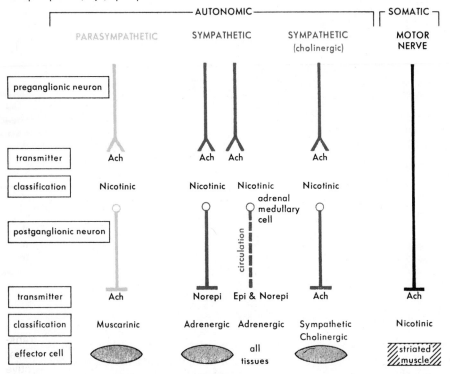

	AUTONOMIC			SOMATIC
	PARASYMPATHETIC	SYMPATHETIC	SYMPATHETIC (cholinergic)	MOTOR NERVE
preganglionic neuron				
transmitter	Ach	Ach Ach	Ach	
classification	Nicotinic	Nicotinic Nicotinic	Nicotinic	
postganglionic neuron			adrenal medullary cell / circulation	
transmitter	Ach	Norepi Epi & Norepi	Ach	Ach
classification	Muscarinic	Adrenergic Adrenergic	Sympathetic Cholinergic	Nicotinic
effector cell		all tissues		striated muscle

thetic nerve ending is almost exclusively *l*-norepinephrine, and from the adrenal medulla, a mixture of *l*-epinephrine and *l*-norepinephrine. In Figure 14–4, the efferent neurons and the principal neurohumoral transmitters of the peripheral nervous system are represented schematically. There is one notable exception: Fibers to sweat glands and to certain blood vessels (e.g., in skeletal muscle) liberate acetylcholine, although they are anatomically part of the sympathetic nervous system. Other exceptions to this seemingly simple arrangement are under experimental investigation. Other possible transmitters include histamine, serotonin, γ-aminobutyric acid, purines and possibly some amino acids and polypeptides. A role of some of these substances in modulating transmission has been proposed.

Principal Events in Transmission

Vesicles (secretory granules) are aggregated in neuronal terminations or in the plexi formed by

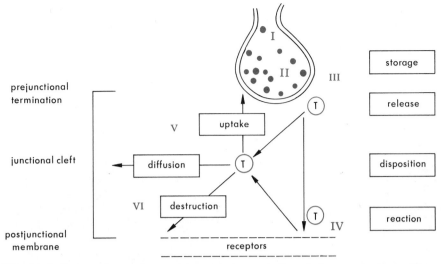

FIG. 14–5. Stages of neurohumoral transmission and sites of pharmacologic modification. See text discussion under Classification by Mode of Action, **T**, transmitter.

their terminations. These are storage sites or organs for the transmitter. During nervous activity, the vesicles appear to migrate toward the neurilemma and release their contents into the extracellular space probably by exocytosis. The released transmitter diffuses across the synaptic or junctional cleft which is generally around 200–400 A in width but sometimes may be as great as 10,000 A. There it combines with specific receptors probably found on the axonal membrane of the postganglionic neuron or the cell membrane of the effector cell. In some cells, such as skeletal muscle, the postjunctional membrane is specialized into a receptor containing area or **end plate.** In other cells, e.g., vascular muscle, the receptors are probably distributed more widely over the cell surface. The precise nature of the reaction of the transmitter with its receptors and the subsequent events leading to excitation or inhibition are not unequivocally established.

Vesicles are manufactured in the cell body and pass along the axon to its terminal areas. At each junctional site, special mechanisms exist for the synthesis, release and disposition of the transmitters. There are a number of feedback systems that regulate each of these processes and which insure precise control of response. There are three possible disposition mechanisms: 1) diffusion from the junctional cleft, 2) destruction by enzymatic activity or 3) reuptake of the transmitter into the nerve endings (Fig. 14–5). The relative importance of these pathways varies from one junction to another.

CHOLINERGIC TRANSMISSION. In the nerve ending acetylation of choline transported into the synaptic vesicle is catalyzed by **choline acetyl-**

ase. The acetylcholine formed is stored within the synaptic vesicles. The rate of synthesis of neuronal acetylcholine is linked to the level of neuronal activity. Within a few milliseconds of its release from the nerve ending probably by exocytosis into the synaptic cleft, and its subsequent reaction with cholinergic receptor, the transmitter is hydrolyzed mainly by **acetylcholinesterase** found at the neuromuscular junction. At cholinergic sites, transmitter inactivation by metabolism is the dominant mechanism. Acetylcholine often causes a local depolarization or hyperpolarization of the postsynaptic membrane (Ch. 15), e.g., in skeletal muscle at the end plate, the released acetylcholine causes depolarization, an end plate potential (Ch. 21), which if of sufficient magnitude initiates a regenerative or action potential.

ADRENERGIC TRANSMISSION. Although some *l*–norepinephrine is present in the synaptic vesicles that pass from the cell body to nerve endings, the main site of amine formation is in or near the nerve endings. Phenylalanine or tyrosine is taken up via a special transport mechanism into the axoplasm of the nerve terminal and there synthesized into either *l*-Norepinephrine or epinephrine. The pathways and the enzymes that regulate these processes are shown in Figure 14–6. The initial steps in this process leading to the synthesis of dopamine are carried on in the cytoplasm from where the amine must enter a synaptic vesicle before being finally converted into norepinephrine. Dopamine β-hydroxylase is the only biosynthetic enzyme in the storage organelle. The rate limiting step in biosynthesis is the conversion of tyrosine to dopa. The rate of synthesis of transmitter is dependent mainly

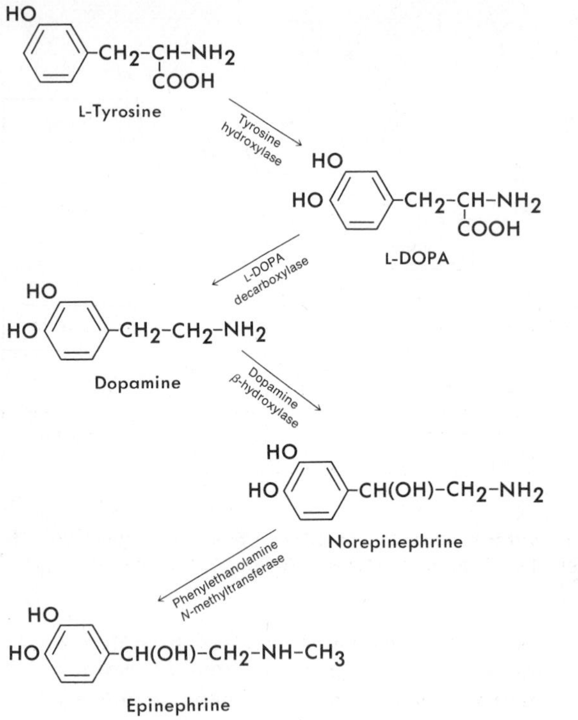

FIG. 14–6. Synthetic pathway of sympathetic transmitters.

upon the level of autonomic activity and is regulated by a local feedback system.

The *l*-norepinephrine released from the terminal plexus by neuronal activity derives from that which is taken up into the terminal from the extracellular space (see below) and that which is locally synthesized. Release is intimately regulated by local norepinephrine concentrations. The released amine is disposed of mainly by reuptake into the nerve terminals. Small amounts are metabolized, taken up and or bound in non-neural tissues, or else diffuse away from the site of release into the extracellular space. The biologic activity of the transmitter on the effector cells of a number of tissues is terminated almost entirely by reuptake, in others these additional mechanisms are relatively important. The two enzymes that catalyze the degradation of norepinephrine and epinephrine are monoamine oxidase and catechol-O-methyl transferase. It is impossible to generalize concerning the role of these enzymes in peripheral systems, except to affirm that their role is of secondary importance. Circulating catecholamines, on the other hand, are metabolized rapidly by these enzymes present in the liver through a complex degradative pathway.

PHARMACOLOGY

The drugs that modify the activity of the peripheral nervous system are described in succeeding chapters. These agents are classified according to their site of action (Fig. 14–4) and the mechanism whereby they exert their principal effects.

Classification by Site of Action

Drugs that act in the region of the postganglionic sympathetic nerve ending are known as **adrenergic drugs. Sympathomimetic drugs** mimic at least some of the actions of the sympathetic nervous system (mimetic means simulating or imitating); **sympatholytic drugs** (lysis means dissolution) block sympathetic activity. As would be expected drugs that act in the region of the postganglionic parasympathetic nerve endings are **cholinergic.** The terms **parasympathomimetic** and **parasympatholytic** are self explantory. Since sympathetic and parasympathetic ganglia are pharmacologically identical, the simple terms **ganglionic stimulating** or **ganglionic blocking** are applied to drugs that act at these sites.

Since acetylcholine is the mediator at autonomic ganglia, the postganglionic parasympathetic endings and the neuromuscular junction, and since drugs with actions specific to each are known, distinguishing names are necessary. Early pharmacologists were aware that mus-

carine, derived from the poisonous mushroom *Amanita muscaria,* stimulated specifically cholinergic receptors at the postganglionic parasympathetic junctions. Consequently, these are commonly referred to as **muscarinic** receptors or sites. Since small doses of nicotine act on cholinergic receptors in the ganglia and the neuromuscular junction, these sites are often referred to as **nicotinic.**

Classification by Mode of Action

Autonomic drugs exert their effects by modifying one or more of the steps or stages of neurohumoral transmission and may be classified on this basis (Fig. 14–5); see also Chapter 23 where this same classification is extended to CNS synapses.

1. *Interference with transmitter biosynthesis.* There are no drugs of therapeutic value which cause their effects exclusively by interfering with transmitter biosynthesis. α-methyl-p-tyrosine and hemicholinium are experimentally used drugs which interfere with adrenergic and cholinergic transmission respectively.

2. *Interference with transmitter storage.* Certain sympathomimetic amines, such as amphetamine, ephedrine and tyramine, act in part by displacing the transmitter from its storage

sites. The released transmitter in turn reacts with the receptor in the normal way causing sympathomimetic effects (Ch. 18). Reserpine causes the liberation of the adrenergic transmitter and, by preventing its reaccumulation, depletes the transmitter stores at the nerve ending (Ch. 20).

3. *Interference with release of transmitter.* The only drugs of therapeutic value in this category act on the postganglionic sympathetic neuron, e.g., bretylium (Ch. 20).

4. *Stimulation of receptors on postjunctional membranes.* Many drugs mimic autonomic activity by reacting with the same receptors on postjunctional membranes as the physiologic transmitters. They are frequently related chemically to the transmitter. Muscarine, nicotine in small dose and the choline esters react with cholinergic receptors. Certain sympathomimetic amines, epinephrine, isopropyl-norepinephrine and phenylephrine react with adrenergic receptors (Ch. 18).

Interference with interaction of transmitter with postjunctional receptors. Some drugs by reacting with the receptors of the effector cells prevent or block the normal effects of the transmitter. These are commonly referred to as blocking agents and are classified according to their site of action as neuromuscular (Ch. 21), adrenergic (Ch. 19), ganglionic (Ch. 20), muscarinic (Ch. 15) or parasympathetic (Ch. 17) blocking agents.

5. *Interference with disposition of the transmitter by reuptake.* Drugs such as cocaine and imipramine are considered to act by inhibiting the reuptake of the adrenergic transmitter. Thus they prolong its local effect within the synapse (Chs. 22 and 24).

6. *Interference with disposition of the transmitter by metabolism.* Anticholinesterases act by inhibiting the hydrolytic action of acetylcholine esterases. The result is an increase in the local concentration of acetylcholine in the synaptic cleft and an increase in the effector response (Ch. 16). Inhibitors of monoamine oxidase and catechol-O-methyl transferase affect adrenergic transmission in peripheral synapses in a variable and relatively minor degree.

FURTHER READING

Iverson LL (ed) (1973): Catecholamines. Br Med J 29:91–178

Bennett MR (1972): Autonomic Neuromuscular Transmission. Cambridge, University Press

Triggle DJ (1971): Neurotransmitter-Receptor Interactions. New York, Academic Press

THOMAS C. WESTFALL

15. MUSCARINIC AGENTS

The primary action of muscarinic agents is at cholinergic receptors located at parasympathetic postganglionic junctions (smooth muscle, cardiac muscle and various glands). This can cause activation or inhibition of the various effector systems. Parasympathetic innervation of a particular organ is not a prerequisite for the presence of muscarinic receptors, however. Other names given to muscarinic agents are parasympathomimetics or cholinomimetics (Ch. 14). The prototype drug of this group is acetylcholine which serves as the transmitter at the postgan-glionic parasympathetic junction. Various muscarinic drugs differ from acetylcholine in being more resistant to inactivation by cholinesterase and therefore in having a more prolonged and useful action. These drugs are primarily directly acting agents, which implies that they combine directly with muscarinic receptors on the effector cells. This is in contrast to cholinesterase inhibitors (Ch. 16) which act indirectly and, in addition to their muscarinic action, have prominent effects at other sites.

ACETYLCHOLINE

Acetylcholine is of no important therapeutic value because of its diffuse action on cholinergic sites throughout the body and its susceptibility to hydrolysis by acetylcholinesterases. A knowledge of its pharmacologic actions forms the basis for our understanding of the pharmacology, toxicology and therapeutic usefulness of muscarinic agents, and for this reason it is the prototype drug.

CHEMISTRY

Acetylcholine is a quaternary ammonium compound (Fig. 15–1) containing three spatially separated centers of importance for its biologic activity: the positively charged nitrogen, the carboxyl oxygen carrying a relative negative charge and the relatively electron—poor esteratic oxygen. Although acetylcholine possesses three reactive sites, only two of these are necessary for the various actions of the compound. The quaternary nitrogen is necessary for the activation of all Ach receptors, but it must be coupled with either the positive or the negative oxygen.

For muscarinic activity, the combination of the quaternary nitrogen and the positive oxygen separated by a particular distance predicted by molecular orbital studies is necessary. This type of binding and spatial orientation is present in the alkaloid muscarine (Ch. 15) whose effects were originally used to distinguish the various actions of acetylcholine. Another combination of sites is found in nicotine. When acetylcholine is in this spatial configuration, it can activate nicotinic receptors (autonomic ganglia and skeletal—neuromuscular junctions, Chs. 14, 21).

PHARMACOLOGIC ACTIONS

The pharmacologic effects produced by acetylcholine and other muscarinic agents can to a considerable extent be deduced from a knowl-edge of the physiology of the autonomic nervous system. A brief discussion follows.

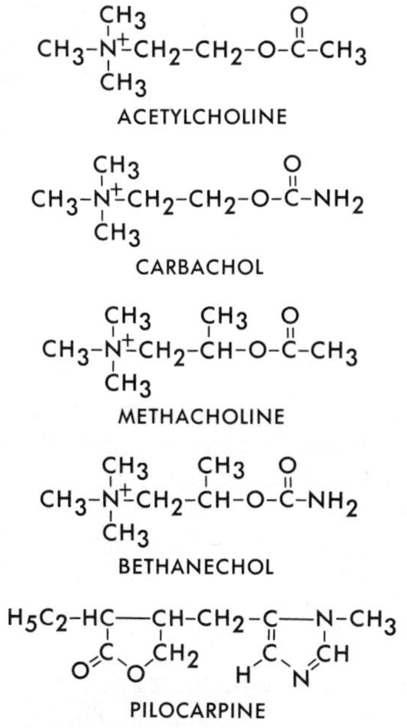

Figure 15-1 structures

$$CH_3-N^{\pm}(CH_3)_2-CH_2-CH_2-O-\overset{O}{\overset{\|}{C}}-CH_3$$

ACETYLCHOLINE

$$CH_3-N^{\pm}(CH_3)_2-CH_2-CH_2-O-\overset{O}{\overset{\|}{C}}-NH_2$$

CARBACHOL

$$CH_3-N^{\pm}(CH_3)_2-CH_2-CH(CH_3)-O-\overset{O}{\overset{\|}{C}}-CH_3$$

METHACHOLINE

$$CH_3-N^{\pm}(CH_3)_2-CH_2-CH(CH_3)-O-\overset{O}{\overset{\|}{C}}-NH_2$$

BETHANECHOL

$$H_5C_2-HC\!\!-\!\!CH-CH_2-C\!\!-\!\!N-CH_3$$

PILOCARPINE

FIG. 15-1. Principal muscarinic agents.

CARDIOVASCULAR SYSTEM.

Acetylcholine lowers arterial pressure as a result of vasodilation of vascular smooth muscle and decreased cardiac function. This response is potentiated by a cholinesterase inhibitor and blocked by atropine. In the presence of both drugs, acetylcholine may raise arterial pressure by stimulating sympathetic ganglia (nicotinic effect) and releasing catecholamines from the adrenal medulla.

Acetylcholine appears to have a greater effect on small resistance vessels, arteries and arterioles than it has on larger vessels and veins.

On the heart, acetylcholine resembles vagal stimulation, causing bradycardia, prolongation of atrioventricular conduction and a negative inotropic effect on the atria and ventricle. The drug shortens the atrial action potential, and conduction velocity may actually increase. Acetylcholine increases the permeability of cardiac fibers to potassium. This increase, relative to the change in permeability to sodium, decreases the rate of discharge of sinoatrial pacemaker fibers. There is a decrease in the conduction velocity and an increase in the refractory period in the atrioventricular node. High concentrations of drug produce complete heart block. Acetylcholine decreases the slope of the diastolic prepotential.

In addition to direct effects of acetylcholine on the vascular system, indirect reflex effects are produced. The fall in arterial pressure produced by acetylcholine reflexly activates sympathetic activity via pressor receptive mechanisms, resulting in an increase in heart rate.

SMOOTH MUSCLE.

Smooth muscles of the gastrointestinal urogenital and respiratory tracts, as well as the eye, are stimulated by acetylcholine. In the gastrointestinal tract, there is an increase in both tone and motility. With high concentrations, spasm and tetanus can occur. The motility of the gall bladder and bile ducts is also increased. The smooth muscles of the ureters and urinary bladder are contracted and their sphincters relaxed, leading to voiding of urine. In the bronchial smooth muscle, contraction by acetylcholine results in bronchospasm. In the eye, acetylcholine produces pupillary constriction (miosis), spasm of accommodation and a transitory rise in intraocular pressure, followed by a more persistent fall.

At all these sites acetycholine produces an increase in permeability of the muscle cell to all ions with a resultant depolarization of the cell membrane. In addition to this partial depolarization, acetylcholine increases the frequency of the spontaneous action potentials presumably by increasing pacemaker activity.

GLANDS.

Acetylcholine causes an increase in the secretions from lacrimal, salivary (profuse and watery) nasopharyngeal, bronchial, gastric, intestinal, pancreas and sweat glands. At these sites acetylcholine causes an increasaed permeability leading to an inward flux of calcium which in turn activates the specific cellular function. Acetylcholine also increases the release of catecholamines from the adrenal medulla by activation of either nicotinic or muscarinic receptors.

MECHANISM OF ACTION

Acetylcholine and other muscarinic agents exert their principal action at the cell membrane by combining with specific receptors. This action results in alterations in membrane permeability. In the presence of the drug the membrane becomes more permeable to one or more of various ions (i.e., potassium, sodium and calcium). The preexistant flux equilibrium is disturbed and the membrane potential altered. The direction of the change depends on the magnitude of the membrane potential and on the ratio between the increase in sodium and potassium conductance. Under the influence of acetylcholine the membrane permeabilities for potassium and sodium increase unequally, so that the ratio of permeability for potassium to that of sodium may either increase resulting in hyperpolarization or decrease leading to depolarization. The final result can be either depolarization (as in smooth muscle cells) or hyperpolarization (as in myocardial pacemaker cells).

METHACHOLINE (MECHOLYL)

This drug differs from acetylcholine only by the addition of a methyl group to the β-methyl position of choline (Fig. 15–1). It is hydrolyzed by acetylcholinesterase but not by butyrocholinesterase (Ch. 16). As the rate of hydrolysis is considerably slower than that of acetylcholine, its actions are more persistent. This drug acts principally on muscarinic receptors and is essentially devoid of nicotinic effects. The muscarinic actions of methacholine are qualitatively the same as acetylcholine. The drug is administered orally but is poorly and irregularly absorbed from the gastrointestinal tract. It is partly destroyed by gastric secretions.

CARBAMYLCHOLINE (CARBACHOL)

This drug is one of the most powerful of the choline esters (Fig. 15–1). The acid component is carbamic rather than acetic, and the carbamic ester linkage is not readily susceptible to hydrolysis by acetylcholinesterase or butyrocholinesterase. Carbachol has both muscarinic and nicotinic actions, but the muscarinic actions predominate. Its pharmacologic actions are similar to acetylcholine.

BETHANECHOL (URECHOLINE)

This drug has structural features common to both methacholine and carbachol (Fig. 15–1). It is not hydrolyzed by acetylcholinesterase or butyrocholinesterase. It is principally a muscarinic agonist with a somewhat more selective action on the gastrointestinal tract and urinary bladder, and it is preferred to other cholinergic drugs for stimulation of these systems. This drug is administered orally, never by IV or IM route.

PILOCARPINE

In contrast to the above drugs, this agent is not a choline ester but a naturally occurring muscarinic alkaloid with additional nicotinic actions. It is obtained from the leaves of tropical American shrubs, belonging to the genus *Pilocarpus.* The hydrochloride salt is hygroscopic and is inactivated by light. The nitrate salt is not hygroscopic and therefore offers some advantages.

Pilocarpine has a direct effect on muscarinic effector cells and stimulates autonomic ganglia. It very markedly stimulates the secretion of sweat and saliva. As much as 2–3 liters of sweat and 350 ml of saliva can be secreted in a few hours. Pilocarpine produces similar effects on smooth muscle and glands as acetylcholine. On the cardiovascular system, however, hypertension and tachycardia may result from its nicotinic actions on the sympathetic ganglia and the adrenal medulla. Despite this, it is the standard drug used in treating various forms of glaucoma and has great usefulness in these conditions.

THERAPEUTIC USES

GASTROINTESTINAL AND UROLOGIC DISORDERS. Muscarinic agents, in particular bethanechol, are used in the treatment of nonobstructive urinary retention and gastrointestinal atony by virtue of their ability to stimulate the smooth muscles of the gastrointestinal and urinary tracts. They are used to restore normal micturition in patients with urinary retention related to surgery, parturition, trauma or psychic factors. It is also useful for the treatment of postoperative gastrointestinal atony, including postvagotomy atony and adynamic ileus secondary to trauma, infection or neurogenic disorders.

OPHTHALMOLOGICAL DISORDERS. Muscarinic agents are used as miotics in the treatment of glaucoma but have also been applied in accommodative estropia or convergent strabismus. When applied directly to the eye, these drugs cause miosis, spasm of accommodation and a persistent fall in intraocular pressure that may be preceded by a transitory rise.

PRIMARY ANGLE-CLOSURE (ACUTE CONGESTIVE OR NARROW ANGLE) GLAUCOMA. In this form of glaucoma, these drugs are used to reduce the intraocular pressure prior to iridectomy, the treatment of choice. They can also be used to control residual glaucoma if present following surgery. The fall in intraocular pressure is brought about by constriction of the pupil which pulls the iris away from the filtration angle and thus improves the outflow of aqueous humor.

PRIMARY OPEN-ANGLE (CHRONIC SIMPLE) GLAUCOMA. Pilocarpine is the standard drug used for initial and maintenance therapy in primary open-angle glaucoma, and this or other muscarinic drugs may have to be given indefinitely. The mechanism of the lowering of intraocular pressure in this form of glaucoma is not known. It may be the result of contraction of the ciliary muscle resulting in a spreading of the trabecular interspaces, thereby increasing the facility of outflow of aqueous humor. Vasomotor factors may also be involved. Miotics are generally not used in the treatment of secondary glaucomas.

ADVERSE EFFECTS AND CONTRAINDICATIONS

Since muscarinic agents produce ubiquitous effects on numerous organ systems, all the effects except the desired one can be considered adverse. These are likely to be particularly serious if the drug is given IV, and consequently this route should never by employed. The more common adverse effects include severe gastrointestinal cramping, profuse sweating, generalized or localized paresthesia, shock, bladder pain, salivation and diarrhea. When used in ophthalmology as miotics, these drugs may produce ciliary spasm, browache, headache, false myopia and undesirable rises in intraocular pressure. In addition, patients may become hypersensitive or refractory to the effects of the drug.

Muscarinic agents are contraindicated in any condition in which one or more of their actions is likely to be particularly dangerous, including patients with myasthenia gravis who are receiving neostigmine, progressive muscular atrophy or bulbar palsy, mechanical intestinal or urinary retention, severe cardiac disease, peptic ulcer and asthma.

FURTHER READING

Carrier O Jr (1972): Pharmacology of the Peripheral Autonomic System. Chicago, Year Book Med Publishers

Crossland J (1971): Peripheral cholinergic systems. Practitioner 206:836

Kosterlitz HW (1967): Effects on choline esters on smooth muscle and secretions. Physiological Pharmacology. Root WS, Hoffman FG (eds). New York, Academic Press

Rand MJ, Stafford A (1967): Cardiovascular effects of choline esters. Physiological Pharmacology. Root WS, Hoffman FG (eds). New York, Academic Press

THOMAS C. WESTFALL

16. CHOLINESTERASE INHIBITORS

Cholinesterase inhibitors represent a second major group of drugs that produce effects similar to acetylcholine. These actions are the result of inhibition of the enzymes (acetylcholinesterase and butyrocholinesterase) which are involved in the hydrolysis of acetylcholine. **Acetylcholinesterase** (specific cholinesterase, true cholinesterase) is the enzyme responsible for the destruction of acetylcholine involved in synaptic transmission. This represents the principal mechanism for the disposition of the transmitter following its liberation from nerve terminals. Pharmacologic evidence indicates that acetylcholinesterase is also active presynaptically and plays a role in regulating acetylcholine levels in cholinergic nerve terminals. The enzyme is found in high concentrations at all sites at which acetylcholine serves as a transmitter including: the skeletal-neuromuscular junction, autonomic ganglia, postganglionic parasympathetic neuroeffector sites and at certain synapses in the CNS. **Butyrocholinesterase** (nonspecific cholinesterase, pseudocholinesterase), plasma cholinesterase) is a related enzyme with less substrate specificity found in plasma, intestine, glial cells and other organs. The function of this enzyme is less clear.

The pharmacologic effects of cholinesterase inhibitors are principally due to their action on acetylcholinesterase, the inhibition of which results in the accumulation of excessive amounts of the acetylcholine transmitter in the synaptic region. The action of acetylcholine released from nerve terminals is potentiated and prolonged, resulting in increased skeletal muscle contraction, increased activity of organs and tissues receiving postganglionic parasympathetic innervation (glands, smooth muscle, heart), increased ganglionic transmission and cholinergic effects in the CNS. In addition, some of these drugs have a direct cholinomimetic action by directing stimulating cholinergic receptors.

Cholinesterase inhibitors are useful in the treatment of myasthenia gravis, in the management of glaucoma and in atony of the gastrointestinal and urinary tracts. They are active ingredients of many potent insecticides and thus of toxicologic importance. They are extensively used as investigative tools. Finally, they represent a potential hazard as chemical warfare agents.

CHEMISTRY AND MECHANISM OF ACTION

Acetylcholine binds to acetylcholinesterase at two sites, one specific for the quaternary ammonium moiety of acetylcholine, the anionic site, and the other for its esteratic site. The anionic site is negatively charged, stereospecific, and is most likely a carboxyl group of a decarboxylic amino acid such as glutamic acid. This site attracts the positively charged nitrogen atom of acetylcholine and binds the attached methyl groups by Van der Waal's forces. The esteratic site of the enzyme is made up of two basic groups, serine and histidine, and one acid group, most likely the hydroxyl of tyrosine. The esteratic site combines with the carbonyl carbon atoms of the acetyl group and forms a covalent bond with the enzyme. This results in the acetylation of the enzyme, rupture of the ester linkage and the elimination of choline.

The hydrolysis of acetylcholine, or any other substrate, takes place in three steps presented schematically in Figure 16–1.

The first step consists of the reversible formation of a complex between acetylcholine and the enzyme in which the principal bonds are formed with the cationic site of acetylcholine and the carbonyl atom of the ester group.

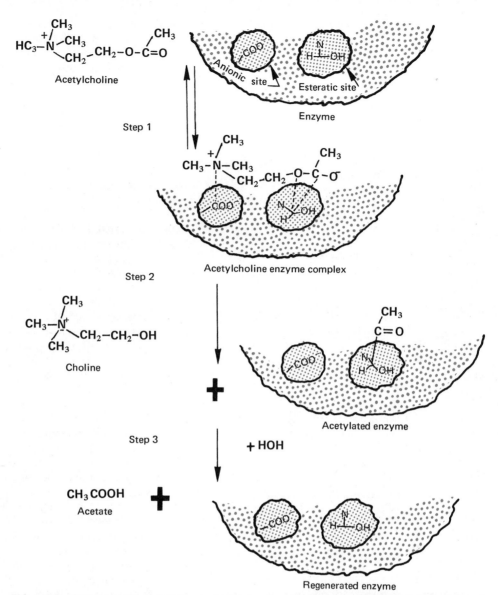

FIG. 16-1. Sequence of reactions involved in the cholinesterase-catalyzed hydrolysis of acetylcholine.

The second step results in an acyl transfer through nucleophilic attack on the ester carbonyl by a serine residue in the enzyme releasing choline and forming an acyl-enzyme intermediate.

In the third step there is hydrolysis of the acyl-enzyme (rate limiting step) yielding acetate and hydrogen ions and regenerating the enzyme.

The hydrolysis of acetylcholine occurs extremely fast. Each active site in a purified sample of ox red blood cell acetylcholinesterase is capable of hydrolyzing 3×10^5 molecules of acetylcholine per minute.

Cholinesterase inhibitors prevent the above reactions by forming inhibitor-enzyme complexes in competition with acetylcholine. These inhibitor-enzyme complexes are more stable than the acetylcholine enzyme complex and therefore delay the hydrolysis of acetylcholine. The most convenient way of classifying the cholinesterase inhibitors is based on the type of chemical interaction occurring between the inhibitor and the enzyme. Drugs are classified as **reversible** or **nonreversible** cholinesterase inhibitors. Reversible cholinesterase inhibitors delay the hydrolysis of acetylcholine from 1–8 hr. The breakdown of the inhibitor-enzyme complex in the case of nonreversible agents is much slower.

REVERSIBLE INHIBITORS. Reversible cholinesterase inhibitors can interact with acetylcholinesterase in two ways.

First, a reversible complex between the en-

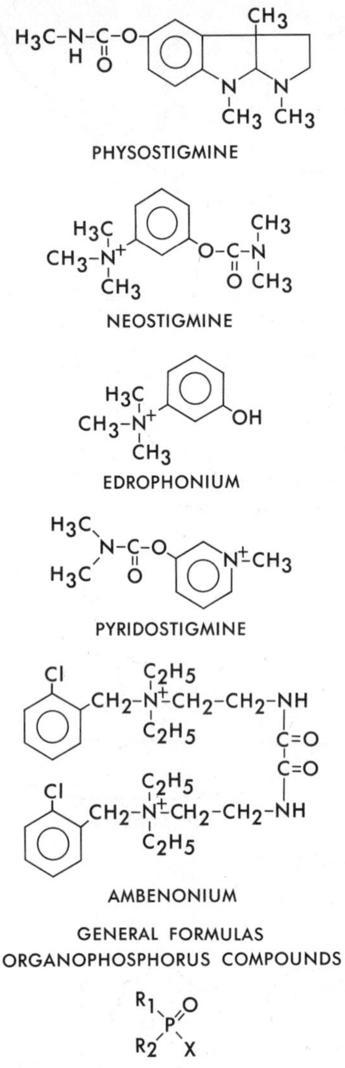

PHYSOSTIGMINE

NEOSTIGMINE

EDROPHONIUM

PYRIDOSTIGMINE

AMBENONIUM

GENERAL FORMULAS
ORGANOPHOSPHORUS COMPOUNDS

FIG. 16–2. Principal cholinesterase inhibitors.

zyme and the inhibitor is formed (step I), but steps analogous to steps II and III do not occur. Edrophonium (Fig. 16–2), an example of this type of inhibition, binds only with the anionic site of acetylcholine to form a rapidly reversible enzyme-substrate complex.

Second, a reversible complex between the inhibitor is formed, and steps analogous to II and III occur very slowly. **Physostigmine** and **neostigmine** (Fig. 16–2) are examples of this type of inhibitor. Both are substituted carbamate esters, and the enzyme-inhibitor complex decomposes to yield the corresponding alcohol and carbamylated enzyme. Unlike the acetylated enzyme, the carbamylated enzyme is relatively stable, and free enzyme is only slowly regenerated by hydrolysis.

In addition both **edrophonium** and **neostigmine** have a direct stimulating action at cholinergic sites.

NONREVERSIBLE CHOLINESTERASE INHIBITORS. Nonreversible cholinesterase inhibitors are mostly organophosphate compounds. These are widely used as the active ingredients of many insecticides and war gases (Fig. 16–2). With the organophosphate cholinesterase inhibitors, steps corresponding to I and II are very rapid, but step III does not occur at any appreciable rate. These agents form a stable phosphorylated enzyme intermediate resulting from nucleophilic displacement by the enzyme at its esteratic site.

These drugs produce an essentially permanent inactivation of the enzyme because the organically substituted phosphoryl enzyme that is formed is extremely resistant to attack by water. The phosphorylated enzyme cannot hydrolyze acetylcholine and so is inhibited. Eventually there is hydrolysis of the ester bond by water, but this hydrolytic step is extremely slow and for some agents the reaction is not measurable. Most members of this class lack a cationic group and therefore attack only the esteratic site of the enzyme. Both types of cholinesterase are inactivated. Some drugs, such as *echothiophate,* are quaternary compounds containing a cationic group and appear potent and selective inhibitors of acetylcholinesterase. The duration of action of these drugs is longer than cholinesterase inhibitors containing no cationic group and is determined principally by the rate of synthesis of new enzyme, and may be several weeks.

PHARMACOLOGIC ACTIONS

The administration of cholinesterase inhibitors results in generalized cholinergic responses. The most prominent effects are those originating from the parasympathetic postganglionic nerve terminals, due to activitation of muscarinic receptors. These include decrease in heart rate, vasodilation with resultant decrease in arterial pressure; increase in skin temperature, and in gastrointestinal activity; bronchial constriction and spasm; pupillary constriction; increase in the secretions of salivary, sweat, gastric and mucosal glands. A local action restricted to the eye may be achieved by conjunctival instillation. This results in miosis, conjunctival hyperemia, spasm of the ciliary muscle which may be painful and accommodation for near vision.

In low doses, cholinesterase inhibitors have little effect at the skeletal neuromuscular junction. However, at higher doses muscle fasiculations associated with augmentation of miniature end plate and excitatory postsynaptic potentials, conversion of twitch to tetanus and ultimately depolarizing block may be seen. If neuromuscular transmission has been impaired by antidepolarizing blocking agents such as d-tubocurarine, protection of the liberated acetylcholine against destruction by cholinesterase may cause a significant improvement (Chap. 21). A similar improvement may be seen in myasthenia gravis, a disease in which local or general muscular weakness is produced by a disorder in neuromuscular transmission (see below). Inhibition of acetylcholinesterase and accumulation of acetylcholine can lead to repetitive antidromic firing.

Ganglionic stimulant and subsequent blocking effects can be demonstrated only after high doses of cholinesterase inhibitors, and for the most part these effects are of no practical importance. A considerable proportion of the acetylcholinesterase in autonomic ganglia seems to be in excess. In the superior cervical ganglion of the cat, for instance, at least 50% of the acetylcholinesterase must be inhibited before a potentiation of the effects of preganglionic stimulation can be demonstrated. It is possible that an effect on the nerve plexus of the gastrointestinal tract plays a part in the increased gastrointestinal motility seen after cholinesterase inhibitors.

A variety of central effects may be produced after high doses of those cholinesterase inhibitors that cross the blood-brain barrier. These include drugs which contain a tertiary nitrogen such as physostigmine but not a quaternary nitrogen like neostigmine. These effects are characterized by stimulation followed by depression and include disturbances of sleep, tremor and ataxia, hallucinations and desynchronization of the electroencephalogram. Death from cholinesterase inhibitors is usually due to respiratory paralysis secondary to depression of the respiratory centers.

REVERSIBLE CHOLINESTERASE INHIBITORS
PHYSOSTIGMINE (ESERINE). This drug was the first specific cholinesterase inhibitor. The importance of its discovery is twofold. First, it was the first instance in which the mechanism of action of a drug was defined in relatively simple chemical terms. It is the active ingredient of the calabar bean (the nut of Etu Esére), extracts of which were used in the trial by ordeal of Nigerian women suspected of witchcraft. If the accused could save her life by vomiting the poison, she was deemed innocent of the charge brought against her. The properties of this drug were studied as early as 1855. Second, it proved to be an important tool with which evidence was secured to support the theory of chemical neurotransmission.

The drug is a tertiary ammonium alkaloid (Fig. 16–2). It is well absorbed from the gastrointestinal tract and enters the CNS. Physostigmine appears about equally effective against acetylcholinesterase and butyrocholinesterase.

The principal use of this drug is as a miotic and is used for this reason to treat narrow angle glaucoma and to reverse the mydriasis caused by atropine. It is also the antidote of choice to treat atropine poisoning.

NEOSTIGMINE (PROSTIGMINE). This drug is a synthetic, reversible quaternary (Fig. 16–2) cholinesterase inhibitor. It differs from physostigmine in that because it is a quaternary ammonium nitrogen compound and is poorly and irregularly absorbed from the gastrointestinal tract, it does not cross the blood-brain barrier (Ch. 2). This irregular absorption produces some problems in therapy but minimizes CNS toxicity. The presence of the quaternary nitrogen enables the drug to have a direct action on both nicotinic and muscarinic receptors which makes it particularly useful for its effect at the neuromuscular junction.

Neostigmine has a very powerful anticurare action; it increases the amount of acetylcholine liberated from nerve terminals, preserves the liberated acetylcholine by blocking acetylcholinesterase and has a direct action on the skeletal-neuromuscular end plate. The neuromuscular action of the neostigmine has made it very beneficial in the management and diagnosis of myasthenia gravis. It has also been used as a miotic and in treating postoperative atony of the intestine and urinary bladder.

PYRIDOSTIGMINE BROMIDE (MESTINON). Mestinon is a reversible cholinesterase inhibitor with pharmacological properties similar to neostigmine, but it is about 100 times less potent. It has less severe, though typical, side effects and a longer duration of action.

AMBENONIUM (MYTELASE CHLORIDE). Ambenonium is a bis-quaternary compound with anticholinesterase activity about six times greater than neostigmine. It facilitates transmission at the neuromuscular junction, has anticurare actions and at high doses exhibits neuromuscular blocking activity. The drug is generally given orally when treating myasthenia gravis and has fewer side effects and a longer duration of action than neostigmine. It is very useful in treating patients who cannot tolerate neostigmine bromide or pyridostigmine bromide because of sensitivity to bromide ion. Overdosage can result in all of the typical cholinergic effects.

EDROPHONIUM (TENSILON). This agent is a synthetic cholinesterase inhibitor but is unique in having a much shorter onset and duration of action than neostigmine. The absence of the carbamate group results in a marked reduction in its ability to inhibit acetylcholinesterase. It acts only at the anionic site to form a rapidly reversible enzyme substrate complex. It has a direct stimulant action on the motor end plate and probably stimulates the skeletal-neuromuscular junction by this direct action. This agent is more effective at the skeletal neuromuscular junction than at postganglionic parasympathetic neuroeffector sites.

Edrophonium is very important in establishing the diagnosis of myasthenia gravis and in differentiating between "myasthenia weakness or crises" and "cholinergic crises." To diagnose myasthenia gravis, small amounts of edrophonium are injected IV in divided doses. An improvement in muscle strength within 1–3 min is diagnostic in myasthenia patients. A smaller IV dose will produce a brief remission of symptoms if they are caused by inadequate anticholinesterase therapy ("myasthenia crisis") but will further weaken patients suffering from an overdose of medication ("cholinergic crisis").

Edrophonium has a very powerful anticurare action and is used to reverse curare paralysis of skeletal muscle. This action does not appear to be due to a cholinesterase inhibitor action but rather to a facilitation of transmitter release and a direct displacement of curare from the motor end plate. This action of edrophonium is prolonged.

Because the drug has a short duration of action, side effects are not as severe as other cholinesterase inhibitors. Most muscarinic symptoms can be seen after IV administration and are readily reversed with atropine.

THERAPEUTIC USE OF CHOLINESTERASE INHIBITORS

MYASTHENIA GRAVIS. One of the principle uses of the reversible cholinesterase inhibitors is in the diagnosis and treatment of myasthenia gravis. This disease is characterized by the weakness and rapid fatigability of skeletal muscle. The pattern of the disease is variable and may be diffused or limited to specific muscles. Often muscle weakness is severe and widespread and during an exacerbation typically begins in the face and neck and then spreads progressively to involve the upper limbs, the abdomen and muscles of respiration. The underlying etiology of myasthenia gravis is still unknown. Both the presynaptic nerve terminals and the postsynaptic receptors are involved. Presynaptically there is evidence suggesting a decreased synthesis and release of acetylcholine from vesicles, while postsynaptically the sensitivity of the motor end plate appears to be decreased. An autoimmune response involving the thymus gland may be implicated. Regardless of the underlying mechanism, however, the disease presents as a failure in neuromuscular transmission, and the rational treatment of the disease is to increase the amount of available acetylcholine.

Reversible cholinesterase inhibitors are used for both the diagnosis and treatment of myasthenia gravis. For diagnosis, both edrophonium and neostigmine are used. In the majority of cases dramatic improvement in muscle strength can be observed shortly after the administration of either of these two drugs. Physostigmine, the first cholinesterase inhibitor used to treat myasthenia gravis, has now been replaced by the more effective quaternary ammonium compounds, neostigmine, ambenonium and pyrido-stigmine. These drugs are given orally, but in severe cases neostigmine can be give parenterally. The maximal muscle strength attained following optimal doses of these agents is about the same, but the effectiveness of therapy varies among patients. In addition there are differences in onset and duration of action. There are major problems regulating the dosage to maintain a uniform level of strength throughout the day and yet minimize the production of side effects. With insufficient drug a "myasthenia crisis" results; if there is too much, a "cholinergic crisis" may be precipitated. The most common adverse effects are muscarinic and include excessive salivation, perspiration, abdominal distress, nausea and vomiting.

OPHTHALMOLOGICAL DISORDERS. Cholinesterase inhibitors may be used together with or in place of directly acting muscarinic agents (Ch. 15) to treat glaucoma as well as for other opthalmological indications. These agents are applied directly to the eye and produce conjunctival hyperemia, miosis, spasm of accommodation and a reduction in intraocular pressure. When administered locally, systemic adsorption is minimal but can take place with high doses of the drugs.

Short acting agents such as physostigmine or neostigmine are occassionally used in the emergency treatment of primary angle-closure glaucoma, usually in conjunction with pilocarpine. They are also sometimes used in treating primary open-angle glaucoma but are not usually as well tolerated as pilocarpine and may cause local irritation or allergic reactions.

Long lasting cholinesterase inhibitors such as **demecarium** (Humorsol) and the organophosphate compounds **isoflurophate** (Floropryl) and **echothiophate** (Phospholine) are used in the treatment of primary open-angle glaucoma. Because of their much longer duration of action, these drugs have a clear advantage when long-continued medication is necessary. Owing to their toxicity, they are generally reserved for use when shorter acting miotics have failed. In such situations, these long lasting cholinesterase inhibitor drugs should be used because the risk of visual loss due to uncontrolled open-angle glaucoma is greater than the potential toxicity of the compounds. Because of the possibility of precipitating an attack, these long acting inhibitors are not advocated prior to iridectomy in angle-closure glaucoma; however, they may be used after iridectomy.

GASTROINTESTINAL AND UROLOGIC DISORDERS. Quaternary cholinesterase inhibitors such as neostigmine may be used to treat postoperative abdominal distention or urinary retention by virtue of their ability to stimulate the smooth muscle. They may also be used to counteract the constipating effect of morphine. They should not be used in the presence of a mechanical obstruction.

ORGANOPHOSPHATE ANTICHOLINESTERASE POISONING

As mentioned above, organophosphate cholinesterase inhibitors such as isoflurophate (DFP), echothiophate (Phospholine), **parathion,** etc. (Tables 16–1, 16–2) are highly toxic compounds that produce nonreversible inhibition of acetylcholinesterase and butyrocholinesterase. These drugs were developed as potential chemical warfare agents because of their extreme toxicity and free absorption through the intact skin. Although they have some therapeutic application, their principle interest is toxicologic because a number of organophosphate anticholinesterases are widely used as agricultural insecticides and because of their potential as warfare agents (Table 16–2). For these reasons, the diagnosis and treatment of poisoning by organophosphate anticholinesterases are of considerable practical importance.

When these agents are administered, the clinical picture is a combination of peripheral cholinergic and CNS effects. The most pronounced systemic effects are profuse salivation, sweating, diarrhea, muscular weakness and fasciculations, mental confusion and ataxia and disturbances of ventilation culminating in respiratory paralysis and death. Severe dehydration may also develop. Depending on the route of administration, a variety of local effects may also be observed; bronchoconstriction and increased bronchial secretion are prominant after inhalation, while nausea, vomiting and intestinal cramps occur earliest after ingestion.

If the outcome is not immediately fatal, the effects may persist for several days or weeks. The rate of recovery depends on the rate of synthesis of new cholinesterase.

Delayed neurotoxic effects may begin three months or more after exposure to certain organophosphate agents, including the triaryl phosphates, which may be metabolized to form cholinesterase inhibitors. The latter are extensively used commercially as hydraulic fluids and gasoline additives. Symptoms consist of polyneuritis with flaccid paralysis of the upper and lower extremities and degeneration of myelin sheaths and axons in the spinal cord sciatic nerve and medulla. The mechanism is not understood.

TREATMENT OF ANTICHOLINESTERASE POISONING

Atropine provides a specific and effective antidote to the muscarinic effects of cholinesterase inhibitors and to some degree is also active against the CNS effects. It must be given in large and repeated doses until the muscarinic effects are controlled. Supportive measures including artificial ventilation, if this is necessary, must also be applied. It must be emphasized that atropine only antagonizes the effects of cholinesterase inactivation and does not restore the cholinesterase. Because of the prolonged inactivation of cholinesterase, atropine treatment may have to be continued for several days or weeks.

Although attack by the organophosphate cholinesterase inhibitors upon the enzyme yields a phosphorylated enzyme which is resistant to attack by water, spontaneous hydrolysis of phosphorylated acetylcholinesterase and butyrocholinesterase is accelerated by nucleophilic reactivators such as hydoxamic acids and oximes. These are capable of displacing the phosphoryl group and reactivating the enzyme. Inclusion of a quaternary ammonium group in the reactivator may greatly increase its potency, although diminishing its ability to penetrate into the CNS.

The most commonly employed reactivator is **pralidoxime** (pyridine-2-aldoxime-methiodide; PAM) which is effective principally at the neuromuscular junction and to some extent at mus-

TABLE 16–1. Principal Cholinesterase Inhibitors Used Therapeutically

Drug	Trade name	Source	Type of inhibition*	Dose	Route of administration	Duration of action	Major therapeutic indications
Ambenonium	Mytelase	Synthetic	2	10–30 mg	Oral	4 hr	Myasthenia gravis
Demecarium	Humorsol	Synthetic	2	0.2–0.5%	Conjunctival	3–5 days	Glaucoma
Echothiophate	Phospholine	Synthetic	3	0.25%	Conjunctival	3–7 days	Glaucoma
Edrophonium	Tensilon	Synthetic	1	2–8 mg	IV	1–2 hr	Diagnosis of myasthenia gravis; *d*-tubocurarine overdose
Neostigmine	Prostigmine	Synthetic	2	0.022 mg/kg (for diagnosis) 0.5–2 mg 30 mg	IM IM Oral	 3–6 hr 2–4 hr	Diagnosis and management of myasthenia gravis
Pyridostigmine	Mestinon	Synthetic	2	60–300 mg	Oral	4 hr	Myasthenia gravis
Physostigmine	Eserine	Calabar bean (physostigma venenosum)	2	0.2–1%	Conjunctival	6–12 hr	Ophthalmologic applications

*The numbers 1, 2 and 3 refer to the types of cholinesterase inhibition discussed in text under Chemistry and Mechanism of Action

TABLE 16–2. Representative Organophosphate Cholinesterase Inhibitors

Drug	Use	Comment
Diisopropyl fluorophosphonate (isoflurophate, DFP)	Investigative, medical	First organophosphate cholinesterase inhibitor discovered. Rarely used therapeutically. Water soluble
Malathion	Insecticide	Relatively safe to mammals because of rapid metabolism in liver
Parathion	Insecticide	Highly toxic to higher animals. Frequent cause of accidental poisoning
Sarin (GB)	Chemical warfare	Extremely toxic. No commercial use
Tabun	Chemical warfare	Extremely toxic. No commercial use

carinic sites, but ineffective in the CNS. Pralidoxime must be administered parenterally, usually by IV infusion. The agent has some depolarizing effect of its own in addition to enzyme reactivation. As a supplement to atropine and general supportive therapy, pralidoxime is of value in the treatment of poisoning by both organophosphate and carbonyl ester cholinesterase inhibitors. Sometimes a process of aging takes place which renders the phosphorylated enzyme refractory to reactivation by agents like pralidoxime, presumably because the anionic site of acetylcholinesterase is occupied. In this case treatment is restricted to general supportive measures and atropine.

FURTHER READING

Carrier O, Jr (1972): Pharmacology of the Peripheral Autonomic System. Chicago, Year Book Med Publishers

Koelle GB (ed) (1963): Cholinesterases and Anticholinesterase Agents. Springer, New York

THOMAS C. WESTFALL

17. ANTIMUSCARINIC AGENTS

Antimuscarinic agents antagonize the muscarinic actions of acetylcholine and related compounds. They act at the receptors of organs innervated by cholinergic postganglionic autonomic nerves by blocking the effects of liberated acetylcholine. Like acetylcholine, these drugs possess a high affinity for these receptors, but unlike acetylcholine, they have zero intrinsic activity or ability to stimulate or inhibit the tissue through these receptors. In general, the doses required to block the effects of nerve stimulation are greater than those which block the effects of injected acetylcholine or choline esters. The terms cholinolytic, anticholinergic or cholinergic blocking have often been applied to this group of drugs. Since they imply antagonism of the effects of acetylcholine at all sites, they are imprecise and broad.

The principal actions of these drugs include inhibition of secretions from lacrimal, salivary, nasopharyngeal, bronchial, gastric, intestinal and sweat glands and the pancreas; increase in heart rate, depression of the tone and motility of the stomach and intestines, relaxation of bronchial and tracheal smooth muscle; dilation of the pupil (mydriasis) and paralysis of accommodation (cycloplegia). All postganglionic autonomic neuroeffector junctions are not equally sensitive to antimuscarinic agents, although the order of sensitivity of various organs to blockade by these agents varies little.

In higher doses antimuscarinic agents have antinicotinic actions, blocking cholinergic transmission at motor nerve endings and ganglionic synapses. Muscarinic actions on autonomic ganglia are also antagonized. Several drugs in this group have important actions on the CNS which result in part from actions on cholinergic synapses which are pharmacologically similar to the postganglionic cholinergic junction. In addition, these drugs have central actions apparently unrelated to their antimuscarinic properties.

The most important and best known of the antimuscarinic drugs are **atropine** (*dl*-hyoscyamine) and **scopolamine** (*l*-hyoscine). For this reason this group of drugs is often referred to as atropinic (Fig. 17–1). Atropine and scopolamine have widespread actions and have been used in the treatment of a large number of clinical conditions. In attempts to obtain atropine-like drugs with a greater selectivity, with a different duration of action or with fewer side effects, a large number of related synthetic or semisynthetic drugs have been introduced. Because the actions and effects of the antimuscarinic agents differ only quantitatively from those of atropine or scopolamine, these two drugs will be discussed as prototypes and their properties considered in detail. Differences between these and other agents are discussed subsequently.

SOURCE AND CHEMISTRY

Atropine (*dl*-hyoscyamine) and scopolamine (*l*-hyoscine) are found in a number of plants belonging to the potato family, the order Solanacea. These include *Atropa belladonna* (deadly night shade), *Hyoscyamus niger* (black henbane) and *Datura stramonium* (thorn apple, Jamestown weed or Jimson weed). The major active ingredients in these plants are *l*-hyoscyamine, with smaller quantities of *l*-scopolamine (hyoscine). Atropine is *dl*-hyoscyamine. It may be prepared by racemization of the L-rotatory hyoscyamine after extraction from plants, or it may be manufactured synthetically. The *l*-isomer is more potent both peripherally and centrally than the

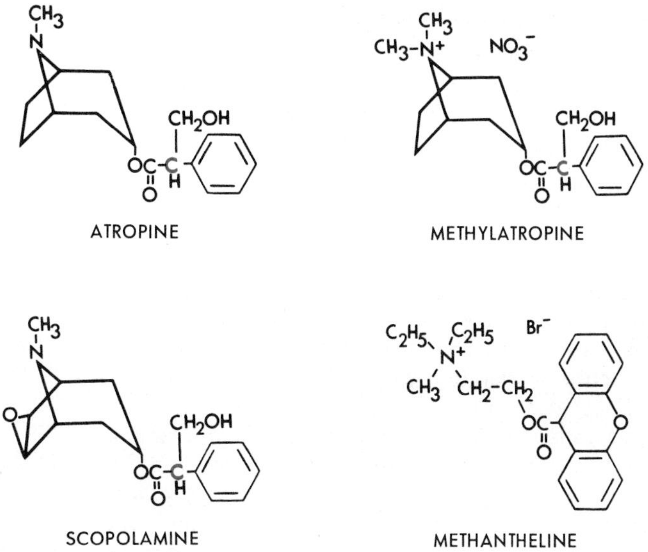

FIG. 17–1. Some representative antimuscarinic compounds. **Red C** indicates asymmetric carbon atom responsible for natural isomers of Belladonna alkaloids.

D-form, which is almost inert, but the racemic form is preferred because it is more stable chemically. *l*-Hyoscine is more active peripherally than *d*-hyoscine, but the actions of the isomers on the CNS are similar.

Atropine, scopolamine and most synthetic antimuscarinic agents are esters of complex organic bases with tropic acid. Atropine is *dl*-tropyl tropine and is an ester of tropic acid and the organic base tropine. Scopolamine is *l*-tropyl-α-scopine and is an ester of tropic acid and the organic base scopine. These two drugs differ only by the presence of an epoxide bridge on the amino acid moiety of scopolamine. Many of the synthetic antimuscarinic agents are quaternary ammonium compounds; these are generally more potent than the corresponding tertiary amines, having some ganglionic blocking activity, but lack effects on the CNS. They are also less well absorbed after oral administration and tend to have a shorter duration of action.

MECHANISM OF ACTION

Atropine, scopolamine and most synthetic antimuscarinic agents are competitive or surmountable antagonists of acetylcholine at muscarinic receptor sites in smooth muscle, cardiac muscle, exocrine glands and the CNS. Their blocking action can be overcome by increasing the local contraction of acetylcholine or choline ester. They do not react chemically with acetylcholine, nor do they affect the release or rate of hydrolysis of acetylcholine. The effectiveness of antimuscarinic agents is greater against the muscarinic effects of injected cholinergic drugs than to stimulation of cholinergic postganglionic nerves. This difference in sensitivity is most likely due to release of the chemical mediator in an area in which it has much greater proximity to the receptor and therefore in higher concentration than is capable by exogenous administration. With some drugs the antagonism of muscarinic receptors is preceded by a brief agonist action.

Atropine and similar drugs produce a highly selective antagonism of muscarinic receptors. This antagonism is so selective that atropine blockade of a drug's actions have been taken as evidence that the drug is acting on muscarinic receptors. The selectivity for muscarinic receptors is not absolute however, and in very large doses and with intraarterial administration, these drugs can antagonize ganglionic as well as neuromuscular transmission. In addition, in a concentration about 1000 times the muscarinic blocking dose, atropine also antagonizes 5-hydroxytryptamine (serotonin), histamine and norepinephrine receptors.

It is thought that atropine, scopolamine and similar drugs form a three-point attachment to the receptors: on the onium nitrogen, on the tropyl hydroxyl group and on the benzene ring. Structure activity studies support this concept.

PHARMACOLOGIC ACTIONS

CARDIOVASCULAR EFFECTS. The administration of atropine produces complex effects on the heart rate in man. Soon after its administration, atropine produces a transient slowing of the heart more noticeable than with small doses. This bradycardia is due to the stimulation of the medullary cardioinhibitory center. The main effect of atropine however, particularly with larger doses (1–2 mg), is to produce an increase in heart rate due to blockade of the normal action of the vagus nerve at the postganglionic neuroeffector junction. Vagal tone, hence the cardioaccelerator effect of atropine, varies considerably. In man this tone is most marked in the trained athlete and the young adult, whereas in children and old people it is slight. Tachycardia produced by atropine would be fairly marked in the former but quite small in the latter group. Atropine and similar drugs can reverse all the cardiac effects of acetylcholine and vagal stimulation; therefore, it reverses the shortening of the refractory period, prolongation of the P-R interval, decreased conduction and the decreased cardiac output and oxygen consumption (Ch. 16). The effect on cardiac output is generally slight because of compensatory circulatory mechanisms. Atropine also reduces or abolishes cardioinhibitory reflexes, though some cardiac slowing can occur owing to reduction of sympathetic tone. Atropine will frequently stop atrial fibrillation induced by acetylcholine during vagal stimulation. In addition, it has a quinidine-like action on the heart and has local anesthetic properties, equivalent to one-half the activity of procaine (Ch. 22). This is seen only at doses greatly in excess of those required to block muscarinic receptors. With such doses, atropine can prevent cardiac arrhythmias produced by epinephrine in the presence of cyclopropane anesthesia (Ch. 18). Cardiac contractility is generally unaffected by atropine except at high doses where it produces depression.

Because few blood vessels receive cholinergic innervation, the effect of atropine on arterial pressure in man is small. At higher doses a slight decrease in systolic arterial pressure may be seen and may be due to reduced filling of the heart during tachycardia. Atropine can block the muscarinic receptors on blood vessels and thereby block the depressor response to acetylcholine and other muscarinic agents.

Large doses of atropine cause vasodilation of cutaneous blood vessels, unrelated to its muscarinic blocking properties. This is due to a direct action on blood vessels or to local histamine release. Flushing of the skin, the result of this vasodilation, may be very noticeable following moderately high doses of atropine. In addition, in warm environments atropine can cause cutaneous vasodilation secondary to blockage of the sweat glands resulting in a rise in body temperature.

OCULAR EFFECTS. When atropine or related drugs are administered systemically or locally into the conjunctival sac of the eye, they produce dilation of the pupil (mydriasis), paralysis of accommodation of the lens (cycloplegia) and a rise in intraocular pressure. All these effects can be deduced from an understanding of the autonomic innervation of the eye. The circular smooth muscle of the iris and the ciliary muscles are innervated by parasympathetic neurones in the third cranial (oculomotor) nerve. The radial muscles of the iris are innervated by sympathetic adrenergic fibers originating from the superior cervical ganglion. Under normal circumstances, the parasympathetic system is tonically active. Atropine causes pupillary dilation by blocking the effects of tonic vagal activity on the muscarinic receptors in the circular muscle and leaving unopposed the influence of the sympathetic dilator fibers. An atropinized pupil does not respond to light.

Accommodation for near vision is dependent upon the contraction of the ciliary muscles, which slackens the suspensory ligament, reducing tension on the lens and allowing it to become more convex. Atropine prevents contraction of the ciliary muscle, paralyzing accommodation (cycloplegia). Distant vision remains good, but near vision is indistinct.

The effects of antimuscarinic agents differ from those of sympathomimetic amines in that the latter have no effect on the ciliary muscle and cause mydriasis by stimulation of the radial muscle of the iris. Accommodation therefore is not lost, and the pupillary responses to light and accommodation are retained.

Atropine also increases intraocular pressure. This is a purely mechanical effect resulting from pupillary dilation which causes thickening of the peripheral part of the iris with a consequent narrowing of the iridocorneal angle. This restricts the drainage of aqueous humour which is normally continuously secreted by the ciliary processes. The rise in intraocular pressure rarely does harm in the normal eye of young adults. However, when the intraocular pressure is raised, particularly in people over 40, an attack of glaucoma may be precipitated. This constitutes a serious hazard.

GASTROINTESTINAL, BILIARY AND GENITOURINARY TRACTS. Atropine, scopolamine and related drugs antagonize the increase in smooth muscle tone and activity that follows activation of cholinergic nerves and muscarinic drugs in the gastrointestinal, biliary and urinary tracts.

In general they decrease tone and the amplitude and frequency of peristalsis of all segments of the intestinal tract. The degree of inhibition depends on the level of the existing cholinergic (vagal) nerve activity, since intestinal movements and tone of intestinal muscle are under predominantly parasympathetic control.

The bladder has a very complex but predominantly parasympathetic innervation. In general, atropine reduces tone and spontaneous activity of the fundus and contraction of the sphincter, thus favoring urinary retention. The bile ducts and gall bladder are slightly relaxed by atropine. The parasympathetic nerves appear to play an unimportant role in the control of the uterus and in consequence atropine has little effect.

RESPIRATORY SYSTEM. Bronchial smooth muscle is under predominantly parasympathetic control. Following the administration of atropinic drugs, bronchial and tracheal smooth muscles relax, particularly when parasympathetic tone is high or muscle tone has been increased by muscarinic agents. The bronchodilation produced by atropine results in a larger vital capacity and decreased bronchial resistance. These drugs also inhibit secretions from bronchial glands.

GLANDS. Atropine and related drugs reduce or abolish secretions from glands which receive cholinergic innervation. This includes tears, sweat, saliva, mucous and digestive juices. The flow of saliva and mucous from the glands lining the respiratory tract is reduced, and drying of the mucous membranes of the mouth, nose and bronchi occurs. Complaints of a dry mouth (Xerostomia) and of difficulty in swallowing are very common. Eccrine sweat gland activity which depends upon cholinergic sympathetic nerve fibers is suppressed, and the skin becomes hot and dry. After large doses of atropine, the body temperature rises. The apocrine sweat glands found in the axilla, around the nipples and labia majora and mons pubis are not blocked. Both thermal and emotional sweating is reduced by atropinic drugs. The secretions of the stomach, the actions of the hormone gastrin and the exocrine secretion of the pancreas are at least partly blocked by atropine (Ch. 36). There is no inhibition of the secretion of milk, urine or bile.

Suppression of the secretion of tears by atropine results in drying of the conjunctiva and exposes the eye to a greater risk of superficial injuries from dust and other particles in the atmosphere.

CENTRAL NERVOUS SYSTEM. The principal difference between atropine and scopolamine exists in their central action. In doses usually used in man, atropine has slight effects on the CNS. It produces a mild stimulation. This is generally seen as a slight bradycardia resulting from stimulation of medullary centers with increased vagal outflow. With higher doses, the central effects are more pronounced, and restlessness, irritability, disorientation, hallucinations and delirium can occur. If the dose is further increased, stimulation is followed by depression, and respiratory paralysis follows, causing death. Scopolamine has a more pronounced central effect and at therapeutic levels causes drowsiness, euphoria, amnesia, fatigue and sleep. Restlessness and other signs of central stimulation occur only after high doses of the drug. Scopolamine has been found to have a central potency 8–9 times that of atropine. Physostigmine (Ch. 16) is highly effective in reversing these central effects. Other central effects of these prototype and similar acting drugs are utilized in the treatment of motion sickness and Parkinson's Disease (Ch. 31).

ABSORPTION, EXCRETION AND METABOLISM

Atropine and scopolamine are well absorbed from the gastrointestinal tract and from other mucosal membranes but only to a limited extent from the eye or intact skin. Quaternary derivatives are poorly adsorbed from all routes but are still effective as cycloplegics or mydriatics. Distribution occurs throughout the body and across the placenta. Approximately 85–90% is excreted in the urine within 24 hr. Metabolism is still incompletely understood, but about half of the drug is excreted unchanged and the rest as tropic acid esters or tropine.

THERAPEUTIC USES. Because of the multitudinous pharmacologic effects of the belladonna alkaloids, they have been employed in a great variety of therapeutic applications. However, regardless of the particular effect sought therapeutically, side effects invariably occur. Whether an effect of the drug is termed adverse or therapeutic depends upon the reason for drug administration. More than 600 pharmaceutical preparations and combinations containing atropine or scopolamine are available as well as more than 60 atropine-like synthetic substitutes. These have been introduced in an attempt to achieve greater specificity and hence fewer side effects. Despite aggressive advertising claims that particular drugs are selective for various organ systems, etc., all these drugs produce dose-dependent muscarinic blockade identical to that produced by atropine or scopolamine. The two naturally occurring alkaloids are still the drugs of choice and the most commonly employed for most therapeutic measures calling for an antimuscarinic agent.

Central Nervous System Disorders

VESTIBULAR DISTURBANCES. Anticholinergics and antihistaminics (Ch. 49) are effective in the treatment of nausea and vomiting resulting from vestibular disturbances such as motion sickness. These disorders are most commonly treated with antihistaminics which are probably no more effective than scopolamine, particularly when administered by the IM route. They are more effective when given prophylactically. The major disadvantage is sedation.

PARKINSON'S DISEASE. Belladonna alkaloids have long been used and are beneficial in the treatment of Parkinson's disease (Ch. 31).

OPHTHALMOLOGIC USE. Antimuscarinic agents are applied topically to the eye to produce cycloplegia and mydriasis. They are used primarily as an aid for the measurement of refractive errors and for other diagnostic purposes, pre and postoperatively in intraocular surgery and in the treatment of anterior uveitis and some secondary glaucomas. Although only a brief duration of action is required when these agents are used for most diagnostic purposes, prolonged mydriasis is required in the treatment of iritis and certain other conditions. The principal antimuscarinic agents used to produce mydriasis and cycloplegia are listed in Table 17–1 and include atropine, scopolamine, **homatropine, cyclopentolate** (Cyclogy), **tropicamide** (Mydriacyl) and **eucatropine.**

In diagnostic work it is usual to employ cyclopentolate, homatropine, eucatropine or tropicamide because they produce the same effects as atropine but for a much shorter period of time. The affects of one or two drops of atropine, for instance, may persist for a week or more. Short acting antimuscarinic agents are often combined with a sympathomimetic amine such as phenylephrine or hydroxyamphetamine to ensure a more rapid effect and faster recovery with minimal cycloplegia.

Muscarinic agents such as pilocarpine or physostigmine are frequently employed by topical application to terminate the mydriatic and cycloplegic effects of antimuscarinic agents more rapidly.

Although these agents are applied topically in the form of eyedrops and their systemic absorption is minimal, antimuscarinic eyedrops are important household poisons. Accidental ingestion of very small quantities can produce a severe atropine psychosis and is particularly dangerous in children (Ch. 13).

Gastrointestinal Tract

ANTISPASMODICS. Because the antimuscarinic drugs reduce the tone and motility of smooth muscle, these drugs have been widely promoted as antispasmodics. (For details see Ch. 37.) Table 17–2 lists some commonly used antimuscarinic antispasmodics. Many of these drugs are packaged in pharmaceutical preparations which also contain antianxiety agents or antacids in addition. The routine use of such mixtures is generally frowned upon because of the problem of regulating the dosage of each component of the mixture.

PEPTIC ULCER. The rationale for the use of antimuscarinic agents in the treatment of peptic ulcer is discussed in Chapter 37.

PREANESTHETIC MEDICATION. The administration of an antimuscarinic agent as a preanesthetic medication is a time honored and universally accepted procedure. Its use originated because some inhalation anesthetics stimulate bronchial secretions, and this effect can be prevented by atropine or scopolamine. In addition, the sedative action of scopolamine is useful in calming patients before surgery. The routine use of antimuscarinic agents preoperatively is now questionable, since newer anesthetic gases are far less irritating to the bronchial mucosa. In addition, noninhalation anesthesia has become more common. It is wise to limit preoperative antimuscarinic medication to patients where there is a specific indication.

CARDIAC DISEASE. Atropine has been found beneficial in the treatment of patients with severe bradycardia complicated by excessive hypoten-

TABLE 17–1. Antimuscarinic Agents Commonly Used in Opthalmology

Drug	Concentration	Duration of action	Cycloplegia
Atropine sulfate	1–4%	6–12 days	+++
Cyclopentolate hydrochloride	1–2%	12–24 hr	++
Eucatropine hydrochloride	5–10%	2–4 hr	−
Homatropine hydrobromide	2%	12–48 hr	+
Scopolamine hydrobromide	0.25%	1–3 days	+++
Tropicamide	0.5–1%	1–2 hr	++

TABLE 17—2. Antimuscarinic Agents Used as Antispasmodics and/or to Treat Peptic Ulcer

Drug	Trade name	Dose (mg)	Duration (hr)
Belladonna alkaloids:			
atropine sulfate	—	1	6
hyoscyamine hydrobromide	—	0.25	6
Quaternary ammonium derivatives of belladonna alkaloids:			
homatropine methylbromide	(many trade names)	6	6
methscopolamine bromide	Pamine	5	6
methylatropine nitrate	Metropine	2	6
Synthetic substitutes:			
anisotropine methylbromide	Valpin	10	6
diphemanil methylsulfate	Prantal	100	6—8
glycopyrrolate	Robinul	2	8
hexocyclium methylsulfate	Tral	25	6
isopropamide iodide	Darbid	5	12
mepenzolate bromide	Cantil	25	6
methantheline bromide	Banthine	50	6
oxyphencyclimide hydrochloride	Daricon	10	12
oxyphenonium bromide	Antrenyl bromide	10	6
pentapiperium methylsulfate	Quilene	10—20	8
pipenzolate bromide	Piptal	5	6
poldine methylsulfate	Nacton	4	8
propantheline bromide	Pro-Banthine	15	8
tridihexethyl chloride	Pathilon	25	8

sion or excessive ventricular activity which develops in the first few hours after acute myocardial infarction. Such treatment can restore adequate ventricular rates and cardiac output while reducing ectopic activity. This often obliviates the need for adrenergic agents, external pacing or antiarrhythmics. Therefore, the use of atropine for this indication, particularly in the setting of the coronary care unit, appears well founded, the potential benefit of the routine use of atropine in patients with acute myocardial infarction remains controversial. In fact there is evidence to suggest that the administration of atropine increases the heart rate and may actually increase the incidence of arrhythmias. The criteria for using atropine as well as the appropriate dose and route of administration of the drug in the therapy of bradycardia is under active debate and investigation.

Atropine is the choice of drug in treating heart block due to digitalis toxicity.

ANTICHOLINESTERASE AND MUSCARINE POISONING. Anticholinesterases are the active ingredients of many insecticides commonly used by the agricultural industry (Ch. 16). Poisoning by these substances produces cholinergic hyperactivity including bradycardia, sialorrhea, bronchospasm and depolarizing neuromuscular block. The muscarinic effects of these indirectly acting cholinergic toxins can be promptly antagonized by atropine. The neuromuscular paralysis is treated with cholinesterase reactivators such as prolidoxime. Recovery from anticholinesterase intoxication is enhanced if the antidotes are given soon after exposure to the toxin.

A second use of antimuscarinic agents is in treating intoxication by mushrooms (Amanita muscaria) containing muscarine (Ch. 14). Poisoning by these mushrooms is likewise manifested by signs and symptoms of cholinergic hyperactivity which can be successfully neutralized by the administration of atropine or similar compounds.

MISCELLANEOUS USES. The antisecretory effect of belladonna alkaloids is utilized in numerous combinations with antihistamines and sympathomimetics and widely promoted as proprietary (over the counter) cold remedies. These should be used with caution in patients with asthma or respiratory tract infection. The principal side effect is a dry mouth.

Scopolamine has been used in a large number of sleep inducing proprietary preparations and is frequently used in combination with a sedative antihistamine. The hypnotic efficacy of these preparations is of questionable value.

ADVERSE EFFECTS

The principle adverse effects of antimuscarinic agents may be deduced from a consideration of their total pharmacologic properties in relation to the therapeutically desirable effect. As mentioned earlier, the use of these drugs is coupled with widespread side effects, and whether these effects are termed adverse or therapeutic depends upon the reason for drug administration. The most common troublesome effects are dry mouth, blurred vision, tachycardia, constipation and urinary hesitancy and are not really adverse effects but reflect the primary pharmacologic action of antimuscarinic drugs (Ch. 7). Tolerance is lower in subjects with glaucoma or prostatic hypertrophy. Mention has already been made of the danger of precipitating acute glaucoma in susceptible individuals by conjunctival application and the danger of hyperthermia in hot climates as a result of inhibition of sweating. Central nervous effects of these drugs are much less tolerable, less predictable and more variable. It has been reported that up to 20% of patients receiving antimuscarinic drugs for Parkinson's disease experience CNS toxicity.

POISONING BY BELLADONNA ALKALOIDS

Acute poisoning by belladonna alkaloids may result from the accidental ingestion of berries or seeds, from dosage errors and occasionally from systemic absorption of a drug applied to the conjunctiva after it has transversed the nasolacrimal duct. Although an alarming reaction may occur, a fatal outcome is uncommon, for atropine has one of the widest margins of safety of all commonly used drugs. Ingestion of 1 g of atropine has been survived. Patients poisoned with atropine or scopolamine rapidly develop the following symptoms: dryness of the mouth, blurred vision and photophobia and hot and dry skin; fever occurs in about one-fourth of the patients and may reach dangerously high levels, weak but rapid pulse and rise in arterial pressure. The mental state is abnormal, fluctuating unpredictably from unresponsiveness and coma to an agitated, confused, combative, delirious or psychotic state.

Dry mucous membranes, widely dilated unresponsive pupils, tachycardia, hot skin and fever should produce immediate suspicion of atropine toxicity. The diagnosis of antimuscarinic poisoning may be confirmed by administration of a dose of 10–30 mg of methacholine given parenterally. Failure to elicit bradycardia, rhinorrhea, salivation, sweating and abdominal distress unequivocally indicates that an atropine-like substance is involved.

Intoxication is usually of short duration and relatively benign, but recovery may take a week or more and is usually followed by amnesia. Diazapam or chlordiazepoxide are often used to treat the psychotic effects if reassurance alone is ineffective. Phenothiazines are contraindicated because of their anticholinergic properties. Physostigmine, a nonquaternary cholinesterase inhibitor (Ch. 16), is the specific antidote producing reversal of delirium and hyperpyrexia. Other cholinesterase inhibitors such as neostigmine do not cross the blood-brain barrier and are ineffective. Except for counteracting the central effects of atropine poisoning, cholinesterase inhibitors are of doubtful value, and treatment is mainly supportive.

FURTHER READING

Greenblatt DJ, Shader RI (1973): Anticholinergics. N Engl J Med 288:1215

Rumack BH (1973): Anticholinergic poisoning: treatment with physostigmine. Pediatrics 52:449

JOHN A. BEVAN

18. SYMPATHOMIMETIC DRUGS

The term **sympathomimetic,** if used strictly, should be reserved for drugs that mimic the peripheral effects of sympathetic nervous activity. By general assent, however, this term is applied to all drugs chemically related to the sympathetic transmitter that act on the peripheral nervous system and its effector organs to cause similar effects. Many of these do not produce the identical peripheral responses as norepinephrine or epinephrine, and some have additional actions on the CNS which are more prominent than their peripheral sympathomimetic effects.

Although many dozens of sympathomimetic amines are in existence, many used clinically, only the prototype, epinephrine and four others—**norepinephrine, isopropylnorepineph-rine, ephedrine** and **amphetamine** (Fig. 18–1)—will be described in detail. All sympathomimetic amines may be described in terms of these five classic compounds.

Some aspects of the physiologic role and pharmacologic effects of **dopamine** will be mentioned.

MECHANISM OF ACTION

Epinephrine, norepinephrine and isopropyl-norepinephrine differ chemically only in the group substituted on the amine N atom (Fig. 18–1). Because they combine directly with postjunctional adrenergic receptors of effector cells to cause their pharmacologic effects (Ch. 14), they are known as "directly acting amines." In contrast, ephedrine and amphetamine are described as "indirectly acting amines," since they cause most of their pharmacologic effect by releasing the sympathetic transmitter from the terminations of the postganglionic sympathetic neurons and the adrenal medullary cells. This distinction between directly and indirectly acting amines is

rarely absolute. Most amines act predominantly by one mechanism or the other. However, **phenylephrine** is almost exclusively directly acting, and small doses of **tyramine** are indirectly acting. There are a number of consequences of this difference in mechanism of action of the two classes of sympathomimetic amines. Drugs that block the uptake of norepinephrine into the nerve terminal and those that deplete stored norepinephrine (Chs. 14,20) will tend to inhibit effects of indirect but not direct sympathomimetic action.

Structure-action relationships of the sympathomimetic amines have been extensively studied. A few important generalizations can be made; substitution in the amine N will alter the relative α and β receptor potency, and in the α C atom, duration of action. The hydroxyl substitution in the β C atom is necessary for storage in the vesicles of the nerve terminals.

Postjunctional adrenergic receptors are classified as α and β on the basis of analytic pharmacologic methods, a distinction first introduced by Ahlquist in 1948. In general, stimulation or reaction with α receptors leads to excitation or elevation of basal activity, stimulation of β receptors leads to inhibition or depression of basal or ongoing activity. Norepinephrine preferentially stimulates α receptors, isopropylnorepinephrine, β receptors. Epinephrine acts on both. Specific α and β receptor-blocking drugs are known (Ch. 19). Most organs contain both types of receptors, although one is invariably preponderant. Provided the most common receptor in each tissue is known, the actions of a predominantly α or β stimulating amine can be predicted (Table 14–1).

There are a number of important exceptions to this classification:

1. Myocardial receptors. Isopropylnorepinephrine, a drug which might be expected to have

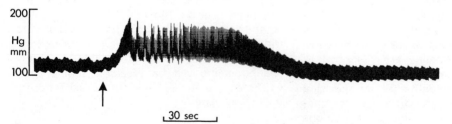

		H	H	H
		C_β	C_α	N

EPINEPHRINE	HO	HO	OH	H	CH₃	
NOREPINEPHRINE	HO	HO	OH	H	H	
ISOPROPYLNOREPINEPHRINE	HO	HO	OH	H	CH(CH₃)₂	
EPHEDRINE	H	H	OH	CH₃	CH₃	
AMPHETAMINE	H	H	H	CH₃	H	

FIG. 18–1. Sympathomimetic drugs.

negative inotropic and chronotropic actions, is probably the most potent cardiac stimulant known. Since its pharmacologic effects are blocked by the β blocker propranolol, and not by the α blocker phenoxybenzamine (Ch. 19), cardiac receptors, although excitatory, are classified as β.

2. Intestinal smooth muscle receptors. The gut contains α and β receptors. Stimulation of either type of receptor using norepinephrine or isopropylnorepinephrine leads to inhibition of tone. Both α and β blocking agents are needed to block the inhibitory effect of epinephrine on this organ.

3. Receptors for metabolic and CNS effects. These receptors are neither typically α nor β. Furthermore, there are marked species and tissue differences.

EPINEPHRINE

The naturally occurring *l*-isomer of epinephrine, also known by its official British name, **adrenaline,** is as much as 50 times more active pharmacologically than the *d*-isomer.

Epinephrine is found in nervous tissue, in the adrenal medulla and scattered throughout the body in chromaffin cells. Activation of the adrenal medulla leads to the secretion of varying proportions of epinephrine and norepinephrine. The importance or significance of "extra-neuronal" epinephrine in the chromaffin cells is unknown.

ACTIONS

Although epinephrine is considered to possess both α and β stimulating properties, in small doses it causes a predominantly β effect, since β receptors are more sensitive to epinephrine than α receptors. The effect of higher doses depends upon the relative importance of α and β responses in any one organ.

The effects described below are those which result from an IV injection of epinephrine into an *experimental animal.* The words experimental animal are italicized to emphasize (see below) that because of potential adverse effects, IV injections of epinephrine are given to man only as heroic treatment. The effects are listed because they best illustrate the pharmacologic action of the drug.

Cardiovascular Effects

A characteristic series of changes in arterial pressure follows the IV injection of epinephrine into an experimental animal. Usually a rise in arterial pressure is followed by a moderate fall before normal levels are resumed (Fig. 18–1).

HYPERTENSION (FIG. 18–2). There is an increase in both systolic and diastolic arterial pressures. The causes are *cardiac* and *vascular.* Cardiac output increases due to an increased

FIG. 18–2. Arterial pressure response to IV injection of epinephrine in an experimental animal.

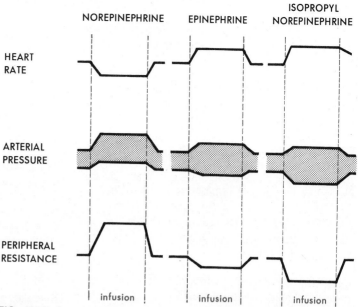

NOREPINEPHRINE   EPINEPHRINE   ISOPROPYL NOREPINEPHRINE

HEART RATE

ARTERIAL PRESSURE

PERIPHERAL RESISTANCE

infusion   infusion   infusion

FIG. 18–3. Cardiovascular effects of infusions of norepinephrine, epinephrine and isopropyl norepinephrine in man. (Allwood MJ, Cobbold AF, Ginsberg J (1963): Peripheral vascular effects of noradrenaline, isopropylnoradrenaline, and dopamine. Br Med Bull 19:132)

heart rate (β effect) and stroke volume (β effect), the result of direct myocardial stimulation. At the same time the myocardium becomes more susceptible to arrhythmias (β effect) (Ch. 34). Total peripheral resistance is increased. Epinephrine constricts resistance and capacitance vessels in the skin, mucosa, splanchnic organs and kidney because α effects predominate over β effects in these regions. It dilates vessels in the coronary and skeletal muscle beds (β effect). In some species splenic constriction (α effect) increases the circulating blood volume. Probably the direct action of epinephrine on the coronary and skeletal muscle vessels is small compared with the increased flow in these beds secondary to the rise in systemic arterial pressure and metabolic changes. Alterations in the cerebral, renal and pulmonary beds are initially passive following the arterial pressure, but flow tends to return to control levels as a result of local autoregulatory mechanisms. Veins are constricted, decreasing venous volume and increasing venous return and, as a result, cardiac output.

These direct effects of the drug are modified by compensatory mechanisms in the circulation. Homeostatic pressoreceptor reflexes tend to reduce the drug-induced hypertension by reflex bradycardia and vasodilation as evidenced by early hypotensive "notch" in the arterial pressure record. If these homeostatic reflexes were abolished, the hypertensive and hypotensive response to the drug (see below) would be considerably greater and more prolonged.

In summary, after epinephrine administration, blood circulates faster and is redistributed to the vital organs. It is diverted away from the skin and splanchnic regions to the heart, skeletal muscles, brain and lungs.

HYPOTENSION (FIG. 18–2). As the extracellular concentration of epinephrine falls, β effects predominate. The decrease in peripheral resistance outweighs the cardiac excitatory effects of epinephrine, and arterial pressure in particular, diastolic pressure falls. This resembles the effect produced in man by a slow IV infusion or subcutaneous injection of epinephrine (Fig. 18–3). Under these circumstances, the tachycardia and small rise in systolic pressure are the consequence of cardiac stimulation (β effect). The fall in diastolic pressure is the result of a decreased peripheral resistance due to the effect, predominantly β of small doses of epinephrine on the blood vessels. Small doses of epinephrine in animals produce a similar picture.

Effects on the Bronchi

Bronchial muscle is relaxed (β effect) and the microcirculation in the bronchial mucosa constricted (α effect), mucosal edema, if present, tends to diminish. All changes contribute to a decreased bronchial resistance. Owing to a CNS effect, ventilatory stimulation is preceded by transient apnea in man and some animals.

Other Effects

EYES. Provided the dose is sufficient, the radial muscles of the iris contract, resulting in mydriasis (α effect).

GASTROINTESTINAL TRACT. Tone, frequency and amplitude of peristalsis are reduced (α and β effects). Sphincters are constricted (α effect).

GLANDS. Saliva becomes sparse, thick and mucoid; other secretions are inhibited (α effect). Although sweat glands receive a cholinergic innervation, they are stimulated by epinephrine.

URINARY TRACT. The detrusor muscle is relaxed (β effect); the trigone and sphincters constricted (α effect).

UTERUS. Effect varies with dose, species, pregnancy and stage of estrous cycle.

CENTRAL NERVOUS SYSTEM. A feeling of anxiety, apprehension and restlessness, and sometimes tremor and weakness, are experienced.

Metabolic Effects

Glycogenolysis in the liver and skeletal muscle leads to hyperglycemia. Oxygen consumption may increase up to 25%. Lipolysis in adipose tissue results in lipemia. Both effects are the consequence of an increased rate of synthesis of cyclic AMP. An increase in basal metabolic rate and cardiovascular effects cause a rise in body temperature (calorigenic effect).

USES

ALLERGIC DISORDERS. Epinephrine is the drug of choice in the treatment of an acute moderate to severe attack of **bronchial asthma.** The symptoms and signs of this condition are the result of increased bronchial resistance. Epinephrine causes bronchodilation (reduces bronchial resistance) by relaxing bronchial muscle, constricting or shrinking the bronchial mucosa and inhibiting mucoid secretions. Other potentially serious manifestations of acute allergic reactions, e.g., urticaria and angioneurotic edema, may be treated similarly. Epinephrine given orally as droplets or aerosol may not always reach its site of action; however, when given parenterally, it invariably does.

LOCAL ANESTHETICS. The vasoconstrictor action of epinephrine is used to decrease absorption of local anesthetics from their injection sites. This prolongs their local action, limits their spread, minimizes their absorption and therefore their systemic toxicity (Ch. 22).

CONTROL OF BLEEDING. Local arteriolar constriction caused by epinephrine soaked packs or sprays is sometimes used to control superficial hemorrhage from the skin and mucous membranes.

CARDIAC ARREST. In cardiac arrest after external physical methods have failed and before manual cardiac massage is attempted, an intracardiac injection of epinephrine may be made. If ventricular fibrillation is induced, this may be controlled by electrical defibrillation.

PREPARATIONS AND DOSAGE

Since epinephrine is destroyed in the gastrointestinal tract and that which is absorbed is detoxified in the liver, it is ineffective by mouth and must be administered parenterally, as a nebula, or applied locally. Many preparations are available.

Epinephrine Injection, *U.S.P., B.P.,* is a 1/1000 solution of epinephrine base. The dose is 0.1–0.5 ml by subcutaneous injection. The IV or intracardiac route is used only in extreme conditions. During routine use it is mandatory to be absolutely certain that the needle is not in a vein; an IV injection must not be given in error.

Epinephrine Inhalation, *U.S.P.,* is a nonsterile 1/100 solution of epinephrine base, for oral inhalation from a nebulizer.

Great care must be exercised in distinguishing the two preparations. The parenteral use of the inhalation concentration is an established cause of accidental death.

ADVERSE EFFECTS

These are seen most frequently in the very young and very old, in patients who because of hyperthyroidism or hypertension are hypersensitive and following inadvertent IV injection or overdosage.

CENTRAL NERVOUS SYSTEM. The effects of even therapeutic doses can sometimes be very disturbing and cause considerable alarm but are not generally dangerous. They include a sense of uneasiness, anxiety, tension and sometimes tremor.

CARDIOVASCULAR SYSTEM. An excessive rise in arterial pressure can result in cerebral or subarachnoid hemorrhage and myocardial infarction. The concomitant increase in cardiac work can lead to coronary insufficiency and angina pectoris. The increased myocardial irritability may lead to palpitations, atrial and possibly ventricular arrhythmias. Inhalation anesthesia using cyclopropane or the halogenated hydrocarbon anesthetics appear to sensitize the heart to this effect (Ch. 27).

CYCLIC AMP

In a series of brilliant studies, Sutherland, Rall and colleagues showed that some of the metabolic changes produced by epinephrine, in particular glycogenolysis, are associated with an accumulation of cyclic 3′5′-AMP (cAMP). Epinephrine acts on a membrane bound **adenylcyclase** which catalyses the conversion of ATP to cAMP. This in turn via several protein kinases converts a less active liver phosphorylase to an active form, or in the case of muscle phosphorylase b to phosphorylase a. Glycogenolysis is augmented.

There is good evidence that hyperlipidemia is the consequence of the activation of a specific triglyceride lipase found in body fat and is the result of the accumulation of cAMP. cAMP also seems to be a physiologic mediator of hormonal effects including insulin, thyroxine, steroids and growth hormone, in a number of body tissues.

cAMP is broken down to an inactive 5′-AMP by phosphodiesterase, an effect that is inhibited by the xanthines (Ch. 32). Phosphodiesterase may be involved in a feedback regulation of cAMP concentration in the cell.

There is still active controversy regarding the specifics of the role of cAMP in many tissues. Most, however, are agreed that cAMP is a versatile, comparatively universal mediator, probably forming an essential link in most β adrenergic effects.

LEVARTERENOL (NOREPINEPHRINE)

Nor is derived from the German N(itrogen) O(hne) R(adikal)—nitrogen without radical. Levarterenol, or norepinephrine, differs chemically from epinephrine in that the "nitrogen is without" the methyl substitution (Fig. 18–1). The *l*-isomer is the neurohumoral transmitter at the postganglionic sympathetic nerve ending. There is some evidence that there may be an alteration in norepinephrine metabolism and/or release in essential hypertension.

ACTIONS

Norepinephrine has a predominant action on α adrenergic receptors: it has only minimal effects on β adrenergic receptors.

CARDIOVASCULAR. In contrast to epinephrine, norepinephrine causes a rise in both systolic and diastolic pressures due to an increase in total peripheral resistance, which is independent of dose. Cardiac output is either unchanged or reduced. The weak β stimulating effect of the drug on the heart is antagonized by reflex cardiac inhibitory changes secondary to the hypertension mediated via the aortic and carotid pressoreceptors. The bradycardia seen in Figure 18–3 is secondary to the hypertension.

OTHER EFFECTS. Other effects in man in doses clinically employed are minimal and clinically unimportant. They may be accurately forecast by reference to Table 14–1.

USES

SHOCK. Norepinephrine has been used as a vasopressor agent in the treatment of hypotension occurring as a result of myocardial infarction (cardiogenic shock). It was reasoned that it raises arterial pressure by an action on blood vessels, not on a diseased or damaged heart. Norepinephrine raises arterial pressure almost exclusively by increasing peripheral resistance. Unfortunately, however, even though the damaged myocardium is not stimulated pharmacologically, the increased peripheral resistance per se inevitably increases the work load on the heart. Because of the pharmacologic vasoconstriction, there is not always a parallel increase in either coronary blood flow or blood flow to other important areas. Particularly when there has been blood loss, the opposite is often the case. Restoration of arterial pressure with a vasopressor agent is therefore not always the best procedure. The important consideration under these circumstances apart from the heart is not the absolute level of arterial pressure but the adequacy of local blood flow. Norepinephrine is used to raise arterial pressure in other types of shock with circulatory depression.

PREPARATIONS AND DOSAGE

Levarterenol Bitartrate Injection, *U.S.P.,* is a 1/1000 solution of norepinephrine base. It is administered by IV infusion in a concentration of 4 mg in 1000 ml of solution. The rate of infusion is adjusted to maintain the desired level of arterial pressure. Ascorbic acid (0.5 g/liter) is added to prevent breakdown of the amine in the infusion system.

ADVERSE EFFECTS AND TOXICITY

CARDIOVASCULAR. If an excessive rise in arterial pressure is permitted, cardiovascular effects similar to those described for epinephrine occur.

LOCAL NECROSIS. Extravasation of the IV infusion at the site of injection produces intense cutaneous vasoconstriction which may lead to necrosis and sloughing of the skin. In addition to more careful infusion techniques, the local infiltration of an α adrenergic blocking agent or its inclusion in the infusion medium is prophylactic; this latter technique is rarely used.

ISOPROTERENOL (ISOPROPYLNOREPINEPHRINE)

The formula of isoproterenol (isopropylnorepinephrine or Isuprel) is shown in Figure 18–1.

ACTIONS

Isopropylnorepinephrine acts almost exclusively on β adrenergic receptors.

CARDIOVASCULAR EFFECTS. The change in arterial pressure is the net result of the drug's positive inotropic and chronotropic cardiac actions and its vasodilator effects, which tend to increase and decrease arterial pressure, respectively. The latter are most marked in skeletal muscle and mesenteric vascular beds. The doses commonly used in man usually cause a slight drop in mean arterial pressure (Fig. 18–3). Usually there is an increase in pulse pressure, a rise in systolic and a fall in diastolic pressure. Higher doses cause a more dramatic fall in mean arterial pressure.

BRONCHIAL EFFECTS. Bronchial muscle contains a predominance of β receptors; isopropylnorepinephrine decreases muscle tone. Unlike epinephrine, isopropylnorepinephrine does not constrict the mucosal circulation (α effect) nor inhibit mucous secretion (α effect).

OTHER EFFECTS. Other effects of isopropylnorepinephrine in doses commonly used clinically are not important, but may be predicted by reference to Table 14–1.

USES

BRONCHIAL ASTHMA. In the treatment of a moderate to severe attack of bronchial asthma, isopropylnorepinephrine may be administered by sublingual tablet or by oral inhalation. The latter route is usually preferred as the incidence of palpitation is lower. Isopropylnorepinephrine is sometimes effective in patients resistant to epinephrine.

HEART BLOCK. Isopropylnorepinephrine, the most potent cardiac stimulant in the *Pharmacopeia,* is useful in the **immediate** treatment of heart block. Heart rate is increased, and the incidence and severity of syncopal seizures associated with extensive cardiac slowing (Stokes-Adams syndrome) are reduced. Usually a cardiac pacemaker is implanted.

PREPARATIONS AND DOSAGE

Isoproterenol Hydrochloride Inhalation, *U.S.P.,* is a 1/100 solution of the amine base. Other concentrations are dispensed.

Sublingual tablets of 10 and 15 mg are available in sustained action form.

ADVERSE EFFECTS AND TOXICITY

Adverse effects are associated with the drug's action on the heart and are minimal after inhalation. The drug must be used with caution in patients with coronary artery disease and hypertension. Under these circumstances its use is associated with palpitation and possibly angina and various arrhythmias.

DOPAMINE

In the past few years dopamine, the third endogenously occurring catecholamine, has been the subject of increasing interest. There is evidence that dopamine is not only a precursor of norepinephrine (Ch. 14) but is itself a transmitter in the CNS (Ch. 23). Alteration in dopaminergic neuronal mechanism in the substantia nigra is linked with parkinsonism (Ch. 31).

Although dopaminergic nerves have not been demonstrated in the peripheral nervous system of animals, there is evidence that dopamine receptors, as distinct from α and β adrenergic receptors, occur in peripheral organs. Small doses of dopamine dilate mesenteric and renal vascular beds by an action on these receptors. This effect is blocked by haloperidol, among other drugs. Large doses of dopamine have additional effects attributable to two actions equivalent to that of a combined direct and indirectly acting sympathomimetic amine. Dopamine is a mixed amine, acting directly on receptors and also indirectly by releasing the adrenergic transmitter.

The hemodynamic response to an infusion of dopamine is different from any other amine; cardiac output is increased, peripheral resistance decreased, mean arterial pressure and heart rate are unaltered. These hemodynamic effects have lead to the clinical trial of dopamine as a treatment of shock, congestive heart failure, and liver and renal failure.

EPHEDRINE AND AMPHETAMINE

Ephedrine and amphetamine are typical members of two classes of therapeutically valuable amines. Although these drugs are classified as sympathomimetic amines, in contrast to the preceding agents, they are orally active, relatively stable in the body and, therefore, of longer duration of action (measured in hours rather than minutes) and of lower absolute potency. They act not only *directly* on the adrenergic receptors but *indirectly* by liberating the adrenergic transmitter from its peripheral stores. In addition, they stimulate the cerebrospinal axis.

If a second dose is given too soon after the first, the response is smaller. The response to a third injection may be absent. This phenomenon in which the biologic responses to repeated doses become progressively smaller is known as **tachyphylaxis.** Its cause is different for different drugs. Since ephedrine acts indirectly by releasing the sympathetic transmitter, ephedrine tachyphylaxis is probably the result of transmitter depletion. The mechanisms of transmitter synthesis do not keep pace with loss through release.

EPHEDRINE

For many centuries, ephedrine extracted from a variety of plant sources has been used for medicinal purposes. It is now obtained entirely by chemical synthesis. As both the α and β carbon atoms are asymmetric (Fig. 18–1), six isomers or isomeric mixtures exist. Although subtle differences of action between these isomers are described, their pharmacologic properties are practically identical.

ACTIONS

CARDIOVASCULAR. Ephedrine causes typical adrenergic or sympathomimetic changes. In comparison with norepinephrine, the changes are slow in onset and persist for a longer period of time. With the doses used in man, the drug's action on the myocardium leading to an increase in cardiac output is more important than increased peripheral resistance in causing the hypertension.

BRONCHIAL. The bronchodilator effect of ephedrine is weaker, slower in onset but more persistent than that of epinephrine.

OCULAR. When ephedrine is put into the conjunctival sac, the pupil is dilated (mydriasis) but not paralyzed. Accommodation is unaffected. The drug is relatively inactive in heavily pigmented irises, presumably because it is inactivated rapidly.

CENTRAL NERVOUS SYSTEM. The central stimulant effects of ephedrine are similar to, but less marked than, those of amphetamine. Doses of the drug that have appreciable central effects also cause peripheral changes of significance. In therapeutic doses, ephedrine causes insomnia, restlessness, tremor, alertness and feelings of tension, anxiety and agitation. It is a weak analeptic (Ch. 32).

USES

ALLERGIC DISORDERS. Ephedrine is the preferred prophylactic, and is also used therapeutically, in mild or moderate cases of **bronchial asthma.** It is limited by its slow rate of onset, modest pharmacologic potency, tachyphylaxis and CNS effects. It has the advantage of a long duration of action. Ephedrine is commonly employed to relieve **nasal congestion** of allergic origin (hay fever) and following viral or bacterial infection of the upper respiratory tract and to prevent barotrauma. The small vessels in the mucous membranes are constricted and mucous secretions inhibited. This provides not only subjective relief by permitting breathing through the nose but better drainage of sinuses and eustachian passages.

Nasal decongestants, as a class, should be effective causing only minimal local and systemic side effects, be nonirritant and not induce secondary or rebound congestion of the mucosa. Spray application is usually preferred to drops. Ephedrine is effective at first, tachyphylaxis subsequently minimizes its value; central stimulant effects occur especially in babies, due to systemic absorption. Medication should therefore be avoided late in the evening if a night's sleep is to be achieved. Transistory stinging and burning of the mucosa is sometimes experienced. In comparison with some other amines, ephedrine is nonirritant, but even so often causes sufficient rebound congestion to necessitate repetition of use. This process can become a vicious circle. Rebound congestion may in part result from tissue anoxia or ischemia following intense vasoconstriction. Because of these disadvantages, nose drops are now less popular and have been somewhat superceded by oral vasoconstrictors sometimes combined with an antihistamine and often dispensed in a prolonged action form.

HEART BLOCK. The incidence of syncope in the Stokes-Adams syndrome is reduced by ephedrine. More reliable and effective electric pacemaker devices are superseding long-term pharmacologic treatment in this condition.

OTHER. Ephedrine can be used to produce mydriasis without cycloplegia in the treatment of enuresis in children, as a mild central stimulant, for a condition such as narcolepsy and as a pressor agent during spinal anesthesia. In general, however, other drugs have superseded ephedrine in the management of these conditions. The pharmacologic basis for its use is self-evident.

Preparations and Dosage

Ephedrine Sulfate, *U.S.P.,* and Ephedrine Hydrochloride, *N.F.,* preparations of the *l*-isomer, are available in a variety of forms and dilutions for oral administration, nose drops and as sprays. The oral dose varies 15–50 mg. Ephedrine sulfate (and hydrochloride) injection, rarely used, contains 25–50 mg/ml.

Adverse Effects and Toxicity

Apart from its adverse cardiovascular effects, which are essentially the same as those described for epinephrine, the other adverse effects of ephedrine are due to CNS stimulation. The drug does not cause addiction. It may cause urinary retention in elderly men, glucogenolysis in diabetics and general systemic effects in children. The tolerance developed after several weeks of continuous use disappears if the drug is discontinued for 3 or 4 days.

AMPHETAMINE

Amphetamine (Benzedrine) is a powerful general stimulant of the cerebrospinal axis. In therapeutic doses this action overshadows its peripheral sympathomimetic effects. The term amphetamine refers to the racemic form of the drug, dextroamphetamine (Dexedrine), to the *d*-isomer. Both are of synthetic origin.

ACTIONS AND USES

PERIPHERAL NERVOUS SYSTEM. In general, the peripheral effects of amphetamine are similar to those of ephedrine. In common with other sympathomimetic amines, the *l*-isomer is more active at peripheral sites.

CENTRAL NERVOUS SYSTEM. The central stimulator effects of amphetamine are dramatic and best described in terms of the clinical uses of the drug. The *d*-isomer is most potent in causing central excitation. Amphetamine causes an improved or elevated sense of well being, confidence, self-satisfaction and self-esteem—a general elevation or improvement of mood. These actions underlie its use in some psychoses and neuropsychoses (Chs. 24, 25). Amphetamine is usually of value in reducing the incidence of attacks of narcolepsy.

It has been repeatedly shown that the performance of dull, repetitive tasks and athletic prowess are temporarily improved by amphetamine. Physical fatigue is allayed. In contrast, intellectual effort or creativity, although subjectively improved, by objective assessment deteriorates. Errors are more common and self-criticism less censorious, especially if the subject is mentally fatigued. These apparently beneficial effects of amphetamine are lost upon repeated use and replaced by depression, apprehension, agitation and panic. Amphetamines are sometimes used as an aid in the management of minimal brain dysfunction in children, e.g., hyperkinetic behavior disorders.

BARBITURATE POISONING. Because of its general stimulatory properties, amphetamine is a useful physiologic nonspecific antagonist of the central depression caused by mild barbiturate poisoning. It is a particularly powerful stimulant of the ventilatory center.

OBESITY. Because amphetamine reduces the desire for food and diminishes the hunger drive, it has been considered a useful adjunct in the treatment of obesity. It is classed as an anorexiant or anoretic. The small changes in basal metabolic rate induced by the drug are not responsible for this effect. Unfortunately, tolerance develops and because of its addictive properties, its use is not without danger (Ch. 9). Other amines claimed to be more specific in this anoretic effect are listed in Table 18–1.

TABLE 18-1. Sympathomimetic Amines Not Discussed in Text

Drug	Trade name	Dose	Comment
Compounds resembling l-norepinephrine (predominantly α stimulating; causing minimal central stimulation)			
Metaraminol bitartrate	Aramine Bitartrate	5–10 mg IM	Orally active, less potent, longer acting vasopressor agent. May be given IV. Has little action on the heart
Methoxamine hydrochloride	Vasoxyl hydrochloride	10–20 mg IM	Longer acting vasopressor agent. Can be used to inhibit cardiac irregularities by reflex increase in vagal tone. Nasal decongestant
Phenylephrine hydrochloride	Neo-Synephrine	0.25%–10% topically; 5 mg IM	Orally active, less potent, longer acting vasopressor. May be given IV. By local application, nasal decongestant and mydriatic
Mephentermine sulfate	Wyamine sulfate	0.5% topically; 10–30 mg IM	Long-duration vasopressor agent. Nasal decongestant
Compound resembling l-epinephrine			
Nordefrin hydrochloride	Cobefrin hydrochloride	1:10,000 solution	Used with local anesthetics
Compounds resembling isopropylnorepinephrine (predominantly β stimulating; causing minimal central effects)			
Isoxsuprine hydrochloride	Vasodilan hydrochloride	5–10 mg PO	Orally active, long-duration vasodilator, especially in skeletal muscle. Myocardial stimulant
Nylidrin hydrochloride	Arlidin hydrochloride	6 mg PO	Orally active, long-duration vasodilator, especially in skeletal muscle. Myocardial stimulant
Protokylol hydrochloride	Caytine	1% inhalant; 2–4 mg PO	Orally active, persistent bronchodilator
Compounds resembling ephedrine (causing peripheral sympathomimetic and central stimulation)			
Hydroxyamphetamine hydrochloride	Paredrine hydrochloride	1–3% topically; 20–60 mg PO	Similar to ephedrine in uses but with less central stimulant action
Phenylpropanolamine hydrochloride	Propadrine	25 mg PO	Similar to ephedrine in uses but with less central stimulant action
Compound resembling amphetamine (causing predominantly central stimulation)			
Methamphetamine hydrochloride	Methedrine hydrochloride	2.5–5.0 mg PO	Probably more pronounced central stimulant action. Vasopressor agent
Miscellaneous anoretic drugs			
Benzphetamine	Didrex		
Chlorphentermine	Pre-Sate		
Diethylpropion	Tenuate, Tepanil		
Phenmetrazine	Preludin		
Phentermine hydrochloride	Wilpo		
Phentermine Resin	Ionamin		
Miscellaneous bronchodilator drugs			
Ethylephedrine	Nethamine		
Methoxyphenamine	Orthoxine		
Pseudoephedrine	Sudafed		
Racemic Ephedrine	Racephrine		
Miscellaneous nasal decongestants			
Cyclopentamine hydrochloride	Clopane		
2-Methylaminoheptane	Oenethyl		
Methylhexaneamine	Forthane		
Phenylpropanolamine hydrochloride	Propadrine hydrochloride		
Phenylpropylmethylamine hydrochloride	Vonedrine hydrochloride		
Propylhexedrine	Benzedrex		
Tetrahydrozoline hydrochloride	Tyzine		Volatile for inhalation
Tuaminoheptane sulfate	Tuamine		

OTHER. Amphetamine is often used to counteract some undesirable sedative side effects of other medication such as antiepileptic agents (Ch. 30).

Preparations and Dosage

Amphetamine Sulfate, *N.F.,* Amphetamine Phosphate, *N.F.,* and Dextroamphetamine Sulfate, *U.S.P.,* are available in many forms. Tablets usually weigh 5 or 10 mg. The usual initial oral dose is 2.5–5.0 mg.

Adverse Effects

Amphetamine **addiction** is discussed in Chapter 9. Adult patients with amphetamine in their possession for legitimate purposes should be warned to guard against the morbid curiosity of the adolescent. In certain personalities, amphetamine precipitates **acute psychotic epidoses,** during which suicide may be attempted. Its continuous use over a period of time may mask an underlying progressive chronic fatigue, and severe depression may follow withdrawal of the drug.

High doses of amphetamine produce typical **peripheral sympathomimetic effects,** mainly cardiovascular, together with signs of **exaggerated central stimulation:** insomnia, confusion, hallucinations, panic, tremor and even syncope and collapse.

OTHER SYMPATHOMIMETIC AMINES

Other clinically useful sympathomimetic amines are described briefly in Table 18–1. They are described in terms of the compound discussed above that they most closely resemble pharmacologically, not chemically. Brevity of description does not imply clinical or therapeutic inferiority. Reference sources should be consulted when further details are required.

FURTHER READING

Aviado DM, Jr (1959): Cardiovascular effects of some commonly used pressor amines. Anesthesiology 20:71

Cotten MdeV, Moran NC (1961): Cardiovascular pharmacology. Annu Rev Pharmacol 1:261

Second symposium on cathecholamines (1966). Pharmacol Rev 18:1

Sutherland EW, Rall TW (1960): The relation of adenosine 3',5'-phosphate and phosphorylase to the action of catecholamines and other hormones. Pharmacol Rev 12:265–300

Zaimis E (1968): Vasopressor drugs and catecholamines. Anesthesiology 29:732–762

JOHN A. BEVAN

19. ADRENERGIC RECEPTOR BLOCKING DRUGS

Adrenergic receptor blocking agents inhibit the response of effector cells to either sympathetic nerve activity or sympathomimetic amines by their action on adrenergic receptors. Drugs are known that block either α or β receptors but not both (Chs. 14, 18). Their primary site of action is distal to the neuroeffector or synaptic cleft and must be clearly differentiated from adrenergic *neuron* blocking agents, such as guanethidine, that act proximal to the cleft on the terminations of the postganglionic adrenergic neurons (Ch.

20). Drugs in this latter class prevent both α and β responses to sympathetic activity by interfering with the release of the adrenergic transmitter. Thus they block the effects of indirectly but not directly acting sympathomimetic amines (Ch. 18).

If the predominant adrenergic receptor and the influence of tonic sympathetic activity on the various organs are known, the pharmacologic effects of these drugs may be deduced (Table 14–1).

ALPHA ADRENERGIC RECEPTOR BLOCKING AGENTS

These drugs block most of the effects of norepinephrine. The predominantly hypertensive response to epinephrine given in high dose to an experimental animal (Ch. 18) is changed after α receptor blockade to a mainly hypotensive reaction. The latter is the result of β receptor stimulation; the β dilator effects on the blood vessels overshadow the β stimulation actions on the heart (Ch. 18).

Alpha adrenergic receptor blocking agents are classified as irreversible and reversible, on the basis of their duration of action.

IRREVERSIBLE AGENTS. Phenoxybenzamine (Dibenzyline) is the classic example of this group. It is related to the nitrogen mustards and forms a stable covalent bond with the α receptor (Ch. 1) which results in an insurmountable, nonequilibrium block of the α adrenergic receptor. Its pharmacologic effects persist for a number of days. Doses not much greater than those that block the adrenergic receptor block serotonin receptors as well (Ch. 50).

REVERSIBLE AGENTS. A heterogeneous miscellany is included in this category. The **ergot alkaloids, tolazoline** (Priscoline), **phentolamine**

(Regitine) and **azapetine** (Ilidar) are best known. All agents in this class are of low pharmacologic specificity, and consequently only doses that produce a modest level of α receptor blockade can be tolerated clinically.

USES

With the exception of the ergot alkaloids, α adrenergic blocking agents have been used in the treatment of **peripheral vascular spastic disease** for such conditions as thromboangiitis obliterans (Buerger's disease) and Raynaud's syndrome. It is assumed that sympathetic hyperactivity contributes in part to these conditions and that this component is eliminated by α receptor blockade (Ch. 35). As the vessel wall is often rigid and narrowed by pathologic change, this precludes a satisfactory dilator response. Furthermore, the fall in perfusion pressure caused by the general vascular effect of these agents often offsets their therapeutic value. Obviously they are of little use in vascular beds dominated by autoregulatory or β adrenergic receptor dilator mechanisms.

Alpha receptor blocking agents have a rational place in the control of **pheochromocytoma,** a tumor of the adrenal medulla (chromaffin tissue) which is associated with a periodic hypersecretion of catecholamines. In certain types of **shock,** when reflex neurogenic vasoconstriction due to the hyperactivity of compensatory mechanisms is a prominent feature, the judicial use of α receptor blocking agents can increase local blood flow to important areas, in particular the mesenteric bed. It is claimed that under these circumstances local anoxia is relieved and recovery facilitated.

ERGOT ALKALOIDS

Although traditionally the ergot alkaloids are classified as α adrenergic blocking agents, their clinical uses depend upon their *other* pharmacologic properties.

SOURCE AND CHEMISTRY

The ergot alkaloids together with many other substances are obtained on extraction of a fungus (*Claviceps purpurea*) parasitic to rye and other grains. Even today in the United States, infected rye is fairly common. The substances derived from ergot which are commonly used in medicine are all related to lysergic acid (Fig. 19–1). The most important are **ergotamine** and **ergonovine.** Hydrogenation of one of the double bonds in the lysergic acid nucleus enhances the adrenergic blocking properties of these compounds and reduces their other actions. Lysergic acid diethylamide (LSD) is an easily prepared congener (Ch. 9).

ACTIONS

In addition to their α adrenergic blocking activity, ergot alkaloids constrict smooth muscle, particularly vascular and uterine, and cause endothelial damage in the small peripheral blood vessels. The increase in smooth muscle tone is due to a direct action of the drug on the muscle cells, independent of adrenergic mechanisms. In addition, by an action on the cardiovascular centers in the medulla, there is mild hypotension and depression of reflex compensatory mechanisms.

USES AND EFFECTIVENESS

Use in Migraine

The pain of migraine headaches is associated with vasodilation, edema and sometimes visible pulsation of extracranial blood vessels. This is possibly associated with the local release of serotonin (Ch. 50) in periarterial tissues. The prodromal symptoms or aura which precede the headache, on the other hand, are associated with excessive constriction of the same vessels. The ergot alkaloids are effective in migraine because of their vasoconstrictor, or smooth muscle stimulant, properties. They should not be administered more than once a week, avoided during pregnancy and used with care in patients with peripheral vascular disease.

Ergotamine is effective in almost 90% of migraine attacks if given early, preferably during the prodromal period (the phase of vasoconstriction). In nonmigraineous attacks, only 15% claim relief. Attacks are not prevented.

Dihydroergotamine, a weaker vasoconstrictor but a more potent adrenergic blocking agent, is generally less effective than ergotamine in the treatment of migraine, although it is preferred by some patients.

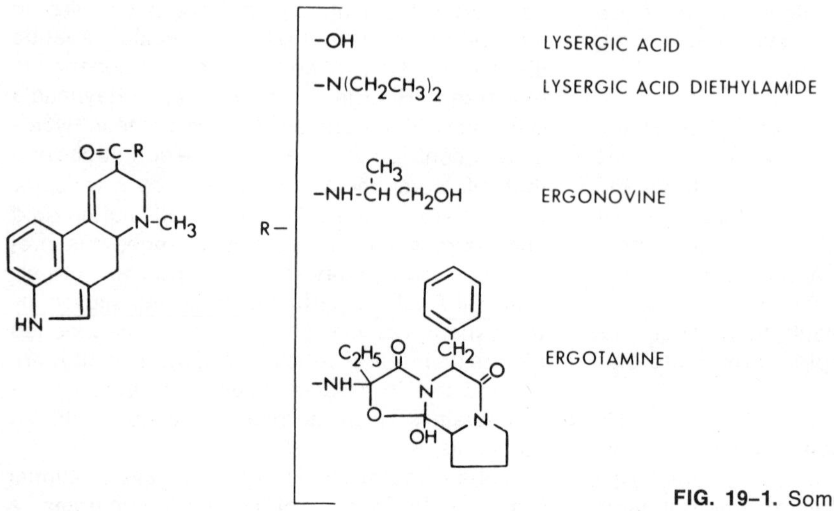

FIG. 19–1. Some derivatives of lysergic acid.

The combination of caffeine with these alkaloids enhances their therapeutic properties, probably because of the additive direct vasoconstrictor action of the xanthine molecule (Ch. 32).

Methysergide (Sansert), a congener of ergonovine, is closely related to LSD and is a potent serotonin antagonist. It is effective only after several days; protection persists for some time after its withdrawal and is the only prophylactic therapy available. Unfortunately, in about 20% of patients the frequency of adverse effects often limits its use (Ch. 49). These effects include nausea, vomiting and cramps and central effects somewhat reminiscent of its hallucinatory congener LSD, although very considerably weaker. In addition, a variety of effects attributable to excess vasoconstriction, angina and peripheral vascular insufficiency occur. Retroperitoneal fibrosis has been reported.

It is available in 2 mg tablets.

Use as an Oxytocic

Ergonovine and its derivative, **methylergonovine,** are oxytocics; they increase the frequency and duration of uterine contractions and consequently shorten the periods of relaxation, within 3–5 min of subcutaneous and 30 sec of IV injection. In addition, the basal level of uterine tone is increased. The effect is most marked on the uterus at term. **Ergotamine,** after a latent period of up to 30 min exerts a qualitatively similar but more prolonged effect (Ch. 43).

These alkaloids are used routinely toward the end of labor after delivery of the fetus, to promote a firm and persistent contraction of the uterus. This closes off the uterine sinuses and reduces the incidence and severity of postpartum hemorrhage. Ergonovine and ergotamine may be combined and administered IM. The former ensures a rapid action and the latter a persistent effect. They may be given IV if a rapid effect is desired.

PREPARATIONS AND DOSAGE

Ergotamine Tartrate, *U.S.P.* (Gynergen), is available in sublingual tablets. The dose is 3–4 mg stat, then 0.5–1.0 mg hourly to a total of 10 mg. The course is not to be repeated within a week. Dose by injection is 0.25–0.5 mg stat, IM or subcutaneously, to be repeated once if ineffective. It is also effective in an inhaled form.

Ergotamine tartrate (1 mg) plus caffeine (100 mg) (Cafergot) is a commonly used mixture. The dosage is as above.

Ergonovine Maleate, *U.S.P.* (Ergometrine Maleate, *B.P.*), may be given intramuscularly, orally or sublingually. The dose for injection is 0.2 mg. The oral or sublingual dose is 0.5 mg.

ADVERSE EFFECTS

Acute effects such as headache, nausea, vomiting, diarrhea, weakness, muscle pain, confusion, depression, convulsions and various neurologic symptoms are experienced by approximately 15% of patients. Other symptoms, such as hypertension, especially in patients with toxemia and angina, are probably the result of direct vasoconstriction. Many of these effects may be minimized by symptomatic treatment with other agents (vasodilators, antiemetics), permitting the continued use of the drug in migraine.

The dramatic **chronic effects** of ergot ingestion, sometimes of epidemic proportions, witnessed in the past from eating bread prepared from infected rye are seldom seen today. This condition in its extreme is characterized by convulsions, abortion and peripheral vascular stasis and gangrene, the result of the intense vasoconstriction and toxicologic damage to the vascular endothelium of the small peripheral blood vessels. Sporadic reports of these effects still appear, due presumably to accidental overdosage, a hypersensitive response to the drug or preexisting vascular disease.

BETA ADRENERGIC BLOCKING AGENTS

All β adrenergic blocking agents are synthetic. The dichloro derivative of isoproterenol, **dichloroisoproterenol,** was the first specific and effective drug of this class (Fig. 19–2). Unfortunately, in addition to its β receptor blocking action, it exhibited β receptor stimulating activity. Recently **pronethalol** (Nethalide) and subsequently **propranolol** (Inderal), both related to isoproterenol, were developed. Pronethalol was found to produce lymphosarcoma in mice, and its use has been discontinued. Propranolol appears to be without this undesirable property and, as can be seen from its inclusion in a variety of chapters (see below) is proving to be of considerable value.

ACTIONS

Propranolol is a reversible, competitive antagonist of sympathomimetic amines at the β adrenergic receptor. Its effects on the body can be deduced from a knowledge of those physiologic consequences of adrenergic tone which are mediated through the β adrenergic receptor. For example, the sympathetic nervous system to some degree at rest, and particularly under

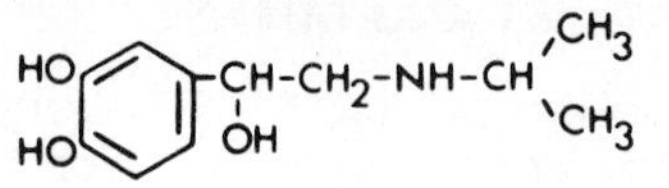

FIG. 19–2. A β receptor stimulating agent (isoproterenol) and a β receptor blocking agent (propranolol).

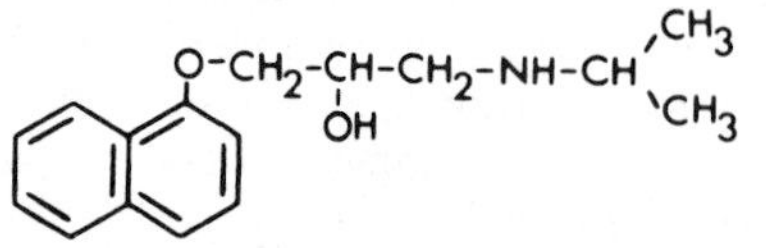

stress, exerts a positive inotropic and chronotropic effect on the myocardium. Thus, propranolol has a small negative inotropic and chronotropic effect at rest and depresses these normal responses to stress. It has little effect on the vasculature, since the sympathetic drive to this system is mediated predominantly by α adrenergic receptors.

A variety of studies in animals and man using a large series of sympathomimetic amines and some new experimental adrenergic receptor blocking agents suggest that the β receptor is not uniform throughout the body. A number of subdivisions have been suggested, but none are entirely satisfactory. However, the recognition of significant differences between the β adrenergic receptors in different organs has prompted a determined search for new highly specific β receptor agonists and antagonists. A number of workers have suggested that the β receptor of the heart and those for lipolysis (β_1) should be differentiated from those found in bronchial muscle and blood vessels (β_2). A number of relatively specific blocking agents are under active investigation. Of these, **practolol** appears to be fairly specific for the cardiac β adrenergic receptor and has only minimal effects on those in bronchi or blood vessels.

Propranolol is rapidly absorbed from the gastrointestinal tract. Maximum effects are realized within 90 min. Its half-time in the plasma is 2.5–3.0 hr. As yet unidentified metabolites are claimed to have a similar but prolonged action and may be responsible for the extreme variation in the required dosage.

USES AND EFFECTIVENESS

ANGINA PECTORIS. The pain of angina (see also Ch. 35) is due to a relative ischemia of the myocardium. Propranolol is effective in reducing the incidence and severity of attacks in some patients. By depressing the sympathetic drive to the heart, myocardial work and in consequence myocardial oxygen requirements are reduced (see Ch. 35). It may also be responsible for redistribution of intramyocardial blood flow. The cardiac response to exercise is blunted.

CARDIAC ARRHYTHMIAS. Propranolol is of value in the treatment of a variety of arrhythmias, including those that result from digitalis toxicity (Chs. 33, 34). Since propranolol can depress myocardial contractility and atrioventricular conduction, it should be used with care; however, under some circumstances advantageous use can be made of these actions. Presumably because of its antiarrhythmic properties, propranolol reduces the mortality associated with myocardial infarction.

HYPERTENSION. Although still under investigation in the U.S., propranolol is widely used in Europe in the treatment of essential hypertension (Ch. 20).

In pheochromocytoma it is sometimes combined with an α adrenergic receptor blocking agent and used in the pharmacologic premedication of the patient prior to surgery.

HYPERTROPHIC SUBAORTIC STENOSIS. Propranolol, by its negative inotropic effect, improves this condition and the tolerance of the patient to exercise.

ADVERSE REACTIONS

General symptoms, such as nausea, malaise, skin changes, visual changes and insomnia, are seen in approximately 2% of patients. More serious effects are associated with blockade of sympathetic β receptor mediated drive. Heart failure may be exacerbated by blocking compensatory and supportative sympathetic hyperactivity. High doses of propranolol directly depress the heart. Concomitant administration of digitalis, however, can often minimize this problem. Propranolol must be used with care in patients with asthma; its use can result in bronchial spasm. In diabetic patients, propranolol interferes with the normal response to hyperglycemia—palpitations, sweating and glucose release. These are warning symptoms and protective reactions mediated by β adrenergic receptors. For similar reasons there is an increased risk in patients during general anesthesia and major surgery.

Other adverse effects include, in the cardiovascular system, bradycardia, congestive heart failure, increased AV block and hypotension; in the CNS, lightheadedness, depression, hallucinations, visual disturbance, short-term memory loss and various psychologic disturbances. In addition, it can cause increased activity of the gastrointestinal tract, various allergenic phenomena, reversible alopecia and agranulocytosis and purpura.

FURTHER READING

Barger G (1931): Ergot and Ergotism. London, Gurney

Epstein SE, Braunwald E (1966): Beta adrenergic receptor blocking drugs. N Engl J Med 275:1106

Nickerson M (1949): The pharmacology of adrenergic blockade. Pharmacol Rev 1:27

Wolff HG (1948): Headache and Other Head Pains. London, Oxford

JOHN A. BEVAN

20. ANTIHYPERTENSIVE DRUGS

It has been estimated that approximately 23 million Americans suffer from a raised arterial pressure and that one-third of these have pressures within the range where antihypertensive therapy has been demonstrated to be therapeutically valuable. The danger of hypertension is related by and large to the level of the arterial pressure. The object of therapy is to lower pressure and a variety of pharmacologic agents are effective in accomplishing this.

A diagnosis of **essential hypertension** can be made only after known causes of raised arterial pressure, primary aldosteronism, renal vascular disease, pheochromocytoma, etc., have been excluded. Its cause is unknown and recent studies suggest that there are a number of specific disease entities grouped under the same title. In early uncomplicated essential hypertension, total peripheral resistance is elevated and cardiac output is normal. Urinary aldosterone, plasma renin, sympathetic nervous activity, are within normal range. The increase in resistance of vascular beds following the injection of norepinephrine is greater than in the normal subject. The study of experimental models of hypertension has shown that there may be an alteration of the adrenergic innervation of the blood vessel associated with changes in adrenergic transmitter mechanism together with an alteration in the amount, sensitivity and contractility of vascular smooth muscle cells. Homeostatic mechanisms are altered. The clinical disease, however, is rarely simple and is often associated with complex alteration of regulating mechanisms, together with blood vessel and target organ damage and altered hemodynamics.

RATIONALE OF THERAPY

Drug therapy is suppressive not curative. It is not specifically directed towards the underlying cause since this is unknown. The therapeutic objective is to reduce the absolute level of arterial pressure while maintaining an adequate blood flow to the vital organs and maintaining, as far as possible, normal circulatory compensatory mechanisms. Whereas for many patients a standardized drug regime will suffice, there are a sufficient variety of drugs available that vary in their mode and pattern of action, that therapy can to some extent be tailored to the particular and individual manifestations of the disease. To be satisfactory, treatment must be acceptable to the patient, particularly since once initiated it will most likely be continued throughout life. Essential hypertension is rarely cured even after many years of therapy.

A number of long-term controlled prospective studies have demonstrated reduced mortality and morbidity associated with effective antihypertensive therapy, specifically in those with an arterial pressure greater than 105 mm Hg. In one such study, 143 patients had diastolic pressures greater than 115 mm Hg. After 20 months, just less than 20% of the untreated group of patients developed severe complications and four died. Among the treated patients there was only one moderately severe complication. Although the results of all studies are not so dramatic as this, they point in the same direction. Antihypertensive therapy is particularly effective in reducing the complications of congestive heart failure, malignant hypertension and renal damage, less so, the incidence of stroke. The frequency of cardiac disease associated with coronary artery disease is little altered. It is important to remember that effective therapy also includes changes in life style, minimizing those factors found to influence the course of the disease; es-

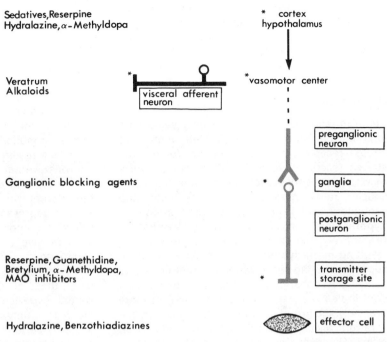

Sedatives, Reserpine
Hydralazine, α-Methyldopa

* cortex
hypothalamus

Veratrum
Alkaloids

*vasomotor center

visceral afferent
neuron

preganglionic
neuron

Ganglionic blocking agents

ganglia

postganglionic
neuron

Reserpine, Guanethidine,
Bretylium, α-Methyldopa,
MAO inhibitors

transmitter
storage site

Hydralazine, Benzothiadiazines

effector cell

FIG. 20–1. Sites of action of antihypertensive drugs. **Asterisks** indicate the sites of action of nicotine.

tablishing a regular exercise pattern, taking sufficient rest, a reduction in weight, a decrease in salt intake, stopping tobacco consumption and the minimizing of life's stresses.

Drugs used in the treatment of hypertension act in a variety of ways. Many reduce neurogenic vascular tone, i.e., the influence of the sympathetic nervous system on the resistance and capacitance blood vessels. Others cause dilation of blood vessels by an action on the smooth muscle cell itself. Some alter the size of the vascular and extravascular fluid compartments.

Ideally, a decrease in arterial pressure should be achieved without a reduction in cardiac output and without significant effect on the distribution of this output to various body regions. Blood flow to the brain, heart and kidneys must not be endangered. Should this occur, the possibility of organ failure or thrombosis of the arterial bed is real and dangerous. Since antihypertensive drugs depress the sympathetic efferent pathways used by the homeostatic reflexes, the adaptive capacity of the circulation is always reduced to some degree by their actions. The most common and most troublesome consequence of

this is **orthostatic** or **postural hypotension.** On changing position, e.g., from a horizontal to a vertical stance, marked transient hypotension occurs after administration of most antihypertensives, since the compensatory capacity of the circulation is depressed. This is associated with dizziness, faintness and even loss of consciousness.

In this chapter, drugs used in the treatment of hypertension—the antihypertensive drugs—are discussed systematically, without reference to their importance, efficacy or popularity. At the conclusion of this chapter these various agents are discussed from the perspective of contemporary practice. There is no single ideal drug or combination of drugs, and views are continually and rapidly changing as a result of discovery and clinical experience. A knowledge of the pharmacology of each antihypertensive agent is considered essential. One important therapeutic objective is to suit the therapy to the manifestations of the disease in a particular patient. This can only be achieved by making optimum use of the variety of possible therapeutic agents available. The major sites of action of these drugs are summarized in Figure 20–1.

VERATRUM ALKALOIDS

Although the use of the alkaloids extracted from the *Veratrum* species (Hellebore) are now almost

therapeutically obsolete, they are of some historic importance. Extracts have been used since antiquity to treat circulatory disorders and other diseases. The interest in the last one or two decades in using these as antihypertensive agents has markedly declined. A variety of mixtures, galenicals, pure alkaloids and semisynthetic derivatives have been prepared, all of which produce hypotension by essentially similar mechanisms.

Mechanism of Action

Veratrum alkaloids sensitize sensory vagal endings in the heart (specifically left ventricular stretch receptors) and in the lungs (pulmonary stretch receptors) to their natural stimuli. As a result, the sensory input to the brain is increased, causing reflex inhibition of the vasomotor and ventilatory centers leading to **vasodilation and hypotension** and **depression of ventilation,** respectively, and stimulation of the vagal center, resulting in **bradycardia.** Experimental evidence suggests that the sensitization of other vagal and some glossopharyngeal sensory endings also contributes to these changes. The reflex (or more precisely, the group of reflexes) stimulated by the veratrum alkaloids is called the Bezold-Jarisch reflex. Compensatory chemoreceptor and other adaptive mechanisms rapidly restore ventilatory movement. Consequently, hypotension and brady-

cardia are the predominant changes seen with long-term administration of these alkaloids. Cardiac output is not altered significantly.

Clinical Pharmacology and Adverse Effects

The reflex hypotension caused by veratrum alkaloids in doses that can be tolerated clinically is usually small. In man, dosage is limited by nausea and vomiting, the result of a reflexogenic action of the drug on sensory endings in the nodose ganglion of the vagus. Other effects of the drug resulting from its action on sensory neurons are paresthesia, a burning sensation in the mouth and epigastrium, and hiccups. Since the efferent sympathetic pathways to the vessels are not depressed (sympathetic drive is inhibited reflexly), compensatory mechanisms are generally effective and postural hypotension is not experienced.

After an initial period of enthusiastic endorsement, these alkaloids are now rarely used in essential hypertension. Pure alkaloids still have much to commend them for the control of the acute hypertensive crises of toxemia of pregnancy. Emesis is not a great problem following IV injection.

RESERPINE

Reserpine is the prototype of the therapeutically valuable alkaloids obtained from *Rauwolfia serpentina,* a small shrub indigenous to India. The main pharmacologic actions of this drug on the CNS are described in Chapter 25. Only its use as an antihypertensive agent is described below.

Actions

The ability of reserpine to lower arterial pressure is attributed to three actions:

1. Sedation or tranquilization. All sedative drugs, including the barbiturates, lower arterial pressure. They are particularly effective in tense, anxious, irritable and hyperdynamic individuals.
2. Depression of the sympathetic centers in the hypothalamus. This effect is associated with overactivity of centers controlling parasympathetic function.
3. Depletion of the peripheral stores of adrenergic transmitter. The entry of norepinephrine or its precursors into the amine storage granules is prevented. This effect, combined with a deficiency of storage function, leads to a depletion of the amine as the norepinephrine is released spontaneously or as a re-

sult of nerve activity. Not only does the stored transmitter leak away from the nerve ending, but its replenishment from circulating catecholamine is inhibited (Ch. 14).

Clinical Pharmacology and Adverse Effects

After oral administration, there is a delay of several days before a significant hypotensive effect is produced. A maximum effect is not achieved for up to 3 weeks. Because reserpine is a weak hypotensive drug and a significant part of its effect is due to a central inhibition of sympathetic drive, postural hypotension is not a prominent feature of its use. Cardiac output is often slightly increased and peripheral resistance reduced.

Adverse effects limit its usefulness, particularly

RESERPINE

if high doses are required. Most of these effects are either extensions of the drug's therapeutically valuable actions or the logical consequence of its mode of action. They include **mental changes**—drowsiness, lethargy, apathy and, most serious, depression, despondency, anxiety associated with suicidal tendencies; paradoxically, delirium, excitement and nightmares also occur. **Increased parasympathetic, associated with decreased sympathetic, activity** leads to an increase in gastric acid secretion, peptic ulceration, and an increase in gastrointestinal tone and motility resulting in diarrhea. Nasal stuffiness, ectopic heart beats and flushing occur. In addition, fluid retention, weight gain and extrapyramidal syndromes are described. Precipitous falls in arterial pressure occur in reserpinized patients during general anesthesia. Recent studies suggest that long term administration is associated with an increased risk of developing breast cancer.

Preparation and Dosage

Reserpine, *U.S.P.*, is available in a multiplicity of forms. The daily dose is 0.25–1.0 mg orally; owing to its long duration of action, the dose need not be divided.

HYDRALAZINE

Hydralazine (Apresoline) is a fairly potent hypotensive agent, which increases cardiac output despite a fall in arterial pressure. Its therapeutic usefulness is limited by the adverse effects it can cause.

Mechanism of Action

Hydralazine causes a fall in systolic and diastolic pressures mainly by a **direct relaxant** action on the vascular smooth muscle of the resistance and capacitance vessels. **Adrenolytic** and **central depressant** effects contribute to its antihypertensive activity.

Clinical Pharmacology and Adverse Effects

Hydralazine is unique among antihypertensive drugs in that hypotension is associated with an increased heart rate, cardiac output and blood flow to all organs, including the kidney. Blood flow to skeletal muscle is the exception to this generalization. Because of its mechanism of action, orthostatic or postural hypotension is less prominent than with drugs that interrupt directly the sympathetic nervous discharge. Hydralazine is frequently used in combination with other antihypertensive agents, especially those that reduce renal blood flow and decrease heart rate. By such a combination, advantage may be taken of the desirable properties of hydralazine without the disadvantage of the adverse effects that might attend its sole use at high dosage.

Because hydralazine acts directly on the arterial wall, its effectiveness in decreasing peripheral resistance is limited by a reflex increase in sympathetic activity via the pressor receptors leading to an increase in heart rate and cardiac output and two effects which seem to be associated with all drugs that lower arterial pressure, an increase in plasma renin and sodium water retention. The consequences of the first two effects can be minimized by the concomitant use of propranolol. Diuretics may be used to minimize the latter.

Hydralazine causes a depressing galaxy of adverse reactions. General toxic effects (headache, malaise, fatigue), gastrointestinal irritation (nausea, vomiting, epigastric distress, diarrhea), myocardial stimulation (palpitation, aggravation of angina and even coronary thrombosis) due, presumably, to reflex sympathetic activation, hyperesthesia and paresthesia, regional edema, sensitivity reactions, psychotic effects and reversible depression of one or more cellular blood components have been recorded. Long-term administration of high doses can lead to a reversible acute rheumatoid–like state and a clinical picture indistinguishable from that of lupus erythematosus.

HYDRALAZINE

Preparation and Dosage

Hydralazine Hydrochloride, *N.F., N.N.D.* (Apresoline), is available in oral or parenteral form. The oral dose starts at 10–25 mg every 6 hours, but this is usually slowly increased to 25–50 mg every 6 hours. Doses of 200 mg/day and over are rarely used without the occurrence of serious adverse effects.

Two new directly acting vasodilator drugs are under investigation, **gyancydine** and **minoxidil.** Like hydralazine, these relax vascular smooth muscle by an action independent of the adrenergic system. They are more effective and longer lasting but must be administered with a diuretic. Minoxidil appears to be associated with the over-production of hair, which limits its acceptance by women.

GANGLIONIC STIMULATING AND BLOCKING AGENTS

Ganglionic stimulating agents enhance or initiate activity in the postganglionic autonomic neurons. Ganglionic blocking agents depress or interrupt tonic and reflexly induced changes in activity in the efferent limbs of both parasympathetic and sympathetic nervous systems. The pharmacology of the sympathetic and parasympathetic ganglia is identical.

GANGLIONIC STIMULATING AGENTS: NICOTINE

A variety of drugs, including nicotine, are known which stimulate autonomic ganglion cells. None of these drugs are truly specific, nor do they have essential clinical value. Because of its general interest, particularly in relation to the effects of smoking, the pharmacology of nicotine, is briefly outlined here.

Pharmacology and Mechanism of Action

Nicotine, an alkaloid obtained from the leaves of the shrub, *Nicotiana tabacum,* has a complex multiplicity of pharmacologic actions. The net effect of the drug on any one organ is the result of

NICOTINE

its pharmacologic action at many sites. The action of nicotine at any one site differs with different doses and with different levels of tolerance.

Nicotine stimulates and, provided the dose is sufficient, subsequently depresses autonomic centers in the central nervous system; autonomic ganglia; sensory endings, especially vagal endings within the thorax; and the chemoreceptor cells of the carotid and aortic bodies. In addition, it releases *l*-norepinephrine and *l*-epinephrine from the adrenal medulla and the terminations of postganglionic sympathetic neurons. In Figure 20–1, the main sites of action of nicotine influencing the tone of a "typical" arteriolar cell are illustrated.

Nicotine, in small doses, stimulates ganglion cells by causing a transient depolarization of the ganglion cell membrane, an action presumably similar to that caused by the physiologic transmitter, acetylcholine. Nicotine and acetylcholine probably act on the same group of phar-macologic receptors. In higher doses, the ganglion cells are persistently depolarized by the drug, causing blockade of ganglionic transmission. It is presumed that nicotine acts by similar mechanisms at other sites.

GANGLIONIC BLOCKING AGENTS

Most clinically valuable ganglionic blocking agents are competitive inhibitors of the physiologic transmitter, acetylcholine. They are analogous, therefore, to atropine and *d*-tubocurarine at the postganglionic parasympathetic ending and the neuromuscular junction, respectively. Although atropine-sensitive cholinergic and adrenergic transmitter mechanisms in ganglia have been demonstrated, their role in normal ganglion transmission has not yet been defined.

Actions

All ganglionic blocking agents cause essentially the same effects, since they all interrupt the autonomic efferent discharge. Their effects can be anticipated, provided the division of the autonomic nervous system which exerts dominant tonic control on each end organ or tissue and the major efferent pathway of each autonomic reflex are known (Table 14–1).

CARDIOVASCULAR EFFECTS. Inhibition of the tonic sympathetic influence on arterioles and venules and of the vagal influence on the heart results in hypotension and tachycardia. Since all compensatory reflexes are interrupted or depressed, postural hypotension is marked. If the same dose of a ganglionic blocking agent is administered to a standing and a recumbent subject, hypotension is considerably more marked in the former. Cardiac output is generally reduced as a result of venous pooling of blood, and total peripheral resistance is decreased. All adaptive changes of the circulation to varying external and internal environments are depressed.

Changes in the regional distribution of blood flow are variable. Splanchnic, cerebral and usually, renal and coronary flow are reduced, although the proportion of the output distributed to the brain and heart is usually increased. Since the relative importance of tonic sympathetic activity in regulating the flow to the various regions differs from one individual to another, it is easy to understand the inconsistent changes in regional flow following use of these drugs. This is particularly true when the arterial disease itself shows a predilection for different regions in different individuals.

OTHER ACTIONS. The tone, motility and most secretions of the gastrointestinal tract are depressed, causing dryness of the mouth (xerostomia), indigestion and constipation. Difficulty in voiding urine and impotency are experienced. Bronchi are dilated. Secretions of the nasopharynx and respiratory systems are inhibited. The skin is dry and warm due to dilation of cutaneous vessels. The pupil is dilated (mydriasis) and accommodation paralyzed.

Clinical Pharmacology and Adverse Effects

Ganglionic blocking agents are extremely potent hypotensive agents which, until the discovery of equally potent but more specific adrenergic neuron blocking agents (see below), were lifesaving in the treatment of the severely hypertensive patient. They block all autonomic efferent activity—sympathetic and parasympathetic. Parasympathetic blockade contributes little to hypotension, and most adverse effects not due to hypotension itself result from this action. Such effects include constipation and urinary retention. Irregular gastrointestinal activity can result in the irregular absorption of the drug itself and occasionally in temporary overdose, due to the absorption of several doses of the drug over a short period of time. This results in excessive hypotension with all its associated dangers. A reduction in renal blood flow may cause uremia, especially in severe hypertension. **Mecamylamine,** unlike most other ganglionic blocking agents, is a secondary amine. It can pass the blood-brain barrier and cause a variety of CNS effects.

Preparations and Dosage

Many ganglionic blocking agents have been used clinically. Tetraethylammonium, the first clinically useful agent, because of its low specificity is now obsolete. **Hexamethonium chloride** (C-6), the prototype of many newer ganglionic blocking agents, is the homolog of decamethonium (C-10, Ch. 21). The differing distance between the positively charged nitrogen atoms in these two molecules is considered responsible for their specificity of action. Owing to its irregular and unpredictable absorption from the gastrointestinal tract, hexamethonium has been superseded. Both **pentolinium tartrate** (Ansolysen Tartrate) and **chlorisondamine chloride** (Ecolid Chloride) are more potent and longer lasting than hexamethonium, but have the same disadvantage of erratic absorption.

Mecamylamine Hydrochloride, *U.S.P.* (Inversine Hydrochloride), in contrast to other agents, is a secondary amine and in consequence is well absorbed by mouth. It causes a smooth and prolonged hypotension. Mecamylamine crosses the blood-brain barrier and exerts central effects which probably contribute to its total hypotensive action. Because of these features, it is the most popular clinical agent in this class. An initial oral dose of 2.5 mg twice daily is given, which may be slowly increased until a desirable therapeutic effect is obtained, usually at a dose level of 12.5–15.0 mg twice daily.

Trimethaphan camphorsulfonate (Arfonad Camphorsulfonate) has an extremely short duration of action. When given by a continuous infusion it can be used to control the level of arterial pressure and in consequence arterial hemorrhage during surgery. It is used to produce the so-called "bloodless" surgical field.

ADRENERGIC NEURON BLOCKING AGENTS

Adrenergic neuron blocking drugs act at the terminals of postganglionic sympathetic neurons to prevent in one way or another the release of effective quantities of adrenergic transmitter in response to sympathetic activity. They do not interfere with the action of exogenous directly acting sympathomimetic amines, i.e., do not block the α and β adrenergic receptors (Chs. 18, 19). In sharp contrast to ganglionic blocking agents, they do not interfere with tonic parasympathetic activity. Signs and symptoms of the overactivity of this latter division, presumably the consequence of the pharmacologic depression of its physiological antagonist, is characteristic of this group of drugs. Reserpine owes some of its hypotensive effect to its adrenergic neuron blocking ability.

GUANETHIDINE

Guanethidine (Ismelin), a comparatively recent discovery, has displaced ganglionic blocking agents as the pharmacologic mainstay of the control of severe hypertension. It is equally as potent as the ganglionic blocking drugs; yet is relatively free from serious adverse effects.

GUANETHIDINE

Mechanism of Action

In Chapter 14, guanethidine is classified as a drug that interferes with the terminal neuronal stores of sympathetic transmitter. Transmitter uptake, storage and release mechanisms are affected, and this results in a reduction in transmitter release from the nerve terminal following nervous activity (Fig. 20–2). This may be associated with a local depolarization block of the sympathetic nerve terminal resulting in diminution of transmitter release. Since guanethidine interferes with transmitter storage, norepinephrine leaks away from its storage sites causing circulatory changes immediately following guanethidine administration. As might be expected after guanethidine, indirectly-acting sympathomimetic amines are ineffective in releasing the adrenergic transmitter. There is evidence that before action, guanethidine must be taken up into the nerve terminal. Drugs that block norepinephrine uptake, e.g., cocaine (Ch. 22), tricyclic antidepressants (Ch. 24), etc., prevent the action of guanethidine on the sympathetic nerve terminal. As would be expected, indirectly acting sympathomimetic amines lose their effectiveness after guanethidine administration (Ch. 18). After continuous use of guanethidine, the effector cells become hypersensitive to either exogenous or endogenous catecholamines. Since guanethidine can completely inactivate the sympathetic motor neurons, this is the pharmacologic equivalent to **denervation sensitivity.** Hypersensitivity of the effector cells is due to changes in the cells themselves as well as the result of the blockade or removal of neuronal norepinephrine uptake

mechanisms. In some circumstances, after the administration of guanethidine, transient sympathomimetic effects are seen, due presumably to the local effects of transmitter release.

Clinical Pharmacology and Adverse Effects

Although the hypotension caused by guanethidine sometimes takes 2–3 days to become manifest, reaching a peak in 2 weeks, it is smooth and prolonged. The effect of a single dose may last for several days. Tolerance is slow to develop. Heart rate and cardiac output are commonly decreased, associated with the decreased sympathetic drive and decreased venous tone and therefore increased venous capacity, and since peripheral resistance is generally unchanged, blood flow to all regions is reduced. As expected from its mode of action, **postural hypotension,** although important, is not so disabling as that associated with ganglionic blocking agents. **Exertional hypotension,** however, is a common complaint. Guanethidine causes sodium and fluid retention as well as an increase in plasma renin and should be used for maximum effectiveness in combination with a diuretic (see below).

A number of the adverse effects of guanethidine are due to the unopposed activity of the parasympathetic nervous system and/or the reduced activity of the sympathetic nervous system. Diarrhea, activation of preexisting peptic

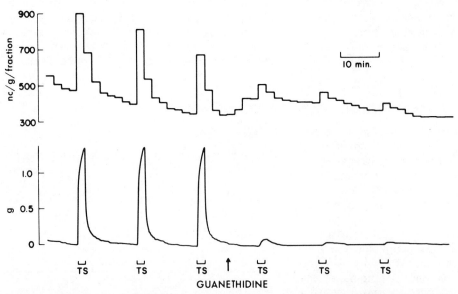

FIG. 20–2. Effect of guanethidine on the release of norepinephrine from nerve endings in an isolated artery. Electrical stimulation of the vasoconstrictor nerves (**TS**) resulted in arterial contraction (*bottom*) and a sharp rise in release of norepinephrine (the transmitter stores had been previously loaded with tritiated norepinephrine). Guanethidine (4 × 10⁻⁵M) caused an increase in spontaneous release of the transmitter and inhibited release and contraction following nerve stimulation. (Used by permission of Dr. Che Su.)

ulceration, parotid pain, nasal stuffiness, failure of ejaculation, nocturia and lowering of intraocular pressure occur. In addition, patients complain of weakness and water retention. Because of the increased sensitivity of the circulation to vasoconstrictor amines after guanethidine, it is contraindicated in pheochromocytoma.

Preparations and Dosage

Guanethidine Sulfate, *U.S.P.* (Ismelin), is available as tablets. Patients vary widely in their sensitivity to this drug. After an initial dose of 10 mg/day, dosage is increased slowly until effective or toxic levels are reached. This may vary from 25–500 mg/day.

Bethanidine, a drug with a mode of action similar to that of guanethidine but not used at the moment in the United States, is claimed to cause fewer adverse effects.

BRETYLIUM

Bretylium (Darenthin) produces a pharmacologic effect similar to that of guanethidine, but by a different mechanism. In Chapter 14 this drug is classified as one that interferes with transmitter release. It differs from guanethidine in not depleting the adrenergic transmitter store. There is some evidence that bretylium may substitute for norepinephrine in the normal transmission process and become a false transmitter (see below). Because of its short and irregular action, rapidly developing tolerance and toxic manifestations, it has been superseded.

ALPHA METHYLDOPA

Methyldopa (Aldomet) is a moderately potent hypotensive drug whose action is often associated with an increased renal blood flow. Although alpha methyldopa inhibits an important step in the synthesis of *l*-norepinephrine, this particular action is probably not responsible for its hypotensive effect. Unfortunately, patients tend to become tolerant to its action.

METHYLDOPA

Mechanism of Action

Methyldopa, an analog of dihydroxphenylalanine, inhibits dopa decarboxylase in vitro. As this enzyme is normally responsible for the decarboxylation of dopa, an essential step in the synthesis of norepinephrine (Ch. 14), this has been proposed as the mechanism of its hypotensive action, since by such an action, effective amounts of the adrenergic transmitter at the postsynaptic receptors would be reduced. That its effect on arterial pressure is not due to this action is shown by the following observations; its hypotensive effect is longer than that of enzyme inactivation; its action on dopa decarboxylase in a series of individuals does not parallel its hypotensive effect, and other decarboxylase inhibitors do not lower arterial pressure.

It has been proposed that the depression of dopa decarboxylase results in the formation of an abnormal metabolite **methyldopa,** which in turn is transformed into **alpha methyl norepinephrine.** This compound blocks the uptake of norepinephrine and is actively stored in the adrenergic vesicles of the nerve terminal. From there it is released in place of norepinephrine. Since its pharmacologic potency is lower than norepinephrine, the effectiveness of transmission is diminished and hypotension results. Such a substance is called a **false transmitter;** a substance not normally present in the nerve ending, accumulating at the same site as norepinephrine and released from that site by apparently normal mechanisms. In addition, methyldopa has an action on the CNS similar to that of reserpine causing tranquilization and depression. Methyldopa is known to inhibit or depress the synthesis of other physiologically important amines in the body, including serotonin. This may be responsible for its tranquilizing effect.

Clinical Pharmacology and Adverse Effects

The effect of a single dose of methyldopa lasts about 1 day. Cardiac output, heart rate and total peripheral resistance are variably affected. In almost two-thirds of patients, renal blood flow is increased. Postural hypotension is less marked than with guanethidine and ganglionic blocking agents. The patient's response is unpredictable: For some it appears to be the ideal drug, while others are almost completely resistant to it. With chronic use there is salt and water retention necessitating the administration of a diuretic.

The incidence of other undesirable effects is low. They include such CNS changes as sedation, depression and tiredness. Auditory symptoms, heart failure, liver damage, drug fever, granulocytopenia and hemolytic anemia have been recorded.

Preparations and Dosage

Methyldopa (Aldomet) is available in tablets and also in a form for parenteral use. Because of individual variation, the drug must be assayed separately on each patient beginning with 250 mg twice daily. The dose may be adjusted sometimes to a maximum of 2000 mg/day.

MONOAMINE OXIDASE INHIBITORS: PARGYLINE

Monoamine oxidase (MAO) is important in the metabolic inactivation of *l*-norepinephrine and some other physiologically active amines, such as serotonin. Drugs that inhibit this enzyme as a class have important actions on the CNS (Ch. 25) and are potent hypotensive agents. Because of their potential risk and the availability of other effective drugs, this class of antihypertensive agents is now obsolete.

DIURETICS

Diuretics possess weak antihypertensive properties and are useful on their own in mild hypertension. When used in combination with other antihypertensive drugs, they significantly reduce the dose needed to produce a given effect. When these drugs are used as adjuvants in antihypertensive therapy, the incidence of adverse effects is reduced. The use and mode of action of these compounds as diuretics are described in Chapter 38.

Mechanism of Action

Arterial pressure is lowered as a result of a decrease in peripheral resistance, mainly because of the direct action of the diuretics on arterial smooth muscle. Alteration of the ionic content of the cells reduces their intrinsic tone, possibly their thickness and their reaction to adrenergic stimuli. In addition, these agents alter extracellular fluid volume. As stated above, they tend to minimize the disadvantageous effects of the prolonged use of antihypertensive drugs, sodium retention and fluid expansion. Thus they serve to potentiate the therapeutic value of these other agents. Antihypertensive effectiveness is exhibited by all members of the diuretic group although furosemide and ethacrynic acid have possibly greater maximum therapeutic effects than the others.

The adverse effects of various diuretics are described in Chapter 38 and include blood volume depletion, and sodium and potassium loss. Mild potassium depletion is common when diuretics are used in the hypertensive patient and is usually only of concern if the patient is receiving digitalis concomitantly (Ch. 33). Under these circumstances, potassium sparing diuretics, triamterene and spirolactone can be prescribed. The latter drug is an effective agent in the treatment of hypertension associated with primary aldosteronism.

Clinical Pharmacology and Adverse Effects

When used in long-term therapy, a benzothiadiazine such as **chlorothiazide** decreases total peripheral resistance but has little effect on heart rate and cardiac output. Coronary and renal blood flow may be slightly decreased. Presumably because of the absence of any effect on capacitance vessels, postural hypotension is not a prominent feature.

The adverse effects of these drugs and the various preparations and dosages are described in Chapter 38. The daily dose of chlorothiazide is of the order of 500 mg twice daily.

PROPRANOLOL

This β adrenergic receptor blocking agent (Ch. 19), still under investigation in this country, has been found to be an effective antihypertensive agent in many patients. It lowers arterial pressure by decreasing cardiac output by a variety of pharmacologic actions, including blocking the sympathetic drive to the myocardium, by reducing the secretion of renin from the kidney and by an as yet undefined action on central adrenergic neurons. Because of the complexity of action, the pattern of response and magnitude of its effectiveness varies remarkably from patient to patient.

THERAPY OF HYPERTENSIVE CRISES

Although a number of drugs have been used, including ganglionic blocking agents, hydralazine and the veratrum alkaloids, two agents **diazoxide** and **sodium nitroprusside** are currently favored. Diazoxide is a nondiuretic thiazide and probably the drug of choice in the immediate control of raised arterial pressure, as occurs in malignant hypertension, in the hypertensive crises of eclampsia, etc. By a direct action on arteriolar but not venular muscle, total peripheral resistance and thus arterial pressure is reduced. Sodium nitroprusside, still under investigation, is an alternative agent, particularly if the diazoxide is ineffective. It is administered as an infusion and is almost immediately effective. A fresh solution of 16 mg of sodium nitroprusside per liter of dextrose is infused at a rate determined by the arterial pressure response.

PROGRAMS OF DRUG THERAPY IN HYPERTENSION

A detailed account of the use of drugs in the clinical management of essential hypertension is out of place in a textbook of pharmacology. A simple comprehensive account is precluded by the variety of drugs available; the varying severity, time course and pattern of the disease; semantic difficulties among physicians in describing the different stages of the disease; and varying therapeutic goals.

Most physicians are agreed that patients with diastolic arterial pressure greater than 100–105 mm Hg should be treated. There is not a unanimous agreement concerning patients with lower pressures. Decisions to institute treatment in this group depend on such considerations as, positive family history, evidence for target organ damage, age, blood cholesterol, etc. It is agreed that such patients should receive regular medical examination.

For those requiring therapy, a "stepped-use" program is instituted. A single drug is instituted in small dose and increased slowly until a maximum therapeutic effect or an adverse effect is achieved. If this is insufficient to control pressures, other drugs are substituted or added. Regular periodic reevaluation is essential. Most are agreed that the diuretics usually the thiazides, should be the common denominator, the mainstay or background of all therapy. Any diuretic is admissable as long as it is effective. If potassium loss is important, then potassium sparing diuretics should be used. When diuretics alone are insufficient, additional drugs, reserpine, methyldopa and hydralazine can be used. All three have advantages and disadvantages. In severe cases, guanethidine, and if that is ineffective, ganglionic blocking agents may be employed.

Hypertension, although a killing disease, is in many asymptomatic and for this reason patient compliance with drug therapy is frequently poor. Thus, patient participation should be actively sought, his drug regime constantly adjusted to minimize discomfort and kept simple. With an explanation of his condition, "at home" pressure monitoring can be introduced. All these will optimize the value to the patient of the drug therapy.

Antihypertensive drug combinations provide a number of advantages to the clinician. The same antihypertensive effect may be achieved using smaller doses of the individual drugs. This reduces the incidence or severity of adverse reactions and delays the development of tolerance. Sometimes, when the adverse or side effects of one drug are particularly undesirable, e.g., the reduction in renal blood flow caused by ganglionic blocking agents, the additional use of a drug having an opposite side effect, e.g., hydralazine, may be beneficial.

Generally speaking, the prescription of fixed-dose mixtures is undesirable, since the degree to which therapy may be adjusted by the physician to individual needs is curtailed.

FURTHER READING

Brest AN, Mayer JH (eds) (1965): Cardiovascular Drug Therapy. New York, Grune & Stratton

Laragh JH (ed): Hypertensive Manual. New York, Yorke Medical Bldg

National high blood pressure educational program (1973): DHEW publication # (NIH) 74–593

Pardo EG, Vargas R, Vidrio H (1965): Antihypertensive drug action. Annu Rev Pharmacol 5:77

DERMOT B. TAYLOR

21. MUSCLE RELAXANTS: PERIPHERAL AND CENTRAL

There are three distinct classes of clinically useful relaxants of voluntary muscle: Those that act centrally in the brain and spinal cord, those that act peripherally at the postjunctional membrane of the neuromuscular junction and those that act on the contractile mechanism of the muscle itself.

PERIPHERALLY ACTING (QUATERNARY AMMONIUM) NEUROMUSCULAR BLOCKING AGENTS

The neuromuscular junction of voluntary muscle (Ch. 14) is a synapse with important characteristics, some of which it has in common with many synapses in the CNS. It is the focus through which the disease myasthenia gravis manifests itself (Ch. 17) and the site of action of a group of valuable muscle-relaxing drugs with a long and interesting history.

Primitive, prescientific man in South America knew of three substances of sufficient potency and availability to be used on the tips of his blow-pipe darts as disabling or poisonous agents for hunting small game. Two of these extracts both paralyzants, were obtained from distinct plant species (d-tubocurarine from *chondodendron tomentosum* and C-toxiferine I from *Strychnos toxifera*) and the third from the skin of a species of Colombian tree frog.

About 150 years ago, Brodie and Waterton showed that a preparation of crude curare killed animals by paralyzing the muscles of ventilation. Since artificial ventilation preserved life even after very large doses, the drug clearly lacked other serious toxic or adverse effects.

In 1856 Claude Bernard applied curare to a voluntary muscle preparation of the frog and found that although the muscle did not contract following nerve stimulation, it still responded to a direct electrical stimulus. When he restricted the curare to the nerve itself, it had no effect. He correctly concluded that curare acts at the neuromuscular junction.

After an adequate source of plant had been secured and a satisfactory biologic assay developed, a highly purified preparation of d-tubocurarine was introduced into clinical practice by Griffith and Johnson in 1942. The pure crystalline d-tubocurarine soon became available, and its medicinal value led to the preparation of a series of synthetic analogs from which several clinically useful compounds have emerged.

The introduction of the neuromuscular blocking agents into anesthesiology and surgery has facilitated and increased the safety of many procedures, especially in certain high-risk surgical patients, and has made possible new clinical techniques.

PHYSIOLOGY OF THE NEUROMUSCULAR JUNCTION (CH. 14)

A motor unit consists of an anterior horn cell, its processes (lower motor neuron) and the voluntary muscle fibers it supplies (Fig. 21–1). The quaternary ammonium neuromuscular blocking drugs disrupt the continuity of this unit by preventing the transmission of excitation from nerve ending to muscle fiber.

As the motor nerve approaches the muscle, it divides repeatedly and sends a single branch to each muscle fiber in the motor unit. As each nerve fiber comes in contact with its muscle fiber, it forms a small multiprocessed ending which is partly recessed into the muscle fiber surface, so that the surface membranes of both nerve and muscle are in close apposition. The space between the nerve ending (prejunctional membrane) and the muscle fiber surface is the junctional, or synaptic cleft. The muscle fiber

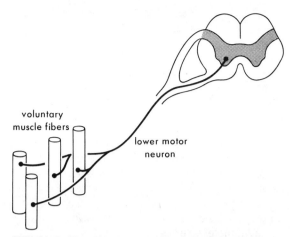

FIG. 21–1. The motor unit, consisting of the lower motor neuron and the muscle fibers it supplies. (Based on an original drawing by Siroun Ariyan.)

membrane in this area is folded and called the postjunctional membrane (Fig. 21–2).

The nerve ending contains a large number of transmitter-containing spherical synaptic vesicles which tend to be concentrated near the inner surface of the presynaptic membrane, ready to discharge into the junctional cleft. The enzyme acetylcholinesterase is localized at the postjunctional membrane.

Although the transmission of a nerve impulse along its fiber is similar to the transmission of the muscle membrane impulse, there are a break and a change in transmission mechanism at the neuromuscular junction, as there are at many other synapses.

Arrival of the nerve impulse at the nerve ending causes the presynaptic granules to liberate the positively charged organic ion acetylcholine (for formula, see Fig. 15–1) into the junctional cleft, where it almost instantly activates the postsynaptic muscle membrane and is then destroyed by acetylcholinesterase.

EVIDENCE FOR ROLE OF ACETYLCHOLINE IN TRANSMISSION AT NEUROMUSCULAR JUNCTION

There are several distinctive characteristics of transmission at the neuromuscular junction of voluntary muscle which must be emphasized. The general evidence for neurohumoral transmission is presented in Chapter 14.

ACETYLCHOLINE SYNTHESIS, STORAGE, LIBERATION AND DESTRUCTION. The presynaptic nerve endings can synthesize and store acetylcholine, which in turn is liberated into the synaptic cleft by nerve stimulation. The liberation of acetylcholine can be prevented by botulinum toxin and by hemicholinium.

Histochemical methods have shown that the enzyme acetylcholinesterase is localized at the postsynaptic membrane. Kinetic studies indicate that it can inactivate in milliseconds the acetylcholine liberated by nerve impulses.

ACETYLCHOLINE SENSITIVITY OF THE POST-JUNCTIONAL MEMBRANE. The sudden liberation of acetylcholine from a micropipette placed close to the endplate region imitates the effect of nerve fiber stimulation and causes the muscle fiber to contract. Normally the rest of the fiber membrane is insensitive to acetylcholine, but shortly after denervation, the excitable region at the end plate spreads and eventually extends over the whole fiber surface. The depolarizing actions of applied acetylcholine can be prevented by d-tubocurarine and related agents (see below).

ACTION OF ACETYLCHOLINE. The insertion of the tip of a glass ultramicroelectrode into a muscle fiber shows that there is a potential difference across the muscle membrane of approximately 90 mV. This potential difference is the same all over the fiber. Considering the thickness of the muscle membrane, this is an intense electrical gradient. It plays an essential role in transmission at the junction and in the subsequent spread of the muscle impulse along the fiber.

Using a microelectrode with its tip placed just under the postjunctional membrane, it has been shown that acetylcholine liberated by a nerve impulse (or from a micropipette) depolarizes the postjunctional membrane. The region of depolarization spreads around the fiber to form a short cylinder of depolarized membrane that divides into two which travel in opposite directions along the fiber to its end. Contraction follows.

MOLECULAR PHARMACOLOGY OF DEPOLARIZATION. The classic method of representing a drug receptor reaction is simply

$$D + R \rightleftharpoons DR$$

FIG. 21–2. Cross section of the junctional region between nerve terminal and postsynaptic membrane of voluntary muscle. (Based on an original drawing by Siroun Ariyan.)

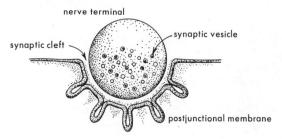

The neuromuscular blocking agents both non-depolarizers and depolarizers including acetylcholine are all positively charged ions, and when they unite with receptors they add positive charge to the receptor structure. To preserve electric neutrality the receptors loose an equivalent of magnesium or calcium ions. This process of ion exchange may be represented by

$$(R^-)_2Mg^{++} + 2ACh^+ \longrightarrow 2R^-ACh^+ + Mg^{++}$$

$$\begin{array}{c} \ominus \\ \diagup \\ \diagdown \\ \ominus \end{array} Mg^{++} + 2ACh^+ \longrightarrow \begin{array}{c} \ominus ACh^+ \\ \ominus ACh^+ \end{array} + Mg^{++}$$

where R is the receptor protein consisting of several loosely bound sub units. Sodium and potassium ions do not appear to be involved in these drug receptor exchange reactions. The displacement of the electrically bivalent magnesium or calcium ions by two monovalent acetylcholine ions may initiate depolarization by destroying the protein monomer binding provided by the divalent ions and lead to a change in the quaternary structure of the receptor protein. This change in turn opens the ion channel to the depolarizing sodium ions in the extracellular fluid.

The peripheral neuromuscular blocking agents are divided into the **nondepolarizers,** typified by d-dtubocurarine (curare), and the **depolarizers,** of which decamethonium and succinylcholine are the prototypes.

NONDEPOLARIZING NEUROMUSCULAR BLOCKING AGENTS

Primitive man knew that curare was not absorbed when given by mouth, for he ate the game he killed and invented the blowgun to put the drug through the skin. He also knew that the action of curare in low doses was reversible, for an animal which did not get an adequate dose would recover and escape. He knew that curare caused muscular weakness or paralysis and tested its ability to do so by noting the reduction in length of a frog's jump. This may have been the first bioassay.

Mode of Action

When d-tubocurarine is injected IV, it is dispersed throughout the extracellular body water but does not cross the blood-brain barrier. A small part of the injected dose combines locally and reversibly with the acetylcholine receptors on the surface of the voluntary muscle fibers in the region of the end plate and blocks transmission (Ch. 1). A much larger portion of the drug combines with "acceptors" or "sites of loss" throughout the body and produces no direct pharmacologic effects.

The union of curare with its receptors may be written as the reversible reaction

curare + receptors $\leftrightarrows$ curare-receptor complex

The union of d-tubocurarine and other non-depolarizers with acceptors, however, is slower than with receptors. It can be seen that the slower binding of curare to sites of loss has a "redistributing" effect which leads to shortening of the duration of action of this class of agent. Acceptor binding and excretion reduce the blood concentration, the curare dissociates from the neuromuscular junction and transmission gradually recovers. The amount of curare which causes paralysis is only about one-thousandth of the administered dose.

By combining with the acetylcholine receptors, curare prevents the postjunctional action of the transmitter. It does not affect liberation of the transmitter. Since curare prevents the depolarization of the postjunctional membrane by the transmitter, it is called a **nondepolarizer,** as are other compounds which act in this way. The only other nondepolarizers in regular clinical use at present are **gallamine triethiodide** and **pan curonium bromide** (Fig. 21–3).

In spite of its apparent complexity, the most important features of the curare molecule are the two positive charges on its nitrogen atoms. These charges bind the molecule to two negatively charged receptors or to one receptor and an inactive binding site (acceptor). Because of molecular flexibility, gallamine is able to fit the same receptors. In its extended configuration, the interquaternary distance in d-tubocurarine is 12.5 A.

Actions of d-Tubocurarine

Curare is a specific drug but not a particularly safe one unless the principles governing its administration are properly understood and a means of artificial ventilation is available to deal with the partial or complete respiratory paralysis that can follow its use.

EFFECT ON THE NEUROMUSCULAR JUNCTION. In man, the extraocular muscles and the hands and feet are first affected, then the muscles of the head and neck, followed by those of the abdomen and limbs. The muscles of ventilation, especially the diaphragm, are the most resistant. Although there are a few exceptions, the muscles supplied by the cranial nerves tend to be the most sensitive, the muscles of ventilation the least and other muscles intermediate.

The increased resistance to paralysis of the diaphragm and of other ventilatory muscles is important and is related to the shapes of the

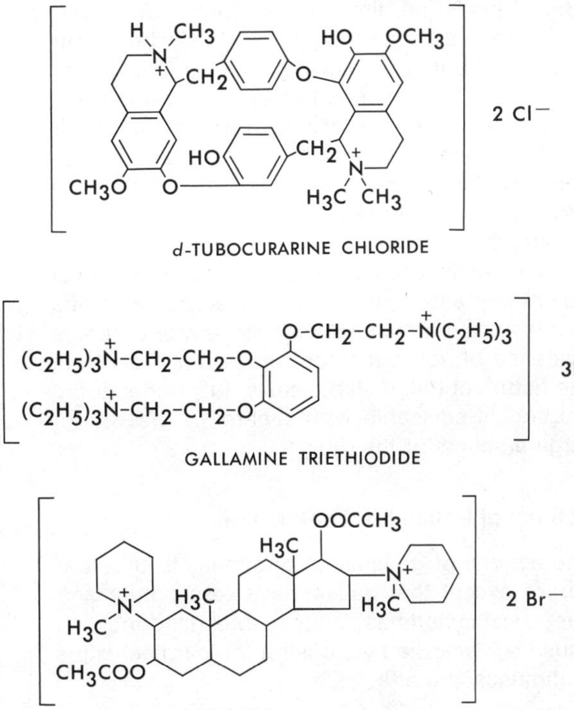

$2 Cl^-$

d-TUBOCURARINE CHLORIDE

$3I^-$

GALLAMINE TRIETHIODIDE

$2 Br^-$

PANCURONIUM BROMIDE

FIG. 21–3. The nondepolarizing quaternary ammonium neuromuscular blocking agents.

dose-response curves of different muscles (Fig. 21–4). The curve for the diaphragm is flatter than that for nonventilatory muscles. Consequently, a dose of curare that relaxes the muscles of the abdominal wall has already begun to encroach on the response of the diaphragm. *The use of curare, therefore, almost always requires some ventilatory assistance.* The dose of curare which will completely paralyze the diaphragm is about two to three times the amount that will block a nonventilatory muscle.

EFFECT ON AUTONOMIC GANGLIA. Curare can block all autonomic ganglia in doses above those needed for muscular relaxation. Such autonomic blockade may occasionally contribute to undesirable hypotension during operative procedures.

EFFECT ON OTHER SYSTEMS. Other than the consequences of autonomic blockade, curare has no action on the antonomic nervous system or on cardiac and smooth muscle.

Pancuronium Bromide

Pancuronium is a typical nondepolarizing agent that was introduced into clinical medicine in

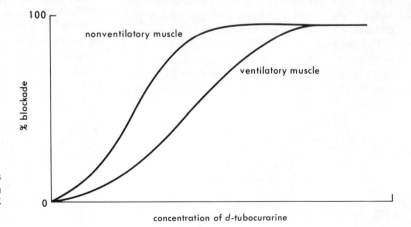

FIG. 21–4. Dose-response curves for the effect of d-tubocurarine on isolated ventilatory and nonventilatory muscle.

1967. Since that time it has found increased acceptance as a safe agent relatively free from side effects. It is about four times more potent than d-tubocurarine and has about the same rate of onset and duration of action. Unlike curare, it does not release histamine or have any significant ganglion blocking activity. It does not cause any fall in arterial pressure and may even raise it a little. It seems to have no undesirable actions on the cardiovascular system. It has no effects commonly associated with the steroid nucleus and is excreted mainly by the kidney, but there is evidence of some metabolism in the liver. Until the nature of this metabolism is fully understood, caution is advisable with regard to the use of large amounts of the drug.

Actions of Gallamine Triethiodide

The actions of gallamine are similar to those of curare except that gallamine is less potent and has the sometimes undesirable tendency to cause tachycardia by blocking the cardiac vagus (antimuscarinic effect, Ch. 17).

Antagonists

Anticholinesterases (Ch. 16), by prolonging the life of the liberated acetylcholine, have a decurarizing action. Their effect is limited, however. They cannot reverse supraparalytic doses of the nondepolarizers, since doses of anticholinesterase beyond those which block the enzyme completely have no further useful effect. Potassium ions also antagonize the nondepolarizers but are not used clinically because of adverse cardiac and other effects (Ch. 33).

DEPOLARIZING NEUROMUSCULAR BLOCKING AGENTS

The drugs of the methonium series were among the first clinically useful peripherally acting agents related to d-tubocurarine to be synthesized. They are simple, slender, flexible bis-quaternary ammonium positively charged ions of the general structure shown in Figure 21–5.

The series reaches maximal activity on voluntary muscle when n is 10. Consequently, the compound is called **decamethonium** or **C-10** (Ch. 20). In the extended form, the interquaternary distance, like that for d-tubocurarine, is approximately 12.5 A.

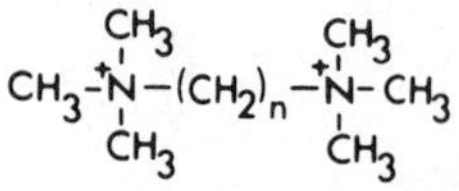

$$CH_3-\overset{+}{\underset{\underset{CH_3}{|}}{\overset{\overset{CH_3}{|}}{N}}}-(CH_2)_n-\overset{+}{\underset{\underset{CH_3}{|}}{\overset{\overset{CH_3}{|}}{N}}}-CH_3$$

FIG. 21–5. The methonium series of drugs.

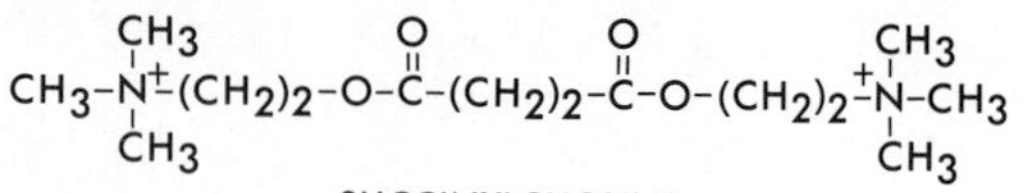

$$CH_3-\overset{+}{\underset{\underset{CH_3}{|}}{\overset{\overset{CH_3}{|}}{N}}}-(CH_2)_2-O-\overset{\overset{O}{\|}}{C}-(CH_2)_2-\overset{\overset{O}{\|}}{C}-O-(CH_2)_2-\overset{+}{\underset{\underset{CH_3}{|}}{\overset{\overset{CH_3}{|}}{N}}}-CH_3$$

SUCCINYLCHOLINE

Succinylcholine is the dicholine ester of succinic acid. The compound resembles decamethonium in being a long, slender, flexible bis-quaternary positively charged ion and is equivalent to two acetylcholine ions joined back to back. For the purposes of this discussion decamethonium and succinylcholine are considered together as the **depolarizers.** Although, like the nondepolarizers, they cause paralysis by an action at the neuromuscular junction, they differ from the nondepolarizers in several important respects.

Mode of Action

Decamethonium and succinylcholine resemble acetylcholine in that they depolarize the postjunctional muscle membrane at the motor end plate. Because these two compounds are much more stable at the neuromuscular junction than acetylcholine, the depolarization they produce is prolonged. It spreads to a small area of muscle membrane around the nerve ending. Since the depolarized membrane is inexcitable, conduction is interrupted.

In contradistinction to the nondepolarizers, which act at the muscle fiber surface and do not enter, *the depolarizers enter muscle fibers* in small amounts, especially at the end-plate region. This entry can be blocked by the nondepolarizers. In fact, these effects reflect the mode of action of curare and the nondepolarizers at the molecular level. In rats given tritium labeled decamethonium, the drug can be detected inside the muscle fibers 2 weeks later.

TWO-PHASE BLOCK. If the concentration of curare or one of the nondepolarizers around a muscle is kept constant, the degree of paralysis remains steady until the drug is removed. This is not true for the depolarizers.

When a constant concentration of a depolarizer is applied to an isolated muscle, paralysis progresses (phase 1 block) to some maximum value (Fig. 21–6) and then declines again in spite of the presence of the depolarizer. The recovery of transmission marks the end of phase 1 block but not the end of the process of paralysis. The recovery from phase 1 is followed by a second slowly increasing paralysis (phase 2) that reaches a steady value only after several hours and from which there is no recovery as long as the depolarizer is present. Phase 2 block differs from phase 1 not only in its slow onset but also in its response to antagonists. It is a nondepolarizing

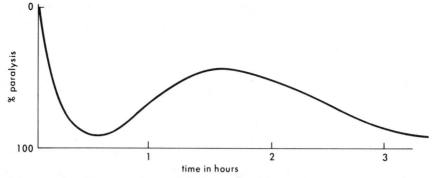

FIG. 21–6. Relation between time and degree of paralysis for the effect of a depolarizer (decamethonium) on isolated voluntary muscle.

type of block and resembles that produced by curare in that it is antagonized by anticholinesterases.

This dual block is a characteristic feature of the action of depolarizers on all voluntary muscle, animal or human, and there is evidence that the onset of phase 2 block is associated with the entry of depolarizers into the muscle fibers. Phase 2 block is seen in man and manifests itself initially as an increasing resistance or tachyphylaxis to repeated injections of decamethonium or succinylcholine. It occurs clinically in response to a high dose or to prolonged administration of both decamethonium and succinylcholine. In the case of the latter drug, phase 2 block readily appears in patients with atypical or reduced cholinesterase (Chs. 8,16). The safest treatment for a prolonged phase 2 type of block is ventilation and patience. Although an anticholinesterase may be helpful, it may delay the ultimate hydrolysis and disposal of succinylcholine.

Actions of Decamethonium and Succinylcholine

In man, the rapid injection of any of the depolarizers is liable to produce some muscular fasciculation. As the effect of the drug progresses, the fasciculations are replaced by increasing paralysis, with relaxation of the muscles of the neck and limbs preceding those of the abdomen and trunk. The muscles of ventilation are most resistant, as in the case of the nondepolarizers. There is no significant difference between the ventilatory muscle sparing ability of the depolarizers and the nondepolarizers. The fibrillation associated with rapid injection is greater after succinylcholine than after decamethonium and can be minimized by the slow administration of the well-diluted drug or by prior administration of a small dose of a nondepolarizer.

Succinycholine is clinically the most important depolarizer because of its short duration of action and the lack of toxicity of its breakdown products, succinic acid and choline, both normal metabolites. But it may produce postoperative muscle pain, which can be reduced by slow administration of the agent or bed rest.

The drug is first hydrolyzed by plasma cholinesterase into the pharmacologically inactive succinylmonocholine and choline. Later, the succinylmonocholine is further hydrolyzed into succinic acid and choline. The duration of action of succinylcholine is about one-third that of d-tubocurarine (Table 21–1). If an overdose is given, metabolism of the drug rapidly restores transmission.

Antagonists

Since acetylcholine also depolarizes, the anticholinesterases do not antagonize decamethonium induced or succinylcholine induced paralysis and must not be used clinically in an attempt to do this. There are no clinically effective antagonists for the depolarizers.

METABOLISM AND EXCRETION OF NEUROMUSCULAR BLOCKING AGENTS

There is no evidence that d-tubocurarine, gallamine or decamethonium are metabolized in man but they are chiefly excreted in the urine.

CLINICAL PHARMACOLOGY AND USES OF NEUROMUSCULAR BLOCKING AGENTS

The peripherally acting neuromuscular blocking agents are virtually restricted to professional

TABLE 21–1. Dosage and Recovery Time for Commonly Used Neuromuscular Blocking Agents

	Initial dose (mg)	Time for recovery (min)
Gallamine	40–100	20–35
Succinylcholine	10–50	8–12
d-Tubocurarine	6–18	20–35
Pancuronium	2–4	30–35

medical use and are not given to patients for personal administration. Their therapeutic use requires trained personnel and the immediate availability of complete facilities for artificial ventilation because of the danger of ventilatory paralysis.

These agents are used chiefly by anesthesiologists to relax voluntary muscle in preference to deepening the level of general anesthesia. Without good muscular relaxation, it is virtually impossible for the surgeon to gain access to the abdominal cavity. The stimulation of the operation causes intense reflex muscular contraction and rigidity of the abdominal wall. Consequently, operative procedures are greatly facilitated by the muscle relaxants. Relaxants also facilitate endotracheal intubation and the reduction of dislocations and fractures.

In ophthalmic surgery, the great sensitivity of the extracular muscles to the nondepolarizers makes these agents the drugs of choice when it is necessary to mobilize the eyeball. The depolarizers, especially succinylcholine, are not used because they may cause undesirable contracture of the extraocular muscles and mechanically raise the intraocular pressure.

In thoracic surgery, muscle relaxants are used to relax the chest wall and paralyze the diaphragm, so reducing movement of the mediastinum. Relaxants are also used in electroconvulsive therapy to protect the patient from the violence of his own muscular contractions.

Selection of Muscle Relaxant

The choice of muscle relaxant and its dosage is made chiefly, but not exclusively, on the basis of the needed duration of relaxation. The site and requirements of the operation, the anesthetic and other agents used and any pathologic conditions which alters the patient's sensitivity to these agents are also relevant.

A single dose of succinylcholine is the most suitable agent for procedures not exceeding 3 min such as endotracheal intubation, the reduction of dislocations and fractures and shock therapy. For procedures not exceeding 15–20 min, a single dose of d-tubocurarine or gallamine will suffice. For prolonged procedures, relaxation can be maintained in several ways. Succinylcholine can be given by continuous infusion, or relaxation may be induced by d-tubocurarine or gallamine and maintained by small repeat doses of these agents.

Dosage and Related Problems

Since many factors influence sensitivity to neuromuscular blocking agents, the initial dose for a given patient is difficult to estimate. Furthermore, the proper assessment of the effect of the initial dose is important in deciding on the size of repeat doses. Since it takes approximately 5 min for the nondepolarizers to produce their maximal effect, it is necessary to wait for this period before assessing the effect and before giving any further dose. The maximal effect of succinylcholine is seen after 2–3 min.

Although all the factors determining individual sensitivity are not known those discussed below are important.

PHYSICAL CHARACTERISTICS. The correct dose is related to body weight. It is higher for muscular than for nonmuscular individuals, higher for males than for females and higher for the young than for the aged.

INFLUENCE OF GENERAL ANESTHETIC. Some inhalation anesthetics potentiate nondepolarizers but not depolarizers. Under ether anesthesia the dose of d-tubocurarine can be reduced to about a third to a quarter of the usual dose. Practical advantage can be taken of this so that at the end of the procedure, when the anesthetic is discontinued, there will be less likelihood of ventilatory depression due to persistence of the action of curare. Fluroxene, methoxyflurane, halothane and cyclopropane (Ch. 25) also potentiate d-tubocurarine and, to a lesser extent, gallamine.

ALTERED PATIENT SENSITIVITY. Patients with myasthenia gravis are exquisitely sensitive to nondepolarizers and are somewhat resistant to depolarizers. Fortunately, relaxants are seldom needed in these patients.

CONCOMITANT PATHOLOGIC AND METABOLIC DISTURBANCES. Dehydration, by raising plasma drug levels, by reducing renal excretion, and by decreasing cellular excitability, increases sensitivity to relaxants and may prolong their effects. Excessive loss of extracellular potassium due to chronic diarrhea, renal disease, chlorothiazide therapy or other causes also increases the effects of the antidepolarizers.

By impairing excretion, severe renal disease may prolong the effects of the stable muscle relaxants, although this effect is seen only after high doses of the drugs. After low doses, the effects of the nondepolarizers are largely terminated by the slow distribution of the drugs to acceptors or sites of loss. Renal excretion becomes a limiting factor in terminating relaxant effects only when the sites of loss have been saturated by large or repeated doses.

An approximate dosage range is indicated in

Table 21–1. Repeat doses of *d*-tubocurarine and gallamine are a third to a quater of the initial dose, but depend on the effect of the initial dose and the time elapsed since it was given.

Muscle relaxants are administered in dilute solution and should be given slowly. A sudden large dose of relaxant may stop breathing and cause a fall of arterial pressure.

THE USE OF ANTAGONISTS TO THE NONDEPOLARIZERS

Antagonists are needed chiefly for postoperative management and (less frequently) in the event of accidental overdose of nondepolarizers. The terminal stages of some operative procedures, notably peritoneal closure, may require the use of relaxants, so the patient may remain paralyzed at the end of the operation. Consequently, it is helpful to be able to accelerate effective and lasting recovery. Present antagonists (anticholinesterases) are effective against the nondepolarizers, but only against the phase 2 block of the depolarizers; they may actually potentiate phase 1 block.

In the treatment of ventilatory depression, there is no substitute for artificial ventilation. If the duration of action of the antagonist is shorter than that of the paralyzant, the patient may again become paralyzed and die if antagonists are solely relied on. Furthermore, the ventilatory depression may not be due to the relaxant, in which case artificial ventilation and other appropriate measures are indicated. Since the state of neuromuscular transmission can be monitored postoperatively by transdermal stimulation of the ulnar nerve, the contribution of relaxants in ventilatory depression can be unequivocally determined.

Although **neostigmine** is the most commonly used antagonist, **pyridostigmine** is also suitable. Neostigmine adminstered in a dose of 0.5–2.0 mg should inactivate all cholinesterase. Nothing is gained by increasing the dose over 5 mg. It should be given slowly after atropine (0.4 mg) to prevent undesirable parasympathomimetic effects (Ch. 16).

ADVERSE EFFECTS OF NEUROMUSCULAR BLOCKING AGENTS

The margin of safety between the dose of a neuromuscular blocking agent which produces a useful relaxation and the dose which stops ventilation is not large. This represents the chief source of danger in the use of these agents.

There is clinical evidence that curare may occasionally liberate histamine, although this has never been conclusively demonstrated in man. Since gallamine and pancuronium do not liberate histamine, they are the drugs of choice for asthmatics. Gallamine may cause tachycardia by blocking the cardiac vagus. In high doses, curare may contribute to hypotension by blocking autonomic ganglia.

Succinylcholine, injected IV, causes contractions, muscular fasciculations and often postoperative muscle pain. Its most important, if occasional, adverse effect is prolonged apnea which may be associated with a congenital deficiency of plasma cholinesterase or the presence of an atypical cholinesterase enzyme (Ch.8).

The neuromuscular blocking agents should be well diluted and administered slowly to avoid sudden ventilatory arrest and/or severe fasciculations and contractions of voluntary muscle.

Fatal ventilatory depression has occurred in anesthetized patients following the peritoneal and immediate postoperative administration (Ch. 56) of such antibiotics as neomycin, streptomycin, dihydrostreptomycin and polymyxin B (Chs. 56, 58), which have neuromuscular blocking activity.

PROMOTION OF SAFETY IN USE OF NEUROMUSCULAR BLOCKING AGENTS

When neuromuscular blocking agents are used, it is important not only to avoid trouble but also to cope with it should it occur. Appreciation of the following general points will help ensure useful and safe relaxation:

1. Use the most appropriate relaxant in the minimum dose necessary to achieve the desired result.
2. Do not attempt to achieve prolonged relaxation by increasing the dose of relaxant.
3. Do not give a repeat dose until the effect of the first has been determined.
4. Discontinue the administration of depolarizer if desensitization to its effects develop.
5. Do not change from one type of relaxant to another arbitrarily. Always use well-known, well-tried procedures.
6. Never use an antagonist as a substitute in circumstances where assisted or supported ventilation is the real need.

DIRECTLY ACTING MUSCLE RELAXANT

Dantrolene sodium is a synthetic agent that acts directly on the contractile mechanism of voluntary muscle without actions on nerve conduction or transmission of excitation at the neuromuscular junction. It has the advantages of being orally active and has a long duration of action.

$$O_2N-\text{(ring)}-O-CH=N-N-C\overset{O}{\underset{NNa}{}}$$
$$H_2C-C\overset{O}{}$$

DANTROLENE SODIUM

The effects of a single dose may begin 1–2 hr after administration and last for several hours. Recently introduced, this agent has an extensive and complex list of adverse side effects, and its use must be carefully evaluated against its adverse actions. Patients must be monitored with respect to both its useful actions and side effects.

Indications

The chief indication for dantrolene sodium is disabling skeletal muscle spasticity resulting from serious chronic disorders such as spinal cord injury, stroke, cerebral palsy and multiple sclerosis. The drug is not used for rheumatic spasm.

Dosage

Dosage should start low and be increased gradually to meet individual patient's needs. Beneficial effects are slow in onset and may take a week or more to develop. Complete information on precautions, adverse reactions and contraindications should be studied before administration. An exhaustive list is beyond the scope of this account.

Precautions

Impaired pulmonary or hepatic function or myocardial disease require caution. Liver function tests should be done before and during therapy. Dantrolene may cause photosensitivity and impair performance in driving motor vehicles. It should not be given to pregnant women, nursing mothers or children under five.

Adverse Reactions

The majority of adverse reactions are reversible, and some are transient and may decrease with use. In general, a low initial dose, gradually increased, minimizes undesirable effects.

Tumors both benign and malignant have been produced in rats by dantrolene, and the benefits of chronic administration to humans must be weighed against this.

CENTRALLY ACTING MUSCLE RELAXANTS

The first centrally acting compound (antodyne) to relax voluntary muscle without loss of consciousness was synthesized in 1910. This lead, in spite of its potential clinical value in various types of spasticity, was not followed up until 1946, when a search for better compounds was started. Antodyne was a simple ether of glycerol. Later relaxants were developed from other polyhydroxy compounds, and recently the ability to relax voluntary muscle by central action has been found in compounds of quite different structures (Fig. 21–7). Although the effects of these agents on experimental animals are impressive, they leave something to be desired in human practice. Moreover, these agents do not produce the rapid profound relaxation characteristic of the neuromuscular blocking agents.

Actions

The centrally acting muscle relaxants are not a sharply defined pharmacologic group but a heterogeneous collection of agents with other actions. Several compounds originally introduced for other purposes have subsequently shown muscle relaxant properties.

MUSCLE RELAXATION. Low doses tend to reduce spontaneous activity and muscle tone. As the dose is raised, ataxia, flaccid paralysis and even ventilatory depression and death may occur. There is no preparalytic excitement.

EFFECTS ON REFLEXES. In clinically useful doses, the knee jerk is unaffected because there is no internuncial neuron between the afferent and efferent pathways. However, reflexes such as the crossed extensor, involving multiple connecting neurons, are depressed or blocked. Decerebrate rigidity is reduced. There is evidence that neurons in the brain stem, thalamus and basal ganglia may also be depressed.

STRYCHNINE ANTAGONISM. Animals can be protected from strychnine poisoning by nonparalyzing doses. This characteristic emphasizes that the chief site of action of these centrally acting muscle relaxants is the spinal cord, where strychnine has its main action. On the molecular level, the mechanism is unknown.

OTHER EFFECTS. Some sedative, local anesthetic, antipyretic and anticonvulsant actions

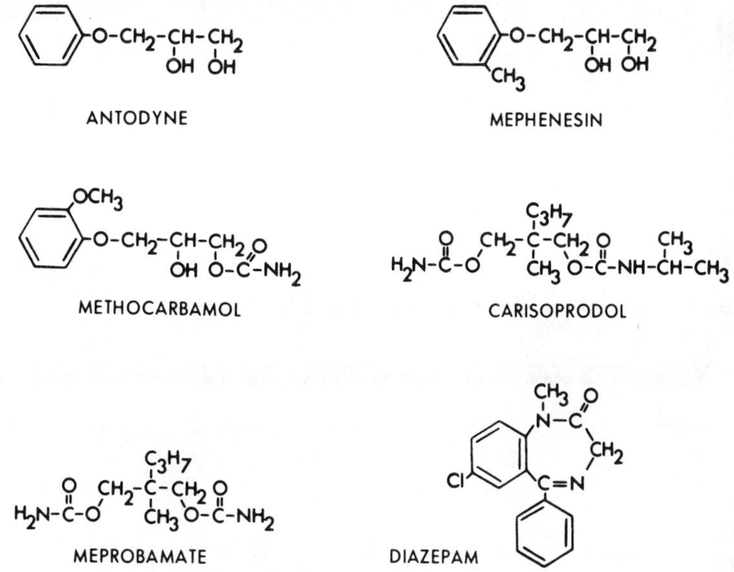

FIG. 21-7. Some centrally acting muscle relaxants.

have been encountered in the group but are not important. No effective degree of analgesia has been detected. Some component of muscle relaxation has been noted among certain antihistamines (orphenadrine) and minor tranquilizers (meprobamate).

Clinical Pharmacology and Uses

The low efficacy of the centrally acting muscle relaxants following oral administration in human practice is accentuated by the definite clinical need for such agents. They have been used for virtually all conditions of painful muscle spasm or spasticity. In acute painful spasm associated with trauma, when the spasm is resistant to extension and where splinting may contribute to a vicious cycle, the breaking of the cycle with an adequate dose of relaxant may achieve real and lasting relief. The chronic spasticity that is a major and disabling consequence of neurologic disorder is harder to treat.

FURTHER READING

Foldes FF (1957): Muscle Relaxants in Anesthesiology. Springfield, Ill. Thomas

Foldes FF (ed) (1966): Muscle Relaxants. Philadelphia, Davis

Taylor DB (1959): The mechanism of action of muscle relaxants and their antagonists. Anesthesiology 20:439

Taylor DB (1973): The role of inorganic ions in exchange processes at the cholinergic receptor of voluntary muscle. J Pharmacol Exp Ther 186:537

Wylie WD, Churchill-Davidson HC (1966): A Practice of Anesthesia. (2nd ed) London, Lloyd-Luke

PETER LOMAX

22. LOCAL ANESTHETICS

Local anesthetics are drugs that block conduction in nerve tissue when applied in appropriate concentrations. Many compounds have this property but often cause permanent neural damage or else are too toxic following systemic absorption from their site of application. With clinically useful local anesthetics, the blocking effect is completely reversible, no functional damage to the nerve occurs and serious systemic effects are rare.

A good local anesthetic should be nonirritating to the tissues, cause no permanent damage, have a low systemic toxicity, be effective both topically and when injected, have a short latent period before onset and an adequate duration of action,

LIDOCAINE

be soluble in water and stable in solution and be sterilizable without deterioration.

The naturally occurring alkaloid cocaine was the first local anesthetic used clinically. A chemical search for substitutes led to the discovery of procaine (1905). Subsequently, an extremely large number of local anesthetics has been synthesized. The local anesthetics in common use are described in Table 22–1.

CHEMISTRY

The useful local anesthetics are structurally similar and consist of a lipophilic aromatic group, an intermediate chain and a hydrophilic amine group. The general formula is shown in Figure 22–1 together with that of procaine. The amino group is always either a tertiary or a secondary amine. The link between the aromatic and the intermediate group is either an ester link —CO—OCH$_2$, as in procaine, or an amide link —NH—COCH$_2$, as in lidocaine.

Changes in any part of the molecule may change the potency or toxicity of the drug. Increasing the length of the intermediate chain leads to greater potency and toxicity. A compound with an ethyl ester link, such as procaine, is usually the least toxic. The toxicity and potency of synthetic local anesthetics are always compared with procaine as the standard.

All local anesthetics are bases with a pK$_a$ in the range 7–9 and are only sparingly soluble in water. These compounds form salts with strong acids and most often are supplied for clinical use as the hydrochlorides. The salts are freely soluble in water and give rise to solutions with a pH of 6 or less. When these salts are injected into the tissues (pH 7.4), the buffering effect of the tissue fluids leads to the release of free base (Fig. 22–2).

The products of infection in inflamed tissues tend to lower the pH, and if a local anesthetic is injected into such sites, less base is liberated and consequently less effective anesthesia results.

MECHANISM OF ACTION

The sequence of changes in the nerve fiber following local application of the anesthetic agent

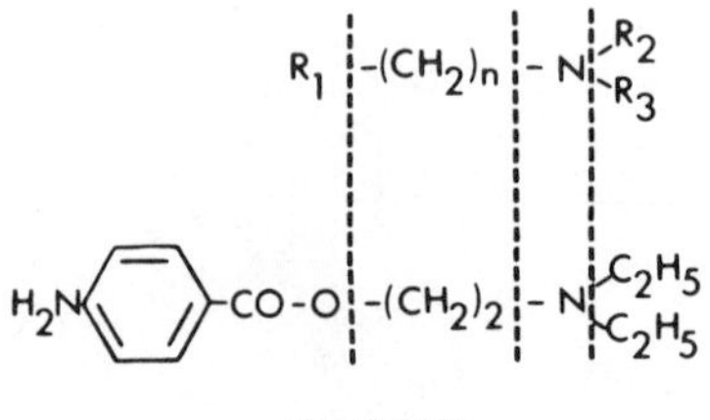

PROCAINE

FIG. 22–1. General structural formula of local anesthetics and procaine.

TABLE 22-1. Common Local Anesthetics

Drug	Trade name	Concentration %	Latency (min)	Duration (hr)	Comment
Dibucaine hydrochloride	Nupercaine	0.1	10	3	Fifteen times potency and toxicity of procaine
Lidocaine hydrochloride	Xylocaine	0.5—2.0	1	4—5	About equal toxicity to procaine. Best surface anesthetic. Effective without epinephrine in patients sensitive to epinephrine. So dissimilar to procaine (is an amino acyl amide) that it can be used in patients sensitive to former. Causes sleepiness
Mepivacaine hydrochloride	Carbocaine	1—2			Similar to lidocaine with slightly faster onset and longer duration
Procaine hydrochloride	Novocaine	1—2	2—5	1	
Tetracaine hydrochloride	Amethocaine, Pontocaine	0.25	5—10	2	Ten times potency and toxicity of procaine. Good surface anesthetic

can be followed by electrophysiologic methods. Changes consist of an increase in the threshold for electric stimulation, slowing of the rate of propagation of the impulse, reduction in the rate of rise of the action potential and eventual complete block of conduction.

The fundamental process in nerve conduction is the large transient rise in sodium permeability of the neural membrane, which is triggered by a slight depolarization of the membrane. The changes enumerated above can be explained as the result of increasing blockade of this process. The end effect of these changes is that the nerve membrane becomes stabilized and cannot be depolarized by the potentials reaching the blocked region. Thus conduction is blocked.

The local anesthetic must enter the nerve fiber in order to reach its site of action. The anesthetic crosses the nerve membrane in the uncharged form. Inside the fiber a large proportion returns to the charged form, and it may be this cationic state of the drug which is responsible for its action. pH differences on each side of the neural membrane may lead to a higher concentration of local anesthetic inside than outside the fiber (Ch. 2). The intimate processes concerned in the transient depolarization of the membrane are still poorly understood. There is some evidence that calcium ions are involved in the sodium transport mechanism and that the removal of these is the initial step. It has been suggested that the primary effect of local anesthetics is to interfere with this release.

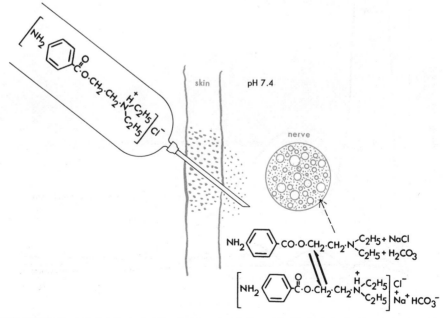

FIG. 22-2. Procaine injected subcutaneously as the chloride salt is buffered by the extracellular fluid, and free procaine base is liberated and enters the nerves.

PHARMACOLOGIC ACTIONS
AND THERAPEUTIC APPLICATIONS

Whatever the mechanism of action of local anesthetics, a critical concentration must be built up inside the nerve fiber in order to block conduction. To achieve this, the concentration around the nerve must be many times the level that would be toxic systemically. Thus local application is necessary.

One of the major factors governing the time taken to reach this particular axoplasmic concentration is the ratio of volume to surface area of the fiber. Small fibers tend to be blocked before large fibers. This sequence can sometimes be seen clinically when the small autonomic fibers are blocked before the larger diameter sensory or motor fibers to voluntary muscle.

Increasing the concentration of the local anesthetic injected increases the amount that enters the nerve fiber. This does not alter the degree of block in an individual fiber once the threshold level is reached, but since the time taken for the greater amount of anesthetic to diffuse out of the nerve is longer, the duration of blockade will be increased. However, the higher the concentration, the greater the chance of systemic intoxication.

In the case of topical application of local anesthetics to mucous membranes, there appears to be an optimal concentration, and further increases in concentration not only fail to prolong the duration of anesthesia but may even reduce it.

There is a latent period, which may amount to several minutes, between administration of the anesthetic and onset of blockade. The longer acting local anesthetics have longer latent periods, e.g., dibucaine > tetracaine > procaine (Table 22–1). Failure to allow for this latency, and the application of unnecessary further quantities of the drug to shorten it, can lead to severe or lethal toxic reactions.

All the local anesthetic is eventually absorbed into the blood stream, regardless of its site of application. If this absorption is slow, then dilution, storage and metabolism prevent toxic blood levels from occurring.

After perineural infiltration in quantities normally employed, the concentration of the drug in blood is barely perceptible. Rapid absorption occurs from the mucous membranes following topical application, and the blood levels approach 50% of those found after rapid IV injection of the same dose. For anesthetizing mucous membranes, the dose should be divided into several fractions, and a few minutes should elapse between each application. The relative blood levels of a local anesthetic after various methods of administration are shown in Figure 22–3. Ab-

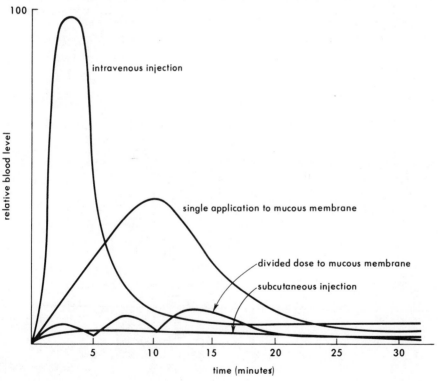

FIG. 22–3. Relative blood levels of a local anesthetic following various methods of administration.

sorption from mucous membranes varies considerably. It is more rapid from the trachea than from the larynx and pharynx, for instance, and gravitation into the trachea can be avoided by anesthetizing the larynx with the patient in a head-down position. No appreciable absorption occurs from the stomach or from the bladder and urethra. Instrumental trauma at these latter sites, however, may allow absorption through the damaged epithelium. Local anesthetics are not absorbed through the unbroken skin or from the denuded areas of first- or second-degree burns.

In order to slow absorption and prolong the duration of action, vasoconstrictors are frequently added to local anesthetic solutions. Epinephrine is most effective. Norepinephrine may cause sloughing of the tissues. Vasoconstrictors can be used effectively when the anesthetic is perfused around nerve fibers, infiltrated under the skin or used intrathecally for spinal anesthesia. However, vasoconstrictors do not alter the duration of action or rate of absorption of local anesthetics applied to mucous membranes.

Effective constriction of the vessels is achieved with a concentration of, for epinephrine, 1:200,000. Generally about twice this concentration is mixed with the anesthetic initially to allow for deterioration and losses during sterilization.

Most local anesthetics are vasodilators owing to direct paralysis of the muscle of the vessel wall. Cocaine is the only true vasoconstrictor. It blocks the uptake of catecholamines released from the vasoconstrictor nerve terminals and so enhances the sympathetic effect (Ch. 14). Owing to its high toxicity, cocaine is now little used except for shrinking the mucous membranes before antrostomy. This constrictive action of cocaine does not, however, retard its rate of absorption from the mucous membrane.

Norepinephrine may be responsible for delayed wound healing, as it not only reduces the blood supply but it also increases tissue oxygen consumption. Trials have been initiated using vasopressin (Ch. 43) or a synthetic analog (felly-pressin) as the vasoconstrictor since it does not have this metabolic effect.

ADVERSE EFFECTS

The ester and amide types of local anesthetics undergo hydrolytic cleavage, and the products are excreted in the urine. Detoxification takes place mainly in the liver, and little or no destruction of the drug occurs in the perineural tissues. Data on the metabolic fate of many of the drugs in man are lacking. Cholinesterases are involved in the degradation of the ester-linked compounds. The rate of removal varies with the metabolic state of the patient, and esterase activity may be reduced in certain diseases such as toxic goiter, severe anemia, hepatic dysfunction and any debilitating condition.

Paraminobenzoic acid is produced from metabolism of procaine and other anesthetics, and this could possibly interfere with the action of sulfonamides. Amide-linked local anesthetics should be used during sulfonamide therapy.

The value of a local anesthetic is most dependent on its toxicity, although potency and duration are important characteristics. Potency and toxicity are not clearly related. The type and severity of toxic reactions to local anesthetics depend upon many factors, including the inherent toxicity of the drug, the susceptibility of the patient and the blood level. This latter depends upon the rate of absorption from the injection site, the rate of diffusion through the tissues and the rate of inactivation. Certain precautions can be taken to ensure that the concentration of the anesthetic in the blood is kept at a low level. The amount used should be kept to a minimum; the most dilute effective solution should be used; vasoconstrictors should be employed where possible and care should be taken to avoid intravascular injection.

Toxic reactions are referable to either CNS or the cardiovascular system. The onset of toxic effects is generally heralded by prodromal symptoms and signs. Epinephrine may cause tachycardia, palpitations, restlessness and anxiety. Such symptoms and signs may be confused with toxic reactions to the anesthetic. It is better not to use epinephrine in patients with severe myocardial disease.

CENTRAL NERVOUS SYSTEM. Initially there are signs of central stimulation which may be due to depression of inhibitory areas. Depression follows if the blood levels of the drug continue to increase. Prodromal signs are excitement, apprehension, disorientation, nausea and vomiting. The condition may then progress to twitching, convulsions and finally respiratory paralysis and circulatory failure. The convulsive phase is treated by giving an ultra short-acting barbiturate, administering oxygen and providing general supportive therapy. Pretreatment with a barbiturate has been recommended for procedures involving extensive nerve block in hospitalized patients.

CARDIOVASCULAR. The onset of toxic effects may be heralded by pallor, tachycardia and syncope. The drug may have a toxic effect directly on the myocardium and circulation, and gradual or sudden general circulatory failure results. Drowsiness and coma can occur. Vasopressor agents such as ephedrine, methoxamine or phenylephrine are used to treat the circulatory collapse. Oxygen, artificial respiration and cardiac massage should be used without delay if required.

Local anesthetics are frequently used preferentially in so-called "poor-risk" patients. It should be remembered, however, that these same patients are also more likely to develop adverse reactions to local anesthetics.

TECHNIQUES FOR LOCAL ANESTHESIA

SURFACE. For application to wounds, ulcers and burns the local anesthetic bases can be dissolved in ointments. A 2% solution of lidocaine in carboxymethylcellulose can be used to anesthetize the mucous membranes of the mouth and pharynx, e.g., before subcutaneous infiltration or the passage of gastric tubes. Solutions are usually sprayed onto the mucous membranes of the larynx and nasal passages. Many local anesthetics such as procaine are ineffective as surface anesthetics unless applied in extremely high concentrations and are therefore not used in this manner.

INFILTRATION. The nerve endings in the infiltration area are blocked directly.

BLOCK. The main nerve trunks (e.g., the occipital nerve) or a plexus (e.g., brachial plexus) are infiltrated so that the field of distribution of the nerves is anesthetized.

SPINAL. The spinal nerve roots are anesthetized by injecting the local anesthetic into the subarachnoid space (into the cerebrospinal fluid). The injection is generally made into the fourth lumbar intravertebral space. The level of anesthesia attained depends on many factors, mainly the position of the patient and the specific gravity of the injected solution, which is adjusted by the addition of glucose.

EPIDURAL. The anesthetic is introduced into the epidural space below the second lumbar segment. The mixed nerves in the paravertebral space and nerve roots are blocked.

CAUDAL. The anesthetic is introduced into the epidural space of the sacral canal.

FURTHER READING

Adriani J (1960): The clinical pharmacology of local anesthetics. Clin Pharmacol Ther 1:645

Adriani J (1960): The Pharmacology of Anesthetic Drugs. Springfield, Ill, Thomas

Ritchie JM, Greengard P (1966): On the mode of action of local anesthetics. Ann Rev Pharmacol 6:405

DRUGS ACTING ON THE CENTRAL NERVOUS SYSTEM

ROBERT H. ROTH

23. CENTRAL NERVOUS SYSTEM

TRANSMITTER MECHANISMS

The brain is composed of a complex collection of millions of nerve cells and processes that are functionally interconnected but anatomically independent. Information in the form of an impulse originating in a single neuron can propagate throughout the CNS over a wide variety of neuronal pathways. The actual route taken by any given impulse is determined largely by the inborn organization of the brain, but ongoing neuronal events can establish new circuits as a result of the neuronal plasticity of the CNS. In this manner numerous variations in circuitry and associated behavioral patterns can be established. For meaningful activity to occur, impulses must be transmitted from one nerve to the next. This transmission process, believed to be a chemical phenomenon in the majority of mammalian synapses, is therefore an essential part of neural function since it is the means by which neurons communicate with one another. Thus the highest processes of neural activity, i.e., behavior, memory, emotion, etc., have a chemical basis that is related at least in part to the interneuronal transmission process. The chemical substances that are responsible for transferring nerve impulses from one neuron to the next are referred to collectively as **neurotransmitters.**

In recent years the major emphasis of neuropharmacologic research has been upon presumptive transmitter substances, their life cycles and the substances that modify these cycles. Since chemical transmission of impulses across synaptic junctions is the major means by which neurons communicate with each other, alteration in such communication could represent key mechanisms through which drugs might influence neuronal function. Probably the ultimate action of the majority of psychotropic drugs will turn out to involve modulation of ongoing activity in one neuronal system or another by interfering with the life cycle of transmitter agents. The spec-

ificity of action of any given drug would then depend primarily upon which transmitter or which synapse was affected and the nature of the change produced, whether it was inhibition or facilitation. It is not difficult to imagine that psychotropic drugs can alter neuronal function by altering the disposition of one or perhaps several neurotransmitter agents. What is more difficult to comprehend is the contrast between the action of a drug on a simple neuronal system causing it either to fire or not to fire or altering its rate of firing and the wide diversity of CNS effects including subtle changes in mood and behavior which such a drug will induce.

At first sight, the concept that a given psychotropic drug acts at a given synapse by interfering with a given transmitter agent seems quite simple. On a more practical level, however, the study of synaptic transmission and the life cycle of transmitter substances in the mammalian CNS poses a number of formidable technical problems for the pharmacologist. In the first place, the total amounts of transmitter present in the CNS are quite small and the actual amount involved in the transmission process almost impossible to measure. In addition, the neurons under study are usually exceedingly small, only 10–20 μ in diameter, and the synapses themselves, approximately 200 Å wide, are very difficult to isolate and study.

Although the cellular organization of the brain and spinal cord has been studied for many decades by classic histologic and silver impregnation techniques, neuronal systems defined on the basis of their chemical transmitter have only recently been mapped out. This has been made possible by the recent development of histochemical techniques based upon the presence of a given transmitter substance or upon specific enzymes involved in the synthesis of a given transmitter. For example, by using the formaldehyde fluorescence histochemical method of Falck and Hillarp, it has been possible to map out **norepinephrine, dopamine** and **5-hydroxy-tryptamine** containing systems in mammalian brain. Immunohistochemical fluorescent techniques have made it possible to begin to define other chemical transmitter systems, such as **cholinergic** (acetylcholine containing) and **gabaergic** (γ-aminobutyric acid containing) on the basis of the presence of their synthetic enzymes, choline acetylase and glutamic acid decarboxylase, respectively. Although in use for only a few years, it is already becoming clear that the distribution of these chemically defined neuronal systems do not necessarily correspond to systems described earlier with classical techniques.

At present, the monoamine systems (norepinephrine, dopamine and 5-hydroxytryptamine) have been most extensively studied. Fluorescence histochemical localization of neuronal perikarya, axonal pathways and terminal areas has provided a clear circuit diagram of many central systems (see Ungerstedt, 1971). With this information, fundamental anatomic, biochemical and physiologic correlations can be made. Knowledge of the anatomy of these systems allows for, among others, the following types of investigations: electrical stimulation of specific monoaminergic pathways with a concomitant measurement of changes in transmitter turnover and monitoring the response of postsynaptic cell; electrothermic or mechanical destruction of specific pathways and the measurement of biochemical, physiologic or behavioral consequences and single unit recordings from histochemically identified monoaminergic neurons and their postsynaptic follower cells. This permits the analysis of physiologic function and drug effects at a cellular level and constitutes a relatively new approach to the study of the relationship between monoamine turnover and impulse flow within monoaminergic systems. The histochemical localization of certain monoamine neuronal perikarya within well-defined nuclei permits a high degree of assurance that the recordings in such cases are from bona fide monoamine cells. In addition, it has recently become possible to apply drugs directly to these neurons by microiontophoresis and thus determine whether a given drug is having a direct or indirect effect on the activity of a specific neuronal type. By recording the electrical activity of single monoaminergic neurons, it is possible to test directly hypotheses derived from biochemical studies of the effects of drugs and other treatments on neuronal activity.

Many of the proposed mechanisms of actions of the drugs described in Chapters 24 and 25

have been derived in part from such experiments. In addition to these studies on the monoamines, dopamine, norepinephrine and serotonin, some attention is now being devoted to the action of psychoactive drugs upon other putative transmitter substances in the brain such as acetylcholine, γ-aminobutyric acid, glutamic acid and glycine. Since in most cases these substances as well as their synthetic enzymes are unique to selective neuronal systems, it is often possible to analyze drug induced changes in specific chemically defined neuronal pathways.

The basic criteria which must be established for a substance to qualify as a neurotransmitter in the peripheral nervous system have been discussed in Chapter 14. They are essentially the same in the CNS and can be summarized as follows: the chemical should be synthesized and stored in the presynaptic neuron, be released from the terminals of that neuron upon depolarization, produce the same physiologic action (inhibition or excitation) upon the postsynaptic neurons as produced by activation of the presynaptic neuron and have its action blocked by agents or drugs which block the effects of activation of the presynaptic neuron. Finally, some mechanism for terminating the action of the transmitter must be available. As would be anticipated from the foregoing discussion, each of these steps in the life cycle of various transmitter candidates is presently undergoing very careful scrutiny as a possible site of drug action.

A diagrammatic illustration of a hypothetical central synapse which summarizes the events believed to occur at a typical synapse and also indicates a number of potential sites of drug intervention is shown in Figure 23-1. The ultimate goal in the evaluation of the mechanism of action of a given drug is to determine what effect the drug has on synaptic transmission and on the output of the postsynaptic or follower cell.

In this idealized synapse, information in the form of action potentials is propagated or conducted along the neuron. When the action potential arrives at the nerve terminal region, the terminal becomes depolarized, and there is a transient synchronous release of the transmitter. Once the transmitter is released from the presynaptic neuron it diffuses across the synaptic cleft and interacts with the postsynaptic neuronal receptor sites. This combination initiates a change in membrane permeability of the postjunctional neuron. In the case of an excitatory transmitter, this change in permeability to ions can result in a depolarization of the postsynaptic cell. The summed effects of several excitatory inputs may generate an action potential in the postsynaptic neuron and in essence integrate the message originating from several presynaptic neurons

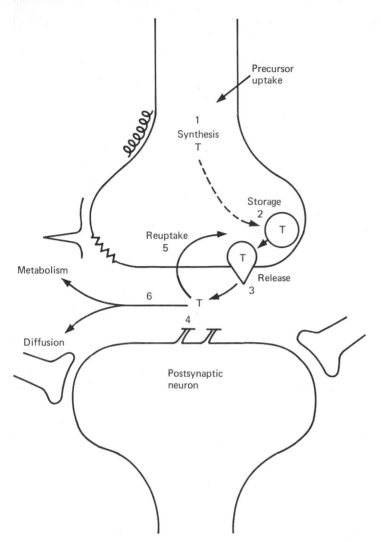

FIG. 23–1. Schematic illustration of a central synapse indicating possible sites of drug intervention in transmitter dynamics. **T** indicates the transmitter and the number of potential sites of drug intervention.

which impinge on it. In the CNS, in some instances, an inhibitory rather than an excitatory transmitter may be released. Instead of increasing the permeability of the postjunctional membrane to all ions, an inhibitory transmitter usually causes a selective increase in the permeability of the membrane to either potassium or chloride. The net result is an increase in the resting potential and a hyperpolarization or stabilization of the postsynaptic membrane. Thus, the end result of release of an inhibitory transmitter is a reduction in the excitability of the postsynaptic neuron. Once the transmitter substance, either excitatory or inhibitory, has exerted its effects on the postsynaptic cell, its action is terminated. Transmitter actions are terminated mainly by enzymatic destruction, reuptake into presynaptic nerve terminals or diffusion away from the receptor and synaptic cleft (Ch. 14).

Let us turn for a moment from the events of synaptic transmission to those involved in the life cycle of a typical transmitter substance. The life cycle of the transmitter will be traced from its initial formation until it is destroyed or reutilized to indicate potential sites for drug intervention.

BIOSYNTHESIS. The uptake of precursors into the neuron followed by their conversion to the transmitter substance is the first step in the transmitter life cycle which can be influenced by drugs. A drug may have a direct effect on the synthetic enzymes or may alter the availability of substrate to the enzyme. The general assumption is usually made that effective inhibition of the synthesis of a transmitter will lead to an inhibition of transmission at synapses where it is utilized. Similarly, if the synthesis of the transmitter is enhanced, a facilitation of transmission would be expected. At the present time none of the major drugs used therapeutically in psychiatry appear to produce their primary effects by interfering with transmitter synthesis. However, there are available a number of substances which can influence transmitter biosynthesis whose actions are currently being explored both in animal and human studies.

STORAGE. Most neurotransmitter substances are stored in small vesicular structures, synaptic vesicles, located in the presynaptic terminals. Despite the fact that only a small percentage of the total storage supply of transmitter is released with each nerve impulse, drugs which can effectively deplete the stores of transmitter will interfere with synaptic processes involving that transmitter substance. Depletion of stores from within the nerve terminals is sometimes referred to as intraneuronal release, whereas transmitter released physiologically or by drugs from nerve terminals onto a postsynaptic cell is termed extraneuronal or, more appropriately, synaptic release.

RELEASE. The transmitter is released from the presynaptic terminals into the synaptic cleft where it migrates to and ultimately interacts with the receptors on the postsynaptic cell. Drugs could conceivably interact at this site and block or facilitate release of transmitter. A potent action in either direction could produce a profound effect on neuronal function.

RECEPTOR INTERACTION. The interaction of the transmitter with the postsynaptic receptor initiates the permeability changes in the postsynaptic cell which lead either to depolarization or hyperpolarization of the postsynaptic neuron. Drugs that stimulate or block those receptors have potent effects on the action of the postsynaptic follower cell.

TERMINATION OF ACTION. Transmitter action can be terminated by removal from the synaptic cleft by reuptake into the presynaptic neuron, by metabolism or by diffusion away from the postsynaptic receptor. Drugs, by inhibiting the reuptake or metabolic breakdown of a transmitter, should potentiate the effects of the transmitter since it now lingers for a longer period of time in the vicinity of the receptor.

CLASSIFICATION OF PSYCHOTROPIC DRUGS

Numerous schemes have been suggested for the classification of psychotropic drugs. Schemes based upon their chemical structure, their neuropharmacologic activity or their major therapeutic effect have been proposed. In many cases chemical classification can be quite misleading. Sometimes the activity of a given drug molecule can be drastically altered by only minor structural changes. For example, the addition of a carbon bridge in place of the sulphur of the phenothiazine molecule (Ch. 25) converts an antipsychotic drug to a molecule which has potent antidepressant activity. In addition, the activity of separate portions of a drug molecule may have little or nothing to do with the activity of these molecules when they are combined. A classic example is the antipsychotic drug, perphenazine, which consists of two moieties, a phenothiazine and a piperazine, both of which alone are effective anthelminthics. Plainly, this action has nothing to do with the antipsychotic properties of this drug, despite the fact that the Greek philosopher Paracelsus believed that madness was caused by the presence of worms in the brain.

Unfortunately, a neuropharmacologic classification of drugs also has many drawbacks. Many of the known actions of the psychotropic drugs have nothing to do with their efficacy in the treatment of mental illness. For example, the antipsychotic drug, chlorpromazine, has been shown to possess every conceivable action from stimulating motility in protozoans to altering the pecking behavior of pigeons. On the mammalian CNS, chlorpromazine also has a wide spectrum of actions, and it is probable that few if any of these actions are associated with its efficacy in the treatment of psychosis. It has thus become the practice to classify these substances according to their clinically useful effects. By and large this scheme has been adopted in the chapters that follow. However, in some instances subclassifications based on chemical structure and neuropharmacologic activity have also been used.

The psychotropic drugs alter behavior, mood, affect and perception in man and behavior in animals. They can be subdivided into the psychotoxic agents and the psychotherapeutic drugs. The psychotherapeutic drugs are dealt with in Chapters 24–26, the psychotoxic drugs in Chapter 9. The psychotherapeutic drugs can be further subdivided into antipsychotic, antidepressant, antianxiety drugs and the sedative-hypnotics.

No specific factors have been etiologically incriminated in psychiatric disorders. Of necessity, a multitude of factors enter into their etiology, and thus experimentally it is extremely difficult to establish with certainty the mode of action of psychotherapeutic drugs. Nevertheless, these agents do seem to decrease the frequency of recurrence of affective disorders or curtail the expression of schizophrenic symptoms. In both cases the end result is invariably a better adjustment of the patient in the community setting.

The cause of mental disease is unknown, and

the field of psychopharmacology is in its infancy. It more or less began in 1952 when chlorpromazine was first introduced for the treatment of mental disorders. Despite the newness and incompleteness of our knowledge, the physician needs a frame of reference within which he can seek answers to the problems he faces in the use of the various psychotherapeutic agents in his armentarium. In the chapters that follow a frame of reference based upon the pharmacology of these drugs will be presented. Where possible, a working, although highly speculative, model will be formulated to explain their modes of action based upon an interaction with chemically defined neuronal systems in the CNS.

FURTHER READING

Cooper JR, Bloom FE, Roth RH (1974): Biochemical Basis of Neuropharmacology. New Jersey, Oxford University Press

Iversen SD, Iversen LL (1975): Behavioral Pharmacology. New Jersey, Oxford University Press

Ungerstedt U (1971): Stereotaxic mapping of the monoamine pathways in the rat brain. Acta Physiol Scand Suppl 367:1–47

MARGARET C. BOADLE-BIBER

ROBERT H. ROTH

24. ANTIDEPRESSANT AND ANTIMANIC DRUGS

Depression and mania are extreme conditions of mood or affect. Of the two, depression is by far the more widespread and debilitating. The severely depressed individual is overwhelmed by sadness and feelings of worthlessness. Characteristically, he withdraws into himself and becomes both mentally and physically inactive. He gives the impression that nothing is worth attempting any longer. Although the condition often disappears spontaneously, it may be so life threatening (the incidence of successful and attempted suicides is high) as to warrant immediate therapeutic intervention and often hospitalization. Drugs used in the treatment of severe depressions fall into two main groups: the so-called **tricyclic antidepressants** and the **monoamine oxidase inhibitors.** In addition, the condi-tion often responds to electroconvulsive therapy.

Another group of compounds, the **psychomotor stimulants** have had limited usefulness in mild forms of depression but are of no value in its severest and most incapacitating forms. Occasionally, the antianxiety drugs are employed in treatment of mild anxious depression (Ch. 26).

In contrast to the severely depressed patient, the manic patient has a tremendous sense of well being, is immensely talkative and overactive and may indulge in the most unrealistic projects. His condition responds to **lithium carbonate** as well as to the antipsychotic agents such as chlorpromazine (Ch. 25). Lithium is also used prophylactically to reduce the mood swings in manic depressive syndrome.

TRICYCLIC ANTIDEPRESSANTS

Chemistry

This is the most widely used class of antidepressants. **Imipramine,** (Tofranil) a dibenzazepine

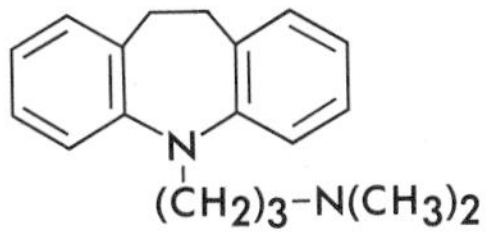

$(CH_2)_3-N(CH_3)_2$

IMIPRAMINE

derivative, is the prototype drug. The name tricyclic originates from the three membered ring which is characteristic of this group of drugs as well as the structurally related phenothiazines (see Chapter 25 for comparison of structures). Other members of the class include **desmethylimipramine** or **desipramine** (Norpramin; Pertofrane), **amitriptyline** (Elavil), **nortriptyline** (Aventyl), **protriptyline** (Vivactil) and **doxepin** (Sinequan).

History

The antidepressant properties of imipramine were discovered accidentally in 1958 when it was tested for antipsychotic activity on a group of depressed schizophrenic patients. The depression but not the psychosis improved. Although a variety of congeners are now available for clinical use, they all have basically the same spectrum of action.

Actions

CENTRAL NERVOUS SYSTEM. In normal individuals, imipramine has a sedative-like action. In depressed patients, however, there is a remarkable improvement in mood after 2–3 weeks of drug treatment. The reason for the delay in onset of beneficial effects is unclear but may be related to some slowly induced change in monoamine metabolism in the CNS. In some patients depression is occasionally succeeded by mania and euphoria.

INTERACTION WITH MONOAMINE NEURONES.

Imipramine and the other tricyclic antidepressants block the reuptake of norepinephrine at the sympathetic neurone (Chs. 14,23) and at monoaminergic neurones, particularly those containing norepinephrine and serotonin in the CNS. Since the reuptake by the sympathetic neurone of norepinephrine released from the nerve ending is important in terminating the action of the transmitter, any drug which blocks this reuptake process will potentiate the effects of sympathetic nerve stimulation. By analogy, inhibition of the reuptake process in the CNS is believed to prolong or potentiate the effect of monoamine neurotransmitters released from central neurones. Such an interaction has been proposed as the basis for the therapeutic effect of these drugs in depression. Implicit in such an hypothesis is the idea that in depression there is a deficiency of certain monoamine neurotransmitters at particular synapses in the CNS. The tricyclic drugs presumably allow the transmitter to linger in the synapse for longer periods and to accumulate so that more transmitter reaches the postsynaptic receptor. This is the same end result as an increased release of transmitter.

AUTONOMIC NERVOUS SYSTEM. Imipramine

has potent anticholinergic effects (Ch. 17). The most prominent effects seen in patients include tachycardia and even palpitations (due to block of vagal imput) dizziness, blurred vision, dry mouth, constipation and urinary retention (this side effect has been exploited in the treatment of severe enuresis in children which has failed to respond to other forms of treatment, e.g., psychotherapy). In addition, imipramine may directly enhance sympathomimetic effects because of its ability, in therapeutic doses, to reduce the reuptake of norepinephrine at the sympathetic neurone. The effects of any directly acting sympathomimetic amines (Ch. 18) will also be potentiated by tricyclic drugs, since their action will no longer be terminated as rapidly by neuronal reuptake. On the other hand, indirectly acting sympathomimetic amines will be ineffective, since they can no longer enter the sympathetic neurone and release endogenous transmitter.

CARDIOVASCULAR SYSTEM. Hypotension is a

frequent and troublesome effect seen during initial drug therapy. Its origin is not known.

Absorption, Metabolism and Excretion

Imipramine is well absorbed from the gastrointestinal tract and is bound to plasma protein. It is metabolized in the liver, undergoing aromatic hydroxylation, demethylation and oxidation. Demethylation converts imipramine to another pharmacologically active species desmethylimipramine. Imipramine is excreted primarily as the 2-hydroxyl and N-oxide metabolites.

Adverse Reactions

The most pronounced and troublesome side effects are very largely anticholinergic (Ch. 17). These include tachycardia, dry mouth, blurred vision, urinary retention and constipation. In addition, fine muscle tremor, dizziness and headache are quite common. In higher doses, imipramine can precipitate convulsions. Among reported cardiovascular difficulties is an increased prevalence of arrythmias, particularly in cardiac patients. This may be associated with enhanced levels of free norepinephrine in the heart and the heightened susceptibility of damaged myocardial tissue to arrythmias. The drug has also been implicated in myocardial infarction, congestive heart failure and abnormalities of conduction. Clearly, the status of cardiac patients should be evaluated before prescribing a tricyclic antidepressant. Blood dyscrasias do occur but only rarely.

The consequences of a large overdose of imipramine are dangerous and very often life threatening. They include hyperpyrexia, hypertension, tachycardia, arrythmias, disturbances of cardiac conduction, seizures and coma. Children have died from as little as 250 mg imipramine or the equivalent of twice the average adult daily dose. Gastric lavage may be helpful, but more important is supportive therapy to assist respiration and to control blood pressure, temperature, convulsions and any cardiac abnormalities.

Drug Interactions

Imipramine modifies the action of many drugs which interact at the sympathetic nerve terminal (Chs. 4,74). For example, it blocks the action of the antihypertensive drug, guanethidine, that must first be taken up into the sympathetic nerve terminal in order to produce an effect on arterial pressure (Ch. 20). It potentiates the effects of many directly acting sympathomimetic amines (e.g., phenylephrine) which are inactivated at least in part by the reuptake mechanism (Ch. 18). Doses of pressor substances should therefore be reduced when administered to individuals receiving these antidepressants. Imipramine also produces a very dangerous reaction characterized by hyperpyrexia if given concurrently with or immediately following monoamine oxidase inhibitors. Since the outcome of this combination may be fatal, 10 days to 2 weeks should be allowed to elapse between stopping a monoamine oxidase inhibitor and switching to a tricyclic antidepressant.

Clinical Uses

The tricyclic antidepressants are used for treating severe forms of depression and usually take anywhere from one to three weeks to produce any improvement in mood. For this reason they should be taken continuously and never prescribed on an "as needed" basis. In addition to their use as antidepressants, they are increasingly being used to treat enuresis which is unresponsive to other forms of treatment.

Preparations and Dosage

The tricyclic antidepressants are usually taken orally but are available for IM injection. In view of the wide variation in response to these drugs, it is usual to start therapy with small doses and gradually build up to a maintenance dose over a 2 week period. The usual ranges for daily maintenance doses are: imipramine, desipramine and amitriptyline 75–300 mg, nortryptyline 50–100 mg, protryptyline 15–60 mg and doxepin 75–150 mg.

MONOAMINE OXIDASE INHIBITORS

Chemistry

This is a diverse group of compounds which share the property of irreversibly inhibiting **monoamine oxidase** (MAO), a mitochondrial enzyme found in a wide variety of tissues such as intestine, kidney, liver, exocrine glands as well as both the central and peripheral nervous system. The drugs of this class currently available for clinical use as antidepressants include **isocarboxazid** (Marplan), **nialamide** (Niamid) and

PHENELZINE

phenelzine (Nardil), three hydrazine derivatives, and **tranylcypromine** (Parnate), which is structu-

TRANYLCYPROMINE

rally related to amphetamine. Their target enzyme MAO has a very broad substrate specificity, oxidatively deaminating a great variety of naturally occuring primary and secondary monoamines in which the amino group is attached to a methylene residue. (Any substituents on this methylene carbon, e.g., a methyl group, as with amphetamine prevents the removal of the amino group.) The fact that MAO is such a widespread enzyme which plays an important detoxifying role in the body has important consequences for the clinical use of MAO inhibitors as antidepressant drugs.

History

Iproniazid (Marsilid), a MAO inhibitor which was removed from the market because it caused severe liver toxicity, was originally developed as a congener to the tuberculostatic drug isoniazid (Ch. 61). Its central stimulant effects were discovered accidentally when it was being tested clinically for treatment of tuberculosis. Only later was it found to be a MAO inhibitor. This led to the synthesis and testing of many other MAO inhibitors as potential antidepressant drugs.

Actions

CENTRAL NERVOUS SYSTEM. The MAO inhibitors improve the mood of depressed patients, the beneficial effect being seen anywhere from one to several weeks after treatment is started. Tranylcypromine has the shortest onset of action probably because of its additional amphetamine-like effects. In some instances, the improvement may progress to a state of euphoria, hypomania or even mania. Central stimulatory effects are seen with these drugs in normal individuals as well as in depressed patients.

EFFECT ON MONOAMINES. Inhibition of MAO leads to a very pronounced increase in the levels of norepinephrine in the sympathetic nervous system and of the monoamines serotonin, norepinephrine and dopamine in the monoamine containing neurones of the CNS. Under normal circumstances, only small amounts of a given monoamine are present in the cytoplasm of the nerve terminal because unbound amine which originates largely from synthesis or reuptake is either rapidly sequestered in the amine storage vesicles or is metabolized by MAO (Ch. 14). In the presence of a MAO inhibitor, large amounts of amine now accumulate in the cytoplasm, the storage sites rapidly become saturated, and the nerve terminal finally becomes filled to capacity with the transmitter. This enhanced accumulation of monoamines within the neurones is presumed to be the basis for the antidepressant action of the MAO inhibitors. Excess amine leaks out of the neurons, ultimately reaching the postsynaptic receptors. Alternatively, more amine may be available for release during nerve activity. Just as with the tricyclic antidepressants, the hypothesis explaining the therapeutic effectiveness of these drugs is based on the assumption that in depression there is a critical lack of availability of certain monoamines.

While it is true that most of the monoamines in the body are found within the nervous system, there are a number of other systems in which monoamines accumulate. Examples of these are the blood platelets and the enterochromaffin cells of the gut, both of which bind serotonin. It should be added that the presence in the urine of large amounts of unmetabolized serotonin and 3-0-methylated catecholamines is characteristic of patients on MAO inhibitor antidepressants.

In addition to affecting the metabolism of endogenously produced amines, inhibition of MAO permits amines either already present in food or generated from amino acids by the bacterial flora in the intestine to be absorbed and to enter the circulation. Under normal conditions such amines are inactivated before they reach the general circulation by MAO present in the intestine, or, failing this, by MAO in the liver and also kidney. It is the combined effects of the increased levels of monoamines in the nervous system, particularly norepinephrine in sympathetic nerves innervating the vasculature, and the removal of the normal detoxification mechanisms in the intestine that produces many of the dangerous drug and food incompatibilities discussed below.

EFFECTS ON SLEEP. MAO inhibitors suppress REM sleep, and this property is the basis for their use in the treatment of narcolepsy.

CARDIOVASCULAR EFFECTS. MAO inhibitors lower arterial pressure, an effect which has been exploited in the use of one of this group of drugs, pargyline, as an antihypertensive (Ch. 20). In general, however, the orthostatic hypotension associated with administration of MAO inhibitors is an inconvenient and unwanted side effect.

EFFECTS ON OTHER ENZYME SYSTEMS. In addition to inhibiting MAO, these drugs inhibit a variety of other enzymes to a greater or lesser extent, the most notable being the microsomal drug metabolizing enzymes of the liver (Chs. 4,74). Thus, the effects of an enormous variety of drugs are greatly potentiated in the presence of a MAO inhibitor.

Absorption Rate and Excretion

The MAO inhibitors used clinically are well absorbed from the GI tract. Drugs containing a hydrazine moiety must be metabolized before they can react with MAO, in contrast to tranylcypromine which interacts with the enzyme unchanged. The turnover time of these compounds corresponds to the turnover time of the enzyme (several weeks), since the binding is irreversible.

Adverse Reactions

The most serious adverse effect seen when these drugs are taken in **therapeutic doses** is an allergic reaction affecting the liver. Fortunately, the frequency is very low. Other effects that occur more often include excessive central stimulation typified by very excitable behavior, sleeplessness and agitation, orthostatic hypotension which can be controlled by reducing the dose of the drug, dizziness and finally a number of anticholinergic type symptoms (Ch. 17).

OVERDOSAGE. Perhaps the most dangerous aspect of poisoning with the MAO inhibitor is the complete and misleading absence of symptoms sometimes for many hours prior to the sudden onset of severe fever (which can prove fatal), agitation, hallucinations, hyperexcitable reflexes and increased or decreased arterial pressure. Extreme caution must be used before other drugs are administered to control symptoms such as decreased or increased arterial pressure and central stimulation, since serious interactions can occur (see below).

Interactions With Other Drugs and Foreign Substances

Basically, two types of drug interaction occur in the presence of MAO inhibitors. One involves sympathomimetic amines and related compounds present in food or taken as medication. Since these amines are no longer oxidatively deaminated, they circulate in the blood with a very long half-life and produce prolonged pressor effects by acting either directly on the vascular smooth muscle or indirectly by releasing the norepinephrine present in the sympathetic nerve terminals in greater than usual amounts (Ch. 20). This type of interaction is characterized by a so-called **hypertensive crisis** which may be accompanied by tremendous headache and can be fatal in the event of intracranial bleeding. The commonest culprits are indirectly acting sympathomimetic amines such as tyramine found in cheese, wine and herrings, amino acids such as tryptophan or dopa which can be converted to the corresponding amines and sympathomimetic amines, e.g., phenylpropanolamine used in over-the-counter preparations for the common cold. The second type of interaction arises because the microsomal drug metabolizing enzymes are inhibited by MAO inhibitors. The action of any substance normally metabolized by these enzymes may be dramatically potentiated. Among the drugs involved are many anaesthetics, narcotics, barbituates, alcohol and anticholinergic compounds (Chs. 3,75). This means that, barring an emergency, surgery should be postponed for several weeks in such patients until the effects of the MAO inhibitor have worn off.

A severe reaction often follows the use of a tricyclic antidepressant concurrently with or following a MAO inhibitor (see preceding section).

Clinical Uses

The MAO inhibitors are used to treat severe depression, but because of their potential toxicity they are usually reserved for those who have failed to respond to the tricyclic antidepressants. They have limited use in narcolepsy and as antihypertensives (pargyline).

Doses and Preparations

The MAO inhibitors are available in tablet form for oral ingestion. The average maintenance dose is as follows: isocarboxazid *N.F.* (Marplan) 10–50 mg phenelzine sulfate *N.F.* (Nardil) 15–75 mg nialamide (Niamid) 50–200 mg tranylcypromine (Parnate) 10–40 mg.

LITHIUM CARBONATE

Chemistry

Lithium carbonate is the salt of a monovalent cation belonging to the alkaline earth series of metals.

History

Lithium was used in the 1940s as a salt substitute for cardiac patients on a low salt diet, a practice which proved disasterous since lithium ions cannot be excreted as readily as sodium ions, and many individuals died of lithium poisoning.

This experience undoubtedly slowed the introduction of this substance into the United States for treatment of mania, even though it was being widely and successfully used for this disorder in Scandinavia. It is now approved by the FDA.

Actions

CENTRAL NERVOUS SYSTEM. Lithium abolishes the excitement, euphoria and insomnia of mania, without producing sedation. In this respect it is superior to the phenothiazines. Its effects, however, take several days to develop.

The basis for the beneficial effect of lithium in mania is not understood. It produces a large number of biochemical changes in the CNS, which are probably all related to their interaction with the distribution of sodium and potassium ions across the cell membrane. Lithium can replace sodium ions in the extracellular fluid. It can also replace sodium in the inward sodium current of the nerve action potential. However, lithium, unlike sodium, is not pumped out of nerve axons in exchange for potassium by the sodium-potassium activated ATPase (sodium pump). Thus, lithium ions tend to accumulate within neurones at the expense of potassium ions, and there is a net loss of intracellular potassium. In cases of severe lithium toxicity, so much potassium is lost that the resting membrane potential falls and eventually action potentials can no longer be generated. In the presence of therapeutic levels of lithium (0.9–1.4 mEq/liter), these drastic alterations in intracellular ion concentrations are not seen. However, there is probably a change in the proportions of sodium and potassium ions which in turn may modify many sodium/potassium dependent processes at cell membranes such as glucose and amino acid uptake and the reuptake of transmitters like norepinephrine, dopamine and serotonin. Many other processes are probably also affected in subtle and as yet undetermined ways by the presence of lithium ions.

Absorption Rate and Excretion

Lithium carbonate is readily absorbed from the gastrointestinal tract, with plasma levels reaching a maximum in 1–3 hr. Lithium is excreted by the kidneys with a half-life of about 24 hr in the presence of normal sodium concentrations. However, with low plasma sodium levels, lithium is much less effectively cleared from the body, and toxicity can result. Thus, lithium is contraindicated in individuals who must restrict their salt intake. Therapeutically effective plasma levels of lithium lie between 0.9–1.4 mEq/liter plasma. Above 2 mEq/liter serious toxicity can ensue. Because of this low safety margin, it is essential to monitor serum lithium levels during initiation of therapy and to continue this monitoring at regular intervals thereafter. Renal function tests should be carried out before instituting therapy.

Adverse Effects

During the first week or two of therapy, patients may show signs of sleepiness and tiredness and may experience muscle weakness and tremor. Other symptoms may include nausea, vomiting, diuresis, diarrhea and an intense thirst. While most of these effects disappear during continued therapy, the diuresis, tremor and thirst may not. Initially, toxic levels of lithium produce marked fatigue, ataxia, muscle twitching and tremor. In severe cases, kidney failure, cardiac arrythmias, coma and convulsions may ensue. Therapy is largely supportive, although administration of sodium chloride may hasten the elimination of lithium.

Clinical Uses

Lithium is used to treat manic episodes and also on a prophylactic basis to control the mood swings characteristic of manic depressive illness.

Preparations and Dosage

Lithium carbonate *U.S.P.* is available in 300 mg tablets. The average maintenance dose is about 1200 mg/day. During manic episodes, doses of 1800 mg may be used.

Psychomotor Stimulants

This class of drugs includes amphetamine (Benzedrine, Biphetamine), dextroamphetamine (Dexedrine), methamphetamine (Desoxyn, Fetamin), methylphenidate (Ritalin) and pipradrol (Meratran) (Ch. 18). These stimulants, regardless of chemical class, have similar pharmacologic properties characterized by excitement, sleeplessness, euphoria and hyperactivity in adults but which tend to quiet the behavior of preteenage hyperactive children who are otherwise unable to concentrate for any extended period of time. The main clinical use of these and related drugs nowadays is in the treatment of hyperkinetic children, in narcolepsy and as appetite suppressants. They are of no benefit in severe forms of depression and should never be used. They are absolutely contraindicated when a patient is on an MAO inhibitor. In view of their significant potential for abuse (Ch. 9), their only short term anorectic effect and the rapid development of tolerance, these drugs should be employed therapeutically only with extreme caution.

FURTHER READING

Byck R (1975): The Pharmacological Basis of Therapeutics. (5th ed) LS Goodman, A Gilman, (eds). New York, Macmillan

Hollister LE (1971): Clinical use of psychotherapeutic drugs. II. Antidepressant and antianxiety drugs and special problems in the use of psychotherapeutic drugs. Drugs 4:361–410

Singer I, Totenberg D (1973): Mechanisms of lithium action. N Engl J Med 289:254–260

Schildkraut JJ (1973): Neuropharmacology of the affective disorders. Annu Rev Pharmacol 13: 427–454

BENJAMIN S. BUNNEY

ROBERT H. ROTH

25. ANTIPSYCHOTIC DRUGS

HISTORY

In 1952 the French surgeon Laborit used a newly synthesized drug, chlorpromazine, as an adjuvant to anesthesia and noted its ability to sedate patients without causing a loss of consciousness. Persuaded by Laborit's enthusiasm for the unique properties of this new drug, several French psychiatrists treated psychotic patients with chlorpromazine and reported its ability to make an aggressive paranoid patient "charming and docile" in 3 days. Within the year physical restraints were a thing of the past. The atmosphere on the wards for disturbed patients had been transformed. Thus, with the discovery of chlorpromazine, a new era of psychopharmacology began—an era which would see not only the development of numerous drugs to treat a wide variety of mental disorders, but also a shift of emphasis away from the psychological aspects of mental illness and toward an investigation of possible organic factors involved in their pathogenesis. This new field of "biological psychiatry" is now one of the most rapidly advancing areas in science today.

NOSOLOGY

Psychopharmacologic agents can be divided into two broad categories: **Psychotherapeutic**—those drugs that prevent or help ameliorate symptoms of mental illness and **psychotoxic**—agents that have adverse affects on the CNS. The antipsychotic drugs belong to the former category. Several terms commonly used for these drugs include major tranquilizers, neuroleptics, psycholeptics and psycholytics. The term antipsychotic will be used, as it most clearly suggests the primary use of these drugs.

Unfortunately, diagnostic terms in psychiatry are not nearly as well defined as in other branches of medicine. Even the definition of mental illness varies from subculture to subculture. Since, in almost every case, the cause of mental illness is unknown, etiology cannot be used as a criterion for diagnosis. Consequently, when the clinical uses of antipsychotic drugs are discussed, emphasis will be placed on specific treatable symptoms rather than on trying to match a given treatment to a given diagnostic category.

Despite classification difficulties, a few broad diagnostic terms such as psychosis have commonly accepted definitions. A patient is described as psychotic when he evidences profound alterations in mood and disorganization of thinking, both of which are frequently associated with withdrawal into an unreal world of highly personalized preoccupations. The impairment of function resulting from these symptoms often interferes with his ability to meet the ordinary demands of life. Hallucinations and delusions may contribute to the impairment. In addition, the patient may experience loss of control which manifests itself in agitation and aggressive behavior. It was the ability of antipsychotic drugs to sedate (or "tranquilize") patients with these latter symptoms that fostered their immediate widespread use. Prior to chlorpromazine, the only sedative drugs available were the hypnotics, such as barbiturates (Ch. 26). Chlorpromazine had a great advantage over these in that it calmed the patient while still allowing him to function. Sedatives were only effective in doses that clouded consciousness—an undesirable side effect in patients for whom the other major therapeutic modality is psychotherapy. Fortunately, the antipsychotic drugs were also found to be effective in treating many of the primary symptoms of psychosis, including the underlying thought disorder.

PHARMACOLOGY

Antipsychotic drugs currently used clinically can be divided into four major categories according to the structural class of compound from which they are derived: **phenothiazines, butyrophenones, thioxanthenes** and **dibenzodiazapines.** The phenothiazines have been the most thoroughly studied and will be described in the most detail.

PHENOTHIAZINES

Chemistry

Phenothiazine is a three-ring structure in which two benzene rings are attached to each other by a sulfur and a nitrogen atom in the 5 and 10 position, respectively (Table 25–1). Substitutions usually occur at the 2 and 10 position. Substitution of a chlorine, methoxy, thiomethyl, acetyl or trifluoromethyl group in the 2 position increases the antipsychotic potency of these drugs. The nature of the side chain substituent at the 10 position influences both the potency and pharmacological activity of the compound. Antipsychotic properties are only present if there are three carbon atoms between the nitrogen in the 10 position of the phenothiazine nucleus and the amine group of the side chain. The presence of a fourth carbon atom in the chain causes a loss of antipsychotic activity. Reduction of the side chain to 2 carbon atoms can change the antipsychotic activity to antihistaminic or antiparkinsonian, depending on the nature of the substitution on the basic amino group. Antipsychotic phenothiazines can be divided into three groups based on the nature of the side chain attached to the 10 position: dimethylamino-alkyls, piperazinyl-alkyls and piperidyl-alkyls. The dimethylamino derivatives, of which **chlorpromazine** (Thorazine) is the best known example, are characterized by significant sedative properties making them particularly useful in the treatment of psychotic patients who are agitated and/or experiencing sleep disturbances. The piperazine derivatives are the most potent antipsychotic compounds and possess significantly less sedative action than the amino-alkyl phenothiazines. However, they have a greater tendency to produce extrapyramidal side effects. Antipsychotic compounds in this group include **fluphenazine** (Permitil, Prolixin), **perphenazine** (Trilafon) and **trifluoperazine** (Stelazine). **Thioridazine** (Mellaril), the most important member of the piperidine derivatives, resembles chlorpromazine in potency and sedative effects but has a significantly lower incidence of extrapyramidal side effects.

Absorption, Distribution and Metabolism

The aromatic group of the antipsychotic phenothiazines is lipophilic and is the major determinant of their solubility properties. At the pH of the gastrointestinal tract beyond the stomach (Ch. 2) these drugs exist largely in their uncharged free form and thus are readily absorbed. Because of their lipid solubility, these drugs pass through the blood-brain barrier to the areas of the CNS, where their specific effects are elicited. (Ch. 2).

Most of the antipsychotic phenothiazines can be administered either orally or parenterally. When given orally, highest plasma levels are reached when the drug is given in an elixir form and on an empty stomach. Because of its lipid solubility, chlorpromazine is stored in lipid containing tissues throughout the body, including the lung, liver and brain. Its extensive storage may explain why its clinical effects last up to several weeks and why metabolites of chlorpromazine are found in urine up to 18 months after cessation of administration.

Chlorpromazine is metabolized primarily in the liver, and the parent compound, as well as its metabolites, are excreted in both urine and feces. Over a hundred possible metabolites have been postulated, and many have been found in human urine. Over 80% of the total daily drug content in the urine consists of metabolites hydroxylated in the 7 and/or 3 position. The second most common metabolic pathway of chlorpromazine appears to be the formation of sulfoxides. Both animal and clinical evidence suggests that 7-hydroxychlorpromazine is an active metabolite, whereas chlorpromazine sulfoxide is inactive. It has been suggested that the difference between patients who do or do not respond to chlorpromazine may reside in the different ways individual patients metabolize the parent compound.

Mechanism of Action

Although our knowledge of the mechanism of action of the antipsychotic drugs is far from complete, it is no longer a total mystery. The antipsychotic phenothiazines are very active com-

TABLE 25-1. Representative Structural Interrelationships of Phenothiazines

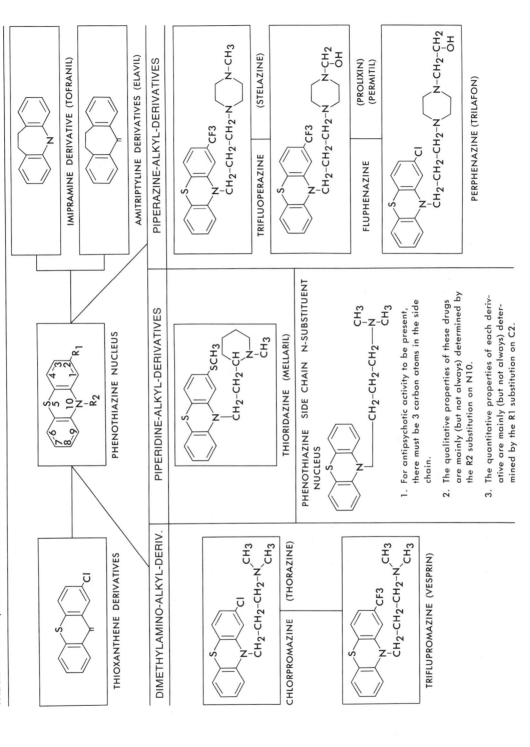

pounds with a wide variety of effects on biologic systems. However, of their many actions only one effect has been shown to correlate with their antipsychotic efficacy: they increase the rate of dopamine turnover (synthesis and destruction) in the brain. Based on biochemical findings, Carlsson and Lindqvist suggested that antipsychotic phenothiazines may increase dopamine turnover by blocking postsynaptic dopamine receptors. They further hypothesized that this blockade of dopamine receptors might lead to a compensatory increase in the firing rate of dopaminergic neurons mediated via an as yet unidentified neuronal feedback pathway. The increase in dopamine turnover would thus be due to an increase in the activity of dopaminergic neurons.

Coyle and Snyder, using X-ray crystalography have demonstrated that part of the three-dimensional configuration of the chlorpromazine molecule can be exactly superimposed upon a three-dimensional model of the dopamine molecule, thus lending some support to the idea that a postsynaptic dopamine receptor might recognize and accept part of the chlorpromazine molecule and be blocked by it. Recently it has been possible to record extracellularly from single dopaminergic neurons in the CNS previously identified anatomically by Dahlström and Fuxe using fluorescent histochemical methods. It was found that many antipsychotic drugs do indeed increase the firing rate of dopamine-containing cells. In addition, all antipsychotic drugs which were tested reversed amphetamine-induced depression of these cells. The latter finding is of significance because at high doses d-amphetamine produces an acute paranoid psychosis that many feel is indistinguishable from acute paranoid schizophrenia. Antipsychotic phenothiazines are extremely efficacious in reversing this drug-induced psychosis. Drugs lacking antipsychotic properties do not increase dopamine turnover, increase the firing rate of dopamine-containing cells or reverse amphetamine-induced depression of these neurons.

One of the two major dopamine systems in the brain consists of cell bodies located in the zona compacta of the substantia nigra with terminals in the neostriatum. It is these cell bodies that are destroyed in Parkinson's disease. Based on this observation L-Dopa, the immediate precursor of dopamine, has been used to treat Parkinsonian symptoms with remarkable success (Ch. 31). Many antipsychotic drugs produce extrapyramidal side effects indistinguishable from some of the symptoms of Parkinson's disease. Since antipsychotic drugs block dopamine receptors, they produce a functional depletion of dopamine in the neostriatum. Absence of dopamine at the postsynaptic receptor site for whatever reason

would be expected to produce a common clinical syndrome. This reasoning has led some investigators to suggest that the extrapyramidal side effects of the antipsychotic drugs are elicited through their action on dopamine receptors in the neostriatum. Evidence for the site of action of the antipsychotic properties of these drugs is not nearly as convincing. One candidate for such a site is another dopaminergic system which has cell bodies in the ventral tegmental area of the midbrain and terminals in parts of the limbic system and frontal cortex.

Some of the antipsychotic phenothiazines also affect the norepinephrine-containing systems of the brain but only in doses significantly larger than those demonstrated to produce an effect on the dopamine system.

THIOXANTHENES

Thioxanthenes are similar in structure to the phenothiazines except that the central nitrogen in the 10 position is replaced with a carbon atom (Table 25–1). The side chain in thioxanthenes is connected to this carbon atom by a double bond rather than a single bond as in the phenothiazines. There are thioxanthene analogs of many of the phenothiazines [i.e., chlorpromazine—**chlorprothixene** (Taractan), fluphenazine—**flupenthixol**, perphenazine—**clopenthixol**]. This group of antipsychotic drugs has been less widely studied than their phenothiazine analogs. Nevertheless, in well-controlled studies, chlorprothixene has been shown to be more effective than placebo in the treatment of schizophrenia. Their mechanism of action is thought to be similar to that of the antipsychotic phenothiazines (i.e., they affect dopamine turnover in the same way). Clinically their actions are very similar to their phenothiazine analogs, both in terms of potency as antipsychotic agents and in terms of their side effects. The same considerations apply in the clinical management with these drugs as apply to other antipsychotic drugs (see section on Clinical Uses). At the present time there is no good evidence suggesting that these drugs provide any advantages in the treatment of psychosis over the more intensely studied antipsychotic drugs (phenothiazines and butyrophenones).

BUTYROPHENONES

Chemistry

Haloperidol (Haldol) is the only antipsychotic drug from this class of compounds used in the United States. First synthesized by Janssen, it consists of a ketonic phenyl ring with a straight propylene side chain and a piperidine nucleus. A fluorine atom is substituted in the para position of the ketonic phenyl ring and a tertiary alcohol group with a phenyl ring is substituted in the 4 position of the piperidine nucleus.

HALOPERIDOL

Although structurally different, haloperidol resembles the piperazine phenothiazines in its antipsychotic action and side effects. Its mechanism of action is presumed to be identical to that of the antipsychotic phenothiazines since it also increases dopamine turnover and appears to block dopamine receptors.

Absorption, Distribution and Metabolism

Haloperidol is rapidly and nearly completely absorbed from the gastrointestinal tract. Plasma levels are highest 2–6 hr after ingestion and remain elevated for approximately 72 hr. Plasma concentration then decreases slowly, detectable levels being present weeks after ingestion of a small dose. The highest concentration of haloperidol is found in the liver, and approximately 15% of a given dose is excreted in the bile. Approximately 40% of a single dose is excreted by the kidney during the first 5 days.

DIBENZODIAZEPINES

Although no drugs of this class are presently being used in the United States, one derivative, **clozapine** (Leponex), is reported in Europe to be an effective antipsychotic agent. This drug is of considerable research and therapeutic interest because it has almost no extrapyramidal side effects. In addition it does not appear to meet any of the usual animal test criteria for antipsychotic drugs, such as the ability to produce catalepsy or antagonize apomorphine-induced stereotyped behavior. It does, however, increase the turnover of cerebral dopamine and reverses the amphetamine-induced depression of dopaminergic cell activity.

Recently, it has been reported that several

CLOZAPINE

patients have developed agranulocytosis while taking clozapine. Whether the agranulocytosis was caused by clozapine has yet to be determined.

Chemistry

Clozapine is 8-chloro-11-(4-methyl-1-piperazinyl)-5H-dibenzo[b,e,][1,4]-diazepine.

In terms of dose range and clinical effects, it appears to be most similar to chlorpromazine.

RAUWOLFIA ALKALOIDS

Rauwolfia alkaloids were first used in Hindu medicine to treat a variety of ills including insanity. They began to be used in Europe as psychotherapeutic agents in 1953, shortly after the introduction of chlorpromazine. In 1954, Schlittler isolated **reserpine** as the active agent responsible for the sedative properties of these drugs. In the same year, the use of reserpine in psychiatry was begun simultaneously in Europe and the United States. Reserpine and its derivatives act by blocking the intraneuronal storage of monoamines, thereby depleting stores of dopamine, norepinephrine and serotonin. Although widely used as an antihypertensive agent (Ch. 20) and valuable as a research tool, both reserpine and its synthetic analog tetrabenazine were found to be unsuitable as antipsychotic agents. Not only are they much less effective in treating psychosis than chlorpromazine, but they produce adverse effects. By far the most serious is depression. Occurring in approximately 6% of patients treated with reserpine, it is often serious enough to necessitate hospitalization and/or electroconvulsive therapy. Other adverse effects are described in Chapter 20. For these reasons the rauwolfia alkaloids are no longer used in this country to treat mental illness.

CLINICAL PHARMACOLOGY

CLINICAL USES

Psychosis

Numerous well-controlled studies have shown that the antipsychotic drugs are markedly better than placebo in the treatment and prevention of

psychotic episodes. However, they do not cure psychosis, they only ameliorate symptoms. Psychotic patients manifest a wide variety of symptoms which students of human behavior have tried to categorize in different ways. One major contribution in this regard was made by

TABLE 25–2. Selected Properties of Representative Antipsychotic Drugs

| Drug | Antipsychotic Dose | | | Extra Pyramidal Effects | Sedative Effects | Hypotensive Effects |
| | Oral (mg/day)* | | IM* | | | |
	Usual	Extreme	mg			
Phenothiazines						
Chlorpromazine	300–800	50–3000¶	25-100 q 2-6h	Moderate	High	Moderate
Fluphenazine	4–8†	1–25†¶	12.5–100 q 2 wk‡	High	Low	Low
Perphenazine	20–40	8–120¶	5–10 initial dose then 5 q 4–6h	High	Low	Low
Thioridazine	400–800	50–1000††¶		Low	Moderate	Moderate
Trifluoperazine	15–30	2–50¶	1–2 q 4h	High	Low	Low
Thioxanthenes						
Chlorprothixene	200–600	100–1000¶	25–50 q 6h	Moderate	Moderate	Moderate
Butyrophenones						
Haloperidol	4–15	1–100	3–5 initial dose then q 2–4h	High	Low	Moderate
Dibenzodiazepines						
Clozapine	300	150–600		Low	High	Low

*These are only rough guide lines. The optimum dose must be established for each patient starting with small doses
 and increasing as rapidly as clinical condition necessitates
†Fluphenazine Hydrochloride
‡Fluphenazine enanthate or decanoate
††Higher doses have been used but are not recommended because of the increased risk of pigmentary retinopathy
 ¶Exceeds FDA recommended limits

Bleuler who introduced the concept of primary and secondary symptoms. Primary symptoms included thought disorder, flattened affect and autistic behavior. Secondary symptoms included hallucinations, delusions, belligerence and agitation. Antipsychotic drugs modify all of these symptoms to varying degrees in different people. Symptoms such as anxiety, depression, guilt, somatization and disorientation are less likely to respond to antipsychotic medication.

CHOICE OF DRUG. Although the potency of antipsychotic drugs varies over a wide range (Table 25–2), no one antipsychotic drug has been demonstrated to be more effective in treating a particular symptom complex than any other. Other criteria must be used in the selection of a specific drug for a particular patient. Criteria used include the following: Is there a drug to which the patient has responded well in the past? If so, that is the drug of choice. Does the patient's physician have experience in the use of a specific drug and therefore skill and confidence in its use? This may be the most important consideration. Are there specific side effects that are less desirable for a given patient? One would rather give haloperidol or a piperazine phenothiazine to patients with a history of cardiovascular or cerebral vascular disease because hypotension would be less likely to occur than with chlorpromazine. Is patient resistance to taking medication a consideration? In this case a long acting phenothiazine, such as fluphenazine enanthate or decanoate, given on a biweekly injection schedule would be the drug of choice.

Whatever drug is chosen, the average patient can be expected to obtain two-thirds to three-fourths of his maximal therapeutic gain within the first 6 weeks of treatment. It is important to know how long it should take for a particular drug effect to occur, as approximately 10% of psychotic patients will not respond at all. Therapy is often required for 3 weeks or more before an antipsychotic effect is seen. Some patients show rapid improvement in a single day, whereas others may gradually improve over months or even years. In contrast, the ability of antipsychotic drugs to calm agitated patients can be noted within minutes to a few hours after parenteral administration. If a patient fails to respond after 6 weeks of treatment with an adequate dose (see later section), his diagnosis and status should be re-evaluated. Before deciding, however, that the patient is not responding to treatment, it is important to determine whether or not he is taking his medication (Ch. 7). If patient failure is suspected, a different form of the medication, such as liquid or injection, may be indicated. If this is not the problem, another antipsychotic drug may be tried.

DURATION OF TREATMENT. Well-controlled studies have shown a significantly greater rate of relapse in patients whose antipsychotic medication has been switched to placebo compared to those maintained on their original medication. However, it is impossible to predict who will relapse and who will not. Relapse is often a gradual process occurring over several months after medication is stopped. If and when antipsychotic medication should be discontinued is, therefore, a clinical judgment that must take into consideration both the increased risk of relapse if discontinued and the increased risk of permanent side effects (tardive dyskinesia) if maintained for a longer period of time.

DOSAGE. Each patient differs in the amount of antipsychotic medication needed to obtain optimal therapeutic results and in the type and severity of the side effects that may develop. In addition, there is great variability in the potency of different antipsychotic drugs (Table 25–2). Therefore each patient must be titrated for his specific response to the particular medication being used. Once a maximal or optimal effect has been achieved, it is often possible to establish a maintenance dose considerably lower than that needed in the initial stages of treatment. Ideally when initiating treatment of acute psychosis one should start with a low dose and build up rapidly over 2–3 days. By this time the patient is often more comfortable, manageable and able to function, at least at a minimal level. It must be remembered, however, that the underlying psychotic symptoms may not begin to subside until 3 weeks or longer after the initiation of therapy.

In the acutely agitated patient, it is often necessary to begin with parenteral medication immediately. Typically, chlorpromazine 25 or 50 mg IM is given and may be repeated every hour until the desired effect is obtained. Since chlorpromazine has a local irritating effect, it should be injected deep into large muscle masses such as the buttocks, and the site of injection rotated. As soon as the patient's clinical status permits, oral medication should replace parenteral. However, the patient should be watched closely for exacerbation of his symptoms and the oral dose increased as necessary. The range of dosage used for a given drug is large and depends on the individual patient's needs. Since the dose range between therapeutic efficacy and toxic overdose is wide it is better to err in the direction of too high a dose in the initial stages of drug therapy.

The antipsychotic drugs are supplied in a wide variety of forms and dosages. Most are prepared as tablets, liquid concentrate and injectable solutions. Fluphenazine is unique in that it is available in a long acting depot form (fluphenazine enanthate or decanoate) that when injected produces a sustained therapeutic effect over a period of 2–3 weeks. Chlorpromazine and prochlorperazine, in addition to the usual forms, are available in rectal suppositories for administration to patients suffering from nausea and vomiting. Thioridazine is the only frequently used antipsychotic drug that is *not* injectable. This limitation is unfortunate since it has the lowest incidence of neurologic side effects of all the antipsychotic drugs currently used in this country. Some drug combinations are also available (e.g., perphenazine plus amitriptyline). Although this decreases the total number of pills a patient has to take, the dosage ratio of the two drugs is fixed and often is not optimal for a given patient.

Organic Brain Syndromes

Antipsychotic drugs are used to treat the agitation sometimes associated with either acute or chronic organic brain syndromes. The choice of drug often depends upon the supposed *etiology* of the syndrome. Thus, in older people with cerebral vascular disease, an antipsychotic agent with the least hypotensive effect should be chosen. If seizures are likely to occur, antipsychotic medication should be administered with caution, as these drugs lower the seizure threshold.

Mania

Chlorpromazine and haloperidol are the antipsychotic drugs most often used in the treatment of mania. Large doses are usually required and can range as high as 3000 mg/day of chlorpromazine. Lithium is often begun concomitantly with antipsychotic medication when treating this disorder.

Childhood Psychosis

The efficacy of antipsychotic drugs in this disorder is problematic. Some children appear to respond, while others become worse.

Anxiety

Unless there is an underlying psychosis, the use of antipsychotic drugs in the treatment of anxiety states is inappropriate. There are good antianxiety agents available that lack the serious side effects of antipsychotic drugs.

Miscellaneous

GILLES DE LA TOURETTE DISEASE. This is a rare neurologic syndrome consisting of facial grimacing, violent muscular jerks involving the torso and the extremities and coprolalia (explosive, repetitive shouting of foul expletives). Haloperidol is the most effective treatment now available for this disorder.

HUNTINGTON'S DISEASE. A hereditary disorder characterized by choreiform movements and progressive mental deterioration, this disease sometimes first manifests itself as a psychosis indistinguishable from schizophrenia. Recent evidence suggests that the symptoms of this disease are due to the degeneration of interneurons in the basal ganglia which in turn may lead to an imbalance between gabaergic, cholinergic or dopaminergic systems of the brain. Interestingly, some of the antipsychotic drugs including fluphenazine and haloperidol are helpful in the treatment of this disease. Unfortunately, however, their therapeutic effects are sporadic and often minimal.

VOMITING; INTRACTABLE HICCUPS. In low doses some phenothiazines, e.g., **prochlorperazine** (Compazine), are effective in preventing specific types of nausea and vomiting, depending upon their etiology. They are useful in the treatment of vomiting associated with radiation sickness, gastroenteritus, uremia, carcinomatosis and vomiting induced by drugs such as morphine, estrogens, nitrogen mustards, disulfiram and folic acid antagonists. Phenothiazines with antiemetic properties are less effective in the treatment of motion sickness (Chs. 37, 49). Paradoxically, nausea can occasionally be seen as a side effect of this drug.

Phenothiazines (e.g., chlorpromazine) have also been shown to be useful in the control of intractable hiccups. Their mechanism of action is not known.

ANTIPRURITICS. Some nonantipsychotic phenothiazines with antihistaminic properties such as **trimeprazine** (Temaril) and **methdilazine** (Tacaryl) are effective antipruritics. These drugs are administered orally in doses of 2.5 and 8 mg, respectively, 2–4 times daily.

ADDICTION AND TOLERANCE

The antipsychotic drugs are not addictive in that physiologic dependence to these drugs does not develop. Occasionally mild withdrawal symptoms such as nausea, vomiting, malaise and headaches occur after abrupt discontinuation. They should therefore be withdrawn slowly at a rate of 10–25%/day.

ADVERSE EFFECTS

The antipsychotic drugs are extremely safe. Their margin of safety is so great that deaths from overdose are very rare. However, all produce a wide variety of adverse effects as might be predicted from their extensive and diverse pharmacological actions. Only the most common and/or dangerous adverse reactions will be discussed.

Hypersensitivity Reactions

These reactions usually occur within the first 3 months of therapy and are not dose related. They are most commonly associated with the phenothiazines and thioxanthenes.

JAUNDICE. The incidence is low, between 2–4%. It is usually a temporary reaction and not necessarily a reason to discontinue treatment. Obstructive in nature and usually mild, it is felt to be a hypersensitivity reaction. If not observed within the first month of therapy, it is unlikely to occur later. Cross reaction between antipsychotic drugs has not been demonstrated, and therefore a patient may be shifted from one drug to another when the jaundice is worrisome and the patient's psychiatric condition necessitates uninterrupted therapy.

BLOOD DYSCRASIAS. Several blood abnormalities can occur with phenothiazine treatment including leukopenia, leukocytosis and eosinophilia. However, the only serious side effect is the rare occurrence of agranuolcytosis reported to occur in 1 out of 10 thousand patients treated with chlorpromazine. This potentially fatal complication usually occurs during the first 6 weeks of treatment. Despite the rarity of this complication, some experts recommend that a complete blood count precede all antipsychotic therapy. Periodic blood counts are not necessary, but the physician should be alert to the sudden appearance of infections concomitant with the start of antipsychotic drugs and to the occurrence of prolonged illnesses that would normally be expected to be of short duration.

Neurologic Effects

These adverse effects are common to all antipsychotic drugs, although incidence varies considerably between specific agents. Piperazine phenothiazine derivatives and haloperidol have a relatively high incidence, particularly those involving the extrapyramidal system. The piperidine phenothiazine derivatives such as thioridazine and the dibenzodiazapine derivatives such as clozapine have a much lower incidence of acute extrapyramidal side effects.

The extrapyramidal syndromes produced by the antipsychotic drugs can be divided into four groups. Three of these appear concomitantly with initiation of drug therapy, and one (tardive dyskinesia) may not manifest itself until after drug therapy has stopped or after prolonged treatment with high doses.

PARKINSONIAN SYNDROME. This syndrome usually appears within 5–20 days after initiation of therapy. Clinically it is indistinguishable from idiopathic Parkinson's disease and classically consists of akinesia—decrease or slowing of voluntary movement associated with masked facies and a decrease in reciprocal arm movements during walking; tremor at rest, including pill rolling movement—most marked in the upper extremities, and rigidity. The severity of this syndrome is dose related and can readily be treated either by decreasing the dose (preferable if feasible) or by adding an anticholinergic drug, such as benztropine methanesulfate (Cogentin), 2–4 mg daily or trihexyphenidyl (Artane), 4–8 mg daily, to the therapeutic regime. There is a tendency for this adverse effect to decrease spontaneously with time so that periodic trials without anticholinergic medication are indicated to determine whether it is still necessary.

DYSTONIC REACTIONS. These effects most commonly occur between 1 hr and 5 days after initiation of therapy and are not dose related. Facial grimacing and torticollis are the most common effects and may be accompanied by oculogyric crises. Uncoordinated spastic movements of the body and limbs may also occur. This syndrome is sometimes misdiagnosed as an hysterical reaction and responds rapidly to the administration of parenteral antiparkinson medication or diphenhydramine (Benadryl).

AKATHISIA. Most commonly occurring 5–40 days after antipsychotic drug therapy has begun, this is frequently misdiagnosed as anxiety or an exacerbation of the patient's psychosis. It consists of involuntary motor restlessness characterized by fidgeting, constant pacing and lip movements, foot tapping and an inability to sit quietly. A correct diagnosis is essential because the treatment of choice is a reduction in dosage. When misdiagnosed as agitation, the patient is often treated by increasing the dosage which leads to an exacerbation of his already distressful condition. These patients usually respond dramatically to IM injections of benztropine. Response to benztropine can therefore be used to help in the differential diagnosis between drug induced akathisia and psychotic agitation; in the latter case, benztropine has no effect. There are, however, some patients whose akathisia appears refractory to antiparkinson medication. Changing to another antipsychotic drug is often helpful in this case.

TARDIVE DYSKINESIA. Although reported in a few patients who have received phenothiazines for only 4 months, this syndrome commonly occurs in chronic psychotics who have received antipsychotic therapy for prolonged periods of time. Unrecognized until relatively recently, it has been variously estimated to occur in 6–20% of chronically institutionalized patients. It is most frequently seen in older psychotic patients with concomitant organic brain disease. However, advanced age and organic pathology are by no means requirements for the appearance of this disorder. Tardive dyskinesia is characterized by involuntary bucco-facio-mandibular or bucco-lingual movements consisting of steryotyped sucking and smacking of the lips, lateral movements of the jaw and backward and forward movements of the tongue. Less frequently, choreiform-like movements can occur, characterized by jerky, quick purposeless movements of the extremities. By far the most serious of the neurologic syndromes produced by antipsychotic drugs, tardive dyskinesia may persist indefinitely after discontinuation of medication, and no effective treatment has yet been devised. Increasing the dose or switching to another drug will often temporarily mask the symptoms. However, inevitably they reappear, often in a more severe form than before. The etiology of this syndrome is unclear, and it is impossible to predict who will develop these particular symptoms.

As there is some tentative evidence and much theoretical concern that antiparkinson drugs may actually facilitate the appearance of tardive dyskinesia, it is recommended that these drugs not be administered routinely with antipsychotic medication. Perhaps the best way to avoid this neurologic side effect is always to determine the minimal effective dose for each patient and to discontinue medication as soon as it is clinically warranted. For those patients with a high risk of developing tardive dyskinesia (i.e., older patients who have received long term drug therapy), it may be wise temporarily to discontinue medication periodically, in an effort to determine as early as possible the onset of this syndrome.

Autonomic Nervous System Effects

ADRENERGIC. Orthostatic hypotension that usually occurs within the first five days of therapy is due to the adrenergic receptor blocking activity of these drugs. Tolerance usually develops rapidly. Phenothiazines with an aminoalkyl side chain are the worst offenders, whereas piperazine derivatives are much less likely to produce hypotension. This side effect is potentially hazardous in older patients who may have advanced cardiac or cerebral arteriosclerosis.

ANTICHOLINERGIC. The antipsychotic phenothiazines, thioxanthenes and haloperidol exhibit weak antimuscarinic properties (Ch. 17) that cause a variety of unpleasant side effects. These include: A dry mouth which can lead to difficulty with dentures in older patients and an increased incidence of oral infection, especially moniliasis;

decreased tearing with increased propensity to corneal abrasions in patients wearing contact lenses; nasal congestion and blurred vision. The latter is particularly bothersome for patients whose jobs depend on visual acuity or prolonged use of their eyes.

OTHER. Both the phenothiazines and thioxanthenes can cause menstrual irregularities and weight gain. Constipation can occur with these drugs as well as haloperidol, especially in the elderly patient. Two adverse effects are particularly associated with thioridazine therapy—inhibition of ejaculation without interference with erection and pigmentary retinopathy. The latter has only been seen in patients receiving thioridazine in excess of a 1000 mg/day.

Cautions and Counterindications

Antipsychotic drugs may have a synergistic effect in patients with brain damage that can result in respiratory paralysis or circulatory collapse. Patients with cardiovascular or cerebrovascular disease should be treated with caution owing to the hypotensive effects. The antipsychotic drugs lower the convulsive threshold and although not definitely contraindicated should be carefully used in patients with epilepsy. As they are detoxified in the liver and excreted in the urine, they should be administered with discretion to patients with liver or kidney disease. Their anticholinergic effects may also cause a relative paresis of the bladder which in the presence of prostatic hypertrophy can lead to urinary retention or cause an increase in intracular pressure in patients with glaucoma. Chlorpromazine has a synergistic effect with a number of CNS depressants including alcohol and the barbiturates. In addition, it is known to increase the sedative effect of morphine and the respiratory depression caused by meperidine. Chlorpromazine should not be combined with guanethidine, as it may block the antihypertensive effect of the latter.

Many antipsychotic drugs produce undesirable neurological side effects. These side effects are treated by administration of anticholinergic drugs such as benztropine or trihexyphenidyl. Unfortunately, these drugs intensify the undesirable anticholinergic effect of the antipsychotic drugs. In addition they can occasionally produce a toxic psychosis. Thus, the psychotic symptoms of a patient treated with antipsychotic medication may improve, while at the same time he develops disturbing extrapyramidal side effects. An anticholinergic drug is added to the regimen, and the patient's psychosis becomes worse. If the clinician is not aware of this syndrome, he may then increase the dosage of antipsychotic medication and add more anticholinergic drug to combat the side effects. This can become a vicious circle that has been known to result in death. The toxic psychosis induced by the anticholinergic drugs can often be differentiated from the endogenous psychosis by a careful mental status examination. In the toxic psychosis the patient will often be found to be confused and disoriented, whereas the endogenous psychosis usually occurs in a clear sensorium.

FURTHER READING

Gardos G, Cole JO, Orzock MH (1973): The importance of dosage in antipsychotic drug administration: A review of dose response studies. Psychopharmacologia 29:221

Klein DF, Davis JM (1969): Diagnosis and Drug Treatment of Psychiatric Disorders. Baltimore, Williams and Wilkins, pp. 1–173

JUDITH R. WALTERS

ROBERT H. ROTH

26. SEDATIVE-HYPNOTIC AND ANTIANXIETY DRUGS

Some of the oldest, some of the newest and some of the most widely used drugs in psycho-pharmacology are included in the sedative-hyp-notic, antianxiety category. CNS depressants have been in use for a long time in the form of opiates and alcohol, but these are neither safe nor reliable as hypnotics. In the mid-1800's, the sleep-inducing effects of the **bromide** salts were discovered; and bromides were used exclusively until the turn of the century. At that time more ef-fective sedative-hypnotics became available with the introduction of **chloral hydrate** and the **bar-biturates.** These continue to be used, together with the newer nonbarbiturate sedative-hyp-notics, in low doses as sedatives and in some-what higher doses for the induction and mainte-nance of sleep.

For a long time, drugs that produced drows-iness and sedation were also the only agents available for the treatment of manic and psy-chotic patients. In 1952, the specific antipsychotic effect of chlorpromazine was discovered, and the phenothiazines replaced the sedative-hyp-notics for the treatment and tranquilization of psychotic and schizophrenic patients. The pheno-thiazines, however, did not effectively produce "daytime sedation" or relieve anxiety and tension in individuals who were not psychotic. The classic sedative-hypnotics are still used for this purpose, but less frequently now than the **propanediols** and **benzodiazepines.**

The newest class of sedative-hypnotics, the benzodiazepines, were introduced in the early 1960's as more specific antianxiety agents with a wider margin of safety than their predecessors.

They immediately found a large market, which has been growing ever since. Although still CNS depressants, the benzodiazepines seemed able to relieve anxiety and tension at doses that cause less actual drowsiness and sedation than the other sedative-hypnotics.

The benzodiazepines, the barbiturates and the nonbarbiturate sedative-hypnotics, however, all have effects ranging from antianxiety and seda-tion to sleep and coma, depending upon the amount administered. Their classification as sed-ative-hypnotics or antianxiety agents may say less about their specific properties than it does about their dosage. Moreover, classification by use is far from satisfactory, since many of these agents have multiple uses. Some are anticonvul-sants and muscle relaxants. Nevertheless, those drugs used primarily for the relief of anxiety and daytime sedation, such as the benzodiazepines and propanediols, are termed **antianxiety agents, anxiolytics** or **minor tranquilizers.** The specific antipsychotic agents (Ch. 25) such as the phenothiazines and butyrophenones (sometimes referred to as major tranquilizers) have different mechanisms of action from the antianxiety agents, and do not cause progressive increases in CNS depression with increasing dosage.

The term **sedative-hypnotic** generally refers to drugs used primarily for the induction and/or maintenance of sleep. In contrast to the gaseous anesthetics that are commonly used for the pro-duction and maintenance of anesthesia and which are also CNS depressants, the drugs used as sedative-hypnotics are either liquid or solid and have much longer lasting effects.

SEDATIVE-HYPNOTICS

The prescription of drugs for the induction and maintenance of sleep is widely practiced in clin-ical medicine today. There is also a market for over-the-counter preparations advertised to pro-mote sleep. It is easy to understand the demand for such drugs. No one would argue that there is subjective discomfort involved in sleep deprivation, whether it is voluntary or involuntary. Moreover, the psychologic and physical discomforts and disorders which can cause insomnia may also be further aggravated by the loss of sleep. However, there are drawbacks to the use of these drugs, and it is important to keep the following two points in mind when deciding whether drug intervention for the promotion of sleep is indicated.

First, the prescription of the sedative-hypnotics generally represents the treatment of a symptom rather than a disease. Such treatment should only be used in addition to, rather than as an alternative to, concern and treatment of the primary disorder. Second, the advantages to be gained should be weighed against the potential disadvantages. The ideal hypnotic would consistently induce a rapid onset of natural sleep which would be maintained throughout the night so that the subject would awaken in the morning refreshed. However, none of the sedative-hypnotics currently available produce a state that is identical to normal sleep, and many have effects which persist into the morning leaving the individual with a groggy, "hung-over" feeling. The ideal drug should continue to be effective if used several nights in a row and withdrawal should not leave the subject worse off than he was originally. In fact, tolerance develops to the effect of many of the sedative-hypnotics, and withdrawal can itself precipitate sleep disturbances. The drug should be taken by mouth and be palatable and nontoxic. It should not produce dependency, and overdose should not seriously endanger health and life. All sedative-hypnotics available to date, however, have been shown to have some liability for dependence and addiction.

For a while thalidomide was felt to come close to being an ideal hypnotic. The extraordinary margin of safety claimed for this drug and its low incidence of side effects led to its unrestricted availability in West Germany in 1958, and then elsewhere. It was 3 years before Lenz discovered that the increasing numbers of infants born with deformed limbs and other organs were associated with the ingestion of as little as 100 mg of thalidomide between the 28th and 42nd day of pregnancy (Ch. 7). Fortunately, this drug was never approved in the United States.

Mechanism of Action

The therapeutically useful hypnotics exhibit a wide variety of chemical structures. Their common property of inducing CNS depression in both man and animals depends upon certain physiochemical characteristics that they share rather than upon the possession of any special chemical structure. This lack of structural specificity, and the fact that no specific antagonists exists for any class of hypnotics, makes it quite unlikely that these drugs exert their effects by interaction with specific "hypnotic receptor sites." At present there is no satisfactory explanation for the ability of such a group of diverse compounds to cause sedation and CNS depression.

Effect on Sleep

Our understanding of the characteristics and stages of sleep has increased rapidly over the past 15 years. The effects of drugs on normal and abnormal sleep cycles have been studied in sleep laboratories where the EEGs of sleeping subjects are monitored throughout the night. All of the drugs used to induce sleep have been found to alter the normal sleep cycle in some way. More information is needed about the function of the various stages of sleep before the significance of some of these alterations can really be assessed, but sleep deprivation studies in both animals and man have provided some clues.

On the basis of the EEG changes that occur during the night, sleep has been divided into two main phases, variously referred to as **REM (rapid-eye-movement)** or paradoxical sleep; and **NREM (nonrapid-eye-movement,** or slowwave sleep). An average night's sleep consists of alternating periods of REM and NREM sleep.

NREM SLEEP. This phase is characterized by synchronized cortical EEG activity composed of spindles and/or a high voltage slow wave pattern. NREM has been divided into 4 stages, each with increasing degrees of the characteristic synchronized high voltage slow wave EEG activity. Upon falling asleep, a person normally passes through these 4 stages, until after approximately 70–100 min, the first period of REM occurs. These cycles repeat themselves at approximately 90 min intervals throughout the night. It is generally assumed that NREM sleep serves in some way to allow the brain as well as the body to recuperate from its daily activity. Sleep walking and "night terrors" have been associated with this phase of sleep. Most drugs affect REM sleep more than NREM, but the benzodiazepines seem to be an exception. Sleep laboratory studies have suggested that in hypnotic doses, the benzodiazepines have their greatest effect on stage 4 sleep, causing a significant decrease in the amount of time spent in this phase.

REM SLEEP. The onset and cessation of REM sleep can be determined quite precisely from behavioral events. REM sleep is characterized by rapid eye movements and a complete abolition of muscle tone. A low voltage, fast, cortical EEG activity similar to that seen during arousal is characteristic. As the periods of NREM and REM repeat throughout the night, increasing periods of time are spent in REM sleep and decreasing time in the lower stages of NREM with each cycle. Approximately 20–25% of the night is normally spent in REM sleep.

Dreaming is associated with the REM phase of sleep and some evidence suggests that deprivation of REM sleep may lead to emotional distortion and personality changes. Sleep laboratory studies have indicated that when people are specifically deprived of REM sleep, but allowed to sleep in NREM periods, a "REM debt" is built up. When the individual is then permitted to sleep undisturbed, a *REM rebound* period will be observed and, during the following nights, relatively more time will be spent in REM sleep.

Unfortunately, all drugs used for the promotion and maintenance of sleep have, to some extent, the effect of decreasing the relative amount of time spent in REM sleep. Depending on the length of action of the drug and the dose, this may lead to a "REM rebound" in the later part of the night, or on subsequent nights. An increase in the length of the REM periods has been associated with the subjective feeling of not sleeping well, or of having a light and troubled night's sleep. It is easy to understand how this can promote a vicious cycle where the withdrawal of sleep medication leads an individual to feel that he needs "something" to help him sleep.

Classification

The clinically useful sedative-hypnotics are often classified as short, intermediate and long acting, although some of the implied differences are dose related (Table 26–1). In addition to dosage, the duration of action of a sedative-hypnotic is determined by its rate of absorption, distribution and metabolism. These variables are affected by the degree of ionization, water-lipid solubility coefficient and protein binding characteristics of the drug.

These drugs are also commonly referred to as either barbiturate or nonbarbiturate sedative-hypnotics. In the following discussion the barbiturates will be considered as a group and the nonbarbiturate sedative-hypnotics will be considered individually. A section is also included on nonprescription preparations advertised to promote sleep. Specific information on the drugs described in this chapter are shown in Tables 26–1 and 26–2.

NONPRESCRIPTION SEDATIVES

Bromides

In the 1850's, the bromide salts were found to have significant CNS depressant properties and were widely utilized in a variety of preparations. The bromides have since been replaced by safer and more efficacious drugs, but they are still found in over-the-counter nerve tonics and headache remedies. Indiscriminant use of such preparations may require specific treatment.

BROMIDE TOXICITY. Large doses of bromide causes GI irritation and vomiting, making acute intoxication rare. However, chronic intoxication is not at all uncommon. The half-life of the bromide ion in the body is 12 days and daily injection of bromide salts can lead to the accumulation of toxic levels over a period of just a few weeks.

Over-the-counter preparations containing the compound **carbromal** is another source of bromide poisoning. This ureide has CNS depressant effects of its own but also liberates bromide ions when metabolized. Carbromal is used in countless proprietary remedies for nervousness and insomnia, and has led to many cases of chronic poisoning throughout the world.

The toxic effects of the bromide ion consist of mental and emotional disturbances and psychotic behavior which can be misdiagnosed as schizophrenia.

Other effects include drowsiness, dizziness, irritability, delirium and coma. Dermatitis, often called the bromide rash or acne, and GI disturbances, manifested by anorexia, constipation and foul breath may also occur. The excretion of bromide from the body is accelerated by increased excretion of chloride ions. The administration of NaCl in large quantities (at least 6 g/day in divided doses) shortens the biologic half-life of bromide to 3–4 days. In serious cases of "bromism," it may be necessary to administer a mercurial or thiazide diuretic to remove the drug more rapidly.

Other Over-the-Counter "Sedatives"

Nonprescription compounds, such as Sominex, Sleep Eze, Dozoff, Proquil and Nyquil contain antihistamines and sometimes anticholinergics, such as scopolamine. The efficacy of these compounds in inducing and maintaining sleep has not been established. Unlike the other sedative-hypnotics discussed in this chapter, increasing the dosage of these drugs does not intensify their hypnotic effects. Instead, high doses can cause excitation, restlessness, agitation and occasional convulsions. Cases of severe toxic psychosis have been reported, resulting from

TABLE 26–1. Nonbarbiturate Sedative-Hypnotics

Drug	Trade name	Structure	Hypnotic dose	Preparations available
Short acting Chloral hydrate	Noctec	CCl_3-CH(OH)$_2$	500–1000 mg	Capsules—250 and 500 mg Syrup—500 mg/5 cc Suppositories—300, 500 and 275 mg
Chloral betaine	Beta-Chlor		870–1740 mg	Tablets—870 mg
Trichlorethyl phosphate	Triclos		1500 mg	Tablets—750 mg
Paraldehyde			5–10 mg	Vials—2, 5, 10 and 30 mg
Ethchlorvynol	Placidyl	CH_3-CH_2-C(OH)(CH=CHCl)-C≡CH	500–750 mg	Capsules—100, 200 and 500 mg
Ethinamate	Valmid		500 mg	Capsules—500 mg
Intermediate acting Glutethimide	Doriden		250–500 mg	Tablets—125, 250 and 500 mg Capsules—500 mg Suppositories—8, 15, 30 and 60 mg
Methyprylon	Nodular		200–400 mg	Capsules—200 and 300 mg Tablets—50 mg
Methaqualone	Quaalude Parest Sopor		150–300 mg	Tablets—75, 150, 200, 300 and 400 mg
Flurazepam	Dalmane		15–30 mg	Tablets—15 and 30 mg

TABLE 26–2. Barbiturates

$$\begin{array}{c} R_3 \\ \diagdown N-C \diagup O \\ X=C \qquad \diagdown C \diagup R_1 \\ \diagup N-C \diagdown R_2 \\ H \qquad O \end{array}$$

Name	Trade name	R_1	R_2	R_3	X	Use and dosage
Long acting (longer than 8 hr)						
Barbital	Veronal	Ethyl	Ethyl	H	O	Hypnotic — 300–500 mg
Mephobarbital	Mebaral	Ethyl	Phenyl	H	O	Antiepileptic
Phenobarbital	Luminal	Ethyl	Phenyl	H	O	Antiepileptic
						Hypnotic — 130–200 mg
						Sedative — 30–60 mg, 2–4 times/day
Short To Intermediate Acting (up to 8 hr)						
Amobarbital	Amytal	Ethyl	Isoamyl	H	O	Hypnotic — 100–200 mg
						Sedative — 30–50 mg, 2–3 times/day
Pentobarbital	Nembutal	Ethyl	1-methylbutyl	H	O	Hypnotic — 100 mg
						Sedative — 30 mg, 3–4 times/day
Secobarbital	Seconal	Allyl	1-methylbutyl	H	O	Hypnotic — 100 mg
Ultra Short Acting						
Thiamylal	Surital	Allyl	1-methylbutyl	H	S	Anesthetic
Thiopental	Pentothal	Ethyl	1-methylbutyl	H	S	Anesthetic

suicide attempts with preparations containing scopolamine.

BARBITURATES

Chemistry

The barbiturates are derived from the condensation of malonic acid with urea, forming malonyl urea, or barbituric acid. This parent compound is not itself a CNS depressant. However, when certain alkyl or aryl groups replace the two hydrogens on C_5, compounds with hypnotic activity are produced. The structures of the most important barbiturates are shown in Table 26–2. The compounds that have a sulfur group replacing the oxygen are referred to as thiobarbiturates, those without the sulfur group are called oxybarbiturates.

The anticonvulsant properties of the barbiturates seem to be somewhat independent of their sedative-hypnotic properties (Ch. 30) from a structural point of view. The phenyl group on C_5 of phenobarbital is important for its anticonvulsant, but not its hypnotic effects. Too long an alkyl group on this carbon will decrease the hypnotic effects of the drug and convert it into a convulsant.

Absorption, Metabolism and Excretion

The barbiturates are weak acids and largely unionized at physiologic pH (Ch. 2). The pKa's of the clinically effective barbiturates fall within a fairly narrow range. Lipid solubility is also important in determining the rate of absorption, distribution and metabolism of a specific barbitu-

rate (Ch. 3). There is a strong correlation between the partition coefficient, the degree of binding to both plasma and brain proteins and the duration of action of these drugs.

The ultra short acting barbiturates penetrate the brain very rapidly due to their high lipid solubility and the relatively large blood flow to this organ. They are then rapidly redistributed to other parts of the body. The barbiturates are not selectively concentrated at particular sites within the brain and the CNS depression caused by these drugs is dependent upon the amount of barbiturate which reaches the brain and remains there. In the first 15–20 min after the administration of a small single dose of an ultra short acting barbiturate, the decline in brain concentration is due largely to the redistribution of the drug from brain to lean body mass or muscle. Plasma concentrations then decline slowly due to uptake into fat and gradual metabolism. Especially in the case of the short acting barbiturates, metabolism rate is less important in determining duration of action than the rate of redistribution. The fact that thiopental remains in the body after its effects appear to have terminated accounts for the cumulative effects of repeated doses of this drug.

Longer acting barbiturates are more ionized at the plasma pH and are less lipid soluble so that they penetrate the brain and are redistributed more slowly. The barbiturates are metabolized by the liver to more polar compounds that can be more effectively excreted in the urine (Ch. 3). The longer acting, less lipid soluble drugs, such as phenobarbital and barbital, are also, to some extent, excreted unchanged in the urine.

The barbiturates are metabolized by oxidation

of the side chains on carbon 5, N-dealkylation, desulfuration of thiobarbiturates and destruction of the barbituric acid ring (Ch. 3). Side-chain oxidation is the most important metabolic pathway. The larger of the substituted groups on C_5 is usually oxidized to produce relatively polar alcohols, ketones, phenols and carboxylic acids. These are either excreted directly or as conjugates with glucuronic acid. N-dealkylation of the N-alkyl barbiturates can, in some instances, result in the production of an active metabolic product. Mephobarbital, e.g., is converted by this process into phenobarbital. Desulfuration of the thiobarbiturates results in the corresponding oxybarbiturates, but this route of metabolism probably accounts for only a small portion of the administered dose in man. Hydrolytic cleavage of the barbituric acid ring is also only of minor importance.

Clinical Uses

The barbiturates are classified as ultra short, short, intermediate and long acting, and the preferred use of an individual barbiturate is related to its duration of action. The short acting compounds such as **thiopental** (Pentothal) are generally used as IV anesthetics (Ch. 27) and occasionally as sleep-inducing agents. The long acting barbiturates are preferred as daytime sedatives, antianxiety agents and anticonvulsants (Ch. 30).

The barbiturates most commonly used as sedative-hypnotics are intermediate acting; **secobarbital** (Seconal), **pentobarbital** (Nembutal) and **amobarbital** (Amytal). In hypnotic doses, these drugs produce a decrease in sleep latency and an increase in total sleep time, and are thus useful for those who have trouble either falling asleep, staying asleep or both.

Adverse Effects

EFFECT ON SLEEP. Hangover and drowsiness may sometimes occur in the morning after barbiturate use. Sleep studies have shown that the barbiturates cause a significant decrease in time spent in the REM phase of sleep. Continuous use of the barbiturates seems to be accompanied by a tolerance to their therapeutic effects and a "REM rebound" period when the drug is withdrawn, which is sometimes accompanied by poor sleep and nightmares.

ENZYME INDUCTION. Use of the barbiturates causes the induction of the hepatic microsomal enzymes (Chs. 3,4). This has the effect of increasing the rate of metabolism, and thus limiting the activity, of many drugs including the barbiturates themselves and the oral anticoagulants. This phenomena contributes to the tolerance that develops with continued use of the barbiturates. Stimulation of liver enzymes is also responsible for the ability of barbiturates to precipitate attacks of acute, intermittent porphyria in individuals suffering from this disorder. These attacks may culminate in paralysis and death. They are due to an increase in the rate limiting enzyme, Δ-aminolevulinic acid synthetase, which results in an increase in porphyrin biosynthesis.

PARADOXIC EXCITATION. In some individuals, these drugs may cause paradoxic restlessness, excitement and delirium. Elderly people are also prone to hangover effects associated with confusion and agitation.

OVERDOSE. The term "automatism" refers to the state in which an individual takes repeated doses of barbiturates without recalling the previous doses, until, eventually, potentially lethal amounts are ingested. The simultaneous use of alcohol makes the danger of this state considerably worse. The toxic depressant effects of the barbiturates are potentiated by alcohol and many cases of serious overdose and accidental suicide have been attributed to the simultaneous ingestion of large but individually nontoxic amounts of these two drugs. Barbiturate overdose also occurs all too frequently as a result of a suicide attempt. While lethal doses vary with the individual, ten times the normal therapeutic dose is considered life-threatening. Treatment of barbiturate and hypnotic drug overdose in general is largely supportive (Ch. 13). One of the most successful protocols, the Scandanavian method, involves gastric lavage and dialysis, in combination with constant attention to the maintenance of an adequate airway and blood volume. Alkalinization of the urine is effective in facilitating the elimination of some of the barbiturates.

ADDICTION. The most serious problem with the barbiturates is their addictive liability. These drugs can produce both psychologic and physical dependence, and barbiturate abuse is a very real problem today. Abrupt withdrawal from barbiturates after physical addiction can result in grand mal seizures and death (Ch. 9).

CONTRAINDICATIONS. The barbiturates should be given very cautiously in the presence of hepatic disease and severe pulmonary insufficiency. Patients with chronic emphysema are often very sensitive to respiratory depressant actions of ordinary hypnotic doses. Hypersensitivity reactions sometimes occur usually involving the skin, urticaria, angioneurotic edema and a generalized morbilliform rash or bullous erythema. These drugs should not be given to individuals with the history of such a reaction.

Finally, as indicated above, they should be avoided in patients with acute intermittent porphyria, suicidal tendencies and a predilection to drug abuse.

NONBARBITURATES

CHLORAL HYDRATE

Chemistry

Chloral hydrate (Noctec) is a crystalline solid with a pungent odor and a somewhat caustic taste. Its metabolite, trichlorethanol, is one of a group of halogenated aliphatic alcohols that also have hypnotic effects.

Absorption, Metabolism and Excretion

After administration, chloral hydrate is rapidly reduced to trichloroethanol, which in itself is an effective hypnotic. Both compounds probably contribute to the hypnotic action. The reduction occurs in all tissues including the brain. In the liver, the alcohol is further metabolized and conjugated with glucuronic acid to urochloralic acid. In alkaline urine, this compound decomposes to yield products which reduce Fehling's and Benedict's reagent and can be responsible for a false positive reaction for glucose. Chloral hydrate is also metabolized in the liver and kidney to trichloroacetic acid that is slowly excreted in the urine.

Clinical Uses

Chloral hydrate was introduced into medicine in 1869 and it is still a widely used and highly regarded hypnotic. It is a short acting drug with a rapid onset of action, making it more suitable for inducing sleep than maintaining or prolonging it. This drug is especially useful in pediatric and geriatric populations, as in these individuals it is associated with a lower incidence of paradoxic excitation than is barbiturate medication. Hangover and depressant after effects are less frequent than with longer acting hypnotics. REM suppression occurs with this drug but has been reported to be less than that observed with the barbiturates. Chronic use of chloral hydrate is accompanied by the development of tolerance to its effects.

This drug has a caustic taste and is irritating to the gastric mucosa, and should be administered well diluted with water or milk to avoid nausea or vomiting. To eliminate the undesirable effects of chloral hydrate a variety of derivatives of this agent have been introduced (chloral betaine, trichlorethyl phosphate). These compounds lack the strong odor and unpleasant taste, and do not produce gastric irritation.

Adverse Effects

The chloral hydrate therapeutic ratio is similar to that of the barbiturates. However, chloral hydrate overdose is less frequently reported than barbiturate overdose. When toxic doses are taken, respiratory depression and hypotension occur (Ch. 13). Treatment should be supportive and similar to that used for barbiturate overdose. Alcohol potentiates the depressant effects of this hypnotic and both intended and accidental suicide has been associated with simultaneous ingestion of these two drugs. Chloral hydrate is the extra-added ingredient in the legendary Mickey Finn knock-out drink.

Addiction to chloral hydrate is also far less common than addiction to barbiturates, probably because of the gastric irritation caused by chronic administration of large doses. Withdrawal is similar to withdrawal from alcohol.

The drug metabolizing enzymes of the liver are not stimulated by chloral hydrate in humans. The drug does, however, interfere with plasma protein binding of the coumarin type anticoagulants, increasing both their bioavailability and metabolism, suggesting caution when these drugs are coadministered. Allergic reactions may occur with chloral hydrate as with any of the sedative hypnotics. The drug is not recommended for those with gastritis, ulcers or severe heart disease. As with all sedative-hypnotics, patients should be cautioned against trying to drive or operate potentially dangerous machinery after taking this drug.

PARALDEHYDE

Chemistry

Paraldehyde is a trimer of acetaldehyde. It is a colorless liquid that on exposure to light and air, decomposes readily to acetaldehyde and acetic acid.

Absorption, Metabolism and Distribution

Paraldehyde is easily absorbed, has a rapid onset of action and is largely metabolized by the liver. However, a portion is excreted by the lungs, and the breath of someone who has taken paraldehyde has a very disagreeable odor. This together with the drug's unpleasant taste diminish its abuse potential. In the presence of liver damage, paraldehyde remains in the body longer and more is excreted by the lungs.

Clinical Uses

This drug is not often prescribed for ambulatory patients because of its unpleasant odor and taste. In the past it has often been used as a sedative for conditions involving excitement and delirium such as delirium tremens, tetanus, etc. Other drugs, however, such as the benzodiazepines, have been shown to be as good if not better. Moreover, paraldehyde has two main disadvantages: First, it is not recommended for parenteral administration, a route often necessary if the patient is quite ill. Second, if the drug preparation is old, has been exposed to sun or heat or has been previously opened, it is likely to contain toxic decomposition products.

Because it has irritating effects on gastric mucosa, paraldehyde should not be administered orally to patients with esophagitis, gastritis or gastric or duodenal ulcers. Its rectal administration should be avoided in the presence of inflammatory conditions of the anus or lower bowel. Paraldehyde is also contraindicated for patients taking disulfiram.

ETHCHLORVYNOL AND MEPARFYNOL

Chemistry

The CNS depressant effects of tertiary alcohols have been known since the end of the last century. In the 1950s, it was found that tertiary alcohols with unsaturated groups have greater hypnotic activity than the corresponding alcohols with saturated groups. Two of these compounds are currently available as sedative-hypnotics. **Meparfynol** (Oblivon, Dormison) has hypnotic activity, although its clinical value is questionable because of its long half-life. **Ethchlorvynol** (Placidyl) is a tertiary alcohol with a β-chlorovinyl group which contributes to its hypnotic potency.

Absorption, Metabolism and Excretion

Meparfynol is adequately absorbed from the GI track but is slowly metabolized. The drug can be detected in patients 48 hr after its administration. Therefore, repeated doses present the danger of cumulative toxicity. Ethchlorvynol, on the other hand, is rapidly metabolized by the liver and is no longer detectable 3 hr after administration.

Clinical Uses

Ethchlorvynol is an effective short acting hypnotic with less profound effects than those produced by chloral hydrate or the barbiturates. The incidence of after effects is low. The drug has some anticonvulsant and muscle relaxing properties. Adverse effects include unpleasant after taste and interference with oral anticoagulants.

Physical dependence to ethchlorvynol has been reported to occur with doses of 1.5 g daily. The therapeutic ratio of this drug is similar to that of the barbiturates. Overdose can result in prolonged coma that may be shortened by emptying the bowel.

ETHINAMATE

Chemistry

The esterification of alcohols with carbamic acid increases their sedative-hypnotic activity and produces a class of compounds referred to as **urethanes.** The best known urethane is **meprobamate,** a dicarbamate. This drug is most commonly used as an antianxiety agent (see below). Ethinamate (Valmid), introduced in Germany in 1953, is the only carbamic acid derivative used primarily as a sedative-hypnotic in current clinical practice.

Absorption, Metabolism and Distribution

Ethinamate is hydroxylated by the liver to 4-hydroxyethinamate and excreted both as such and as the glucuronide conjugate. Within 4 hr it is completely inactivated.

Clinical Uses

Ethinamate has a rapid onset and brief duration of action, making it a reliable agent for the induction, but not the maintenance of sleep. Because it is a short acting drug, it has a low incidence of hangover. The effects of ethinamate overdose are also of short duration.

Addiction to ethinamate has been reported. The use of this drug has also been associated with a few cases of thrombocytopenia.

GLUTETHIMIDE

Chemistry

Glutethimide (Doriden) is a solid with a high lipid-water partition coefficient. It is structurally similar to phenobarbital. This drug and methyprylon (see below) are piperidinedione derivatives that were introduced as sedative hypnotics in the mid-1950s.

Absorption, Metabolism and Distribution

As glutethimide is not very water soluble, its absorption from the GI track is unpredictable and its onset of action is slow when the drug is taken orally. Due to its high lipid solubility, it is rapidly distributed to the brain when given IV, and then redistributed to other parts of the body. The *d*- and *l*-stereoisomers of this drug are metabolized by different routes. The products are largely excreted in the bile into the intestine. This drug is similar in structure to thalidomide, but metabolized differently. No teratogenic effects have been reported.

Clinical Uses

Glutethimide is an intermediate acting sedative-hypnotic, similar to secobarbital or pentobarbital and with no apparent advantages over these drugs. Even when this drug is taken at bedtime some patients report a "hangover effect" the following morning, and it should not be taken within 4 hr of rising. Glutethimide has as great a potential for tolerance and addiction and is more toxic than the barbiturates. It is a potent cardiovascular depressant and because of its marked lipid solubility, the use of dialysis for the treatment of overdose is not effective. Toxic psychoses and convulsions have been associated not only with withdrawal, but with continuous use. Glutethimide stimulates the drug-metabolizing enzymes and antagonizes the action of oral anticoagulants.

METHYPRYLON

Chemistry

Unlike glutethimide, this piperidinedione derivative is quite water soluble.

Absorption, Metabolism and Distribution

Methyprylon (Nodular) is excreted in the bile and urine, largely conjugated to glucuronic acid. One of the metabolites of methyprylon is structurally analogous to a tetrahydropyridine which has been implicated as a causative factor in agranulocytosis. Methyprylon has not been associated with the production of blood dyscrasias, but if used repeatedly blood counts should be made.

Clinical Uses

This drug is similar in action to the intermediate acting barbiturates and to glutethimide. It is not widely used nor has it been widely investigated. Tolerance and addiction have been reported.

Like the barbiturates, methylprylone stimulates Δ-aminolevulinic acid synthetase, and is contraindicated in patients with intermittent porphyria.

METHAQUALONE

Chemistry

Methaqualone (Quaalude, Sopor), introduced in the mid-1960s, was derived from a class of compounds developed as potential antimalarial agents and then found to have significant sedative-hypnotic properties. It is a disubstituted quinazolone.

Absorption, Metabolism and Distribution

This drug is metabolized by the liver and excreted rapidly in the urine and feces. Its use is contraindicated in the presence of hepatic disease.

Clinical Uses

Methaqualone is a fast acting sedative-hypnotic with a duration of about 4–8 hr. A hypnotic dose can produce hangover effects in the morning, as well as dizziness, urticaria and parethesias. Like most other sedative-hypnotics, it has been reported to cause a significant depression of REM sleep. Although originally advertised as having no addictive liability, methaqualone is currently quite a popular drug of abuse. Addiction is not infrequent and the popularity of "luding out" is becoming a matter of concern; some countries have withdrawn the compound from the market. A combination of methaqualone and diphenhydramine, called **mandrax** has also been shown to have strong addictive potential.

Methaqualone overdose is clinically different from barbiturate overdose. Hypertonia, muscle spasm and convulsion occur in addition to coma. Recommended treatment is supportive; forced diuresis or dialysis are not very effective in treating methaqualone overdose.

FLURAZEPAM

Chemistry

Flurazepam (Dalmane), a member of the benzodiazepine family, was introduced in the United States in 1970 as a sedative-hypnotic. The diethylaminoethyl group on the N-1 nitrogen of the 7-membered ring distinguishes this drug chemically from the other clinically available benzodiazepines which will be discussed under the antianxiety section.

Absorption, Metabolism and Distribution

The difference between flurazepam and the benzodiazepines that are more commonly used as antianxiety agents may be mostly pharmacokinetic. Unlike drugs such as diazepam and chlordiazepoxide, flurazepam is metabolized quite rapidly and its metabolites have no sedative-hypnotic activity. The drug is largely dealkylated and oxidized, and excreted in the urine. Blood levels are undetectable within a few hours after ingestion. Initial absorption of the drug from the GI track seems to be rapid and efficient.

Clinical Uses

Flurazepam has been around for a relatively short time. In the past it has been common for new sedative-hypnotics to have a honeymoon period when grand, but generally short lived, claims are made about their safety and efficacy. However, there are some indications that flurazepam may really be a significant addition to the list of useful sedative-hypnotics. Several laboratories have reported that flurazepam has less effect on REM sleep than most other sedative-hypnotics, although it causes a significantly greater decrease in the amount of time spent in stage 4 NREM. The clinical significance of this is unclear. However, it has also been reported that flurazepam continues to be effective in inducing sleep when used chronically, while tolerance develops to most of the other sedative hypnotics. It has also been found, in contrast with other hypnotics, that the improvement in sleep parameters achieved with flurazepam are maintained for several days after discontinuation.

It is well established that the benzodiazepines are less toxic than the barbiturates. Habituation and addiction have been reported, but deaths attributed specifically to benzodiazepine overdose are very rare or nonexistent. As sedative-hypnotics are often used in suicide attempts, the relative safety of the benzodiazepines in this regard may be an important consideration when prescribing a drug of this type for some individuals.

Induction of liver metabolizing enzymes and interference with anticoagulant therapy are not clinically significant with chronic use of flurazepam. The effects of alcohol and flurazepam are additive; it is not recommended that these drugs be used together.

ANTIANXIETY DRUGS

The use of drugs for the treatment of anxiety has increased tremendously during the last 10 years. Recent surveys indicate that 5–15% of American adults take antianxiety agents at some time during a year. The benzodiazepines account for the majority of these prescriptions. **Diazepam** (Valium) and **chlordiazepoxide** (Librium) were estimated to be, respectively, the first and third most commonly prescribed drugs in 1972.

Anxiety is a ubiquitous state and there is little objective criteria with which to describe the situations where drug treatment is indicated. Anxiety reactions may be mild, panicy, acute, free-floating, appropriate or out of proportion to reality. They may be associated with depression or other illnesses, or transformed into a variety of seemingly unrelated signs and symptoms. Anxiety is also often a constructive and desirable reaction. The extent of warranted drug treatment in any of these conditions is debated by many, and the extent to which such treatment will be therapeutic will depend on the role of anxiety in an individual's functional disability. As with insomnia, anxiety is a symptom rather than a disease, and it should not be treated without primary attention to the underlying problem. The prescription of an antianxiety agent is not a valid substitute for a physician's time and concern.

The difficulties encountered in trying to define the conditions best treated by these drugs are reflected in the problems involved in assessing their antianxiety effects. Anxiety often responds to placebo or remits spontaneously. The ability of a drug to induce sleep in animals or man is a relatively easy parameter to measure, compared with its ability to reduce anxiety. The current demand for these drugs may be an indication of their efficacy. A more objective criterion is called for, however, but there is no single method for the measurement of anxiety that is completely satisfactory. Taken together, however, the results of many different animal and clinical studies have shown that the drugs commonly used as antianxiety agents, the barbiturates, the propanediols and the benzodiazepines, have significant antiaggression and disinhibitory effects in animals and anxiety-reducing effects in man. Whether the present popularity of the benzodiazepines is related to their lower incidence of adverse side effects or to a significantly different mechanism of action from the other sedative-hypnotics remains to be determined.

PROPANEDIOLS

Chemistry

The most important antianxiety agent of this class is **meprobamate** (Miltown, Equanil), a substituted dicarbamate with a simple aliphatic structure. It is a derivative of mephenesin, a short acting muscle relaxant (Ch. 21). **Tybamate** (Tybatran) is a shorter acting analog of meprobamate with a butyl group on one of the carbamyl nitrogens. Because of its short duration of action, it has limited usefulness in the treatment of chronic anxiety states.

Absorption, Metabolism and Excretion

Meprobamate is readily absorbed from the GI tract. Its maximal effect and peak blood levels occur about 2–3 hr after ingestion and its half-life is 10 hr. The half-life of tybamate is about one-third that of meprobamate. Meprobamate is hydroxylated and conjugated to glucuronic acid in the liver and excreted in the urine. Hydroxy-meprobamate, the major metabolite that accounts for about 60% of the oral dose, is pharmacologically inactive.

Clinical Uses

In 1955 meprobamate was introduced as the first specific antianxiety agent, a drug able to reduce anxiety and tension without drowsiness. At this time the remarkable success of the phenothiazine antipsychotic agents had generated a demand for drugs that would be equally effective in providing tranquilization for individuals who were not psychotic. Meprobamate was well advertised and became very popular and widely prescribed. Within a couple of years, however, it became evident that this drug was no more effective than the barbiturates in providing relief from anxiety without causing other sedative side effects. Its actions are very similar to those of amobarbital and phenobarbital. It is still frequently used although the benzodiazepines have become much more popular.

Meprobamate has significant muscle relaxing properties due to suppression of interneuronal synaptic transmission in the spinal cord.

The toxicity of meprobamate is equal to or greater than that of the barbiturates. Overdose can cause respiratory depression, hypotension, CNS depression, coma and death. In a survey of 16 fatalities, the average ingested dose was 28 g. Tolerance, habituation and physical addiction can occur at doses as low as 2.4 g daily. The effects of sudden withdrawal range from insomnia to convulsions and death.

Meprobamate can occasionally cause allergic reactions, including urticaria, erythematous cytopenia and nonthrombocytopenic purpura. Aplastic anemia has been reported. Meprobamate causes induction of the liver microsomal enzymes.

BENZODIAZEPINES

Chemistry

In 1955, Sternbach at Roche Laboratories synthesized a series of compounds by treating quinazolines, 6-membered ring structures, with various amines. When one of the products was investigated 2 years later, it was found to have an unexpected 7-membered ring structure and equally unexpected pharmacologic effects. Since that time a great many benzodiazepines have been synthesized and studied.

Structurally, the active compounds fall into two groups. Within the first group, the 2-amino-4-oxides, **chlordiazepoxide** (Librium) is the most pharmacologically potent member (Table 26–3). The 2-methyl amino group is the most effective

substitution on C_2. Activity is reduced when either no group or longer chains are attached to this carbon. An electronegative group at the 7 position is important for antianxiety efficacy and a decrease in potency results from a substitution at position 3. Chlordiazepoxide is a colorless solid existing as a hydrochloride conjugate. It is water soluble, but unstable in solution. Parenteral preparations should be freshly prepared. This drug should be protected from light as ultra violet light isomerizes the compound.

The rest of the available benzodiazepines are 1,3-dihydro-2-ketones. These include **diazepam** (Valium), **oxazepam** (Serax), and **clorazepate** (Tranxene). The electronegative group at the 7 position on the molecule is also important in these compounds. A methyl group on nitrogen 1 is optimal as is either no substitution or a methyl group on C_3. These compounds are relatively insoluble in water.

Absorption, Metabolism and Excretion

Chlordiazepoxide is well absorbed from the GI tract reaching maximum blood levels within 2–6

TABLE 26—3. Antianxiety Agents

Drug	Trade name	Structure	Dose	Preparations available
Meprobamate	Miltown Equanil	$CH_3-(CH_2)_2-C-CH_3$ with $CH_2-O-C-NH_2$ (O) groups	1200—1600 mg, 3—4 times/day	Tablets - 200, 400 mg
Tybamate	Tybatran	$H_2N-C-O-CH_2-C-CH_2-O-C-NH-(CH_2)_3-CH_3$; CH_3 , $(CH_2)_2-CH_3$	250—500 mg, 3—4 times/day	Capsules - 125, 250 and 350 mg
Chlordiazepine	Librium	(benzodiazepine structure, Cl, N-CH3, N→O, phenyl)	5—10 mg, 3—4 times/day	Capsules - 5, 10 and 25 mg Tablets - 5, 10 and 25 mg Injectable - 5 mg ampul + 2 ml ampul diluent
Diazepam	Valium	(benzodiazepine structure, CH3, Cl, phenyl)	2—10 mg, 2—4 times/day	Tablets - 2, 5 and 10 mg Injectable - 5 mg/1 ml
Oxazepam	Serax	(benzodiazepine structure, OH, Cl, phenyl)	10—30 mg, 3—4 times/day	Capsules - 10, 15 and 30 mg
Chlorazepate	Tranxene	(benzodiazepine structure, OH, O^-K^+, $C-O^-K^+$, Cl, phenyl)	30 mg/day in divided doses	Capsules - 3.75, 7.5 and 15 mg

hr after ingestion. Its half-life ranges from 7–28 hr in different individuals. Two important metabolic products of chlordiazepoxide, desmethylchlordiazepoxide and its oxidized derivative, demoxepam, are also pharmacologically active and have longer half-lives than chlordiazepoxide. Daily use of this drug could lead to cumulative sedation due to the slow rate of elimination of these metabolites. Small amounts of oxazepam are also formed. These metabolites are either excreted unchanged in the urine or further metabolized by conjugation to glucuronide or by cleavage of the 7-membered ring.

Diazepam is rapidly absorbed after oral administration. Peak blood levels are reached within 2 hr. Its disappearance from the blood is biphasic. The initial phase has a half-life of a few hours and the second phase, 20–50 hr. It is more tightly bound to plasma proteins than chlordiazepoxide. For parenteral administration, this drug is dissolved in a nonaqueous solvent that may affect its availability. Most often this is propylene glycol which has some CNS depressant effects of its own. After IV administration of a 10–20 mg dose, profound sedation is achieved in about 4 min accompanied by a short period of anteriograde amnesia. Recovery occurs in about 1 hr coincident with declining blood levels.

The metabolites of diazepam also have antianxiety and sedative activity. Desmethyldiazepam, the most important metabolite, has a half-life of 96 hr. Repeated oral administration leads to the accumulation, first of the drug itself and then, after a few days, of this metabolite. At equilibrium, desmethyldiazepam levels are similar to, or greater than those of diazepam. Two other active metabolites, the 3-hydroxylated derivative, temazepam and the demethylated, 3-hydroxylated derivative, oxazepam are also formed. These compounds are either excreted free, as glucuronides, or to a small degree, as sulfates.

Oxazepam is insoluble in water. It is sold as the water-soluble sodium salt of the succinic acid conjugate. The d-isomer of this conjugate is more potent than the l- as it is more rapidly deconjugated. Oxazepam has a shorter half-life than diazepam and 80% of the drug is excreted in the urine within 72 hr, mostly as oxazepam glucuronide. The repeated administration of this benzodiazepine, therefore, does not lead to accumulation of either the drug itself or of any active metabolites.

Chlorazepate, available in the United States since 1972, is also metabolized to desmethyldiazepam and would be expected to have long lasting effects.

Actions

When chlordiazepoxide was first tested in various animal models, it was found to have calming and taming effects similar to those observed with the barbiturates, but unlike the barbiturates, these effects occurred at doses significantly lower than those that cause a decrease in activity, sleepiness and ataxia. The effects of punishment or lack of reward on animal behavior are consistently attenuated by the benzodiazepines. They reduce both evoked and spontaneous hostility and aggressive behavior. When aggressive behavior has been suppressed by punishment, however, the disinhibitory effects of these drugs produce paradoxical increases in aggression.

The benzodiazepines are effective antianxiety agents in humans. The effects of the benzodiazepines on other aspects of human behavior and performance, such as intellectual function, motor performance, coordination and reaction time are not established.

The benzodiazepines have muscle relaxing properties and prevent drug or shock induced convulsions in animals. Diazepam is several times more potent than chlordiazepoxide in this regard. Clinical studies have suggested that the muscle relaxing effects of these drugs are supraspinal, unlike those of the propanediols.

Clinical Uses

In a recent comprehensive review, Greenblatt and Shader (1974) concluded that benzodiazepines are clinically superior to placebo in the treatment of anxious neurotic patients. They are more efficacious than the barbiturates and meprobamate in reducing anxiety. The benzodiazepines are useful in the treatment of depression if anxiety or agitation is an important aspect, but they have no specific antidepressant actions. There is no indication that any one benzodiazepine is more effective than the others. Oxazepam is metabolized more rapidly and does not lead to cummulative effects, and it may therefore be less toxic in use.

The benzodiazepines are also useful in spastic musculoskeletal disease and in a variety of seizure disorders (Ch. 30). Diazepam is currently the drug of choice for tetanus, status epilepticus and strychnine poisoning. It is also used for muscle strain.

The benzodiazepines have become widely used as psychosedative premedication for direct current cardioversion, gastroscopy, bronchoscopy, and dental procedures. They are also the most commonly used tranquilizing agents in the treatment of acute alcohol withdrawal, delirium tremens and hallucinogenic drug crises.

The benzodiazepine most commonly used as a hypnotic is flurazepam (see Sedative-Hypnotics). This drug is rapidly metabolized and no longer detectable in the blood 4 hr after ingestion. Because of their longer half-lives, the hypnotic doses of the other benzodiazepines taken at bedtime will continue to produce sedative and antianxiety effects throughout the next day. This is beneficial if these effects are desired and it is recommended that these drugs be given in two doses; the larger at bed time, and a smaller one in the morning.

Adverse Effects

In 3–10% of the people using chlordiazepoxide or diazepam, drowsiness and ataxia have been reported. These effects are dose dependent, and may be relieved by a gradual reduction of the dose as the levels of the drug and its metabolites accumulate and reach equilibrium in the blood. Occasionally, the benzodiazepines produce stimulation and increase aggressive behavior. This may be especially true when this behavior has been repressed by fear and anxiety about the results of its expression. Performance and motor control may be impaired by these drugs under some conditions.

Outside the CNS, the benzodiazepines have relatively little effect. They do not cause an induction of human liver microsomal enzymes nor affect the reproductive cycle in females. Like all sedative-hypnotics, however, the benzodiazepines are potential respiratory depressants and should be used with caution in the presence of pulmonary disease and other drugs, such as the opiates and alcohol, that have similar depressant effects.

Dependence and addiction can occur. Withdrawal is not usually serious however, probably because of the slow rate of decline of the blood levels. Overdose also has less serious effects than with the other sedative-hypnotics and antianxiety agents. Very rarely do large doses produce coma. Deaths specifically attributable to the benzodiazepines have not yet been reported.

BARBITURATES

In low doses, several of the barbiturates are satisfactory for the treatment of anxious, agitated and overactive patients. Most commonly used for this purpose are **pentobarbital** (Nembutal), **phenobarbital** (Luminal), and **amobarbital** (Amytal). These are more toxic than the benzodiazepines and are associated with a greater incidence of excessive sedation and drowsiness. Tolerance develops rapidly to barbiturates such as phenobarbital, so that much of their action is lost in 2–3 weeks unless the dose is increased. Moreover, if used for 2–3 months or more, addiction can occur if the daily dosage of the barbiturate is sufficiently high (i.e., 0.4–0.6 g). These drugs are not recommended for a prolonged period of administration. The barbiturates, however, are much less expensive than any of the other antianxiety drugs and are the drugs of choice when cost is a major consideration.

MISCELLANEOUS DRUGS

Hydroxyzine (Atarax), **benactyzine** (Suavitil) and **phenaglycodol** (Ultran) have been claimed to have some clinical usefulness as antianxiety agents. Numerous other drugs, many with antihistaminic properties, have been suggested to be useful as antianxiety agents but significant efficacy has not been established.

FURTHER READING

Blackwell B (1973): Psychotropic drugs in use today: The role of diazepam in medical practice. JAMA 225:1637–1641

Greenblatt DJ, Shader RI (1974): Benzodiazepines in Clinical Practice. New York, Raven Press

Greenblatt DJ, Shader RI (1972): The clinical choice of sedative hypnotics. Ann Intern Med 77:91–100

Kales A, Kales J (1974): Sleep disorders. N Engl J Med 290:487–499

Katz RL (1972): Sedatives and tranquilizers. N Engl J Med 286:757–760

Lasagna L (1972): Drug therapy: Hypnotic drugs. N Engl J Med 287:1182–1184

McNair DM (1973): Antianxiety drugs and human performance. Arch Gen Psychiatry 29:611–617

JORDAN D. MILLER

RONALD L. KATZ

27. ANESTHETIC AGENTS

The earliest use of drugs for the suppression of pain during surgery cannot be easily identified. Alcohol and opiates were known in antiquity, and some even point to the removal of Adam's rib while he was asleep as an early example of general anesthesia. Prior to the use of anesthetics, operations were torturous, and the length and success of the surgery were related more to the patient's constitution than to any other factor. Speed during surgery was essential. Mortality rates of 50% or greater were common. Predictable and relatively safe relief from the pain of surgery awaited the use of ether, chloroform and nitrous oxide in the mid 19th century. Though the use of these and a host of other agents spread rapidly, the science of anesthesia progressed slowly. It is only in the last 50 years that major changes have occurred. The use of sodium pentothal as an induction agent in the 1930s and the introduction of the muscle relaxants in the 1940s date the modern era of anesthesia. The medical specialty of anesthesiology developed after World War II, partly out of the realization for the need which arose during the war. Although the modern era began in the 1930s, the regular use of open drop ether continued into the 1960s.

It is fair to say that many of the major advances in surgery had to wait the development of anesthetic techniques. A simple example is the development of the endotracheal tube which made feasible positive pressure ventilation and therefore intrathoracic surgery.

GENERAL ANESTHESIA: A DEFINITION

General anesthesia can be divided into five components: amnesia, loss of consciousness, analgesia, loss of reflexes (both sensory and autonomic) and finally, muscle relaxation. Though all of the drugs used during an anesthetic are aimed at producing at least one of these ef-

fects, the agent termed the "general anesthetic" is the one that produces amnesia, analgesia and loss of consciousness. A complete anesthetic agent is one that can produce all of the effects by itself. The extent to which a general anesthetic possesses each of the above characteristics will vary among agents. Modern anesthesia combines a variety of drugs in an attempt to utilize the best properties of each and to minimize the unnecessary or harmful side effects. Thus ether, that will produce all of the above effects is generally not used alone. Modern anesthesia would combine ether, nitrous oxide, muscle relaxants and drugs to suppress some of the autonomic reflexes, all in an attempt to produce the smoothest and least detrimental depression of the patient.

At present, there are two classes of general anesthetics, those administered by inhalation and those given by injection. The largest class by far are inhalational general anesthetics.

MECHANISM OF ACTION

The specific site of action in the CNS on which anesthetics work is uncertain. Some general anesthetics inhibit the reticular activating system before blocking other areas. The reticular activating system is that portion of the CNS which receives nonspecific sensory input and is responsible for initiating and maintaining alert wakefulness. The production of unconsciousness may be related to the suppression of this system. It is known that synaptic transmission is slowed by general anesthesia and, since the reticular activating system has a great number of synapses, it would be most susceptible to blockade.

The cellular site of action of anesthetics is unknown. Pauling and Miller proposed that all inhalational anesthetics act as a nidus for "water crystals" or "clathrates." The crystal formation interferes with neural transmission. This theory remains to be proven, since clathrates have never been demonstrated to exist under conditions likely to be found in the body.

It has been shown that the more soluble an agent is in a lipid, the lower the concentration necessary for it to produce general anesthesia. Although this parameter may be related to the need of an anesthetic agent to cross lipid membranes, it does not indicate the cellular site of action of the anesthetic. Recently evidence has been presented which supports the hypothesis that anesthetics act by expanding lipid layers (i.e. cell membrane) in which they dissolve. Pressure can counteract this effect. The lipid solubility does not predict or guarantee which agents will be anesthetic.

SIGNS AND STAGES OF ANESTHESIA

The depth of ether anesthesia was divided by Guedel into sequential stages and planes of anesthesia. Though not used in its entirety by modern anesthesiologists, this classification of the sequence of events is useful. **Analgesia** and **amnesia (stage 1)** precede the loss of consciousness. This is followed by **delirium** or **stage 2.** It is during this period that vomiting and violent combative behavior can occur. In order to avoid this excitement stage, short acting barbiturates, such as sodium pentothal, are given intravenously prior to most anesthetics. (Ch. 26). (The use of sodium pentothal has gained wide acceptance for this purpose.) Barbiturates, though technically general anesthetics, have too narrow a therapeutic ratio to be used as the sole agent.

Stage 3 is surgical anesthesia. This has been subdivided into four planes which will not be discussed since they are no longer relevant. For example, muscle relaxation or apnea were formerly used to define different planes. Today, these effects are produced by specific drugs, thus making the plane concept outdated. Another reason for abandoning the plane concept is that the effects of general anesthetics are dependent upon the sensory input as well as upon the concentration of the agent being used. Thus, respiratory and cardiovascular depression are much greater with low sensory input when the patient is anesthetized but surgery has not begun. After surgical stimulation, both of these parameters tend to be less depressed, and the patient appears to be in a lighter plane. Therefore, a patient's level reflects a balance between anesthetic depression and surgical stimulation.

The stages described above for general anesthesia can apply to any depressant of the CNS. Hypoxia, or decreased cerebral blood flow, can produce each of the stages but with more permanent damage. During a cardiac arrest, the adequacy of external cardiac massage can be evaluated by that stage of "general anesthesia" the patient appears to have achieved. The return of reflexes, corneal and respiratory in particular, are signs of improving cerebral perfusion.

The awakening from general anesthesia is the reverse of the process of induction. Patients first regain reflexes, may then go through a short excitement stage, and finally come to analgesia and full wakefulness. The shorter the recovery the safer it is for the patient.

The minimum goals of anesthesia are amnesia, analgesia and ideal operating conditions for the surgeon. This frequently requires the use of muscle relaxants that may make evaluation of somatic reflexes difficult. However, autonomic reflexes, such as blood pressure and heart rate, are a good guide to the depth of anesthesia. Increases in blood pressure and heart rate with surgical stimulation indicate inadequate depth of anesthesia, and so the concentration of the anesthetic is increased. If, on the other hand, the blood pressure falls, the anesthetic concentration is decreased.

Recently, the therapeutic concentration or ED_{50} for inhalational anesthetics has been assessed by Eger, et al. Minimum alveolar concentration (MAC) is the alveolar tension at which 50% of the patients move when a surgical stimulus is applied. The conditions under which this is measured require that patients receive no premedication, no barbiturate for induction and no supplementation at any time. All of these factors would tend to decrease the concentration of anesthetic necessary for adequate surgical anesthesia. Thus, under clinical circumstances MAC may be an overestimate. The concept of an ED_{50} or MAC is useful in comparing pharmacologic effects of different anesthetic agents.

It has been found that MAC is additive; thus, if 0.5 MAC halothane (0.38%) and 0.5 MAC nitrous oxide (50%) are used, the patient appears to be at 1 MAC. MAC is also age dependent, the younger the patient, the higher the concentration of anesthetic necessary. Finally, the patients' temperature is important. *Hyperthermic* patients require more anesthetic. Those who are hypothermic require less. MAC values for general anesthetics are found in Table 27–1. It must be remembered that MAC is only a guideline and represents the concentration at which 50% of the patients will be too lightly anesthetized for surgery. Furthermore, MAC is the alveolar concentration, not the delivered concentration. As can be seen in Figure 27–1, the alveolar concentration may be much lower than the concentration delivered from the anesthesia machine. This

TABLE 27—1. Physical Contents and Formula of Anesthetic Agents

	Blood Gas	MAC %	MAC mm Hg	Fat/ blood	P Vapor 20° C	Formula
Nitrous oxide	0.43	100	760	3	—	N_2O
Halothane	2.3	0.76	6	60	243	$CF_3 CH Br Cl$
Enflurane	1.9	1.68	13	55	174	$CHF_2 -O-CF_2 CHFCl$
Methoxyflurane	10	0.16	1.2	38	24	$CH_3 - OCF_2 CHCl_2$
Trichloroethylene	9	0.22	1.7	—	—	$CHCl = CCl_2$
Fluroxene	1.4	3.4	26	—	286	$CF_3 CH_2 -O -CH = CH_2$
Chloroform	9.1	0.37	2.7	26	160	$CH Cl_3$
Isoflurane	1.4	1.3	10	—	260	$CHF_2 -O - CHClCF_3$
Diethyl ether	12	2	15	5	443	$(C_2H_5)_2O$
Cyclopropane	0.46	10	76	21	—	C_3H_6
Ethylene	0.14	80	610	9	—	C_2H_4

is particularly true for agents with high solubility or those delivered for a short period of time. The concentration listed applies to an atmospheric pressure equal to 760 mm of mercury. Whereas MAC is commonly reported in concentration, it is actually the anesthetic tension or partial pressure that is important. Therefore, when atmospheric pressure differs significantly from 760 mm of mercury, as may occur in a hyperbaric chamber or at altitude, the partial pressure expressed in millimeters of mercury is the correct value. Thus, at 2 atm, nitrous oxide MAC is 760 mm of mercury, or 50%. At 1 atm it is still 760 mm of mercury, but it requires 100% nitrous oxide and this is an unobtainable goal. Conversely, at a higher altitude, where atmospheric pressure is 600 mm of mercury, halothane MAC is still 6 mm Hg but 1% rather than 0.76% at sea level.

UPTAKE

The depth of anesthesia depends on the tension or partial pressure (expressed in millimeters of mercury) that reaches the brain. This in turn depends on the arterial tension that is at equilibrium with the alveolar tension. The higher the tension in the alveoli, the more rapid the induction. The tension in the alveoli is dependent both on the administered tension and solubility of the anesthetic. The more soluble the anesthetic is in blood, the more agent is removed from the alveoli and the *lower* the alveolar tension. The less soluble the agent is in blood, the more rapidly the alveolar tension approaches that of the inspired gas. As a result, the less soluble the agent, the more rapidly the brain (which again is in equilibrium with the blood) will reach the

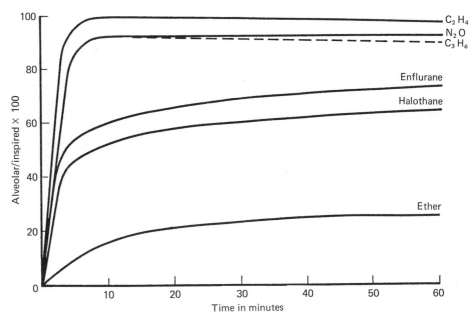

FIG. 27—1. Alveolar concentration of anesthetics as a fraction of the inspired tension during the first 60 min of anesthesia.

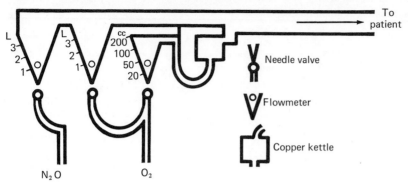

FIG. 27–2. Diagramatic representation of the flowmeters and copper kettle of an anesthetic machine.

anesthetic tension. It is important when giving anesthetics to realize that it is not the dose which matters. Thus, ether, which is very soluble, will have many more molecules in the blood before reaching an anesthetic level or (tension) than a less soluble agent, even though both agents have the same MAC.

A second factor determining uptake is ventilation. The greater the ventilation of the alveoli, the more anesthetic is delivered to the alveoli and the more rapid the induction. This factor is most important early in the induction of anesthesia, when uptake by the blood is most rapid. It is also more important for soluble agents than for the insoluble ones.

A third important factor is blood flow. The higher the flow through the lungs, the more agent is removed from the alveoli and so initially the tension is low. However, as time passes, the tissues become saturated more rapidly, and so the rate of approach to equilibrium is hastened.

The initial inspired tension is a fourth factor influencing uptake. If the tension is higher than that necessary for maintenance anesthesia, the brain will reach anesthetic levels more rapidly. This is called overpressure, and, though used for most agents, it is of greatest importance with those which are soluble. Thus, ether, that requires a brain tension of approximately 14 mm Hg, may initially be administered at an inspired tension of 140 mm Hg to allow for its great solubility and uptake into the blood. Nitrous oxide needs almost no overpressure since its solubility is so low. Halothane may initially be administered at 2–3 times the maintenance concentration to speed its onset of action.

Awakening from anesthesia is the reverse process. The less soluble an agent, the more completely it is removed from the blood in one passage through the lungs and thus the more rapid the awakening.

Anesthetics are metabolized, in some cases as much as 35% of the administered dose. However, this process is slow and of no clinical significance as far as induction or awakening is concerned. The metabolic products, however, may be toxic which will be discussed later under methoxyflurane and halothane. Appreciation of the fact that inhalation anesthetic agents are metabolized is relatively recent. For years the classic concept was that these agents were eliminated unchanged.

The solubility of most anesthetics in tissues is equal to that in blood. The only exception to this is fat. Fat acts as a storehouse for anesthetics and may account for a delay in awakening of patients from agents with high solubility.

ANESTHESIA MACHINE

Flowmeter

The anesthesia machine diagramed in Figure 27–2 is composed of several gas sources which can be either tanks of compressed gas, such as oxygen or nitrous oxide, or, in modern operating rooms, wall sources of these two gases. The pressure is reduced from these sources, and the final pressure supplied to the flowmeters is approximately 6 lb/sq in. The most common flowmeter is controlled by a needle valve. An indicator or float sitting in a carefully calibrated tube indicates the rate of flow of the gas. Each tube is calibrated for a specific gas. The gases are then collected and leave the machine at a common site. Volatile anesthetics, those that are liquid at room temperature, can be accurately vaporized by one of several means. The simplest is the copper kettle. Oxygen from a flowmeter is bubbled through the liquid in the kettle. The vapor reaches equilibrium and is collected in the common outflow from the machine. The concentration of vapor leaving the kettle is dependent on the vapor pressure of the liquid. The formula is:

$$cc \text{ vapor} = \frac{P_{vap} \times cc \ O_2}{P_{atm} - P_{vap}}$$

where P_{vap} — vapor pressure of liquid (mm Hg)
            P_{atm} — atmospheric pressure (mm Hg)

Since the evaporation of the vapor requires energy in the form of heat, the liquid tends to cool. To prevent large changes in the temperature of the liquid, the copper kettle is attached to the metal of the anesthesia machine that acts as a large heat sink and stabilizes the temperature of the liquid. The advantage of a copper kettle is that it can be used with any volatile anesthetic and does not require frequent calibration. However, it is temperature dependent, and if the temperature changes rapidly, it can deliver concentrations of an anesthetic very different from the one expected (e.g., if enflurane is used at a temperature of 18°C, vapor pressure = 198, but at 28°C, it is 357). Once the vaporizer output is calculated for the oxygen flow, the final anesthetic concentration is this figure divided by the diluent gases coming from the oxygen and nitrous oxide flowmeters. Thus 100 cc of oxygen into the copper kettle filled with enflurane yields 26 cc of enflurane vapor at 18°C. If the oxygen flow is 1 liter/min and nitrous oxide flow is 1.5 liters/min, the final enflurane concentration is 1%.

Temperature and Flow Compensated Vaporizer

A simpler system which does not require these calculations is the temperature and flow compensated vaporizer. There are several of these available (Fig. 27–3). In this system, the total gas flow from the machine is passed through the input, then divided into two streams, one passing through the anesthetic liquid and the other bypassing the chamber holding the liquid. As the temperature increases and, thus, the vapor pressure of the liquid increases, a bimetallic strip acts as a valve and decreases flow through the volatile anesthetic. As a result a steady output concentration is maintained. These systems suffer from several disadvantages. First, they can only be used with one specific anesthetic vapor. In addition, they must be calibrated very frequently, and any mechanical defect might lead to a massive overdose. For instance, if the bimetallic strip is stuck in the open position, the patient might receive an unacceptably high concentration. They are, however, growing in popularity because of the ease with which they can be used. There are many other types of vaporizers, but the two kinds listed above are the most frequently used.

ANESTHESIA CIRCUITS

Closed System

A variety of anesthetic circuits are available. The most commonly used circuit is diagrammed in Figure 27–4. Gas leaving the anesthesia machine enters a circle with two one-way valves. An inflatable bag allows the patient to breathe spontaneously or to be ventilated by the anesthesiologist who squeezes the bag. A simple pop off valve allows excess gas to leave the circuit. A cannister containing soda lime absorbs carbon dioxide that is present in any rebreathed gas. If the gas flow into the circuit just equals the uptake of oxygen and the anesthetic agent, the system is called "closed." The exact concentration that the patient is breathing is not known, since the uptake of each gas occurs independently. Cyclopropane is almost always administered by a closed system, as the anesthetic is extremely explosive as well as expensive. The danger of explosion is significantly decreased because little of the cyclopropane enters the room.

Semiclosed or Partial Rebreathing System

A semiclosed or partial rebreathing system is one in that more gas enters the circle than is taken

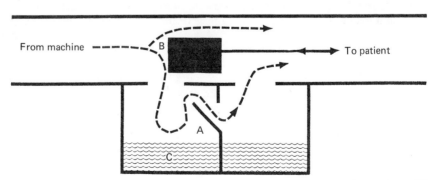

FIG. 27–3. Path of anesthetic gases in a temperature compensated vaporizer. (**A**) Bimetalic strip; (**B**) slide to occlude path of gases through vaporizer; (**C**) anesthetic liquid.

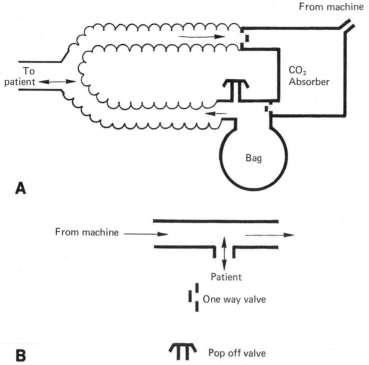

From machine

To patient

CO₂ Absorber

Bag

A

From machine

Patient

One way valve

B

Pop off valve

FIG. 27–4. (A) Diagramatic representation of a circle system; (B) Diagram of an Ayre's T-piece.

up by the patient. Generally 2–6 liters/min are used. The patient does rebreathe some previously exhaled gas, but the inspired concentration approaches that which the machine delivers. Absorption of CO_2 is important to prevent increased CO_2 in the inspired gas. The advantage of the closed and semiclosed systems is that dry gas which comes from the machine gains moisture both from the CO_2 absorber and from water vapor in the tubing. Thus, secretions in the tracheobronchial tree do not get as thick and tenacious and are less likely to cause obstruction. This is particularly important in infants and children, especially when an endotracheal tube is used that bypasses the normal humidifiers of the upper airways.

Nonrebreathing System

The nonrebreathing system does not use a circle or CO_2 absorber. It depends on an extremely high fresh gas flow to keep the patient from accumulating CO_2. There are many such systems, but probably the simplest one used is an Ayre's T piece. In its most basic form the fresh gas must enter at 2–3 times the patient's minute ventilation to prevent rebreathing of exhaled gas or inhalation of room air. This tends to dry the patient's

respiratory tract and at the same time is extremely wasteful of anesthetics and is a pollutant of the operating room environment. The advantages, however, of this system are that it is simple, and it allows rapid changes in inhaled concentration and therefore a more rapid change in anesthetic depth. To avoid the high flows necessary for this system, various nonrebreathing valves have been designed to permit one to use flows that just match the ventilation of the patient and still prevent rebreathing. However, the flows are still larger than those necessary in the semiclosed circle. This and other difficulties tend to make nonrebreathing valves less commonly used than the circle absorption system.

At present, anesthesiologists are attempting to prevent the buildup of anesthetic vapors in the operating room. Recently, several papers have discussed the increased incidence of spontaneous abortion in pregnant women working in operating rooms. In addition, a decreased attention span and other signs of depressed mental function have been observed in the operating team after prolonged inhalation of anesthetics. Most of the systems for removing anesthetic agents from the operating room pass the excess vapors into a suction that carries them away.

FLAMMABLE AGENTS

It is common to classify anesthetic agents in terms of flammability. In general, the use of flammable agents has decreased markedly as new, more satisfactory, nonflammable agents have become available. The flammable agents require special care in handling, not only during transport and storage but also during administration in the operating room. In the operating room all possibility of sparks either from electrical equipment or static electrical discharges must be eliminated. All switches must be at least 5 ft above the floor or of special construction. All electrical outlets must have special design to prevent a spark during connection of equipment. Electric cautery may not be used. This requirement has handicapped many surgeons. All personnel and equipment must be interconnected through conductive flooring so that no static electric charges may build up. All high voltage equipment must be 5 ft above the floor or in specially constructed cases. Many hospitals are unwilling to spend the extra money for these precautions as well as the increased insurance costs. Many anesthesiologists, because they are unwilling to accept the extra risk to their patients and themselves, and in the absence of well-documented advantage, have given up the flammable agents.

In the following classification of anesthetic agents, we will start with those most commonly used and progress to those least commonly used.

NONFLAMMABLE AGENTS

Nitrous Oxide—MAC 100%; Blood/Gas Ratio 0.43

One of the oldest agents available, it is the only inorganic substance presently used for anesthesia. Nitrous oxide is one of the least soluble anesthetics, and so its onset of action is extremely rapid and awakening is similarly fast. A primary limitation is the concentration that can be administered and still allow an adequate concentration of oxygen (note, MAC of 100%). Therefore, it is not used alone, except when the patient is very ill and MAC may be 70–80%. However, it is an ideal supplemental anesthetic. In the "balance technique," barbiturates with or without narcotics and/or neuromuscular blocking agents (muscle relaxants) are used to supplement nitrous oxide. Balanced anesthesia can produce adequate anesthesia for all forms of surgery. The nitrous oxide provides primarily amnesia and analgesia, while the barbiturate and narcotic add depression of reflexes as well as analgesia and

sleep. The neuromuscular blockers add muscle relaxation.

Nitrous oxide is also used along with other more potent inhalation agents, allowing a lower concentration of the latter to be used. This may offer several advantages over the use of the more potent agent alone. If nitrous oxide is used to supplement a slower inhalational agent, both onset of surgical anesthesia and awakening are more rapid. In addition, nitrous oxide is less depressant to both the cardiovascular system and respiratory system than most of the inhalational agents currently available. As a result, combining nitrous oxide with other inhalational agents produce less cardiovascular and respiratory depression than an equal depth of anesthesia produced by a single inhalational agent.

Because it is used in such high concentrations (50–70%), and because its solubility in blood is greater than that of nitrogen, it will replace nitrogen in any air pockets in the body. This generally is of no consequence, but in bowel obstructions the volume of gas in the bowel may increase twofold in only 2 hr of administration of nitrous oxide, making it difficult to replace the bowel in the abdomen. Similarly, after injection of air into the ventricles of the brain during a pneumoencephalogram, nitrous oxide inhalation may dangerously raise the cerebral spinal fluid pressure and cause decreased blood flow to the brain or even herniation of the brain stem.

Halothane (Fluothane)—MAC 0.76%; Blood/Gas Ratio 2.3

Since its introduction in 1956, halothane has become one of the most widely used anesthetics and is a potent agent producing total anesthesia on its own. However, muscle relaxation is poor at normally used concentrations. When muscle relaxation is needed, neuromuscular blockers must be used. While depressant to the cardiovascular system and capable of lowering the blood pressure, there is a fall in peripheral resistance before a decrease in cardiac output. The addition of nitrous oxide (and hence a lowering of the concentration of halothane required for anesthesia) makes for less depression of the blood pressure at equal depths of anesthesia. Awakening is rapid and usually uneventful. Laryngeal reflexes are obtunded early, and laryngospasm (reflex closure of vocal cords) is rarely a problem.

Respiration under halothane becomes rapid and shallow, but the Pco_2 may be only minimally elevated, especially if light anesthesia is maintained. The addition of nitrous oxide to supplement halothane will also help to maintain a normal Pco_2. However, controlled ventilation is frequently necessary to maintain a normal Pco_2 and certainly is needed for deeper anesthesia or if muscle relaxants are used. Narcotics decrease the rate and increase the depth of respiration under halothane, but the overall alveolar ventilation is decreased and Pco_2 increased. Halothane exerts potent relaxant effects on smooth muscle. The bronchospasm of asthma is diminished by deep halothane anesthesia, and if bronchospasm occurs under anesthesia or is an expected problem, halothane is an excellent choice. It will also relax the smooth muscle of the pregnant uterus, having the undesirable side effect of excessive blood loss during delivery.

A potential problem with halothane is that it sensitizes the myocardium to the arrhythmogenic properties of catecholamines (Ch. 18). Thus, there may be cardiac arrhythmias secondary to exogenous catecholamines (injected by surgeon or anesthesiologist) or by endogenously released catecholamines due to increased carbon dioxide tensions. This limits the amount of catecholamines or local anesthetics with catecholamines which may be used during operations.

A rare complication of halothane anesthesia is halothane hepatitis and is thought to be a sensitization hepatitis produced after repeated administration of halothane and is at present totally unpredictable. There have been no reports of its occurrence in children. The onset of hepatitis is preceded by fever frequently occurring between 3–10 days postoperatively and unfortunately, deaths are common. It is believed by many that the sensitization is not due to halothane but rather to one of its metabolites. If an individual is sensitized, halothane should not be used, but in nonsensitized patients halothane may be repeated as frequently as necessary, with no limit on the interval between administrations. Although the prevailing view is that this is a sensitization phenomenon, there are two other schools of thought. One is that there is no such thing as halothane hepatitis, and the other is that halothane is a direct hepatotoxin. Supporters of these two views are presently few in number.

The occurrence of nodal rhythm under halothane is very common and usually presents no undesirable effects to the patient. The patient reverts spontaneously to normal sinus rhythm with the end of the anesthetic, if not before.

Enflurane (Ethrane)—MAC 1.68%; Blood/Gas Ratio 1.9

Introduced clinically in 1972, it is similar in effect to halothane. However, enflurane is less potent, soluble and it produces better muscle relaxation

than halothane, even at light level of anesthesia. Not infrequently a muscle relaxant is necessary for intraabdominal operations, though in smaller doses than with halothane. Again, nitrous oxide is almost always used to allow a lower concentration of enflurane and thus diminish cardiovascular and respiratory depression which is similar in extent to that seen with halothane. Sensitization to catecholamines appears to be similar to that of halothane, but the magnitude of sensitization is less. In addition, increased Pco_2 does not produce cardiac arrhythmias as it does with halothane. Hepatitis has not been reported with this agent, but only further experience will establish this difference. Metabolism of the agent is very low, leading to the prediction that sensitization may be less frequent. Inorganic fluoride as a product of metabolism does not seem to be sufficient to cause renal problems (see methoxyflurane). Seizures (both physical and on EEG) have been seen during the use of this agent. The deeper the anesthetic and the lower the Pco_2, the more frequent is their occurrence. However at commonly used concentrations and with close to normal Pco_2 this is not a problem. The mechanism of the seizure activity is unknown. Awakening is usually rapid and uneventful, though nausea appears to be somewhat more common than after the halothane.

Methoxyflurane (Penthrane)—MAC 0.16%; Blood/Gas Ratio 10

Methoxyflurane is the most potent agent presently available, but has a high blood solubility. Because of the extreme solubility, overpressure is needed during induction. The use of nitrous oxide and frequently doses of barbiturates early in the anesthetic also help to produce a rapid onset of surgical anesthesia. Awakening, however, cannot be similarly facilitated and is therefore quite slow. Methoxyflurane is a complete anesthetic producing good muscle relaxation at usual levels of anesthesia. In addition, it sensitizes the myocardium minimally to the effects of catecholamines. The analgesic effect is quite marked, and even before loss of consciousness it produces profound analgesia. Patients awaken relatively free of pain. It has been used in labor to decrease pain over prolonged periods of time by periodic breathing of its vapor. The major and at present the main reason for its lack of favor is that it is metabolized to inorganic fluoride over many days. This is due to the fact that it is stored in fat to a large extent. If the fluoride level is high enough, it causes a high output renal failure which may progress to total renal failure. Though usually reversible, this is too high a price to pay for its limited advantages. Obese patients under deep anesthesia and undergoing long procedures are most susceptible to the renal failure as they receive a large total dose and take a long time to excrete the agent.

Fluroxene (Fluomar)—MAC 3.4%; Blood/Gas Ratio 1.5

This agent was introduced shortly before halothane and has been eclipsed by it. The compound is flammable at concentrations greater than 4%. If used with nitrous oxide, which decreases the amount of fluroxene necessary, it may be possible to use this agent below the explosive range. However this entails a risk that most anesthesiologists feel is unacceptable and therefore this agent is treated as flammable. Fluroxene does offer certain advantages. First, it does not sensitize the myocardium to catecholamines or to increased Pco_2. Blood pressure is better maintained than with the other halogenated agents, and respiratory depression seems to be less marked. If sensitivity hepatitis exists in man, it is much rarer than with halothane. Awakening is rapid, but nausea is quite common.

Trichloroethylene (Trilene or Trimar)—MAC 0.22%; Blood/Gas Ratio 9

This agent is rarely used in this country except as an inhalational analgesic during labor. This compound is metabolized in the body to trichloracetic acid, but it is not produced in enough quantity to be toxic. If used in a circle system in the presence of soda lime to absorb exhaled carbon dioxide, it is decomposed to phosgene and carbon monoxide, both extremely toxic agents. The decomposition is facilitated by increased temperature. Cranial nerve palsies were reported before the problem was appreciated and were probably due to the breakdown products. When trichloroethylene is used, it is not used with soda lime. Instead, a nonrebreathing system that does not require carbon dioxide absorption is used. At excessively deep levels of anesthesia, cardiac arrhythmias may occur. However, at the levels required for light anesthesia, arrhythmias are rare.

Chloroform—MAC 0.37%; Blood/Gas Ratio 9.1

Its hepatotoxicity plus the availability of better agents have virtually eliminated its use from anesthesia.

Isoflurane (Forane)—MAC 1.3%; Blood/Gas Ratio 1.4

This agent is currently available for research only. Isoflurane is said to have better muscle relaxing ability than any other halogenated anesthetic. It markedly potentiates the action of neuromuscular blocking agents, and minimal doses are necessary. Because of the low blood-gas solubility, it has an extremely rapid onset and recovery. It does not sensitize the heart to catecholamines and produces less depression of the cardiovascular system than other halogenated hydrocarbons. It is a respiratory depressant. It has an extremely low degree of metabolism, and as such it is thought to be the least likely agent to produce hepatic toxicity through a sensitization mechanism. Barring problems not yet apparent, this agent may find widespread use.

FLAMMABLE AGENTS

Diethyl ether—MAC 2.0%; Blood/Gas Ratio 12

This agent is now rarely used alone primarily because of its extremely slow induction and recovery. Secretions can be copious, and belladonna drugs are necessary for preanesthetic medication. The cardiovascular system is less depressed than with the halogenated agents, and in this respect it is similar to fluroxene. Respiration is initially increased but is depressed at deeper anesthetic levels. Muscle relaxation is good, and it can be used without muscle relaxants. However, to allow for faster recovery, it is generally used along with nitrous oxide. Only small amounts of neuromuscular blockers are needed to produce adequate muscle relaxation for intraabdominal surgery. Nausea and vomiting occur over a prolonged period, even with light levels of ether. As a result, it has poor public acceptance. Properly managed, however, it is at least as safe an agent as any other, and some anesthesiologists feel that it still has some qualities which make it superior to other agents currently available.

Cyclopropane—MAC 10%; Blood/Gas Ratio 0.47

This agent has gone out of favor recently because of its explosive nature. It supports the blood pressure and may even cause moderate hypertension, even at deep levels of anesthesia. This, along with increased skin blood flow, may appear to produce more than usual blood loss during the skin incision and may tend to slow down the operation, but otherwise the total blood loss is not significantly increased. The pulse rate generally falls as a baroreceptor response to the hypertension. If atropine is given to increase heart rate, multifocal ventricular premature contractions frequently occur. It is the most potent sensitizer of the myocardium to catecholamines. In the presence of an increased Pco_2, cardiac arrhythmias frequently occur.

Spontaneous respiration with this agent will result in an increased Pco, so controlled ventilation is often necessary except at the lightest levels of anesthesia. Because of its high cost and its extreme flammability, it is administered in a closed-circle system.

Ethylene—MAC 80%; Blood/Gas Ratio 0.14

This agent is similar to nitrous oxide, but its flammability far outweighs any small benefits obtained by the slightly lower solubility and greater potency. It is rarely used today.

Divinyl Ether

This agent is primarily used for rapid induction prior to ether anesthesia. Prolonged administration leads to hepatic necrosis, and thus limits its use to less than 30 min. It is rarely used.

INTRAVENOUS AGENTS

Ketamine (Ketalar or Ketaject)

This is the only true general anesthetic that is administered by means other than inhalation. It produces profound somatic anesthesia, no muscle relaxation and most reflexes are maintained. Patients will exhibit protective reflexes, maintain their own airway and normal respiration and display corneal reflexes. The patient seems awake but disconnected from the environment. The term dissociative anesthesia is used to describe this state. The agent produces variable hypertension and tachycardia that can potentially cause problems. It seems particularly useful during diagnostic procedures, as it permits a well-maintained airway. When a patient is hypotensive and hypovolemic, it maintains the blood pressure while other measures are being instituted to correct the primary problem. However, problems inheritant in its use include the production of hallucinations which may be remembered by the patient as extremely unpleasant, a long sleep time relative to the length of the surgical anesthesia, inadequate anesthesia for deep pain such as intraabdominal surgery and, finally, it is not readily reversible. The dose is 2–4 mg/kg, IV, or 5–10 mg/kg, IM. Repeated doses are given when the patient shows signs of responding to pain.

Morphine—Oxygen

In some cases, primarily open heart surgery, large doses of morphine, (1–3 mg/kg, IV) may be used with oxygen with or without neuromuscular blocking agents. It is felt that this regimen is least depressant to the myocardium, though it does cause some vasodilitation and the blood pressure may fall. With this technique, amnesia is not guaranteed. The patients do not experience discomfort during surgery and will not be uncomfortable as long as they are properly prepared preoperatively. Ventilation is mandatory intraoperatively and usually 24–48 hr postoperatively until the morphine has been metabolized.

For detailed descriptions of agents used to supplement anesthesia, see the chapters on barbiturates (Ch. 26), neuromuscular blocking agents (Ch. 21), narcotics (Ch. 29) and tranquilizers (Ch. 25).

PREANESTHETIC MEDICATION

It is the goal of the anesthesiologist to bring the patient to the operating room in a state of carefree wakefulness. To reach this goal, many agents have been given for preoperative medication. Combinations of barbiturates, narcotics and minor tranquilizers, even antihistaminics with sedative properties, have been used. Since there is no one best agent, the most commonly used agents are barbiturates, such as secobarbital, tranquilizers, such as diazepam, droperidol, hydroxyzine, and agents of mixed properties, such as promethazine.

Belladonna alkaloids (atropine or scopolamine) (Ch. 19) are used less frequently now that salivary secretions are less of a problem with new agents as compared to ether or cyclopropane. When used, the dose in adults is 0.4–0.6 mg of scopolamine and 0.6–0.8 mg of atropine.

Narcotics are frequently used for preanesthetic medication and may be useful in the early postoperative period to prevent pain upon awakening from the anesthetic.

FURTHER READING

Dripps RD, Eckenhoff JE, Vandam LD (1972): Introduction to Anesthesia the Principle of Safe Practice. Philadelphia, WB Saunders

Schwartz H, Ngai SH, Papper EM (1962): Manual of Anesthesiology for Residents and Medical Students. Springfield, Ill, Charles C Thomas

Wylie WD, Churchill-Davidson HC (1971): A Practice of Anesthesia. Chicago, Year Book Publishers

HAROLD E. PAULUS

28. ANALGESIC, ANTIPYRETIC, ANTIINFLAMMATORY AGENTS*

The group of drugs that are used to moderate the pain, swelling, heat and general discomfort of acute and chronic inflammatory conditions are called the analgesic, antipyretic, antiinflammatory agents. These compounds differ from the narcotic analgesics (discussed in Ch. 29) in that they are not addicting and have little effect on the central recognition of painful stimuli by the brain; instead they appear to act peripherally, suppressing inflammatory processes that trigger the pain receptors of peripheral nerve endings. They are particularly useful for the treatment of musculoskeletal discomfort and headaches but are ineffective for severe pain or pain of cardiac or visceral origin. Most of these nonsteroidal antiinflammatory drugs also tend to restore an elevated body temperature toward normal, hence their designation as antipyretic. They are most frequently prescribed for patients with chronic inflammatory arthritis, e.g., rheumatoid arthritis, ankylosing spondylitis, osteoarthritis, gout, and it is primarily in this context that the **salicylates, acetaminophen, phenylbutazone, indomethacin and colchicine,** will be discussed in this chapter. Except for acetaminophen, each has significant gastrointestinal toxicity which may be considered to be a general characteristic of this class of drugs. Although they have no analgesic or antiinflammatory activity, the drugs that are used to decrease plasma uric acid concentrations in patients with gout, **probenecid, sulfinpyrazone** and **allopurinol,** are also included in this chapter.

TARGETS OF DRUG THERAPY IN CHRONIC INFLAMMATION

Inflammation is the normal protective response to tissue injury, restoring the host to its former healthy state. Normally, the tissue damaging stimulus initiates a series of biochemical, immunologic and cellular events that proceed through apparently well-regulated steps, culminating in tissue repair and restoration of function. When healing is completed, the inflammatory response ceases until it is needed again. The sequence of events in inflammation can be pictured as follows (Table 28–1): the prime cause of the inflammation either directly or through mediators (such as antigen-antibody-complement complexes) produces the initial injury to the tissue. The injured tissue then releases mediators which initiate the complex cellular and biochemical events of normal inflammation. Usually, these events result in the elimination of the prime cause, followed by healing and restoration of

function. However, if the prime cause cannot be eradicated, the various mediators of inflammation enhance tissue injury and magnify the damage produced by the prime cause. The consequence is chronic inflammation, which results in the manifestations of disease and ultimately in loss of function. This formulation of chronic inflammatory disease suggests that treatment may be directed at four targets (Table 28–1).

1. **Eradication of the prime cause** could be expected to result in healing or scar formation. This may occur even if the disease has been present for many years, as is seen when tuberculosis or syphilis is adequately treated with an effective antibiotic. When dealing with diseases of unknown etiology, it must be noted that a so-called "disease" may merely be a common clinical expression of injury that may be produced by any one of a number of prime causes; e.g., the disease "pneumonia" may be caused by *Diplococcus pneumoniae, Staphy-*

* The author gratefully acknowledges the support of the United States Public Health Service (GM 15759).

TABLE 28–1. Targets for Therapy of Chronic Inflammatory States

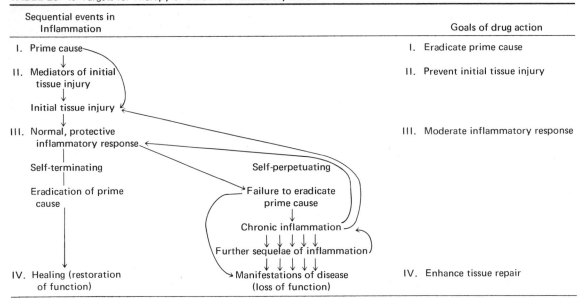

Sequential events in Inflammation	Goals of drug action
I. Prime cause	I. Eradicate prime cause
II. Mediators of initial tissue injury	II. Prevent initial tissue injury
Initial tissue injury	
III. Normal, protective inflammatory response	III. Moderate inflammatory response
Self-terminating — Self-perpetuating	
Eradication of prime cause — Failure to eradicate prime cause	
Chronic inflammation	
Further sequelae of inflammation	
IV. Healing (restoration of function) — Manifestations of disease (loss of function)	IV. Enhance tissue repair

lococcus aureus or one of a number of other microorganisms. If treatment is aimed at the prime cause, it must be specific. None of the drugs currently available for the management of inflammatory arthritis even remotely approaches the goal of eradicating the prime cause, but if such a drug were found, it might be effective in only a minority of patients with a particular diagnosis.

2. The second possible target for drug therapy is **prevention of initial tissue injury.** A drug of this type might be unable to eliminate the prime cause but in some way would completely prevent it from producing tissue injury and thus would circumvent the events of the normal inflammatory response. Such a drug could not be expected to "cure" the disease and indeed might permit wider dissemination of the prime cause since it masks the prime cause from the effects of the normal inflammatory response. As a corollary to this, however, it would not interfere with established inflammatory responses, nor would it suppress the body's response to ordinary environmental challenges. Tetanus antitoxin is an example of a therapeutic agent acting on this target; it prevents tetanus without destroying the causative bacterium or interfering with the normal immune or inflammatory mechanisms. For the inflammatory arthritides, the investigational cytotoxic immunosuppressive drugs (Ch. 74) may fall in this category. They appear to interfere with the normal immunologic response (that in this case is misguided and results in tissue damage) against the prime cause, preventing the initia-

tion of the inflammatory sequence by these immunologic mediators. There is some suggestion that cyclophosphamide may prevent the progression of destructive joint erosions in patients who are undergoing effective treatment with it. However, as might be expected, if there is no effect on the prime cause, the disease recurs when the immunosuppressive therapy is discontinued. The gold salts (Ch. 74), for that minority of patients who achieve complete remission while taking them, may also fall in this category.

3. If it is impossible to eradicate the cause of the disease or to prevent tissue injury and the resultant inflammatory response, attempts may be made to **moderate the inflammatory response** in order to suppress at least some of the manifestations of established inflammation. Aspirin, indomethacin, phenylbutazone, the gold salts in most situations, corticosteroids and all of the new investigational antiinflammatory agents are included in this category. They may be expected to relieve, in varying degrees, some of the symptoms and signs of inflammation, regardless of its cause. A major advantage of these drugs is that they do not interfere with the normal immunologic response, although a truly effective antiinflammatory drug, such as high doses of corticosteroid (Ch. 46), substantially disarms the recipient in his daily battle to protect himself against his environment. Despite treatment with these agents, tissue injury continues, the disease progresses and disability continues to become more severe. The available drugs cover a wide spectrum of effectiveness,

varying from almost complete suppression of inflammation by large doses of prednisone to minor symptomatic improvement by small doses of salicylates. Each of the available drugs may have serious side effects that prevent its use in a substantial number of patients. A large number of new drugs of this type are currently undergoing controlled clinical evaluation, and many of them should become generally available within the next 10 years. They should give the clinician more flexibility in many patients in whom the conventional drugs are contraindicated, e.g., those with peptic ulcer disease.

4. Lastly, treatment of chronic inflammation may be directed at the reparative and healing process which occurs as the terminal event in normal inflammation; drug therapy might be used to **enhance tissue repair.** Drugs of this type might be particularly useful in degenerative processes. Unfortunately, so little is known about the regulation of these reparative processes that this problem has not even begun to be approached by pharmaceutical chemists and experimental pharmacologists. No drugs that act in this area are available at the present time, and none are under active investigation.

The rapidly acting nonsteroidal antiinflammatory compounds have no effect on the causes of inflammation, but their importance as symptomatic therapy is attested to by the huge quantities of these drugs that are used. They moderate the activity of inflammation within the first few days of administration and are effective only while blood levels are sustained. Unless the underlying inflammatory condition has already subsided spontaneously, their withdrawal is soon followed by a recurrence of signs and symptoms. They appear to act late in the events of the inflammatory cascade and have little or no discernible effect on immune defenses. Since inflammation appears to be a multifaceted defense system with many mechanisms for arriving at the same end state, it is likely that they interfere with all of the mediators in the more distal aspects of the inflammatory process, rather than specifically affecting only one or two mediators. Evidence for this conclusion is supplied each time a new mediator is discovered. Thus, the clinically useful antiinflammatory drugs have been found to uncouple oxidative phosphorylation, inhibit the release of hyaluronidase and β-glucuronidase from isolated rat liver lysosomes, inhibit phosphatase and cathepsins, inhibit the induction of inflammation by kinins and inhibit the production of inflammatory prostaglandins from arachidonic acid. Each of these effects has been considered to be their mode of action, but it might be anticipated that as additional mediators of inflammation are described in the future, the clinically useful antiinflammatory agents will also be active against them.

ANTIINFLAMMATORY ANALGESICS

SALICYLATES

Willow and poplar barks that contain salicin have long been used to treat sepsis, pain, gout and fever. Salicylic acid was first synthesized in 1860 and acetylsalicylic acid (aspirin) in 1899. Today, aspirin is one of the least expensive and most widely used drugs in the world. About 30 tons of aspirin are consumed daily in the United States. Even though salicylates have such an ancient heritage and are so casually used, they continue to be the prototype of the nonsteroidal, antiinflammatory, antirheumatic drug and are still the yardstick that newer agents are assessed against. The fairly frequent occurrence of fatal salicylate intoxication in children emphasizes that salicylates are potent drugs which deserve the same careful administration as other potentially dangerous pharmacologic agents.

Chemistry

The parent compound, salicylic acid, and its methyl ester, methyl salicylate (oil of wintergreen), are local irritants and are used only as keratolytic agents or as counter irritants for topical application to the skin. **Sodium salicylate** and acetylsalicylic acid (**aspirin**) are useful analgesic antipyretic antiinflammatory agents, and aspirin is the prototype compound for this group.

Pharmacology

Aspirin has a broad spectrum of pharmacologic activities. In therapeutic concentrations (0.5–2.0 mM) salicylates uncouple oxidative phosphorylation in the mitochondria, and at much higher concentrations they may inhibit cellular oxidative enzymes, prevent the activation of kinin forming

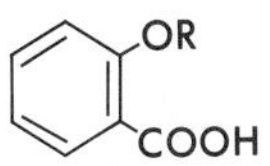

'SALICYLATES'
R=H. SALICYCLIC ACID
R=COCH3, ASPIRIN

FIG. 28–1. Salicylates.

enzymes and antagonize peripheral effects of kinins. In sensitized animals, they inhibit the release of histamine and modify the effects of intradermal histamine injections; in addition, the response to serotonin is inhibited, both in experimental animals and in man. In experimental animals, high doses of salicylates may suppress antibody production, interfere with antigen-antibody aggregation and stabilize capillary permeability in the presence of immunologic insults. Blood coagulation may be inhibited by increasing the prothrombin time, and aspirin decreases platelet adhesiveness. Since salicylate is an organic acid that is tolerated in rather high plasma concentrations, it competes with other organic acids in the renal tubules.

Aspirin also is an effective antagonist of the enzyme prostaglandin synthetase, that is responsible for the production of prostaglandin E_1 from arachidonic acid (Ch. 51). Because prostaglandin E_1 inhibits gastric acid secretion, the inhibition of prostaglandin synthesis by antiinflammatory drugs may be the common factor responsible for their gastric toxicity. Salicylates decrease blood glucose concentrations in diabetic patients, but high levels may elevate blood glucose levels in normal subjects. Very high doses stimulate the release of corticoids from the adrenal cortex. Aspirin is thought to irreversibly acetylate a lysyl residue of human serum albumin.

Salicylates bind rather tightly to albumin and also to erythrocytes. They may displace other drugs from albumin binding sites and are known to increase protein free levels of coumarin, thus enhancing its anticoagulant effects. Salicylates may also interfere with the binding of thyroxin by thyroxin binding prealbumin, thus decreasing plasma protein bound iodine levels without decreasing normal concentrations of free circulating thyroxin.

ANALGESIA. Salicylates are particularly effective for relieving pain due to headache, myalgia and arthralgia but are relatively ineffective for visceral pain. Their major analgesic effect probably is related to their peripheral antiinflammatory activity or to an effect on pain receptors, although a subcortical CNS site of analgesic action has been suggested but not conclusively demonstrated. In any event, in contrast with the narcotic analgesic agents, analgesic doses of aspirin do not cause disturbances in mentation, nor are they addicting. However, for pain of musculoskeletal origin they are much more effective than narcotics; indeed, patients with chronic inflammatory arthritis rarely become addicted to narcotic drugs.

ANTIPYRESIS. Salicylates lower the body temperature in febrile patients but have no effect on normal body temperature. The antipyretic effect of salicylate is due to normalization of temperature sensitive neurons in the hypothalamus, whose function appears to be depressed by pyrogens in the febrile patient. Sweating generally is associated with reduction of fever in salicylate treated patients. Paradoxically, salicylate poisoning may cause fever when increased oxygen consumption is caused by uncoupling of oxidative phosphorylation.

ANTIRHEUMATIC AND ANTIINFLAMMATORY ACTIONS. Salicylates are the most widely used therapeutic agents in rheumatoid arthritis and rheumatic fever. They markedly reduce painful joint swelling and fever but do not affect the ultimate course of the disease. The degree of suppression of inflammation increases with the plasma concentration of salicylate even beyond the point of toxicity. Thus, patients with severe inflammatory arthritis often tolerate tinnitus and other mild toxic manifestations in order to obtain the increased antiinflammatory effects associated with plasma levels of about 30–35 mg/100 ml, although the usual optimal subtoxic plasma level is in a range of 20–30 mg/100 ml. The mechanism of their antiinflammatory action is probably related to a number of the factors discussed at the beginning of this section. Currently, the inhibition of prostaglandin biosynthesis by salicylates is considered to be one of the primary reasons for their antiinflammatory activity. The antiinflammatory activity of salicylates has been demonstrated in induced inflammation in experimental animals and documented in patients with rheumatoid arthritis.

URICOSURIC ACTION. Salicylates affect renal tubular reabsorption and secretion of uric acid. In low doses (1–2 g/day) tubular secretion of uric acid is inhibited, and serum uric acid concentrations are increased. In doses that cause serum salicylate concentrations of greater than 20 mg/100 ml, salicylates also inhibit tubular reabsorption of uric acid. The net effect of inhibition of tubular secretion and reabsorption is an enhanced excretion of uric acid; hence, uric acid concentrations decrease. However, because more effective and less toxic uricosuric drugs are available, salicylates are no longer used for this purpose.

DECREASED PLATELET ADHESIVENESS. Aspirin inhibits platelet aggregation. As little as 300 mg of aspirin may produce an antiaggregation effect that is still detectable 4–6 days after ingestion. The prophylactic use of this anticoagulant effect is being explored in patients predisposed toward myocardial infarctions and cerebrovascular accidents.

Absorption and Metabolism

Aspirin is readily absorbed from the stomach and the small intestine. It is rapidly and completely hydrolyzed to salicylate by a plasma esterase, and within 90 min acetylsalicylic acid concentrations in the plasma are insignificant because all of the aspirin has been converted to salicylate. Plasma salicylate levels are not a simple function of the dose ingested because several of the major pathways of drug metabolism (conversion to salicylurate and formation of a glucuronide) become saturated at higher doses. Therefore, the time required to excrete half of a large dose of salicylate is longer than that needed to excrete half of a small dose. In addition, above a certain point, there is a sharp rise of the blood concentration of salicylate with small increments in the dose. Further, the renal excretion of unmetabolized salicylate is increased when the urine is alkaline and decreased when the urine is acid, approaching zero when its pH is five or less. Because of genetically determined variations in the metabolism of salicylate, serum concentrations attained by different individuals taking the same weight adjusted dose of aspirin may vary widely; fivefold differences have been observed. As the serum salicylate concentration associated with optimal antiinflammatory effect is rather critical, therapeutic doses of salicylate must be determined individually for each patient.

Adverse Effects

Gastric intolerance, in the form of epigastric discomfort, nausea, anorexia or heartburn, is common in patients who take fairly large doses of aspirin chronically. Increased **occult fecal blood loss** during salicylate administration is well documented. It can be reduced or prevented by administering aspirin in a solution of sufficient buffer capacity to completely neutralize the acidity of the gastric juice. The important role of acid in the gastric irritation produced by aspirin has been confirmed by studies in achlorhydric subjects who had fewer mucosal erosions and less occult blood loss than normal subjects given the same aspirin dose. These studies suggest that the toxic effects are predominantly local and are supported by animal studies which were unable to relate gastric toxicity to plasma salicylate concentrations. Ethanol ingestion may increase the occult blood loss induced by aspirin.

Tinnitus and **decreased auditory acuity** are reliable early signs of salicylate toxicity in the adult. In individuals with normal hearing, persistent tinnitus is present only when serum salicylate concentrations are greater than 20 mg/100 ml, and this has been used as a guide for individualization of aspirin dosage. Unfortunately, many older patients have preexisting hearing loss and cannot perceive tinnitus, while children may fail to appreciate it. In these two age groups, serum salicylate concentration should be used to individualize drug dosage. Both the tinnitus and deafness associated with high salicylate concentrations are readily reversible when the drug is discontinued.

Reversible **hepatocellular toxicity** has been observed in a small number of children and in a few patients with systemic lupus erythematosus who had therapeutic plasma salicylate concentrations. These abnormalities of liver function apparently are rather unusual and disappear when the drug is discontinued. Because salicylate binding to plasma proteins is quite avid, it may enhance the effect of drugs that are displaced from their protein binding sites by salicylate (Ch. 2); examples include coumarin anticoagulants, diphenylhydantoin, the oral hypoglycemic agents and phenylbutazone. Nephrotoxicity has been observed with chronic ingestion of combinations of salicylate and phenacetin, but there is no convincing evidence that prolonged use of aspirin alone has any clinically important effect on the kidney. Serious **allergic reactions** to aspirin may be manifested as asthma, hypotension and hives. The syndrome of rhinitis and nasal polyposis has also been attributed to aspirin hypersensitivity.

SALICYLATE POISONING. Because of their ubiquity, salicylates frequently cause serious intoxication in children (Ch. 13). Hyperventilation, severe acidosis, irritability, psychosis, fever, coma and cardiovascular collapse may occur with salicylate poisoning and may be complicated by gastrointestinal hemorrhage due to local gastric irritation and the hypoprothrombinemic and antiplatelet activities of aspirin. Gastric lavage, alkalinization, diuresis and intensive supportive measures are necessary to treat salicylate poisoning. Because of the peculiarities of salicylate metabolism, elevated plasma levels may fall very slowly.

The characteristic **disturbance of acid base balance** by salicylate toxicity may be explained as follows. Therapeutic concentrations of salicylate increase oxygen consumption and CO_2 production by uncoupling oxidative phosphorylation. Increased ventilation compensates for the increased CO_2 production. With slightly higher salicylate concentrations of greater than 35 mg/100 ml, the respiratory center is stimulated, causing hyperventilation and respiratory alkalosis; if these concentrations persist, renal excretion of bicarbonate, sodium and potassium returns the blood pH toward normal, resulting in compensated respiratory alkalosis but also decreasing the reserve buffering capacity of the system. With further increase in salicylate concentrations above 50 mg/100 ml, the medullary respiratory center is depressed. Hypoventilation, combined with increased CO_2 production, causes respiratory acidosis with increased plasma P_{CO_2} and pH, but this cannot be adequately buffered because of the earlier compensatory excretion of cations (to correct the respiratory alkalosis). Acidosis is enhanced by the substantial concentrations of the organic acids of salicylate and acetylsalicylate and the accumulation of lactic, pyruvic and acetoacetic acids due to salicylate induced disturbance of carbohydrate metabolism. Coma, cardiovascular collapse, impaired tissue oxygenation and impaired renal function all add to the acidosis and contribute to a fatal outcome in severe salicylate poisoning.

Preparations and Dosage

Aspirin is the most commonly used salicylate. Buffered preparations may dissociate more readily in the stomach, but do not contain sufficient buffer to neutralize the gastric contents. Enteric coated aspirin tablets are often better tolerated, but in some individuals may be incompletely absorbed. The usual dosage form is the 300 mg tablet. Combinations with propoxyphene, codeine or phenacetin (acetophenetidin) are often used for the treatment of headaches and pain syndromes. Salicylamide has little or no antipyretic, analgesic or antiinflammatory effect but shares the potential for gastrointestinal irritation with other members of the salicylate family.

For the relief of mild pain, aspirin and other forms of salicylate are effective in doses of 0.3–0.9 g every 3–4 hr. Fever usually can be relieved with similar doses. For intensive antiinflammatory therapy, plasma concentrations of 20–30 mg/100 ml should be maintained as discussed above.

PARA-AMINOPHENOL DERIVATIVES

PHENACETIN AND ACETAMINOPHEN. The parent compound for this group of drugs is acet-

PHENACETIN · ACETAMINOPHEN

anilid, but it is no longer used because of excessive toxicity. Phenacetin and acetaminophen are useful for their **antipyretic and analgesic effects** but have no antirheumatic or antiinflammatory activity. Their major advantage is their lack of gastrointestinal side effects. Phenacetin was widely used in combination with aspirin and caffeine as a mild analgesic, but its use has been largely abandoned owing to occasional occurrence of chronic interstitial nephritis and papillary necrosis in association with chronic use of high doses of the combination product. Acetaminophen is used as a substitute for salicylates in patients who have peptic ulcer disease or who for other reasons are unable to tolerate aspirin. It is bound to plasma protein to a much smaller extent than are the salicylates. A minor metabolite may cause the formation of methemoglobin. This is seen more frequently with phenacetin than with acetaminophen and rarely causes clinical problems.

PYRAZOLON DERIVATIVES

Antipyrine and aminopyrine are phenylpyrazolon derivatives that were first used during the Nineteenth Century. Although they are effective analgesic antipyretic antiinflammatory drugs, they are no longer used because they occasionally cause fatal agranulocytosis.

PHENYLBUTAZONE

Phenylbutazone is a pyrazolon derivative that has been available since 1949 for the treatment of inflammatory musculoskeletal conditions. Although it has analgesic and antipyretic effects, its major virtue is its **potent antiinflammatory activity.** Because of its occasional serious toxicity, it is generally used as a secondary drug in patients who are unresponsive to or unable to tolerate aspirin or indomethacin. It is particularly effective in patients with ankylosing spondylitis, psoriatic arthritis, Reiter's syndrome and bursitis, tendonitis or tenosynovitis. It is also somewhat effective in the treatment of thrombophlebitis, pericarditis and pleurisy and is especially effective in the treatment of acute gout.

Pharmacology

The analgesic and antipyretic effects of phenyl-butazone are less marked than those of salicy-lates, and it is not used for these purposes. It is nearly as potent as the corticosteroids in its antiinflammatory effects in experimental models of inflammation. The mechanism of its antiinflammatory action is probably similar to that of the salicylates. It is rapidly and completely absorbed from the gastrointestinal tract, with peak plasma levels being obtained in about 2 hr. It is slowly metabolized in the liver to **oxyphenbutazone** and a **metabolite with moderate uricosuric properties.** Its biological half-life in man is about 72 hr owing to marked reabsorption of the un-ionized molecule in the distal tubules of the kidney. Both phenylbutazone and its metabolites are strongly bound to plasma proteins. With maximum therapeutic doses of 400–600 mg daily, the albumin binding sites for phenylbutazone become saturated. Further increases in the dose considerably increase the unbound fraction of the drug in plasma and increase the frequency of untoward side effects. In addition, the potency of coumarin anticoagulants is increased by displacing plasma protein bound coumarin. Chronic administration of phenylbutazone or phenobarbital **induces hepatic microsomal enzymes** (P450 cytochrome system) and increases the rate of metabolism of the drug, shortening its effective half-life. **Sodium retention** occurs frequently and occasionally causes clinically apparent edema. This can be minimized by use of a low salt diet, but this drug should be avoided in patients with borderline cardiac function.

Adverse Effects

Gastrointestinal side effects are fairly frequent. These may consist of nausea, epigastric discomfort or vomiting, but peptic ulcers may occur or may perforate or bleed during phenylbutazone therapy. Renal or hepatic dysfunction occurs rarely. Although it is said to occur in less than one in 50,000 patients treated with this drug, the abrupt occurrence of **bone marrow failure** has resulted in a number of deaths from aplastic anemia or agranulocytosis. Because of its fairly common less serious side effects and its rare association with lethal bone marrow failure, phenylbutazone is generally used only for relatively short courses of therapy, and blood counts should be followed closely.

Preparations and Dosage

Phenylbutazone is available in 100 mg tablets. For treatment of acute gout or acute bursitis, the usual dose is 100 mg 4–6 × daily. For ankylosing spondylitis, 100 or 200 mg daily often suffices.

Oxyphenbutazone is also available in 100 mg tablets. It has the same properties as phenylbutazone, and its dosage is similar.

INDOMETHACIN

A systematic study of indole acetic acid compounds resulted in the development of in-

INDOMETHACIN

domethacin as an antiinflammatory drug, and it has been available for prescription since 1965. Its therapeutic spectrum is similar to that of phenylbutazone, to which it is preferred because it has not caused fatal bone marrow suppression.

Pharmacology

Indomethacin was originally synthesized as a potential antiserotonin drug. It is an effective **antipyretic** agent and is especially useful in the treatment of fever due to lymphoma or other malignancies. It has little or no intrinsic analgesic activity and relieves pain only in inflammatory conditions. It is an exceptionally potent **antiinflammatory** agent and, in animals, inhibits carrageenin induced edema and exudate formation, adjuvant induced polyarthritis and urate induced synovitis. Its exact site of action is not known, but, in common with other acidic antiinflammatory drugs, it uncouples oxidative phosphorylation in isolated liver mitochondria. It is one of the most effective inhibitors of prostaglandin synthetase that is clinically available.

Absorption, Excretion and Metabolism

In man, indomethacin is rapidly absorbed and excreted. Peak blood levels are reached in 30–60 min in fasting subjects, but a prior meal slows absorption and flattens the peak. The rate at which it is eliminated from the blood is quite rapid, and serum concentrations decrease by 50% within 1½–2½ hr. Indomethacin serum concentrations are higher on the second day of administration but thereafter do not continue to increase with continued administration of the same dose. It is 90–95% bound to plasma proteins. Indomethacin is primarily excreted by the kidney as several inactive conjugation products that are formed in the liver. The administration of probenecid substantially decreases the rate of urinary excretion and results in higher serum indomethacin concentrations.

Adverse Effects

Indomethacin shares the problem of **gastric toxicity** with aspirin and phenylbutazone but causes somewhat less gastrointestinal blood loss than aspirin when evaluated by Cr^{51} labeled red blood cell studies. It is unique among the antiinflammatory drugs in its **CNS effects** and produces the feeling of "muzziness" in some patients, while severe drug related headaches prevent other patients from continuing to take it. Serious hypersensitivity to the drug, neutropenia or hepatotoxicity are very rare. However, several deaths due to hepatitis in children who were taking indomethacin have prompted the recommendation that the drug not be given to children. Some side effects occur in nearly half of the patients taking indomethacin, and about 20% are unable to continue to use it.

Therapeutic Uses

Indomethacin is moderately effective in the treatment of rheumatoid arthritis, but salicylates are usually preferable. It is as effective as phenylbutazone for the treatment of ankylosing spondylitis, the rheumatoid variants, acute gout and the bursitis and tendonitis syndromes. It is also useful for treating patients with osteoarthritis of the hip, and occasional patients with classic rheumatoid arthritis find it exceptionally effective.

Preparations and Dosage

Indomethacin capsules contain 25 or 50 mg of the drug. For the acute inflammation of gout or bursitis, up to 200 mg daily in divided doses may be used for a few days. For the chronic inflammation of ankylosing spondylitis or rheumatoid arthritis, 25 mg 1–4 × daily are used. Side effects are less frequent if the drug is given with meals and if the dose is increased gradually.

COLCHICINE

Symptomatic antiinflammatory therapy of gout was practiced long before hyperuricemia and urate crystal deposition were first described by Garrod in 1848. Extracts of the autumn crocus were recommended for articular pain in the Sixth Century A.D., and the alkyloid colchicine was isolated in 1820 by Pelletier and Coventou.

COLCHICINE

Colchicine is used primarily in **gouty arthritis** and is of little use in other conditions. Its antiinflammatory effect is apparently due to its action on the polymorphonuclear leukocyte. It suppresses the oxidation of glucose in phagocytizing and nonphagocytizing leukocytes, diminishes phagocytosis and interferes with the chemotactic response of leukocytes. It inhibits the adherence of polymorphs to glass beads and interferes with kinin generation by granulocytes, thus decreasing the emigration of leukocytes into the crystal containing synovial fluid and diminishing the metabolic and phagocytic activity of those polymorphs already present. The net effect is a decrease in local lactic acid production and lysosomal enzyme liberation, thereby interrupting part of the inflammatory process of gout.

Colchicine is not analgesic and has no effect on the metabolism, excretion or solubility of urate, but it abolishes the pain of acute gout entirely by its antiinflammatory action. It may be given IV in a dose of 1 or 2 mg in 15 ml of 5% glucose in water—with a maximum of 5 mg in any 24 hr period, or it may be given orally in a dose of 0.6 mg/hr until symptomatic relief is obtained or gastrointestinal toxicity occurs. Dramatic improvement in the exquisite pain, swelling and inflammation of acute gout usually occurs within 6–12 hr after initiating intensive therapy; complete recovery of joint function occurs within 24–48 hr. Colchicine 0.6 mg 1–3 times daily is frequently given prophylactically to prevent gouty attacks, even though the underlying hyperuricemia is not altered by this drug.

The primary symptoms of colchicine overdosage are abdominal pain, nausea, vomiting and diarrhea that may become bloody due to a hemorrhagic gastroenteritis. With severe toxicity, paralysis develops and death is usually due to respiratory arrest. Significant amounts of colchicine are excreted in the bile and reabsorbed in the intestine, perhaps partly explaining the prominence of intestinal symptoms with overdosage.

Preparations and Dosage

Colchicine tablets: 0.5 or 0.6 mg oral tablets. Colchicine sterile solution 0.5 mg/ml. Dosage as described above.

INVESTIGATIONAL ANTIINFLAMMATORY DRUGS

Many new antiinflammatory agents have been developed by the pharmaceutic industry during the past decade. Some of these have been undergoing intensive clinical investigation for at least 5 years but have not yet been released for general prescription. Undoubtedly a number of useful new agents will become generally available during the next 4 or 5 years. The clinical activity of these new drugs is similar to that of the salicylates, phenylbutazone and indomethacin, although they vary somewhat in their ratio of analgesic to antiinflammatory activity. Most of them seem to cause somewhat less gastric irritation than aspirin, and selected patients may respond better to them than they do to the currently available drugs.

URATE LOWERING DRUGS

The hyperuricemia responsible for gout may be pharmacologically controlled by increasing uric acid excretion or by decreasing uric acid production.

URICOSURIC DRUGS

Urate is filtered by the renal glomeruli, reabsorbed in the proximal tubule and then secreted by the distal tubule. Substances that decrease distal tubular urate secretion produce hyperuricemia; examples are organic anions such as lactate or salicylate in low doses, and most diuretics. Substances that decrease proximal tubular reabsorption increase renal uric acid clearance and lower serum uric acid levels. Salicylates in high doses, phenylbutazone, sulfinpyrazone and probenecid are among the drugs that have been found to inhibit the renal tubular transport of urate. Small doses of these agents decrease urate clearance, presumably by inhibiting its secretion, but larger doses also block reabsorption and thus have a uricosuric effect. Probenecid and sulfinpyrazone are the two most frequently used uricosuric agents.

Probenecid is available as 0.5 g oral tablets. Dosage is regulated by following the serum uric acid concentration and may vary from 0.5–2.5 g daily in divided doses. The drug is readily absorbed, and peak plasma levels are achieved in 2–4 hr, while the half-life varies from 6–12 hr. It is generally well tolerated, but it must be given for many years because it has no effect on the underlying cause of the patient's hyperuricemia. Gastrointestinal discomfort and hypersensitivity are the most common side effects, but are rarely serious. Uricosuric drugs should be avoided in patients who have renal calculi since the increased clearance of urate tends to exacerbate stone formation. Probenecid also effectively blocks renal tubular secretion of penicillin, thus enhancing penicillin blood levels; although the drug was originally developed for this purpose, it is now most frequently used to control hyperuricemia.

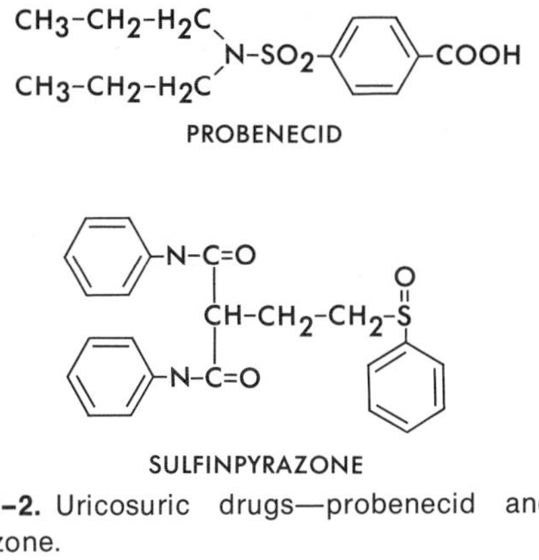

Sulfinpyrazone is a modification of the uricosuric metabolite of phenylbutazone. Its action is similar to that of probenecid, and it has no antiinflammatory or analgesic properties. It is available in 100 mg tablets. One tablet is usually given 1–4 times daily depending on the response of the serum uric acid concentration. Gastrointestinal irritation is somewhat less frequent, and bone marrow suppression has not been reported with sulfinpyrazone, despite its ancestry.

INHIBITORS OF URATE SYNTHESIS

The immediate metabolic precursor of uric acid is xanthine. Xanthine is formed from hypoxanthine by the enzyme xanthine oxidase and is also oxidized to uric acid by the same enzyme. **Allopurinol** is a structural isomer of hypoxanthine. It competitively inhibits these metabolic reactions and thus reduces the production of uric acid. Inhibition of xanthine oxidase increases the concentrations of xanthine and hypoxanthine in the urine, but these two oxypurines are somewhat more soluble than uric acid, and there have been few reports of xanthine crystal deposition in patients treated with allopurinol. The dose is 100–500 mg daily in divided doses; the drug is available as 100 mg tablets. It is particularly useful in patients with impaired renal urate clearance due to renal failure or chronic diuretic ingestion and is in-

FIG. 28-2. Uricosuric drugs—probenecid and sulfinpyrazone.

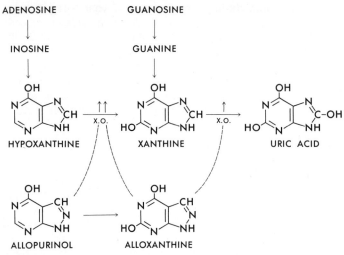

FIG. 28-3. Purine metabolism by xanthine oxidase (XO) and its inhibition by allopurinol.

dicated in patients with renal calculi. The drug is generally well tolerated and rarely causes hypersensitivity rashes or mild gastrointestinal toxicity.

Neither the uricosuric agents nor allopurinol have any antiinflammatory or analgesic effect, and they are not useful for treating the inflammation of gouty arthritis. Thus, in gout there is a complete separation of the therapy for inflammation from the therapy for the underlying cause of the inflammation. Effective treatment of gout necessitates the use of an antiinflammatory agent and a uric acid lowering agent. Unless both are used, the patient with gout cannot be optimally treated.

FURTHER READING

Klinenberg JR (1969): Current concepts of hyperuricemia and gout. Calif Med 110:231–243

Melmon KL, Morrelli H, Rowland M (1969): The clinical pharmacology of salicylates. Calif Med 110:410–422

Mills JA (1974): Drug therapy: nonsteroidal antiinflammatory drugs (Parts 1 and 2). N Engl J Med 290:781–784 and 1002–1005

Paulus HE, Whitehouse MW (1973): Nonsteroid antiinflammatory agents. Annu Rev Pharmacol 13:107–125

LOUIS S. HARRIS

WILLIAM L. DEWEY

29. NARCOTIC AND OTHER STRONG ANALGESICS, NARCOTIC ANTAGONISTS AND ANTITUSSIVES

NARCOTIC AND OTHER STRONG ANALGESICS

Pain is a universal syndrome with which almost everyone has had some personal experience. Those in the health professions are constantly faced with the problem of treating pain be they general practitioners, specialists or research workers. The mild or antipyretic analgesics (Ch. 28) are not effective in the treatment of severe pain. The narcotic or strong analgesics are capable of relieving severe pain and represent the best first line of therapy in this regard. While these drugs do have adverse effects, their proper use make their hazards relatively insignificant in relationship to their benefit.

In 1680, Sydenham, the celebrated English physician, wrote "Among the remedies which it has pleased Almighty God to give to man to relieve his sufferings, none is so universal and so efficacious as opium." This statement still has a ring of truth. Opium is the dried exudate obtained from the seed pods of the poppy plant *Papaver somniferum.* Opium has been in medical use for millennia. From it are obtained **morphine** and its methyl ether **codeine,** which are mainly responsible for its analgesic activity. Opium also contains a large number of other alkaloids such as **thebaine, papaverine** and **noscapine** that have different pharmacologic properties.

The narcotic analgesics have a great deal in common. They share major structural features (Fig. 29–1). They are all effective analgesics, depress the respiratory center, cause constipation and most of their effects are reversed or prevented by the specific narcotic antagonists such as **nalorphine** and **naloxone.** Their prolonged use leads to the development of tolerance to most of their pharmacologic actions as well as to physical dependence (Ch. 9).

The morphine structure (Fig. 29–1) was first completely elucidated by Sir Robert Robinson early in this century. Although its total synthesis has been accomplished, it is not practical and our total supply of morphine and codeine is derived from plant material. From the basic structure of morphine has come a wide variety of new drugs which share, to a greater or lesser extent, both its therapeutic utility and side effect liability. There are few drug classes for which such an extensive structure activity relationship is known or where the chemists have been so successful in producing new compounds with clinical efficacy and relative safety.

ACTIONS

The pharmacologic properties of morphine are typical of the whole class of narcotic analgesics. For this reason, only the actions of morphine will be discussed in any detail. Where significant differences occur they will be mentioned with the description of the specific drug.

In general, the main effects of the narcotic analgesics are confined to the CNS and the gastrointestinal tract.

Central Nervous System Effects

In man, morphine produces **analgesia, drowsiness** and **sleep.** The extremities feel heavy and the body warm, the face and nose itch and the mouth is dry. **Hunger is abolished** and when **nausea and vomiting** occur, they are not accompanied by the usual unpleasant emotional reactions. **The respiration is depressed** and the **pupils constricted.** In other words, morphine has a mixed depressant and stimulatory action on the CNS.

The analgesic effects of morphine are not due to interference with the conduction of pain im-

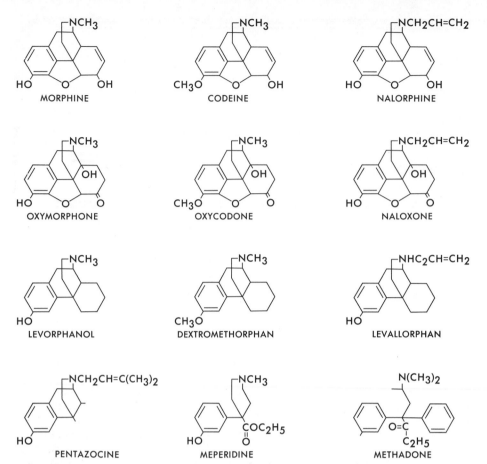

FIG. 29-1. Structures of strong analgesics, narcotic antagonists and antitussives.

pulses from the periphery such as occurs with the local anesthetics (Ch. 22). Most commonly patients will indicate that they still feel pain but that it no longer bothers them. Thus, the analgesics in some way interfere with the perception of pain. The precise details of the mechanisms involved have not been worked out but it appears that specific receptors and neurochemical systems in the brain may be implicated.

The word morphine is derived from *Morpheus*, the Greek god of sleep. It is not surprising that drowsiness and sleep are prominent actions of the narcotic analgesics. They do not, however, account for the analgesia, nor does the euphoria which often accompanies their administration. The evaluation of pain relief is extremely complex. Approximately one-third of patients with severe pain will regularly report good to excellent relief after receiving a placebo. Because of this, carefully designed double-blind studies are necessary to ascertain the clinical efficacy of any drug or other treatment purported to produce analgesia.

The nausea and vomiting commonly produced by morphine is a result of its direct stimulatory action on the medullary chemoreceptor trigger zone leading to activation of the vomiting center. The emetic effects of morphine are tempered, however, by its direct inhibitory action on the vomiting center.

Pulmonary ventilation is depressed by morphine and all the other narcotic analgesics. This phenomena is dose related and is the principal cause of death from acute overdose. Morphine produces a reduction in the sensitivity of the respiratory center in the medulla to carbon dioxide. This leads to an increase in the levels of carbon dioxide in blood and expired air which, by reflex action, tend to increase respiratory rate. Thus, until high doses of narcotic are given, the effects on ventilation may not be readily observed. Morphine has little effect on the response of the respiratory center to chemoreceptor stimulation by hypoxia. Since high O_2 levels inhibit ventilation, the administration of oxygen to a patient with an overdose of narcotic may lead to apnea. For this reason, the use of oxygen must be carefully monitored and is not usually advised. This is especially true since very specific narcotic antagonists are available for use in the treatment of narcotic induced respiratory depression.

Morphine and the other narcotic analgesics constrict the pupils. This miosis is brought about by stimulation of the nuclei of the third cranial nerve. Pin-point pupils, along with needle tracts, are a useful sign of narcotic addiction since it is one of the few actions of the narcotics to which tolerance does not develop.

The narcotic analgesics **depress the cough reflex,** thus some enjoy widespread use as antitussive agents (see below).

Although sedation and general depression are the predominant overt signs of morphine in man, general **excitatory effects** can also occur. These are characterized by restlessness, delirium, mania and a "strychnine-like" stimulation of the spinal cord. For this reason, the use of analeptics such as picrotoxin and metrazol are contraindicated in the treatment of the respiratory depression produced by the narcotics. In some species, such as cats and horses, the excitatory effects are predominant. This has led to the illicit use of narcotics in an attempt to "fix" horse races.

Gastrointestinal Effects

The **constipating action** of opium was among the first recognized and led to its widespread use in the treatment of diarrhea. The effects of morphine on the gastrointestinal tract are complex. Constipation can be accounted for by three factors; The first is a delayed emptying time of the stomach caused by contraction of the pyloric sphincter and an increased tone of the antral portion of the stomach and duodenum. Second, there is a delayed passage of the intestinal contents due to markedly decreased propulsive contractions of the small bowel along with increased amplitude of the nonpropulsive contractions, and an increased tone of the large bowel. Biliary and pancreatic secretions are also diminished thus interfering with digestion. Third, there is an increased tone of the anal sphincter that, combined with inattention to the normal sensory stimuli for defecation, completes the picture of morphine produced constipation. Although morphine has a direct inhibitory effect on cholinergic systems in the gut, the complex pattern described above demonstrates that this cannot fully account for the constipation. Tolerance does not develop to the constipating actions of the narcotics.

Other Effects

Other smooth muscles are also effected by morphine. The bile duct is constricted and there is a spasm of the sphincter of Oddi. This action is not reversed by atropine. The ureters are also constricted by morphine and this effect is blocked by atropine. In any case, morphine should advisedly be used for the pain associated with biliary and renal colic.

The narcotic analgesics produce a marked degree of **tolerance.** After repeated medication at appropriate intervals, dosage must be increased to maintain the same effect. Carried to extreme, doses many times greater than those which produce death can be attained. Accompanying the development of tolerance is the development of **physical dependence** that is manifested by a specific "withdrawal syndrome" when the drug is discontinued. It is not entirely known whether the phenomena of tolerance and physical dependence are related or if they are, how. Continued use of the narcotics also may lead to psychologic dependence and a complete picture of addiction (Ch. 9).

OTHER STRONG ANALGESICS

The observation in the mid 1950s that the narcotic antagonist **nalorphine** was approximately as potent as morphine in relieving pain in man accelerated the search for new nonaddicting strong analgesics. The reason for this lay in the fact that nalorphine had little or no analgesic activity in the animal test procedures in use at the time and the low abuse potential of the drug. However, nalorphine produces dysphoria and other psychotomimetic effects in man which preclude its usefulness as an analgesic. In the ensuing years a weaker narcotic antagonist was sought based on the hope that it would have low addiction liability and not have dysphoric effects at analgesic doses in man. **Pentazocine** (Fig. 29–1) is the result of this search. Pentazocine is effective in the treatment of severe pain, has markedly lower abuse potential but does produce occasional "nalorphine-like" adverse effects, especially at elevated doses.

The major tranquilizers (Ch. 25) have potent antinociceptive activity in a variety of animal test procedures despite the fact that they are not analgesic in man. These findings led to the development of **methotrimeprazine,** a phenothiazine derivative with potent analgesic properties in man. This drug does not produce physical or psychologic dependence. It does, however, share most of the adverse effects associated with the phenothiazine tranquilizers. These compounds are discussed more fully below.

THERAPEUTIC APPLICATION

The most important use of the narcotic analgesics is for the symptomatic relief of **severe pain.** Because of their possible serious adverse effects and their abuse potential, the narcotics should not be used where the mild or nonaddicting analgesics will suffice. On the other hand, the withholding of adequate pain relief in a patient with terminal carcinoma because of a concern about addiction is also poor medicine. Care must be exercised in the use of strong analgesics lest the masking of pain interfere with proper diagnosis of the underlying condition producing the symptom. The symptomatic treatment of pain is no substitute for the treatment of the underlying disease process.

The strong analgesics are commonly used to treat the pain arising from surgery, severe trauma, carcinoma, delivery, and renal and biliary colic. In obstetric pain, care must be taken to select and properly use an analgesic because of the danger of respiratory depression in the infant. **Meperidine** is the drug most commonly used for this purpose. As indicated above, the use of morphine in biliary and urinary colic should be tempered with the knowledge that the drug produces a constriction of the smooth muscle involved and may thus exacerbate the painful condition.

Morphine is quite useful in the treatment of the pain and apprehension associated with myocardial infarction. Acute pulmonary edema produces pain and many unpleasant sensations associated with the air hunger accompanying the pathologic state. Morphine produces a dramatic relief of these symptoms. The narcotics are potent suppressors of the cough reflex. **Codeine** is particularly useful especially if the cough is severe and accompanied by pain (see antitussive agents). The opium alkaloids are quite useful in the treatment of diarrhea. A newer drug, a meperidine derivative, **diphenoxylate,** has less abuse potential and is currently widely used for this purpose (Ch. 37).

The narcotic analgesics are also widely used as a **preanesthetic** medication because of their analgesic, sedative and antianxiety properties. Their use provides a smoother induction and maintenance of anesthesia. However, in the absence of pain these purposes might better be served by a sedative hypnotic or mild tranquilizer (Chs. 25, 26). In recent years the narcotic analgesics have also been used IV along with a major tranquilizer to produce a type of anesthesia known as **neuroleptanalgesia,** i.e., as in general anesthesia (Ch. 27). This procedure has proven useful in certain types of high risk surgical patients.

CHOICE OF DRUGS

Over the last three decades there has been a massive search for new, safer analgesics with a lessened abuse potential. Thousands of compounds have been synthesized and hundreds studied in animals and man. Some success has been achieved but the ideal analgesic still does not exist and the search continues. This has, however, created some problems for the practitioner. Which drug is the proper choice? In general, the mildest analgesic with the least potential for adverse effects should be chosen first. If this does not afford good pain relief, a more effective and potent drug should then be used. The most widely used drugs are listed in Table 29–1 along with some information concerning their use.

Let us look at some of the drugs in a little more detail. First the natural products. Camphorated tincture of opium, *U.S.P.* (paragoric) has little use as an analgesic. It is given by mouth and is the most commonly used drug in the treatment of diarrhea. **Morphine** is an excellent analgesic. Indeed, no other drug has been demonstrated to be more efficacious than morphine. Morphine is available as the sulfate salt and is given parenterally usually by the IM or subcutaneous route. Occasionally morphine is given IV, but it should be given cautiously since sudden profound respiratory depression and hypotension may ensue. This is true for the IV use of any narcotic analgesic. Morphine is rapidly inactivated by the liver after oral administration making proper dosage by this route difficult. **Codeine** is not as effective an analgesic. When given subcutaneously, 120 mg of codeine is approximately equivalent to 10 mg of morphine. The incidence of adverse effects markedly increases at this dose. Because of this, the usual dose of codeine is 30–60 mg. Codeine is, however, effective when given orally and has considerably less abuse potential than morphine. It is often combined with aspirin and other mild analgesics to provide good relief of moderate pain. Codeine is also often used in the treatment of cough (see below). No compound with as low an abuse liability has yet been found that combines the analgesic, antitussive and sedative effects provided by codeine.

A number of drugs are available that are semisynthetic derivatives of morphine. These include diacetyl-morphine or **heroin,** which is approximately three times more potent than morphine but has never been shown to provide greater pain relief. Heroin is not a legal drug in the United States although it is the narcotic analgesic most often prescribed for severe pain in England. **Oxymorphone** and **oxycodone** are related as morphine is to codeine. They have similar pharmacologic properties but are approximately ten times more potent than their respective congeners. Oxycodone, however, has a higher abuse liability than codeine. Finally, in this group is **hydromorphone** (dilaudid).

TABLE 29—1. Principal Analgesics, Antagonists and Antitussive Agents

Drug	Trade name	Dose (mg)	Preferred route of administration	Duration (hr)	Comment
Narcotic analgesics					
Codeine	—	30–60	PO	4–6	Used primarily for moderate pain or as antitussive. Less addicting than morphine.
Dextropropoxyphene	Darvon	30–60	PO	2–4	Chemically related to methadone, but similiar as an analgesic to codeine. Less gastrointestinal effect and no antitussive action. Little significant addiction potential.
Heroin	—	3–5	—	3–4	Drug preferred by most addicts; cannot be legally used in United States.
Meperidine	Demerol, Pethidine	75–100	IM	2–4	Less constipating than morphine. No antitussive or miotic action. Overdosage causes CNS excitation. Less well antagonized by nalorphine than is morphine.
Methadone	Dolophine	10–15 7–10	PO IM	4–6	Less sedation, euphoria, emetic action than morphine; used in controlled narcotic withdrawal.
Morphine	—	10	IM, SC	4	See text.
Oxycodone	Percodan	10–15 15–20	IM PO	4	Similar to morphine in potency and addiction potential.
Oxymorphone	Numorphan	1–2	IM	4–6	Similar actions to morphine.
Hydromorphinone	Dilaudid	1–2	PO	3–4	Better oral absorption than morphine.
Levorphanol	Levo-Dromoran	2–3	IM	4–6	Similar pharmacology to morphine.
Other strong Analgesics					
Methotrimeprazine	Levoprome	10–30	IM	4–6	Not to be used for ambulatory patients due to orthostatic hypotension and sedation.
Pentazocine	Talwin	30	IM, PO	3–4	Shorter duration and faster onset than morphine. Not a controlled substance.
Narcotic antagonists					
Naloxone	Narcan	0.4	IV, IM, SC		Pure narcotic antagonist.
Nalorphine	Nalline	5	IV		Its agnoist properties make it less desireable than naloxone in the treatment of heroin overdose.
Levallorphan	Lorphan	0.5	IV		
Antitussive agents					
Codeine		8–15	PO	4	All new centrally acting antitussives are compared to codeine.
Dextromethorphan	Romilar	15–30	PO	4	Most widely used antitussive. A prescription is not needed.

A number of other agents are available as antitussives but clear objective evidence of their efficaciousness is lacking. They include noscapine, L-propoxyphene, benzonatate, chlophedianol, glyceryl guaiacolate, pipazethatae and pholcodine.

This compound is approximately eight times more potent than morphine but offers no advantage other than better oral absorption.

The purely synthetic compounds include **levorphanol,** a morphinan derivative about four times more potent than morphine. It is considerably more effective than morphine by mouth and shares all the useful and adverse actions of morphine. The optical isomer of the methyl ether of levorphanol is **dextromethorphan,** a very useful nonaddicting antitussive agent (see below). **Meperidine** was the first totally synthetic strong analgesic; discovered in Germany during a search for atropine-like antispasmotics. Meperidine is only one-tenth as potent as morphine parenterally and is somewhat less effective than morphine in relieving severe pain. Meperidine does depress the respiration, but tidal volume is more effected than rate which may increase after subcutaneous or IM administration. Meperidine is the drug most commonly used for obstetric analgesia. Although it may produce less respiratory depression in the newborn than do equianalgesic doses of morphine, ventilation is significantly depressed: an action that should not be ignored. The differences between these drugs may be due to the shorter duration of action of meperidine so that by the time of delivery, the effects of the drug may be dissipating. This drug was hailed in its early introduction as being nonaddicting. This is not so. Indeed, it is the narcotic physicians, nurses and dentists most commonly become dependent on. A number of meperidine derivatives are commercially available but offer little advantage over the parent compound. However, mention should be made of **Fentanyl** that is approximately 100 times more potent than morphine and is used, in combination with the potent butyrophenone tranquilizer, droperidol, to produce neuroleptanalgesia (see above).

Methadone was synthesized in Germany during World War II and soon became widely available as a morphine substitute. It is somewhat more potent than morphine parenterally and has a considerably better oral to parenteral ratio. This property has made the drug quite useful for the treatment of chronic pain where an oral medication was preferred. Methadone has a longer duration of action than morphine. The withdrawal symptoms in a person physically dependent on methadone develop more slowly, are less intense but more prolonged. This led to the use of oral methadone in the detoxification of narcotic dependent patients. More recently, oral methadone has been widely used in a maintenance type of therapy for the management of morphine-like physical dependence (Ch. 9). This use of the drug and the problems it has created has led the FDA to strictly control its use and dis-tribution. Methadone may now be used only for severe pain, detoxification and temporary maintenance of narcotic addicts, and maintenance treatment in approved methadone programs. Routine use for severe pain must be justified and the drug is currently only available in approved pharmacies. **Propoxyphene** is a methadone analog that is a less potent and effective analgesic. It cannot be used parenterally because of its irritant properties, although when it is given IV, it exhibits most of the typical properties of a narcotic. Results of controlled studies indicate that 65 mg of propoxyphene is no more effective than 650 mg of aspirin. Propoxyphene is available in a variety of combinations with mild analgesics. In these combinations, proproxyphene can be quite useful in the treatment of mild to moderate pain. Since the abuse potential of propoxyphene is relatively low, it is not subject to narcotic controls.

Two other strong analgesics, pentazocine and methotrimeprazine, with low abuse potential are also available (see above). **Pentazocine** is available for both parenteral and oral administration. When compared to morphine in the treatment of severe pain, pentazocine is about one-third as potent but just as efficacious except in very severe pain where adverse effects prevent large increases in dose. Pentazocine has a more rapid onset and shorter duration of action than morphine. The use of the drug in patients with a history of narcotic use is contraindicated because of its weak narcotic antagonist properties. When used orally, pentazocine has been shown to be as effective as codeine in the treatment of mild to moderate pain. Although the abuse potential of pentazocine is low and the drug is not covered by the Controlled Substances Act, it can produce physical dependence and has been abused. For this reason, care should be exercised in the use and prescription of this drug especially for self-administration of parenteral preparations. **Methotrimeprazine** is a phenothiazine derivative closely related to the major tranquilizers. It is about one-half as potent as morphine, but just as effective in most types of pain. Methotrimeprazine produces neither psychic nor physical dependence and thus is not subject to narcotic controls. However, like the phenothiazine tranquilizers (Ch. 25), methotrimeprazine is a potent α-adrenergic blocking agent. For this reason, it often produces a profound orthostatic hypotension. This, coupled with its marked sedative effects, makes its use in surgical, obstetric and ambulatory patients hazardous. Methotrimeprazine should be used with great caution in elderly patients, those with heart disease or in patients receiving anticholinergics such as atropine or scopolamine. The drug should not be given to patients in premature labor or those receiving antihypertensive medication.

ADVERSE REACTIONS

The most consistent and serious adverse reaction is **psychic and physical dependence.** All analgesics including pentazocine and propoxyphene, that do not come under the Controlled Substances Act, have been abused by some patients.

The most life endangering effect of the narcotics is their **respiratory depressant** activity. Some respiratory depression is seen either at or slightly above therapeutic analgesic doses. The therapeutic ratio between analgesia and respiratory depression is not large. An overdose of a narcotic produces severe respiratory depression, which like most other effects of the narcotics, can be reversed by **naloxone** or another narcotic antagonist. As a result of the depressed ventilation and hypercapnia there is an attendent dilation of the cerebral vessels and an increased intracranial pressure. Therefore, the narcotic analgesics are contraindicated in patients with head injury or other conditions associated with an elevated intracranial pressure.

The narcotics produce constipation at therapeutic doses. Although few cardiovascular effects are seen in man at therapeutic doses, higher doses can depress the cardiovascular system, although these effects are usually much less serious than the respiratory depression. The narcotics as a class cause a release of histamine and this accounts in part for the itching and hypotension which is seen particularly after intravenous administration. Allergic or idiosyncratic reactions, however, are rare.

The narcotic analgesics should not be used in patients with Addison's disease, myxedema or hepatic cirrhosis since they may cause stupor or frank coma. The narcotics may decrease urine production and lead to urinary retention by causing a release of antidiuretic hormone and spasm of the bladder sphincter and ureters. Because of this, the narcotics should be used cautiously in patients with renal or urinary tract disease. For adverse reactions of individual drugs see above in Choice of Drugs.

NARCOTIC ANTAGONISTS

Narcotic antagonists are only approved for the treatment of **opiate overdosage.** The narcotic antagonists reverse both the central and peripheral effects of the narcotics including general CNS and respiratory depression, analgesia, miosis and constipation. The duration of action of the narcotic antagonists is usually much shorter than the duration of the narcotic. Therefore, when treating narcotic overdosage, the narcotic antagonist must be given repeatedly to maintain the antagonistic effect and prevent respiratory depression due to the prolonged action of the narcotic. One injection of a narcotic antagonist will not ordinarily suffice to treat an overdose of heroin. Obviously, should a patient who is suffering from an overdose of heroin be dependent on a narcotic, an abrupt withdrawal syndrome could be induced by the antagonist, which would not be in the best interest of the patient. For this reason, the narcotic antagonists should be used cautiously in patients with evidence of narcotic addiction. The narcotic antagonists are specific in that they only reverse the CNS and respiratory depression produced by narcotics. They are not generally useful analeptic agents, and will not shorten the duration of anesthesia nor reverse respiratory depression induced by barbiturates or other sedatives and hypnotics. This specificity of action is most probably due to their structural similarities with the narcotics (Fig. 29–1). Allyl substitution on the nitrogen in the morphinan and other narcotic series also leads to compounds with antagonist activity. In general, the more potent the parent analgesic, the more potent is the N-allyl derivative as an antagonist.

As a group, the narcotic antagonists are devoid of antinociceptive activity in classic laboratory animal experiments. However, many of the antagonists do have analgesic activity in man. These compounds are referred to as narcotic-antagonist analgesics of which pentazocine and nalorphine are most noteworthy (see above).

Recently, **naloxone** (Narcan), a relatively pure narcotic antagonist without analgesic activity in man has been marketed. It is also devoid of analgesic activity in laboratory animals and will induce abrupt withdrawal signs when injected into an opiate dependent animal or person. Naloxone does not produce euphoria, respiratory depression or other effects characteristic of the opiates in man. Because of its specificity of narcotic antagonist effect, naloxone is the drug of choice in the treatment of narcotic overdosage.

Recently, clinical trials have begun to determine how efficacious the narcotic antagonists are as a treatment regimen in the rehabilitation of past narcotic addicts. These investigations are based upon the fact that following complete opiate withdrawal, the administration of an antagonist will block the euphoria produced by a subsequent opiate injection. It is postulated that the absence of euphoria will discourage additional injections of opiate. Although some success has been attained, at least two problems remain that need to be resolved before this treatment plan gains broad acceptance. The first issue is whether the antagonist should contain some agonist properties in order to induce the addict to take the drug or would a pure antagonist like naloxone be the drug of choice. Second, the duration of antagonistic action is quite short, less than 24 hr for most drugs. A new antagonist or a new preparation of an existing antagonist which will have activity in the order of at least a few weeks would be desirable.

ANTITUSSIVES

The **cough reflex** is a protective mechanism which is initiated by chemical or mechanical stimulation in the tracheobronchial tree. Although it is feasible for drugs to block the cough at either the sensory, central or motor portion of the arc, the majority of useful antitussive agents work by depressing this reflex centrally, at the cough center in the medulla. The most potent antitussive agents are found among the narcotic analgesics. **Morphine** is an efficacious antitussive agent but its addiction potential at therapeutic doses precludes its use for this purpose. **Codeine** is the antitussive of choice among the narcotics. It has antitussive properties at one-fourth to one-half of its analgesic dose. The addiction potential of codeine at antitussive doses, although still present, is less than at analgesic doses or antitussive doses of other narcotics. Codeine has the additional advantage over morphine of being an active antitussive when taken orally. The dextrorotatory isomer of many of the narcotics do not possess signifi-

cant analgesic properties or addiction potential but many are orally effective antitussives. **Dextromethorphan** is the prototype drug in this class and has a potency as an antitussive agent comparable to that of codeine.

Antitussives are often indicated to allow the patient to obtain rest and sleep rather than to inhibit the pathologic condition. Therefore, a sedative is often combined with a nonnarcotic antitussive agent, not because it blocks or potentiates the blockade of the cough reflex, but to prolong sleep. In addition, the centrally acting antitussive agents may be mixed with a demulcent which decreases the irritation of the mucous membranes and/or an expectorant which increases sputum volume or alters its character and aids in its expulsion.

A variety of other antitussive agents with a low abuse potential are also available (see Table 29–1), but these lack good objective proof of their efficacy.

FURTHER READING

Eddy NB, Friebel H, Hahn KJ, Halbach H (1970): Codeine and its alternates for pain and cough relief. Bull WHO 3–253

Fraser HF, Harris LS (1967): Narcotic and narcotic antagonist analgesics. Annu Rev Pharmacol 7:277

Lasagna L (1964): The clinical evaluation of morphine and its substitutes as analgesics. Pharmacol Rev 16:47

Lewis JW, Bentley KW, Cowan A (1971): Narcotic analgesics and antagonists. Annu Rev Pharmacol 11:241

Martin WR (1967): Opioid antagonists. Pharmacol Rev 19:463

MARK A. GOLDBERG

30. ANTICONVULSANT DRUGS

Epilepsy is a common disorder of the CNS with a prevalence rate of approximately 5/thousand. If untreated it may be socially, psychologically and physically devastating to the patient. Fortunately, 70–85% of all patients can be adequately controlled by drug therapy. The term epilepsy, used synonymously with convulsive disorder or seizure disorder, is generally applied to a syndrome characterized by brief, recurrent, paroxysmal episodes of disturbed CNS function, usually with alteration in the state of consciousness. This definition does not fully account for some of the manifestations which may occur in epilepsy. For example, although the usual seizure lasts seconds or minutes, occasionally patients may have repetitive seizures lasting for hours or, rarely, even days. While loss of consciousness is usual, in certain forms of epilepsy the patient may remain alert and awake throughout the attack.

Epilepsy should not be considered a disease, but is a complex syndrome of disordered central nervous system function which can occur as a symptom of a wide variety of pathologic processes that affect the brain. A tumor or laceration of the brain, a defect in a single enzyme or a metabolic disturbance elsewhere in the body all can manifest themselves by seizures. Therefore, all patients with seizures require a careful neurologic evaluation to seek out any possible causes of seizures that lend themselves to correction.

CLASSIFICATION OF SEIZURES

A number of classifications of epileptic seizures have been proposed; however, the World Health Organization (WHO) classification is most widely accepted and will be used in this text. Classification is of great importance in drug therapy inasmuch as certain drugs are effective against certain types of seizures while they are totally ineffective against other seizure categories. This point must be borne in mind because unless the correct seizure diagnosis is made rational drug therapy becomes impossible.

Generalized Seizures Without Focal Onset

GRAND MAL SEIZURES. This is the most common type of seizure encountered clinically and represents a common response of the CNS to many pathologic processes. This is the type of seizure usually associated with epilepsy in the public mind. Characteristically, the patient has no warning or recollection of preceding events. The patient may stiffen briefly or fall to the ground if standing. Initially there is generalized tonic activity with flexion of the upper extremities and forced extension of the lower extremities. Urinary incontinence may occur. The tonic phase is followed by a clonic phase in which there is generalized tremulousness followed by rhythmic contraction of the arms and legs. This gradually subsides and the patient lies quietly and gradually recovers consciousness. Characteristically the patient is somewhat confused and feels sleepy following a seizure. The entire event usually lasts several minutes. During the seizure the patient frequently becomes cyanotic, has apneic periods interspersed with normal respiratory patterns, blood pressure rises, heart rate increases and the pupils become widely dialated and unresponsive to light. These responses are the result of discharge of the sympathetic nervous system. They return to normal soon after the seizure.

ABSENCE (PETIT MAL). This type of seizure occurs characteristically in young children above the age of 6 and frequently terminates spontaneously following adolescence. The seizures are very brief in duration, lasting only a few seconds and are characterized by a staring spell during which the patient is unaware of his surroundings. There may be some movement of the eyelids or tremor of the lips but there is no gross motor activity. The patient usually recovers and continues his previous activity, and may not be aware that a seizure has occurred. These attacks can occur up to hundreds of times a day and may be overlooked by parents and teachers and the child merely thought to be inattentive or "day dreaming." However, these attacks do represent brief periods of unconsciousness during which time a child is unable to learn or interact socially, and can therefore result in apparent personality changes and learning difficulties. There are no known structural abnormalities of the CNS associated with petit mal epilepsy.

Focal Seizures (partial seizures)

FOCAL MOTOR SEIZURES. These are seizures which begin and may be entirely limited to movement of one side of the body or even one extremity. They may begin on one side and then gradually spread to the other side becoming a generalized seizure. This type of seizure represents more limited cortical pathology or indicates that inhibitory mechanisms are present which limit the spread of the seizure. Consciousness will not be lost if the seizure does not spread. Focal sensory seizures may also occur, although they are extremely rare. All partial seizures have the potential of becoming generalized, but the term partial seizure is maintained if a focal origin is discernible.

PSYCHOMOTOR OR TEMPORAL LOBE SEIZURES. These are partial seizures with extremely varied and complex symptomatology. The anterior temporal lobe is the most common site of origin of these seizures. Usually there is a preceding aura which may be an olfactory hallucination. Other typical warning symptoms may be a feeling of epigastric discomfort, a sense of warmth or a very poorly definable sense that something is going to happen. During the attack the patient may continue standing or continue with some semi-purposeful activity. He is out of contact with his environment and does not understand if spoken to. He may perform relatively complex activities during the attack or simply stare vacantly into space. If restrained, he may exhibit aggressive behavior. Following the attack the patient may be confused and totally unaware of what took place during the seizure. These spells may last for a number of minutes. Symptomatology of temporal lobe epilepsy is extremely varied and complex and is frequently misinterpreted as abnormal behavior rather than an event of cortical origin. Because autonomic phenom-

ena are common, patients are frequently evaluated for systemic illnesses before the nature of the attacks becomes obvious.

A number of other seizure types are recognized, especially in young children. These are frequently unresponsive to the usual anticonvulsants and are relatively rare and beyond the scope of the present discussion.

Status Epilepticus

This term refers to acute repetitive generalized seizure activity in which the patient has a subsequent seizure before recovering from the initial seizure. These repetitive seizures may, if untreated, last for hours or even days. Grand mal status represents a medical emergency in that if uncontrolled it may result in significant CNS damage or even death.

THE ELECTROENCEPHALOGRAM (EEG)

Recording electrical activity of the brain by electrodes placed on the scalp has become a standard diagnostic procedure, and is especially useful in the evaluation of patients with epilepsy. In petit mal a characteristic 3/sec "spike and wave" pattern may be seen during an attack and this pattern is virtually diagnostic of this type of epilepsy. A number of other abnormal electrical discharges can be recorded from patients which are strongly suggestive of an underlying convulsive disorder. The EEG is also frequently useful in localizing the focus of seizure discharges. However, it is important to keep in mind that at any given time the patient with epilepsy may have a completely normal EEG and the absence of electrical abnormalities does not rule out the diagnosis of epilepsy. Abnormal EEGs may also be found in individuals who have never had seizures.

EDUCATION OF THE PATIENT AND HIS FAMILY

It is extremely important that the patient understand the nature of his illness at a level appropriate to his educational background. His family too should learn to accept the illness without excessive limitation of activities or unnecessary attention. Unfortunately in the minds of many laymen epilepsy is synonymous with insanity or mental retardation and only through education of the patient and his family will he be able to accept the social problems which may arise because of the seizure disorder. Patient cooperation and understanding are of critical importance in the management of epilepsy because a physician will rarely witness even a single seizure and must depend on reports of the patient and his family for a description of the seizure and for keeping records of seizure frequency.

PRINCIPLES OF DRUG THERAPY

The underlying principle of drug therapy is to select the appropriate anticonvulsant for the type of seizure the patient is having and then to gradually increase the dose of medication until seizure control is achieved or toxicity prevents further increases in dose. The dose should be increased by small increments with sufficient time between dosage adjustment to fully evaluate the effectiveness of the preceding change. Measurement of serum levels of anticonvulsants, a relatively new clinical procedure, can serve as a useful guide to predicting therapeutic effect and toxicity, but ultimately clinical criteria are the most useful. If seizure control is not obtained and toxicity is approached, the usual procedure would be to add a second anticonvulsant drug to the patient's therapeutic regime without withdrawing the first anticonvulsant agent. Occasionally it may be necessary to add further anticonvulsants in order to effect good control. Careful monitoring of serum levels is especially important in the early stages of therapy to insure that the patient is complying with the physician's instructions and to identify any patients with unusual patterns of drug metabolism. Failure to take medications properly is perhaps the most common single cause of drug failure in patients with epilepsy, and is frequently due to inadequate education of the patient. Unusual metabolic patterns may occur on a genetically determined basis or may be the result of the addition of other drugs to the patient's therapy which can affect the metabolism of anticonvulsants.

Hematopoietic depression and renal damage are the most serious toxic effects associated with the use of anticonvulsants. For this reason blood counts and urine analysis should be obtained at regular intervals, especially when a new drug is added to the patient's therapy.

The practice of using combinations of anticonvulsants at the outset is not recommended because adverse effects that occur after initiation of two new drugs cannot accurately be ascribed to either and may lead to the necessity of discontinuing both drugs. Fixed drug combinations available as a single dosage form have a similar disadvantage as well as limiting the physician's flexibility in prescribing the proper dose of each agent.

The ideal anticonvulsant agent will be one that is effective in controlling the patient's seizures without producing adverse effects such as sedation or ataxia which will interfere with his normal daily activity. The drug should have a low degree of long term toxicity, since patients may be required to take anticonvulsants for years or even throughout their lifetimes. It should have a relatively long duration of action so that the patient need not take many doses a day and if a dose is occasionally missed adequate blood and tissue levels can be maintained. The price of the medication is important because the long term of treatment makes it imperative that maintenance of good health not place a financial burden on the patient.

INTRODUCTION OF NEW ANTICONVULSANTS. Several laboratory methods have been useful in the development of newer anticonvulsant agents. One is the prevention of seizures induced in animals by electroshock or the drug pentylenetetrazol. The latter agent has been particularly useful in evaluating drugs for the treatment of absence attacks. New anticonvulsant agents have also been developed by making changes in the chemical structure of previously recognized agents, e.g., the benzodiazapine group.

Experimental epilepsy can also be induced in animals by making a lesion in a small area of cerebral cortex, either by trauma or with an irritating chemical substance. This results in a small focus of abnormal seizure activity known as the epileptogenic focus. A similar focus may occur in human seizure disorders but frequently the site of origin of the seizure is unknown. Nevertheless, the concept of the epileptogenic focus is useful in studying the mechanism of action of these agents.

SPECIFIC ANTICONVULSANT AGENTS

The first effective anticonvulsant agents to be used in clinical medicine were the salts of hydrobromic acid introduced in the mid-nineteenth century. Although bromides are effective to a limited degree, serious toxic problems occur and there is no indication for their use today. Most of the agents useful in controlling seizures in use today are organic substances with relatively similar molecular structure (Fig. 30–1).

PHENYTOIN*

Introduced into clinical medicine by Merritt and Putnam in 1938, this compound has proved remarkably effective in the treatment of several types of epilepsy and is considered the drug of choice for grand mal seizures. Although a number of potential toxic side effects have been described, it is a relatively safe agent which

* Phenytoin is referred to as diphenylhydantoin elsewhere in this book. This chapter was changed in proof to conform to the new name.

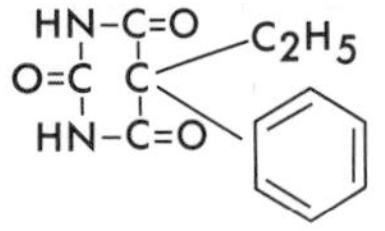

$HN-C=O$ C_2H_5
$O=C$ C
$HN-C=O$

PHENOBARBITAL

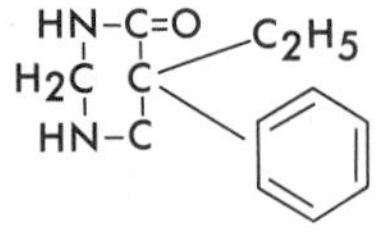

$HN-C=O$ C_2H_5
H_2C C
$HN-C$

PRIMIDONE

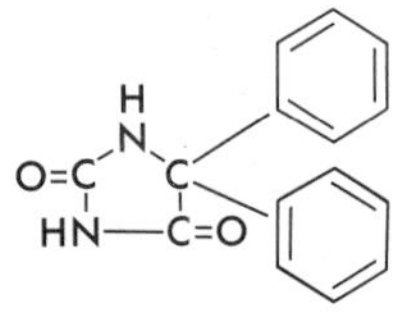

$O=C$ N C
$HN-C=O$

PHENYTOIN

$O=C$ C C_2H_5
CH_3
$HN-C=O$

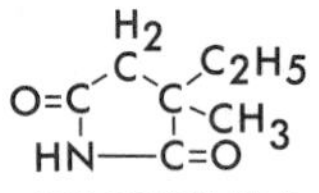

ETHOSUXIMIDE

FIG. 30–1. The most effective anticonvulsants are substituted derivatives of closely related synthetic heterocyclic compounds.

meets many of the criteria of the ideal anticonvulsant (Table 30–1).

Actions

Phenytoin is highly effective in the treatment of grand mal, focal motor and psychomotor epilepsy, and in addition has been found useful in several other neurologic conditions unrelated to epilepsy. It is of no value in petit mal epilepsy. A number of theories concerning the molecular basis of phenytoin's action have been proposed, but none are fully acceptable. In general it ap-

pears to act as a stabilizer of excitable cellular membranes including peripheral nerves and skeletal and cardiac muscle membranes, as well as in central neurons. Under certain experimental conditions phenytoin stimulates the enzyme Na^+–K^+–ATPase, and reduces sodium conductance in membranes with a consequent decrease in intracellular sodium ion. It also limits membrane permeability to calcium ion. Both of these actions tend to lower the excitability of neural membranes and could prevent seizure discharges from spreading. Its action on the CNS is to reduce the spread of the seizure from the epileptogenic focus to normal surrounding neurons, preventing their activation and therefore the spread of the seizure. Phenytoin inhibits posttetanic potentiation and prevents development of chains of rapidly firing neurons. It has little suppressant effect on the epileptogenic focus itself and produces little change in normal neurons. In usual therapeutic dosage it does not impair consciousness nor produce significant mental changes.

Clinical Pharmacology

In recent years the development of gas chromatographic and other analytic techniques has enabled the measurement of serum levels of most anticonvulsants, and a much better understanding of the requirements for clinical control of seizures has emerged. When a patient begins the usual dosage of 300–400 mg daily (5 mgm/kgm in children) adequate serum levels may not be achieved for 7–10 days and effective seizure control cannot be expected before then. A blood level of 1.0–2.0 mg/100 ml correlates best with anticonvulsant activity and minimal toxicity. Between 2.0–3.0 mg/100 ml some evidence of toxicity may be apparent but this is only occa-

TABLE 30–1. Commonly Used Anticonvulsant Agents

Generic name	Common trade name	Dosage units available
Phenytoin	Dilantin	Susp 30 mgm/5 ml, 125 mgm/5 ml; Caps 30 mgm, 100 mgm; Tabs 50 mgm; Inj 50 mgm/ml
Mephenytoin	Mesantoin	Tabs 100 mgm
Phenobarbital*	Luminal	Tab 15–100 mgm; Elix 20 mgm/5 ml; Inf 50–150 mgm/ml
Mephobarbital	Mebaral	Tabs 30, 50, 100 and 200 mgm
Primidone	Mysoline	Susp 250 mgm/5 ml; Tabs 50, 250 mgm
Ethosuximide	Zarontin	Caps 250 mgm
Methsuximide	Celontin	Caps 150, 300 mgm
Phensuximide	Milontin	Susp 300 mgm/5 ml; Caps 250, 500 mgm
Trimethadione	Tridione	Solu 200 mgm/5 ml; Caps 150, 300 mgm
Diazepam	Valium	Tabs 2, 5, 10 mgm; Inj 5 mgm/ml
Acetazolamide	Diamox	Tabs 125, 250 mgm
Carbamazepine	Tegretol	Tabs 200 mgm

*Available from many manufacturers under a variety of brand names in many dosage forms and sizes

sionally of clinical importance. Above 3.0 mg/100 ml toxicity is present in a majority of patients and may become severe enough to limit the patient's functioning and require a lowering of the dose. Once adequate levels are achieved they tend to remain fairly stable as long as the patient maintains the same daily intake of phenytoin. If rapid seizure control is required, loading doses of up to 1000 mg in divided doses may be used the first day, 500 mg on the second day and then usual maintenance levels of 300–400 mg/day instituted. Drug levels in the therapeutic range will be achieved in 3–5 days. As the half-life in the serum is 22–30 hr it is possible to take the medication only once a day after therapeutic levels are achieved. Although there will be small fluctuations in serum levels, most patients will remain within the therapeutic range. Because of this long half-life it must be remembered that the drug will remain in serum for several days after intake has been discontinued, a factor that is of some importance in toxic reactions. Intramuscular phenytoin is slowly and irregularly absorbed and reliable blood levels may not be achieved and therefore the use of this agent intramuscularly is not recommended. Phenytoin can be given IV in emergency circumstances, but its use has been associated with severe cardiotoxic reactions and even death, so its use by this route must be limited to extreme emergencies and then given by very slow infusion at a rate no greater than 50 mg/min.

Metabolism

Phenytoin is metabolized by hepatic microsomal enzymes with the parahydroxyphenyl compound being the principal metabolite in man. This metabolite is very soluble and rapidly excreted by the kidney. It is thought not to have any anticonvulsant activity of its own. Other drugs which stimulate hepatic microsomal enzymes may stimulate the detoxification of phenytoin resulting in lower serum levels and poor antiepileptic control (Ch. 3). Conversely, drugs which compete with phenytoin for detoxification may result in diminished metabolism and higher serum levels. Phenobarbital, although it induces microsomal enzymes, rarely affects serum levels in patients on chronic phenytoin therapy. Conversely, phenytoin stimulates the rate of metabolism of other drugs. These drug interactions can be extremely complex and vary greatly in individual patients. Therefore, it is important to determine the serum level of phenytoin in patients who are given other medications. Approximately 90% of phenytoin in the serum is bound to plasma proteins, principally albumin. Patients with liver disease or other conditions causing hypo-albuminemia may require smaller doses of this drug.

Toxicity

The toxic effects of phenytoin can be divided into three groups: allergic, acute toxicity and chronic toxicity.

ALLERGIC REACTIONS. A small number of patients will manifest severe allergic reactions to phenytoin. Characteristically symptoms begin 2–3 weeks after the institution of therapy and pruritis, fever and skin rash are the commonest complaints. Eosinophilia is usually present. In some individuals severe allergic reaction may occur with exfoliation of the skin, hepatic toxicity and bone marrow depression with pancytopenia. Because of the severe nature of some allergic reactions to this agent it is imperative that the drug be withdrawn immediately after symptoms appear. Because of the long half-life symptoms may continue to progress for a short time after withdrawal, which is usually the only therapy necessary. Occasionally patients require antihistamines for symptomatic relief and, rarely, glucocorticosteroids are necessary in cases of severe allergic toxicity.

ACUTE TOXICITY. More commonly experienced are acute, dose-related toxic symptoms. These include nystagmus with blurring of vision or diplopia, ataxia, dysarthria and, with blood levels of 4.0 mg/100 ml or greater, stupor or coma may occur. Occasionally there is an increase in seizure frequency when toxic levels are achieved. Acute ataxic symptoms are usually reversible by lowering the serum level of phenytoin to the range of 1.0–2.0 mg/100 ml. In addition, with the initiation of therapy patients may have transient sedation.

CHRONIC TOXICITY. As more and more patients have taken this agent for over 20 years a number of chronic toxic effects have been described. Most of these are relatively rare and usually require no special treatment; however, the physician must be aware that occasionally severe problems can arise. A very common toxic effect, especially in children, is gingival hyperplasia, which in some instances may cause painful bleeding gums. It is the result of fibroblastic proliferation in gingival tissues induced by phenytoin. In most patients good oral hygiene will prevent this from becoming a serious side effect, but occasionally surgical intervention is necessary. Hirsutism occurs frequently, especially in young girls, and while this is not a serious effect, it is aesthetically disturbing. More serious chronic toxic side effects include folic acid deficiency due to interference with absorption of folic acid from the small intestine; hypocalcemia and osteomalacia occur, probably due to interference with absorption of calcium from the intestine and perhaps due to increased metabolism of vitamin D by the liver. A syndrome resembling systemic lupus erythematosus has been described in patients taking anticonvulsants. This syndrome is indistinguishable from the spontaneously occurring disease except that renal involvement is less common and the syndrome is usually completely reversible within several months of withdrawal of anticonvulsants. The induction of lymphoid hyperplasia and even lymphoma in patients taking phenytoin has been described but at present it is not known whether the incidence of these changes is directly related to drug usage. Although these toxic effects are potentially serious, they are rarely encountered clinically.

Finally, there is a statistically higher incidence of birth defects, especially cleft palate, in children of mothers taking phenytoin during their pregnancy. The clinical significance of these findings is as yet undetermined, but it is best if patients not receive this drug during pregnancy if the seizures can be controlled with other drugs.

Several other hydantoin derivatives, for example mephenytoin, are effective in controlling seizures, but they are associated with a number of adverse reactions and they are no longer recommended for use.

BARBITURATES

Many of the commonly used barbiturates (Ch. 26) possess some anticonvulsant activity, but in general produce too much sedation at therapeutic dosage levels to be clinically useful. Phenobarbital is the principal exception and has emerged as one of the safest and most widely used anticonvulsant agents.

Action

Phenobarbital is effective in the treatment of grand mal, focal motor and psychomotor seizures, but not petit mal. Phenobarbital is particularly useful in the control of febrile convulsions in children and convulsions associated with withdrawal from sedative agents such as barbiturates and alcohol. In contrast to other barbiturates it has a selective depressant action of the motor cortex and can suppress seizure activity at an epileptogenic focus at a concentration which does not produce generalized sedation. In contrast to phenytoin, it increases the threshold of normal cells and can prevent seizures induced by both pentylenetetrazol and electroshock. It is thought to increase presynaptic inhibition and therefore decrease repetitive firing of neurons in the epileptogenic focus. It has no effect on cells outside of the central nervous system or on sodium and calcium transport.

Clinical Pharmacology

Absorption of phenobarbital upon oral ingestion is slow and steady state blood levels are reached in approximately 3 weeks after onset of therapy. Its half-life in adults is approximately four days and is somewhat shorter in young children. Clinical anticonvulsant activity is best correlated with serum levels of 1.5–3.0 mg/100 ml, but many patients can tolerate higher serum levels. Toxic manifestations occur regularly above 4 mg/100 ml. Once adequate blood levels are reached they tend to remain fairly constant as long as oral intake is maintained. Traces of phenobarbital may be found in patient serum several weeks after discontinuation. Usual oral starting dose in adults is 100 mg/day and 100–150 mg/day is usually adequate to achieve therapeutic serum levels. In children approximately 4 mg/kg will achieve therapeutic serum levels. As a consequence of its long half-life, this amount can be taken as a single daily dose. Intramuscular phenobarbital is absorbed into the blood more rapidly than phenytoin and can be used when oral intake is limited. Intravenous phenobarbital can be used safely if slow injection is employed.

Metabolism

Phenobarbital is a potent stimulator of hepatic microsomal enzymes and can affect the metabolism of other drugs, e.g., anticoagulants. As was noted previously it does not appreciably alter blood levels of phenytoin when both drugs are given. Phenobarbital is metabolized in man to the parahydroxyphenyl derivative which may then be conjugated with glucuronic acid and excreted by the kidney. The hydroxylated metabolite is extremely water soluble, does not pass the blood brain barrier and has no anticonvulsant activity. Phenobarbital is bound approximately 50% by plasma proteins, principally albumin, and serum levels of this substance may affect the clinical effectiveness and toxicity.

Toxicity

Phenobarbital is an extremely safe agent and while many patients develop mild sedation initially, tolerance rapidly develops to this side effect but not to the anticonvulsant activity. At higher blood levels of phenobarbital (greater than 4 mgm/100 ml), ataxia and blurring of vision may occur but can easily be reversed by lowering the dosage of phenobarbital. Toxic serum levels of phenobarbital can result in a paradoxic increase in seizures, especially in children.

Allergic reactions to phenobarbital can occur, usually manifested by pruritis and urticarial skin eruptions. The severe dermatologic, hematologic and hepatic complications encountered with phenytoin rarely occur with phenobarbital. Chronic toxicity is relatively rare although some of the syndromes encountered with hydantoin derivatives may occasionally be found with this drug.

Mephobarbital differs from phenobarbital by the addition of one methyl group, and it is partially metabolized to phenobarbital. It is unknown whether the intact molecule has anticonvulsive activity of its own, but its actions and toxicity are quite similar to the parent compound. It is much more expensive than phenobarbital.

PRIMIDONE

This agent, although not an authentic barbiturate, is structurally very similar. It is effective in psychomotor epilepsy, and is also useful in grand mal and focal motor seizures. Recent evidence has indicated that it is partially metabolized to phenobarbital and phenylethylmalonamide, both of which have anticonvulsant activity. Patients on usual doses of primidone may achieve serum levels of phenobarbital similar to those encountered when that drug is used alone, and there is little indication for the use of primidone and phenobarbital in the same patient. The presence of primidone and its active metabolites have made clinical correlation between serum level and clinical control difficult. The exact blood levels of each component required for control of seizures has not as yet been established, but measurements of phenobarbital levels may provide an estimate of patient compliance.

The initial use of the agent is associated with sedation and so it is best to start with low doses of 125 mg/day, gradually increasing the dose to 500–750 mg/day, the usual dose required for seizure control in adults. In children the dose requirements are quite variable, but 5–10 mgm/kg daily is recommended. In most patients tolerance develops to the sedative effect of this agent but not to the anticonvulsant activity. Occasionally sedation is a limiting factor in the use of this agent and in such patients the addition of a central nervous stimulant such as dextroamphetamine in small doses can be considered. Toxicity of this agent is similar to that of phenobarbital.

Other barbiturate derivatives commercially available do not have the specific anticonvulsant properties of the agents discussed above and produce their anticonvulsant effect only at hypnotic dosage levels and, therefore, have no place in the treatment of epilepsy.

SUCCINIMIDES

Several substituted succinimides have been introduced in recent years for the treatment of petit mal epilepsy (absence).

Ethosuximide is generally considered the drug of choice in petit mal seizures controlling 80–90% of symptoms. It is ineffective in grand mal and focal motor epilepsy but occasionally is of value in psychomotor seizures.

Actions

Electrophysiologic studies have suggested that petit mal seizures result from the synchronization of both excitatory and inhibitory neurons within the brain stem and mesial reticular activating system. These agents may act by increasing postsynaptic inhibition and preventing the propagation of seizure activity by way of the thalamocortical projection. They have no effect on posttetanic potentiation or cellular ion movement. The succinimides have little effect on electrically induced seizures in experimental animals but are potent antagonists to the seizures produced by pentylenetetrazol.

Clinical Pharmacology

Ethosuximide is rapidly absorbed from the gastrointestinal tract. Peak serum levels are achieved in 1–2 hr and fall off very slowly thereafter. Its biologic half-life is approximately 30 hr in children and 60 hr in adults. This drug is converted by hepatic microsomal enzymes into two metabolites resulting from the oxidation of the ethyl side chain of the parent molecule. Maximum clinical control is achieved with doses of approximately 10–20 mg/kg and clinical control is correlated with serum levels of 4–8 mg/100 ml. Clinical control in petit mal may be related to the severity of the disorder and, unlike other types of seizures, monitoring of the electroencephalogram has proven to be a useful way to evaluate seizure control. Because of its relatively long half-life ethosuximide can be given in two divided doses daily to children and in adults a single dose will suffice. Treatment is usually begun with a single capsule (250 mg) a day and increased gradually by one capsule every 3–4 days until seizures are controlled or toxic symptoms develop.

Toxicity

Ethosuximide is a relatively safe drug although transient leukopenia occurs occasionally. Although usually of a minor nature, more severe pancytopenia has been reported. Dose related symptoms of toxicity include gastrointestinal upset, sedation, headache and occasional allergic manifestations.

Methsuximide and Phensuximide are effective in suppressing petit mal seizures, but are less efficacious than ethosuximide. Side effects such as nausea, vomiting and headache occur more frequently than with ethosuximide. Renal dysfunction may occur with phensuximide and anorexia is a prominent side effect of methsuximide. Because of the higher incidence of serious side effects with these two agents they are less commonly used in the treatment of petit mal and are reserved for refractory cases.

Oxazolidinediones

These agents, of which trimethadione is the only commonly used example, are specific for absence seizures. They are effective, but their usefulness is limited by serious toxic side effects. The mechanism of action of trimethadione is similar to that of the succinimides, including the specific antagonism to pentylenetetrazol-induced convulsions. Their toxicity includes dose related sedation, ataxia and hemeralopia. The latter symptom, sometimes called light blindness, represents a decreased visual acuity in the presence of bright light and is thought to be due to an effect on the retinal ganglion cells. More serious toxic effects include bone marrow depression, and the nephrotic syndrome, which may not be reversible upon withdrawal of the drug and can be fatal. Because of the severe toxicity associated with these agents, they should be reserved for treatment of resistent cases of petit mal. Patients receiving these agents should have frequent monitoring of blood count and urine analysis to prevent the development of severe bone marrow or renal dysfunction.

MISCELLANEOUS AGENTS

Acetazolamide

This agent is a potent inhibitor of carbonic anhydrase, the enzyme which catalyzes the hydration of carbon dioxide. Originally introduced as a diuretic, it was found to be effective in the treatment of petit mal epilepsy. It may act by producing an elevation of intraneuronal carbon dioxide with consequent depression of neuronal activity. It is useful as a secondary drug in the treatment of petit mal epilepsy when ethosuximide does not produce complete relief of symptoms. In addition, because of its naturetic action, it is used for seizures associated with sodium retention, e.g., those associated with the premenstrual period of the menstrual cycle or during pregnancy. This agent is relatively nontoxic, although occasional hypersensitivity reactions can occur. Acetazolamide is a sulfonamide and should be used with caution in patients known to be allergic to this group of drugs.

Carbamazepine

This agent originally was introduced for the treatment of trigeminal neuralgia and recently released for use as an anticonvulsant. It has been used extensively in Europe and is reported to be especially useful in the treatment of psychomotor or temporal lobe epilepsy which is refractory to other drugs. Chemically it is a tricyclic compound structurally related to the antidepressant agents and unlike most of the other anticonvulsant drugs.

Carbamazepine is available in 200 mg tablets. The initial dose is usually 600 mg daily. Its half-life is approximately 12 hr and at least 2 doses a day are necessary. Therapeutic serum levels have not been determined with certainty but are approximately 1.0 mg/100 ml. The daily dosage will vary in individual cases but should not exceed 1200 mg a day. Approximately 80% of carbamazepine is bound to serum protein. It is metabolized in the liver and a number of metabolites have been identified but their activity as anticonvulsants is unknown.

Initial treatment is associated with sedation and gastrointestinal irritation but in general long term use of this drug is well tolerated by patients. However, a number of cases of pancytopenia and aplastic anemia have been reported, occasionally with fatal results. Therefore, it is necessary to monitor hematological status of patients very carefully, especially during the first 6 months of therapy.

Benzodiazepines

A large number of compounds of this class have been introduced as antianxiety agents and hypnotics (Ch. 26). Diazepam has been employed in the treatment of petit mal epilepsy and a number of related agents are currently undergoing investigational trials as anticonvulsants. One of these, Clonazepam, has been found to be effective in the treatment of a variety of seizure disorders. The usefulness of diazepam in treating status epilepticus is discussed below.

A number of other agents including quinacrine, ACTH and prednisone are occasionally used as secondary agents in the treatment of refractory epilepsy or for treatment of specific unusual types of seizures. Their use should be reserved for the special conditions for which they have been reported to be helpful. They are of no value in most forms of epilepsy.

TREATMENT OF STATUS EPILEPTICUS

Status epilepticus or acute repetitive grand mal seizures is a medical emergency, resulting from continuous or repetitive grand mal seizures. Serious brain damage occurs with untreated status epilepticus and the degree of potential danger is related to the duration of the seizures. Several methods of treating this condition have been used, all of which have advantages and disadvantages. The essential principle of therapy is that the patient should be given large doses of the appropriate anticonvulsant by the IV route. The use of IM or oral drugs in small doses is usually ineffective and only serves to complicate therapy.

Three anticonvulsants are used extensively:

1. Intravenous **diazapam** in doses of approximately 10 mg administered slowly will usually stop the seizures. However, the half-life of this agent following IV administration is extremely short and recurrence of seizures within 30 min to an hr is common. Its usefulness therefore is limited to emergency care until more definitive therapy can be undertaken.

2. Large doses of **phenobarbital** given by slow IV infusion are usually effective in controlling status epilepticus. In practice an adult can receive 250 mg of phenobarbital over a period of 2–3 min and this dose can be repeated in 30 min if control is not achieved. Higher doses are rarely necessary. This procedure is usually safe, but respiratory depression may occur and physicians should be prepared to treat this complication. The principal disadvantage of this therapy is that it produces deep sleep in most patients which may persist for 24 hr.

3. Intravenous **phenytoin** can be effective in controlling grand mal seizures in some patients. However, as was noted above, large doses of the agent are required to achieve therapeutic blood levels and there is the potential for cardiac toxicity and hypotension from the rapid IV injection of this drug. When used, a loading dose of 1000 mg is given very slowly at the rate of 50 mg per min, preferably with EKG and blood pressure monitoring. If hypotension or changes in cardiac rhythm occur the administration of drug should be immediately discontinued. This therapy has the advantage of producing relatively little sedation, but its effectiveness in stopping seizures is variable.

It should be recalled that these therapies are aimed at stopping the acute repetitive phase of seizures, but maintainance therapy will usually be required and should be instituted soon after the acute phase has subsided. Patients who are refractory to the above treatment have a rather dire prognosis and therefore if seizures persist over a period of several hours in spite of vigorous IV therapy. they should be placed under general anesthesia with thiopenthal or ether. It is rarely necessary to maintain general anesthesia for more than 60–120 min and longer acting anticonvulsants should be administered in addition. The halogenated general anesthetics are potentially harmful to the patient with status epilepticus because they may produce EEG abnormalities and seizures.

FURTHER READING

Woodbury DM (1969): Role of pharmacological factors in the evaluation of anticonvulsant drugs. Epilepsia 10:121–144

Schmidt RP, Wilder BJ (1968): Epilepsy. Contemporary Neurology Series. Plum F, McDowell FH (eds) Philadelphia, Davis

Woodbury DM, Penry JK, Schmidt RP (eds) (1972): Antiepileptic Drugs. New York, Raven Press

CHARLES H. MARKHAM

ROBERT D. ANSEL

31. ANTIPARKINSON DRUGS*

In the last 5 years, a great stride forward has been made in the treatment of Parkinson's disease. This has been due to the use of **levodopa** (L-dopa) and to a lesser extent **amantadine hydrochloride** (Symmetrel) and older **anticholinergic** medications. In order to understand how these medications work, we have to look at the disease itself and anatomical and biochemical processes in the basal ganglia.

The main symptoms of Parkinson's disease are: a 3–6/sec tremor of a limb, when that part of the body is at rest; rigidity, a relatively unremitting low grade muscular contraction which the patient feels as stiffness or awkwardness, and the physician detects as an increased tone as he moves the involved limb; and akinesia, a hesitancy in initiating a movement, changing its speed or direction and carrying it to completion. Other symptoms include flexed posture and a soft voice with disturbed rhythm.

While these very different symptoms have different and poorly defined pathophysiologic substrates, they do have one lesion in common. This is loss of the large pigmented cells in the substantia nigra. Other changes in the substantia nigra and elsewhere in the basal ganglia depend on the particular etiology of the parkinsonism.

SOME ANATOMY AND BIOCHEMISTRY

It is now known that the large pigmented nigral neurons contain melanin, manufacture dopamine and have unmyelinated axons 0.1–0.2 microns in diameter, which project to two nearby nuclei, the caudate and putamen. These structures, together termed the striatum, have much the highest concentration of dopamine in the CNS (Ch. 23). Striatal dopamine is contained in irregular varicose presynaptic terminals whose axons arise from cell bodies in the substantia nigra.

In Parkinson's disease, dopamine content in the striatum and in the nigra is very low. L-dopa decarboxylase (Ch. 14), the dopamine synthesizing enzyme, and homovanillic acid, the main dopamine metabolite, are also diminished in the striatum in Parkinson's disease. This led to replacement therapy with large oral doses of L-dopa, the precursor of dopamine which crosses the blood-brain barrier.

The main steps in dopamine neurotransmission are as follows. Dopamine is decarboxylated from L-dopa within the nigrostriatal neuron and is held in storage vesicles in the synaptic terminal. Free dopamine within the nigrostriatal neuron is apparently degradated by the mitochondrial enzyme monoamine oxidase (MAO). The nigrostriatal neuron releases dopamine, a probable inhibitory transmitter, into the presynaptic cleft. Multiple branching of the dopaminergic axons suggest one nigral cell acts on many striatal neurons, probably the middle-sized spiny neurons (see below). After presumably causing a hyperpolarization of the receptor cell, the dopamine is released from the receptor site to be either taken up into the presynaptic terminal or inactivated (O-methylated) by catecholamine methyl transferase (COMT).

The striatum contains other neurotransmitters which are either altered in Parkinson's disease or in the course of its treatment: acetylcholine (Ach), gamma amino butyric acid (GABA) and serotonin. Ach concentration in the striatum is significant, as is the activity of acetylcholines-

---

* The drug therapy of Parkinson's disease is presented in more detail than most other topics, because it is an example of the successful rational application of the findings of basic medical research to a human disease process in the CNS.

terase (AchE) and choline acetylase (Chs. 14–17). It now seems likely that all or almost all the Ach is formed and released within the striatum by one group of interneurons. Choline acetylase activity is reduced about 50% in Huntington's chorea, a disease with major loss of striatal neurons. While Ach, or its forming or inactivating enzyme, has not been conclusively shown to be abnormal in Parkinson's disease, it is clear that anticholinergic drugs benefit parkinsonian symptoms (Ch. 17). This suggests that decreased striatal dopamine in this disease may allow a class of striatal Ach interneurons to be relatively overactive, and anticholinergic agents partially correct this imbalance.

GABA, an inhibitory neurotransmitter, and its forming enzyme, glutamic acid decarboxylase (GAD), are also important in striatal function. In untreated Parkinson's disease, GAD activity is reduced in the striatum to less than 50% of the control mean, whereas in Parkinson's disease chemically treated with L-dopa, it is normal. In Huntington's chorea, a disease with massive degeneration of striatal neurons, GABA is low in the striatum, globus pallidus and substantia nigra, and GAD activity reduced to 10–20% of control in the striatum. This, coupled with recent anatomic findings in the striatum (see below) suggests that GABA may be formed and released in another class of interneurons in the striatum, and that parkinsonian nigrostriatal dopamine deficiency may lead to the lowered GAD activity.

Serotonin is still another neurohumor in the striatum which is mildly decreased in Parkinson's disease. Serotonin is concentrated in nerve cell terminals and is converted there from its precursor by 5-hydroxytryptophan decarboxylase, which is apparently the same enzyme as dopa decarboxylase. The cell bodies of the serotonin containing neurons lie in the midbrain and pontine raphé nuclei not far from the dopaminergic neurons in the midbrain. It is not known why serotonin is decreased in the striatum in Parkinson's disease, but it may be from death of some of these cells. Administration of 5-hydroxytryptophan, the precursor of serotonin, does not significantly change human parkinsonian symptoms.

It is now possible to look a little closer at the cellular makeup of the striatum, keeping in mind that in most cases of Parkinson's disease, cells die in the substantia nigra but that many symptoms are attributable to failure of dopamine to be delivered to specific sites in the striatum. The striatum has several morphologic cell types, described in Kemp and Powell's series of articles. The medium spiny, short axon cell has many spines on its branched dendrites. The dendritic spines constitute the most frequent type of

postsynaptic contact, but there are also synapses on proximal dendrites (bare of spines), the cell body and the initial segment of the axon. The axons are branched and very short, and do not extend beyond the arborization of the dendritic tree. These cells are interneurons. The medium spiny cell constitutes about 96% of the striatal cells. There are also 1–2% of other cells with short axons.

The medium sized long-axon cell and the giant cell are the only efferent cells of the striatum and constitute about 2% of the striatal cells. It is not clear how the many medium spiny cells presumably converge on the striatal efferent cells. The axons from the striatum project to the globus pallidus (which in turn projects to the nigra, other midbrain sites, and to the thalamus) and to the substantia nigra (Fig. 31–1). The striatonigral neurons send collaterals into the globus pallidus, cause inhibition of both nigral and pallidal cells, and apparently contain GABA.

Electron microscopic and Golgi studies combined with lesions of the thalamus, cortex or both showed the cortex and the thalamus have afferents to the striatum which terminate predominantly on dendritic spines of the same medium sized spiny cells. Another study using electron microscopy combined with autoradiography showed dopaminergic terminals ending on dendritic spines (and thus on a probabilistic basis these were likely medium sized spiny cells).

At the risk of oversimplification one might conclude:

1. There are at least four inputs to the striatum (from the cortex, thalamus, the raphé nucleus of the midbrain and the substantia nigra). Dopamine is the neurotransmitter for the nigrostriatal path, and serotonin for the ascending fibres from the midbrain raphé nuclei.

2. The cortical and thalamic efferents terminate largely on dendrites of the medium spiny cells, often on the same cells. The dopaminergic cells in the nigra send axons to the striatum which branch repeatedly before terminating on cells with dendritic spines. These cells may be the same as those receiving thalamic or cortical terminations.

3. The medium sized spiny neurons are interneurons and constitute about 96% of the striatal cells. Some striatal interneurons produce and release GABA while others release Ach. It is not known how these cells interact or in turn act on the long-axoned striatal efferent cells.

4. Striatal efferents, at least one class of which contains GABA, project to the globus pallidus and substantia nigra.

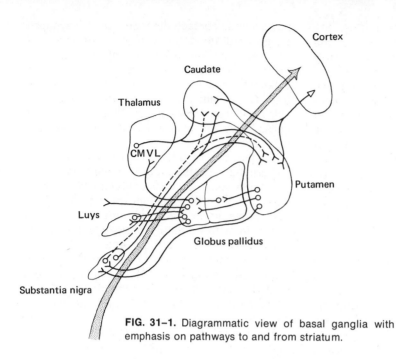

FIG. 31–1. Diagrammatic view of basal ganglia with emphasis on pathways to and from striatum.

RESPONSE TO INJURY OF THE SUBSTANTIA NIGRA

When a lesion is made in the substantia nigra in an experimental animal, some cells die, axons going to the striatum and elsewhere are severed and striatal dopamine content decreases.

Several changes occur:

1. Vigorous sprouting of the remaining and/or possibly damaged dopaminergic cells takes place in the region of the injury. Nearby areas, including such aberrant sites as capillaries and scar tissue, receive many terminals filled with dopamine.

2. With loss of some striatal endings following death of their distant cell bodies in the nigra, some postsynaptic terminals clearly become vacated and neighboring intact nigrostriatal presynaptic endings may sprout and cover them. Dependent on the pattern of loss of presynaptic terminations, there might be postsynaptic sites with either too few or too many new presynaptic terminations. Depending on the pattern of new growth in the nigrostriatal path, therapeutic elevation of brain dopamine could either do little good, help certain symptoms or produce signs of local overdosage (choreoathetosis, see below).

3. Adrenergic and serotoninergic neurons in the CNS have also been shown to sprout vigorously in response to injury, and also to have grown into postsynaptic sites previously covered by presynaptic endings with entirely different transmitters. If similar aberrant reinnervation took place in Parkinson's disease, striatal terminals, formerly dopaminergic, might be reinnervated by Ach or serotoninergic endings. Some of the variations in clinical symptoms or in therapeutic response to different drugs may be due to such variations in regrowth (see below).

4. Some terminals may make the "wrong" neurotransmitter. For example, regenerating dopaminergic terminals seem to make norepinephrine. Further, serotoninergic terminals, regenerating or not, appear to be able to convert dopa to dopamine.

5. When there is partial degeneration of dopaminergic nigrostriatal pathways in the rat, there is hyperactivity of the remaining dopaminergic neurons. This compensating mechanism may also be a factor in human parkinsonism.

6. Lastly, denervated dopamine receptors may become hypersensitive to dopamine.

DRUGS

Several drugs are known to improve the symptoms of human Parkinson's disease. These are L-dopa, anticholinergic medications and amantadine hydrochloride (Symmetrel). Certain other drugs are occasionally helpful. Still others can produce a state resembling naturally occurring Parkinson's disease. The latter include the phenothiazines and haloperidol (Ch. 25) (possibly by blocking the postsynaptic dopamine receptor site); and reserpine (by interfering with dopamine storage in the presynaptic terminal).

DOPA

The rationale for using L-dopa has been presented above. About 20% of orally administered L-dopa reaches the peripheral circulation intact. Some is destroyed in the stomach. Decreasing gastric acidity, or increasing gastric and upper intestinal motility or even gastrectomy favor greater absorption. Passage through the small intestinal wall is enhanced by dopa decarboxylase inhibitors, suggesting that this enzyme is in the intestinal mucosa. In the first passage through the liver, more dopa is degradated, mainly by catechol-O-methyltransferase (COMT). In the peripheral circulation dopa is free in the plasma or bound to plasma protein, and/or in red blood cells. Following a single IV injection, L-dopa is maintained at reasonably stable blood levels for many hours.

In order to enter the CNS, dopa must cross the blood-brain barrier, and much is destroyed by dopa decarboxylase in the capillary endothelium. It is estimated that only 1–2% of orally administered L-dopa enters the CNS. There dopa is converted to dopamine within both the cell bodies and synaptic terminals of the nigrostriatal cells. However, when large doses of L-dopa are given, or when some of the nigral cells have died, it is possible some dopamine is formed in serotoninergic terminals or elsewhere.

Since 1967 there has been considerable clinical experience with L-dopa in Parkinson's disease. It is the best therapeutic agent for this disease, but it is difficult to use, largely because of its side effects. Fortunately the latter are neither lethal nor permanent.

Initially the oral dose of L-dopa should be low, 0.5 g/day in 3–4 divided doses. Higher doses considerably enhance the likelihood of nausea and vomiting, or of postural hypotension. Every few days the total daily dose is increased by 0.5 g increments until side effects occur, or until the patient is receiving about 3.0 g/day. This medication is then increased more slowly until either a level of 8.0–9.0 g/day is reached, or (more likely) nausea or vomiting or other side effects occur. In the latter instance the dosage is reduced by 0.5–1.0 g/day. The optimum dose ranges from 1.0–9.0 g/day with a mean of a little over 4.0 g/day. It usually takes 3–6 weeks to establish this dose level. Dosage should be adjusted every few months to maintain the best balance between therapeutic benefits and side effects.

The parkinsonian symptoms usually start improving after 3–4 weeks and improvement may continue for as long as a year. Of the major parkinsonian symptoms, akinesia and rigidity are helped most, and tremor less frequently. At a year about 10% of patients are symptom-free (as long as they take their medication daily), 50% are markedly improved and 10% are worse or have little improvement. By 5 years, many patients are more disabled, some because of clear progression of parkinsonian symptoms and others because of old age. However at 5 years, 9% are still nearly symptom-free and about another 50% are much better than before L-dopa was started. This is the first time any medical treatment has interrupted the progressive worsening of Parkinson's disease. Up to 1967, people with primary Parkinson's disease had about three times greater likelihood of dying at a given age than did the average individual. Present figures obtained from relatively few deaths suggest that patients with primary parkinsonism who take L-dopa daily on an optimum schedule have the same life expectancy as their nonparkinsonian contemporaries.

The side effects of L-dopa are troublesome. Nausea and vomiting may be present even after years of use. Administration of L-dopa with dopa decarboxylase inhibitors which act outside the CNS virtually eliminates the problem of nausea and vomiting, probably because they permit a reduction in L-dopa dosage to one-fifth or so of the previous amount.

Postural or orthostatic hypotension is occasionally an early side effect but is rarely a persistent problem. It is well controlled by concomitant use of peripherally acting dopa decarboxylase inhibitor.

Choreoathetosis, involuntary movements consisting of pulling of the head to one side, or facial grimacing or restless movements of a limb may also accompany L-dopa therapy. It makes its appearance after the patient has been on L-dopa for 3–12 months and usually occurs at a dosage just above that needed to control the parkinsonian symptoms, so is easily dealt with by reducing the daily intake. In a few patients, choreoathetosis is present at the same dosage needed to treat the parkinsonian symptoms and then constitutes a real therapeutic challenge. It is not benefited, or is made worse, by peripherally acting dopa decarboxylase inhibitors. It is probably due to too much dopamine activity on some striatal receptors. It occurs always, or almost always, when there is partial loss of either nigrostriatal terminations (as in Parkinson's disease) or of some striatal cells (as in Huntington's chorea).

Behavioral alterations from L-dopa are relatively infrequent except in those patients who have preexisting organic dementia. They may become more confused, or euphoric, or may become less inhibited including in their sexual behavior. L-dopa has been reported to improve depression, or to make it worse, but probably does neither.

ANTICHOLINERGIC MEDICATIONS

Belladonna alkaloids and certain synthetic preparations, e.g., trihexyphenidyl (Artane), benztropine (Cogentin), procyclidine (Kemadrin), chlorphenoxamine (Phenoxene), ethopropazine (Parsidol), etc. have long been known to improve parkinsonian tremor and rigidity (Ch. 17). Usually this improvement is modest, but in a patient with severe Parkinson's disease, withdrawal may lead to a significant increase in invalidism and even death from pneumonia.

As noted earlier, the striatum has very high concentrations of Ach. Since striatal Ach does not diminish following lesions of the cortex, thalamus and midbrain, the major inputs to the striatum, it seems likely its source is some striatal interneuron.

In Parkinson's disease, there appears to be a relative or absolute increase in striatal Ach, and an absolute decrease in striatal dopamine. Either elevating the dopamine concentration or interfering with Ach utilization helps parkinsonian symptoms. Over half the patients do best on a combination of the two approaches.

The main adverse effects of the anticholinergic medications are organic confusion, hallucinations and delirium, and urinary retention. The former group of symptoms is more common in the patient with some degree of preexisting organic dementia, and is especially likely to occur in the individual recovering from an operation or intercurrent illness. Urinary hesitancy or retention almost exclusively occurs in the middle aged or elderly male with a narrowed bladder neck due to prostatic hypertrophy. Urinary retention and organic confusion can usually be dealt with by reducing the daily dosage of the anticholinergic, or changing to another anticholinergic preparation. Benztropine and ethopropazine are more likely to produce these side effects and procyclidine somewhat less so.

AMANTADINE HYDROCHLORIDE (Symmetrel)

Amantadine hydrochloride was originally prescribed as an antiviral against the A_2 influenza virus (Ch. 65). One such patient with the flu also had Parkinson's disease and the tremor and rigidity improved while amantadine was being taken. Since this initial observation amantadine has been shown to be helpful in many patients in decreasing parkinsonian symptoms, particularly tremor. It is most useful as an adjunct to L-dopa.

The mode of action of amantadine is uncertain. Clinical observations of adverse effects such as decreased salivation and urinary hesitancy suggest it has a mild anticholinergic action. However, experimental evidence shows it releases dopamine from synaptic storage sites, and also increases GABA in the striatum and substantia nigra.

The adverse effects of urinary hesitancy and decreased salivation are usually mild enough to allow the drug to be continued. Other side effects include livido reticularis and grand mal convulsions. The latter is a rare complication and has only been reported to occur at 2–3 times the recommended upper dosage limit of 300 mg/day. Incidentally, these last two effects clearly indicate amantadine has an action other than anticholinergic.

SURGERY

It should not be forgotten that operations may occasionally help certain parkinsonian symptoms. Stereotaxic thalamotomy, in which surgical lesions are made in the ventrolateral thalamus, has largely been replaced by L-dopa therapy. This was because thalamotomy and other operations did not help akinesia, the most disabling parkinsonian symptom. However, a few cases have persistent or progressive tremor and may be best treated by a one-sided operation opposite to the side of the most severe tremor.

FURTHER READING

Kemp JM, Powell TPS (1971): Series of papers on the neuroanatomy of structures related to Parkinson's disease. Phil Trans R Soc Lond B 262:383–457

McDowell FH, Markham CH (eds) (1971): Recent Advances in Parkinson's Disease. Philadelphia, Davis

JOHN A. BEVAN

32. CENTRAL NERVOUS SYSTEM STIMULANTS

A heterogeneous group of drugs stimulate the CNS. These are grouped or subdivided on the basis of their dominant site of action—the cerebrum, brainstem or spinal cord. However, this classification is artificial in that none of these drugs act specifically on one part of the brain and as a result of interconnecting pathways, their effects never remain localized. The CNS stimulants are classified in Table 32–1.

Drugs that are considered to act predominantly on the cerebrum, in small dose increase wakefulness and spontaneity of ideas and words. With increasing dose these effects are exaggerated and uncoordinated movement, hallucinations and eventually convulsions, hyperthermia and death occur. With all these drugs, stimulation is invariably succeeded by depression.

The brainstem is the main site of action of an extremely diverse group of agents. Their pharmacologic effects are most apparent when administered after brainstem depression, e.g., by barbiturates, when the depression may be reversed. This is the **analeptic** action of these drugs. Excessive dosage employed in the treatment of barbiturate poisoning, can lead to convulsions which in turn is followed by central depression. The basis of central depression after analeptics must be recognized since its treatment with further analeptic agents would only worsen the condition.

Stimulant activity on the spinal cord is usually associated with tonic convulsions. Such drugs that cause this are of historic and experimental value only. In general, the therapeutic value of pharmacologic cerebral stimulation is declining. There are some who question whether they have any use whatsoever in human therapy.

It would seem natural to use a central stimulant to counteract the effect of a central depressant, since the pharmacologic actions of each drug alone are apparently opposite. In practice, however, it is exceedingly difficult to treat a severely pharmacologically depressed patient with a central stimulant. Some treatment centers claim that supportive treatment alone—the maintenance of adequate tissue oxygenation and electrolyte balance, the prompt treatment of infections, and the use of hemodialysis—is the regimen of choice.

CEREBRAL STIMULANTS

Most of the drugs included in this group are discussed elsewhere (see Table 32–1). Their action on the cerebrum only rarely represents a primary therapeutic objective and in almost all circumstances is an undesired adverse action. **Caffeine** is included with Xanthines (see below).

Camphor and **menthol** are both nonspecific CNS stimulants and also affect sensory nerve endings. Menthol produces a sensation of coolness on the mucous membranes and skin. Camphor is used as a counterirritant.

BRAIN STEM STIMULANTS

Bemegride (Megimide) is chemically related to the barbiturates (Ch. 26), but is not a specific barbiturate antagonist. It is a general CNS stimulant with an action similar to that of pentylenetetrazol but with a wider margin of safety. Its effect is rapid in onset and of short duration.

Pentylenetetrazol (Metrazol) is a general CNS stimulant. Its latency of action is short. The use

253

TABLE 32-1. Classification of CNS Stimulants

Cerebral	Brainstem	Spinal
Amphetamine (Ch. 18)	Bemegride	Strychnine
Atropine (Ch. 15)	Pentylenetetrazol	
Caffeine		
(Xanthines, Ch. 32)	Picrotoxin	
Cocaine (Ch. 14, 22)	Nikethamide	
Ephedrine (Ch. 18)	Ethamivan	
Methylphenidate		
(Ch. 18)	Doxapran	
Camphor and menthol		

of this drug as a convulsant in shock or convulsive therapy is obsolescent.

Picrotoxin is obtained from an East Indian shrub. After a latency of 25–30 minutes, it exerts a powerful analeptic action which is difficult to control clinically. It is claimed that picrotoxin interferes with presynaptic inhibitory mechanisms that result in a decreased transmitter release.

Nikethamide (Coramine) is a weak analeptic of low toxicity. Its effect is fairly rapid in onset following IV injection, but is short-lived. It is not a direct cardiac stimulant, although it may stimulate medullary cardiovascular centers. Its popularity may be derived from the belief that because of its low toxicity, its use will do no harm.

Ethamivan (Emivan) is a fairly recent analeptic related to nikethamide. Its value awaits final assessment. It is claimed to be of some value as a respiratory stimulant in hypoventilatory states, e.g., in barbiturate poisoning.

Doxapran is claimed to be particularly effective as a respiratory stimulant although higher doses stimulate the spinal cord and brain stem. The therapeutic index is probably higher than with other analeptics.

SPINAL CORD STIMULANTS

Strychnine obtained from the seeds of *Strychnos nux-vomica,* produces convulsions of spinal origin. Since it is an active constituent of rat poison, it is not an infrequent cause of accidental poisoning. The normal inhibitory effect of the small Renshaw cells on the motor neurons in the spinal cord are inhibited by strychnine, leading to an increase in their excitatory state. Thus normal reflex action is converted to convulsive activity. Although this particular effect on the spinal cord may represent only part of the action of strychnine leading to convulsions, it may mirror its mode of action at other sites in the nervous system.

Lobeline, a nicotine-like drug, stimulates chemoreceptor and other sensory endings and for this reason has been used as a respiratory stimulant in the newborn. Its value however is debatable. This drug, like the veratrum alkaloids (Ch. 20), owes most of its action to the stimulation of specialized sensory nerve endings.

A number of these drugs can be used diagnostically to activate latent epileptic foci in the brain.

XANTHINES

Xanthines occur naturally. **Caffeine** is found in the coffee bean (*Coffea arabica*), in the leaves of tea (*Thea sinensis*), in the bean of cocoa (*Theobroma cacao*). The kola nut (*Cola acuminata*), the basis of the cola drinks, also contains caffeine. In addition, **theophylline** is found in tea and **theobromine** in cocoa.

Chemistry

These naturally occurring substances are methylated xanthines and are related to the purines and uric acid (Fig. 32–1).

Actions

Although the methylxanthines have common multiple pharmacologic actions, the various xanthine derivatives exhibit small quantitative differences in pharmacologic effect.

CENTRAL NERVOUS SYSTEM EFFECTS. Caffeine, theophylline and theobromine, in order of decreasing potency, stimulate the CNS. Provided dosage is not excessive, they cause no secondary depression. Mental activity, performance and association of ideas are facilitated. Fatigue and drowsiness are allayed. Effects on the brainstem and spinal cord are also evident, but not so important.

CARDIOVASCULAR EFFECTS. The methylxanthines stimulate the myocardium increasing coronary artery flow, cardiac output and thus myocardial work and oxygen consumption. They also stimulate the vasomotor center. With the exception of the cerebral vessels, they relax vascular smooth muscle. This complexity of action probably explains the variable effects of the drugs on arterial pressure and heart rate.

OTHER EFFECTS. All smooth muscle, especially that in the bronchi, is relaxed. Diuresis occurs mainly as a result of a reduction in tubular reabsorption. Gastric secretions are stimu-

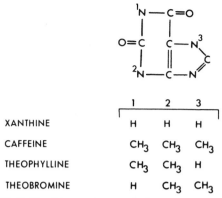

	1	2	3
XANTHINE	H	H	H
CAFFEINE	CH_3	CH_3	CH_3
THEOPHYLLINE	CH_3	CH_3	H
THEOBROMINE	H	CH_3	CH_3

FIG. 32–1. Xanthine and some derivatives.

lated. In higher doses, respiration is stimulated.

Mechanism

The xanthines are competitive inhibitors of phosphodiesterase, an enzyme that inhibits the breakdown of cyclic **3'5'-AMP** (cAMP). This direct action of the drug is augmented by its indirect sympathomimetic effects resulting from the facilitation of adrenergic transmitter release. The adrenergic transmitter acts on membrane-bound adenylcyclase that catalyses the conversion of ATP to cAMP. This increase in cAMP in the myocardium is associated with a positive inotropic effect.

Uses and Effectiveness

USE IN ACUTE HEART FAILURE. The xanthine salt, **aminophylline** (theophylline ethylenediamine), is used to relieve the consequences of acute exacerbations of left heart failure. Myocardial stimulation, resulting in a lowered venous pressure and bronchial dilation, provide the rationale for its use. In addition to aminophylline, rapid-acting cardiac glycosides, morphine, oxygen and physical procedures designed to lower the central venous pressure are employed in the treatment of this condition.

OTHER USES. For reasons apparent from their pharmacologic actions, xanthines are occasionally used in bronchial asthma, as analeptics and diuretics, and because of their cerebral vasoconstrictor properties, as adjuncts to ergotamine in migraine therapy (Ch. 19).

The popular social use of xanthine-containing drinks reflects their pleasurable central stimulant properties. The problems and difficulties caused by their sudden complete withdrawal illustrates the degree of habituation that develops to their long-term administration. They establish a sense of well-being and increase mental performance. All their effects, however, are not so pleasing. Especially after excessive indulgence, many people become tense, nervous, restless and hyperexcited. Cardiac stimulation results in extrasystoles, palpitation and tachycardia; hypertension may be exaggerated. The irritant oils contained in most xanthine-containing beverages can cause gastritis and even diarrhea and activate a latent peptic ulcer. Decaffeinated beverages still retain these irritant substances.

Preparation and Dosage

Aminophylline, *U.S.P.*, is available for IV, oral and rectal use. The IV dose is 250–500 mg in 20 ml administered over a 5 min period.

FURTHER READING

Clemmesen C, Nilsson E (1961): Therapeutic trends in the treatment of barbiturate poisoning. Clin Pharmacol Ther 2:220

Hahn F (1960): Analeptics. Pharmacol Rev 12:447

Koppanyl T, Richards RK (1958): Treatment for barbiturate poisoning with or without analeptics. Anesth Analg (Cleve) 37:182

Nash H (1962): Alcohol and Caffeine: A Study of Their Psychological Effects. Springfield, Ill, Thomas

DRUGS ACTING ON THE CARDIOVASCULAR SYSTEM

JOHN A. BEVAN

33. CARDIAC GLYCOSIDES

The term "cardiac glycosides" is used to describe a group of compounds of common basic chemical structure, which increase the work generated by the heart muscle. As this action is most remarkable on the "failing heart," these compounds are used clinically in heart failure with dramatic effect. Additional pharmacologic actions make the cardiac glycosides of benefit in the control of certain cardiac irregularities. As the best known members of this group are derived from plants of the genus *Digitalis,* the terms **digitalis** or **digitalis-like glycosides** and **cardiac glycosides** are used interchangeably.

SOURCE

PLANT. Digitalis leaf, digoxin, digitoxin and deslanoside are derived from the purple and the white foxglove (*Digitalis purpurea* and *D. lanata*); ouabain and strophanthin, from various species of *Strophanthus.* The sea onion or squill, the lily of the valley, the oleander and *Helleborus* species are botanic sources of other clinically useful but less popular glycosides.

ANIMAL. The skin secretions of some toads (toad poison) contain glycosides.

HISTORY

Although digitalis-like glycosides have been used for various purposes for over 3000 years, an English physician and botanist, William Withering, was the first to describe the main indications and actions of an extract of digitalis leaf. His monograph, *An Account of the Foxglove and Some of Its Medical Uses, with Practical Remarks on Dropsy and Other Diseases* (1785) contains a surprisingly accurate account of the main effects of digitalis extracts on the patient with heart failure.

CHEMISTRY

A cardiac glycoside molecule can be considered to be made up of an **aglycone,** or **genin,** which possesses the same pharmacologic activity as the parent combined chemically with one or more sugars. These sugars are specific to each glycoside (Fig. 33–1). An aglycone consists of a steroid-like complex with an α, β, unsaturated 5- or 6-member lactone ring attached at the C-17 position. The basic pharmacologic properties of all aglycones are similar. The attached sugars seem to be important in determining the absolute potency, solubility, absorbability, rate of onset, duration of action and plasma and tissue protein-binding properties of the glycosides.

ACTIONS

The pharmacologic actions of all glycosides are very similar. The agents differ from each other only in the properties ascribable to their sugar moieties (see above). Their main actions are on the heart.

Action on Myocardial Contraction

Digitalis has a positive inotrophic effect on the heart. It alters the relationship between ventricular function and size, so that for any given atrial pressure (ventricular filling pressure) there is a greater output of work by the ventricle. The maximum tension developed by the heart muscle and its rate of development are increased. This increase in work is achieved without a proportionate increase in oxygen consumption. This represents the most important property of cardiac glycosides. The effect is not dependent upon extracardiac factors, such as level of autonomic nervous activity, venous return and heart rate. The effect of digitalis on a normal heart is

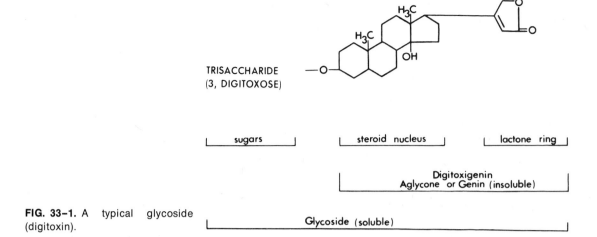

TRISACCHARIDE
(3, DIGITOXOSE)

| sugars | steroid nucleus | lactone ring |

Digitoxigenin
Aglycone or Genin (insoluble)

Glycoside (soluble)

FIG. 33–1. A typical glycoside (digitoxin).

relatively small in comparison to that on the failing heart, partly because in the normal circulation, reflex or compensatory adjustments mask the change. The efficacy of the glycosides in heart failure is due solely to these actions (see below).

The positive inotropic effect of digitalis may be most conveniently demonstrated using a fatigued papillary muscle from the cat's heart (Fig. 33–2). It has been shown that the maximum developed isometric force and velocity of shortening are increased. These effects have also been demonstrated in preparations of human myocardium.

Actions on Other Myocardial Properties

The other myocardial effects of digitalis are complex (Table 33–1). They vary not only with dosage but between different parts of the heart. The action of the glycosides on the myocardial cells is referred to as its **direct action.** In addition, digitalis increases parasympathetic (vagal) and also sympathetic tone. The ongoing continuous efferent discharge in these systems is increased due presumably to a central effect of the drug. Consequently, the direct effects of digitalis on the myocardium are complicated by its **indirect actions** through the autonomic nervous system.

In the following discussion, **excitability** may be defined in terms of myocardial threshold to electrical excitation. The lower the threshold, the greater the excitability. **Automaticity** is the property of initiating intrinsic spontaneous pacemaker activity.

ACTION ON THE ATRIOVENTRICULAR NODE AND THE VENTRICULAR CONDUCTION SYSTEM.

The effective refractory period of the node is prolonged and the rate of conduction in the atrioventricular bundle is reduced. This is the result of both the **direct** and **indirect** (vagal) ac-

tions of the drug which are additive. There is a decrease in the amplitude, duration and maximum velocity of the upstroke of the membrane action potential. This effect of digitalis on the atrioventricular conduction or transmission system of decreasing conduction, lengthening refractory period and increasing likelihood of decremental or abortive conduction, underlies its usefulness in the treatment of atrial fibrillation.

ACTION ON THE ATRIA AND THE SINUS NODE.

The spontaneous rate of the sino-atrial node is decreased by a **direct** and **indirect** action of the glycosides. The **direct** and **indirect effects** of digitalis on the effective refractory period and site of conduction on the atrial muscle **are opposite** and tend to cancel each other (see Table 33–1). In the average patient, the **indirect,** or

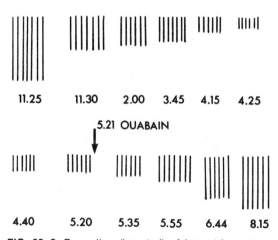

11.25   11.30   2.00   3.45   4.15   4.25

5.21 OUABAIN

4.40   5.20   5.35   5.55   6.44   8.15

FIG. 33–2. Recording (inverted) of isometric contraction of cat papillary muscle on electrical stimulation. The addition of ouabain to the fluid surrounding the muscle almost restored the original force of contraction. Figures refer to times of recording. (Gold H, Cattel M (1940): Mechanism of digitalis action in abolishing heart failure. Arch Intern Med 65:263)

TABLE 33–1. Summary of Effects of Cardiac Glycosides on the Heart

Effect	Atria	AV node and bundle	Ventricles
Direct digitalis effects	**Contractile force increased** Refractory period lengthened Conduction velocity decreased Automaticity slightly increased	**Refractory period lengthened** **Conduction velocity decreased**	**Contractile force increased** Refractory period shortened Marked increase in automaticity
Indirect digitalis effects (increased vagal tone)	Refractory period shortened Conduction velocity increased	**Refractory period lengthened** **Conduction velocity decreased**	No effect
Electrocardiographic changes	P changes	PR interval increased	QT shortened; T and ST depressed
Adverse irregularities	Extrasystoles Tachycardia	AV depression or block	Fibrillation Extrasystoles Tachycardia

Therapeutically important actions are set in **bold face type.**

vagal, **effects are dominant.** The refractory period is shortened, and conduction velocity increased. Automaticity is increased more in the atria than in the ventricles.

ACTION ON THE VENTRICLES. Since the vagi do not innervate the ventricular muscle, **indirect parasympathetic influences** do not extend to the ventricles, except when secondary to supraventricular changes. Digitalis still exerts a **direct effect.** The refractory period is shortened, and the Purkinje cells in particular show increased automaticity. This latter effect may be associated with an increase in sympathetic tone, and is concurrent with an increase in the rate of spontaneous diastolic depolarization.

MECHANISM OF ACTION

The present concensus is that digitalis increases the concentration of calcium ion in the region of the myocardial muscle fiber during contraction. During diastole the concentration of calcium ions in the cytoplasm surrounding the myofilaments is low, about $10^{-7}M$; it is maintained at this concentration by a pump located in a complex cellular tubular system, the sarcoplasmic reticulum, which takes up calcium against a concentration gradient. The myofilaments shorten when calcium ion concentrations are increased by influx from the sarcoplasmic reticulum during an action potential. Activity of the calcium pump subsequently lowers calcium ion concentration, an effect associated with relaxation. The transfer of calcium ions is a process requiring energy derived from the hydrolysis of ATP.

For some time the inhibitory effect of cardiac glycosides on $(Na^+ + K^+)$-ATPase, a sodium and potassium activated enzyme that hydrolyzes ATP and which plays an integral role in the transfer of sodium and potassium across membranes has been known. The evidence for this action is so strong that it has been postulated that this enzyme may be a receptor for digitalis. If this is the case, there must be a relationship between the effect of the glycoside on ATPase, intracellular calcium ion concentration and the positive inotropic effect of the agent. A number of mechanisms have been proposed. After digitalis, measurements show that Na^+ is increased and K^+ decreased. Inhibition of Na^+ transport by ATPase inhibition would result in the accumulation of intracellular Na^+. A variety of mechanisms have been proposed that would relate this effect to the amount of calcium ion available to the myofilaments. For example, by reducing nonspecific sites of ion binding more calcium would be made available. Alternatively, the reduction of Na^+ efflux could reduce calcium ion efflux and thus the concentration of this ion might increase in available pools.

On the other hand, the effect of cardiac glycosides on the ATPase might not be related to the change in the activator calcium concentration during contraction. Evidence has been obtained that these agents might directly increase calcium ion efflux and decrease calcium ion uptake from the sarcoplasmic reticulum.

Changes in the electric properties of the cardiac cells appear to be associated with $(Na^+ + K^+)$-ATPase inhibition. This results in the loss of intracellular potassium ions and a gain of intracellular sodium ions with a consequent decrease in the membrane potential. Other changes in the electric properties of the heart muscle cells, e.g., in the action potential, may be related to this effect.

CLINICAL PHARMACOLOGY

Heart Failure

Digitalis may be used with advantage in congestive heart failure, no matter what the cause, except when failure is associated with digitalis overdose or ventricular tachycardia. Clinical improvement can almost always be expected, although adjuvant therapy is often needed to obtain the optimal effect. The improvement is greater in failure due to some causes (e.g., hypertensive heart disease) than to others (e.g., thyrotoxicosis). It is emphasized that cardiac glycosides, despite their extremely valuable therapeutic actions, are potentially dangerous and must be used with caution in the old patient and in the patient with recent cardiac infarction.

The effects of digitalis in heart failure are the result of one primary action—improvement in the work and energy utilization of the myocardium. Continued use of the drug once the heart has recovered will often prevent recurrence of failure, especially if every effort is made to remove or reduce causative factors. Cardiac glycosides are commonly used prophylactically before cardiac surgery to prevent dangerous arrhythmias and failure.

In congestive heart failure, contractility is diminished, cardiac output is less than optimal and there is no cardiac reserve. The body initially involves a number of compensatory mechanisms, an increase in sympathetic tone associated with tachycardia, an increased maximum systolic tension development, velocity of shortening and hypertrophy of the heart wall which provides additional contractile material. Eventually, because of poor contractility, the end diastolic pressure rises resulting in increased venous pressure and heart enlargement. Soon blood "piles up" in the venous side of the greater and lesser circulations. Many of the symptoms and signs of congestive heart failure are the result of this venous engorgement. Invariably, venous pressure is increased, altering the hydrostatic forces that control water reabsorption at the venous end of the capillary bed. These changes lead to dyspnea, cyanosis, edema, ascites and pleural effusions. The increased hydrostatic pressure in the renal capillaries and the diminished renal blood flow reduce urinary output, causing fluid retention. The reversal of these changes following digitalization is solely the result of the positive inotropic effect of the glycoside. The myocardial contractile state improves, cardiac output increases and diastolic pressure falls.

Although other theories about the action of digitalis in heart failure have been by and large discountenanced, they are briefly mentioned below, since they still have some adherents and are instructive.

1. Action on veins. It has been proposed that the primary action of digitalis in heart failure is to cause venoconstriction. This would increase the venous return and in consequence, provided the myocardium were capable, cardiac output. Digitalis has been shown to cause venous (and also arteriolar) constriction, by a direct action on vascular smooth muscle and also probably by increasing sympathetic outflow by a central effect. However, many experimental studies carried out using a variety of cardiac preparations, when all known extracardiac factors, in particular venous return and venous filling, are rigorously controlled, have all demonstrated the positive inotropic effect of the glycosides. The effect on the vessels must be considered a secondary action of the drug.

2. Action on the kidneys. Withering believed that the cardinal action of digitalis in congestive heart failure was directly on the kidney, promoting diuresis. Current research has demonstrated that the diuretic effect of digitalis in heart failure is secondary to a decrease in net capillary hydrostatic pressure, allowing the resorption of fluid from the extracellular space and the amelioration of renal hemodynamics. The increased aldosterone secretion associated with failure (Ch. 38) which is partly responsible for some sodium and fluid retention is also the consequence of circulatory change. These effects are reversed by the improved tissue blood flow that follows the cardiotonic action of digitalis. It seems unlikely that the small effect of digitalis on tubular $(Na^+ + K^+)$-ATPase has significant consequences.

3. Action on heart rate. After digitalization, heart rate is usually slowed. Restoration of the stroke volume and cardiac output removes the various causes of reflex compensatory tachycardia, and heart rate falls toward more normal values. The heart is further slowed by the direct depressant action of digitalis on the sinoatrial node and indirectly as a result of the increase in vagal tone. The restoration of a more normal heart rate is not sufficient to account for the increase in output caused by the drug. In atrial fibrillation, the heart rate is reduced by additional actions of digitalis (see below).

Atrial Fibrillation

The cardiac cycle is initiated normally from, and its rate controlled by, the cardiac pacemaker—the sinoatrial node. Activity spreads across the atria, initiating activity in the atrioventricular transmission system which leads to ventricular excitation. In atrial fibrillation, the sinoatrial node loses control and the atrioventricular node is bombarded irregularly (up to 500 times/min) by impulses originating from abnormal or ectopic foci in the atria (Ch. 34). Most of these impulses are extinguished because they arrive at the atrioventricular node during the refractory period of previously conducted excitation. The ventricular rate may be as high as 180 beats/min. The pulse is irregular in rhythm and force.

Digitalis is used to control the mean ventricular rate in atrial fibrillation, irrespective of any associated conditions. It prolongs the refractory period of the conduction system by the additive effect of its indirect (vagal) and direct actions on the Purkinje cells of the conduction system. Consequently, fewer impulses from the atria reach the ventricles. Because of its complex effect on the resting membrane and action potential, impulses initiated in the conduction system more frequently abort. Digitalis is not curative: It controls ventricular rate and allows the heart to function more effectively as a pump. The digitalized patient with atrial fibrillation is often able to live a comparatively normal life in spite of his condition. After digitalis, the refractory period of atrial muscle is shortened and the fibrillary rate of the atria increases. The atrioventricular node is bombarded more rapidly than before. This is not usually important, since the depressant action of the drug on the atrioventricular system overrides any change in the atrial condition.

Atrial Flutter

Digitalis is used in the treatment of atrial flutter. The heart block usually present in this condition is increased and then maintained by the use of digitalis, frequently in large doses. Sometimes the heart spontaneously reverts to normal sinus rhythm or to well-controlled atrial fibrillation. If neither occurs, quinidine therapy (Ch. 34) or direct-current electrical cardioconversion may be tried.

Paroxysmal Tachycardia

Rapid digitalization is one of a number of procedures that may be effective in paroxysmal atrial or supraventricular tachycardia. Its effectiveness is probably the result of its vagal stimulating effects on the sinoatrial node and the atrioventricular bundle. It is essential to establish that the condition is not the result of digitalis overdose.

ELECTROCARDIOGRAPHIC CHANGES

Therapeutic doses of digitalis (one-third to one-half the lethal dose) cause characteristic electrocardiographic changes. These are listed below in the order of most common occurrence. The EKG is sometimes useful in determining if a patient has received recent glycoside therapy.

T-wave changes in which the T wave becomes small, isoelectric or inverted, occur. At the same time the ST segment frequently becomes depressed and often falls below the isoelectric line. These changes have no relation to the adequacy of the therapeutic dose or the imminence of toxicity.

Lengthened PR interval is associated with slower or delayed atrioventricular conduction.

Shortened QT interval is the result of the shortening of the plateau phase of the transmembrane action potential.

P-wave changes are presumably caused by the complex action of the glycosides on the atria.

With higher doses of digitalis, the above changes are exaggerated and electrocardiographic patterns appropriate to the drug-induced irregularities seen.

PREPARATIONS, ASSAY, ADMINISTRATION, AND DOSAGE

Only a few examples of the many clinically used glycosides are discussed. These are either the most popular compounds or compounds whose special properties make them extremely desirable on certain occasions. Since the therapeutic ratio of all glycosides is the same, selection must be based upon such criteria as rate of onset, duration, purity, absorbability and bioavailability.

Preparations

Digitalis Leaf, *U.S.P.* (*D. purpurea*), is unquestionably the standard drug for oral use. Digitoxin *U.S.P.*, its main active principle, may be administered either orally or parenterally. Since it is almost completely absorbed by mouth, oral and parenteral dosage is identical (Table 33–2). Digoxin, *U.S.P.*, the main active glycoside in *D. lanata,* is another widely used preparation, for both oral and parenteral administration. Since digoxin is *not* completely absorbed by mouth, the dosage for the two routes is not the same. Ouabain, *U.S.P.,* from *Strophanthus gratus,* is probably the most rapidly acting parenteral glycoside. Deslanoside, *N.F.* (desacetyllanatoside-C, cedilanid-D), is a little slower but is the most popular.

Equivalents of the glycoside preparations from *D. purpurea* are shown in Table 33–3.

Assay

A number of galenical preparations of glycosides are in common use. These are assayed biologically against the international Digitalis Standard Powder. The assay involves the intravenous infusion of the glycoside into lightly etherized pigeons and measurement of the time taken to

TABLE 33—2. Characteristics of Common Cardiac Glycosides

Drug	Gastrointestinal absorption	Route of admin- istration	Latency	Time to maximum effect	Half-life	Digitalizing dose	Maintenance dose
Ouabain	—	IV	5—10 min	½—2 hr	21 hr	0.25—0.50 mg	—
Deslanoside	—	IV	10—30 min	1—2 hr	36 hr	1.2 —1.6 mg	—
Digoxin	—	IV	10—30 min	1½—5 hr	36 hr	0.75—1.25 mg	—
Digoxin	50—75%	PO	1½—4 hr	6—8 hr	36 hr	2.0 —3.0 mg	0.25—0.5 mg
Digitoxin	—	IV	½—2 hr	8 hr	4—6 days	1.0 —1.5 mg	—
Digitoxin	90—100%	PO	2—6 hr	4—12 hr	4—6 days	1.0 —1.5 mg	0.1 —0.2 mg
Digitalis leaf	40%	PO	2—6 hr	½—1 day	4—6 days	1.0 —2.0 g	0.12g

cause death. Since this estimation has all the disadvantages of a biologic assay made in one species for use in another, attempts have been made to assay galenical preparations in human patients. Specific electrocardiographic changes are used as criteria of effect. Considerable variation in the bioavailability of various commercial preparations of cardiac glycosides is experienced by practicing physicians. This emphasizes the need to assay individually the effectiveness of digitalis on each patient, to use a preparation with which the physician is experienced, and for the patient not to switch from one particular form of medication to another.

Plasma concentrations of glycosides can now be routinely and accurately measured. The various methods available provide similar information relating plasma levels and therapeutic and toxic manifestations. For example, digoxin plasma concentrations in patients with toxicity are several times greater than those without. Although variation in levels associated with particular effects is considerable, they have been used to follow the course of treatment, particularly in patients with alteration in absorption and/or excretory mechanisms and to differentiate digitalis-induced toxicities from others.

Administration

Except in an emergency, when speed rather than maximum safety is the prime consideration, or when poor absorption is expected, cardiac glycosides should be given **orally.**

When minutes are vital, a crystalline glycoside, well diluted, may be given very slowly by **IV injection.** Absorption from subcutaneous and IM sites is irregular.

As the therapeutic ratio of the cardiac glycosides is small, optimal dosage is particularly desirable. A detailed knowledge of the pharmacokinetics and other factors influencing dosage is important to insure this. It has been demonstrated that the incidence of adverse effects significantly declines when a special digitalis dosage program, sometimes computer based, is initiated. A detailed study of such an approach is

however, out of place in this textbook. Some of the more important features to be considered in determining dose are shown in Table 33–2. Gastrointestinal absorption is unreliable and incomplete with all glycosides except with digitoxin. The biologic half-life varies from under 1 day to 4–6 days. Furthermore, plasma binding varies considerably from one glycoside to another. The principal route of excretion is renal for deslanoside, ouabain and digoxin. Although gastrointestinal excretion has some importance for the latter two glycosides, digitoxin and digitalis leaf are involved in an entero-hepatic circulation; their metabolites are excreted by the kidney. Binding of the glycoside is influenced by various drugs (Ch. 4), plasma ion levels and by various disease states including those of the thyroid.

Glycosides are administered orally in two stages. For **initial digitalization** (of a patient who has not recently received the drug) the glycoside is administered at a rate designed to cause its accumulation within the body. This dosage scheme is continued until the desired therapeutic aim is attained or serious toxic effects emerge. Since the dose that causes the same therapeutic effect varies widely from one individual to another, the procedure of initial digitalization is essentially equivalent to an individual biologic assay. Once the desired effect is obtained, **maintenance dosage** is initiated. This dose also varies widely and is selected to maintain optimal therapeutic effect. Rate of drug absorption must equal rate of elimination.

Dosage

Many fixed dosage schemes are in use. The total oral initial digitalizing dose of Powdered Digitalis Leaf, given over a period of 1–2 days is of the

TABLE 33—3. Approximate Equivalents of Glycoside Preparations from *D. purpurea*

Powdered Digitalis, *U.S.P.* (leaf of *D. purpurea*), 0.1 g ≡ 1.0 *U.S.P.* unit
Digitalis Tincture, *N.F.,* 1.0 ml ≡ 0.1 g digitalis leaf
Digitoxin Injection, *U.S.P.,* 0.1 mg ≡ 0.1 g digitalis leaf

order of 12–20 *U.S.P.* units or 1.2–2.0 g. Frequently, the dose is divided into four parts and given every 6 hr. However, this regimen may be varied according to urgency and other circumstances. The average maintenance dose is 1.0–1.5 *U.S.P.* units/day. However, wide variations are encountered, and the dose must always be matched to the clinical effect in each individual. As pointed previously, knowledge of the pharmacokinetics of a particular glycoside and some of the relevant features of a particular patient can be used to design optimal dosage schedules. Average doses of other glycosides are given in Table 33–2.

ADVERSE EFFECTS AND TOXICITY

The therapeutic index of cardiac glycosides is between two and three, one of the lowest indexes of all commonly used therapeutic agents. Consequently, adverse effects are not rare. Even in hospitalized patients, it has been reported that up to 30% of those treated with cardiac glycoside experience some potentially serious toxicity. In the discussion that follows, the figures in parentheses indicate the percentage of patients who complain of the adverse effect. Absence of a parenthetical figure indicates that data are not available.

Gastrointestinal Effects

Anorexia (50), nausea, and vomiting (35) are frequently the first signs of intoxication. Although galenicals cause gastric and intestinal irritation, most of these effects are the result of a direct action of the drug on the vomiting center. In addition, abdominal discomfort, pain, diarrhea (10) and cramps may be experienced.

Neurologic Effects

Many diverse adverse effects have been described, including headache, malaise, drowsiness and neuralgic pain; mental symptoms include delirium, convulsions and confusion. Visual effects are fairly common: blurred vision, white, yellow, green or red colored perception have been reported.

Cardiac Effects

Digitalis overdose can simulate every known cardiac irregularity. Some occur more commonly than others. In the following discussion, the parenthetical figures refer to the approximate incidence of the irregularity among total diagnosed cardiac irregularities. In one study, 124 abnormal rhythms were found in a total of 88 patients.

EXTRASYSTOLES (25). Automaticity of the ventricles is increased by the direct action of the glycosides enhancing spontaneous diastolic depolarization. Premature junctional or ventricular beats are often seen. Since glycosides do not influence ventricular and Purkinje cells quantatively to the same degree, increased automaticity may progress through reentry or local circuit mechanisms. The terms "coupling" and "bigeminy" are used to describe a common variant in which a normal heart beat alternates with an extrasystole (12). Multifocal ventricular premature beats are serious and probably prelude ventricular fibrillation.

ATRIOVENTRICULAR BLOCK (40). Partial or complete heart block (dissociation of atria and ventricles) occurs presumably due to an extension of the therapeutically useful effects of digitalis on the atrioventricular bundle. Propagation in the atrioventricular bundle ceases. Atrial tachycardia with heart block is a classic rhythm of digitalis intoxication.

TACHYCARDIA (10). Tachycardia, both atrial and ventricular, occurs and is usually considered an indication to discontinue treatment. The latter is more dangerous since it may prelude ventricular fibrillation. This latter arrhythmia is the usual cause of death following an overdose of digitalis, particularly its rapid intravenous administration.

A digitalis dosage adequate to control fibrillation or flutter may be toxic to the myocardium controlled by sinus rhythm. To prevent the emergence of adverse effects, digitalis is stopped a few days before elective electrical conversion.

Treatment of Intoxication

Because the therapeutic index of the glycosides is low and their duration of action long, and because treatment involves a clinical compromise between an effective therapeutic dose and one causing adverse effects, intoxication is fairly common. Mortality among those with demonstrable adverse effects has been reported to be as high as 20%. Discontinuation of treatment must be considered as soon as the first adverse effects appear. For many this is the only "treatment" required, and once these adverse effects disappear, the glycoside may be resumed at a lower dose. Careful clinical observation during the period of initial digitalization is crucial.

Serious adverse effects are often seen in the patient who, without the physician's and perhaps even his own knowledge, has had digitalis therapy within the previous 10 days. Standard digitalization under these circumstances may be fatal.

The electrocardiogram is often helpful in deciding this problem, although it is sometimes difficult to distinguish the effects of prior digitalization and underlying cardiac disease.

Toxicity that impedes the output of the heart or that may progress to ventricular fibrillation must be taken extremely seriously.

A reduction in serum potassium sensitizes the myocardium to digitalis. If hypopotassemia occurs, e.g., as a result of coincidently pursued diuretic or steroid therapy, toxic effects may become manifest following standard digitalis dosage. Under these circumstances the carefully controlled oral or, if necessary, parenteral administration of potassium may be effective in reducing intoxication within an hour. Parenteral injections must be made with extreme caution, since too rapid injection can cause asystole. The administration of potassium is contraindicated when disturbances of conduction are detected. Elevated calcium levels have similar consequences. They may be reduced with chelating agents such as disodium versenate.

Drug therapy includes diphenylhydantoin, lidocaine and propranolol (Ch. 34). The first two agents have little or no effect on conduction, whereas propranolol may depress conduction in the atrioventricular bundle system. The sympatholytic effect of propranolol may have undesirable consequences in some circumstances.

FURTHER READING

Braunwald E, Ross J, Jr, Sonnenblick EH (1968): Mechanisms of Contraction of the Normal and Failing Heart. Boston, Little Brown

Marks BH, Weissler AM (eds) (1972): Basic and Clinical Pharmacology of Digitalis. Springfield, Ill, Charles C Thomas

BERTRAM G. KATZUNG

34. ANTIARRHYTHMIC DRUGS

Antiarrhythmic drugs are used to control or cure cardiac arrhythmias. Arrhythmias are defined as disorders of rate, rhythm, origin or conduction of impulses within the heart. They are common manifestations of functional and anatomic cardiac disease. Various studies have estimated their incidence at 10–25% during digitalization of hospitalized patients, 20–50% in general anesthetic procedures and 80–90% in patients with acute myocardial infarction. In fact, ventricular arrhythmias are the major cause of death following myocardial infarction.

PATHOPHYSIOLOGY OF ARRHYTHMIAS

The factors which precipitate arrhythmias may include ischemia with resulting hypoxia and pH and electrolyte abnormalities, excessive fiber stretch, excessive discharge of or sensitivity to autonomic regulator substances and exposure to foreign chemicals such as digitalis and other potentially toxic substances. However, all arrhythmias result from one or a combination of the following fundamental conditions:

1. abnormal impulse formation: *automaticity* defects.
2. abnormal propagation of impulses: *conduction* defects.

The quantitative description of these defects requires an understanding of the electrical activity of cells in the different parts of the heart, and the way this electrical activity is propagated (Fig. 34–1).

Determinants of Automaticity

As suggested by Figure 34–2, rate of discharge of a spontaneously discharging cardiac cell is determined by the *slope of phase 4* of the trans-

membrane electrical potential as well as several other factors. Normally, the phase 4 slope of cardiac cells outside the normal pacemaker, the sinoatrial (SA) node, is less than that of SA nodal cells. Under conditions conducive to arrhythmias, Purkinje or other cells may develop a much steeper phase 4 slope and take over pacemaker function, i.e., they become *ectopic* pacemakers. Increased catecholamine concentration, depolarization, hypoxia, inadequate extracellular potassium and toxic amounts of digitalis are a few of the potential causes of increased automaticity, especially in Purkinje fibers. Common arrhythmias resulting from ectopic automaticity include ventricular escape rhythms, premature ventricular beats and probably some ventricular tachycardias.

Determinants of Conduction

The *excitability* of electrically excitable cells is inversely proportional to the stimulus current required to change the membrane potential from its resting level to the threshold potential at which an all-or-none spike occurs. The *effective refractory period* is that period of time which must elapse after an action potential before a second propagated action potential can be elicited.

Once an action potential has been elicited, the ability of a cardiac cell to propagate the impulse can be estimated from the slope of phase 0—the maximum rate of depolarization—and the amplitude of the action potential. Both of these parameters are measures of the *sodium* ion current flowing into the cell. As shown in Figures 34–3,4 these quantities are controlled by two major variables: The level of resting membrane potential preceding the action potential, and the time allowed for recovery of the sodium mechanism following previous activity.

266

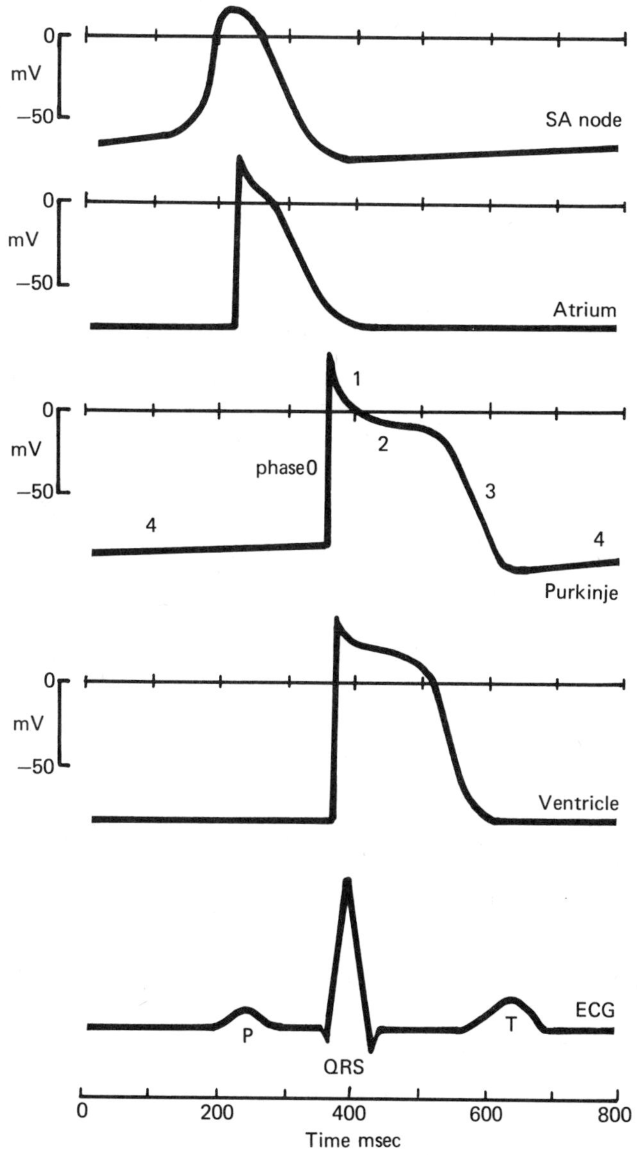

FIG. 34–1. Schematic drawing of typical transmembrane potential recordings from several areas of the heart and their relation in time to the electrocardiogram (ECG). The sinoatrial (SA) node recording is characterized by a slow action potential upstroke, low overshoot at the peak of the depolarization, and relatively rapid depolarization between action potentials (diastolic depolarization). The atrial action potentials differ primarily in their faster upstroke and flat (nonpacemaker) diastolic potential. The Purkinje fiber recording shows the conventional numbering for identifying the various phases of cardiac action potentials. Note that this fiber demonstrates a slow but definite pacemaker depolarization during phase 4, i.e., it is a *latent* pacemaker. The ventricular pattern differs from that of a Purkinje fiber in having a stable diastolic potential and a somewhat shorter action potential duration. The ECG record illustrates the correlation of the P wave with atrial activity, the P-R interval with the A-V conduction delay, the QRS complex with ventricular depolarization and the Q-T interval with the ventricular action potential duration.

Depression of conduction can lead to significant cardiac malfunction. Simple slowing or block results in such recognized arrhythmias as AV blockade and bundle-branch block. More complex arrhythmias such as paroxysmal atrial tachycardia, AV nodal tachycardias and many ventricular tachycardias seem to result from the phenomenon of *reentry* (Fig. 34–5). In reentry, the arrhythmia is dependent on an intermediate degree of conduction depression; either normalization or further depression abolish the unidirectional block upon which re-entry depends.

EFFECTS OF IONS. The level of extracellular *potassium* ion (K_o) is of crucial importance in modulating both automaticity and conduction. Ectopic automaticity is suppressed by adequate or elevated K_o because it tends to reduce the slope of phase 4 (diastolic depolarization), especially in Purkinje fibers. Conduction velocity is usually depressed by elevated K_o since increased K_o tends to reduce the resting membrane potential (Fig. 34–3) and to prolong the recovery time for the sodium conductance mechanism (Fig. 34–4). Normal cardiac rhythm implies minimal automaticity (outside of the normal SA nodal pacemaker) but optimal conduction velocity. Thus it can be expected that increasing K_o might reduce ectopic automaticity but impair conduction.

MODES OF THERAPY IN THE ARRHYTHMIAS

The major modes of therapy include: electrical pacemakers and DC electroshock ("cardioversion"), autonomic manipulation through drugs

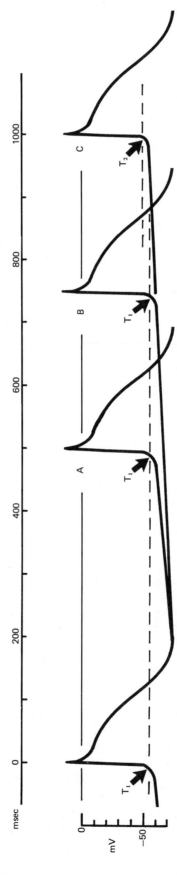

FIG. 34–2. Schematic representation of pacemaker activity in a Purkinje fiber. Trace A indicates the pretreatment condition in which diastolic depolarization causes threshold (T_1) to be reached every 500 msec, corresponding to a rate of 120 beats/min. Under the influence of a drug which slows diastolic depolarization (Trace B), the threshold is reached every 750 msec, corresponding to a rate of 80 beats/min. Trace C shows the effect of a drug such as quinidine which changes the threshold to a more positive potential (T_2) in addition to slowing diastolic depolarization. The combination of these two effects results in further slowing of the ectopic rate to 1 beat/sec or 60/min. Other variables also influence pacemaker rate but phase 4 slope (diastolic depolarization) and threshold potential are the most important ones in determining antiarrhythmic drug effect on pacemakers.

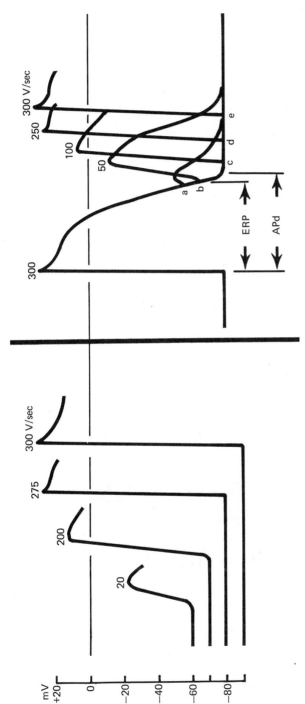

FIG. 34–3. Dependence of action potential upstroke velocity (numbers at each action potential peak, volts per second) and amplitude on the prior level of resting potential. Note that at resting potentials more negative than −80 mV, upstroke velocity stabilizes at a maximum level. At resting potentials less negative than −80 mV, there is a steep fall in upstroke velocity, declining to zero at −45 to −50 mV.

FIG. 34–4. Dependence of action potential upstroke velocity and amplitude on recovery time following the preceding action potential. Stimuli arriving before completion of the effective refractory period (ERP) produce only a small, nonpropagated response (trace A). A stimulus arriving immediately after completion of the ERP results in a very small, slowly conducted response (trace B). Both of these early responses may occur before complete repolarization and are therefore depressed by the low "resting" potential at the time they are elicited according to the mechanism shown in Figure 34–3. However, even after full repolarization, an early extrasystole, e.g., trace C, will be associated with slow upstroke and low amplitude showing that these variables are dependent on recovery time as well as on membrane potential. In normal tissue, recovery requires only 10–20 msec. However, in depressed tissue, recovery may require 100 msec or more.

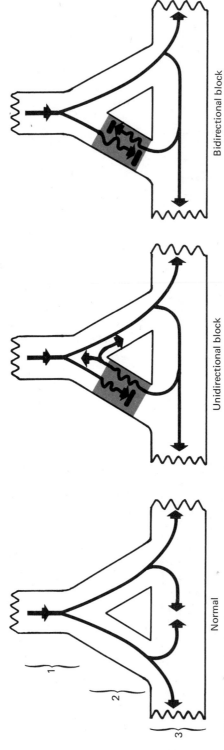

FIG. 34–5. Conduction patterns in a main Purkinje fiber (1), terminal Purkinje branches (2) and ventricular wall (3). Diagram on the left shows how a normally conducted impulse would spread in the myocardium. Disease or drug toxicity may cause *unidirectional* conduction block (Center Diagram). In this case the descending impulse in the left hand branch enters a partially blocked or refractory area (color) and is extinguished. The impulse from the right hand branch, arriving somewhat later in time, is able to traverse the region and therefore *reenters* both the main fiber and the right branch. Reexcitation and an arrhythmia is the result. More severe depression of the Purkinje branch may result in *bidirectional* conduction block (Diagram on right). Now the depressed area (color) will not conduct in either direction so reentry is prevented.

Normal

Unidirectional block

Bidirectional block

TABLE 34–1. Major Cardiac Effects of Antiarrhythmic Drugs

Drug	Action	EKG changes
Quinidine and procainamide	Atria: decreased automaticity	Increased P-P
	AV node: increased refractory period (direct)	
	Decreased conduction velocity (direct)	Increased P-R
	Increased conduction velocity (antivagal)	Decreased P-R
	His-Purkinje system: decreased automaticity	Decreased ectopic rate
	Ventricles: increased action potential duration	Increased QT
	Decreased conduction velocity	Increased QRS
Propranolol	Atria: decreased SA automaticity	Increased P-P
	AV node: decreased conduction velocity	Increased P-R
	His-Purkinje system: decreased automaticity	Decreased ectopic rate
Lidocaine and phenytoin	Atria: decreased automaticity (high doses or high serum K)	
	AV node: no effect, facilitation, or depression of conduction	No effect, decreased, or increased P-R
	His-Purkinje system: decreased automaticity	Decreased ectopic rate

which stimulate or suppress normal autonomic regulatory mechanisms in the heart (Chs. 14–19) and direct pharmacologic manipulation of cardiac cell membrane properties. The major antiarrhythmic agents act via the last mechanism. These drugs include quinidine, procainamide, propranolol, lidocaine and phenytoin.* Bretylium, an agent still under study for its effects on arrhythmias following myocardial infarction, probably acts by reducing the release of catecholamines in the heart (Ch. 20) and will not be discussed further in this chapter.

MODE OF ANTIARRHYTHMIC DRUG ACTION. Since all the standard antiarrhythmic agents reduce ectopic automaticity (Table 34–1), one clear mechanism for their beneficial effects is suppression of ectopic pacemakers. Arrhythmias caused by a reentry mechanism might be abolished in several ways (Fig. 34–5). Purely depressant effects such as decreased excitability or increased refractory period could convert unidirectional conduction block to bidirectional conduction block. Improvement of conduction on the other hand, might convert the unidirectional block to normal conduction. Both effects would abolish reentry.

Conduction velocity can be modified in several ways by the antiarrhythmic drugs. Some agents may depress the steady state sodium conduc-

tance system at all membrane potentials (mechanism of Fig. 34–3), independent of recovery time. This would result in a decrease in conduction velocity at all heart rates. Other drugs appear to prolong recovery time of the conductance mechanism without major effects on steady-state sodium conductance. This action would selectively depress conduction of extrasystoles and beats occurring at high rates since recovery time is limited under these circumstances.

Most antiarrhythmic agents increase the duration of the effective refractory period relative to the action potential duration (*ERP/APd* ratio). The result of this action is to prevent action potentials from occurring very close to a preceding one. Such "closely coupled" extrasystoles are more likely to be abnormally conducted and are therefore more likely to set up reentry circuits. Thus an increase in the ERP/APd ratio would reduce the incidence of reentry arrhythmias.

Finally, some evidence suggests that hypoxic or damaged myocardium is much more sensitive to the depressant effects of these drugs than is normal tissue. Assuming that the total mass of damaged tissue is not too large, complete suppression of both automaticity and conduction in a localized area could result in abolition of arrhythmias of both the ectopic pacemaker and reentry type.

QUINIDINE

Quinidine, the optical isomer of quinine (Ch. 61) is obtained from the bark of the cinchona tree indigenous to South America and Indonesia. The use of cinchona extracts in cardiac disease re-

* Phenytoin is referred to as diphenylhydantoin elsewhere in this book. This chapter was changed in proof to conform to the new name.

sulted from the observation that the treatment of malaria with cinchona occasionally brought about relief of coexisting cardiac arrhythmias.

ACTIONS

CARDIAC EFFECTS (Table 34–1). The major effects of quinidine on automaticity and conduction are depressant; the depression of automaticity is more marked in ectopic pacemakers, e.g. Purkinje fiber, than in the SA node. Quinidine depresses excitability and increases the ERP/APd ratio. These actions are *direct* ones, exerted on the cardiac cell membrane.

Quinidine also has *indirect* effects on the heart resulting from anticholinergic and antiadrenergic actions. Of these two autonomic effects, the anticholinergic one is more commonly seen. The only significant manifestation of this anticholinergic action is the occasional appearance of cardiac vagal blockade with increased AV conduction velocity and sinus tachycardia.

In the presence of atrial fibrillation, AV conduction time cannot be directly measured but an antivagal effect on this variable is easily detected from the increase in ventricular rate. These effects are readily prevented by prior administration of digitalis (see Ch. 33).

When given in higher doses, and especially if given parenterally, quinidine can *depress cardiac contractility.*

EXTRACARDIAC EFFECTS. Quinidine has no therapeutically useful extracardiac effects. It mimics its isomer, quinine, in having antimalarial, antipyretic and oxytocic properties as well as modest stabilizing effects on the end plate of skeletal muscle. However, in each of these effects it is weaker than quinine.

I-QUININE, D-QUINIDINE

MECHANISM OF ACTION

Quinidine reduces phase 4 depolarization slope in pacemaker cells, probably through reduction of diastolic sodium influx. The result is reduction or abolition of ectopic pacemaker function. The drug also appears to reduce the transfer of sodium across the cell membrane during phase 0 of the action potential. This action occurs at all resting membrane potentials and only extremely long recovery times can alleviate the depression.

As a result conduction velocity is decreased and refractory period is prolonged. The effects on sodium influx are associated with a decreased efflux of potassium and suggest a rather nonspecific "stablilizing" effect on the cardiac cell membrane. The reduction in potassium efflux may be responsible for the increase in the action potential duration that is commonly observed after quinidine.

ABSORPTION, METABOLISM AND EXCRETION

Quinidine is well absorbed from the gastrointestinal tract. It is strongly bound (80%) to plasma proteins and is finally excreted in the urine, largely in the form of hydroxylated metabolites. The half-life of the parent compound in the plasma is 4–7 hours and is more likely to be prolonged in patients with congestive heart failure than in those with renal disease.

PREPARATIONS AND DOSAGE

Quinidine is almost always administered orally. The sulfate (*U.S.P.*) salt is usually used although gluconate and polygalacturonate salts are also available. After a test dose of 0.2 g to detect idiosyncrasy, doses of 0.2–0.6 g may be given 4–6 times/day depending on the therapeutic goal or the appearance of serious toxicity. The therapeutic plasma concentration is 3–5 μg/ml. Quinidine gluconate injection *U.S.P.,* is soluble quinidine for IV use. Its administration is rarely justified since it is accompanied by a high incidence of untoward effects and better parenteral antiarrhythmic agents are available.

ADVERSE EFFECTS AND TOXICITY

CARDIAC. In large doses, and especially when used parenterally, quinidine is a powerful cardiac depressant. It may cause pacemaker arrest, conduction block and depression of contractility, resulting in significant reduction of cardiac output. Through nonhomogeneous impairment of conduction it may even precipitate cardiac arrhythmias, including ventricular fibrillation. These adverse effects are much more likely to occur at high serum potassium levels (greater than 5 mEq/liter) than at low ones.

EXTRACARDIAC. The most common side effects of quinidine are gastrointestinal (nausea, vomiting, diarrhea). Along with quinine (and aspirin), quinidine may cause *cinchonism* (headache, dizziness, tinnitus). Finally, this drug is associated with occasional hypersensitivity reactions which may take the form of skin rash, angioneurotic edema or thrombocytopenic purpura.

PROCAINAMIDE

Early in the development of local anesthetics it was found that procaine, an ester, had significant antiarrhythmic effects. Because procaine is so rapidly metabolized, the amide derivative, procainamide, was developed for cardiovascular applications.

PROCAINAMIDE

ACTIONS

In almost every respect, procainamide can be considered identical to quinidine (Table 34–1). It reduces ectopic pacemaker rate, slows conduction velocity and may increase the ERP/APd ratio. Like quinidine, it is sometimes associated with accelerated AV conduction or sinus tachycardia; these effects can be prevented by digitalis.

ABSORPTION, METABOLISM AND EXCRETION

Procainamide is well absorbed after oral administration and is excreted primarily by the kidneys. About 50% of the administered dose is metabolized. It has a half-life of 3–6 hr.

PREPARATIONS AND DOSAGE

Procainamide hydrochloride *U.S.P.* (Pronestyl) is usually given orally in doses of 0.25–0.5 g, 3–4 times/day. A parenteral preparation is available, administered intramuscularly or intravenously. The therapeutic plasma level is 5–10 μg/ml.

ADVERSE EFFECTS AND TOXICITY

The adverse cardiac effects of procainamide, like its therapeutic effects, resemble those of quinidine. The extracardiac effects include gastrointestinal upsets, hypotension (especially if given parenterally) and dizziness. Occasionally, a lupus erythematosis-like syndrome and agranulocytosis have been reported.

PROPRANOLOL

Propranolol is an important β-adrenergic receptor blocking agent (Ch. 18). It is listed here because one of its approved applications is in the therapy of arrhythmias. Probably a direct membrane stabilizing action augments the β-adrenergic receptor blocking effect in causing a net antiarrhythmic effect. As indicated in Table 34-1 most of propranolol's direct effect are similar to those of quinidine and procainamide. It lacks the anticholinergic (indirect) effect of the two latter agents.

LIDOCAINE

Lidocaine has been an important local anesthetic for many years (Ch. 22). It is now one of the most popular antiarrhythmic drugs for the acute treatment of ventricular arrhythmias and for arrhythmias caused by digitalis.

ACTIONS

In ordinary clinical use, the cardiac actions of lidocaine are more marked on the ventricles than on the atria. In general, the SA and AV nodes are relatively resistant to depression by lidocaine although occasional reports of severe bradycardia or AV blockade have appeared. Under some circumstances, facilitation of AV conduction has been reported. Experimentally, one can demonstrate both facilitation (low drug concentration, low potassium concentration) and depression of conduction (higher drug concentration, normal or high potassium concentration) in

Purkinje fibers and ventricular myocardium (Table 34–1). Like the previously described agents, lidocaine effectively reduces pacemaker activity in the ventricles.

MECHANISMS OF ACTION

The mechanism of the depressant action of lidocaine is similar but not identical to that of quinidine. The cell membrane is stabilized by inhibition of sodium influx. However, the inhibition of phase 0 sodium conductance is much greater at high rates (short recovery times) and is much more marked at low membrane potentials than at high ones. The ERP/APd ratio is increased. Therefore, lidocaine has minimal effects on conduction velocity of normal beats at slow heart rates. Early extrasystoles on the other hand, especially in partially depolarized tissue, are very slowly conducted or abolished by the drug.

PREPARATIONS AND DOSAGE

Lidocaine hydrochloride *U.S.P.*, (Xylocaine), lignocaine *B.P.*, is inactive by the oral route (Ch. 22) and is always given parenterally. The drug has a short half-life (cardiac effects last 15–30 min) and is therefore given either intermittently or by continuous infusion. When given intermittently, IV doses of 1–2 mg/kg every 5–10 min usually yield effective plasma levels (1–5 μg/ml). Continuous infusions of 20–60 μg/kg/min may be used to achieve the same result.

ADVERSE EFFECTS AND TOXICITY

When limited to total doses of less than 300 mg and plasma levels of 5 μg/ml, serious toxicity from lidocaine is rare. While electrical and contractile cardiac depression may occur (especially in the presence of high serum potassium concentration), most of the reported toxicity is restricted to the CNS (Ch. 22).

PHENYTOIN

This anticonvulsant agent (Ch. 30) has clear antiarrhythmic effects and though not officially approved for such use, is frequently prescribed for its cardiac effects.

ACTIONS

The major cardiac effects of phenytoin resemble those of lidocaine (Table 34–1). At low concentrations, the drug appears to be less depressant on atrial function (including SA and AV nodes) than quinidine, and at plasma potassium concentrations less than 4 mEq/liter, it also appears to depress contractility less than the prototype agent. It is more effective in arrhythmias caused by digitalis than in other types of arrhythmias.

PREPARATIONS AND DOSAGE

Phenytoin sodium *U.S.P.* (diphenylhydantoin, Dilantin), can be given orally or parenterally. The antiarrhythmic plasma concentration is 5–15 μg/ml. When used parenterally, doses of 100 mg are given IV every 5 min until the arrhythmia is abolished or until 10 doses have been given unless toxicity occurs first. The half-life of a single dose is 6–10 hr.

ADVERSE EFFECTS AND TOXICITY

The most common acute adverse effects of phenytoin are due to its action on the CNS (Ch. 30). However, cases of cardiovascular collapse and cardiac arrest have been reported following the IV use of this drug as an antiarrhythmic agent.

CLINICAL CONSIDERATIONS

THE EFFECTS OF ANTIARRHYTHMIC DRUGS ON THE ELECTROCARDIOGRAM

Since the electrocardiogram (ECG) provides a convenient measure of some of the electrical properties of the heart, it is an important tool for diagnosing arrhythmias and monitoring the effects of therapy. Some of the ECG effects of the antiarrhythmic drugs are summarized in Table 34–1.

The ECG manifestation of the cardiac effects of quinidine include increased P-P or R-R interval (slowing of rate), increased QT (prolonged action potential duration), increased QRS duration (slowing of intraventricular conduction), and if the direct effects predominate, a prolongation of the P-R interval (slowing of AV conduction). If the indirect (antivagal) effect happens to dominate, a decreased P-R interval may be observed. The effects of procainamide on the ECG are very similar to those of quinidine. With both drugs, prolongation of the QRS interval by more than 30% is associated with an increased incidence of drug induced arrhythmias and is avoided by stopping or decreasing the dosage.

The ECG effects of propranolol differ from those of quinidine and procainamide because AV conduction is uniformly depressed by propranolol and the ventricular action potential is not prolonged at low doses. Therefore propranolol consistently prolongs the P-R interval but has little effect on the QT interval.

The effects of lidocaine and phenytoin on the ECG are quite similar. Neither drug has notable effects on the ECG of normal sinus rhythm when given in low doses. In ventricular tachycardia, on the other hand, a reduction in the ectopic rate or conversion to normal sinus rhythm may be expected. In some cases of depressed AV or intraventricular conduction, these agents may improve conduction and thereby normalize the ECG.

CLINICAL USE OF THE ANTIARRHYTHMIC DRUGS

As noted previously, antiarrhythmic drugs are only one of several modes of treating arrhythmias. In selecting a specific antiarrhythmic drug, the following guidelines are usually followed: Quinidine remains the drug of choice in atrial arrhythmias other than those caused by digitalis. Quinidine is also used chronically to prevent recurrence of ventricular arrhythmias after conversion to normal rhythm since it is orally effective.

Procainamide is useful for chronic therapy in those patients who do not respond well or cannot tolerate quinidine. It is also recommended for the treatment of lidocaine-resistant arrhythmias following myocardial infarction.

Lidocaine is the most popular agent for the management of acute ventricular arrhythmias, especially those due to myocardial infarction. Since it must be given parenterally, it is used almost exclusively in hospitalized patients.

Propranolol is only occasionally used because of the hazard of excessive cardiac depression. However, it is extremely effective in controlling ventricular rate in the presence of very high atrial rates owing to its ability to depress AV conduction.

Phenytoin is still considered an investigational antiarrhythmic drug. Therefore, it is reserved for those arrhythmias which are refractory to all other therapies. For the same reason, its use as an antiarrhythmic is usually restricted to hospitalized patients.

INTERACTIONS ENCOUNTERED IN THE USE OF ANTIARRHYTHMIC DRUGS. Quinidine and

procainamide are organic bases excreted primarily in the urine. Therefore they are removed more rapidly from the body when the urine is acid than when it is alkaline. The phenothiazine tranquilizers and droperidol, a haloperidol derivative, have quinidine-like effects (Ch. 25). Therefore, patients receiving any of these agents should be started with smaller doses of the antiarrhythmic drugs. Quinidine may increase the effects of oral anticoagulants like warfarin (Ch. 40), therefore prothrombin levels should be monitored carefully in patients receiving both drugs.

Propranolol, because of its β-adrenergic receptor blocking effects, predictably interacts with β adrenergic stimulants (Chs. 18,19).

Phenytoin when used chronically accelerates the metabolism of some drugs by the liver. Conversely, isoniazid (INH) has been reported to interfere with the hepatic metabolism of phenytoin. Large doses of phenytoin have been reported to displace coumarin type anticoagulants from plasma protein binding sites.

Finally, most of the antiarrhythmic drugs, including lidocaine, have two interactions in common. First, their depressant actions on both electrical and mechanical functions of the heart are increased when serum potassium is high (greater than 5 mEq/liter). Second, all of these agents are capable of augmenting or prolonging the skeletal muscle paralysis produced by neuromuscular blocking drugs like d-tubocurarine, and succinylcholine (Ch. 21).

FURTHER READING

Gettes LS (1971): The electrophysiologic effects of antiarrhythmic drugs. Am J Cardiol 28:526–535

Mason DT, Spann JF, Zelis R, Amsterdam EA (1970): The clinical pharmacology and therapeutic applications of the antiarrhythmic drugs. Clin Pharmacol Ther 11:460–480

Rosen MR, Hoffman BF (1973): Mechanisms of action of antiarrhythmic drugs. Circ Res 32:1–8

JOHN A. BEVAN

35. ANTIANGINAL AND VASODILATOR DRUGS

In some diseases of the blood vessels, the blood flow and, in consequence, the oxygen supply of certain organs or regions of the body becomes inadequate. Cellular vitality is threatened and serious symptoms and signs occur. In the absence of any therapy specific to the disease process, the condition may be ameliorated pharmacologically in two ways: 1) blood flow to the deprived tissues may be increased by the use of a vasodilator drug, or 2) the metabolic requirements of the cells supplied by the diseased vascular bed may be reduced. Drugs that act by both mechanisms are described in this chapter.

The most important group of drugs described in this chapter, the **nitrites,** are effective in the treatment of angina pectoris, a condition resulting from inadequate myocardial oxygenation. They are effective because they reduce the oxygen demands of the heart. The β adrenergic receptor blocking agent **propranolol** is helpful in angina because it reduces myocardial oxygen re-

quirements and, at the same time, increases coronary blood flow to diseased or ischemic parts of the myocardium. Other vasodilator agents, e.g., the **alpha adrenergic receptor blocking agents,** increase local blood flow by decreasing effective peripheral neurogenic resistance in some vascular beds.

The flow of blood through vessels that run on or near the surface of the heart is little affected by pressure changes within the heart itself. In contrast, blood flow through those vessels that ramify within the heart muscle, especially those subjacent to the endocardium, is greatly influenced by pressure in the ventricle and within the myocardial wall. Flow during systole is small and most occurs during diastole and is related to the difference between diastolic aortic pressure and diastolic intramyocardial pressure. It is the flow in this system that is jeopardized in angina pectoris and which must be increased relative to the needs of the heart by therapy.

NITRITES

A group of inorganic and organic nitrites and organic (but not inorganic) nitrates is known that share qualitatively similar pharmacologic properties: the ability to relax all smooth muscle, particularly vascular. They dilate both resistance and capacitance blood vessels. The various nitrites and nitrates differ only in their rate of onset, duration of action, potency and mode of administration.

Actions

Nitrites relax smooth muscle. This effect is termed "direct" since it is not dependent upon muscle innervation and is not mediated via known types (adrenergic, cholinergic and histaminergic) of pharmacologic receptors. The ni-

trites act as physiologic antagonists to all drugs and nervous influences that increase smooth muscle tone. Fortunately, not all smooth muscle is equally sensitive to nitrites. Doses can be given that reduce the tone of certain regional vascular beds without significantly affecting others.

The most important consequences of the smooth muscle relaxant properties of the nitrites are on the cardiovascular system. The tone of the muscle in the resistance and capacitance vessels is reduced. The consequence of this on the circulation as a whole varies widely and depends not only upon the dose, preparation and rate of administration of the drug but on the patient's compensatory capacity and developed tolerance to the drug. Venous dilation results in decreased venous return, with subsequent reduction in the filling of the heart and in stroke volume. This effect combined with the reduction in arteriolar resistance caused by the nitrites leads to a fall in systemic arterial pressure and activation of compensatory arterial baroreceptor reflexes.

When for example, amyl nitrite is given to the young adult, the heart rate increases and both systolic and diastolic arterial pressures fall. The fall in diastolic pressure reflects the change in total peripheral resistance which occurs mainly in the coronary, cerebral (including meningeal and retinal) and skin vessels. The fall in systolic pressure is the result of the increase in venous capacity and the consequent decrease in venous return. Tachycardia is a compensatory mechanism. The effect of these drugs on the circulation is more pronounced in the vertical than in the horizontal position. Thus the final response to the drug is the net result of many interacting primary and compensatory factors.

Myocardial oxygen consumption is related to cardiac work. The primary effects of the nitrite, decrease in heart size, systolic pressure and subsequently contractility would tend to decrease myocardial oxygen consumption: the reflex sympathetically mediated baroreceptor changes would increase heart rate and contractility leading to an increase in heart oxygen needs.

In addition, the smooth muscle of the bronchi and the gastrointestinal tract, in particular the biliary tract, is relaxed.

Preparations and Dosage

Many preparations are available (Fig. 35–1). Some representative ones are described below in order of decreasing rate of onset and increasing duration of action. Nitrites are explosive and for safety are made up into large bulky tablets with a large amount of excipient.

Amyl Nitrite, *N.F.,* is inflammable and volatile. It is prepared in glass pearls that are crushed and the contents inhaled. It acts within 5–15 sec and lasts for 5–10 min. The dose is 0.1–0.3 ml by inhalation.

Glyceryl Trinitrate, *U.S.P.* (nitroglycerin, trinitrin TNG), is usually administered as a sublingual tablet, since it is well absorbed through the buccal mucosa. It is the drug of choice for the treatment of an anginal attack. Latency of action is 1–2 min; effects last up to 30 min. The dose is 0.2–0.6 mg, sublingually. For maximum rapidity of action the tablet may be crushed between the teeth and flushed around the buccal cavity with the tongue. The drug is less effective when swallowed, since after absorption it must pass through the liver before reaching its site of action.

Sodium Nitrite, *U.S.P.,* is taken orally. It is effective within 5–20 min, and its action is main-

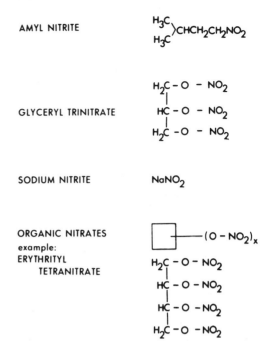

FIG. 35–1. Some representative nitrites.

tained for 1–2 hr. Because of its toxicity (see below), it is rarely used except in the treatment of cyanide poisoning.

Organic nitrates (erythrityl tetranitrate, isosorbide dinitrate, mannitol hexanitrate, pentaerythritol tetranitrate and trolnitrate) are complex organic molecules containing 4–6 nitrate groups. Their effects are slow in onset but persist for 3–4 hours. There is little reason for selecting one over another. All are administered sublingually, except pentaerthritol tetranitrate, which is swallowed.

Uses and Effectiveness

USE IN ANGINA PECTORIS. The pain of angina pectoris is one of ischemia resulting from a relative hypoxia of the myocardium. It is usually associated with coronary artery disease, mainly coronary atherosclerosis. An atheromatous lesion in a large coronary artery is equivalent to a constant narrowing of the blood vessel. This constriction tends to dominate the resistance pattern of the vessel so that flow is not controlled by changes in arteriolar diameter. Consequently adaptation of the vascular bed to extremes of changes in aortic pressure (perfusion pressure) is poor. Pathologic constriction of a larger coronary vessel results over the long term in collateral vessel growth and changes in the overall pattern of blood flow; an area of myocardium receiving its blood supply through a comparatively normal artery may be linked to a poorly vascularized area. One consequence is that the heart is not uniformly vascularized and some parts, e.g., those at rest receiving only a marginal supply might during stress "steal" blood from a normally vascularized section. This hypoxia can be diminished either by increasing blood flow to the ischemic areas or by decreasing the myocardial oxygen requirements of the heart muscle.

Nitrites are used to abort or shorten an impending anginal attack and to prevent or reduce the incidence of attacks. Especially in patients where compensatory changes are not brisk, nitrites decrease oxygen requirements of the heart, i.e., the work done by the heart mainly by reducing ventricular volume and systolic arterial pressure. Many of the factors influencing coronary blood flow are affected by the nitrites. However, in most studies nitrites have been found to cause little change in net total coronary flow. There is evidence, however, because of redistribution effects regional flow through ischemic areas are improved.

The effectiveness of nitrites is obviously dependent on dose. If the noncardiac systemic actions of the nitrites lower aortic pressure too much, many of the advantageous actions of the nitrites are offset by a reduction in coronary perfusion pressure and hence flow. The optimum compromise must be achieved. In practice this depends upon the dose used and the timing of its administration. These are usually worked out by the patient by a process of trial and error. However, since adequacy of treatment is to a great extent in the hands of the patient, he must be well instructed in the objectives of therapy.

Amyl nitrite, taken by inhalation of its vapors from a crushed glass ampoule, or glyceryl trinitrate, chewed and then washed by the tongue over the buccal mucosa, dramatically relieves anginal pain. When taken during the prodromal symptoms or immediately before conditions known to precipitate angina (e.g., exercise), the nitrites may abort an attack. Some patients prefer isosorbide administered sublingually. These preparations are effective and tolerance rarely develops.

Opinion is divided over the value of the long term administration of long acting organic nitrates in the prevention of anginal attacks. It is sufficient to state that well designed clinical trials do not give consistent results.

OTHER USES. Nitrites have been used to relieve spasm of the gastrointestinal tract, in particular **biliary spasm,** to relieve **urinary spasm** and on rare occasions for the relief of **asthma.**

TOLERANCE AND CONTRAINDICATIONS. Prolonged administration leads to tolerance, although tolerance to the adverse effects usually develops before that to the therapeutically useful actions. The original sensitivity returns rapidly when the drug is withheld. Cross tolerance between preparations is not absolute. Nitrites are contraindicated in the acute treatment of myocardial infarction.

Adverse Effects

FAINTING. Particularly in the hypertensive patient and during warm weather, the response to nitrites may be exaggerated or prolonged. The patient faints or exhibits prolonged hypotension. These effects may be looked upon as an exaggeration of the therapeutically useful actions of the drug in a poorly adapting circulation. With practice, however, most patients learn to adjust dosage to their individual needs and circumstances.

HEADACHE. Nitrites may cause a painful throbbing headache associated with the dilation of cerebral or meningeal vessels and an increase in cerebrospinal pressure (Ch. 19, under Migraine). Tolerance to this frequently develops before that to the cardiovascular effects.

METHEMOGLOBINEMIA. Nitrites oxidize the ferrous iron of hemoglobin to the ferric form. The resultant pigment is chocolate brown in color and does not carry oxygen. A functional anemia results.

In cyanide poisoning, cyanide reacts with cellular cytochrome oxidase inhibiting cellular respiration. Cyanide also reacts with methemoglobin, and in the presence of the latter substance, the cytochrome oxidase-cyanide complex dissociates and forms cyanomethemoglobin, restoring cellular respiration. Since sodium nitrite effectively forms methemoglobin, it is given intravenously in cyanide poisoning. It is claimed that this treatment will protect against several lethal doses of cyanide.

PROPRANOLOL

β-Adrenergic receptor blocking agents, in particular propranolol, are now established as part of the pharmacologic armamentarium for the therapy of angina pectoris. Only those features of the action of this drug related to the treatment of angina are described here (Chs. 19, 20).

Actions

Blockade of tonic sympathetic activity to the heart results in a negative inotropic and chronotropic effect reducing oxygen requirements. The augmentation of myocardial activity during stress or exercise is minimized by propranolol. The effect of blockade of the β-adrenergic receptors on the coronary vasculature are complex and are considered to vary with the size of the vessels. However, propranolol is believed to alter the distribution of coronary blood flow within the heart resulting in an improvement of flow to ischemic areas.

Dosage and Administration

Propranolol is usually indicated in patients with angina pectoris due to coronary artery disease who take nitrites daily. It reduces the number of times the patient will need to take the nitrite and lowers the effective dose. The dosage of propranolol varies widely and must be determined in each patient. The drug is usually contraindicated in the treatment of the failing myocardium, since it reduces compensatory supportive sympathetic drive, and thus exacerbates the underlying condition. It also depresses atrioventricular conduction and this limits its use in any condition complicated by some degree of atrioventricular block. Other general considerations are discussed in Chapter 19.

OTHER DRUGS USED IN ANGINA PECTORIS

Many agents have a reputation as effective coronary vasodilators and in consequence are used in the treatment of angina pectoris. These are either ineffective or their effectiveness awaits complete evaluation. In the former group are ethyl alcohol, nicotinic acid, nicotinyl tartrate, theophylline derivatives, androgens and vitamin E; in the latter group are dipyridamole (Persantin) and antithyroid agents.

VASODILATOR DRUGS

α-ADRENERGIC BLOCKING AGENTS

α-Receptors are predominant in the cutaneous vasculature, and the effect of tonic sympathetic neurogenic activity on this part of the circulation may be inhibited by α-adrenergic blocking agents (Ch. 19). Although these agents are of considerable scientific interest, their clinical usefulness is essentially restricted to the treatment of vascular insufficiency of the limbs, particularly the skin. **Tolazoline** (Priscoline), **phentolamine** (Regitine) and **azapetine** (Ilidar) have all been used. These drugs exhibit some additional direct vasodilator properties.

β-ADRENERGIC STIMULATING AGENTS

β-Receptors are preponderant in the vascular bed of skeletal muscles. Although the flow through this bed is regulated in the most part by the metabolic products of muscular exercise, β stimulating agents are used to treat conditions of reduced blood flow. **Isoxsuprine hydrochloride** and **nylidrin hydrochloride,** the best known in this class, are similar in action to isoproterenol but are orally active and have a longer duration of action (Ch. 18). The evidence is not conclusive that these are of clinical value in the acute stage of the disorder. Their long term administration may hinder its rate of progress.

PAPAVERINE

Papaverine is an alkaloid from opium which relaxes vascular muscle, especially muscle in spasm. It is said to inhibit phosphodiesterase, the enzyme involved in the breakdown of cyclic AMP. This in turn is related to the active dilation of the blood vessel wall (Chs. 18, 32). It is used to overcome or relieve spasm of collateral vessels after embolization in the limbs and in the pulmonary circulation, and primary spasm in pulmonary and cerebral vessels.

Hepatic hypersensitivity and a quinidine-like action on the heart are among the reported adverse effects.

FURTHER READING

Braunwald E (1969): Determinance of myocardial oxygen consumption. (13th Bowditch Lecture) Physiologist 12:65–93

Gorlin R (1962): Drugs and angina pectoris. Am J Cardiol 9:419

Melville KI (1970): The Pharmacological basis of antianginal drugs. Pharmacol Physicians 4:1

Winbury WM (1967): Problems in Laboratory Evaluation of Antianginal Agents. Amsterdam, North Holland Publishing

Wolfson S, Gorlin R (1969): Cardiovascular pharmacology of propranolol in man. Circulation 40:501–511

JOHN P. KANE

36. DRUGS USED IN THE TREATMENT OF HYPERLIPIDEMIA

Hyperlipidemia may be defined as a pathologic elevation of content of one or more of the macromolecular complexes of lipid and protein (lipoproteins) of plasma. This is reflected by an elevation of the level in plasma of either cholesterol or triglycerides or both. The clinical importance of hyperlipidemia derives from its repeated identification as one of the most important epidemiologic risk factors for accelerated development of atherosclerosis, most notably, coronary artery disease. Definitive analysis of the effect that normalizing blood lipoprotein levels will have on the rate of atherogenesis must await primary (before the advent of overt arterial disease) intervention studies of long duration. However, the results of several more brief dietary and drug intervention studies indicate that a significant reduction of morbidity or of mortality from coronary vascular disease may be realized by such therapy.

Since hyperlipidemia in man occurs in a number of phenotypic forms which display highly individual responses to therapy, understanding of the fundamentals of the biochemistry of lipoproteins is essential to definitive diagnosis and the selection of a rational therapeutic regimen.

PLASMA LIPOPROTEINS

Essentially all of the lipids of human plasma are bound noncovalently to protein. With the exception of free (unesterified) fatty acids which bind to albumin, they are organized into lipoprotein complexes of large molecular weight containing specific apoproteins. Plasma lipoproteins may be studied analytically either by electrophoresis or by ultracentrifugation, thus, leading to a double nomenclature. Some biochemical characteristics of the principal classes of human plasma lipoproteins are presented in Table 36–1.

Exogenous (dietary) triglyceride is transported in chylomicrons in the lymphatic system from the intestine, ultimately entering the bloodstream via the thoracic duct. Endogenous triglycerides (synthesized within the body) enter the blood, largely from liver, in very low density (pre β) lipoproteins (VLDL). The triglycerides of both these complexes yield fatty acids for utilization or storage in peripheral tissues such as striated muscle, myocardium and adipose tissue after hydrolysis by the **lipoprotein lipase** enzyme system. This enzyme, resident on the capillary endothelium, is capable of hydrolysis of much of the triglyceride content of these lipoproteins. At the same time certain apoproteins of small molecular weight are transferred to high density lipoproteins (HDL). The remaining triglyceride-containing particle, ("remnant particle") is further catabolized by liver, with the production of low density (β) lipoprotein (LDL). Both LDL and HDL appear to have roles in the transport of cholesterol in plasma.

CLINICAL TYPES OF HYPERLIPIDEMIA

The most meaningful schema for classification of disorders of lipoprotein metabolism is based on the class(es) of plasma lipoproteins which are abnormally elevated. Each phenotypic pattern can arise as a primary genetic abnormality or as the result of some other pathologic process (secondary hyperlipidemia). Before consideration of therapy, this distinction must be made, as treatment of the underlying disorder if possible, is indicated in secondary hyperlipide-

TABLE 36-1. Human Plasma Lipoproteins

Electrophoretic mobility	Ultracentrifugal designation	Principal lipids in quantitative order	Approximate diameter (nm)
α_1	High density lipoprotein (HDL)	Cholesterol Phospholipid	8—10
β	Low density lipoprotein (LDL)	Cholesterol Phospholipid	21
Preβ	Very low density lipoprotein (VLDL)	Triglyceride Cholesterol Phospholipid	30—100
No mobility in most systems	Chylomicrons (normally absent from plasma after an overnight fast)	Triglyceride Phospholipid Cholesterol	>100

mia. A nomenclature for the common phenotypic patterns, proposed by the WHO, employing Roman numerals, is indicated in parentheses.

HYPER-β-LIPOPROTEINEMIA (IIA)

This disorder is characterized by elevated plasma levels of LDL (β lipoprotein), and consequently of cholesterol. Forms with moderate elevation of LDL exist which are often responsive to dietary therapy alone. A more severe form, transmitted as a Mendelian dominant, may be accompanied by accumulation of cholesteryl esters in tendons (tendon xanthomata). Hyper-β-lipoproteinemia is generally associated with a significantly increased risk of coronary vascular disease and persons homozygous for this gene are especially severely affected. Major causes of secondary hyperlipidemia presenting with this phenotypic pattern are hypothyroidism and early nephrosis.

HYPERPRE-β-LIPOPROTEINEMIA (IV)

This disorder is characterized by elevations of VLDL (pre-β-lipoprotein) in plasma. Thus, triglyceride levels are increased and the level of cholesterol will be elevated as well if the abnormality is severe, due to the cholesterol content of this class of lipoprotein. The large molecular complexes scatter light, giving a milky appearance to the serum (lipemia). This disorder, too, is associated with an increased risk of coronary vascular disease. Obesity, impaired glucose tolerance and hyperuricemia are frequently present in these patients. Among the more common causes of secondary hyperpre-β-lipoproteinemia are uncontrolled diabetes mellitus, advanced nephrosis and alcohol abuse. Eruptive xanthomata of the skin may be present when lipemia is severe.

COMBINED HYPERLIPIDEMIA (IIB)

This phenotype is characterized by elevations of both LDL and VLDL in plasma. An increased risk of coronary disease is associated with this abnormality and familial aggregation has been demonstrated.

DYS-β-LIPOPROTEINEMIA (III)

In this phenotype an abnormal lipoprotein resembling a "remnant" particle, is present. Characteristically cholesterol and triglyceride levels are elevated to approximately the same extent. There is an increased risk of both coronary and peripheral atherosclerosis. Obesity and abnormal glucose tolerance are frequently present and palmar xanthomata may be observed.

MIXED LIPEMIA (V)

In this phenotype both VLDL and chylomicrons are present in excess in blood drawn after an overnight fast. Thus, triglyceride levels are elevated and a supernatant chylomicron layer will be observed after serum has been refrigerated for a day. Cholesterol levels will usually be increased if the triglyceride levels are markedly elevated. Life threatening attacks of **acute pancreatitis** may occur when levels of triglycerides are very high. Secondary forms occur as with hyperpre-β-lipoproteinemia.

CHYLOMICRONEMIA (I)

This disorder, an increase predominantly of chylomicrons, is associated with extremely high levels of triglycerides and moderate increases in levels of cholesterol in plasma. This rare phenotype is usually due to a genetic deficiency of lipoprotein lipase, transmitted as a Mendelian recessive. As in other forms of severe hypertriglyceridemia this disorder is associated with the risk of acute pancreatitis.

Having excluded secondary hyperlipidemia, the first therapeutic effort of the physician is always directed at diet. With two exceptions a single dietary regimen appears to suffice. This entails caloric restriction to achieve normal body weight, reduction of dietary cholesterol to 300 mg/day, and restriction of saturated fats to 20% of calories. Strict interdiction of alcohol is indicated in hypertriglyceridemia. Polyunsaturated fats may be used, in moderation, to increase palatability. Exceptions are primary chylomicronemia, in which total dietary fat is restricted to a functional minimum, and the hypertriglyceridemic patient with incipient pancreatitis where oral intake is replaced by glucose given IV, to be followed later by a fat restricted diet. In a large percentage of cases, mild hyper-β-lipoproteinemia will respond to diet alone. Triglyceride levels will return toward normal in the majority of patients with endogenous lipemia if body weight is normalized and no alcohol is taken.

Drug treatment of hyperlipidemia is indicated only after a well supervised dietary regimen fails to produce satisfactory reduction of lipoprotein levels. It is important that dietary management be continued during drug treatment. With the exception of patients homozygous for hyper-β-lipoproteinemia the drug treatment of children with hyperlipidemia should be regarded as investigational at this time. In all cases plasma lipid levels must be measured at regular intervals whenever a patient is on a treatment regimen.

DRUGS USED IN TREATMENT OF HYPER-β-LIPOPROTEINEMIA

Bile Acid Binding Resins

MECHANISM OF ACTION. These agents are high molecular weight cationic polymers which have high binding affinity for bile acids. Taken orally, they are not absorbed from the intestine and their metabolic effects appear to result entirely from sequestration of bile acids in the intestinal lumen. Normally about 98% of the bile acid presented to the intestine is reabsorbed, to be excreted again in bile, the so-called enterohepatic circulation of bile acids. In the absence of sequestration about 0.5 g of bile acids are lost in the stool per day. Because depletion of the bile acid pool relieves feedback inhibition of bile acids on the conversion of cholesterol to bile acid in liver, the synthesis of bile acids is increased when sequestrating agents are employed. The daily excretion of bile acids may increase as much as 15-fold while fecal loss of cholesterol is only minimally increased.

The degree to which this effect can induce negative cholesterol balance is sharply limited by increased cholesterol biosynthesis in both liver and gut. The plasma cholesterol level usually declines rapidly during the first 2–3 weeks of therapy and may decrease more slowly for up to a year following the initial fall, usually reaching values 20–40% below pretreatment levels. The decrease of plasma cholesterol levels is attributable almost exclusively to reduction of the content of LDL in plasma. Plasma cholesterol content returns to pretreatment levels within 3 weeks following cessation of therapy.

CLINICAL USE. Bile acid binding resins appear to be the treatment of choice for those disorders in which elevated levels of LDL occur. These agents may be added to the treatment regimen in hyperpre-β-lipoproteinemia in those cases in which levels of LDL increase as pre-β-lipoprotein levels decline in response to dietary or drug management. Bile acid binding resins alone have very limited effectiveness in homozygous hyper-β-lipoproteinemia, however the addition of nicotinic acid (see below) to the regimen may achieve a significant reduction of LDL levels.

PREPARATIONS AND DOSAGE. Cholestyramine *U.S.P.* and **Colestipol** come in the form of granules, in packets of 4 and 5 g, respectively. The usual starting dose is 16–20 g/day in 3 doses, with meals. The therapeutic effect usually increases with dose. While most patients are managed with 24–25 g daily some can tolerate up to 32 g, under close supervision. Patients should be encouraged to mix the granules in fruit juice or other fluid and semifluid foods to increase palatability.

TOXICITY. With a few rare exceptions toxicity is limited to symptoms of gastroenteric irritation, constipation and malabsorption of fat soluble substances. Patients may at first complain of gastric irritation or bloating but these symptoms usually subside, especially if the medication is taken with meals. Magnesium oxide may be given to relieve constipation. Malabsorption of fat soluble vitamins is virtually never encountered with daily doses of 24 g or less. Appropriate vitamin supplementation should be given at higher doses of resin and special attention should be paid to vitamin K intake in subjects receiving coumarin or indandione-type anticoagulants. Hypoprothrombinemia has been encountered in the presence of biliary cirrhosis and preexisting intestinal disease. Steatorrhea which is negligible in most individuals receiving up to 24 g/day, may be severe in patients with underlying intestinal pathology.

DRUG BINDING. The absorption of some drugs can be seriously reduced in the presence of these resins. Binding is not due to the ionic charge of the drugs alone, as the absorption of some apolar or even cationic agents may be affected. Among the most important drugs affected are thyroxin, warfarin and digitalis glycosides. In general these agents may be given successfully if they are taken 1 hr before the morning dose of resin and the effect is monitored closely. Since the resins have a moderate binding affinity for tetracyclines similar interference may be expected with these agents.

Nicotinic Acid

MECHANISM OF ACTION. The mechanisms by which nicotinic acid influences circulating lipoproteins remain obscure, however in many subjects plasma levels of both VLDL and LDL are reduced. The carboxyl group is apparently required for activity as nicotinamide has little effect on lipid metabolism. Nicotinic acid and

NICOTINIC ACID

certain of its congeners acutely inhibit the hydrolysis of triglycerides by the intracellular or hormone sensitive lipase of adipose tissue, resulting in decreased levels of free fatty acids (FFA) in plasma. The reduced flux to liver of FFA, which is the principal precursor of the triglyceride fatty acids of VLDL may contribute to decreased secretion of that lipoprotein into plasma. However, convincing evidence that chronic treatment with nicotinic acid results in sustained reduction of FFA levels in plasma is lacking.

CLINICAL USE. Individual variation in response of LDL levels in patients with hyperbetalipoproteinemia is great, however the average reduction in plasma cholesterol levels is from 20–30%. Nicotinic acid is thus generally somewhat less effective in reducing plasma levels of LDL than bile acid sequestrants but its use is indicated in those individuals in whom the resins are not tolerated well, or in addition to resin in patients who do not have a satisfactory response to the resin alone.

PREPARATIONS AND DOSAGE. Niacin, *N.F.* is available in tablets of 0.1, 0.5 and 1.0 g. Treatment is usually initiated with 3 g daily divided into 3 doses, given with meals. The daily dose may then be increased by 0.5 g each month up to a maximum of 9 g. Whereas most patients experience little gastric irritation at a daily dose of 3 g, nausea may limit the dose at some point below the maximum dosage. A satisfactory clinical response is often achieved with doses between 4 and 7 g. Unabsorbable antacids should be given when gastric irritation is present.

TOXICITY. Biochemical evidence of hepatic parenchymal dysfunction in the form of elevated serum glutamic-oxaloacetic and glutamic-pyruvic transaminase and, less commonly, alkaline phosphatase levels, may be present. These changes are reversible upon discontinuance of the drug. Abnormal retention of bromsulfalein may also be observed. Bilirubin levels are usually normal and no consistent abnormality of hepatic histology is present. The frequency of occurrence of abnormalities of hepatic function appears to be greater in patients receiving aluminum nicotinate.

Mild hyperglycemia is frequently encountered and also appears to be reversible. Patients with latent or overt diabetes mellitus may develop additional requirements for insulin or other hypoglycemic agents, which may not diminish upon cessation of therapy with nicotinic acid. Transient hyperuricemia may occur during the first few weeks of treatment.

ADVERSE EFFECTS. All patients at first experience acute cutaneous vasodilatation, especially of the face and upper thorax, shortly after taking a dose of nicotinic acid. The intensity of this symptom diminishes rapidly over the first few weeks of therapy and it is seldom intolerable to patients. Many patients experience nausea, as noted above, which is often relieved by antacids. Nicotinic acid may potentiate the effect of gangioplegic agents on blood pressure.

Other Agents

CLOFIBRATE (ETHYL CHLORPHENOXYISOBU-TYRATE). This agent which will be discussed in the section on treatment of hypertriglyceridemia is largely ineffective in severe forms of hyper-β-lipoproteinemia. However, an average reduction of plasma cholesterol levels of approximately 15% has been observed in patients with mild hyperbetalipoproteinemia.

***d*-THYROXIN (SODIUM *d*-THYROXIN,** *N.F.*). This agent is thought to effect a reduction in levels of LDL by increasing cholesterol catabolism to bile acids in liver as does *l*-thyroxin. While the effect of *d*-thyroxin on metabolic rate is much less than that of its natural isomer, some hypercalorigenic effect apparently is retained, even in preparations essentially free of the *l*-form. It is employed in an initial daily dose of 2 mg which is increased by 1 or 2 mg/month to a maximum of 8 mg/day. Reduction of plasma cholesterol levels is usually modest.

This agent potentiates the action of coumarin or indandione-type anticoagulants. The use of *d*-thyroxin is contraindicated in patients with coronary vascular disease because of increased risk of ventricular arrhythmia. Glucose intolerance, abnormal hepatic parenchymal function and neutropenia have each occurred during treatment with *d*-thyroxin.

ESTROGEN. Estrogens formerly enjoyed wide use in an attempt to prevent the development or progression of atherosclerotic heart disease. They were prescribed on the assumption that the slower development of coronary disease in premenopausal women must be attributable to these hormones. Recent secondary intervention studies have indicated, rather, an increased risk of coronary disease in men receiving estrogen. These agents appear to increase the risk of thromboembolism and in addition, induce significant increases in VLDL levels and decreased carbohydrate tolerance in certain individuals. There appears to be no role for estrogens in the management of hyperlipidemia.

DRUGS USED FOR HYPERTRIGLYCERIDEMIA

Dysbetalipoproteinemia

This disorder usually responds very well to dietary management, however if the patient cannot adhere to the diet, the addition of clofibrate (see below) will virtually always achieve a dramatic reduction of lipid levels.

Hyperpre-β-lipoproteinemia

CLOFIBRATE. This drug is the ethyl ester of parachlorophenoxyisobutyric acid. The ester bond is hydrolyzed in plasma and body tissues to

CLOFIBRATE

yield the free anion which is bound to proteins, principally albumin. It has a half-life of 12 hr and is largely excreted in urine, principally as the glucuronide.

MECHANISMS OF ACTION. Clofibrate induces a fall in plasma triglyceride levels over a period of 2–5 days, reflecting a decline in the level of

VLDL. Evidence has been adduced in support of several mechanisms of action, however the most important would appear to be an increase in the catabolic rate for VLDL. Clofibrate also decreases cholesterol synthesis, increases the conversion of FFA to ketoacids in liver and increases the excretion of cholesterol from the gut.

CLINICAL USE. Clofibrate therapy is indicated when elevated VLDL levels do not respond to diet. In a significant number of subjects a fall in VLDL levels will be accompanied by an **increase** of LDL, a catabolic product of VLDL. This phenomenon, the so-called "β shift", is to be found where the triglyceride level declines in response to the drug but plasma cholesterol levels remain at approximately the pretreatment value. Subjects showing this phenomenon should either be treated with nicotinic acid, or a bile acid binding resin should be added to the therapeutic regimen to decrease LDL levels.

PREPARATIONS AND DOSAGE. Clofibrate is available in capsules of 0.5 g. The usual dose is 1 g twice daily.

TOXICITY. Rarely, a syndrome of myopathy with elevated levels of creatine phosphokinase and glutamic-oxaloacetic transaminase has been described. Skin eruptions, abnormalities of liver function and cardiac arrhythmias occur infrequently. Some patients experience nausea or diarrhea. Clofibrate potentiates the action of sodium warfarin, presumably by competitive binding to albumin. The dosage of the anticoagulant should be reduced by one-third to one-half when initiating therapy with clofibrate until the appropriate dose for the individual is determined by repeated measurement of prothrombin time. Small but significant increases in the risk of developing thromboembolic disease or cholelithiasis are associated with long-term therapy with clofibrate. Therapy with clofibrate is contraindicated in uremia unless blood levels of the drug can be monitored.

Nicotinic Acid

This agent (see above) frequently produces significant reduction in both VLDL and LDL levels.

TREATMENT OF MIXED LIPEMIA

The response to clofibrate is usually of smaller magnitude than in hyperpre-β-lipoproteinemia whereas nicotinic acid (see p. 283) frequently effects a significant reduction of triglyceride levels. The progestational agent norethindrone acetate (Ch. 48) at a daily dose of 5 mg has been reported to reduce triglyceride levels in women with mixed lipemia.

FURTHER READING

Casdorph MR (ed.) (1971): Treatment of the Hyperlipidemic States. Springfield, Charles C Thomas

Fredrickson DS, Levy RI (1972): Familial hyperlipoproteinemia in The Metabolic Basis of Inherited Disease. 3rd ed. Stanbury JB, Wyngaarden JB, Fredrickson DS, (eds) New York, McGraw Hill, pp. 545–614

Havel RJ, Kane JP (1973): Drugs and lipid metabolism. Annu Rev Pharmacol 13:287

Levy RI, Fredrickson DS, Shulman R, Bilheimer DW, Breslow JL, Stone NJ, Lux SE, Sloan HR, Krauss RM, Herbert PN (1972): Dietary and drug treatment of primary hyperlipoproteinemia. Ann Intern Med 77:267

DRUGS ACTING ON THE GASTROINTESTINAL, RENAL, AND HEMATOPOIETIC SYSTEMS

JEREMY H. THOMPSON

37. DRUGS AFFECTING THE GASTROINTESTINAL SYSTEM

Drugs that affect the gastrointestinal tract act mainly on its muscular and glandular tissues, either directly, or indirectly by way of the autonomic nervous system. Discussion of these drugs is best accomplished by grouping them according to therapeutic indications.

DRUGS AFFECTING APPETITE

Stimulants

Many drugs, mostly alkaloidal in nature, and with no other property than a bitter taste, are occasionally used to stimulate the appetite. Their small success is due entirely to reflex vagal stimulation. Alcoholic drinks, appetizers and highly spiced hors d'oeuvres are more valuable. Vitamin preparations are worthless except in the rare case of true vitamin deficiency, and thyroid hormones and insulin may be of value in anorexia nervosa.

Suppressants (Anorexiants)

There are many causes of obesity. The anorexiant or anoretic drugs, those that lead to loss of appetite, are commonly used as *adjuncts* in the management of overweight due to excessive calorie consumption. Anorexiants elevate the patients' mood and make them more tolerant of the dietary restrictions. They also suppress the feelings of hunger by an unknown action. Among the proposed mechanisms of action are: stimulation of the satiety center in the medial hypothalamus, blockade of impulses reaching the "eating center" in the lateral hypothalamus and elevation of plasma free fatty acid levels which in turn depress the "eating center." The commonly used anorexiants include the **amphetamine** group of drugs and a multitude of other synthetic sympathomimetic agents, among which **diethylpropion hydrochloride** and **phenmetrazine hydrochloride** are most popular (Ch. 18). Although these drugs are used frequently, they are ineffective over long periods of time and are of no value without conscientious food restriction.

DRUGS AFFECTING THE STOMACH

Carminatives

Carminatives are mild mucosal irritants that relieve discomfort of the stomach due to gaseous distention by relaxing the cardiac sphincter. Aniseed, camphor, cinnamon, ginger, glycyrrhiza (liquorice), peppermint, sarsaparilla, sassafrass and spearmint are commonly used, but are of doubtful value. Liquorice preparations (see below) are primarily used in the treatment of gastric ulcer disease.

Emetics

Many drugs, if taken by mouth in too large a quantity or too concentrated a solution, excite reflex nausea and vomiting. The induction of emesis may be a therapeutic necessity, e.g., in the treatment of a child who has ingested a poison (Ch. 13). **Locally acting and centrally acting** emetics are available. Hypertonic salt solutions (usually sodium chloride) and copper and mustard solutions act locally on account of their osmotic pressure or by virtue of their irritant properties. Derivatives of the opium alkaloids (particularly apomorphine) stimulate vomiting by an action on the brainstem (Ch. 13).

Antiemetics

Antiemetics are used in the control of nausea and vomiting. Vomiting may be dangerous. If not controlled, it can lead to exhaustion of the patient, with dehydration, pH and electrolyte abnormalities, aspiration of vomitus into the tracheobronchial tree and esophago-gastric bleeding or rupture. Nausea and vomiting are only symptoms and should not be treated without the underlying cause being determined. **Phenothiazine compounds** depress the medullary chemoreceptor trigger zone; common examples are chlorpromazine hydrochloride, prochlorperazine maleate and promazine hydrochloride (Ch. 25). The nonphenothiazine drugs in common use are buclizine hydrochloride, diphenhydramine hydrochloride and meclizine hydrochloride (Ch. 49). They act centrally on the eighth nerve and its connections, by virtue of their anticholinergic properties. Some nonphenothiazine, nonanticholinergic antiemetics are available which act on the medullary chemoreceptor trigger zone. **Trimethobenzamide hydrochloride** (Tigan) and **Diphenidol hydrochloride** (Vontrol) are popular.

ADVERSE EFFECTS

Adverse effects of the phenothiazine and nonphenothizaine compounds are discussed elsewhere (Chs. 25, 49). **Trimethobenzamide** may produce drowsiness, headache, diarrhea, muscle cramps, dizziness and alterations of mood. Rarely, hypotension, blurred vision, bone marrow depression, jaundice, convulsions and extrapyramidal symptoms may appear. Trimethobenzamide suppositories contain benzocaine, and may produce hypersensitivity reactions in children sensitive to the local anesthetic. **Diphenidol** may produce nausea, indigestion, headache, nervousness and rarely hypotension; urticaria and various other skin rashes may develop in sensitive patients. It may also produce adverse effects of drowsiness and anticholinergic-like symptoms of xerostomia, blurred vision, urinary retention, increased intraocular tension, visual and auditory hallucinations and confusional states.

Diagnostic Agents

Histamine and betazole hydrochloride (Histalog) are dealt with in Chapter 49 and azuresin in Chapter 70.

Digestants

The digestants are a group of replacement drugs which supply a deficiency of a normal component of gastrointestinal secretion. Once popular, their exact place in therapy is now questionable.

Hydrochloric acid can be supplied in two forms. Diluted hydrochloric acid N.F. (Acidulin) is a 10% solution that should be administered by glass, drinking through a tube or straw to avoid contact with the teeth. **Betaine hydrochloride** (Normacid) is a formulation of 400 mg betaine hydrochloride containing the equivalent of 1.0 ml dilute HCl, 32.4 mg pepsin and 110 mg methylcellulose. The formulation is said to release HCl slowly within the stomach, paralleling the release of acid occurring during digestion. **Pepsin** is commonly supplied as a powder prepared from the oxyntic gland area of the fresh stomach of the hog (Pepsin N.F.). **Dehydrocholic acid N.F.** (Decholin) and **sodium dehydrocolate N.F.** (Decholin sodium) increase the volume of bile secreted (choleresis). It has been suggested that their administration may aid the absorption of fat and fat soluble vitamins in those conditions associated with partial biliary obstruction. Both agents are contraindicated in complete biliary obstruction, and they may aggrevate the pruritis associated with poor bile formation. Sodium dehydrocholic acid is also used in the determination of the arm-to-tongue circulation time in certain conditions where the velocity of blood flow may be altered.

Pancreatic extracts may benefit patients with cystic fibrosis, adult pancreatic insufficiency and selected postgastrectomy syndromes. **Pancreatin N.F.** is a cream-colored, amorphous powder, obtained from the fresh pancreas of the hog or ox, containing amylase, lipase and trypsin. **Pancrelipase** (Cotazym) is a concentrate of ox pancreatic enzymes standardized by lipase content. Some proprietary pancreatic extracts are enriched with bile salts, cellulases, collagenase and elastase. In the rare patient who lacks both bile and pancreatic enzyme secretion, it is more logical to supply each component separately. Since release from enteric-coated tablets is capricious, the extracts should be given with food, milk or alkali in an attempt to buffer the gastric contents thereby reducing enzymic inactivation. Dosage is variable, and treatment should be directed at restoring weight and a feeling of well being, and converting the volume, consistency and odor of stools to normal. Children occasionally develop perianal soreness, and on rare occasions, allergy to the animal-derived protein may be seen. **Choline dihydrogen citrate** (Monichol) may be effective as a lipotropic agent in patients with hepatic cirrhosis.

Chenodeoxycholic Acid

Chenodeoxycholic acid is a primary dihydroxy bile acid under clinical investigation to promote solubilization of cholesterol in bile, and the dissolution of cholesterol-containing gall stones. It may also be of value in reducing serum triglyceride levels in patients with hypertriglyceridemia. Formation of cholesterol gall stones may be related to diminished secretion of bile acids resulting in an abnormal ratio of cholesterol to bile acids in bile. Chenodeoxycholic acid, which is normally secreted along with cholic acid in human bile, has been shown to decrease the degree of saturation of bile with cholesterol, presumably by expanding the bile acid pool size. In addition, it may also decrease the synthesis of cholesterol. Dosage varies from 0.5–4.5 g/day.

Doses of chenodeoxycholic acid greater than 1 g/day saturate the capacity of the ileum to absorb the drug and produce diarrhea. Transient elevations of serum alkaline phosphatase and serum glutamic oxaloacetic acid transaminase activity rarely develop. The exact importance of this alteration in liver function is not clear. Chenodeoxycholic acid undergoes 7-α-dehydroxylation in the colon by bacteria with the formation of lithocholic acid, which, although poorly absorbed in man, is absorbed in animals where it produces hepatic injury—proliferation of the bile ducts and periportal infiltration. The potential long-term effects of chenodeoxycholic acid on cholesterol and triglyceride metabolism, or on the development of atherosclerosis or liver damage is not known.

It is a theoretic possibility that partially solubilized gall stones may migrate, producing acute obstruction. Chenodeoxycholic acid is expensive.

DRUGS FOR PEPTIC ULCER DISEASE

The term peptic ulcer refers to an ulcer in the gullet (esophageal ulcer), the stomach (gastric ulcer) or the duodenum (duodenal ulcer). Although the cause of these different ulcers is unknown, it is generally believed that gastric acid and the gastric proteolytic enzyme, pepsin, are required for the maintenance and persistence of an ulcer, and the dictum "no acid, no ulcer" is still valid for the most part. In the case of gastric ulcer disease, additional etiologic factors are impaired mucosal resistance, bile reflux and acid back-diffusion, whereas in duodenal ulcer disease, an increased number of parietal cells and vagal overactivity resulting in augmented acid production, are more important.

Numerous drugs have been used in the treatment of peptic ulcer disease. A full under-

standing of their mechanism(s) of action and their therapeutic applications will be facilitated by an understanding of normal gastric secretion.

Mechanisms and Control of Gastric Secretion

Gastric juice is a highly complex fluid, but for the purpose of this chapter only hydrochloric acid, pepsin(ogen) and mucosubstances will be discussed.

Hydrochloric Acid

The quantity of gastric acid secreted at any moment is dependent upon the interplay of many stimulatory and inhibitory factors. Classically, gastric acid secretion has been divided into two periods, **interprandial** (interdigestive, basal, spontaneous) and **postprandial** (digestive, stimulated) secretion. Postprandial secretion is further separated into **cephalic, gastric** and **intestinal** phases; this is an artificial division indicating only the region in which a given stimulus acts.

In man, interprandial secretion contains varying amounts of HCl. The cephalic phase of postprandial secretion is mediated via the vagus nerves. Vagal impulses generated by the thought, sight, smell, taste or swallowing of food produce acid release by direct cholinergic stimulation of parietal cells, and indirectly via the release of pyloric gland area gastrin. Gastric secretion in the gastric phase of postprandial secretion has the same two components and is activated by both vagal impulses and vago-vagal reflexes. The intestinal phase of postprandial secretion is mediated via gastrin release from the intestine, but it is relatively unimportant.

Recent evidence suggests that cyclic adenosine 3', 5-monophosphate (cyclic AMP) is the final link in gastrin-induced acid secretion (Ch. 51). Histamine (and related agents) induces copious gastric acid secretion, but there is little conclusive evidence that this autacoid plays a role in normal gastric secretion (Ch. 49).

When the parietal cells are stimulated to secrete, they produce isotonic hydrochloric acid (165 mN) in which the concentration of hydrogen ions is a million times that in the plasma. The mechanism whereby this intense concentration occurs is unknown, but the overall change can be represented as follows:

$$H_2O + CO_2 \xrightarrow{\text{Carbonic Anhydrase}} (H)^+ + (HCO_3)^-$$

The H^+ accompanied by Cl^- is transported into the gastric lumen, and the HCO^- passes to the extracellular fluid where it is balanced by sodium. In the small bowel the H^+ reacts with biliary, intestinal and pancreatic bicarbonate as indicated below, and is absorbed:

$$(H)^+ + (HCO_3)^- \rightarrow H_2O + CO_2$$

Since the second equation is the exact opposite of the first, there is no overall alteration in extracellular pH as a result of gastric acid secretion and its subsequent intestinal absorption. However, if gastric juice is lost from the body by vomiting or by gastric section, metabolic alkalosis results.

Pepsin(ogen)

Pepsinogen, the inactive precursor of the proteolytic enzyme pepsin, has a molecular weight of about 43,000 and is synthesized and stored in the chief cells of the oxyntic gland area. Pepsinogen is composed of pepsin and peptide moieties; the terminal moiety is an inhibitor of proteolytic activity. The pepsin-inhibitor complex dissociates about pH 5.4, but it is not until the pH falls to about 4.0 that the inhibitor is gradually inactivated autocatalytically by digestion, with progressive development of full peptic activity. Pepsin (molecular weight about 35,000) is maximally active about pH 2.0. During the basal state, pepsin stores remain intact, and the small continuous secretion is probably an "overflow" from continued synthesis. The most powerful stimuli to pepsin secretion are vagal stimulation, and histamine and gastrin administration.

Mucosubstances

Gastric mucin is the viscous secretion of the stomach which serves to protect the mucosa. It is a heterogenous secretion derived from the surface epithelium columnar cells, and the mucous neck cells of the cardiac, oxyntic and pyloric gland areas. Secretion of alkaline mucous is spontaneous. It is increased by mechanical irritation of the mucosa, and by sympathetic and parasympathetic nervous system stimulation.

Prevention of Parietal Cell Secretion

Attempts to reduce parietal cell secretion have not been entirely successful. The popular concept that "stress" and emotional and physical factors stimulate HCl secretion via the limbic system and the vagal motor nuclei, prompted the widespread use of **sedatives** and **tranquillizers** in the treatment of duodenal ulcer. While sedatives and tranquillizers may reduce emotional tension and worry, they have little effect on acid secretion. Numerous **antihistamine** preparations have been tested for possible antisecretory activity, but to date, only **burimamide,**

metiamide and **cimetidine,** have been found effective (Ch. 49).

In general, two groups of drugs are capable of reducing parietal cell acid secretion: **carbonic anhydrase inhibitors** and **anticholinergic drugs.** Carbonic anhydrase facilitates hydrochloric acid production, but even potent carbonic anhydrase inhibitors (e.g., acetazolamide, Ch. 30) reduce gastric acidity only slightly, presumably since the enzyme is present in excess. Furthermore, there is a theoretic disadvantage to their use in that they may increase pepsin release. **Anticholinergic drugs** have achieved some popularity in reducing inter- and post-prandial secretion, since these phases are partly under cholinergic control. However, to effectively reduce acid secretion they need to be given in doses that produce symptoms of systemic parasympathetic blockade. Thus, there is no drug that effectively prevents hydrochloric acid secretion at the level of the parietal cell, and the majority of drugs used to reduce gastric acidity are **antacids** which **neutralize, buffer** and **absorb** preformed acid.

Prevention of Pepsin Secretion and Stimulation of Mucosubstances

Anticholinergic drugs have been used to reduce pepsin secretion, but the same limitations apply as were discussed above. Some antipepsins are available and are discussed below, but their clinical importance is questionable.

Synthetic estrogens, particularly stilbestrol (Ch. 47) and liquorice preparations (see below) alter gastric mucosubstances qualitatively or quantitatively.

Mechanisms of Action of Antacids

Antacids are drugs which diminish the quantity of free hydrochloric acid in the stomach. They achieve this by three main mechanisms:

DIRECT NEUTRALIZATION OF PREFORMED ACID. This phenomenon has been amply demonstrated both in vivo and in vitro, and is the most important mechanism of action of antacids. The commonly used antacids contain a weak basic moiety, which is sufficient to elevate the gastric pH above 4 (see below), but not strong enough to damage the mucosal surface. Examples of antacids that act by direct neutralization are sodium bicarbonate and magnesium oxide.

BUFFERING OF PREFORMED ACID. Examples of antacids which act thus are magnesium trisilicate and sodium citrate.

ADSORPTION OF HYDROGEN IONS AND ADSORPTION AND INACTIVATION OF PEPSIN. Both have been demonstrated with aluminum antacids and with some anion exchange resins.

In addition to these three mechanisms of action, some new formulations of antacids in colloidal suspension form a *protective coating* over the mucosa and ulcer crater. Thus antacids act locally within the stomach to reduce acidity, and are effective only as long as they remain in the stomach. Antacids have no inhibitory effect on the parietal cells which secrete HCl, and consequently their effects are only temporary.

Principles of Antacid Therapy

Antacids are used to raise the gastric pH to about 4.0 or greater so that peptic activity is reduced, and the intralumenal pH is less irritating to the mucosa and ulcer crater. *Complete neutralization* of gastric acid by antacids is *not desirable,* since this will result in more rapid gastric emptying, and may result in rebound acid secretion due to excessive gastrin release from the pyloric gland area. The average patient with duodenal ulcer secretes approximately 3 mEq of acid/hr in the basal state. It has been shown in vitro that 4 g of calcium carbonate effectively neutralizes 80 mEq of acid. Consequently, this dose of calcium carbonate should effectively neutralize gastric acid secretion for over 1 day. However, such is not the case, because with acid neutralization, the rate of gastric emptying increases, thus lowering the gastric antacid concentration. The efficiency of an antacid therefore depends on the amount of acid secreted per unit of time, the neutralizing capacity of the antacid and the rapidity of gastric emptying. Of these variable factors the rapidity of gastric emptying is by far the most important, but it should be remembered that there is considerable patient variation in the amount of acid secreted. Antacids given in the fasting state will neutralize the gastric contents for about 30–60 min, and consequently, *one of the most important factors in the treatment of acute peptic ulcer disease is adequate hourly antacid therapy.* For maintenance therapy, antacids should be given about 1 hr after meals rather than before, since this regimen yields more prolonged acid neutralization. In general, the frequency of antacid administration is governed by the severity of the pain.

Antacids are given orally, and are conveniently classified into systemic and nonsystemic groups, depending upon their degree of absorption. The only systemic antacid of therapeutic value is **sodium bicarbonate.** The nonsystemic antacids most often used are basic compounds of **cal-cium, magnesium** and **aluminum.** Other less efficient members are **milk, anion exchange resins** and **gastric mucin.**

The cationic fraction of systemic antacids does not form insoluble basic compounds in the bowel lumen but is absorbed, and may produce alkalosis and an expanded extracellular fluid volume. Alkalosis occurring with systemic antacid therapy is enhanced by chloride loss (from vomiting, gastric suction or diarrhea) and by sodium absorption. Nausea, vomiting, diarrhea, abdominal pain, irritability, occipital headaches, insomnia, myalgia and tetany may develop. Acute alkalosis may produce paralytic ileus and electrocardiographic abnormalities. Nonsystemic antacids are either not, or only poorly absorbed, and are therefore therapeutically preferable. The sodium content of most nonsystemic antacids is 3–10 mg/100 ml. Thus, 2–3 g of sodium will be ingested daily during conventional antacid therapy, a situation which may compromise cardiovascular and renal function in patients with disease of these systems. Contamination of antacids (and other nonsterile pharmaceuticals, (Ch. 7) by pathogenic yeasts, molds and bacteria has recently been described as a source of potential infection.

There is a plethora of antacids available, many formulated with sedatives, tranquilizers and other antacids or drugs with questionable pharmacologic properties. Table 37–1 lists the properties, dosage and adverse effects of some common antacids.

Uses of Antacids

Because of its disadvantages and the availability of more effective drugs, the routine use of **sodium bicarbonate** should be limited. Oral administration of sodium bicarbonate is often used in combating systemic acidosis, to produce urinary alkalinization in the treatment of gout or urinary tract infection (Ch. 52), or to prevent crystalluria (Ch. 60).

Magnesium trisilicate, hydroxide and **oxide** are effective but slowly acting hydrochloric acid neutralizers. Magnesium trisilicate is usually considered superior to the other two, owing to the added action of the silicon dioxide.

Calcium carbonate is a popular antacid, but its use should be curtailed since it stimulates gastric secretion (Table 37–1).

Aluminum preparations are slow acting, less effective and more expensive than calcium carbonate, and because of their constipating action, they should be combined with a magnesium preparation. Aluminum phosphate gel should be used if phosphate loss is to be avoided. Aluminum hydroxide, or preferably aluminum car-

TABLE 37-1. Properties, Dosage and Adverse Effects of Some Common Antacids

Antacid	Properties	Dose	Adverse effects
Sodium bicarbonate U.S.P. (Baking soda)	Rapid onset and short duration of action since highly soluble. 1.0 g neutralizes 120 ml 0.1 N HCl. Cheap, but taste, color & cost have been added in proprietary preparations	2.0 g hr	Short duration of action. Sodium loading and systemic alkalosis. Gastric distention (CO_2 production). Rebound acid secretion
Precipitated calcium carbonate U.S.P. (Precipitated chalk)	More prolonged duration of action to sodium bicarbonate. Cheap. 1 g neutralizes 200 ml 0.1 N HCl. $CaCl_2$ formed on HCl neutralization reacts in small bowel with dietary fatty acids to form insoluble soaps which produce constipation	2.0—4.0 g hr	Nausea and chalky taste. Constipation. Calcium absorption leading to gastrin release (rebound acid secretion) and rarely the milk-alkali (Burnett's) syndrome, hypercalcemia with metastatic calcification
Magnesium hydroxide U.S.P. (Milk of magnesia)	Insoluble, 8% aqueous suspension with pH of about 10.6. Magnesium chloride, formed on HCl neutralization is highly soluble, and in the small bowel it acts as an osmotic laxative. 4.0 ml neutralizes 110 ml of 0.1 N HCl	4.0 ml hr	Laxative. Hypermagnesemia (in presence of impaired renal function)
Magnesium oxide U.S.P.	Converted into magnesium hydroxide in the stomach and thus acts slowly. 1 g neutralizes 500 ml of 0.1 N HCl	250 mg hr	Laxative. Hypermagnesemia (in presence of impaired renal function)
Magnesium Trisilicate U.S.P.	Contains 20% magnesium trisilicate and 40% silicon dioxide. 1 g neutralizes 100 ml of 0.1 N HCl. Slow acting. The gelatinous silicon dioxide liberated with formation of magnesium chloride in the stomach protectively coats the ulcer crater and absorbs acid and pepsin	1 g hr	Laxative. Hypermagnesemia (in presence of impaired renal function)
Aluminum hydroxide gel U.S.P.	A varying mixture of aluminum oxide, hydroxide, and carbonate. Since the U.S.P. requires that 1 g shall neutralize between 12.5—25.0 ml of 0.1 N HCl different proprietary preparations may elicit different responses. Aluminum hydroxide neutralizes and absorbs HCl, precipitates and inactivates pepsin, increases gastric mucous production, and is mild astringent and a demulcent. Aluminum chloride formed on HCl neutralization does not depress the gastric pH below 3.5. In the small bowel it reconverts to the hydroxide subsequently forming insoluble complexes with phosphates	400 mg of the dried material or 10 ml of the gel, hr	Nausea and anorexia. Constipation, produced by aluminum phosphate and as a direct smooth muscle relaxant effect of the aluminum ion. Phosphate loss may result in fatigue, muscle weakness and osteomalacia. The gastrointestinal absorption of tetracycline antibiotics, INAH, and chlorpromazine is depressed; a chelate is formed with the tetracyclines. Iron deficiency anemia
Aluminum phosphate gel N.F.	Aqueous suspension of 4—5% aluminum phosphate. Similar to aluminum hydroxide except that it does not bind phosphates	10—20 ml hr	Nausea and anorexia. Constipation
Dihydroxy-aluminum aminoacetate N.F.	Insoluble, but rapid acting. 1 g buffers 200 ml 0.1 N HCl	0.5—1.0 hr	Nausea and anorexia, Constipation
Aluminum carbonate	A varying mixture of 4.9—5.3% aluminum oxide and 2.4% carbon dioxide. Similar to aluminum hydroxide but binds phosphate more readily	600 mg hr	Nausea and anorexia. Constipation
Milk	Poor antacid. Relatively available, palatable		Acid rebound. Taken with calcium carbonate, milk may produce the milk-alkali syndrome (see calcium carbonate)
Anion exchange resins	Poor antacids but effective acid adsorbers. Rarely used		Bulky, costly, and possess an offensive odor and a gritty taste
Gastric mucin	An alcoholic precipitate of hog stomach. Inefficient acid neutralizer.		Costly, and has an offensive odor and taste

bonate, may be used in the treatment of phosphate nephrolithiasis or in controlling the blood phosphate level in renal insufficiency.

Liquorice Compounds

Two separate drugs have been prepared from liquorice, **carbenoxolone sodium** and **deglycyrrhizinated liquorice.**

Carbenoxolone Sodium

Carbenoxolone sodium is the water soluble, disodium salt of the hemisuccinate of β-glycyrrhetinic acid, synthesized from a glycoside extracted from liquorice root.

MODE OF ACTION. Carbenoxolone sodium acts locally on the mucosa, and thus, since absorption occurs primarily in the stomach, poor results were initially obtained in the treatment of duodenal ulcer disease. Carbenoxolone sodium inhibits human pepsins 1, 3 and 5, and inhibits the activation of total pepsinogens in mucosal extracts in vitro. In vivo, the drug increases gastric mucus turnover and discharge, and lengthens the life cycle of the gastric mucosal epithelium, effectively prolonging the synthesis and secretion of mucosubstances.

Carbenoxolone sodium has antiinflammatory activity due to stimulation of 11-hydroxycorticosteroid production by the adrenal cortex. It also retains sodium chloride and water, and produces hypokalemia due to an intrinsic aldosterone-like activity of the drug, and to displacement of aldosterone from plasma binding sites.

ABSORPTION, METABOLISM AND EXCRETION. In spite of its large size, carbenoxolone sodium is absorbed rapidly from the stomach when the pH is two or less. The initial plasma maximum at about 1 hr is followed by a second maximum at about 4 hr due, to intestinal reabsorption following biliary excretion. At therapeutic plasma levels (10–100 μg/ml), the drug is more than 99.9% bound to plasma proteins, with 83% being associated with the albumin fraction, and 17% with the globulin fraction. Binding to serum albumin occurs at two different classes of binding sites with apparent association constants of 10^7 and 3×10^6, respectively. Carbenoxolone sodium is metabolized to inactive glucuronide and sulfuric acid conjugates which are excreted in the bile. Less than 2% of the drug and its metabolites are excreted in the urine.

ADVERSE EFFECTS. Carbenoxolone sodium possesses low toxicity. Salt and water retention

producing edema and mild hypertension can be controlled with thiazide diuretics; aldosterone antagonists should not be used since they antagonize the effect of carbenoxolone sodium on ulcer healing. Elevation of serum transaminases and alkaline phosphatase activity, a decrease in plasma C-reactive protein, and muscle weakness, myopathies and myoglobinuria occur rarely. Salt and water retention, edema, hypertension and hypokalemia with muscle weakness also occur following excessive consumption of liquorice.

CLINICAL USE. Carbenoxolone sodium has been hailed in Europe as the most significant contribution to the treatment of gastric ulcer and reflux (peptic) esophagitis in this century; the effectiveness of duogastrone is controversial.

PREPARATIONS AND DOSAGE. Carbenoxolone sodium is available in the United Kingdom, and under trial in the United States as **Biogastrone** for gastric ulcer disease, **Biogastrone electuary** for peptic esophagitis, and **Duogastrone,** a position release form for duodenal ulcer disease. Duogastrone is formulated in a special gelatin capsule which supposedly releases the active ingredient in the pyloric antrum for discharge into the duodenum. The usual dose is 150–300 mg in divided doses per day. Potassium supplements are required to offset hypokalemia, particularly when thiazide diuretics are also employed.

Gefarnate

Gefarnate (geranyl farnesylacetate) is a terpene containing a number of isoprene units, the basic fragments from which pentacyclic ring structures like steroids can be synthesized and with which the triterpenoid carbenoxolone bears some structural resemblances. Gefarnate may possess the beneficial effects of carbenoxolone on gastric ulcer disease but without the side effects of the liquorice preparation; clinical trials in Europe have been contradictory.

Deglycyrrhizinated Liquorice

Glycyrrhizinic acid is the basic moiety of carbenoxolone sodium responsible for both therapeutic and adverse effects. The efficacy of deglycyrrhizinated (about 1–3% glycyrrhizinic acid) liquorice (Caved-S) is controversial. The drug possesses antispasmodic activity and depresses hydrochloric acid secretion, but has no effect on mucus secretion. In addition to deglycyrrhizinated liquorice 380 mg, Caved-S contains bismuth subnitrate 100 mg, aluminum hydroxide gel 100 mg, light magnesium carbonate 200 mg, sodium bicarbonate 100 mg and powdered frangula bark.

Antipepsins

Antipepsins are drugs that inhibit peptic activity independent of changes in gastric pH. Some **aluminum, magnesium** and **bismuth** antacids may adsorb or inactivate pepsin, and **amylopectin sulfate** (Depepsen), the sodium salt of sulfated potato amylopectin, inhibits pepsin by complexing with the enzyme. The usual dose of depepsen is 500 mg six times a day.

Sedatives and Tranquilizers

Sedation with barbiturates should be reserved for those patients with concommitant anxiety, restlessness or insomnia. Controlled trials have shown no benefit of phenobarbital as the sole agent in the medical treatment of peptic ulcer disease. Ataractics should be given only if indicated by specific symptomatology.

Synthetic Estrogens

Stilbestrol increases the production of gastric mucosubstances probably through stimulation of mucosal cyclic AMP, and enhances the rate of epithelial cell renewal. It accelerates the healing of duodenal (but not gastric) ulcers in men and reduces the relapse rate. Synthetic estrogen therapy is not generally suitable since unpleasant feminizing effects develop. There is a reduced incidence of peptic ulcer disease in women taking oral contraceptives. This difference may be attributed to reduced sexual activity among women suffering from peptic ulceration, rather than to a protective effect of oral contraceptives against the disease.

Miscellaneous Treatments for Peptic Ulcer Disease

Deep x-irradiation may rarely be used as an adjunct to intensive medical therapy with total depth doses of 1800–2000 rDn's over a 10–12 day period. Several hormones, e.g., prostaglandins, secretin, glucagon, cholecystokinin/pancreozymin and calcitonin have been shown to possess potent antiulcer or antisecretory properties, and may soon become important in man.

Medical Treatment of Peptic Ulcer Disease

The aims of medical therapy are similar regardless of anatomic location, viz **relief of pain, promotion of healing, prevention of recurrence** and **prevention or control of complications.** Ulcer healing depends upon chronic drug mediated control of gastric secretions, plus other therapeutic approaches such as hospitalization, bed rest, sedation, tranquilization and dietary control. Treatment regimens should be multifaceted

and individually tailored. Patients should be given some insight into their disease, particularly its tendency to recur. Some points common to both gastric and duodenal ulcers are mentioned first.

Precise dietary manipulations remain controversial, but the traditional Sippy diet is obsolete, and there is little evidence that "bland" diets are more advantageous than "regular" diets. Foods are poor antacids, but they increase the duration of action of antacids; the eating of regular meals is more important than their content. Patients should enjoy the food they like, avoid items that make their symptoms worse and take prescribed drugs regularly. Milk should be used primarily for nutrition rather than as an antacid. If possible, caffeine-containing beverages (coffee, tea, coca cola, etc.) should be omitted, since they increase gastric acid secretion via inhibition of phosphodiesterase activity (Ch. 55). Alcohol stimulates gastric acid secretion and possesses mucosa-irritating properties and should also be eliminated.

Certain drugs are contraindicated in patients with peptic ulcer disease (Table 37–2). Although tobacco smoking impedes the healing of peptic ulcers and increases the incidence of complications, any benefit achieved through cessation of smoking during treatment of an acute attack may not offset the associated anxiety and tension generated by such a change.

Peptic ulcer disease is a disorder with a fairly well accepted emotional component that can be generally handled without psychiatric consultation. Important adjuncts in therapy therefore are psychotherapy, and where necessary, sedation and tranquilization.

GASTRIC ULCER. Ideally, all gastric ulcer patients should be hospitalized initially to insure maximal medical therapy, and to confirm the benignancy of the lesion. In addition, hospitalization and bed rest are exceedingly important

TABLE 37–2. Some Drugs Contraindicated in Duodenal Ulcer Disease

Drug	Reason
Anticoagulants	Ulcer bleeding
Aspirin Phenacetin Para-aminosalicyclic acid	Mucosal irritation, leading to erosion and bleeding
ACTH Corticosteroids Phenylbutazone	Diminished tissue resistance, increased acid secretion and defective mucus production
Reserpine Alcohol Xanthine alkaloids	Gastric acid secretory stimulation; alcohol also produces mucosal irritation
Tobacco smoking	Prevention of ulcer healing

adjuncts to full antacid therapy. Carbenoxolone sodium is considered by some gastroenterologists to be of greater benefit than antacids. The role of deglycyrrhizinated liquorice and depepsen is less clear.

DUODENAL ULCER. Since there are wide differences of opinion among experienced gastroenterologists about the relative value of drugs in the treatment of duodenal ulcer disease, only a few general remarks will be advanced. The present confusion over the treatment of choice is only likely to be solved by more precise methods of assessment of ulcer healing.

Since spontaneous remission is common in duodenal ulcer, the usefulness of antacids is difficult to assess. However, there is a strong theoretic basis for their use, namely, to reduce peptic activity and consequently mucosal digestion. Antacids effectively relieve pain and pylorospasm, but do not necessarily reduce the time required for ulcer healing. It is unknown whether or not antacid therapy reduces the incidence of ulcer perforation, chronicity or recurrence, but experimentally, healed duodenal mucosa is less likely to break down than normal mucosa. Antacids are effective only if taken chronically, and the rapid relief of ulcer pain (usually occurring within days of commencing therapy) is not an indication for reduction in dosage. Antacids are more efficacious in acute ulceration, nonsystemic antacids are preferred over systemic antacids and aqueous drugs over tablets or powders. Patients vary in the proportion of constipating antacid required to offset the effects of a laxative preparation. Thus, fixed dosage ratios should not be used (Ch. 12). Since antacids must be taken chronically, patient acceptance is an important consideration. When antacids are prescribed, dosage should be determined by the milliequiva-

lents of neutralizing capacity rather than by an arbitrary volume or number of tablets.

VALUE OF ANTACIDS IN PANCREATITIS

Antacids are of value in the treatment of acute pancreatitis after the initial treatment with nasogastric suction has been completed. By neutralizing gastric acid, antacids indirectly reduce pancreatic secretion by reducing duodenal secretin release. Carbonic anhydrase inhibitors and anticholinergic drugs reduce pancreatic secretion directly but are contraindicated if paralytic ileus is present.

VALUE OF ANTICHOLINERGIC DRUGS IN DUODENAL ULCER

Because gastric secretion and gastric emptying are under vagal cholinergic control, anticholinergic drugs have been proposed as adjuncts to antacids in the treatment of duodenal ulcer. Oral doses of anticholinergic drugs giving minimal and tolerable systemic side effects fail to produce significant diminution of acid secretion or prolongation of gastric emptying. On the other hand, large doses of many anticholinergic drugs reduce gastric acid output and gastric emptying, but only in the face of varying degrees of systemic parasympathetic blockade (Ch. 17). However, anticholinergics may be of value in controlling nocturnal hypersecretion of acid, since systemic side effects of parasympathetic blockade may be tolerable because they occur during sleep. Anticholinergic drugs do not alter the incidence of duodenal ulcer complications or recurrence. They should only be used combined with antacids if the latter have failed to control symptoms and if no contraindications to their use are present (Ch. 17).

DRUGS ACTING ON THE INTESTINES: CATHARTICS

Cathartics (Greek *katharsis,* purification) are used to promote passage of feces. They are primarily intestinal smooth muscle stimulants, fecal mass softeners, or lubricants; parasympathomimetic agents are not included (Ch. 17). Cathartics are often classified in terms of their chemical structure or source or in terms of their site, time or mode of action. A classification based upon their mode of action is clinically desirable, and subdivides cathartics as 1) intestinal smooth muscle stimulants (acting directly or indirectly); 2) agents that distend the bowel lumen by increased bulk or by osmotic attraction thereby increasing peristaltic activity; and 3) agents that lubricate and soften the fecal mass. The terms **aperient, laxative, purgative** and

drastic are sometimes used to describe the magnitude of cathartic action. Thus a small dose of some cathartics produces an **aperient** or **laxative** effect (a few formed feces without griping), whereas a larger dose produces **purgation** (loose watery feces, usually accompanied by griping abdominal pain). The **drastic cathartics** (croton oil, jalap, colocynth and podophyllum) all produce severe mucosal irritation and gastroenteritis, and are obsolete.

Constipation is not a disease, but a functional disturbance of the gastrointestinal tract. Throughout the ages, man has been obsessed with the possible evils associated with retained feces, and bowel conscious subjects fear that harm will come if they do not defecate daily. The important consequence of this association is that many people, particularly overprotective grandparents and the script writers for television commercials, still believe even transient constipation requires a cathartic. Thus cathartics are widely abused by the laity—so widely abused, in fact, that many people, particularly the elderly, become habituated to their daily dose of "salts." Physicians, therefore, more commonly treat symptoms of cathartic overdose (abuse) than symptoms requiring cathartics. A brief discussion of the physiology of normal defecation will facilitate understanding of the rationale behind the use of cathartics.

PHYSIOLOGY OF DEFECATION

Approximately 300–500 ml of chyme daily reaches the cecum of an adult. It contains undigested and unabsorbed food residues (roughage). In the ascending and transverse colon the intestinal contents are slowly mixed by churning movements, which in man are nonpropulsive, and are slowly concentrated by the absorption of water. Several times a day, and usually as a response to meals, the contents of the transverse colon are transported into the descending colon and proximal rectum by strong colonic contractions (gastrocolic reflex). Here, the semisolid food residue (feces) arouses the defecation reflex, which is a local one involving sacral segments of the spinal cord. If the defecation reflex is inhibited (by higher centers), the rectum gradually relaxes and the defecation stimulus subsides. Although defecation can occur independently of any higher center control, in normal man the act is assisted and usually accompanied by voluntary muscle participation. The diaphragm descends to its position of full inspiration, concomitantly the glottis closes, and contraction of the intercostal muscles increases both the intrathoracic and intraabdominal pressures. These voluntary muscle contractions produce, in sequence, an abrupt rise in arterial pressure, almost total cessation of right heart venous return with a rise in peripheral venous pressure and a fall in arterial pressure. During intense voluntary muscle contraction, the intraabdominal pressure may rise to 200 mm Hg or more.

ADVERSE EFFECTS OF CATHARTICS

Some important effects common to many cathartics are discussed below. Adverse effects specific to individual cathartics are discussed with each drug.

HABITUATION. Though the occasional taking of a cathartic is relatively safe, continued use can lead to a habit not easily broken. After a reason-

ably complete cathartic action, the large bowel from the ascending colon distally may be completely empty of food residue, and several days may pass before a further normal bowel movement can occur. If the patient and physician do not realize the normality of this delay, further cathartic exposure is common, leading, after several weeks, to drug dependence and habituation. With habituation, the normal reflex mechanisms initiating defecation are lost, necessitating continual reliance on cathartics.

WITHDRAWAL. Patients dependent on cathartics exhibit withdrawal symptoms when their stimulant is withheld. Anorexia, bloating, irritability, dizziness, weakness, myalgia, occipital headaches, depression, general malaise and insomnia are typically produced in various combinations. It is not certain whether these symptoms develop primarily from bowel irritation or from "stress." However, in most cases symptoms are relieved by a simple tapwater enema.

MISCELLANEOUS EFFECTS. Chronic cathartic exposure may lead to colonic mucosal injury, with the development of protocolitis and associated water and electrolyte loss. Potassium loss may be severe enough to produce hypokalemic renal tubular necrosis.

STIMULANT CATHARTICS

The stimulant cathartics (the anthraquinones, phenolphthalein, bisacodyl, oxyphenisatin and castor oil) increase bowel activity either indirectly, by virtue of mucosal irritation, or directly, by stimulating the intramural nerve plexus (Table 37–3). They tend to produce griping. With the exception of castor oil, all these cathartics act on the large bowel producing laxation in 5–8 hr; castor oil acts in 2–4 hr.

Anthraquinone (Anthracene, Emodin) Cathartics

ACTIONS. Anthraquinone cathartics (cascara, senna, rhubarb and aloe) obtained from numerous plants contain various oxymethylquinones which are present partly in the free form, but principally as inactive glycosides (Table 37–3). The glycosides are slowly hydrolyzed in the small bowel, and more rapidly in the colon, at least in part by bacterial enzymes, with the liberation of their principal active substances **emodin** (trioxymethylanthraquinone) and **chrysophanic** acid (dioxymethylanthraquinone). Several other active anthraquinones are usually present in each drug and consequently, a wide variation in potency occurs depending upon the

TABLE 37–3. The Major Stimulant Cathartics

Drugs	Source and properties	Adverse effects	Preparations and single dose
Emodin Cathartics			
Cascara sagrada ("Sacred bark")	Bark of *Rhamnus purshiana*. Contains 1–2% emodin	Purgation with large doses. Excreted in human milk. Melanosis coli seen with chronic use	Aromatic Cascara sagrada fluidextract *U.S.P.* (plus magnesium oxide) 1-2 ml, orally. Cascara sagrada fluidextract *N.F.* 1–2 ml orally. Cascara tablets *N.F.* 300 mg orally
Senna	Dried leaves of plants *Cassia acutifolia* (Alexandria senna) and *C. angustifolia* (Trinnevelly senna)	As for cascara	Senna syrup *N.F.* 8 ml orally. Senna fluidextract *N.F.* 2 ml orally. Various costly proprietary preparations (e.g. syrup of figs, castoria, sennokot)
Aloe	Juice of the plant *Aloe perryi*. The most irritating of all emodins	As for cascara	Various costly proprietary preparations (e.g. Carter's Little Pills, Hinkels Pills)
Rhubarb	Dried rhizome and roots of *Rheum officinale*. Not obtained from common garden rhubarb	As for cascara	Rhubarb fluidextract, 0.6–1.2 ml orally
Danthron	A synthetic drug related chemically to emodin	Purgation with large doses	Danthron (Dorbane) 150–300 mg orally
Phenolphthalein	Synthetic cathartic. Partially refined (yellow) phenolphthalein produces greater laxation than refined (white) phenolphthalein since it is more water repellant. Acts in small and large bowel by mucosal irritation. About 20% absorbed, conjugated and renal excreted where it colors alkaline urine pinkish red. Laxation produced in 6–12 hr	See text	Phenolphthalein *N.F.* (white phenophthalein) tablets, 60–180 mg orally. Various costly proprietary preparations for children are formulated in candy or chewing gum
Bisacodyl	Synthetic agent resembling phenolphthalein. Not absorbed and stimulates peristalsis by mucosal irritation. Formed feces produced 1 hr or 8–12 hr following suppository or oral administration, respectively	Purgation with large doses	Bisacodyl (Dulcolax) 5 mg enteric coated tablets and 10 mg suppositories. 10–15 mg orally and 10 mg by suppository
Oxphenisatin	Synthetic agent resembling phenolphthalein which acts by mucosal irritation	Oxyphenisatin acetate has been withdrawn from the market due to its propensity in causing hepatic damage. No adverse effects of note have been reported using oxyphenisatin dihydrochloride	Oxyphenisatin dihydrochloride (Lavema) 10–20 mg as an enema
Castor oil (Oleum ricini)	A fixed oil, a triglyceride of unsaturated ricinoleic acid and glycerol obtained from the castor bean *Ricinus communis*. It should not be confused with the poisonous toxalbumin ricin obtained from the castor bean. Hydrolysed by pancreatic and intestinal lipases to glycerol and ricinoleic acid which forms alkaline ricinoleates. The latter are readily absorbed and act on the small bowel within 2–4 hr. Castor oil is also used on the skin as an emolient	Retards gastric emptying. May produce pelvic congestion and therefore contraindicated during menstruation and pregnancy	Castor oil *U.S.P.*, 15–60 ml orally. Aromatic castor oil *N.F.*, 15–60 ml orally

anthraquinone content, and upon their ease of liberation from the inactive glycoside precursor. For example, two isomeric glycosides, sennosides A and B, have been isolated from senna preparations, the use of which ensures a reasonably standardized preparation. However, purified anthraquinone compounds of other stimulant cathartics are not as potent as the crude preparations usually employed because they may contain other active ingredients, or because they are less soluble in the intestinal lumen.

The emodins reach the large bowel by passage down the intestinal lumen and via the blood stream. The intraluminal emodin stimulates peristalis by mucosal irritation, whereas the blood-borne emodin acts directly on the intrinsic nerve plexus. Chrysophanic acid has little or no cathartic action. It is a pigment which, when excreted, colors alkaline urine red and acid urine yellow.

Phenolphthalein

ADVERSE EFFECTS. Phenolphthalein is relatively nontoxic, but occasionally hypersensitivity reactions occur. With severe hypersensitivity, diarrhea, and cardiovascular and respiratory distress may be seen in association with skin rashes. With mild hypersensitivity, skin rashes only are seen, and these take the form of erythema nodosa, and a polychromatic, deep pink to purple, macular rash, which may be pruritic and burning. The macular rash may progress to ulceration, but usually heals rapidly leaving a residual dusky pigmentation (Fig. 7–1). In some cases pigmentation may persist for years. On reexposure to phenolphthalein, the areas of pigmentation or the nonpigmented sites of previous rashes tend to become involved. A malabsorption syndrome, with atrophic villi demonstrable on intestinal biopsy, is a rare adverse effect of long term phenolphthalein ingestion.

SALINE (OSMOTIC) CATHARTICS

ACTIONS. Saline (osmotic) cathartics comprise compounds which are slowly or incompletely absorbed from the intestinal lumen. Consequently, water is retained in the lumen through osmotic pressure and peristalis is stimulated indirectly by the semifluid fecal bulk. Additionally, some saline cathartics, such as magnesium sulfate, may act by releasing cholecystokinin/pancreozymin. The efficiency of these drugs depends upon their rate and degree of absorption and their osmotic pressure. Osmotic pressure is dependent upon the molecular weight of the drug and the number of ions into which it dissociates in solution. Saline cathartics stimulate the small bowel and usually

TABLE 37–4. Some Popular Osmotic Cathartics

Drug	Properties	Dose
Magnesium sulfate *U.S.P.* (Epsom salt)	Bitter tasting	15 g
Milk of magnesia *U.S.P.*	A 7–8% aqueous suspension of magnesium hydroxide. Slow acting since has to be converted into soluble salts.	15 ml
Sodium sulfate *N.F.* (Glaubers salt)	Cheap but impalatable	15 g
Sodium phosphate *N.F.*	Dibasic sodium phosphate. Pleasant tasting	4–10 mg
Potassium sodium tartrate *N.F.* (Rochelle salt)	Pleasant tasting	10 g
Potassium bitartrate *N.F.* (Cream of tartar)	Pleasant tasting	2 g

act within 3–6 hr. The differences among osmotic cathartics depend on rapidity of action, taste and cost. Some popular preparations are indicated in Table 37–4.

The osmotic effect is not greater if both rather than one of the ions are nonabsorbable, because if the cation is nonabsorbable an equivalent amount of anion is retained in the bowel lumen to maintain balance, and vice versa. Catharsis results irrespective of the tonicity of the administered agent. If the cathartic is given in a hypotonic, or hypertonic solution, excessive intestinal water absorption or loss, respectively, results. Hypertonic saline cathartics may cause nausea and vomiting from pyloric sphincter spasm. Up to 10% of magnesium ions from magnesium cathartics can be absorbed. Symptoms of hypermagnesemia may thus develop in subjects with compromised renal function.

BULK CATHARTICS

Bulk cathartics are natural and semisynthetic polysaccharides and celluloses which stimulate peristalsis indirectly by virtue of their content of unabsorbable, undigestible fiber (Table 37–5). They may also absorb water and swell, and assume an emollient gel-like consistency that lubricates the fecal mass and facilitates its passage. Maximal effect may not be seen for several days.

LUBRICANTS AND FECAL SOFTENERS

There are several effective cathartics which can be classified as lubricants and/or fecal softeners which facilitate fecal evacuation (Table 37–5). They have no direct mucosal or muscle stimulant action. Because of their mode of action, they are of particular value in treating patients who

TABLE 37–5. Some Popular Bulk Cathartics, Fecal Mass Softeners and Lubricants

Drug	Source and properties	Adverse effects	Preparations and dosage
Bran fiber	A biproduct of wheat milling containing 15–25% cellulose	Should be taken with sufficient water to avoid acute esophago-intestinal obstruction	Bran cereal, cookies & muffins are regularly used at breakfast time but usually in homeopathic doses
Celluloses	Greyish-white fibrous powders which swell in water producing an opalescent, viscous solution	See bran fiber	Methylcellulose *U.S.P.* and Carboxymethylcellulose *U.S.P.*, 2–4 g daily.
Plantago seed	Cleaned, dried, ripe seed of *Plantago psyllium*. Contains natural mucilage. Highly effective in psychologic constipation and functional bowel syndromes	See bran fiber	Plantago seed *N.F.*, 1–5 g, three times daily.
Agar (Agar agar)	Dried hydrophilic colloid from *Gelidium cartilagineum* containing hemicelluloses which partially hydrolyse to D-galactose and 3,6-anhydro-L-galactose. At 25°C absorbs 5 times its weight of water	See bran fiber	Agar *U.S.P.*, 4 g, three times daily
Mineral oil (Liquid petrolatum)	A complex mixture of indigestible petroleum hydrocarbons mainly of the methane series. It acts primarily as a lubricant, and also as an emulsifying agent augmenting fecal bulk	Sequesters fat soluble vitamins reducing their absorption, and delays gastric emptying. Dosage is difficult to control resulting in anal leakage, fissure in ano, pruritis ani and reduced healing of ano-rectal wounds (e.g. following hemorrhoidectomy). When inadvertently inhaled into the lungs (particularly in the elderly) produces lipoid pneumonia	Mineral oil *U.S.P.*, 10–50 ml orally. Mineral oil emulsion. *N.F.*, 10–50 ml orally
Dioctyl sulfosuccinate	An anionic surface-active emulsifying and wetting agent, which lowers surface tension allowing water to penetrate the fecal mass. Otherwise inert pharmacologically and is not digested or absorbed. May increase the absorption of concomitantly administered agents. Full effects not seen for 1–3 days	Gastrointestinal irritation	Dioctyl sodium sulfocuccinate *N.F.*, 25–120 mg, 4 times daily. Dioctyl calcium sulfosuccinate *N.F.* 25–100 mg, 4 times daily
Poloxalkol	A nonionic surface-active agent composed of a propylene oxide polymer plus ethylene oxide. Similar to dioctyl sulfosuccinate		

should avoid straining at stool. Furthermore, the soft stool so produced tends to result in the restoration of normal function in terms of fecal consistency and frequency of defecation.

OTHER CATHARTIC PROCEDURES

Enemas and glycerine suppositories have been used in the treatment of constipation.

Enema

Rectal distention by tap water, soapy water, saline, olive oil or cotton seed oil enemas may be

TABLE 37–6. Some Applications of Cathartic Drugs

Preparation of bowel for radiography or surgery
Preparation of bowel for proctoscopy or sigmoidoscopy
Diagnosis and treatment of intestinal parasites
As adjunct agents in toxicology, particularly drug and some cases of food poisoning
Postoperatively, following abdominal and hernia operations
Induction of labor and postpartum
To prevent excessive straining at stool (with associated rise in arterial blood pressure) in patients with hypertension, cerebral or coronary arteriosclerosis, pulmonary embolism, etc.
During convalesence from myocardial infarction, pulmonary embolism, cerebral hemorrhage, etc.
Treatment of hepatic precoma and coma
Cerebral edema (hypertonic magnesium sulfate)

effective in softening feces. Rapid rectal distention is dangerous, and in the elderly may precipitate cardiac failure. A tap water enema should not be larger than 500–1000 ml. An enema, when properly administered, comes closer to imitating a normal bowel movement than any of the cathartic drugs, since it usually empties only the descending colon and rectum.

Glycerine Suppository

Evacuant suppositories containing glycerine induce defecation by rectal mucosal irritation. They are especially helpful in children.

USE OF CATHARTICS

Cathartics should never be given to a patient suffering from an undiagnosed abdominal pain or intestinal obstruction. It is important to remember that many young children with abdominal pain become sulky, irritable and fractious, and because they fear a cathartic, will keep silent. How often are fretful children given a "good dose of salts?"

Functional constipation is by far the most common disease requiring active cathartic administration. Physicians use cathartics frequently for conditions other than constipation. A partial list is presented in Table 37–6.

DRUGS ACTING ON THE INTESTINES: CHELATING AGENTS

Cholestyramine is an insoluble anion resin which has a strong affinity for complexing with cholates (bile salts). Thus, it is of some value in reducing the intense pruritus often accompanying biliary cirrhosis and all types of chronic cholestatic jaundice.

ACTIONS. Following oral administration, the resin exchanges chloride for cholates in the intestinal lumen and forms insoluble bile salt complexes which are subsequently lost in the feces. With the enterohepatic bile salt circulation broken, bile salts are synthesized from cholesterol, and in the majority of patients exposed to cholestyramine, a 20–80% reduction in serum cholesterol levels develops within a few weeks. This cholesterol reduction is usually not maintained, however.

ADVERSE EFFECTS. Gastrointestinal upsets are common, especially during early therapy and patients may balk at the drug's offensive odor.

High doses may produce steatorrhea, and theoretically hyperchloremic acidosis is possible from excessive chloride absorption. Cholestyramine prevents fat-soluble vitamin absorption and may chelate other drugs given orally. It may increase the absorption of calcium.

PREPARATIONS AND DOSAGE. Cholestyramine resin, *U.S.P.* (Questran) is given in a dose of 4 g 3 times daily.

USES. Cholestyramine is of value in the treatment of cholate pruritus occurring in primary biliary cirrhosis and all types of chronic cholestatic jaundice. Its value in controlling hypercholesterolemic states is not yet clear. It is very effective in controlling the diarrhea following ileal resections of less than 100 cm. It may be of some value in the treatment of hyperlipoproteinemias, porphyria cutanea tarda and erythropoetic protoporphyria. Occasionally it is effective in the control of the diarrhea of Crohns disease.

DRUGS ACTING ON THE INTESTINES: ANTIDIARRHEA AGENTS

Diarrhea is a symptom associated with too rapid a passage of fecal material and the frequent passage of semisolid or liquid feces. In all cases of severe or prolonged diarrhea, no matter what the cause, the rapid and complete correction of water and electrolyte loss is of the utmost importance.

Sedatives

The opiates (Ch. 23) have been used for many years in the symptomatic control of diarrhea. **Paregoric** (camphorated tincture of opium), 4 ml as required; **laudanum** (tincture of opium), 0.3–0.6 ml as required; and **codeine sulfate,** 16–32 mg as required are popular. It should be remembered that addiction and tolerance (Ch. 7)

often develop rapidly with the opiates. Furthermore, apart from the usual adverse effects, opiates may produce acute pancreatitis.

Diphenoxylate hydrochloride (Lomotil), is a synthetic opium-like drug. The usual dose is 5 mg 3 times daily.

Antispasmodics

The use of antispasmodic agents in the treatment of diarrhea is discussed in Chapter 13.

Hydrophilics

The hydrophilics may incorporate water, forming a gelatinous mass. **Psyllium hydrophilic muciloid** with dextrose (Metamucil), **psyllium seed** with dextrose (Serutan), and **polycarbophil** plus thihexinol, an anticholinergic (Sorboquel), are of value. A variety of other drugs has been used, largely on an empiric basis.

Demulcents

Some **bismuth, calcium,** and **magnesium** salts may exhibit mild demulcent activity (relieves irritation). Bismuth subcarbonate, *U.S.P.,* 2 g orally as required; calcium carbonate, *U.S.P.,* 2 g orally as required; and magnesium oxide, *U.S.P.,* 1 g orally as required, are popular.

Adsorbents

A variety of adsorbents have been used, but their value is questionable. They supposedly adsorb irritants, reduce mucus secretion and bind water. Activated charcoal, *U.S.P.,* 1–6 g orally as required, and kaolin, *N.F.* (aluminum silicate), 30 g every 3 hr are popular. Kaopectate (a mixture of koalin and pectin) is both a demulcent and an adsorbent. The usual dose is 15 ml as required. Many of these preparations contain neomycin (Ch. 56) in addition. Their value is doubtful. Liberal quantities of pectin are found in apples.

FURTHER READING

Fordtran JS, Morawski SG, Richardson CT (1973): In vivo and in vitro evaluation of liquid antacids. N Engl J Med 288:923–928

Jones Sir FA, Sullivan FM (eds) (1972): Carbenoxolone in Gastroenterology. Reading, MA Butterworths

Piper DW, Heap TR (1972): Medical management of peptic ulcer, with reference to anti-ulcer agents in other gastro-intestinal diseases. Drugs 3:366–403

Thompson JH (1972): Gastrointestinal Disorders—Peptic Ulcer Disease, in Search for New Drugs. Rubin AA (ed) New York, Marcel Dekker Ch 2, pp 116–199

PETER LOMAX

38. DIURETICS

The aim of diuretic therapy is to increase renal excretion of electrolytes and water. Originally a diuretic was defined as a drug that increased the net renal excretion of sodium and water. The term "saluretic" is sometimes used to describe drugs that increase renal output of sodium chloride. Except under most unusual circumstances extra water invariably accompanies extra salt in the urine so that the term "saluretic" would appear to be superfluous.

The major use of diuretics is in conditions in which there is an excess of sodium chloride in the body, usually with edema formation. This syndrome can arise as a result of disorders of a number of different organ systems. There is also a group of conditions not usually accompanied by sodium and water retention in which diuretics may be useful adjuncts to therapy.

Some agents, such as mannitol, urea and various salts, produce diuresis by virtue of their osmotic effect on the renal absorptive processes. In this chapter only those agents are discussed that act directly on the renal tubules to increase the output of sodium salts. In Table 38–1, are listed commonly used diuretic drugs.

RENAL HANDLING OF ELECTROLYTES

In order to understand the changes in body fluids resulting from administration of diuretics an appreciation of the function of the different segments of the nephron is required (Fig. 38–1). Theories of renal physiology have undergone continuous change over the past 20 years. To some extent such changes in concepts of renal handling of electrolytes and water have coincided with the development of three major techniques of investigation: stop-flow techniques, micropuncture methodology and perfusion studies on isolated tubules.

Filtration of the plasma by the glomeruli is the initial step in urine formation. The sodium content of this glomerular ultrafiltrate reflects the plasma levels, and the total amount filtered depends on the state of the glomeruli and the filtration pressure. Depending on the glomerular filtration rate (GFR) 50–70% of the sodium is reabsorbed in the proximal tubule together with an osmotically equivalent amount of water. The lumen of the tubule is at a higher electrical potential level than the interior of the tubular cell. The sodium ions travel along this potential gradient into the cell. The interstitial "nonluminal" border of the cell appears to be the site of a sodium pumping mechanism which actively transfers the intracellular sodium across the membrane into the extracellular fluid of the kidney where it is in equilibrium with the renal blood circulation. Chloride is the major anion which accompanies the sodium in this migration and appears to be transferred passively. These mechanisms are illustrated in Figure 38–2.

Bicarbonate ion accompanies the reabsorbed sodium to such a degree that only a trifling amount of bicarbonate normally appears in the urine. The luminal membrane of the proximal tubular cells is impervious to bicarbonate ion as such. Figure 38–3 illustrates the processes involved in the reabsorption of bicarbonate. Intracellular bicarbonate ion is available from carbonic acid formed from water and carbon dioxide under the influence of the enzyme carbonic anhydrase. The hydrogen ion released is able to diffuse into the tubular lumen and react with the bicarbonate ion to reform carbon dioxide and water, which then diffuse back into the cell and the extracellular fluid.

Filtered sodium (15–30%) is reabsorbed in the thick ascending limb of the loop of Henle. This is not accompanied by reabsorption of water so

TABLE 38–1. Common Diuretic Agents

Drug	Trade name	Preparations	Dose
Organic mercurials			
Chlormerodrin	Neohydrin	10 mg tablet	1–4 tablets, PO, daily
Meralluride	Mercuhydrin	Solution containing 40 mg/ml Hg	1–2 ml, IM, twice weekly
Mercaptomerin	Thiomerin	Solution containing 40 mg/ml Hg	1–2 ml, IM, twice weekly
Mercumatilin	Cumertilin	Solution containing 40 mg/ml Hg	1–2 ml, IM, twice weekly
Mercurophylline	Mercuzanthin	Solution containing 40 mg/ml Hg	1–2 ml, IM, twice weekly
Mersalyl sodium	Salyrgan	Solution containing 40 mg/ml Hg	1–2 ml, IM, twice weekly
Carbonic anhydrase inhibitors			
Acetazolamide	Diamox	250 mg tablet	250–500 mg, PO
Dichlorphenamide	Daranide	50 mg tablet	200 mg, PO
Ethoxyzolamide	Cardrase	62.5 and 125 mg tablets	62.5–125 mg, PO
Benzothiadiazides			
Bendroflumethiazide	Naturetin	2.5 and 5 mg tablets	2.5–5 mg, PO, daily
Chlorothiazide	Diuril	250 mg tablet	500–2,000 mg, PO daily
Chlorthalidone	Hygroton	100 mg tablet (without a thiazid group)	100 mg, PO, daily
Flumethiazide	Ademol	500 mg tablet	500–2,000 mg, PO, daily
Hydrochlorothiazide	Esidrex, Oretic, Hydro-Diuril	25 and 50 mg tablets	25–100 mg, PO, daily
Hydroflumethiazide	Saluron	50 mg tablet	25–50 mg, PO, daily
Polythiazide	Renese	1, 2 and 4 mg tablets	4–8 mg, PO, daily
Others			
Ethacrynic acid	Edecrin	50 mg tablet	50–200 mg, PO, daily
Furosemide	Lasix	40 mg tablet	40–200 mg, PO, daily (also see text)
Spironolactone	Aldactone A	25 mg tablet	100 mg, PO, daily
Triamterene	Dyrenium	100 mg capsule	100 mg, PO, twice daily

that dilution of the tubular fluid occurs ("diluting segment"). Reabsorption of sodium at this site appears to be a consequence of active transport of chloride ion out of the tubule; sodium transport is passive.

In the first part of the distal tubule sodium is actively reabsorbed, together with chloride and water as in the proximal tubule; this accounts for 5–10% of the filtered salt. The ultimate fine adjustment of the body sodium content, however, is carried out by the distal tubule and cortical collecting ducts. This distal mechanism is indirectly regulated by the distribution and volume of the body fluids and by the juxtaglomerular apparatus in the kidneys themselves. These volume receptors control the output of adrenal steroids, particularly aldosterone, which act directly on the distal part of the nephron, where they lead to an exchange of sodium in the tubular fluid for intracellular potassium or hydrogen ion (Ch. 46).

Again this process depends on the formation of hydrogen and bicarbonate ion from carbon dioxide and water under the influence of carbonic anhydrase. The hydrogen ion replaces the potassium ion of the intracellular organic phosphates or else passes into the tubular fluid. The bicarbonate ion passes into the extracellular fluid with the reabsorbed sodium.

The sequence of ionic events occurring in the distal tubules is illustrated in Figure 38–4. The intimate mechanisms which regulate the potassium, hydrogen ion and sodium exchange are still obscure.

DIURETIC ACTION

The excretion of sodium, with accompanying anions and water, can be enhanced by an increase in glomerular filtration of sodium or by a decrease in tubular reabsorption. The common clinically useful diuretics act almost wholly at sites where sodium is removed from the lumina of the tubules.

The sites of action of the different diuretics have been investigated by various techniques, including stop-flow methods, catheterization of the collecting ducts, perfusion of isolated tubules, autoradiography and histochemistry. These studies have failed to yield consistent results.

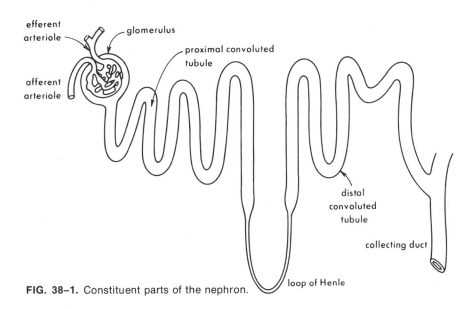

FIG. 38–1. Constituent parts of the nephron.

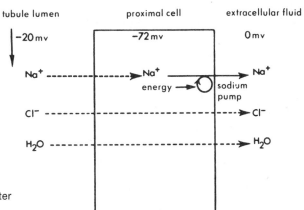

FIG. 38–2. Transport of sodium chloride and water across the proximal tubular cell.

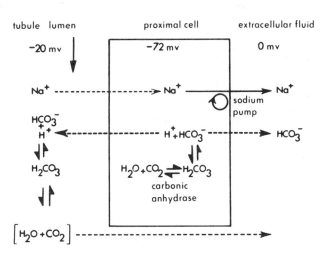

FIG. 38–3. Transport of sodium bicarbonate across the proximal tubular cell.

Drugs that interfere with reabsorption of sodium appear to be active at all sites at which this takes place, although available methods of investigation indicate predominant sites of action.

MERCURIAL DIURETICS

A large number of mercurial diuretic drugs has been synthesized since the original disclosure of the propensity of the antisyphilitic organomercurials to increase urine output.

Chemistry

The clinically useful diuretics are substituted mercuripropyl compounds with the general formula shown in Figure 38–5, together with a commonly used mercurial diuretic, mersalyl (see below). **X** is frequently theophylline (Ch. 32), which, although having some diuretic activity itself, is added to improve absorption of the mercurial compound. **Y** may be hydrogen, methyl, ethyl, etc. The character of this grouping has little to do with the diuretic activity. Substitution at **R** distinguishes the various compounds in potency and toxicity and may vary from urea to coumarin in complexity. The Hg–C bond is stable in neutral or alkaline solutions. This bond is not ionic in vitro, but cleavage may occur in vivo with the liberation of mercury ions.

Pharmacologic Actions

The mercurial diuretics are concentrated in the kidney tubules following administration and exert a prolonged local effect. This accumulation in the renal tissues can lead to toxic levels and cause renal shutdown. The mercurials act directly on the kidney and inhibit the reabsorption of sodium at all sites where the ion is actively transported by blocking either the carrier or the energy supply of the sodium pump mechanism. This inhibition may be due to liberated mercurial ions combining with and inactivating the sulfhydryl side chains of the enzymes of the sodium pump. Also, these drugs seem to inhibit active transport of chloride ion in the thick ascending limb of the loop of Henle and this accounts, in part, for the diuretic effect.

Therapeutic Use and Adverse Effects

With the decrease in proximal reabsorption, greater amounts of sodium are presented to the distal tubules, where there is increased exchange of sodium for potassium. This exchange is further enhanced by the increased circulating aldosterone level which usually accompanies generalized edema (see below). As discussed above, the sodium exchanged for intracellular potassium in the distal tubules eventually passes into the extracellular fluid as the bicarbonate. The inhibition of chloride transport adds to this effect. Thus, the net result is that some sodium chloride initially present in the extracellular fluid before filtration is transformed to sodium bicarbonate, increasing the alkali reserve and producing alkalosis (hypochloremic alkalosis).

The development of alkalosis inhibits the action of the mercurial diuretics, possibly by decreasing the ionization of the mercury. This self-limiting effect of mercurial diuretics can be counteracted by the use of acidifying salts such as ammonium chloride. The ammonium ion is converted to urea, and the chloride displaces bicarbonate in the extracellular fluid, as in the reaction shown in Figure 38–6. Ammonium chloride is taken in the form of enteric-coated tablets. Nausea and vomiting frequently occur with the drug and care must be taken with patients with liver disease, in whom hepatic coma can be pre-

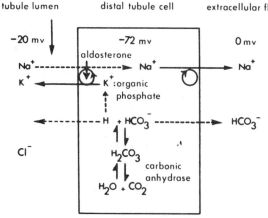

FIG. 38–4. Exchange of sodium for potassium or hydrogen ion in the distal tubular cell.

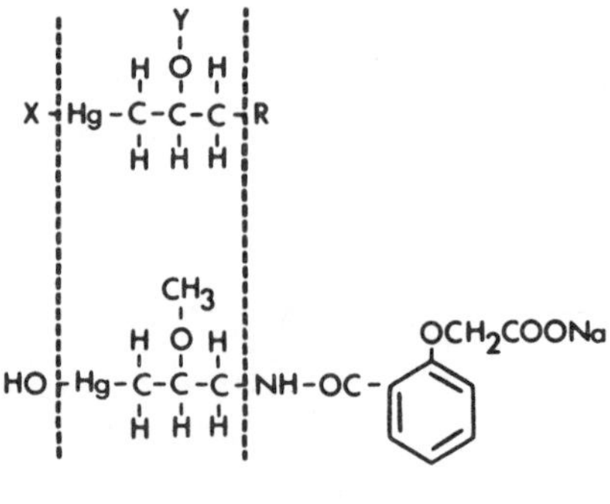

MERSALYL

FIG. 38–5. The organomercurials and mersalyl.

FIG. 38–6. Reaction of ammonium chloride in hypochloremic alkalosis.

$$2NH_4Cl + 2NaHCO_3 \longrightarrow \begin{array}{c} NH_2 \\ NH_2 \end{array}\!\!CO + 2NaCl + 3H_2O + CO_2 \uparrow$$

cipitated, and those with kidney disease, in whom severe acidosis may result. Arginine and lysine hydrochloride may be substituted in patients with liver disease. They are usually injected intravenously so that gastric irritation is avoided.

Mercurial diuretics should be discontinued in patients who do not show a good response, particularly if there is much impairment of renal function. Toxic systemic levels can occur rapidly and irreversible renal damage may develop. The chelating agent dimercaprol (British antiLewisite, BAL) forms a poorly dissociable complex with mercury and can be used in cases of poisoning.

The various mercurial compounds differ mainly in their recommended route of administration. **Chlormerodrin** is usually taken orally and **mer-**

captomerin injected subcutaneously. Other preparations (Table 38–1) are given by deep IM injection. Mercurial diuretics should not be given IV. Injectable preparations are made up to contain approximately 40 mg of mercury/ml, and the usual regime is 1–2 ml twice a week. As adverse effects, in particular hypersensitivity effects, occasionally occur following an initial injection of mercurials in susceptible individuals, it is recommended that a test dose of 0.5 ml be administered 24 hr before a full therapeutic dose is given.

With the advent of modern oral agents mercurial diuretics are now rarely used although they may have a place in therapy where the diuretic response to other agents has been poor.

CARBONIC ANHYDRASE INHIBITORS

When sulfanilamide was introduced as a chemotherapeutic agent, it was noted that metabolic acidosis and diuresis accompanied its use. Subsequent investigation showed that this was due to inhibition of carbonic anhydrase activity in the renal tubules. Since these observations, many sulfonamides, more potent in inhibiting carbonic anhydrase, have been synthesized. **Acetazol-**

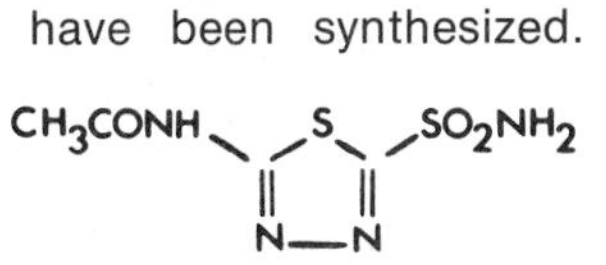

ACETAZOLAMIDE

amide has been the most extensively used. Carbonic anhydrase is a metaloprotein containing zinc; acetazolamide may interact with the metal with resulting inhibition of the enzyme.

Pharmacologic Actions and Therapeutic Use

Carbonic anhydrase influences the tubular reabsorptive processes for sodium at two positions: In the proximal tubules, where bicarbonate absorption occurs (Fig. 38–3), and in the distal tubules, where sodium is exchanged for potassium or hydrogen ion and bicarbonate is formed as the accompanying anion (Fig. 38–4).

The diuretic action of acetazolamide is due to decreased sodium bicarbonate absorption in the proximal tubules and diminished sodium exchange in the distal tubules. The increased output of sodium bicarbonate causes alkalization of the urine, a fall in plasma bicarbonate, and an increase in plasma chloride as more chloride is reabsorbed in the proximal tubules. This metabolic acidosis leads to a reduction in the effec-

tiveness of the drug, since glomerular filtration of bicarbonate falls and sodium is excreted as the chloride, and excess hydrogen ion is now available for exchange for sodium in the distal tubules. Because of this self-limiting action, acetazolamide is generally given on alternate days.

These drugs are effective when taken orally and are generally used in this way. The compound **dichlorphenamide** is one of the most potent carbonic anhydrase inhibitors. The effect of a single dose declines in about 12 hr, and the metabolic disturbance is corrected before the next dose. The drug should be administered every 8 hr in order to sustain a metabolic acidosis.

Carbonic anhydrase inhibitors decrease the activity of the enzyme at other sites in the body, but in the doses usually employed, the effect on, e.g., red blood cell transport of carbon dioxide or secretion of hydrochloric acid in the stomach (Ch. 37) is negligible. The compounds may lead to a decrease in intraocular pressure in acute glaucoma by reducing the production of aqueous humor by the ciliary body. Acetazolamide is also used, somewhat empirically, in the treatment of premenstrual discomfort and obesity, and a favorable effect in some types of epilepsy, particularly petit mal, has been claimed.

Adverse Effects

Like other sulfonamides, the carbonic anhydrase inhibitors can cause fever, allergic skin reactions and more serious side effects such as agranulocytosis and other blood dyscrasias (Ch. 60). Large doses may cause drowsiness and paresthesia.

THIAZIDE DIURETICS

Chemistry

The search for more potent carbonic anhydrase inhibitors led to the synthesis of the benzothiadiazide compounds, and these have proved to be among the most useful therapeutic agents available. **Chlorothiazide** is the prototype of a large number of compounds which appear to have the same mode of action and the same effectiveness in optimal dosage. The benzothiadiazides have the general formula illustrated in Figure 38–7 and are collectively referred to as the "thiazide" diuretics. In chlorothiazide, $R_1 = H_1$, $R_2 = H_1$, the C–N link is unsaturated, and $R_5 = Cl$.

Pharmacologic Actions

Investigation of the renal effects of chlorothiazide revealed that inhibition of carbonic anhydrase is an insignificant feature of the total natriuretic action. The general pattern of electrolyte excretion is, in fact, little different from that of the organomercurials. The thiazide diuretics decrease net reabsorption of sodium, chloride, potassium and bicarbonate by the kidneys.

The sodium osmolality in the early distal tubule rises, suggesting an action on the thick ascending limb of the loop of Henle. Presumably reabsorption of chloride is inhibited. Sodium reabsorption in the early distal tubule is inhibited. The effect of thiazides on the proximal tubule has not been determined. Thiazides increase potassium excretion as a result of increased sodium/potassium exchange in the distal tubule, especially in the presence of excess aldosterone.

Carbonic anhydrase inhibition occurs with some of the thiazides but is 2–3 orders of magnitude weaker than that produced by acetazolamide.

The glomerular filtration rate may be reduced, presumably due to a direct effect of these drugs on the renal vasculature. This effect may be important in patients with diminished renal reserve.

In the treatment of hypertension thiazides are used as diuretic agents, and to counteract the sodium retaining effects of some antihypertensive drugs. They also have an antihypertensive action in their own right (Ch. 20). This antihypertensive effect is not understood; the initial fall in arterial pressure is undoubtedly a consequence

of sodium and water loss and a diminution in the volume of the vascular and extracellular compartments. After several weeks or months hypertensive patients become refractory to the diuretic effect but the arterial pressure remains as low as during the diuretic phase. It has been suggested that the vascular smooth muscle cells become less responsive to norepinephrine during thiazide therapy.

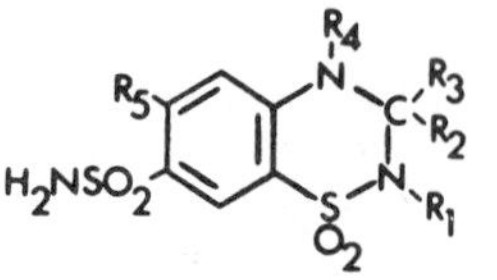

Therapeutic Use

As with the mercurial diuretics, the inhibition of reabsorption at proximal sites leads to an excess of sodium presented at the distal tubule and an increased exchange for potassium. However, the resulting hypochloremic alkalosis does not interfere with the activity of the thiazides, so this exchange can proceed to the stage of serious potassium deficiency, particularly in the presence of increased plasma aldosterone levels. This hypokalemia is of special significance if, as is frequently the case in congestive heart failure, thiazides and cardiac glycosides are administered concomitantly, since the activity of the latter is potentiated by low plasma potassium levels (Ch. 33).

Frequently potassium salts are given orally to combat the loss of the cation. There is some evidence that the administration of potassium chloride in the form of enteric-coated tablets is associated with nonspecific ulceration and stenosis of the small intestine which may lead to obstruction, hemorrhage and perforation. These changes are due to the high localized concentration of the salt achieved upon liberation. Potassium salts ingested orally should be dissolved and diluted to avoid gastrointestinal symptoms. Preparations combining a thiazide diuretic and potassium salts in fixed proportion should be avoided.

The loss of potassium may be combated also by the use of aldosterone antagonists or triamterene (see below).

All the thiazide diuretics are taken orally and are well absorbed from the gut. Peak blood levels appear 2 hr after administration, and the therapeutic effect persists generally 12–24 hr, depending on the preparation used. Daily dosage is usually employed. The prolonged action tends to interfere with the patients' sleep so that more rapidly acting drugs (furosemide and ethacrynic acid) are now often replacing the thiazides.

Two other actions of the thiazide diuretics are of clinical interest. Paradoxically, chronic administration of thiazides produces an antidiuretic effect in patients with diabetes insipidus (Ch. 43).

FIG. 38–7. The benzothiadiazides.

This action is the result of achieving a deficit in body sodium and a decrease in extracellular fluid volume. The glomerular filtration rate falls and more salt and water is absorbed by the proximal tubule so that renal output is diminished. Thiazides may also have a direct antidiuretic hormone-like effect or may increase the sensitivity of the collecting ducts to antidiuretic hormone. These agents should not be substituted for vasopressin, but they offer a therapeutic attack in the management of vasopressin-resistant diabetes insipidus. Thiazides are employed extensively in the treatment of hypertension.

Adverse Effects

Apart from potassium deficiency, other complications may follow chronic administration of thiazides. Acute episodes of gout have been reported and may be related to an influence on the synthesis of purine nucleotides. The thiazides may cause episodes of hyperglycemia and glycosuria in well stabilized diabetic patients and the appearance of diabetic glucose tolerance curves in normal subjects with a family history of diabetes. The diabetes responds to insulin and other antidiabetic agents. These effects cease when thiazide administration is stopped. Thrombocytopenia, neutropenia and acute pancreatitis have also been reported.

Care must be taken in administering thiazide diuretics to patients under lithium for the treatment and prophylaxis of recurrent manic depressive disorders. Serum levels of lithium must be maintained within very narrow limits. Lithium is excreted almost exclusively through the kidneys. Lithium treatment occasionally leads to edema and can induce obesity and thiazides may be prescribed to treat these conditions. Prolonged thiazide treatment can reduce lithium clearance up to 25% and toxic serum levels of lithium may arise. Increased proximal tubular reabsorption of lithium occurs due to extracellular volume contraction.

ETHACRYNIC ACID

Chemistry

Ethacrynic acid is a derivative of aryloxyacetic acid. It was synthesized during a search for compounds which would react with sulfhydryl groups of the enzymes concerned with sodium transport, thus mimicing the action of the potent organomercurial diuretics, and which would be effective by mouth.

Ethacrynic acid has a clinical effectiveness at least equal to that of the organic mercurials and considerably greater than that of the thiazide diuretics. Of the oral diuretics, only furosemide (see below) approaches the same potency.

ETHACRYNIC ACID

Pharmacologic Action

Ethacrynic acid severely impairs the concentrating mechanism of the loop of Henle and virtually abolishes tubular reabsorption of solute free water. This indicates a site of action on the thick ascending limb, reducing the gradient for sodium from the renal cortex to the medulla. Ethacrynic acid forms a complex with cysteine, which may be the active form of the drug. Microperfusion studies indicate that this complex inhibits active chloride transport in the thick ascending limb. Sodium reabsorption in the early distal tubule may also be inhibited. The drug has a marked kaliuretic effect that is independent of the adrenal steroids. This could be partly due to non-reabsorption of potassium at some point proximal to the late distal tubule but is mainly the result of enhanced potassium excretion in the distal tubule. Sodium/hydrogen ion exchange is also greatly enhanced.

Renal blood flow and glomerular filtration rate are increased due to a direct effect on the renal vessels.

Therapeutic Use

A prompt diuresis occurs within 30 min of oral administration, which is maximal in about 2 hr and lasts for 6–8 hr.

The maximum effective dose is in the range 150–200 mg, but the occasional patient may develop a phenomenal diuretic response, even though resistant to other diuretics. In view of the possibility of this hypersensitivity, the initial dose should be limited to 50 mg. Clinical trials have shown ethacrynic acid to be effective in patients who are refractory to other diuretics. The drug can be injected IV in patients with acute pulmonary edema due to left ventricular failure and has been used to prevent pulmonary edema in patients with severe anemia requiring blood transfusion. The diuretic is added to the transfused blood.

Adverse Effects

As with other potent diuretics, ethacrynic acid can induce hypochloremic alkalosis and severe potassium deficiency. Hyperuricemia can occur, but clinical gout is rare. The drug should be used with care in patients with cor pulmonale, as further respiratory depression may result from the induced alkalosis, leading to a dangerous rise in blood pH and partial pressure of carbon dioxide.

Occasional patients complain of gastrointes-tinal discomfort. Transient reversible deafness has been reported after extensive diuresis; this appears to be due to a direct toxic effect of the ethacrynic acid-cysteine complex on the VIII cranial nerve. Neutropenia, thrombocytopenia and hyperglycemia have been reported.

FUROSEMIDE

Chemistry

Like acetazolamide and the thiazides, furosemide is a derivative of sulfanilamide. Its pharmacologic properties are similar to those of ethacrynic acid.

FUROSEMIDE

Pharmacologic Action

Furosemide is a carbonic anhydrase inhibitor in vitro of the same order of potency as sulfanilamide, but is much more effective than the thiazides in promoting excretion of salt and water. In isolated perfused tubules active chloride transport is inhibited in the thick ascending limb of the loop of Henle when furosemide is added to the perfusing fluid. Partial inhibition of sodium reabsorption in the proximal tubules is seen in micropuncture studies.

Increased exchange of sodium for potassium and hydrogen ion occurs in the distal nephron.

Furosemide has a broad dose-response curve so the dose can be graded to avoid prompt and massive changes in fluid balance.

Therapeutic Use

The diuretic response to furosemide commences within 30 min of oral administration and is completed in about 6 hr.

Intravenous administration may be used in the treatment of acute pulmonary edema. This will cause a fall in left ventricular filling pressure within 15 min accompanied by a 50% increase in mean venous capacitance. The increased capacity of the venous system appears to be a direct effect of the drug not related to its diuretic effect.

Marked, serious potassium loss can occur during such therapy and must be prevented.

High doses of furosemide (2000 mg/diem compared to normal doses of 40–200 mg/diem) have been used in the treatment of established acute renal failure. A significant increase in the number of patients attaining a diuresis is seen and the duration of oliguria may be decreased. Provided the dose is kept below 250 mg/hr extrarenal effects are not marked. The beneficial effect of furosemide in such patients may be the result of its action in increasing renal blood flow.

Adverse Effects

When given in large doses to patients with renal failure prominent deafness may occur, sometimes after initial vertigo and tinnitus. This is more common in patients receiving concomitant antibiotic therapy, in particular, streptomycin. Probably the deafness is due to a direct toxic action on the auditory nerves.

Gastrointestinal irritation ("burning" abdominal pain), neutropenia, thrombocytopenia and hyperglycemia have been reported.

INHIBITORS OF SODIUM-POTASSIUM EXCHANGE IN THE DISTAL TUBULES

Aldosterone facilitates the exchange of sodium for potassium in the distal tubules. This action may be due to increased production of enzymes concerned with supplying energy to the carrier mechanism, since protein synthesis is stimulated by aldosterone and the effect of the hormone is abolished by prior treatment with inhibitors of nuclear RNA synthesis, such as actinomycin.

Excessive aldosterone secretion may contribute to the abnormal salt and water retention in certain edematous patients. In congestive heart failure, e.g., impaired liver function may diminish the metabolism of aldosterone (Ch. 33).

Although the drugs discussed below are not powerful diuretics when used alone, they are useful adjuvants to other more powerful diuretics. This is especially the case when aldosterone levels are high and there is a danger of hypokalemia.

SPIRONOLACTONE

Spironolactone is a homolog of aldosterone, and acts as a competitive inhibitor of aldosterone in the distal tubule. Accordingly, the output of sodium is increased and the output of potassium is decreased. A similar action occurs in the sweat and salivary glands.

When first introduced, spironolactone was not well absorbed from the gut, but preparations composed of finely dispersed, smaller particles are better absorbed. The effective dose of this preparation, **Aldactone A,** is 100 mg/day orally in divided doses. The effect of the drug is cumulative, and administration must continue for several days to produce a maximal effect. It is unnecessary to give potassium supplements to most patients receiving spironolactone along with other diuretics. However, careful biochemical regulation of the therapy is required, particularly in patients with hepatic cirrhosis and ascites.

TRIAMTERENE

Triamterene is a pteridine compound related chemically to folic acid and other vitamins. Triamterene increases the excretion of sodium and depresses that of potassium. This effect is mediated at the site of sodium-potassium exchange in the distal tubules, but triamterene is not a competitive inhibitor of aldosterone, nor is its action dependent on the presence of aldosterone. Presumably the effect is directly on the carrier mechanisms leading to sodium reabsorption and potassium excretion so that the action of aldosterone is blocked indirectly. The diuretic effect of triamterene alone is much weaker than that of other diuretics, but it is a useful adjuvant

to therapy, particularly in patients prone to develop severe potassium deficiency. Potassium supplements are not generally required when triamterene is used, and there have been cases where dangerous rises in plasma potassium levels have occurred when supplements have been given. Since the action of triamterene does not involve competitive inhibition of aldosterone and the action of spironolactone does, these agents can be used to identify electrolyte abnormalities due to primary aldosteronism. Triamterene may prevent potassium loss from the myocardium during digitalis therapy, thus protecting against digitalis induced arrhythmias.

The drug is fairly insoluble in water and is administered orally in gelatin capsules. It is rapidly absorbed and the peak effect occurs in 1–2 hr.

There are relatively few side effects although nausea, vomiting, cramps and dizziness have been reported.

AMILORIDE

Amiloride is an organic base whose renal actions appear to be the same as those of triamterene. Usually it is administered orally as 15–25% is absorbed from the gastrointestinal tract. The peak effect occurs in 6 hr and is completed by 24 hr. The drug is used mainly in conjunction with other diuretics to combat potassium loss. The series of changes occurring in the distal tubules during diuretic therapy are illustrated diagramatically in Figures 38–8, 38–9 and 38–10.

DIURETICS IN NONEDEMATOUS CONDITIONS

Diuretics may be used in the treatment of certain conditions not usually accompanied by sodium and water retention. Although the major effect of clinically useful diuretics is on sodium and chloride reabsorption (and therefore water reabsorption) the reabsorption of other filtered substances is also affected. Calcium, magnesium, phosphate, bicarbonate and glucose may follow sodium during conditions of altered reabsorption of the latter.

The use of diuretics in the management of diabetes insipidus has been discussed above.

Renal Tubular Acidosis (RTA)

Two main types are recognized: "Proximal RTA," in which there is a deficit in bicarbonate reabsorption and "distal RTA," characterized by impaired ability to acidify the urine in acidosis. Administration of thiazides may cause blood pH, serum bicarbonate and chloride levels to return to normal in proximal RTA. The main effect of the diuretics is to reduce plasma volume and thus in-

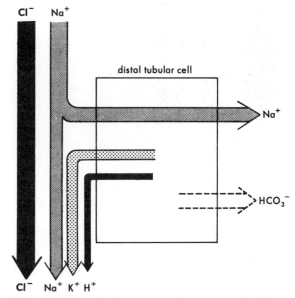

FIG. 38–8. Normal electrolyte exchanges in the distal tubule.

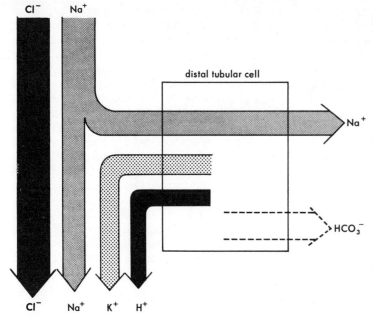

FIG. 38–9. Electrolyte exchanges in the distal tubule during diuretic therapy with benzothiazides in the presence of hyperaldosteronism.

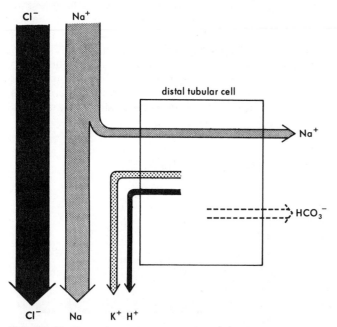

FIG. 38–10. Electrolyte exchanges in the distal tubule during diuretic therapy with benzothiazides in the presence of hyperaldosteronism, but with an aldosterone antagonist.

crease proximal bicarbonate reabsorption. Another factor may be reduced renal excretion of calcium following thiazides (vide infra). Serum calcium rises and reduces the level of circulating parathyroid hormone. Low serum calcium and high PTH levels may contribute to depress proximal bicarbonate reabsorption.

Hypercalciuria and Hypercalcemia

Long term administration of thiazides leads to a fall in urinary calcium excretion. This is useful in the treatment of renal calculi. This effect appears to be due mainly to extracellular volume contraction consequent upon sodium depletion. It has also been suggested that thiazides potentiate the action of parathyroid hormone in increasing calcium reabsorption. The evidence is conflicting, however.

Furosemide and ethacrynic acid increase renal excretion of calcium by inhibiting reabsorption in the ascending limb of the loop of Henle. Urinary losses of sodium, potassium and water must be replaced during therapy to maintain or expand extracellular volume lest contraction leads to enhanced proximal absorption of calcium. This increased calcium excretion is useful in the management of multiple myeloma, massive metastatic disease and in severe primary hyperparathyroidism as in parathyroid carcinoma.

Salicylate and Barbiturate Poisoning

Renal excretion of these drugs depends on serum concentration, urine flow rate and urine pH. Alkalinization of the urine increases clearance of salicylates and barbiturates since the drugs are present in the ionized form and are less readily reabsorbed in the tubules. Acetazolamide, to raise urine pH, and forced diuresis are frequently used in the management of poisoning. Serum potassium should be watched during such therapy.

Hyperuricemia

Serum uric acid levels may rise in lymphoma or leukemia and during therapy with cytotoxic drugs, due to rapid release and metabolism of nucleoprotein (Ch. 67). Urates may precipitate in the tubules and lead to acute renal shutdown. Alkalinization of the urine, which increases the solubility of uric acid, and increased urine flow prevent precipitation. Acetazolamide and osmotic diuresis can be employed to achieve these aims.

Cystinuria

Proximal tubular transport of dibasic amino acids (cystine, lysine, arginine, ornithine) may be defective as a result of a genetic disorder. Since cystine is poorly soluble at acid pH of the urine it precipitates in the urinary tract and forms stones. Obstruction and infection results. Maintenance of high urine volumes by large fluid intakes and alkalinization of the urine with acetazolamide prevents stone formation.

FURTHER READING

Martinez-Maldonado M, Eknoyan G, Suki WN (1973): Diuretics in nonedematous states. Arch Intern Med 131:797–808

Peters G, Roch-Ramel F, Peters-Haefeli L (1972): Pharmacology of diuretics: A progress report, 1968–1971. In Advances in Nephrology, Vol 2 Hamburger J, Crosnier J, Maxwell MH (eds) Chicago, Year Book Publishers, pp. 191–230

Suki WN, Eknoyan G, Martinez-Maldonado M (1973): Tubular sites and mechanisms of diuretic action. Annu Rev Pharmacol 13:91–106

PETER LOMAX

39. DRUGS USED IN ANEMIA

The synthesis of hemoglobin and the formation of red blood cells are normally adjusted to allow for physiologic losses and maintain the body content at a steady level. If the loss of blood is excessive, or the replacement mechanisms become defective, anemia develops.

Many dietary factors important for normal hematopoiesis, including iron, copper, cobalt, vitamin B_{12} and folic acid, are commonly involved in the cause and treatment of anemia. It is important to consider carefully the type of erythropoietic substance required and why the deficiency has arisen before commencing treatment. The precipitate use of an incorrect hematinic may obscure the correct diagnosis and render subsequent treatment difficult.

A list of agents commonly used in the treatment of anemia is presented in Table 39-1.

IRON

Iron is an essential component of the hemoglobin molecule. In most instances, anemia is the result of iron deficiency arising from chronic blood loss or inadequate dietary supplies. Typically, a microcytic, hypochromic anemia results. The mean corpuscular volume falls below the normal 80 cubic μ, and the hemoglobin concentration may be reduced to 5–10 g/100 ml from the normal level of 15 g/100 ml.

Absorption and Metabolism

Many foodstuffs contain iron. This can be adsorbed at all levels of the gastrointestinal tract, although the greatest amount enters through the duodenum. From 5–10% of the dietary iron is absorbed in normal persons and about 20% in iron-deficient patients. Most food iron is in the form of organic complexes. These are mainly broken down by the acid gastric secretions, and ionized iron, in the reduced ferrous state, is liberated Ferrous iron is oxidized to ferric iron in the mucosal cells and is then bound by a protein iron acceptor (**apoferritin**) in the mucosal cell to form **ferritin.** Transport of iron in the body is carried on by a specific iron-binding protein, **transferrin.** The bound iron is carried to its functional sites and free ions liberated.

There do not appear to be any significant mechanisms for clearing the body of excess iron. The total content is regulated by control of the rate of absorption. How this is brought about is not understood. It has been suggested that the rate of absorption depends on the availability of apoferritin or transferrin; this is the mucosal block theory. Alternatively, the active transport of iron across the mucosa may depend upon the level of tissue enzymes regulating absorption. The transport and distribution of iron are summarized in Figure 39-1.

The normal iron stores in the adult are in the range of 0.5–1.5 g. These are mainly in the form of ferritin in the reticuloendothelial cells of the liver, spleen and bone marrow. These stores are rapidly depleted in iron-deficiency anemia.

Preparations, Uses, and Adverse Effects

Iron preparations are available for oral or parenteral administration.

The most common, least expensive oral drug is **ferrous sulfate.** The frequency of adverse effects from ferrous sulfate has led to the marketing of a large variety of iron-containing compounds for oral use. These compounds differ in their degree of absorption, and since, even with the most ef-

TABLE 39–1. Preparations Commonly Used in the Treatment of Anemia

Drug	Trade name	Preparation	Dose
Oral iron preparations			
Ferroglycine sulfate complex	Ferronord	250 mg tablet	250 mg t.i.d.
Ferrous fumarate		200 mg tablet	600 mg daily
Ferrous gluconate		300 mg tablet or capsule; elixir containing 36 mg iron 5 ml	300 mg daily
Ferrous sulfate		300 mg tablet	300 mg t.i.d.
		Syrup containing 40 mg/ml	1 tsp t.i.d. (syrup)
Parenteral iron preparations			
Iron dextran injection	Imferon	Solution containing 50 mg iron/ml	2–5 ml, IM daily
Iron dextrin, dextriferron	Astrafer	Solution containing 20 mg iron/ml	20 mg initial dose increased to 100 mg over several days for slow IV injection
Vitamin B_{12} and folic acid			
Cyanocabalamin injection	Many designations	Solutions of 10, 30, 100, or 1000 μg/ml	30–250 μg, IM (for dosage schedule, see text)
Folic acid		5 mg tablet; solution of 15 mg/ml	0.1–30 mg, orally or parenterally, daily (see text)

FIG. 39–1. Metabolism of dietary iron.

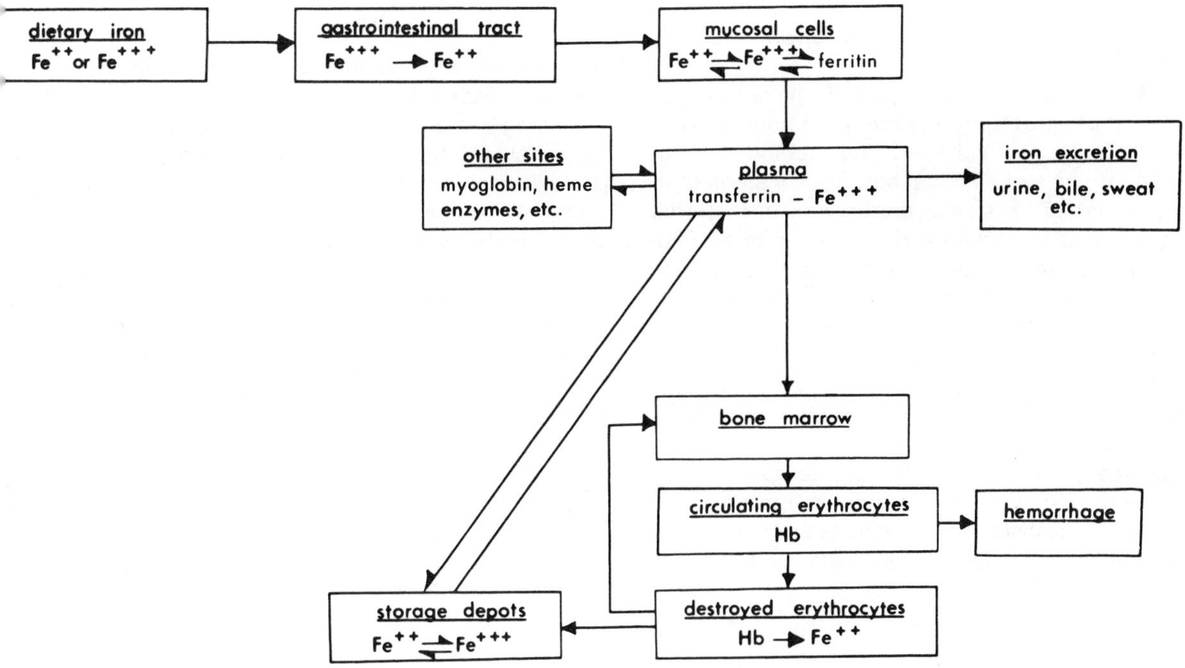

fective preparations, only about 10–15% is absorbed, it is usual to administer an excess of the drug. Oral therapy must be continued for about 6 months in patients with severe anemia. Since iron preparations are incompatible with many other drugs, they should be given alone.

All iron preparations are equally toxic when equivalent amounts of iron are administered. Acute toxic reactions are rare in adults, but serious acute poisoning in infants and children is fairly common. The treatment of acute iron poisoning is discussed in Chapter 13.

With usual doses, gastric distress, colic and diarrhea are frequently related to the total dose administered and to psychologic factors rather than the particular iron salt used. Starting therapy with small doses (e.g., 200 mg of dry ferrous sulfate three times a day) and gradually increasing the daily intake until the limit of tolerance is reached often allows adequate dosage without these adverse effects.

Parenteral therapy is rarely required and should be used only when there are clear indications or there has been no response to oral administration. **Saccharated iron oxide** and **iron-dextran complex** are two of the iron preparations for IV or IM injection.

Local adverse effects near the injection site may occur including pain, discoloration, local inflammation, thrombophlebitis and lymphadenopathy. Systemic intoxication occurs in a small number of patients, giving rise to headache, muscle and joint pain, syncope, nausea, vomiting and dyspnea.

VITAMIN B_{12}

Vitamin B_{12}, or cyanocobalamin, is a cobalt-containing compound with a molecular weight of 1355. There is a group of several cobalamins, all of which exhibit vitamin B_{12} activity. The vitamin is prepared commercially from liver or from the growth of suitable microorganisms and is assayed by a spectrophotometric method.

Absorption and Metabolism

Absorption of dietary vitamin B_{12} from the ileum requires the presence of a specific substance, the **intrinsic factor of Castle,** which is secreted by the gastric mucosa. Intrinsic factor appears to be a glycoprotein and is able to bind to vitamin B_{12} and in some way facilitate its absorption. In the blood the vitamin is bound to an a_1-glycoprotein and is widely distributed throughout the body tissues.

Daily requirements of vitamin B_{12} have been estimated at up to 5 μg, but there are considerable stores in the normal liver. The metabolic functions of the cobalamins have been studied in many biologic systems, particularly in bacteria. They act as coenzymes in a number of biochemical pathways. The systems significantly impaired by vitamin B_{12} deficiency in man are DNA synthesis, proprionate catabolism and the synthesis of methionine methyl groups.

Vitamin B_{12} deficiency arises from inadequate dietary intake or defective intestinal absorption. The most common deficient state is that due to absence of intrinsic factor in the gastric mucosa—Addisonian pernicious anemia. Less common malabsorption syndromes occur following gastrectomy, from overgrowth of abnormal intestinal bacteria associated with conditions producing intestinal stasis, parasitic infestations and disorders of the bowel wall.

The major clinical manifestations of vitamin B_{12} deficiency are: Megaloblastic macrocytic (pernicious) anemia, in which the peripheral blood contains large abnormal erythrocytes with a basophilic cytoplasm (DNA synthesis is impaired so the replication and cell division are blocked and normoblasts fail to form); gastrointestinal symptoms from mucosal atrophy (glossitis, dyspepsia); and degenerative changes of the dorsal and lateral columns of the spinal cord and of the peripheral nerves (subacute combined degeneration).

Preparations and Uses

Administration of vitamin B_{12} restores the blood picture to normal and arrests the development of neurologic damage. Usually the drug must be given by intramuscular or subcutaneous injection. The object of treatment is repletion of the body stores and the maintenance of an intake equal to the daily losses. Intensive treatment for the first 6 weeks leads to rapid clinical improvement. A dosage schedule of up to 250 μg daily for 10–15 days followed by 250 μg weekly for several months is frequently used. Thereafter, monthly injections of 100 μg are continued for the rest of the patient's life.

Oral administration of high doses of vitamin B_{12}, or of vitamin B_{12} plus animal intrinsic factor, has generally proved unreliable.

No toxic effects of vitamin B_{12} are known, and there are no known contraindications to its use.

FOLIC ACID

"Folic acid" is used generally to cover a group of pteroylglutamic acids. The pure compound is **pteroylmonoglutamic acid** and in common usage this is the compound referred to as folic acid.

Absorption and Metabolism

Folates are present in most foodstuffs and are synthesized by many bacteria. Folic acid is readily absorbed from the gut, primarily in the proximal small intestine. The daily human requirement is about 50 μg.

In mammals folic acid is the precursor of coenzymes involved in single carbon transfer reactions and is therefore essential to all metabolic systems in which such transfer occurs. Folic acid and vitamin B_{12} are closely interrelated metabolically.

Deficiency arises in man from malnutrition and from various malabsorption syndromes such as sprue. Malignant disease, hemolytic anemia and pregnancy increase folic acid requirements so that a relative deficiency arises in these conditions. Certain metabolic inhibitors interfere with folic acid, and the megaloblastic anemia during administration of some anticonvulsant drugs may arise in this way.

Folic acid deficiency leads to megaloblastic anemia indistinguishable from that due to vitamin B_{12} deficiency. The gastrointestinal disorders, particularly glossitis and diarrhea, are prominent features of the syndrome. Unlike vitamin B_{12} deficiency, however, neurologic damage does not occur.

Therapeutic Uses

Oral administration of folic acid will correct the hematologic defect in uncomplicated cases. The dose used depends on the severity of the anemia. The drug is administered by intramuscular or deep subcutaneous injection if there is a malabsorption condition. The dose may need to be increased in patients taking chloramphenicol (Ch. 57); in alcoholics; and in patients with uremia, tumors, rheumatoid arthritis or hepatitis.

Initial therapy requires 1 mg daily and this is reduced to 0.1 mg for maintenance. In spite of clinical evidence that this dose level is fully adequate, doses in the range of 10–30 mg/day continue to be recommended. Folic acid is nontoxic in man.

The only therapeutic indication for folic acid is established deficiency. Particular care must be taken in establishing the correct diagnosis before starting therapy. This is especially the case in the patient with pernicious anemia, since folic acid will correct the hematopoietic defect without preventing the neurologic changes, and irreparable cord lesions can develop.

FURTHER READING

Bothwell TH, Finch CA (1962): Iron Metabolism. Boston, Little Brown

Smith EL (1965): Vitamin B_{12}. New York, Wiley

Wintrobe MM (1961): Clinical Hematology. Philadelphia, Lea & Febiger

PETER LOMAX

40. ANTICOAGULANTS

The use of drugs that increase the coagulation time of the blood has become widespread in recent years. These agents have been used in a great many varied pathologic states, including venous thromboembolic conditions, coronary artery disease, cerebral artery disease, polycythemia, pulmonary hypertension and various embolic phenomena, as well as in cardiac and vascular surgery, particularly when an extracorporeal circulation is employed.

In all instances of use other than surgical, there is debate about the indications for, and value of, anticoagulant therapy. Against the claimed efficacy of therapy in patients with coronary thrombosis, for instance, must be weighed the attendant mortality and morbidity resulting from the drugs themselves. On the latter point there is still a lack of reliable statistical information.

Table 40–1 presents a summary of the common anticoagulant agents.

NORMAL COAGULATION MECHANISMS

The arrest of hemorrhage following vascular trauma results from coagulation of the blood and such vascular factors as capillary retraction, arteriolar constriction and the formation of platelet plugs at the puncture sites.

Normal coagulation depends on the formation of fibrin as the basis of the clot. This is the end point of a series of reactions involving all the different components of the clotting system.

Blood coagulation is brought about by activation of either of two mechanisms: an intrinsic or blood mechanism, activated by surface contact of whole blood, and an extrinsic system involving tissue factors. These two systems eventually interact to form a common prothrombin-converting principle. The sequence of events involves a cascade of enzyme reactions of which Figure 40–1 is a useful working model.

The clinically useful anticoagulants act by inhibiting the action, or interfering with the formation, of one or more of these clotting factors.

CONTROL OF ANTICOAGULANT THERAPY

The response of patients to anticoagulants is variable, and the effectiveness of these drugs may even vary at different stages of the condition under treatment. Furthermore, absorption of oral anticoagulants is slow and erratic. These considerations pose a problem in respect to dosage. Anticoagulant therapy is controlled, therefore, by carrying out routine estimations of the ability of the blood to coagulate, and the dose of the agents is adjusted so as to maintain the response within certain limits which have proved optimal in clinical trials. The physician's aim is to obtain an effective therapeutic result without spontaneous hemorrhage.

It should be remembered that the patient undergoing anticoagulant therapy is continually on the brink of a hemorrhagic state and frequent observation is imperative.

Two tests are routinely employed: determination of the whole blood clotting time and determination of the prothrombin time.

WHOLE BLOOD CLOTTING TIME DETERMINATION (LEE-WHITE METHOD). Blood drawn by venepuncture is placed in a clear tube in a bath of 37°C, and the time from withdrawal to clotting is measured. Normally this is between 10–15 min. During therapy with heparin the time is generally held at about three times the normal level.

ONE STAGE PROTHROMBIN TIME DETERMINATION (QUICK METHOD). A sample of blood is placed in a tube containing citrate which chelates the Ca^{++} and prevents coagulation. Under standardized conditions, excess Ca and thromboplastin, obtained from brain tissue, are added

TABLE 40–1. Common Anticoagulants

Drug	Trade name	Time for maximum effect (hr)	Time for recovery (hr)	Preparation	Dose*
Heparin sodium				For injection, solution of 1,000, 5,000, 10,000, 20,000, 40,000 U.S.P. units/ml. Repository form in a gelatin complex containing 20,000 and 40,000 units/ml	
Coumarin derivatives					
Bishydroxycoumarin	Dicumarol	36–48	84–108	25, 50, and 100 mg tablets and capsules	300 mg
Ethylbiscoumacetate	Tromexan	18–30	36– 60	150 and 300 mg tablets	900 mg
Warfarin	Coumadin, Panwarfin, Prothromadin	36–48	84–108	2, 5, 7.5, 10, and 25 mg tablets. Also as powder for preparation of parenteral solutions	50 mg
Indanedione derivatives					
Diphenadione	Dipaxin	48–60	96–168	1 and 5 mg tablets	20 mg
Phenindione	Hedulin, Danilone, Dindevan	36–48	72– 96	20, 50, and 100 mg tablets	200 mg

* See text for detailed discussion of dosage.

to the sample and the time to coagulation is measured. In the same way, a graph of coagulation time against percentage of prothrombin is constructed, using serial dilution of a known normal blood sample (Fig. 40–2). From this graph the prothrombin percentage in the patient's sample is read off. The coagulation time for a normal blood sample is 10–12 sec. The aim of therapy with the oral anticoagulants is to prolong normal coagulation approximately 2–2½ times.

HEPARIN

Chemistry

Heparin is a mucopolysaccharide with a molecular weight between 10,000–12,000. The molecule consists of an alternating sequence of glucosamine and glucuronic acid. The hexose moieties are highly sulfated and carry a dense anionic charge.

The mast cells of the body contain heparin, which accounts for their characteristic metachromatic staining. Lung tissues are rich in heparin, and the drug is prepared commercially from the lungs of cattle. The purified extract is assayed with sheep plasma and must contain at least 120 U.S.P. units of anticoagulant ability per milligram.

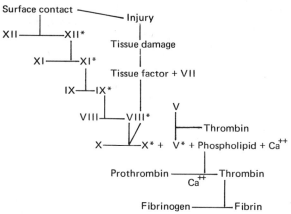

FIG. 40–1. Reactions involved in normal coagulation of the blood. **Asterisks** indicate the activated forms of the coagulation factors.

HEPARIN

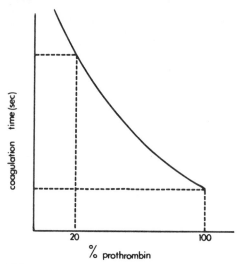

FIG. 40–2. Relation between prothrombin content and coagulation time obtained from serial dilutions of normal plasma. The percentage of prothrombin of test sample is read from the curve. For effective therapy the prothrombin level is held at approximately 20%.

Mechanism of Action

The anticoagulant effect of heparin is probably related to the strong electronegative charge on the molecule. Three effects of heparin on the coagulation process have been described. First, it interferes with the conversion of prothrombin to thrombin. Second, it antagonizes the action of thrombin on fibrinogen, preventing the formation of fibrin. This effect is dependent on the presence of a cofactor in the albumin fraction of the plasma and is the most important effect of heparin. Third, heparin causes a reduction of the agglutination ability of the platelets.

Therapeutic Uses

Heparin is destroyed in the gastrointestinal tract, and attempts at sublingual administration have not been effective. The drug must be given parenterally, and several techniques are available.

1. **Continuous IV infusion.** The anticoagulant effect is achieved immediately following IV injection. With the continuous drip method an initial dose of 5000 I.U. is given and 20,000 to 30,000 I.U. is added to 1 liter of 5% glucose or 0.9% sodium chloride solution and given slowly over the next 24 hr (20–25 drops per min). This method has the advantage of maintaining steady blood levels of the anticoagulant but it requires fairly constant attention, and in some cases, the large fluid volume may be contraindicated by the patient's condition.

2. **Intermittent IV infusion.** A single IV injection of 5000 I.U. is effective for about 3 hr. De-

creased coagulability can be maintained using this dose every 3 hr or larger doses less frequently.

3. **IM injection.** Absorption is slower following IM injection, and the drug is not effective for 30 min, so that an initial IV dose is required (5,000–10,000 I.U.). A dose of 20,000–40,000 I.U. of heparin in 1 ml injected IM lasts 8–10 hr or longer. A repository form of the drug is available for IM injection. Large painful hematomas may occur with both types of preparation.

4. **Deep subcutaneous injection.** From 20,000–40,000 I.U. of heparin injected into the subcutaneous tissues can prolong coagulation for up to 16 hr. An IV priming dose is required initially. Hematoma formation and painful induration of the tissues are frequent occurrences.

Larger than usual doses of heparin may be needed in febrile patients and in those to whom digitalis (Ch 33), antihistamines (Ch. 49), or tetracyclines (Ch. 58) are being given.

Adverse Effects

The usual preparations of heparin are relatively nontoxic and adverse effects are rare. The common danger is of spontaneous hemorrhage, particularly from a previously unsuspected lesion such as a peptic ulcer.

Other uncommon toxic reactions include hypersensitivity and anaphylactoid reactions, thrombocytopenia, fever and alopecia developing 3–4 months later. The latter is usually only transient.

Acute adrenal hemorrhage has been found at autopsy in some patients who have died during heparin therapy, particularly when the drug has been administered for several days. Abdominal pain, nausea, and vomiting are signs of this syndrome. In addition to the checking and correcting of excessive coagulation defects, such patients should be treated with cortisone.

Heparin Antagonists

In the event of minor bleeding during heparin therapy, withdrawal or reduction in dosage is sufficient. When major hemorrhage occurs, specific antagonists such as protamine sulfate are used (Table 40–2). These are able to react with the heparin to form stable compounds.

Protamine sulfate is a low molecular weight protein rich in arginine and carrying a strong basic charge which reacts with the acidic heparin molecule. One mg is equivalent to 1 mg of heparin and is given by slow IV injection as a 1% solution. The dose required is based on the origi-

TABLE 40–2. Anticoagulant Antagonists

Drug	Trade name	Preparation	Dose
Menadiol sodium diphosphate	Synkayvite, Kappadione	5 mg tablet; parenteral solution of 1–75 mg/ml	5–10 mg PO; 10–50 mg, IV (5 mg/min)
Menadione	Vitamin K_3	1 to 10 mg tablets and capsules; oily solution 1 or 2 mg/ml for IM injection	1–2 mg, IM; 2–10 mg, p.O.
Menadione sodium bisulfite	Hykinone	5 mg tablet; parenteral solution of 5–10 mg/ml	5–10 mg, IV; 5–10 mg PO
Phytonadione	Vitamin K_1, Mephyton, Konakion, Mono-Kay	5 mg tablet; emulsion containing 10 or 50 mg/ml for parenteral injection in glucose solution	25–50 mg, IV (slowly); 5 mg, PO
Protamine sulfate		1% sterile solution for injection	1 mg for each 1 mg of heparin

nal dose of heparin (the rate of metabolism of heparin is such that 50% of a given dose is removed in 30 min). Overdosage with protamine sulfate should be avoided since it possesses anticoagulant activity itself.

Other Actions of Heparin

Injection of heparin decreases the turbidity of the plasma normally seen following a fat-containing meal. Absorbed fat is carried in the plasma bound to protein and forms particles of varying size, mainly consisting of protein-triglyceride complexes (the chylomicrons). Heparin is able to release a lipase from the capillary wall which breaks down the chylomicrons, and the free fatty acids liberated dissolve in the plasma (Ch. 36). Heparin probably forms a component of this lipoprotein lipase and may act to bind the lipase to the substrate. Figure 40–3 illustrates these reactions. This lipemia-clearing action of heparin occurs with much lower doses than must be used for effective anticoagulant therapy. The clinical significance of this effect is uncertain at present.

Many other effects of heparin have been described, including antiinflammatory and antiallergic actions. These properties have been investigated for the treatment of bronchopulmonary disease but are not generally used clinically.

COUMARIN ANTICOAGULANTS

Chemistry

The coumarin anticoagulants were discovered in 1941 when it was shown that **bishydroxycoumarin** was the compound present in spoiled sweet clover which led to the development of hemorrhagic disease in cattle. This compound was later synthesized. Since that time many drugs have been investigated for anticoagulant

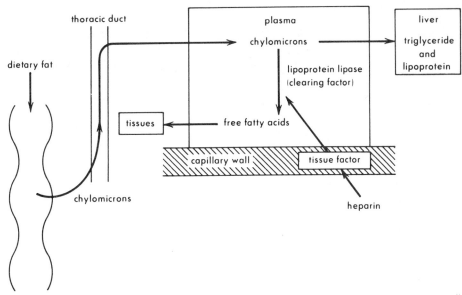

FIG. 40–3. Action of heparin in releasing lipase from the capillary wall.

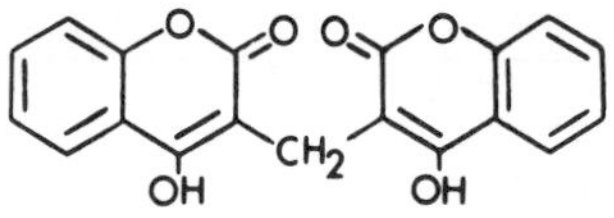

BISHYDROXYCOUMARIN

activity, and the useful compounds fall into two groups: the **coumarin derivatives** and the **indanedione derivatives** (Fig. 40–4).

Mechanism of Action

The basic mechanism of action of all these compounds is the same, but the drugs differ widely in their rate of onset, duration of action and recovery period. Their therapeutic action depends on their ability to suppress the formation of certain clotting factors. Prothrombin and factors VII, IX, and X are synthesized by the liver and their production requires the presence of vitamin K as a coenzyme. Since the coumarins and indanediones structurally resemble vitamin K, they may act as antimetabolites or interfere with uptake of vitamin K by hepatic cells.

There is a delay in onset of the anticoagulant effect of these drugs, since the normal plasma levels of clotting factors must decline before the synthesis deficiency becomes manifest. Since the coumarins have no direct effect on the clotting mechanisms, they are not effective in vitro.

Therapeutic Uses

All the coumarins and indanediones are effective by mouth. There is a wide variation in individual response to their action, however. Factors influencing the dose needed to attain an adequate depression of coagulation include absorption from the gastrointestinal tract, storage in the liver, rate of metabolism (which may vary 10-fold or more from one patient to another), genetically determined resistance to the drug and simultaneous therapy (Ch. 8). Broadspectrum antibiotics (which alter the intestinal flora and influence the production and absorption of vitamin K) and salicylates reduce the required dosage. Patients with decreased liver function show increased susceptibility to anticoagulants.

These many factors render the question of dosage meaningless in terms of "milligrams per day." An average initial dose should be given and the prothrombin activity determined some hours later. Subsequent doses of the drug are based on the results of daily determinations of blood coagulation time. Once a steady daily dose has been established, less frequent blood tests are needed.

Long term therapy is frequently used in patients in whom the dose of the anticoagulant has been stabilized initially in hospital. Such therapy is contraindicated in patients of low intelligence; in those who are unreliable about returning for blood checks; in chronic alcoholics; in pregnant women; in patients undergoing intensive salicylate therapy; and in patients with peptic ulcers, hepatic disease, renal failure or a hemostatic defect.

Owing to the delayed onset of effect of the oral anticoagulants, heparin is administered together with the initial dose and then, as the effect of the oral agent develops, the heparin dosage is tailed off.

Adverse Effects

Side effects, other than hemorrhage, are rare in man. Skin reactions, pyrexia, diarrhea, blood dyscrasias, hepatitis and nephropathy have been reported, and fatalities have occurred.

Hemorrhage during therapy with the oral anticoagulants should be treated by withdrawal of the drug, and this is all that is needed in minor cases. Severe hemorrhage may require the administration of vitamin K, using an intravenous preparation such as **phytonadione sodium diphosphate.** The vitamin competes with the anticoagulant and restores formation of the plasma cofactors. However, the effect of vitamin K persists for up to 2 weeks and there may be difficulty in reinstating coumarin or indanedione therapy.

In more serious hemorrhage attacks the transfusion of whole fresh blood may be indicated.

ARVIN: A DEFIBRINATING AGENT

In patients in whom the bite of the Malayan pit viper had caused systemic poisoning, nonclot-

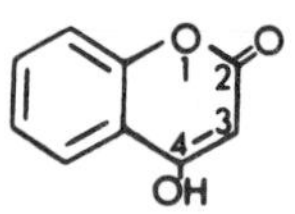

4-HYDROXYCOUMARIN   INDANE-1,3-DIONE

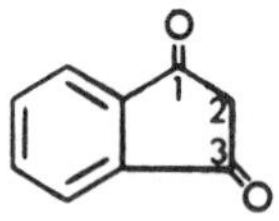

FIG. 40–4. Hydroxycoumarin and indanedione anticoagulants.

ting of the blood was always found, although general intoxication and serious hemorrhage were absent. A purified active fraction of the venom of this snake has now been prepared. This is a low-molecular-weight glucoprotein containing 20% carbohydrate. The name **arvin** has been given to the extract.

Arvin is a coagulant in vitro, but when given IV to animals it reduces the clotting power of the blood without producing serious spontaneous bleeding. The drug is not hemolytic, neurotoxic or hepatotoxic. The anticoagulant effect is primarily due to removal of fibrinogen (defibrination) combined with some antithrombin activity. The action of arvin can be curtailed by administration of specific antibodies.

Preliminary clinical trials suggest that arvin is of value in patients with deep venous thrombosis, arterial lesions, rheumatic heart lesions and coronary disease. Sensitivity reactions may occur owing to the antigenic nature of the molecule.

FURTHER READING

Coon WW Willis PN (1970): Some aspects of the pharmacology of oral anticoagulants. Clin Pharmacol Ther 11:312

Doglass AS (1962) Anticoagulant Therapy. Oxford, Blackwell

Ingram GI (1961): Anticoagulant therapy. Pharmacol Rev 13:279

HORMONES AND DRUGS MODIFYING ENDOCRINE ACTIVITY: AUTOCOIDS

JOHN A. THOMAS

JOHN E. JONES

41. INTRODUCTION TO ENDOCRINE PHARMACOLOGY

Endocrine pharmacology is concerned with the use of hormones, hormone-like substances, or drugs that either inhibit or enhance the metabolic activity of the organs of internal secretion. Hormones can be used in physiologic amounts as in replacement therapy in endocrine deficient states, or in supraphysiologic doses as when adrenocortical hormones are employed in certain inflammatory conditions. Some hormones are important diagnostic tools.

Not only does endocrine pharmacology encompass the therapeutic use of natural and synthetic hormones, but also those drugs which although without inherent hormonal activity create secondary hormonal imbalances. For example, some narcotic analgesics can interfere with the normal menstrual cycle in the female while some of the antineoplastic agents are potent inhibitors of spermatogenesis. Furthermore, drugs that alter hepatic enzymes can produce hormone alterations. Drug-hormone interactions can also occur in the blood and so interfere with a variety of pharmacologic and physiologic mechanisms.

The pharmacologic value of certain hormones, e.g., insulin is clearly established, yet others such as prolactin and thyroid stimulating hormone remain essentially unused. The utilization of some of the larger molecular weight hormones may increase as the biochemist successfully synthesizes these molecules thus avoiding immunologic effects that follow the use of hormones isolated from animal sources. Finally, the recent advances in neuroendocrinology may be very important to the field of endocrine pharmacology since the so-called hypothalamic releasing factors or hormones may provide still another approach to the treatment and/or diagnosis of hormonal disorders.

JOHN A. THOMAS

JOHN E. JONES

42. HYPOTHALAMIC RELEASING HORMONES AND HORMONE TRANSPORTING SUBSTANCES

HYPOTHALAMIC RELEASING FACTORS OR HORMONES

Hypothalamic releasing factors (RFs) or hormones are now recognized as important humoral mediators between the hypothalamus and the pituitary gland. They appear to play a vital role in the regulation and control of various endocrine organs. These RFs do have therapeutic potential, and may someday become very important in the diagnosis and treatment of certain endocrine disorders.

ANATOMIC AND PHYSIOLOGIC CONSIDERATIONS

The anatomic relationship between the hypothalamus and the pituitary gland is seen in Figure 42–1. The hypothalamus comes in contact with the pituitary stalk in a junction region referred to as the median eminence. The stalk connects the hypothalamus to the pituitary gland. The pituitary gland is divided into the anterior lobe or adenohypophysis and the posterior lobe or the neurohypophysis. Certain species also contain an intermediate lobe.

The adenohypophysis unlike the neurohypophysis receives no neural elements from the hypothalamus. The communication is solely by a network of capillaries. This portal system of vessels originates in the median eminence of the tuber cinereum, forms vascular trunks on the pituitary stalk and splits into smaller sinusoids terminating in the pars distalis of the pituitary.

The neurohypophysis is connected to two large nuclei in the anterior hypothalamus. These two nuclei, the paraventricular and supraoptic, contain cells that synthesize the octapeptides **vasopressin** and **oxytocin,** which are transported in their axons to the posterior lobe of the pituitary where they are temporarily stored prior to release by various stimuli.

Each trophic hormone from the anterior pituitary gland is affected by at least one hypothalamic releasing hormone. In most instances the particular trophic hormone is released from its cellular site in the adenohypophysis by the hypothalamic releasing hormones but in the case of prolactin and growth hormones, inhibitory factors or hormones are produced in the hypothalamus. Some trophic hormones may be affected by both an inhibitory and a releasing substance of hypothalamic origin.

A list of hypothalamic hormones and adenohypophysial hormones is shown on Table 42–1. Corticotropic releasing hormone was the first releasing factor to be discovered, but progress in understanding its mechanism of action has been hampered by the fact that there may actually be more than one CRH. It also has been difficult to chemically separate follicle releasing hormone (FRH) from luteinizing releasing hormone (LRH) in some species. These separation difficulties have resulted in the terminology of gonadotropin releasing factor (GnRF) since two distinct releasing factors, namely FRH and LRH, have not always been readily distinguishable. GnRH should not be confused with GRH or growth hormone releasing hormone. The use of the term somatotropin releasing hormone (SRH) would minimize this confusion. The releasing hormone that has been most clearly elucidated is thyrotropic releasing hormone (TRH) for its chemical identity has been established in some species. In fact, synthetic TRH-like molecules mimic the physiologic actions of median eminence-extracted TRH. TRH seems to be the closest among the RFs to be of some therapeutic usefulness (Ch. 44).

In general, most releasing hormones specifically effect the release of a particular trophic hormone. However, until the chemical identity of all

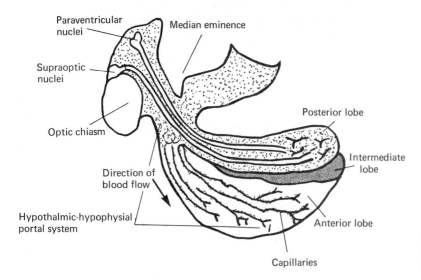

Paraventricular nuclei
Median eminence
Supraoptic nuclei
Optic chiasm
Posterior lobe
Direction of blood flow
Intermediate lobe
Hypothalmic-hypophysial portal system
Anterior lobe
Capillaries

FIG. 42–1. Anatomical relationship between the hypothalamus and the pituitary gland.

the releasing hormones can be firmly established, there is always the possibility of cross-contamination. As TRH can sometimes cause the release of prolactin, there exists some degree of physiologic overlap. This phenomenon of overlap is greater when higher doses are used.

Releasing hormones extracted from a variety of domestic and laboratory animals can evoke responses in humans. The only known exception is SRH which shows some species specificity. Porcine or ovine TRH or LRH are active in mice, rats, rabbits, monkeys, sheep and man. Such a finding is very important if releasing factors are to ultimately take their place as therapeutically or diagnostically useful agents.

TABLE 42–1. The Hypothalamic Releasing and Inhibitory Hormones

Hormone or factor	Trophic hormone affected
Corticotropic-releasing hormone (CRH)	ACTH (adrenocortical tropic hormone)
Thyrotropic-releasing Hormone (TRH)	TSH (thyroid stimulating hormone)
Follicle-stimulating releasing hormone (FRH)	FSH (follicle stimulating hormone)
Luteinizing-hormone releasing hormone (LRH)	LH (luteinizing hormone)
Somatotropin-releasing hormone (SRH) (GRH)	STH (GH) (growth hormone)
Somatotropin-inhibitory hormone (STH) (GIH)	STH (GH) (growth hormone)
Prolactin-inhibitory hormone (PIF)	Prolactin
Prolactin-releasing hormone (PRH)	Prolactin
Melanocyte-stimulating releasing hormone (MRH)	MSH (melanocyte stimulating hormone)
Melanocyte-inhibiting hormone (MIH)	MSH (melanocyte stimulating hormone)

MECHANISM OF ACTION OF RELEASING HORMONES (RH)

The actions of the releasing hormones can be investigated both in vitro and in vivo. CRH, LRH or TRH enhance the secretion of their respective trophic hormone within seconds to minutes following the IV injection of a single dose and are then readily inactivated in plasma, serum and in whole blood by enzymatic degradation.

Insight into the mechanism of action of the RHs have been derived from in vitro experiments. Their action is an oxygen requiring event, and certain ions, e.g., calcium, potassium and sodium, are necessary to affect trophic hormone release. Whether cyclic adenosine monophosphate (cAMP) is involved in their action has not been resolved. RHs do not directly stimulate the biosynthesis of adenohypophysial hormones.

CORTICOTROPIN RELEASING HORMONE (CRH)

While several nonphysiologically occurring substances can affect ACTH release, the physiologic mediator is a polypeptide called CRH. Although vasopressin can also affect the release of CRH, it is doubtful if it is a physiologic mediator. In supraphysiologic amounts vasopressin has been used to determine the pituitary reserves of ACTH.

There are at least two CRHs, one related to α-MSH (α-CRH) and the other to vasopressin (β-CRH). β-CRH can be distinguished from vasopressin. Certain synthetic analogs of vasopressin (e.g., lysine vasopressin derivatives) do, however, possess CRH activity. It is possible that there are two fractions of the α-CRH. The amino acid sequence for β-CRH has been tentatively proposed and appears to consist of about 12 amino acid residues. The tentative structure of β-CRH embodies a terminal amino acid sequence resembling α-MSH and one resembling vasopressin. It seems to have a ring structure similar to vasopressin.

The CRH-like activity of vasopressin in stimulating ACTH release can be increased if cAMP levels in the pituitary gland have been previously elevated. Synthetic glucocorticoids inhibit the ACTH-releasing actions of either vasopressin or dibutyl cAMP. CRH's actions upon the adenohypophysis do not involve protein synthesis.

Whether CRH will play an important therapeutic role in either hyperadrenocorticism or hyposecretory states of the adrenal is not known. As yet, CRH has no pharmacologic use.

THYROTROPIC RELEASING HORMONE (TRH)

TRH will cause a release of TSH both in vivo and in vitro. It has been isolated, purified and its tripeptide amino acid sequence established in at least two domestic animals (Fig. 42–2). The actual chemical synthesis of this tripeptide represents another step in its possible therapeutic usefulness.

Since TRH can be synthesized, sufficient amounts are now available to investigate its actions in humans. The intravenous administration of TRH to normal male volunteers elicits a rapid elevation in the blood levels of TSH. Peak blood levels of TSH occur about 1 hr after injection. The action of TRH in humans is quite specific since most other trophic hormones remain essentially unaffected. Small amounts of bovine TRH administered to human cretins leads to significant increases in the blood levels of TSH. It is orally effective. The only known side effects seem to be nausea and a fleeting bitter taste in the mouth.

TSH may be useful in the diagnosis of thyroidal disorders associated with altered hypothalamic function or with changes in the pituitary gland related to faulty secretory mechanisms associated with TSH release and/or synthesis. Perhaps its most promising clinical use is in the evaluation of altered TSH secretory reserve in

Synthetic Thyrotropic Releasing Hormone

Pyroglu-His-Pro-NH$_2$

Synthetic Luteinizing Releasing Hormone

Pyroglu-Tyr-Arg-Trp-NH$_2$

Synthetic Luteinizing/Follicle Releasing Hormone

Pyroglu-His-Trp-Ser-Tyr-Gly-Leu-Arg-Pro-Gyl-NH$_2$

FIG. 42–2. Amino acid sequence of substances capable of releasing pituitary hormones.

diseases involving the adenohypophysis, the infundibular stalk or the hypothalamus.

LUTEINIZING HORMONE RELEASING HORMONE (LRH)

LRH has been detected in hypothalamic extracts obtained from nearly a dozen different species including humans. The chemical structure of natural occurring LRH has not been disclosed, but it appears to be a polypeptide with a molecular weight of about 2000.

It is now known that certain other peptides will lead to the release of LH or to both LH and FSH. A synthetic tetrapeptide can cause the release of LH (Fig. 42–2). Still another polypeptide, a decapeptide, has been demonstrated in smaller doses to increase both LH and FSH (Fig. 42–2). Limited clinical trials with the decapeptide indicate that it is capable of causing ovulation in women.

FOLLICLE-STIMULATING HORMONE RELEASING HORMONE (FRH)

It has been difficult to separate a distinct chemical entity which can be called FRH. Even the most purified preparations of hypothalamic extracts appear to possess both FRH and LRH activities. It has also been suggested that there is only a single releasing hormone responsible for releasing pituitary gonadotropins (e.g., GnRH). FRH is not a polyamine, but a low molecular weight substance with chemical properties resembling a polypeptide. A synthetic decapeptide contains both LRH and FRH properties (Fig. 42–2). This decapeptide has also been referred to as gonadotropin releasing hormone (GnRH). Whether a so-called GnRH is the only factor responsible for the physiologic release of FSH and LH is not known. Circulating steroids can affect GnRH activity.

In humans, larger doses of GnRH are necessary to elicit the release of FSH than those required to stimulate LH release. GnRH can be administered subcutaneously and produces a stimulation of FSH and LH in about a half-hour following injection.

GROWTH HORMONES INHIBITING OR RELEASING HORMONES (GIH, GRH)

GRH has been purified from at least two domestic animals and is undoubtedly a polypeptide with a molecular weight of about 2500. GRH appears to contain the same number of amino acids as GnRH. The amino acid sequence of a decapeptide with growth hormone releasing action isolated from porcine hypothalami has been reported.

The possible clinical significance of either GRH or GIH (sometime called somatostatin) remains to be established. Certainly the potential usefulness of GRH or GIH lies in the regulation of such growth disorders as dwarfism or giantism.

PROLACTIN INHIBITING OR RELEASING HORMONE (PIH, PRH)

In most mammals, the secretion of prolactin by the adenohypophysis is normally tonically inhibited via Prolactin Inhibitory Hormone (PIH). The chemical nature of PIH remains unknown.

Neither PIH nor PRH have any current clinical usefulness.

It should be noted that both animal and human TRH can stimulate the release of prolactin. Such findings are puzzling in view of the reported specificity of the RH's.

MELANOCYTE-STIMULATING HORMONE INHIBITING OR RELEASING HORMONE (MIH, MRH)

The secretion of MSH is normally under constant inhibition by the hypothalamus. Some progress has been made in disclosing the chemical nature of MIH.

HORMONE TRANSPORTING SUBSTANCES

A universal and characteristic feature of endocrine tissue is the release of a chemical mediator(s) from specific cells into the systemic circulation. Once released into the blood, the chemical mediator (or hormone) is subject to a variety of influences. The particular biologic half-life of a hormone in the blood that varies from several minutes to days is the result of a number of factors including its rate of biotransformation and excretion. Biologic half-life is prolonged when a hormone complexes with larger molecules found in the blood. This binding not only provides a hormonal reservoir, but provides protected transportation. Despite the presence of hormone-transporting proteins, a particular hormone may also exist in a free (i.e., unbound) state. Some hormones will in addition bind nonspecifically to plasma proteins. Generally, if the hormone binding sites on a specific carrier molecule are occupied, then the hormone associates nonspecifically with plasma albumins. The binding of a hormone to its transporting protein is reversible so that the hormone can be released and subsequently assimilated by its target organ.

Most, but not all, hormones have specific carrier proteins which can transport them in body fluids (Table 42–2). Ordinarily, hormones with

smaller molecular weights such as steroids and thyroxine are bound to a carrier protein. Polypeptides of the posterior pituitary gland also appear to be bound to transporting proteins. The binding of smaller hormones to specific transporting proteins unlike that of pituitary hormones is affected by many pharmacologic agents.

SPECIFIC TRANSPORTING PROTEINS FOR THYROID HORMONES

The thyroid hormones circulate in the blood noncovalently bound to transporting proteins. The thyroid gland secretes both thyroxine (T_4) and triiodothyronine (T_3). Three serum proteins transport thyroxine: albumin, thyroxine-binding prealbumin (TBPA) and thyroxine-binding α-globulin (TBG). TBG is found in very small concentrations in the blood, yet it has a very great affinity for T_4 and sizeable amounts of T_3. The affinity of TBPA for T_3 is minimal. Only small amounts of either T_3 or T_4 remain in a free state, but these may be physiologically important.

Both physiologic and pathologic factors can alter the transport of thyroidal hormones. Pharmacologic agents can change thyroid hormone transport (Table 42–3), and also interfere with serum thyroxine (T) and triiodothyronine (T) uptake tests (Table 42–4). In some instances the mechanism of these drug interactions is known (Table 42–4).

STEROID CARRYING PROTEINS

Steroid hormones in the circulating blood are noncovalently bound to serum albumins and globulins. The binding equilibrium is determined by the concentration and by the affinities of the components. The serum proteins that interact with steroid hormones are: 1) albumins (HSA or

TABLE 42–2. Some Hormone Transporting Proteins in the Blood

Hormone	Transporting protein
Cortisol	Corticosteroid binding globulin (CBG)
Testosterone	Sex hormone binding globulin (SHBG)
	Testosterone binding globulin (TeBG)
Estrogen	Sex hormone binding globulin (SHBG)
Progesterone	Progesterone binding globulin (PBG)
Throxine	Thyroxine binding globulin (TBG) and
	Thyroxine binding prealbumin (TBPA)
Oxytocin and/or vasopressin	Neurophysin I and II

TABLE 42–3. Drug-Hormone Interactions and Changes in Thyroid Hormone Transport

Drug	Thyroxin binding globulin	Thyroxin binding prealbumin
Drugs interfering with thyroxine binding affinity		
Diphenylhydantoin	+	
Salicylates		+
Drugs affecting thyroxine binding capacity		
Oral Contraceptives	↑	
Estrogens	↑	
Testosterone	↓	↑
Anabolic Steroids	↓	↑
Corticosteroids	↓	↑

human serum albumin), 2) α-acid glycoproteins (AAG or α-acid globulin-orosomucoid), 3) corticosteroid-binding globulin (CBG or transcortin) and 4) β-globulins (SHBG or sex hormone binding globulin).

Steroid binding proteins vary with respect to their physiochemical characteristics, their affinities for different steroid hormones and their serum concentrations. For example, HSA is found in much higher concentrations than CBG, yet HSA has considerably less affinity for the corticosteroids. The affinity of a carrier protein for a steroid hormone is not absolutely specific. While CBG has a high affinity for cortisol or corticosterone, it will also bind to other steroids such as progesterone.

Hormone-protein complexes may delay the metabolic transformation of steroids by the liver. Steroids that are complexed to a carrier hormone cannot be biotransformed to more polar metabolites. Polar metabolites can be more readily excreted by the kidneys. Although the free unbound form of the hormone is most likely the biologically active form, the free form also is more susceptible to metabolism by the liver or the kidney.

CORTICOSTEROID BINDING GLOBULIN (CBG)

Many of the physiochemical characteristics of CBG have been established for several mammalian species including man. CBG has a higher affinity for most major adrenocortical hormones, but also interacts with progesterone and estrogen. Whereas albumins may contain several active binding sites for a given steroid, CBG possesses only a single site for the interaction of a hormone.

CBG is affected by several factors. Levels of CBG are ordinarily higher in females than in males. Castration causes an increase in the levels of CBG in males. Normal males treated with estrogen exhibit levels of CBG that are comparable to those in females. Pregnancy causes an increase in CBG; a sharp decline is observed soon after parturition. Thyroidectomy results in a loss in CBG activity indicating that thyroxine somehow assists in maintaining the levels of this transporting protein.

Several pharmacologic agents can alter the activity of this transporting protein. Estrogens and progesterone, including oral contraceptives and androgen therapy can alter CBG levels. Similarly, the treatment of hypothyroidism or hyperthyroidism also could be expected to interfere with

TABLE 42–4. Effects of Various Drugs and Hormones on PBI and T_3 Uptake Tests

Drug	Mechanism of interaction	Effect on PBI	Effect on T_3 uptake
Oral contraceptives	Increase thyroxine capacity of serum proteins	+	−
Estrogens	Increase thyroxine capacity of serum proteins	+	−
Testosterone and anabolic steroids	Decreases thyroxine binding capacity of serum proteins	−	+
Courmarin anticoagulants	Unknown	None	+
Phenylbutazone	Unknown	None	+
Diphenylhydantoin	Competes with thyroxine for binding sites on serum proteins	−	+
Salicylates	Competes with thyroxine for binding sites on serum proteins	−	+
Propylthiouracil	Lowers circulating levels of hormone	−	−
Perphenazine	Increases thyroxine-binding capacity of serum proteins	+	−

+Increases values above normal test results.
−Decreases values below normal test results.

CBG activity. Many of the synthetic antiinflammatory steroids have low affinities for CBG. In general, synthetic halogenated adrenocortical-like steroids do not significantly compete with natural corticoids for CBG, but remain free in the sera.

SEX HORMONE BINDING GLOBULINS (SHBG)

Testosterone seems to have a specific plasma binding protein, although this androgen may share a transporting protein with estrogens. Evidence also indicates that progesterone may interact with a specific serum globulin. In the case of estrogens, it is reasonably clear that despite a blood transporting protein, the action of female sex hormones on their target organs can occur in the absence of a transporting substance.

Albumin has a very high capacity for binding testosterone and estrogens. Albumins, however, have a low affinity for sex steroid hormones. The plasma also contains low concentrations of globulins that interact with androgens or estrogens. These globulins have a low capacity for either androgens or estrogens, but a high affinity for the sex steroids.

While a specific transporting protein may have a high affinity for testosterone, evidence indicates that estradiol can displace this androgen from its binding sites on the carrier molecule. Perhaps both androgens and estrogens are bound to the same protein in human plasma. The molecular weight of SHBG has been estimated to be nearly 100,000 or approximately twice the weight for CBG and possesses a single binding site for either testosterone or estradiol. The globulin that appears to specifically transport progesterone may have as many as three distinct binding sites for the steroid. Progesterone also has an affinity for CBG.

Testosterone binding globulin (TeBG) is increased during pregnancy and by the pharmacologic use of estrogens. Similarly, the degree of binding of testosterone or dihydrotestosterone is increased in hyperthyroidism. Oral contraceptives can likewise enhance SHBG levels.

CIRCULATING INSULIN

As yet a specific transporting protein for insulin has not been established. Albeit controversial, a portion of the insulin present in the blood is bound to proteins. Some circulating insulin is also in a free or unbound state. It has been suggested that the free insulin is the physiologically active form of the hormone.

FURTHER READING

Bitensky MW, Gorman RE (1972): Chemical mediation of hormone action. Annu Rev Med 23:263

Burgus R, Guillemin R (1970): Hypothalamic releasing factors. Annu Rev Biochem 39:499

Corvol PL, Chrambach A, Rodbard D, Bardin CW (1971): Physical properties and binding capacity of testosterone-estradiol-binding globulin in human plasma, determined by polyacrylamide gel electrophoresis. J Biol Chem 246:3435

Gay VL (1972): The hypothalamus: physiology and clinical use of releasing factors. Fertil Steril 21:50

Schally AV, Kastin AJ, Arimura A (1972): Follicle stimulating releasing hormone and luteinizing releasing hormone. Vitam Horm 30:84

Westphal U (1970): Corticosteroid-binding globulin and other steroid hormone carriers in the blood stream. J Reprod Fertil Supp 10:15

Wilber JF (1973): Thyrotropin releasing hormone: secretion and actions. Annu Rev Med 24:353

JOHN E. JONES

JOHN A. THOMAS

43. PITUITARY HORMONES AND UTERINE STIMULATING DRUGS

ANTERIOR PITUITARY HORMONES

The therapeutic potential of the anterior pituitary hormones has not yet been fully realized. Endocrine therapy involving trophic hormones has not been widespread because it has been difficult to obtain significant amounts of human trophic hormones. Trophic hormones extracted from domestic animals are often immunologically different and hence tend to be either ineffective in man or else gradually lose their biologic effectiveness. Although some of the trophic hormones have been chemically identified and even synthesized (e.g., ACTH), most have continued to elude the efforts of the biochemist.

Hormonal replacement therapies have usually relied upon the use of the target organ hormone rather than the trophic hormone. Hypothyroidism, e.g., is treated with thyroxine and not TSH. Because the trophic hormones are usually large sized molecules, they are not effective orally. This fact, of course, has not prevented the use of insulin which must be injected, but it did provide the impetus for seeking a suitable replacement in the form of the oral hypoglycemic drugs. Substitutes for trophic hormones have also been sought and have been found in the case of the gonadotropins (e.g., human chorionic gonadotropin and human menopausal gonadotropin).

Trophic hormones are used in the differential diagnosis of endocrine disorders involving either the adenohypophysial-hypothalamic axis or its specific target organ. For example, a single injection of a trophic hormone has been used to distinguish whether the site of disease is primary (pituitary) or secondary (target organ).

Adenohypophysial Target Organ Interactions

The physiologic relationship of a trophic hormone to its specific target cell(s) is well known. Such a relationship is readily appreciated with such trophic hormones as ACTH, TSH, and the gonadotropins, but is poorly understood in the case of prolactin and growth hormone where the concept of specific target cells may not apply.

Under physiologic conditions, but with notable exceptions, the target organ hormone induced by a specific trophic hormone is released into the circulation and carried to the anterior pituitary and/or hypothalamus where it can reduce the secretion of a particular adenohypophysial hormone (Fig. 43–1). This so-called negative feedback effect by the target organ hormone ordinarily exerts a negative or inhibitory action upon the further release of a trophic hormone. This negative or long-loop feedback relationship between the adenohypophysial-hypothalamic areas and a specific target organ is particularly evident in the case of either ACTH or TSH. Short-loop feedback systems between the adenohypophysis and specific areas of the hypothalamus are also known to be operant for some of the trophic hormones. In the case of a short-loop feedback system, a specific trophic hormone secreted by the adenohypophysis could act upon areas of the hypothalamus to inhibit a particular releasing hormone or factor. There are exceptions to this. Certain target organ hormones, e.g., estrogens can cause an increase in the release and/or secretion of trophic hormones. Such positive feedback relationships may be either long-loop or short-loop. At times just prior to ovulation, estrogens stimulate the release of LH. Finally, there are situations where trophic hormones appear to act upon hypothalamic areas to affect their own synthesis and/or release.

It is important that the physiologic relationship between the anterior pituitary gland and its target organ be fully understood before giving

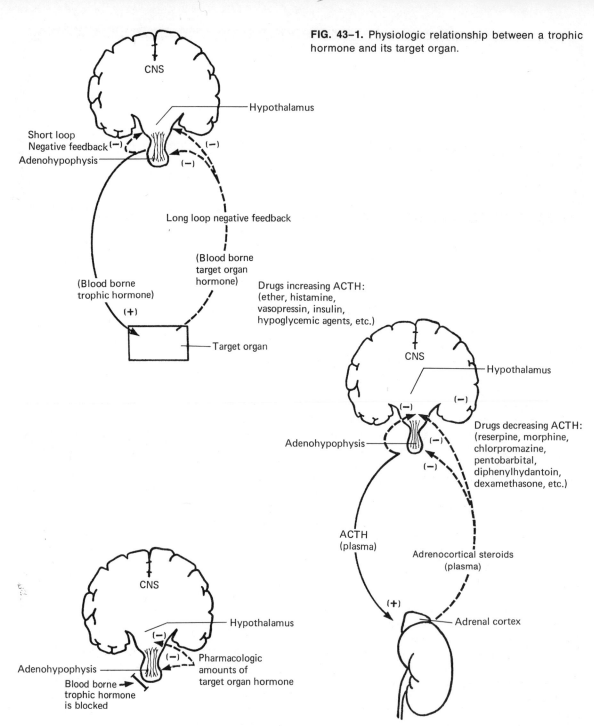

FIG. 43-1. Physiologic relationship between a trophic hormone and its target organ.

CNS

Hypothalamus

Short loop
Negative feedback (−)

Adenohypophysis

(−)

(−)

Long loop negative feedback

(Blood borne
target organ
hormone)

(Blood borne
trophic hormone)

(+)

Target organ

Drugs increasing ACTH:
(ether, histamine,
vasopressin, insulin,
hypoglycemic agents, etc.)

CNS

Hypothalamus

(−)

(−)

Adenohypophysis

(−)

(−)

Drugs decreasing ACTH:
(reserpine, morphine,
chlorpromazine,
pentobarbital,
diphenylhydantoin,
dexamethasone, etc.)

ACTH
(plasma)

Adrenocortical steroids
(plasma)

(+)

Adrenal cortex

CNS

Hypothalamus

(−)

(−)

Adenohypophysis

Pharmacologic
amounts of
target organ hormone

Blood borne →
trophic hormone
is blocked

FIG. 43-3. Effect of certain drugs on ACTH.

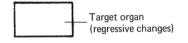

Target organ
(regressive changes)

FIG. 43-2. Effect of administering pharmacologic amounts of target organ hormone on the pituitary target organ axis.

drugs possessing inherent hormonal activity since they can interfere with this basic relationship (Fig. 43–2). For example, the administration of synthetic antiinflammatory steroids can lead to a suppression of endogenous ACTH. Thyroxine-like agents used for their anorexic properties or their cholesterol lowering activities can also produce a reduction in the secretion of TSH. Likewise, the use of pharmacologic amounts of either progesterone or estrogens can suppress the secretion of FSH and LH.

CORTICOTROPIN (ACTH)

Physiologic Considerations

Corticotropin releasing hormone (CRH) and many external stimuli can increase the secretion of ACTH. The physiologic actions resulting from ACTH are due principally to its stimulatory effects upon adrenal steroidogenesis and the release of cortisol, corticosterone and closely related steroids. Adrenal cortical steroids are capable of suppressing the release of ACTH by acting either upon the hypothalamus and/or the adenohypophysis. Several pharmacologic agents can impinge upon the ACTH-cortisol servomechanism leading to either increases or decreases in the levels of circulating ACTH (Fig. 43–3).

Chemical Aspects

ACTH is a single chain polypeptide containing 39 amino acids (Fig. 43–4). The amino acid sequence is slightly different among various species, but the first 23 amino acid sequences are common to many including man. Synthetic ACTH-like molecules are commercially available and contain 18–24 amino acids.

Measurements of ACTH concentrations in plasma were originally carried out using bioassay procedures, but radioimmunoassays are now available. Ordinarily, plasma corticoid determinations provide some index of ACTH activity.

Mechanism of Action

ACTH effects may be mediated by cAMP. ACTH may act by altering the activity of cell membrane bound adenyl cyclase in the adrenal gland. By some as yet unestablished mechanism cAMP enhances the bioconversion of cholesterol to corticosteroids. Cyclic AMP promotes the formation of enzymatic cofactors that are involved in the process of steroidogenesis.

Pharmacologic Uses

Of all the anterior pituitary hormones that are used pharmacologically, ACTH is probably the most extensively employed both therapeutically and diagnostically. Some of its therapeutic effectiveness is derived secondarily by stimulating the secretion of endogenous adrenal cortical steroids. Still other therapeutic uses of ACTH involve its empirical use in the management of certain types of epilepsy that have failed to respond to more conventional therapy (Ch. 30). Most inflammatory states respond better to the synthetic adrenal cortical steroids than to ACTH. (Ch. 46)

Synthetic corticotropin has been useful as a rapid diagnostic test for hypoadrenalism. Either natural or synthetic ACTH must be administered IV, IM or subcutaneously. The duration of action of ACTH can be extended by incorporating it with a zinc phosphate complex, but the principal factor affecting its duration of action is the total dose administered. Hypersensitivity reactions occasionally occur with either natural and rarely synthetic ACTH. Mild fever, anaphylaxis and even death have been reported on rare occasions. ACTH causes sodium retention and hypokalemia, but such actions are caused secondarily by the adrenocorticoids. (Ch. 46) Probably because of chemical similarities between portions of the MSH molecule and the ACTH molecule, increased pigmentation is occasionally observed during corticotropin therapy.

SOMATOTROPIN (STH) (GROWTH HORMONE)

Physiologic Considerations

The hypothalamus exerts an influence on the release or the inhibition of release of growth hormone by the anterior pituitary. A growth hormone feedback system has not been demonstrated despite intensive research efforts.

Growth hormone aids in the regulation of metabolism. It increases the growth of the skeletal system by stimulating the epiphysial plates

Ser-Tyr-Ser-Met-Glu-His-Phe-Arg-Try-Gly-Lys-Pro-Val-Gly-Lys-Lys-Arg-Arg-Pro-Val-Lys-Val-Tyr-
1 2 3 4 5 6 7 8 9 10 11 12 13 14 15 16 17 18 19 20 21 22 23

Pro-Asp-Ala-Gly-Gln-Asp-Glu-Ser-Ala-Glu-Ala-Phe-Pro-Leu-Glu-Phe
24 25 26 27 28 29 30 31 32 33 34 35 36 37 38 39

FIG. 43–4. Amino acid sequence of ACTH.

and enhances chondrogenesis. Growth hormone exerts a protein anabolic action upon many tissues, and effects changes in body calcium, potassium and sodium. It is diabetogenic since it enhances hepatic glucose output and appears to exert an antiinsulin action upon muscles. The action of growth hormone upon blood glucose levels can secondarily promote the release of insulin from the pancreas which contributes to its protein anabolic effect.

The principal physiologic suppressor of growth hormone secretion is glucose. Physical and mental stress, ingestion of a high protein meal, arginine and the onset of sleep can lead to increased levels of plasma growth hormone. Diseases such as acromegaly, diabetes mellitus, certain mammary and endometrial cancers, cirrhosis and starvation states like anorexia nervosa and kwaskiorkor tend to elevate plasma levels of growth hormone. On the other hand hypopituitarism, hypogonadism, hypothyroidism and obesity result in low levels of plasma growth hormone.

Pharmacologic amounts of insulin, glucagon or vasopressin are very effective in elevating plasma levels of growth hormone (Table 43–1). These hormones have been used as diagnostic agents to provoke the release of pituitary growth hormone. Arginine stimulates the release and in general, high doses of the glucocorticoids cause a decrease in levels of growth hormone.

Chemical Aspects

Human growth hormone (HGH) is a polypeptide with a molecular weight of 21,500 containing 188 amino acids. Nonhuman primate growth hormone is chemically similar to HGH, but is less active biologically when used in humans.

Growth hormone can be measured using radioimmunoassay procedures and has proved very useful in the diagnosis of gigantism, hypopituitarism, acromegaly and growth retardation syndromes.

Mechanism of Action

The action of this hormone on protein metabolism appears to be exerted at the ribosomal level, where it may affect either ribosomal translation or attachment. It also stimulates the transport of certain amino acids into cells.

Pharmacologic Uses

HGH is used in the management of growth disorders, particularly dwarfism, however, it is important that the etiology of the growth disorder be properly diagnosed since amounts of HGH are in limited supply. HGH is sometimes effective in increasing the rate of growth in pituitary dwarfism. For optimal therapeutic success, the biweekly injections should be continued for a period of years, usually until skeletal maturity renders further use ineffective. Prior to initiating HGH therapy it is important to confirm a metabolic response to the injected hormone such as a reduction in blood urea and urinary nitrogen excretion. In patients receiving long term HGH therapy there is often a diminishing rate of growth after the first year; occasional resistance to the hormone has been reported.

HGH therapy may be of value during certain phases of renal failure, in bone marrow hypoplasia, in some forms of juvenile spontaneous hypoglycemia, and possibly in the management of the catabolic response to burns and other forms of severe trauma. Because protein anabolic steroids appear to act somewhat synergistically with growth hormone, they are often used together.

Since sensitive assays are now available for HGH, there are several diagnostic applications for this hormone. Assays of HGH are very important in establishing the diagnosis of pituitary dwarfism and acromegaly. Many pharmacologic agents can be administered that will provoke the release of growth hormone (Table 43–1). Insulin increases HGH secretion by inducing hypoglycemia. Other provocative tests for HGH secretion employ arginine, glucagon, vasopressin, L-Dopa and bacterial pyrogens. There is some disagreement as to which provocative test is the most effective.

HGH can produce some adverse side effects. It can be diabetogenic. Severe ketosis with acidosis can develop in diabetic patients receiving only a single dose. It is contraindicated in diabetic dwarfs. Despite the fact that HGH is used in humans, antibodies reportedly affect its therapeutic effectiveness.

TABLE 43–1. Agents Influencing Plasma Levels of Growth Hormone

Agents that may increase growth hormone levels	Agents that may decrease growth hormone levels
Estrogens	Glucocorticoids
Oral contraceptives	Chlorpromazine
Insulin	α-adrenergic
Vasopressin	receptor blocking
Arginine	agents
Glucagon	
Norepinephrine	
Dopamine	
β-adrenergic receptor blocking agents	

THYROTROPIN (TSH)

Physiologic Considerations

The secretion of TSH by the anterior pituitary is controlled principally by a negative feedback system involving thyroxine. TSH causes both morphologic and biochemical changes in the thyroid gland. However, no single metabolic step in thyroxine synthesis or secretion has been demonstrated to be selectively altered by this trophic hormone.

Thyrotropin releasing hormone (TRH) stimulates both the synthesis and release of TSH. As its release is also enhanced by epinephrine, the pituitary thyrotropic cells may possess adrenergic receptors.

Chemical Aspects

TSH is a glycoprotein with a molecular weight of approximately 25,000. Even though human thyroid glands respond to bovine, ovine and whale TSH, immunologic differences exist since antiTSH antibodies are found in heterologous species.

Mechanism of Action

TSH enhances the synthesis, storage and release of iodine-containing thyroid hormones from the thyroid gland. It increases many aspects of intermediary metabolism in the thyroid gland which leads to enhanced oxygen consumption. RNA synthesis and phospholipid metabolism are increased. Some of the actions of TSH can be attributed to increases in cAMP.

Pharmacologic Uses

TSH is not used for replacement therapy in the treatment of hypothyroidal states: thyroxine and its analogs provide suitable therapy. TSH has been used diagnostically to assess the thyroidal uptake of radioactive iodine; ^{131}I uptake by the thyroid is normally increased by TSH. It is inactive orally, has a rather short biologic half-life and is metabolized mainly by the kidney.

FOLLICLE STIMULATING HORMONE (FSH) AND HUMAN MENOPAUSAL GONADOTROPIN (HMG)

Physiologic Considerations

Both FSH and LH act in concert and follow a cyclic pattern in the female (Fig. 43–5). These gonadotropins are required for optimal ovarian estrogen secretion and follicle growth. FSH promotes spermatogenesis and stimulates the metabolic activity of the Sertoli cells in the seminiferous tubules of the testes. Sertoli cells may produce small amounts of testosterone and estrogens when stimulated by FSH.

Chemical Aspects

FSH is a glycoprotein and may be composed of two subunits—α-FSH and β-FSH of somewhat equal molecular weights. One subunit may provide the specific physiologic action important to FSH while the other subunit may simply be a nonspecific portion of the molecule similar to that found in other pituitary glycoprotein hormones.

The chemical properties of human menopausal gonadotropin (HMG) are not entirely known. This substance exhibits principally FSH-like, but not LH-like activity. Commercial preparations of HMG are quite stable. Either human FSH or HMG must be administered parenterally. FSH obtained from animal pituitary glands is antigenic in humans.

Mechanism of Action

The major action of FSH in the female is to enhance young ovarian follicles to develop layers of granulosa and to form antra. Unless FSH and LH act together, estrogen secretion is not sufficient to promote the growth and metabolism of the female reproductive tract. In the male, FSH stimulates spermatogenesis and testicular RNA and protein but has no stimulatory actions upon the testicular production of androgens from the Leydig cells.

FSH, like other protein hormones, probably does not enter the target cell, but exerts its initial actions upon the plasma membrane by interacting with membrane associated adenyl cyclase. The FSH receptors in the testes also have an affinity for HMG, but not LH or HCG. Interstitial cells of the testes will not bind FSH.

Pharmacologic Uses

Human supplies of FSH are limited and animal sources are not suitable for therapeutic uses because of differences in biologic and immunologic properties. Human menopausal gonadotropin (HMG) can be used as a substitute for human FSH.

In females, human FSH (or HMG) is used in conjunction with LH (or HCG) to induce ovulation. Certain cases of infertility respond to sequential regimens of human FSH and LH. Ordinarily the ovary is primed with FSH or HMG. The

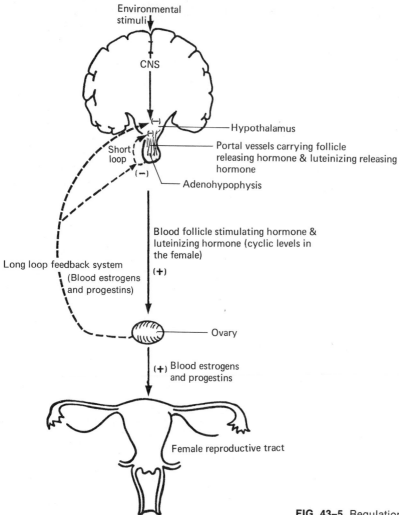

Environmental stimuli

CNS

Hypothalamus

(—)

Short loop

(—)

Portal vessels carrying follicle releasing hormone & luteinizing releasing hormone

Adenohypophysis

Blood follicle stimulating hormone & luteinizing hormone (cyclic levels in the female)

(+)

Long loop feedback system (Blood estrogens and progestins)

Ovary

(+) Blood estrogens and progestins

Female reproductive tract

FIG. 43–5. Regulation of pituitary gonadotropins.

near midcycle injection of HCG or LH may lead to the induction of ovulation. The combined use of FSH and LH (or their substitutes) in women with infertility frequently causes multiple births. It is difficult to determine the proper dose and dosage schedule of FSH and LH in the treatment of infertility.

Another method of inducing ovulation in cases of infertility is to use *clomiphene* (Clomid). Clomiphene acts probably by releasing endogenous FSH and LH. The subsequent release of pituitary gonadotropins causes the ovaries to release ova. Clomiphene, by stimulating the ovaries, causes the overproduction of estrogen. Clomiphene may cause abdominal and pelvic discomfort and an increased incidence of multiple births.

Human FSH has little therapeutic or diagnostic use in the male. Reduced spermatogenesis is more often treated with testosterone than with FSH.

LUTEINIZING HORMONE (LH) AND HUMAN CHORIONIC GONADOTROPIN (HCG)

Physiologic Considerations

The physiologic action of LH (or interstitial-cell stimulating hormone in the male) depends upon FSH to achieve an optimal hormonal response. In the female reproductive cycle, FSH acts to prime the ovaries which are subsequently affected by LH since this latter trophic hormone is responsible for ovulation. In the male, FSH affects principally the process of spermatogenesis whereas LH stimulates steroidogenesis in the Leydig cell or interstitial cells of the testes. Human chorionic gonadotropin (HCG) can be used as a pharmacologic substitute for LH by provoking ovulation in the female and increasing androgen synthesis in the male.

The hypothalamic-adenohypophysial-ovarian axis is a complex feedback system (Fig. 43–5).

Ovarian estrogens and progestins modulate the secretion of pituitary gonadotropins. Generally, estrogens and/or progestins act on receptors located in the hypothalamic and adenohypophysial areas to reduce the secretion of FSH and LH. At critical midcycle intervals these steroids may actually enhance the release of LH resulting in ovulation. Thus, there are both negative and positive feedback receptors involved in gonadotropin secretion. Pharmacologic doses of either estrogens or progestins usually cause an inhibition of the secretion of both FSH and LH. There is little cyclic variation in either FSH or LH in the male.

Chemical Aspects

LH is a glycoprotein and has been separated into an α and a β subunit. The ovulation-inducing actions of LH have been ascribed to the β subunit in certain experimental animals. HCG has been purified and separated into two fractions that exhibit different ratios of FSH and LH activity. Clinically, HCG is used for its LH-like activity.

Mechanism of Action

Since LH and HCG have relatively large molecular weights, they must act at the plasma membrane of the cells of the target organ. HCG and LH must have similar sites of action since they compete with each other for receptors located both in the corpus luteum and the thecal cells of the ovary. LH or HCG binding by ovarian tissues depends upon the priming action of either FSH or an FSH-like hormone such as HMG. Subunits of HCG can bind ovarian receptors, but not with the same affinity as the entire molecule. The β-subunit of HCG appears to compete more readily with the entire molecule than does the α-subunit of HCG.

Interstitial cells of the testes likewise have the ability to bind LH and HCG, but not FSH. LH or HCG can cause a rather rapid increase in steroidogenesis. There is some evidence to indicate that some of the actions of LH or HCG are mediated by increases in either ovarian or testicular cAMP.

Pharmacologic Uses

LH obtained from animal sources is not suitable for use in treating human endocrine disorders since the immunologic and biologic differences are too great. The principal supply of human LH is from pituitary glands obtained at necropsy. Human chorionic gonadotropin (Antuitrin-S, Riogon, Follutein, APL, etc.) is used as a suitable substitute for LH. HCG is extracted from the urine of pregnant women during the first trimester. Only effective after parenteral administration, its biologic half-life may be as long as several hours.

HCG (or human LH if supplies are available) is used in conjunction with human FSH (or HMG) in the treatment of infertility in women. One of the most successful regimens has been to prime the ovary with injections of HMG (for its FSH-like activity) and then inject HCG (for its LH-like activity). HCG sometimes causes the induction of ovulation. Because dosage is difficult to control, multiple pregnancies are a frequent outcome. Unfortunately, this often leads to an increased incidence in stillbirths or abortions.

HCG has been used in an effort to prevent spontaneous abortions associated with insufficient levels of chorionic gonadotropin. Used in conjunction with either FSH or HMG, it may induce ovulation in women suffering from amenorrhea.

HCG is used to induce testicular descent in the treatment of cryptorchidism. It will increase androgen secretion by functional Leydig cells and cause increased virilization.

PROLACTIN

Physiologic Considerations

Prolactin causes milk secretion from the mammary gland, but only after suitable priming by estrogen and progesterone. The increased levels of prolactin secreted during lactation are also capable of producing behavioral changes. Prolactin has no known physiologic role in males.

Chemical Aspects

Prolactin has a molecular weight of approximately 25,000. There are some similarities between the chemical structure of prolactin and growth hormone. There are three homologous subunits in human pituitary growth hormone and ovine prolactin, yet growth and lactation are not controlled by a single molecule in humans.

Mechanism of Action

The mechanism of action of prolactin in lactation is poorly understood. In experimental animals, purified preparations of mammary cell membranes exhibit a high affinity, but a low binding capacity for prolactin.

Pharmacologic Uses

Although the physiologic role of prolactin in the process of lactation is evident, this trophic hormone is of no therapeutic or diagnostic value.

Drugs Affecting Prolactin Levels

Several drugs are known to alter the blood levels of prolactin. Chlorpromazine, reserpine, α-methyl-*para*-tyrosine and α-methyl-*meta*-tyrosine can produce elevations in the blood levels of prolactin and sometimes galactorrhea. These agents appear to act by inhibiting catecholamine metabolism in the hypothalamus (Ch. 18). Under certain conditions, both thyroxine and estrogen can stimulate the secretion of prolactin. Ergocornine and closely related ergot analogs are capable of inhibiting lactation presumably by interfering with hypothalamic mechanisms involved in the release of prolactin.

POSTERIOR PITUITARY HORMONES

The posterior pituitary or neurohypophysis is neither directly innervated by axons from the hypothalamus nor does it receive a rich vascular supply. The posterior pituitary is the site of storage of antidiuretic hormone (ADH or vasopressin) and oxytocin. ADH is synthesized primarily in the cell bodies of the supraoptic nucleus of the hypothalamus and oxytocin in those of the paraventricular nucleus. These hormones are transported to the posterior pituitary by axoplasmic flow and stored in the nerve terminals. ADH and oxytocin are stored in neurosecretory granules complexed with a protein, neurophysin. Both hormones travel with neurophysin down the stalk to the posterior pituitary gland.

epithelium in the renal collecting ducts and allows for the loss of water from the renal tubular fluid into the hypertonic cells of the collecting duct. A deficiency of ADH is the cause of diabetes insipidus which is characterized by the excretion of large volumes of dilute urine and an increased osmolarity of the blood.

Physiologically speaking, the use of the term vasopressin instead of ADH is a misnomer. This hormone will affect vascular smooth muscle only in supraphysiologic doses, although certain species are more sensitive than others to the vasoconstrictor effects of ADH. Injections of supraphysiologic doses of ADH produce elevations in adrenocortical steroids by causing an increase in ACTH.

ANTIDIURETIC HORMONE (ADH)

Physiologic Considerations

ADH is secreted from the nerve terminals in the posterior pituitary in response to a variety of stimuli such as stress, suckling, coitus, parturition and increased osmolarity of the blood, and such drugs as nicotine, ether, barbiturates and morphine. Alcohol inhibits the release of ADH (Ch. 10).

The major physiologic role of ADH is in the regulation of blood osmolarity. When osmolarity is increased, ADH secretion is increased. Conversely, a reduction in the osmolarity inhibits the release. ADH enhances the permeability of the

Chemical Aspects

ADH is a simple polypeptide containing eight amino acids (Fig. 43–6). The cystine moiety of this octapeptide seems to be important for biologic activity. Arginine vasopressin is more prevalent among mammals than is lysine vasopressin. In humans, arginine is essential for maximum biologic activity. Peptides that are more active than naturally occurring ADH have been chemically synthesized. ADH can be administered IV, IM or subcutaneously and by nasal insufflation. The latter route is used in the treatment of diabetes insipidus with *posterior pituitary powder* (*Pitressin*).

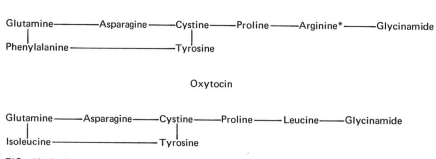

FIG. 43–6. Posterior pituitary hormones. * Arginine is often replaced with lysine to form lysine vasopressin.

Despite the development of radioimmunoassay procedures for ADH, this hormone is still prescribed in posterior pituitary units.

Metabolism and Excretion

Vasopressin preparations are rapidly metabolized by enzymes found both in the liver and the kidney. Its biologic half-life in humans is less than one half-hour. Aminopeptidases are involved in the breakdown of this octapeptide. Amounts of the hormone are excreted by the kidney unchanged.

Mechanism of Action

ADH effects may be mediated through cAMP which is known to enhance the permeability of the renal collecting ducts. Theophylline, an inhibitor of phosphodiesterase, has the same effect. ADH also causes a release of hyaluronidase that digests connective links in the collecting ductile system membranes leading to increased permeability.

Pharmacologic Uses

The major therapeutic indication for vasopressin is in the treatment of diabetes insipidus where it replaces or supplements endogenous levels of ADH. The polyuria is usually reduced. Since *posterior pituitary extract* contains both vasopressin and oxytocin, the latter octapeptide may produce some unwanted side effects when used in this condition. *Vasopressin tannate* is a purified, lipid soluble form of ADH. Not only is this more purified form free of allergic reactions, but it has a longer duration of action. *Lysine vasopressin* (*Lypressin-Diapid*) is also a purified form of ADH and can be administered by nasal insufflation. Patients with diabetes insipidus who become resistant or tolerant to the prolonged use of vasopressin can often be successfully treated with either the thiazide diuretics or with the hypoglycemic agent chlorpropamide.

The smooth muscle stimulatory properties of vasopressin are of little therapeutic value but have been used in the management of distension and incomplete paralysis of the gastrointestinal tract. It is frequently used in conjunction with cholinesterase inhibitory drugs and suction decompression.

Vasopressin has been used to evaluate the pituitary reserve of ACTH. It induces the release of endogenous ACTH and leads to increased blood levels of adrenocorticoids. The availability of exogenous ACTH, and the ability to measure ACTH in the blood, has reduced the diagnostic usefulness of the vasopressin test.

Pure preparations or synthetic vasopressin-like substances have largely replaced less purified pituitary extracts. The less purified the extract, the more likely the allergenic properties. Vasopressin causes constriction of the coronary blood vessels and is contraindicated in angina pectoris. Nausea and intestinal and uterine cramps may result from its administration.

OXYTOCIN

Physiologic Considerations

The major physiologic role of oxytocin is to stimulate the contraction of the smooth muscles of the uterus and the mammary glands by a direct action independent of the autonomic innervation. The myoepithelial cells which line the ductile system of the mammary gland contract and squeeze the milk from the alveoli of the lactating breast into the sinusoids. Many hormones including progesterone, estrogen and prolactin are responsible for mammary gland growth and the secretion of milk into the ductile system, but milk ejection requires oxytocin.

Milk ejection is ordinarily initiated by a neuroendocrine reflex. Many stimuli can initiate this reflex including suckling, coitus and parturition. At coitus, oxytocin stimulates wave-like contractions of the smooth muscles of the uterus. These actions may aid the migration of spermatozoan through the uterus into the oviducts. Prostaglandins (Ch. 51) may also facilitate sperm migration through the female genital tract.

During late pregnancy, the uterine smooth musculature becomes very sensitive to oxytocin. This sensitivity is enhanced by estrogens and inhibited by progesterone. It is possible that oxytocin plays a stimulatory role during parturition as well as in initiating the onset of labor. The nonpregnant uterus is not as sensitive to oxytocin as the pregnant uterus.

Chemical Aspects

Oxytocin is an octapeptide and differs only slightly from vasopressin (Fig. 43–6). This chemical similarity is reflected in an overlapping of biologic activities when used in supraphysiologic doses.

Oxytocin must be administered IV or IM. Sometimes the hormone is administered by slow intravenous infusion to prolong its biologic effectiveness. Synthetic oxytocin can be administered by nasal insufflation. Oxytocin citrate is effective sublingually.

Oxytocin preparations are still bioassayed by their vasodepressor activity in chickens. Thus ADH and oxytocin are often prescribed in *U.S.P.* units rather than milligrams.

Metabolism and Excretion

Oxytocin is degraded by proteolytic enzymes, and therefore, is ineffective when administered orally. It has a very rapid onset of action and a brief biologic half-life in the blood. Oxytocin is metabolized in the liver and the kidneys. During pregnancy, oxytocin inactivating enzymes (oxytocinases) appear in the plasma, placenta and the uterus.

Mechanism of Action

Oxytocin has a high affinity for receptors in the mammary gland. It has been demonstrated to cause the release of cAMP, but whether this biochemical event is an important intermediate in the mechanism of action of oxytocin is not established.

Pharmacologic Uses

Oxytocin is used primarily in obstetrics for its uterine muscle stimulatory properties. There are several therapeutic indications for oxytocin (Table 43–2). It is most widely used in the induction of labor. It increases the force of contraction of uterine muscles but great care must be exer-cised to insure that the increased uterine tone does not harm the fetus. While oxytocin plays an important physiologic role in milk let-down, its pharmacologic use in women experiencing deficient milk ejection has not been very successful.

Oxytocin injection (**Pitocin**) is a mixture of oxytocin and small amounts of vasopressin and is rarely used in obstetrics because it contains significant amounts of vasopressin. Synthetic oxytocin (*Syntocinon*) contains no vasopressin and can be administered by a slow intravenous infusion or sublingually. Oxytocin citrate is more satisfactorily absorbed buccally.

The toxic effects of oxytocin are generally extensions of its ability to induce uterine contractions (Table 42–2). Excessive doses may induce sustained tonic uterine contractions and result in rupture of the uterus and cervix.

Depending upon the purity of the oxytocin preparation and its dose, an antidiuretic action may occur. Oxytocin may produce hypotension, tachycardia and increased cardiac output. It is interesting to note that oxytocin is a potent vasoconstrictor of uterine blood vessels, yet it can dilate cutaneous and renal vessels.

UTERINE STIMULATING DRUGS

Oxytocin cannot be administered orally and has a relatively brief duration of action. The ergot alkaloids (Ch. 19), sparteine and certain prostaglandins (Ch. 51), because of their uterine stimulatory properties, provide pharmacologic substitutes under certain clinical situations.

Sparteine (*Tocosamine*) is a natural occurring alkaloid with an action similar to the ergot alkaloids (Ch. 19). It is administered parenterally or IM for the induction of labor has a rapid onset of action, is readily inactivated but produces somewhat unpredictable results.

Sparteine is seldom preferred to oxytocin as it is not as efficacious.

FURTHER READING

ANTERIOR PITUITARY

deWied D, deJong W (1974): Drug effects and hypothalamic-anterior pituitary function. Ann Rev Pharmacol 14:389

Lefkowitz RJ, Roth J, Pastan, I (1971): ACTH-receptor interaction in the adrenal: a model for the initial step in the action of hormones that stimulate adenyl cyclase. Ann NY Acad Sci 185:195

Malone, DNS, Strong JA (1972): The present state of Corticotrophin therapy. The Practitioner 208:329

Ontjes DA, Ney RL (1972): Tests of anterior pituitary function. Metabolism 21:159

Schwartz NG, McCormack CE (1972): Reproduction: gonadal function and its regulations. Ann Rev Physiol 34:425

Swyer GIM (ed) (1970): Control of human fertility. Br Med Bull Vol 26

Tager HS, Steiner DS (1974): Peptide hormones. Ann Rev Biochem 43:509

POSTERIOR PITUITARY

Knowles JW (1965): Excretion of drugs in milk—a review. J Pediatr 66: 1068

Sawyer WH, Manning M (1973): Synthetic analogs of oxytocin and the vasopressins. Annu Rev Pharmacol 13:5

Schwartz TL, Schwartz WB (eds) (1967): Symposium on antidiuretic hormones. Am J Med 42:651

JOHN E. JONES

JOHN A. THOMAS

44. PHARMACOLOGY OF THE THYROID AND THE PARATHYROID GLANDS

THYROID HORMONE

PHYSIOLOGIC CONSIDERATIONS

The principal function of the thyroid gland is to synthesize, store and secrete triiodothyronine and thyroxine. The thyroid gland is capable of concentrating large amounts of iodine from the blood. Thyroxine and triiodothyronine are synthesized in the colloid by iodination and condensation of tyrosine molecules that are bound in peptide linkage to thyroglobulin. These iodine containing hormones are involved in the regulation of cellular oxygen consumption, cholesterol metabolism, neuromuscular activity and cardiovascular function. Physical growth and development as well as mental development are retarded by a deficiency of these hormones. Thyrotropic hormone (TSH) controls the rate of release of triiodothyronine and thyroxine.

SYNTHESIS, METABOLISM AND EXCRETION OF THYROID HORMONES

The biosynthesis of thyroid hormone entails both an iodination and a condensation reaction involving tyrosine (Fig. 44–1). The concentration of inorganic iodide found in the blood is low relative to that found within the thyroid gland. Iodide must be actively assimilated from the blood into the follicular epithelium of the thyroid gland. In the gland, iodide is readily oxidized by more than one enzyme system to elemental iodine (I_2). Tyrosine bound to thyroglobulin is iodinated initially to monoiodotyrosine (MIT) and then to diiodotyrosine (DIT). Triiodothyronine (T_3) is formed by a coupling reaction between a molecule of MIT and a molecule of DIT. Two DIT molecules are condensed to form thyroxine (T_4). The thyroglobulin, with T_3 or T_4 still attached by peptide linkage, is next assimilated into the cells by endo-

cytosis. Once within the cell, the vacuoles containing thyroglobulin merge with lysosomal proteases and the peptide bonds between T_3 or T_4 and the thyroglobulin are split. Free T_3 or T_4 is released into the blood after this splitting process. T_4 is found in higher concentrations in the blood than is T_3.

Several tissues are capable of metabolizing T_3 and T_4, however, the physiologically important organ seems to be the liver. The kidney is also involved in certain degradative reactions. Some catabolic products include tetraiodothyroacetic acid (TETRAC) and triiodothyroacetic acid (TRIAC). These end products can be conjugated (e.g., glucuronides) and deiodinated in a manner similar to that of either T_3 or T_4. The iodine so removed is nearly all retained by the body.

MECHANISM OF ACTION AND BIOCHEMICAL EFFECTS

Unlike the steroids that possess rather specific target organs for their actions, the effects of thyroxine are not confined to any specific cell or tissue. Also, unlike the steroids, no specific receptor molecule has been elucidated for thyroxine. There are, however, specific anatomic areas located in the preoptic and median eminence regions that appear to be involved in the locus of action of thyroxine feedback. This feedback system in the pituitary, and to a lesser extent the hypothalamus, is involved with the neural regulation of TSH.

The actual mechanism of thyroxine release is poorly understood, but the process is quite rapid and involves TSH. Presumably, TSH attaches to the follicular cell membrane and stimulates adenyl cyclase leading to the production of cyclic AMP or a "second messenger." The exact

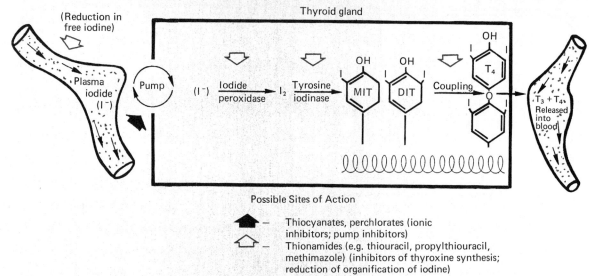

FIG. 44–1. Synthesis of thyroxine and sites of action of antithyroidal agents. Monoiodotyrosine (MIT), Diiodotyrosine (DIT).

role of this second messenger in T_4 and T_3 release into the circulation remains poorly understood. The free hormone that is released from the gland itself is bound to specific transporting plasma proteins.

Thyroid hormones influence a wide variety of important biochemical effects (Table 44–1). The absence of these hormones slows both physical and mental development in children. Thyroxine stimulates the oxygen consumption of most cells and aids in the regulation of both lipid and carbohydrate metabolism. Thyroxine is capable of altering mitochondrial activity as evidenced by an uncoupling of oxidative phosphorylation. Thyroxine administration can lead to increases in protein and nucleic acid synthesis. T_4 has a slower onset of action and a longer duration of action than T_3. T_3 acts quite rapidly and generally causes a greater stimulatory response than T_4.

Both thyroxine and triiodothyronine exert a calorigenic action and lead to an increased metabolic rate. Thyroid gland secretions are increased in a cold environment. Patients suffering from hypothyroidism tend to have subnormal body temperatures.

TABLE 44–1. Changes Caused by Thyroid Hormones

Increased heat production
Increased cellular growth and development
Increased heart rate, contractility and vascular tone
Increased carbohydrate, protein and lipid metabolism
Development of the nervous system
Regulatory actions on water and electrolytes
Increased cholesterol turnover
Increased calcium mobilization from bone
Increased hydrocortisone secretion, particularly in hypothyroidism

Thyroid hormones affect a variety of changes upon the cardiovascular system. Such changes appear to be related to a synergistic action between thyroxine and catecholamines. Pulse pressure and cardiac output are increased by the administration of thyroid hormones. Thyroxine, therefore, enhances the effect of norepinephrine and epinephrine upon the cardiovascular system.

Thyroxine stimulates cholesterol synthesis and enhances the clearance of cholesterol from the blood by the liver. The D-form of thyroxine has been used pharmacologically to reduce blood levels of cholesterol. The D-isomer is less effective than the L-form in causing increases in metabolic activity. There are other nonthyroidal agents that are more effective in lowering blood cholesterol than D-thyroxine.

PHARMACOLOGIC USES OF THYROXINE AND TRIIODOTHYRONINE

The treatment of hypothyroidism usually is carried out effectively by the careful selection and administration of one of the several available commercial preparations (Table 44–2).

Thyroid *U.S.P.* or desiccated thyroid is obtained from dried and defatted thyroid glands of either cows or pigs. It is standardized only on the basis of its iodine content and, therefore, is subject to substantial variation in the actual ratio of T_4 and T_3. Such variations can create some clinical problems in the management of a hypothyroid state. The shelf-life of thyroid *U.S.P.* is limited but it is inexpensive and orally effective.

Thyroglobulin (Proloid), like thyroid *U.S.P.* is also obtained from animal thyroid glands. This partially purified preparation is orally active, but

TABLE 44—2. Pharmacologic Profile of Thyroid Preparations

Drug	Source	Average daily dose	Biologic half-life	Peak action*	Duration of action*
Thyroid U.S.P. (T_3 + T_4)	Animal thyroids	150 mg	1 wk	about 2 wk	3 wk
Thyroglobulin	Animal thyroids	150 mg	1 wk	about 2 wk	3 wk
Sodium L-thyroxine	Synthetic T_4	0.150 mg	1 wk	2 wk	3 wk
Sodium L-thyronine	Synthetic T_3	0.075 mg	1/2 wk	½ wk	1 wk
Liotrix	Synthetic T_3 + T_4 (1:4)		1 wk	2 wk	3 wk

*Related to the dose of the thyroid preparation.

it is somewhat more expensive than thyroid U.S.P. **Thyroglobulin** is not only standardized by its iodine content, but is also bioassayed for its thyroidal potency. Like desiccated thyroid, the T_3/T_4 ratio of thyroglobulin may vary among various preparations. Thyroglobulin offers no therapeutic advantage over thyroid U.S.P.

Sodium L-thyroxine, U.S.P. (Synthroid, Letter) is the sodium salt of synthetic thyroxine (T_4). On a milligram basis, sodium L-thyroxine is more potent than either thyroid U.S.P. or thyroglobulin. This preparation is absorbed reasonably well from the gastrointestinal tract and can also be given IV. The onset and the duration of action of sodium L-thyroxine are very similar to either thyroid U.S.P. or thyroglobulin. Sodium L-thyroxine may well be the drug of choice in hypothyroid disorders. It has a long shelf-life and is not too expensive.

Sodium liothyronine (Cytomel) is the sodium salt of synthetic triiodothyronine (T_3). Like T_4, it has a known potency. Liothyronine has the rapid onset of action, but its duration of action is short. It can reduce serum T_4 or protein bound iodine because it is poorly bound to thyroxine binding globulin. Although this preparation is orally effective, it is expensive. Because of expense and short half-life, there is little justification for its use on a chronic basis. It may, however, be the drug of choice in emergency situations such as myxedema coma.

Liotrix (Euthroid, Thyrolar) is about a 4:1 mixture of the sodium salts of T_4 and T_3. The major advantages of these preparations is their uniform ratios of T_4 and T_3. Liotrix, like thyroid U.S.P. or thyroglobulin, is orally effective. Liotrix offers no therapeutic advantage over L-thyroxine and is much more expensive.

Other pathologic conditions may warrant the use of thyromimetic agents (Table 44–3). Certain types of nontoxic and nodular goiter, depending upon the duration of their existence, regress following the administration of thyromimetic agents. Graves' disease, which recent evidence suggests is a disease of cell-mediated immunity, is often treated with combined antithyroidal agents and thyroxine since the latter can prevent goiter formation.

The toxicity of thyroidal preparations mimics hyperthyroidism. Hyperirritability, nervousness, tachycardia, arrhythmias, angina pectoris and insomnia are manifestations of thyroid hormone overdosage. Increased pulse pressure, hypertension, gastrointestinal disturbances, muscle weakness and anorexia also may be prevalent.

ANTITHYROIDAL AGENTS

The etiologies of hyperthyroidism are usually quite obscure. Only in rare instances can increased levels of TSH be observed. Hyperthyroid states may be characterized by thyroid enlargement, tremors, nervousness or hyperkinetic behavior, smooth and hot skin and excessive sweating. Symptoms such as diarrhea and pruritis are not infrequently encountered. Tachycardia is quite often observed in thyrotoxic diseases. Existing angina pectoris is exacerbated in thyrotoxicosis.

The treatment regimen for thyrotoxicosis may involve the use of antithyroid drugs, radioactive iodine and/or surgery following antithyroidal drug therapy. Combination therapy is sometimes used in the management of hyperthyroid states. A variety of pharmacologic agents are available that will suppress thyroid gland secretions (Table 44–4).

Certain anions can displace iodine from the iodine compartment of the thyroid gland. Of the several anions capable of inhibiting iodide transport, ClO_4 (perchlorate), appears to be the most potent (Fig. 44–1). Perchlorate is selectively concentrated in the thyroid gland, but it cannot be organified like iodide. It competes with iodide

TABLE 44—3. Uses of Thyroxine (T_4) or L-Triiodothyronine (T_3)

Myxedema
Thyroiditis
Myxedema coma
Thyroid suppression test
Nontoxic goiter
Graves' disease*
Thyroid malignancies
Questionable uses (infertility, menstrual disorders)

*Adjunctive therapy

TABLE 44–4. Agents that Inhibit Thyroid Gland Function

Mechanism of action	Example	Average doses*
Inhibitors of iodide trapping (anionic inhibitors):	Potassium perchlorate ($KClO_4$) Thiocyanate (KSCN)	
Inhibitors of Thyroxine Biosynthesis:		
	Methylthiouracil (Methiacil)	50 mg every 6 hr
	Methimazole (Tapazole)	10 mg every 8 hr
	Propylthiouracil (Propacil)	100 mg every 8 hr
	Carbimazole (Neomercazole)	10 mg every 8 hr
	Mercaptoimidazole	
Agents with unknown mechanism of antithyroidal action:	Potassium iodide	
	Sodium iodide	5–10 mg/day
Drugs that destroy thyroidal tissue	^{131}I	2–20 mCi

*Dose will vary somewhat depending upon the severity of the thyrotoxicosis.

and consequently is effective in reversing hyperthyroid states. Perchlorate is therapeutically obsolete in the United States since its usage frequently results in a number of toxic reactions including aplastic anemia. *Thiocynate (KSCN)* is also an anionic inhibitor of iodide transport, but it is not a useful therapeutic agent.

The thionamide antithyroidal agents inhibit thyroid gland activity by interfering with biosynthesis of thyroxine (Fig. 44–1). They also may exert other inhibitory actions upon the thyroid. The antithyroid drugs ordinarily employed in clinical medicine have in common the thionamide structure (S=C$\overset{\displaystyle N}{\diagdown}$); the most active are those agents containing the thiourylene group (S=C$\overset{\displaystyle N}{\underset{\displaystyle N}{\diagup}}$). Of the several thionamide derivatives, *thiorurea* and *thiouracil* have been most often studied, yet *propylthiouracil, carbimazole* and *methimazole* are perhaps the most widely used. The thionamides interfere with the organic binding of iodine. They may block the oxidation of iodides and the condensation of the iodotyrosines to form iodothyronines. The thionamides have little effect on thyroxine that is already synthesized. They do exert a peripheral effect that is poorly understood. The absorption of the various thionamides from the gastrointestinal tract is usually quite rapid. The metabolic fates of all these particular antithyroidal agents are not completely established; there are differences in their distribution. These drugs actually have a goitrogenic action due probably to an increase in TSH secretion secondary to a suppression of T_3 and/or T_4. In addition to the goitrogenic toxicity

caused by the thionamides, they are capable of producing a variety of allergic reactions such as purpuric rash and urticaria. Jaundice, vasculitis, joint effusions, drug fever and suppression of white blood cells also may be observed following the use of the thionamides.

Large oral doses of *iodide* are known to inhibit thyroid hormone synthesis, however, extended administration may lead to a refractoriness in the inhibition of thyroid synthesis. Iodide transport may also be reduced. Thus, organification of iodine probably causes the production of a factor that inhibits iodide transport.

At one time, the therapeutic use of iodides in hyperthyroidism was quite widespread. The use of iodine alone, however, often results in iodine escape (Jodbasedow's disease) resulting in exacerbation of the hyperthyroidism. Their present day usage is principally to prepare patients for surgery. They are also used in combination with antithyroidal drugs to reduce the vascularity within the thyroid.

Radioactive iodine can be used either diagnostically (microcuries) or therapeutically (millicuries). ^{131}I is used extensively in the study of both hyper- and hypothyroidal states. Larger doses are used to selectively destroy thyroidal cells in cases of thyroid carcinoma. The greatest usefulness of ^{131}I lies in its thyroid study capabilities, but other diagnostic tests may be more reliable. The use of radioactive iodine in thyroid cancers has not produced consistent therapeutic results.

Many of the *sulfonamides* and related compounds possess antithyroidal properties. These drugs interfere with the organification of iodine. Sulfadiazine inhibits coupling of iodinated tyrosines more readily than it inhibits iodination of monotyrosine and tyrosine. These agents are not used therapeutically to treat hyperthyroid states, but when used for their antibacterial properties they may cause changes in thyroid gland function.

PARATHYROID HORMONE (PTH)

Physiologic Considerations

The secretion of PTH by the parathyroid glands is regulated by the blood concentration of ionic calcium and not by the total concentration of this cation. PTH is synthesized, stored, and secreted by the chief cells of the parathyroid glands. Following the secretion of PTH, it is reversibly bound to α globulins in the blood.

The chief physiologic role of PTH is to aid in the regulation of calcium homeostasis. Calcium homeostasis is an absolute requirement for normal body function. Calcium is present in high concentrations in several tissues; it is a major constituent of bone. Calcium is associated with the actions of many enzymes, with membrane permeability and with muscle and nerve function. Calcium ion also may be involved in the release of anterior pituitary hormones as well as with the mechanism of action of several target organ hormones. It will enhance the excretion of phosphate.

PTH affects calcium metabolism in bones, kidney, possibly the gastrointestinal tract and in other tissues. This hormone acts to increase blood calcium levels primarily by causing the mobilization of bone calcium. In the kidney, PTH stimulates calcium reabsorption. PTH, along with vitamin D, appears to facilitate the absorption of calcium from the small intestine.

Removal of the parathyroid gland causes serum calcium levels to fall within 24–48 hr. Hypocalcemia gives rise to muscular twitching, spasms and ataxia. With severe hypocalcemia, tetany, convulsions and even death can occur after surgical removal of the parathyroid glands. In mild to moderate hypoparathyroidism, abnormalities such as brittle fingernails, hair loss, anorexia, severe constipation and emotional instability may be manifest.

Chronic hyperparathyroidism that often leads to elevated blood calcium levels can result in decalcification and subsequent spontaneous fracture of bones. This condition may also produce calcification in the kidney, stomach wall and the bronchi. Skeletal and cardiac muscle function are likewise altered by elevated levels of calcium.

Synthesis, Metabolism and Excretion

While there are species differences in PTH, it is a simple polypeptide. The exact chemical structure of human PTH is unknown, but bovine PTH consists of 81 amino acids with a molecular weight of approximately 8500. Apparently only a portion of the PTH molecule is necessary for biologic activity. Human and bovine PTH appear to be immunologically similar.

The normal secretion of PTH from the chief cells of the parathyroid gland is modulated by the concentration of ionized blood calcium. When PTH is first synthesized by the chief cells, it is to a higher molecular weight precursor. This proPTH subsequently is cleaved and stored in the gland as a polypeptide with a molecular weight of about 9500. PTH probably undergoes a second cleavage once it reaches the blood stream resulting in a molecule with a molecular weight of approximately 7500.

The biologic half-life of PTH has been estimated to be about 20 min. The actions of PTH are terminated primarily by metabolic degradation, since very little of the physiologically effective hormone can be detected in the urine. Most likely the kidney and the liver are involved in its degradation.

Biochemical Actions

Nearly all of the body's calcium, most of which is in the form of calcium phosphate, resides in bone in both a stable and labile fraction. Increased PTH secretions results in an increase in blood calcium due principally to the mobilization of bone calcium and phosphate. PTH causes degradation of the central matrix of bone. There is a decrease in collagen synthesis, sulfate uptake and hexosamine and hydroxyproline content of the bone. PTH stimulates RNA synthesis in the osteoclast cell, as well as the release of its lysosomal enzymes. It causes an increase in bone glycolysis leading to an accumulation of acidic metabolites and a degradation of the matrix. The actions of PTH are partially mediated via cAMP which is known to cause a mobilization of bone calcium.

Other hormones besides PTH can affect bone growth and metabolism. Growth hormone promotes bone growth as evidenced by a proliferation of the epiphysial plates prior to the onset of sexual maturity. Likewise, sex hormones are capable of affecting the normal closure of the epiphysial plate at the time of puberty. Furthermore, thyroid hormones can stimulate both the anabolism and the catabolism in bones. Intensive glucocorticoid therapy may produce protein catabolism in bones and cause osteoporosis.

PTH exerts physiologic actions upon the kidney leading to calcium reabsorption by the renal tubules and also acts to enhance the excretion of phosphate by the kidney. Renal mechanisms responsible for magnesium excretion are likewise affected by PTH. The mechanism of action of PTH on various renal ionic transport systems may be influenced by cAMP.

Calcium absorption in the small intestine is probably due to an active transport mechanism. Such a mechanism appears to require vitamin D. Vitamin D deficiency (e.g., rickets) is characterized by a depression of calcium absorption leading to an impairment of processes involved in bone anabolism. The actions of vitamin D on calcium absorption are only slightly enhanced by PTH. It will not enhance the intestinal absorption of calcium in the absence of vitamin D.

Therapeutic Uses

PTH usage is limited primarily to the management of acute hypoparathyroid tetany, however, its therapeutic benefit is questionable since PTH has a relatively long onset of action (about 6 hr). The infusion of calcium salts in an emergency condition such as tetany exerts a more rapid effect and restores the circulating blood levels of this ion much more rapidly than can be mobilized by PTH. Calcium deficient states are often treated not only with high calcium diets, but also with vitamin D.

PTH can be used diagnostically to differentiate between hypoparathyroidism and pseudohypoparathyroidism. This diagnostic test, called the Ellsworth-Howard test, reveals a marked excretion of urinary phosphate after PTH administration in normal subjects or in hypoparathyroidism and a lower than normal response in pseudohypoparathyroidism.

Toxicity

Chronic use of PTH often leads to the development of antibodies against the hormone resulting intolerance and resistance to its biologic actions. Excessive amounts administered acutely can cause disturbances of CNS. Altered skeletal muscle function and myocardial arrhythmias may occur acutely and chronically. With prolonged use, PTH can lead to demineralization of bone. Metastatic calcification may occur in several organs causing such complications as irreversible renal insufficiency.

Preparations

Adequate amounts of human parathyroid extract are not available. Bovine PTH (Paroidin) can provide a therapeutic substitute although it is far from entirely satisfactory. The hormone is usually administered subcutaneously; in emergencies it can be given intravenously. A dose of 50–100 units of PTH may be injected several times daily for about 1 week in the therapeutic management of hypoparathyroid tetany.

CALCITONIN

Physiologic Considerations

In humans, calcitonin (thyrocalcitonin) arises from the parafollicular "C" cells of the thyroid gland. Calcitonin acts to antagonize the effects of PTH on bone tissue. It reduces blood calcium by preventing resorption of this cation from bone. Calcitonin does not directly affect the action of PTH. Calcitonin appears to exert its action(s) by decreasing osteoclastic activity or perhaps by increasing osteoblastic activity.

Synthesis, Metabolism and Excretion

Porcine calcitonin is a single chain polypeptide composed of 32 amino acids and having a molecular weight of about 4000. The chemical composition of human calcitonin has not been completely established, but it does appear to differ from calcitonin found in other species.

The secretion of calcitonin by the parafollicular "C" cells is modulated by the concentration of ionic calcium in the blood. Hypercalcemia produces an increased secretion of calcitonin while low blood calcium levels suppress the release of this hormone. Once calcitonin is released, it is rapidly metabolized. Its half-life is very short, and this may be due to enzymes present in the blood that curtail its biologic actions.

Mechanism of Action and Biochemical Effects

Although the actual mechanism of calcium induced calcitonin release is not understood, evidence suggests that cAMP may serve as an intracellular mediator in the parafollicular cell. Glucagon, as well as high levels of blood magnesium, may stimulate the release of calcitonin.

Calcitonin lowers serum calcium and phosphate; an action due almost completely to the inhibition of bone resorption. It has little effect on calcium metabolism in the kidney or the gastrointestinal tract. This hormone does affect phosphate absorption in the gastrointestinal tract. The action of calcitonin does not depend upon the presence of vitamin D.

Since calcitonin inhibits bone resorption, it exerts a physiologic antagonism upon the action of PTH. The mechanism of antagonism is related to the ability of calcitonin to inhibit osteoclastic activity.

Calcitonin causes an increased urinary excretion of phosphate. This phosphaturia is independent of that caused by PTH. Unlike PTH, calcitonin exerts little effect upon calcium metabolism in the gastrointestinal tract. Calcitonin partially prevents calcification of the kidneys, heart and skin caused by chronic hypercalcemia in such diseases as osteitis fibrosa.

Toxicity

Calcitonin has only a very limited pharmacologic use. Knowledge about its potential toxicity has not really been established, but no serious side effects have been reported. Supraphysiologic amounts of calcitonin may, of course, produce hypocalcemia, but it is unlikely to produce tetany. Porcine calcitonin is allergenic.

Therapeutic Uses

Human calcitonin is not available therapeutically. While pseudohypoparathyroidism may be associated with altered calcitonin, this hormone has not been assigned any specific therapeutic role. Calcitonin is of dubious value in hypercalcemic states. Salmon calcitonin, which has a longer half-life, has been used with limited success in Paget's disease and in osteoporosis.

FURTHER READING

Burrow GN (edit) (1975): Current concepts of thyroid disease. Med Clin North Amer 59:1045

Copp DH (1970): Endocrine regulation of calcium metabolism. Annu Rev Physiol 32:61

Herfindal ET, Hirschman JL (1971): Hypothyroidism. J Am Pharm Assoc 11:493

Hirsch PF, Munson PL (1969): Thyrocalcitonin. Physio Rev 49:548

Liberti P, Stanbury JB (1971): The pharmacology of substances affecting the thyroid gland. Annu Rev Pharmacol 11:113

Potts JT, Keutmann HT, Hall HD, Tregear GW (1971): The chemistry of parathyroid hormone and calcitonins. Vitam Horm 29:41

Raisz LG, Bingham PL (1972): Effects of hormones on bone development. Annu Rev Pharmacol 12:337

Reiss E, Canterbury JM (1973): Blood levels of parathyroid hormone in disorders of calcium metabolism. Annu Rev Med 24:217

Rose E (1966): The clinical use of thyroid hormones. Med Clin North Am 50:1393

JOHN A. THOMAS

JOHN E. JONES

45. INSULIN, HYPOGLYCEMIC DRUGS AND GLUCAGON

INSULIN

Insulin has been used for over 50 years in the treatment of diabetes mellitus. While many factors may be involved, the pancreas is obviously an important organ in its pathogenesis. Several signs and symptoms are characteristic of this disease including hyperglycemia, glucosuria, polyuria, polydypsia, ketonuria and ketonemia. Excessive weight loss and muscular weakness also occur; blood glucagon levels may be elevated. In juvenile diabetes, usually contracted before age 20, the onset of symptoms is quite rapid. This form is frequently characterized by severe ketoacidosis. Only insulin, and not the oral hypoglycemic drugs, will control this severe symptom.

Maturity onset diabetes usually occurs after age 40, most commonly in obese subjects, and is ordinarily less severe and slower in onset than the juvenile form of the disease. Seldom is there a complete absence of pancreatic insulin in maturity onset diabetes. In fact, in some maturity onset obese diabetic patients there may be excessive insulin production, but the body may be resistant to its biologic effects. Therefore, not all forms of diabetes mellitus are characterized by a reduced level of circulating blood insulin. Other factors involved in the genesis of diabetes include substances found in the blood referred to as insulin antagonists. The existence of a genetically altered insulin molecule in humans suffering from diabetes mellitus has been suggested but not established.

Chemistry and Standardization of Insulin

Insulin is a simple protein consisting of two polypeptide chains, an A and a B chain, connected by disulfide bonds. In its monomeric form, it has a molecular weight of about 5700. The insulin molecule is irreversibly inactivated by proteolytic enzymes or by acid hydrolysis and for this reason it is not orally effective.

The insulin used in the treatment of diabetes mellitus is obtained from the pancreas of domestic animals and is biologically standardized by its ability to produce hypoglycemia in rabbits. An international unit of insulin should reduce the blood sugar to 45 mg% when injected into a fasted rabbit. The international standard insulin contains 22 IU/mg.

Insulin Synthesis, Release and Metabolism

Insulin is synthesized in the pancreatic β cells as a single chain polypeptide precursor, proinsulin. Proinsulin has a much larger molecular weight protein than insulin. This larger precursor has very little biologic activity. A small amount of proinsulin can be detected in the blood stream. The cellular site of transformation of proinsulin to insulin takes place in the rough endoplasmic reticulum of the β cell. The Golgi apparatus of the cell is believed to be involved in the sacculation of insulin-containing granules. When an appropriate physiologic or pharmacologic stimuli is presented, the insulin containing granules adjacent to the β cell membrane move toward it, fuse with it and empty their contents into the extracellular space.

Insulin is secreted by pancreatic β cells continuously and in very small amounts. After a meal, insulin levels in the blood may increase several fold. Several physiologic, e.g., secretin, epinephrine etc. and pharmacologic, e.g., sulfonylureas, stimuli will cause the release of insulin from the pancreatic islet cells. After release it circulates in the blood to the peripheral tissues. Much of the released insulin is inactivated almost immediately as it traverses through the liver. The rate of insulin secretion has been estimated to be about 1–2 mg/24 hr. Hepatic degradation of newly released insulin by insulinases may reduce this amount to about half. Insulinase(s) causes a reduction cleavage and hydrolysis of the hormone.

Mechanism of Action and Some Biochemical Effects

Insulin exerts several metabolic effects on responsive cells, altering membrane characteristics, including hexose permeability, amino acid transport and potassium flux. It also affects RNA and protein synthesis within the cell, diminishes levels of cyclic AMP in some tissues, inhibits lipolysis in fat cells and probably proteolysis in muscles. How these intracellular actions can be accomplished by an action in the plasma membrane is not known. Perhaps insulin attaches itself to a plasma membrane receptor and initiates a second messenger(s) activity. Certainly, the initial actions of insulin seem to be at the plasma membrane, the resultant insulin-receptor complex being necessary for initiating subsequent biochemical events. Whether this complex participates directly or indirectly in intracellular metabolism is not known.

The search for an action of insulin upon a key enzyme or enzyme system has not been rewarding. Insulin certainly exerts a profound effect on the rate of membrane transport of glucose and increases the uptake of glucose into a variety of tissues such as skeletal and cardiac muscles, fat cells and fibroblasts. Although the molecular mechanism of hexose transport is not fully understood, it appears that a specific carrier molecule in the membrane is affected by insulin. Insulin accelerates the activity of a specific hexose carrier system. Many of the actions of insulin do not fit in entirely with the hypothesis that the hormone causes an early facilitation of a sugar transport system. Experimentally, it is possible to demonstrate a variety of insulin-induced changes in the absence of glucose.

Insulin can influence the metabolism of fats, proteins and carbohydrates. These overall hormonal effects are well integrated and act in metabolic concert. Insulin functions as a prime storage hormone expediting the conservation of the body's major metabolic fuels. Some of the specific actions of insulin on metabolic processes can be seen by examining its effects upon three primary target tissues, namely, the liver, adipose tissue and skeletal muscles (Table 45–1).

The liver plays an important role in maintaining carbohydrate homeostasis. Insulin acts on the liver cells not only to enhance glucose uptake,

TABLE 45–1. Effect of Insulin on its Target Organs

Metabolism	
Muscle	
Carbohydrate	↑ Glucose transport
	↑ Glycogen synthesis
	↑ Glycolysis
Fat	
Protein	↑ Amino acid uptake
	↑ Protein anabolism
Liver	
Carbohydrate	↑ Glucokinase
	↑ Glycogen synthesis
	↓ Phosphorylase
	↓ Gluconeogenesis
Fat	↑ Lipogenesis
Protein	↓ Proteolysis
Adipose cell	
Carbohydrate	↑ Glucose transport
	↑ Glycerol synthesis
Fat	↑ Triglycerides
	↑ Fatty acid synthesis
	↓ Lipolysis
Protein	↔

but to inhibit intracellular enzymatic processes involved in glucose production and release. Insulin produces several changes in hepatic enzymes involved in carbohydrate metabolism (Table 45–1). The uptake of glucose results in free hexose being phosphorylated to glucose-6-phosphate by glucokinase. A major portion of the phosphorylated glucose is subsequently converted to glycogen through the insulin-induced activation of glycogen synthetase and inhibition of phosphorylase a. The liver is able to affect glycogen breakdown and new glucose production by metabolic processes which differ from those involved in glycogen synthesis and glycolysis. Other enzymes such as those involved in gluconeogenesis may be diminished by insulin thereby providing more optimal conditions for the formation of hepatic glycogen.

Ordinarily, the fat cell membrane can exclude glucose; however, under the influence of insulin its permeability to this hexose is increased and the assimilated glucose synthesized to fatty acids. Substantial amounts of glucose can be converted to α-glycerophosphate and then to free fatty acids and triglycerides. Triglycerides represent a storage form of fat within the adipose cell.

Insulin can also inhibit lipolysis by effectively inhibiting a hormone-sensitive lipase located in the adipose cell. The actions of insulin on the various aspects of lipid metabolism are complex. The net effect of its antilipolytic, fat-synthesizing and glycerogenic actions is to enhance total fat storage.

Insulin facilitates the transport of glucose and amino acids into muscle cells. The intracellular glucose can be either completely metabolized to carbon dioxide or converted into muscle glycogen. Muscle cells lack glucose-6-phosphatase and, therefore, cannot release free glucose from stored glycogen. The breakdown of muscle glycogen leads to an accumulation of lactic acid which must return to the liver to be reconverted to glucose. Insulin also stimulates the incorporation of amino acids into muscle proteins, i.e., it exerts a protein anabolic action.

Uses and Factors Affecting Dosage

Insulin is used chiefly in the management of diabetes mellitus. It is quite effective in controlling either juvenile or maturity onset diabetes. Individuals with juvenile diabetes must be treated with insulin whereas those with the maturity onset form of the disease can often be controlled by diet and/or oral hypoglycemic agents. The choice of therapy depends upon the severity of the disease.

In addition to its use in the management of diabetes, insulin is used in evaluating pituitary growth hormone secretion. It has been used to produce insulin coma in the treatment of certain psychiatric conditions. Insulin can be used therapeutically to rapidly lower serum potassium.

Insulin can interact with other drugs; this can lead to exaggerated hypoglycemic responses, e.g., biguanides, or to an antiinsulin type effect, for example adrenergic agents (Ch. 74). Such interactions require a careful consideration of the insulin dosage and the particular insulin preparation to be used. Physical exercise lowers the requirements for insulin while stress and certain pathologic states may increase the body's demands for the hormone.

Ordinarily insulin is administered subcutaneously. In emergency situations, e.g., in diabetic coma or severe diabetic acidosis, the intravenous route of administration is often used to achieve a more rapid effect. Local allergic reactions associated with the subcutaneous route of adminis-

tration can sometimes be minimized by rotating the site of injection, by selecting a different source of insulin or by injecting the insulin IM.

Preparations

The pharmacokinetic profiles of some insulin preparations on blood glucose levels may be seen in Table 45–2. All preparations cause a reduction in elevated blood sugar levels, but they differ with respect to onset, peak effect and duration of their action. **Insulin injection** U.S.P. (**regular insulin**) and semilente are considered fast-acting preparations while **isophane** (**NPH**) and **lente** (**insulin zinc**) are intermediate acting preparations.

Insulin injection contains small amounts of zinc which may achieve somewhat better chemical stability and also reduce the incidence of allergic reactions. Regular insulin may be reserved for treating diabetic emergencies since it can be administered intravenously.

Isophane insulin suspension is a modified protamine zinc insulin preparation. It generally consists of amounts of a fast acting insulin such as regular insulin and a slow acting insulin, protamine zinc insulin. This combination results in a somewhat intermediate acting preparation. Isophane is very similar to lente insulin in its pharmacokinetic profile (Table 45–2). Lente insulin is a microcrystalline suspension of crystalline zinc insulin.

Protamine zinc insulin (**PZI**) and **ultralente** are considered long acting insulin preparations. Protamine is a basic protein that interacts with insulin rendering it less soluble at body pH. The insolubility is sufficient to delay its absorption and prolong its duration of hypoglycemic action. The combination of protamine and insulin is chemically unstable; the inclusion of zinc restores this stability and renders it more therapeutically useful. PZI is probably prescribed more often than is necessary and frequently causes nocturnal hypoglycemia.

Adverse Effects

The adverse effects of insulin are commonly hypoglycemia, lowering of blood potassium levels and allergic reactions (see Table 45–3). Hypoglycemia due to insulin overdose can lead to nervousness, tremors, enhanced autonomic nervous system activity, convulsions, unconsciousness and even permanent brain damage. Hypoglycemia may cause behavioral changes. Hypopotassemia is associated with alterations in EKG activity. Potassium salts can be administered to correct this untoward reaction.

Mild allergic reactions to insulin are very

TABLE 45–2. Effects of Insulin Preparations on Blood Sugar Levels

Type of insulin preparation	Relative effect (hr)*		
	Onset	Peak	Duration
Regular insulin	½–1	1–2	5–7
Semilente	½–1	1–2	12–16
Isophane (NPH)	1½–2	8–12	20–28
Globin	1½–2		
Lente (insulin zinc)	1½–2	8–12	18–24
Protamine zinc (PZI)	3–4	8–12	about 36
Ultralente	3–4	8–14	about 36

* These times are representative only and will vary depending upon the dose and individual patient response.

common and are not only due to contaminants in the preparations of insulin, but to immunologic differences in the animal insulin itself. Such reactions can be attributed to globin, protamine or to the heterologous insulins.

Insulin can cause a localized atrophy at its site of injection. Insulin lipodystrophy, as it is also called, can be minimized by rotating the sites of injection frequently or by resorting to deeper or IM routes of administration.

Pathologic States Affecting Blood Glucose

Many disease states, as well as a variety of drugs can alter blood glucose levels. Hormones of the anterior pituitary gland, adrenal medulla, adrenal cortex and the thyroid gland exert actions that can alter the requirements of the body for insulin. Supraphysiologic amounts of these hormones can occur pathologically or be administered. For example, epinephrine or norepinephrine used for their actions upon the cardiovascular system can cause hepatic glycogeneolysis and transient hyperglycemia. These neurohormones may also directly inhibit the release of insulin. Growth hormone used to promote growth in dwarfism may also produce hyperglycemia (Ch. 43). Excessive amounts of adrenocortical hormones seen in Cushing's

TABLE 45–3. Adverse Effects of Insulin or Oral Hypoglycemic Agents

Insulin
Prolonged or severe hypoglycemia
Hypopotassemia
Neural and behavioral changes; convulsions
Insulin lipodystrophy

Oral Hypoglycemic Agents
Sulfonylureas:
 Hypoglycemia action
 Allergic responses
 Photosensitivities
 Blood dyscrasias
 Hypersensitivity cholestatic jaundice
 Increased risk of cardiovascular disorder (?)

Biguanides:
 Hypoglycemic action
 G.I. disturbances (nausea and vomiting)
 Anorexia
 Disturbances in lactate metabolism
 Increased risk of cardiovascular disorders (?)

disease can produce a hyperglycemic state by inhibiting the peripheral utilization of glucose. Of course, pharmacologic amounts of either natural or synthetic glucocorticoids or antiinflammatory steroids can also elevate blood glucose levels. So-called "steroid diabetes" is not uncommon in individuals receiving intensive glucocorticoid therapy.

ORAL HYPOGLYCEMIC DRUGS

Insulin remains the therapeutic agent of choice in the management of severe diabetes mellitus. Some forms of mild diabetes can be controlled simply by restricting dietary intake of carbohydrates and/or total calories. Insulin, since it is inactivated when administered orally, must be administered parenterally. Needless to say, the oral route of administration is usually the preferred route of administration of any medication.

The **sulfonylurea** drugs comprise the largest class of oral antidiabetic drugs in current use. The second largest chemical class are the **biguanides.** Their general pharmacologic properties are given in Table 45–4. About half of the known diabetics in the United States are treated with oral hypoglycemic agents.

SULFONYLUREAS

Tolbutamide, chlorpropamide, acetoheximide, and **tolazamide** are the four oral hypoglycemic agents in this class used in the United States (Table 45–5). All are structurally quite similar and presumably act by the same pharmacologic mechanism. They differ in their duration of action (Table 45–5) and other characteristics (Table 45–6). Some of the sulfonylureas are metabolized

by the liver mainly to inactive metabolites. The reduction of acetoheximide, however, produces a metabolite that still possesses some hypoglycemic properties.

Although the sulfonylureas exert their hypoglycemic effect by at least one or more mechanisms, the presence of viable β cells in the pancreas are essential for their action. Juvenile diabetics do not respond to the sulfonylureas since in this condition few insulin secreting cells are viable. The sulfonylureas exert their principal effect by stimulating the pancreas to se-

TABLE 45–4. Pharmacologic Actions of Oral Hypoglycemic Agents

Sulfonylurea-type
 Lowered blood sugar levels
 Decreased glycosuria
 Slight reduction in hepatic glucose output (enchanced liver glycogen)
 Decreased nonesterified fatty acids.

Biguanide-type
 Lowered blood sugar levels
 Decreased glycosuria
 Decreased hepatic glycogen
 Increased blood lactate and pyruvate
 Alteration in lipid metabolism (inhibits lipogenesis)

TABLE 45—5. Estimated Duration of Action of Oral Hypoglycemic Agents

Drug	Approximate duration of action (hr)	Usual dosage range (mg)
Tolbutamide (Orinase)	6—12	500—3000 (divided dose)
Chlorpropamide (Diabinase)	up to 60	100—500 (single dose)
Acetoheximide (Dymelor)	12—24	125—1000 (single or divided dose)
Tolazamide (Tolinase)	10—20	100—1000 (single dose)
Phenformin (DBI) (Meltrol)	4—6	25—150
Phenformin (DBI-TD)	8—12	50—200

TABLE 45—6. Pharmacologic Profile of the Sulfonylureas

	Tolbutamide	Chlorpropamide	Tolazamide	Acetoheximide
Relative potency	1	4	4	2
Metabolic fate	Oxidation	Not metabolized	Oxidation	Reduction
Metabolite	Inactive	None	Inactive	Active
Half-life (approx. hr)	6	36	3	8

crete insulin. It is also possible, particularly at high doses, that they reduce the outflow of glucose from the liver. In normal individuals, but not in diabetics, certain sulfonylureas may increase the peripheral utilization of glucose.

The oral antidiabetic agents enjoy widespread use in the management of maturity onset diabetes mellitus since the pancreas may still contain substantial amounts of insulin. In other words, some β cells are still viable and able to synthesize and secrete insulin. The sulfonylureas are not effective in severe insulin-deficient diabetes.

The adverse effects of the oral antidiabetic agents are listed in Table 45–3. A recent long term study suggests that oral hypoglycemic agents may increase the incidence of cardiovascular deaths.

The sulfonylureas can interact with a number of other classes of drugs, including the salicylates, sulfonamides, MAO inhibitors and the courmarin anticoagulants leading to exaggerated hypoglycemic responses. Ethanol exaggerates their blood glucose lowering action.

BIGUANIDES

Phenformin is perhaps the most widely used. **Metformin** and **buformin** exhibit somewhat similar pharmacologic properties. Their general pharmacologic actions are shown in Table 45–4. Their spectrum of therapeutic usefulness is essentially the same as the sulfonylureas. Phenformin has a somewhat shorter duration of action compared to the sulfonylureas, but timed disintegration tablets containing phenformin (e.g., DBI-TD) cause a slight increase in its duration of hypoglycemic action.

The mechanism of hypoglycemic action of the biguanides is controversial. It is different from the sulfonylureas since they do not stimulate the release of endogenous insulin. Phenformin may exert its effects on glucose metabolism by blocking energy transfer at the cytochrome b site of the respiratory chain. The biguanides may interfere with the binding of insulin to plasma proteins resulting in more free or active hormone. Still other investigations indicate that the biguanides extend the biologic half-life of insulin or even exert an "insulin-like" effect on different cell membrane structures. The biguanides may also increase the peripheral utilization of glucose.

The biguanides are used in the management of maturity onset diabetes mellitus. While they are relatively free from allergic reactions, this feature offers no particular advantage over the sulfonylureas. The reported inherent anorexic properties of the biguanides are minimal and of dubious advantage in the management of the obese diabetic.

Some of the adverse effects of the biguanides are the same as the sulfonylureas (Table 45–3). Gastrointestinal disturbances seem to be related to their accumulation in the gastric juices and the lining of the intestines. These disturbances can be minimized by using formulations that release the drug very slowly and hence tend to minimize accumulation. Phenformin has been associated with severe and rarely fatal disturbances in lactate metabolism. It has also been associated with an increased risk of cardiovascular disorders.

Oral hypoglycemic drugs and insulin are not used concomitantly in the management of diabetes mellitus. Only in selected instances are the sulfonylureas used in combination with the biguanides. Such combination therapy is not universally accepted as good therapeutic practice. Very often, dietary restrictions and low to moderate doses of oral antidiabetic agents will control mild to moderate forms of diabetes mellitus.

Despite the normalization of blood glucose by the oral antidiabetic agents, it is becoming increasingly apparent that diabetes is a very complex metabolic disease and that all of its accompanying pathologic changes are not completely retarded by drug therapy.

GLUCAGON

Glucagon is a polypeptide hormone secreted primarily by the α cells of the pancreas. Physiologically, glucagon will produce hyperglycemia and hypoaminacidemia. It also is a lipolytic agent. Many of the actions of glucagon are mediated by increases in cyclic AMP (Ch. 18).

Glucagon may function physiologically to prevent insulin induced hypoglycemia. Injections of glucagon can elevate blood glucose levels by causing hepatic glycogenolysis, but its therapeutic usefulness in this regard is limited. Hypoglycemic states of a transient nature are best treated by the administration of glucose. Current evidence suggests that glucagon can dilate the coronary vasculature and lower renal vascular resistance. Glucagon exerts a positive inotropic action upon the heart but assessment of its therapeutic valve in the management of congestive cardiac failure awaits further clinical trials.

FURTHER READING

INSULIN

Cahill GF, Jr (1971): Physiology of insulin in man. Diabetes 20:785

Pilkis SJ, Parks CR (1974): Mechanism of action of insulin. Ann Rev Pharmacol 14:365

Porte D, Jr, Bagade JD (1970): Human insulin secretion: an integrated approach. Annu Rev Med 21:219

Levine R (1967): Insulin—the biography of a small protein. N Engl J Med 277:1059

Rubenstein AH, Steiner DF (1971): Proinsulin. Annu Rev Med 22:1

ORAL HYPOGLYCEMIC AGENTS

Davidoff FF (1968): Oral hypoglycemic agents and the mechanism of diabetes mellitus. N Engl J Med 278:148

Desbuquis B, Cuatrecasas P (1973): Insulin receptors. Annu Rev Med 24:233

Holcomb GN (1970): Current concepts in antidiabetics. Am J Pharm Educ 34:648

JOHN E. JONES

JOHN A. THOMAS

46. PHARMACOLOGY OF THE ADRENOCORTICOIDS

PHYSIOLOGIC CONSIDERATIONS

The adrenal glands are situated retroperitoneally over the superior pole of each kidney and are composed of an inner (medulla) and an outer (cortex) region. The adrenal medulla secretes epinephrine and norepinephrine. Physiologically, it resembles a sympathetic ganglion.

The adrenal cortex consists of three concentric cellular layers or zones, the zona glomerulosa, zona fasciculata and the zona reticularis. The zona glomerulosa secretes mineralocorticoids and to a lesser degree glucocorticoids, androgens and estrogens. The latter two zones, zona fasciculata and zona reticularis, do not secrete substantial amounts of electrolyte-influencing steroids.

An important physiologic electrolyte-influencing steroid is the mineralocorticoid *aldosterone.* Aldosterone and other mineralocorticoids are essential for the maintenance of electrolyte balance and extracellular volume. In supraphysiologic amounts, many of the synthetic and endogenous glucocorticoid steroids, also called antiinflammatory steroids, possess an overlapping biologic activity and alter body electrolytes. Pharmacologic inhibitors of aldosterone, aldosterone antagonists, are effective diuretics (Ch. 38).

Physiologically, the glucocorticoids exert a variety of actions upon intermediary metabolism. *Cortisol,* also called hydrocortisone, is a principal glucocorticoid of the human adrenal cortex. Supraphysiologic doses of cortisol and closely related synthetic derivatives possess antiinflammatory actions.

Ordinarily, the secretion of sex hormones by the adrenal cortex is of little significance. Pathologic states, e.g., adrenogenital syndrome, can lead to a reduction in the secretion of glucocorticoids and an increased secretion of virilizing androgens. In the female, the adrenal gland is the primary source of androgens.

Several of the physiologic actions of the adrenal cortical hormones can be readily observed after the gland is surgically removed. Adrenalectomy produces a number of metabolic changes within several organ systems of the body (Table 46–1). Similar changes may be manifest in patients with adrenal insufficiency, but usually are of lesser magnitude. Addison's disease is a form of adrenal insufficiency.

In adrenal insufficiency, the exchange of sodium for potassium and hydrogen ions in the distal tubules of the kidney is sufficiently decreased to induce severe hyponatremia and hyperkalemia. In adrenalectomized states or in patients with Addison's disease, hepatic glycogen or blood glucose levels often remain within normal limits as long as food is continuously available. However, hepatic gluconeogenesis is severely reduced and there is little storage of liver glycogen. Glucocorticoids exert a permissive action on lipolysis. In adrenal insufficiency, lipid catabolism decreases and there is reduction in the transport and storage of fats.

Addison's disease is frequently manifest in a diminished circulating blood volume, reduction in heart size, decreased vasomotor responses and a loss in the contractile force of the myocardium. There may be increased capillary permeability and blood viscosity. These cardiovascular changes can be reversed by the administration of glucocorticoids and mineralocorticoids.

SYNTHESIS, METABOLISM AND EXCRETION

Endogenous glucocorticoids are synthesized by the cells located primarily in the zona fasciculata of the adrenal cortex. Adrenal steroidogenesis, in

356

particular glucocorticoid synthesis, is enhanced and regulated by ACTH (Ch. 43).

The liver is the principal organ involved in the biotransformation of the adrenocortical steroids. The half-life of corticoids in the blood can be correlated with their rate of metabolism by the liver (Ch. 2). In the plasma, most of the corticoids are bound either to albumins or specific transporting globulins, e.g., cortisol binding globulin (Ch. 42). That cortisol which is bound to albumin and that fraction which is unbound in the blood is particularly vulnerable to hepatic biotransformation. The principal metabolic changes catalyzed by the liver include the reduction of certain double bonds in the steroid molecule and the reduction of the important keto groups. The liver can also conjugate these steroids with sulfate or glucuronide (Ch. 3).

There are considerable differences in the plasma half-life of natural and synthetic corticoids (Table 46–2). Steroids that have certain synthetic chemical alterations to their basic structure ordinarily have shorter plasma half-lives. More complex chemical alterations to the cortisol molecule such as halogenation, produce antiinflammatory steroids that remain in the plasma for longer durations.

Corticoids which have been metabolized or conjugated by the liver are more polar and more water soluble and usually do not readily combine with plasma proteins. Because of these changes they can be readily excreted by the kidney. Some of the steroids are eliminated by tubular secretion.

ADRENOCORTICAL RECEPTORS, ACTH REGULATION AND MECHANISM OF ACTION

Although there are specific receptors that bind adrenocortical hormones, the target organ-receptor concept for the corticoids is less firmly established than it is for the sex steroids. The actions of the glucocorticoids, unlike the actions of the sex steroids, are quite diverse and can influence many more organs.

The glucocorticoids appear to bind to specific cytoplasmic and nuclear sites in several tissues responsive to these hormones. A cortisol receptor has been found in the cytoplasm and nuclear fractions of liver cells. The thymus gland contains a specific nuclear binding site for cortisol. The binding of cortisol to this thymic nuclear site requires a cytoplasmic component. The CNS contains receptors. Certain tumor cells contain a cortisol binding receptor or protein.

Specialized binding proteins for the mineralocorticoids are located in the kidney. An aldosterone receptor has been isolated from the nuclear and cytoplasmic fractions of mammalian kidney cells.

TABLE 46–1. Effects of Adrenalectomy

Diminution of glycogen (muscle and liver)
Hypoglycemia and increased sensitivity to insulin
Reduced nitrogen excretion
Diminished lipolysis
Increased inflammatory reaction and scar tissue formation
Excessive loss of sodium by the kidney (hyponatremia)
Retention of potassium by the kidney (hyperkalemia)
Abnormal intracellular fluid volume
Reduction in glomerular filtration rate
Diminished cardiac output and reduced vasomotor responses

The site of action of ACTH on the metabolic pathways of adrenal steroidogenesis is not known, but the biotransformation of cholesterol to pregnenolone seems to be enhanced by this adenohypophysial hormone (Ch. 43). ACTH stimulates the synthesis of cortisol that is released into the blood where it either becomes bound or remains in a free state. Blood cortisol, but not its precursors, is capable of exerting an inhibitory action effect upon the further secretion of ACTH. Potent synthetic glucocorticoids are also capable of exerting this inhibitory action. As a result, adrenal steroidogenesis is commonly suppressed during prolonged antiinflammatory steroid therapy. Blood levels of ACTH and of cortisol exhibit a diurnal rhythm. Usually hormonal blood levels reach their peaks just prior to awakening. The diurnal variation can be masked by pharmacologic amounts of antiinflammatory steroids.

The release of aldosterone is not controlled directly by ACTH. Rather, the hormonal regulation of aldosterone involves an interaction with the renin-angiotensin system. Hypovolemia causes the enzyme renin to be released into the blood from the juxtaglomerular cells of the kidney. This enzyme acts upon angiotensinogen in the serum to convert it to angiotensin I. Converting enzyme transforms angiotensin I (a decapeptide) to angiotensin II (an octapeptide).

TABLE 46–2. Approximate Half-Lives of Corticoids in the Blood

Short acting corticoids
  (Half-life of less than 1½ days)
  Methylprednisolone
  Prednisone
  Cortisol
  Prednisolone
  Cortisone

Intermediate acting corticoids
  (Half-life of about 2 days)
  Paramethasone
  Triamcinolone

Long acting corticoids
  (Half-life of greater than 2 days)
  Dexamethasone
  Betamethasone

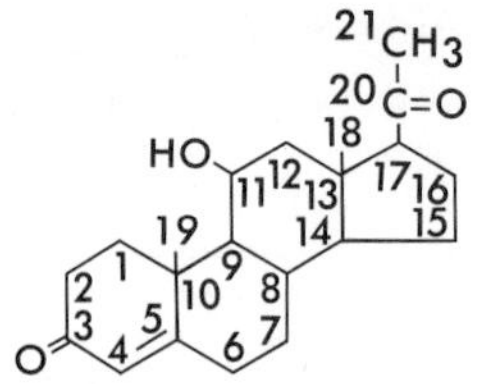

Δ_4-PREGNENE-11-β-oL-3,20 DIONE

Examples of structural modifications of the antiinflammatory nucleus (viz., Δ^4-preg-nene-11-β-ol-3,20 dione) and their effects on pharmacologic activities.

Antiinflammatory and glucocorticoid activity		Mineralocorticoid activity	
Increased	Decreased	Increased	Decreased
Δ^1 double bond	14 α hydroxylation	2 α methylation	16 α hydroxylation
9 α halogenation	16 α hydroxylation	9 α halogenation	16 α methylation
17 α hydroxylation			
21 α hydroxylation			

FIG. 46–1. Basic steroid structure necessary for antiinflammatory activity and its modification.

Angiotensin II can stimulate the release of aldosterone. Since aldosterone induces sodium retention and thereby increases extracellular fluid volume, the further release of renin is inhibited. Angiotensin II is not used clinically to cause the release of aldosterone. Angiotensin II has, however, been used pharmacologically for its unique pressor properties (Ch. 20).

Many chemical modifications of the steroid nucleus render the compound a more useful pharmacologic agent. Often, these synthetic steroids exert a more potent antiinflammatory activity than cortisol. The addition of specific chemical side groups or halogenation can affect antiinflammatory and mineralocorticoid activity (Fig. 46–1). Usually, enhanced antiinflammatory properties are the most desirable therapeutic asset. Only rarely is it desirable to increase mineralocorticoid properties, since excessive mineralocorticoid activity is usually considered an undesirable adverse effect. Unfortunately, increases in antiinflammatory activity and mineralocorticoid activity usually occur in parallel. It has been difficult from a pharmacologic standpoint to completely divorce the mineralocorticoid activity from the antiinflammatory activity.

The mechanism of antiinflammatory activity of adrenocortical steroids is poorly understood. They appear to prevent generalized inflammatory response regardless of the nature of the noxious stimuli whether it be chemical, mechanical or immunologic. They do not cure inflammatory reactions. Rather, the corticoids will suppress such symptoms and signs of inflammation as swelling, redness, heat and local capillary dilation. Stabilization of the lysosomal membrane may be partially involved in this antiinflammatory action.

THERAPEUTIC USES OF ADRENOCORTICAL STEROIDS

Excluding replacement therapy for adrenal insufficiency, the therapeutic use of either the natural or synthetic corticoids and their congeners in most pathologic states is empirical. Their value in certain disease states is very evident, but in other conditions is quite uncertain. Unfortunately, the corticoids are still used in some diseases where their therapeutic efficacy is quite dubious.

The corticoids are used therapeutically in replacement therapy for patients with diminished or absent endogenous secretion of adrenocortical steroids; e.g., in Addison's disease or secondary adrenal insufficiency, and in palliative therapy to suppress certain manifestations of disease as, e.g., in rheumatoid arthritis. Corticoids used for replacement therapy rarely produce toxicity since they are given in physiologic doses. Palliative therapy often necessitates supraphysiologic doses and hence varying degrees of toxicity are anticipated.

Some of the more important clinical indications of the adrenocortical steroids are listed in Table 46–3. More endocrine complications arise from the chronic use of the adrenocortical steroids than if they are given acutely for periods of only 2–3 days. Chronic corticoid therapy should be initiated only when absolutely necessary. In chronic therapy, the dosage is often chosen by trial and error to achieve optimal therapeutic results. Chronic daily corticoid therapy frequently causes suppression of endogenous adrenocortical hormone secretion that may persist up to 9 months (Fig. 43–2). Thus abrupt withdrawal of the pharmacologic corticoid leaves the body with insufficient adrenocortical hormone.

To minimize pituitary-adrenal axis suppression caused by daily corticoid therapy, steroids are often administered on alternate days. With alternate day therapy (ADT), short acting corticoid preparations are administered every other day between the hours of 6 AM and 9 AM. This coincides with the peak levels of endogenous adrenocortical hormones. Since the short acting steroid will readily disappear from the circulation during the day, the time course of blood levels of corticoids mimics to some extent the normal diurnal pattern of adrenal cortical hormone secretion. Because endogenous hormone synthesis is not completely suppressed by ADT, some endogenous corticoids can be released under stress.

TABLE 46–3. Some Indications for the Corticoids

Acute adrenal insufficiency
Chronic adrenal insufficiency
Rheumatoid arthritis
Osteoarthritis (intraarticularly)
Rheumatic carditis
Congenital adrenal hyperplasia
Bronchial asthma
Cerebral edema
Lupus erythematosis
Nephrotic syndrome
Occular inflammations
Skin diseases
Leukemia

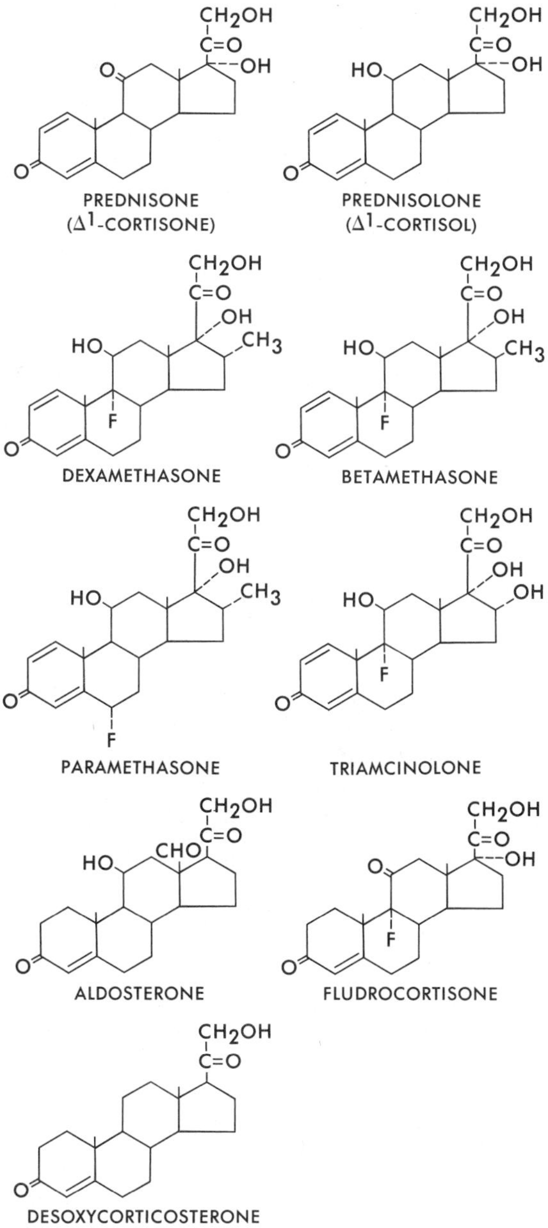

FIG. 46–2. Chemical structures of adrenocortical steroids.

ADT is of value only in those disorders necessitating chronic therapy and in which the hypothalamic-pituitary-adrenal axis is functional. It is of no value in Addison's disease, pituitary failure or in the adrenalectomized patient but may be useful in the management of severe asthma, nephrotic syndrome, lupus nephritis and possibly in rheumatoid arthritis. It has been used in treating pemphigus and other dermatologic diseases.

The corticoids are sometimes used acutely. Large dose regimens for 2–3 days will not usually substantially affect the pituitary-adrenal axis and therefore, withdrawal after an acute regimen will not affect endogenous adrenal steroidogenesis. Adverse effects are usually minimal.

SPECIFIC USES OF CORTICOIDS

Corticoids are used in the treatment of acute adrenal insufficiency, that may result from either pituitary or adrenal disorders. Sometimes when other therapies have failed the corticoids are used chronically in combination with other drugs such as the salicylates to treat rheumatoid arthritis. Not curative, they may provide some relief from the painful symptoms of inflammation. In osteoarthritis, the antiinflammatory steroids may be administered intraarticularly. Antiinflammatory steroids have been prescribed for rheumatic carditis, but again only after intensive salicylate therapy or other measures have failed.

Corticosteroid therapy has been used empirically in both acute and chronic bronchial asthma. They are not the drugs of first choice, and should be used only after conventional bronchiolar dilators, the sympathomimetic amines (Ch. 18) and other measures have failed.

A number of miscellaneous disease states have been treated empirically with corticoids. Antiinflammatory steroids have provided benefit in some cases of cerebral edema. Collagen vascular diseases, certain types of nephrotic syndromes, some nonbacterial or nonviral inflammatory conditions of the eyes, and various skin disorders sometimes respond to corticoid therapy.

The corticoids are used in congenital adrenal hyperplasia which is due to a congenital deficiency of a specific enzyme involved in adrenal steroidogenesis. Any one of at least four steroid hydroxylases may be absent; most commonly the 21-steroid hydroxylase is lacking. Should cortisol levels be low, then excessive secretion of ACTH can proceed unchecked and accounts for the adrenal hyperplasia. Since androgen synthesis by the adrenal is not impaired in the most common forms of this condition and since substantial amounts of glucocorticoid precursors can be shunted into the androgen metabolic pathway, virilization is common. The resulting condition is called the Adrenogenital syndrome. In some congenital adrenal hyperplasia cases there is also a decrease in the secretion of mineralocorticoids such as aldosterone.

Treatment of adrenal hyperplasia requires the administration of cortisol, or a potent derivative, to suppress pituitary ACTH resulting in a reduction in adrenal hyperplasia. This might also relieve the symptoms of adrenal insufficiency as well as slow adrenal androgen secretion.

ADVERSE EFFECTS OF THE ADRENOCORTICAL STEROIDS

There are many precautions associated with the therapeutic use of adrenocortical steroids. Many of the undesirable effects they produce are simply extensions of their therapeutic actions. Supraphysiologic amounts of adrenal cortical steroids can mimic a hypersecretory adrenal gland.

TABLE 46–4. Side Effects Associated With the Chronic Use of Pharmacologic Doses of the Corticosteroids

---

Salt retention, edema formation and hypertension
Hyperglycemia and glycosuria
Increased susceptibility to certain infections
Peptic ulceration
Osteoporosis
Impairment of skeletal and muscular growth
Alteration in fat distribution
Occular complications
Certain psychoses
Acne

The adrenal cortical hormones are often categorized as either mineralocorticoids or glucocorticoids. It is necessary to appreciate that supraphysiologic amounts of either steroid type lead, since there is an overlapping in their biologic activities, to both types of responses. Thus, a potent synthetic antiinflammatory steroid used in supraphysiologic amounts can affect electrolyte balance and salt retention is a common problem associated with pharmacologic amounts of glucocorticoid-type steroids.

Some of the adverse effects associated with the chronic use of corticosteroids are listed in Table 46–4. Fluid and electrolyte disturbances result in a retention of sodium, an increase in extracellular water, edema and subsequently hypertension. Concomitant with sodium retention is often potassium loss. Some of the newer synthetic steroids, e.g., the 16-α substituted corticoids minimize potassium loss by the kidney.

Excessive amounts of corticoids can lead to glycosuria and hyperglycemia. The corticoids antagonize the peripheral utilization of glucose leading to "steroid diabetes." Although the glucocorticoids can still be used in patients with diabetes mellitus, insulin requirements or the dose of oral hypoglycemic drugs must be increased.

Paradoxically, corticoid therapy may sometimes increase susceptibility to, and mask signs and symptoms associated with, certain infectious processes. If an infection is diagnosed while the patient is receiving corticoids, the steroid therapy is usually continued along with suitable antimicrobial therapy.

Corticoids have been indicated in the management of ulcerative colitis. Curiously, the corticoids are also capable of inducing ulceration. Ulceration of the stomach sometimes occurs after the chronic oral ingestion of the corticoids. These steroids decrease the resistance of the gastric mucosa to the effects of gastric secretions. The likelihood of ulceration can be minimized by administering antacids with the corticoid preparation or ingesting the steroid with a meal.

Growth impairment, osteoporosis and myopathy in the adolescent child are extensions of the catabolic actions of the glucocorticoids. Osteoporosis is an exaggerated side effect in postmenopausal women. The antianabolic actions of the glucocorticoids not only precipitate osteoporosis, but they appear to be responsible for ecchymoses and cutaneous, particularly abdominal, striae.

Excessive glucocorticoid therapy can produce alterations in the distribution of body fat. Intensive corticoid therapy may lead to a cushingoid syndrome characterized by a deposition of adipose tissue in the lower abdominal region and upon the nape of the neck. The face may become roundish or moonfaced.

Either the systemic administration of corticosteroids or their topical use in the eyes can produce serious, often irreversible, ophthalmic defects. These complications include exacerbation of herpes simplex keratitis, bacteria and fungal infections of the eyes, posterior subcapsular cataracts and glaucoma. Frequent ophthalmic evaluation should be undertaken in patients receiving prolonged intensive therapy.

Corticoid therapy has been known to induce psychoses such as manic depressive states, schizophrenic-like symptoms and even suicidal tendencies. Under certain conditions, they may produce an elevation in mood and upon rare occasions lead to psychologic dependence.

Certain contraindications of the corticosteroids are reasonably clear, although it is difficult to establish absolute guidelines for all the disease processes for which they have been indicated. Unless an emergency situation exists, the corticoids should not be used in patients with active thoracic tuberculosis, acute psychosis or herpes simplex keratitis. These steroids should be used with great discretion in the presence of ulcers, cataracts, glaucoma or certain cardiovascular disorders. Caution must be exercised if the corticoids are to be used in patients with hypertension, diabetes mellitus or osteoporosis. Growth retardation may occur when using intensive corticoid therapy in children.

Whereas corticoid administration represents replacement therapy in Addison's disease, careful consideration should nevertheless be given in the selection of a specific steroid. Perhaps the very potent steroids such as dexamethasone should be avoided. Instead, cortisol (or prednisone) can be used to manage effec-tively this disease; it is less apt to produce adverse effects if carefully monitored. Furthermore, hydrocortisone and prednisone are less costly than some of the other more potent tailor-made synthetic compounds.

PHARMACOLOGIC PREPARATIONS OF ADRENOCORTICAL STEROIDS

Although there are a large number of adrenocortical steroids available for use, their general properties are quite similar. Many differ only in their potency or absolute dosage. Therapeutic success is more likely if the physician becomes acquainted with the effects of one or two steroids rather than to attempt to use a number of such agents. The corticoids are effective when administered orally or parenterally. Antiinflammatory steroids are often used topically for certain dermatologic disorders.

Although aldosterone is a very important physiologic mineralocorticoid, it is not available for pharmacologic use. Rather, **desoxycorticosterone acetate** (DOCA) or **fludrocortisone acetate** is customarily used for its mineralocorticoid activity (Table 46–5). Fludrocortisone is the preferred agent since it is orally effective whereas desoxycorticosterone must be administered parenterally.

The halogenated synthetic steroids **triamcinolone, dexamethasone, betamethasone** and **paramethasone** are all more potent than either cortisol or cortisone with respect to both their antiinflammatory and mineralocorticoid properties. More water soluble pharmacologic preparations of glucocorticoids are available for certain emergency conditions requiring immediate and massive dosage schedules. The sodium salts or potassium phthalate salts of some of these steroids are suitable for intravenous administration.

TABLE 46–5. Relative Activities of Adrenocorticoids

Steroid	Some common dose ranges* (oral)	Relative mineralocorticoid activity	Relative antiinflammatory activity
Cortisol U.S.P. (hyrocortisone) (Cortef)	5–20 mg	1	1
Cortisone (Cortone)	5–20 mg	1	0.65
Prednisolone (Delta Cortef)	5 mg	<1	3
Prednisone	1–5 mg	<1	3
Methylprednisolone (Medrol)	2–10 mg	0.8	4
Triamcinolone (Aristocort)	1–15 mg	<1	3
Betamethasone (Celestone)	0.5–0.75 mg	<1	20–30
Dexamethasone (Decadron)		<1	20–30
Paramethasone (Haldrone)	1–2 mg	<1	10
Aldosterone		3000	?
Desoxycorticosterone (Cortate)	1–5 mg	100	<1
Corticosterone		15	0.3
Fludrocortisone (Florineff)	0.1–0.3 mg	800	15

*Doses will vary greatly depending not only upon the specific steroid used, but also whether the therapy is for maintenance (replacement) or for palliative indications. Several formulations (e.g., ointments, suspensions, solutions, etc.) are available.

DRUGS AFFECTING ADRENAL STEROIDOGENESIS

The secretory activity of the adrenal cortex can be altered pharmacologically either directly or indirectly (Fig. 43–3). Drugs like morphine, reserpine, chlorpromazine and autonomic agents influence ACTH secretion and secondarily or indirectly affect corticoid secretion. Other drugs such as aminoglutethimide, o,p-DDD and metpyrapone can exert a direct inhibitory effect upon adrenocortical steroid production. These direct acting agents have been used therapeutically in the management of adrenal hyperfunction, but their use is presently experimental. However, **metpyrapone** (Metopirone) is used diagnostically to assess ACTH secretory activity.

The normal response to the so-called metyrapone test is a decrease in the secretion of cortisol and corticosterone as well as an increase in the secretion of 11-desoxycortisol and 11-desoxycorticosterone. This indicates that the drug is a preferential inhibitor of 11-β steroid hydroxylase enzyme systems. Metyrapone prevents the conversion of 11-desoxycortisol to cortisol, and 11-desoxycortisol is unable to inhibit the pituitary secretion of ACTH. In hypopituitarism, metyrapone produces little or no effect upon 11-desoxysteroid secretion. Thus the metyrapone test can be used to determine the pituitary reserve of ACTH when the adrenal is capable of secreting corticoids.

FURTHER READING

Azarnoff DL (ed) (1973): Symposium on steroid therapy. Med Clin North Am Vol 5, No 5

Baxter JD, Forsham PH (1972): Tissue effects of glucocorticoids. Am J Med 53:573

Binder C (1969): The function of the pituitary gland and the adrenal cortex during treatment with glucocorticoids. Acta Med Scand [Suppl] 500:71

Feldman D, Funder JW, Edelman IS (1972): Subcellular mechanisms of action of adrenal steroids. Am J Med 53:545

Mulrow PJ, Forman BH (1972): The tissue effects of mineralocorticoids. Am J Med 53:561

Thorn GW (ed) (1971): Steroid Therapy. New York, Medcom

JOHN E. JONES

JOHN A. THOMAS

47. PHARMACOLOGY OF ANDROGENS AND ESTROGENS

While both androgens and estrogens are used for a variety of endocrine disorders, the estrogens are undoubtedly used more often from a pharmacologic standpoint. There are many more pharmacologic preparations containing estrogens than there are formulations that contain androgens. Often times an estrogen is combined with a progestagen and the two steroids administered in a singular pharmaceutical preparation. Only rarely are androgens combined with other drugs or hormones into a single formulation.

Pharmacologically active androgens are all steroids. Steroid possessing androgenic activity are often synthetically modified (e.g., fluoxymesterone) to render them orally active preparations. Similar chemical additions to the steroid nucleus of the estrogen are also necessary for attaining better oral activity (e.g., ethynylestradiol).

Not all estrogenic substances have a steroid structure. Diethylstilbestrol is not only a potent nonsteroidal estrogen, but a very important orally active agent used in the management of a host of endocrine disorders.

Pharmacologically speaking, androgens can often antagonize many of the biochemical actions of estrogens. Likewise, estrogens can frequently interfere with the pharmacologic actions of androgens. This hormonal antagonism forms the rational basis for the treatment of certain endocrine related diseases. For example, high doses of estrogens can sometimes antagonize androgen dependent tumors of the prostate gland. In certain estrogen sensitive mammary carcinomas, androgen therapy may afford amelioration of tumor growth.

ANDROGENS

Physiologic Considerations

Many organs including the skin, salivary and adrenal glands, and testes in the male synthesize male sex hormones or androgens. The testes are a primary source, but in certain pathologic states, and prior to puberty, the adrenal gland may sometimes secrete significant amounts of androgens.

The testes contain high concentrations of both testosterone (the major circulating androgen) and androstenedione. In sex accessory organs such as the prostate or seminal vesicles, dihydrotestosterone is particularly important. Sexual differentiation in the fetus is regulated by androgens.

Testicular secretion of androgen markedly increases at puberty producing several physiologic changes culminating in the development of the sexually mature male. These alterations include the development of facial and body hair, a lower-

ing of voice tone, and several changes in skeletal and muscle growth. Androgens cause a rapid growth of long bones that is followed by epiphysial closure. Male sex hormones cause a loss of subcutaneous fat and a generalized enhancement of protein anabolic activity leading to increased muscular size and strength. The size of the several reproductive organs increases and spermatogenesis is initiated. Androgen secretion remains quite constant during the life of the adult male and maintains the metabolic integrity of the reproductive organs as well as secondary sex characteristics. Only after about the seventh or eighth decade of life does androgen production begin to decline.

Biosynthesis, Metabolism and Excretion

The enzymes required to synthesize androgens are present in the testes, ovary, adrenal cortex and placenta. Androgen secretion by the female is normally much lower than in the male. Although blood levels of testosterone in the female are considerably less than in the male, levels of androstenedione are higher in the female. The latter steroid originates from the adrenal gland of the female. Androstenedione is androgenic, but less masculinizing than testosterone. Testosterone production in the female is generally extragonadal and may occur in such organs as the liver. Adrenal tumors often times secrete excessive amounts of androgens or androgen-like steroids.

Testicular steroidogenesis occurs in both the sustentacular cells (Sertoli cells) and the interstitial cells (Leydig cells). The germinal epithelium is under the influence of follicle-stimulating hormone, but Sertoli cell androgens may contribute an additional stimulus for spermatogenesis. Interstitial cell androgens produce characteristic physiologic changes in the male reproductive system. The testicular interstitium is richly endowed with lymph and blood vessels so that newly synthesized Leydig cell androgens can readily enter the systemic circulation.

The liver plays an important role in regulating the biologic half-life of androgens. Such hepatic enzymes as the androgen hydroxylases render male sex hormones more polar, more water soluble, and thus more readily excreted by the kidney (Chs. 2, 3). The liver and the kidney may affect further metabolic alterations, e.g., conjugation, and thereby expedite their elimination. Drugs like the barbiturates and certain organochloride insecticides can induce hepatic androgen hydroxylases and hence shorten the biologic half-life of circulating male sex hormones. The principal secretory products of male sex hormones found in the urine are androsterone, etiocholanone and dehydroisoandrosterone.

Mechanism of Action and Biochemical Effects

Androgens are capable of causing several complex and diverse biochemical events in organs such as the prostate and seminal vesicles. While the mechanism of action of androgens still remains to be established, sex accessory organ metabolic responses to these hormones have provided some insight into the complexities of various biochemical events. These sex accessory organs are truly androgen dependent since castration of the mature animal leads to a decrease in metabolic activity and a generalized regression of cellular processes. Injections of androgen to castrate animals leads to a stimulation of most enzymatic and metabolic pathways in the prostate gland or seminal vesicles. Androgens in-

crease RNA polymerase activity to enhance synthesis of protein. RNA directs the synthesis of functional proteins according to the genetic information coded in cellular DNA. They exert some control over tissue differentiation and cell growth by a direct action on DNA synthesis and on the cell mitotic cycle. Some recent evidence also indicates that cyclic adenosine monophosphate (cAMP) may be an intermediary in the action of androgens. Target organ levels of ATP are changed by androgens. Testosterone may cause changes in cellular permeability leading to increased uptake of certain electrolytes, hexoses and amino acids. Several enzymes involved in target organ lipid and carbohydrate metabolism are also stimulated.

Therapeutic Uses of Androgens

The pharmacologic actions of androgens are primarily an extension of their physiologic actions. Those used therapeutically are for their virilizing or masculinizing, protein anabolic, or antiestrogenic actions.

Substances with potential androgenic or protein anabolic actions are frequently tested in castrated animals, usually rodents. Androgenic-like substances, such as testosterone, cause an increase in seminal vesicle weight. The levator ani muscle weight change has been used to assess protein anabolic properties. However, it is difficult to entirely divorce these two primary pharmacologic actions.

Androgens are indicated in a number of pathologic states (Table 47–1). Their use in hormonal replacement therapy often involves long term treatment. In cases of prepubertal hypopituitarism or hypogonadism, testosterone (or a close derivative) is administered to induce puberty and to subsequently maintain secondary sexual characteristics. Replacement therapy must be undertaken with some caution since it will accelerate the closure of the epiphysial plates in long bones and have a stunting effect. To minimize this possibility, lower dose schedules of androgens may be used during critical periods of long bone growth or skeletal maturation.

Potent androgens have also been used in the medical treatment of undescended testes. Human chorionic gonadotropin (Ch. 43) is also used in cryptorchidism followed by orchiopexy. Such treatment is usually delayed until the age of 9 or 10 unless there is an associated hernia or the gonads are ectopic.

Testosterone and its close derivatives are capable of stimulating erythropoeisis and the formation of other cellular elements of the blood. In some instances, androgens have been used

TABLE 47-1. Pharmacologic Uses of Androgens

Indications	Comments on suggested therapy*
Replacement therapy in hypogonadism or castration	Testosterone enanthate (200 mg IM every 3rd or 4th wk) in adults; provide more frequent injections in younger undeveloped males
Induction of delayed puberty	Testosterone enanthate (200–300 mg IM/mo for 4–6 mo. Human chorionic gonadrotropin may be drug of choice
Management of osteoporosis in elderly	Methyltestosterone (5 mg/day) used in combination with estrogens. Higher doses may be necessary in males than in females
Stimulation of erythropoeisis in certain anemic states	Large doses of testosterone preparations (500–1000 mg/day)
Promote growth of long bones in selected cases of dwarfism	Variable dose schedules. Choose anabolic steroid (e.g., oxandrolone 0.1 mg/day). Human chorionic gonadotropin drug of choice
Management of cryptorchidism	Testosterone and/or HCG
Management of menopausal symptoms	In females, a half to full maintenance dose of methyltestosterone (25–50 mg/day) or fluoxymesterone (10–20 mg/day). In males, methyltestosterone (2–4 mg/day)

*Dosages represent guidelines and will vary depending upon the magnitude of hormonal imbalance and incidence of side effects.

in treating marrow erythrocyte deficiencies in aplastic anemia, certain leukemias and in thrombocytopenia.

Adverse Effects of Androgens

There are few immediate adverse effects associated with the use of androgens. Untoward effects are likely to occur only when they are used chronically (Table 47–2). What constitutes an undesirable effect of androgen therapy depends to some extent upon whether the hormone is being administered to the male or female and on the age of the patient. Excessive growth of hair in the female provides cosmetic problems whereas such an action in the male may be only an inconvenience. Excessive virilization in children receiving androgen therapy might also result in undesirable adverse effects whereas similar actions in the adult male would remain unnoticed.

In mature females androgens can lead to excessive facial and body hair. It also may cause a deepening of the voice, masculinization of body configuration and hypertrophy of the clitoris. If vigorous androgen therapy is undertaken in the child, it may impair the growth of long bones by prematurely accelerating epiphyseal closure. Precocious puberty may result from intensive androgen therapy. Steroid-induced edema is more common with the adrenocortical hormones, but intensive androgen therapy can likewise cause edema by causing the retention of electrolytes and water by the kidney.

Although testosterone and testosterone esters cause few changes in liver function, the 17-α

alkyl side group substitutions on the testosterone molecule are most apt to cause impairment of certain hepatic processes. Jaundice is not an uncommon side effect of methyl testosterone toxicity. Most of the 19-nortestosterone derivatives are also protein anabolic agents and are capable of causing varying degrees of liver damage. Such damage ordinarily is reversible. Some synthetic androgens produce creatinuria.

PHARMACOLOGIC PREPARATIONS OF ANDROGENS

Androgens possess varying degrees of both virilizing and protein anabolic pharmacologic actions (Table 47–3). While the 19-nortestosterone steroids are used principally for their protein anabolic actions, some nevertheless possess some virilizing properties.

Pharmacologically active androgens are steroids (Fig. 47–1). Testosterone itself is very poorly absorbed by mouth and has a relatively short biologic half-life. Certain side chain substitutions to testosterone render it orally active. Further, esterification produces a less polar

TABLE 47-2. Adverse Effects of Androgens

Excessive virilization or masculinization, particularly in females (hirsuitism) or children
Precocious puberty (priapism)
Retention of fluids and precordial pain
Creatinuria
Biliary stasis and/or hepatic dysfunction (17α-substituted androgens)

TABLE 47–3. Pharmacologic Preparations of Androgens

Preparation	Common route of administration	Major pharmacologic property*	Common dose range
Testosterone	IM, implantation	Androgenic	
Testosterone propionate	IM	Androgenic	
Testosterone enanthate (Delatestryl)	IM	Androgenic	
Testosterone cypionate (Depo-Testosterone cypionate)	IM	Androgenic	
Methyltestosterone	Sublingual	Androgenic	5—10 mg
Fluoxymesterone (Halotestin)	Oral	Androgenic	
Methandrostenolone (Dianabol)	Oral	Protein anabolic	0.25 mg
Ethylestrenol (Maxibolin)	Oral	Protein anabolic	
Stanozolol (Winstrol)	Oral	Protein anabolic	0.05 — 0.1 mg
Norethandrolone (Nilevar)	Oral	Protein anabolic	0.2 — 0.5 mg
Oxandrolone (Anadrol)	Oral	Protein anabolic	0.1 — 0.2 mg

*All of these compounds possess both androgenic (virilizing) and protein anabolic activities.

steroid with a longer biologic half-life. The 19-nortestosterone-type compounds such as norethandrolone have minimal virilizing properties and are used principally for their protein anabolic properties.

ANTIANDROGENS

An agent that can effectively antagonize the action of testosterone, or its close derivatives, is referred to as an antiandrogen. An antiandrogen does not necessarily have to exert its antagonistic action directly upon an androgen target cell. Rather it might suppress pituitary gonadotropin secretions and thereby indirectly interfere with androgenic responses.

Estrogens and some progestational agents, might be considered to be antiandrogenic when used in special therapeutic circumstances. The chronic administration of estrogens to intact males leads to a castration-like action upon androgen target organs.

Cyproterone acetate is a synthetic steroid that possesses some progestational activities. It is more widely known for its antiandrogenic properties. While this agent will prevent dihydrotestosterone from binding to its receptor, thus far its clinical effectiveness in controlling androgen-dependent tumors has been disappointing.

ESTROGENS

Physiologic Considerations

Female sex hormones or estrogens originate from the ovaries, placenta and the adrenal glands. Except during pregnancy, extragonadal estrogens are of little physiologic significance in the premenopausal woman. Adrenal estrogen secretion is normally quite low, but in certain pathologic states excessive amounts of female sex hormones are produced.

Levels of estrogen fluctuate during the normal menstrual cycle. In the cycling human female, two estrogen surges in blood levels of the hormones are seen: a preovulatory peak and a luteal phase peak. These are due to enhanced hormonal secretion by the ovaries. The preovulatory peak is probably due to increased secretion of estrogens by cells of the membrane granulosa or theca interna of the follicles and may signal the midcycle luteinizing hormone (LH)

secretion peak. The cells of the corpus luteum are responsible for the luteal phase peak of blood estrogens. Estradiol-17-β appears to be the principal estrogen secreted from these cells.

Estrogens are responsible for the increased growth and proliferation of several reproductive organs in the female. Many of these hormone-induced growth responses such as those seen in the uterus or vagina provide the pharmacologic basis for bioassaying substances with estrogenic activity.

Estrogens are responsible for the physiologic changes that occur at puberty in the female and result in changes in body configuration and the development of secondary sex characteristics. They are responsible for musculo-skeletal changes, growth of mammary glands and alterations in skin texture.

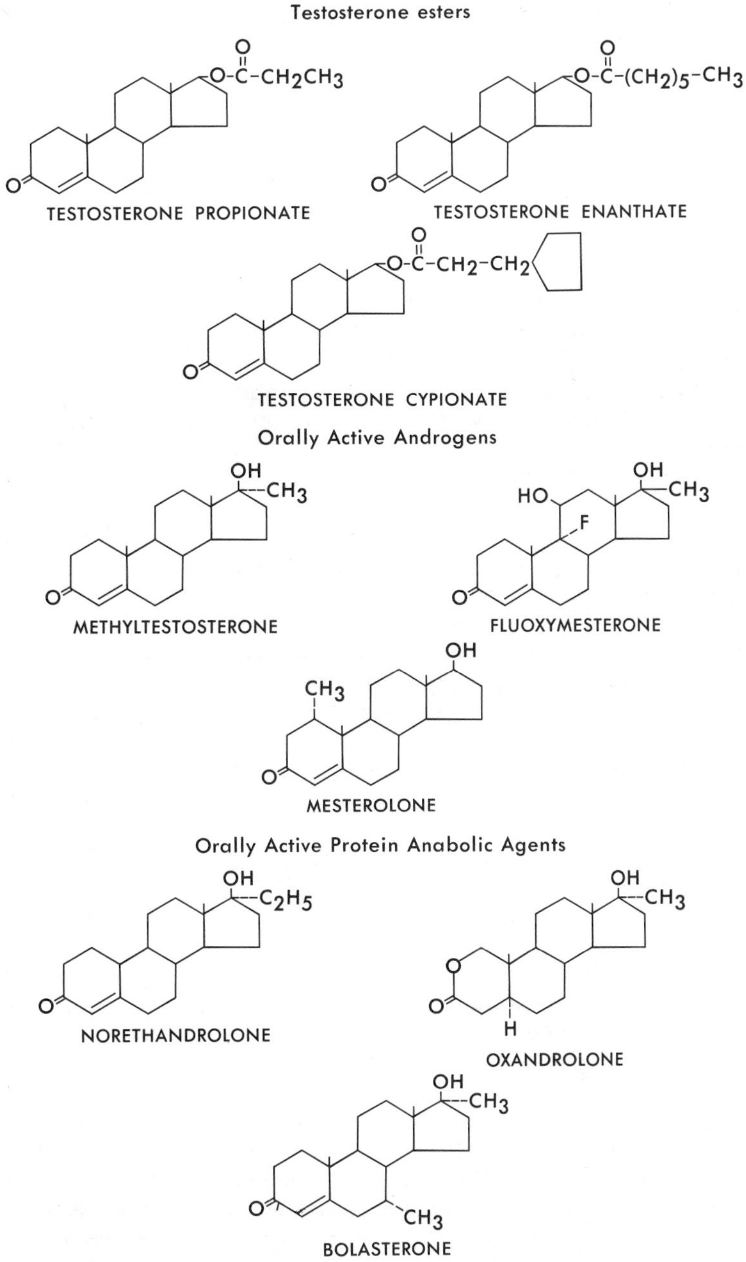

FIG. 47–1. Synthetic androgens.

Biosynthesis, Metabolism and Excretion

The follicular synthesis of estradiol is regulated by the adenohypophysis (Ch. 43). Follicle-stimulating hormone (FSH) and luteinizing hormone (LH) are involved in regulating ovarian estrogen biosynthesis. FSH alone has little effect on the synthesis of follicular estrogen. LH causes a slight stimulation of estrogen biosynthesis; its actions are increased greatly by the presence of FSH. The interaction of these two tropic hormones, however, results in a physiologic environment more suitable for estrogen biosynthesis. Since both tropic hormones are normally present during the follicular phase of the menstrual cycle, and since they act in concert to stimulate estrogen synthesis, both FSH and LH probably are involved in stimulating follicular estrogen production. In the pregnant state, the corpus luteum and the placenta are the principal sources of estrogens.

In the first trimester of pregnancy when the corpus luteum secretes large amounts of estrogens, the steroidogenic activity of the corpus luteum appears to be affected by another hormone, human chorionic gonadotropin (HCG)

(Ch. 43). HCG secretion reaches a peak approximately 1 month following conception. High levels of this hormone are found in the blood and urine of the pregnant woman (also in choriocarcinoma) and form the basis of certain biologic and immunologic tests used in the early diagnosis of pregnancy.

One of the initial biochemical steps in the synthesis of estrogens involves the conversion of acetate to cholesterol. This bioconversion involves several separate metabolic processes. Cholesterol may be metabolized to pregnenolone and progesterone. The stimulatory actions of FSH and LH on estradiol biosynthesis probably occur at the biochemical step between cholesterol and pregnenolone.

Estrogens are subject to a variety of metabolic alterations. The site of metabolic alteration of estrogens is in the liver, although the target organs are also capable of affecting changes in some of the female sex hormones. The liver can metabolize both steroidal or nonsteroidal estrogens. Hepatic conjugation of steroid estrogens results in a molecule that is less active, more polar and hence, more water soluble and more readily excreted. Nonsteroid estrogens are not as readily metabolized. A large fraction of diethylstilbestrol, e.g., is excreted by the kidney in a free or unconjugated state.

A number of hormones and drugs can alter the metabolism of estrogens by the liver. Thyroxine, androgens, adrenocortical steroids and barbiturates can change the rate of estrogen biotransformation by the liver.

The urine contains both free and conjugated estrogens. The amount present will fluctuate according to the menstrual cycle. Postmenopausal women excrete less urinary estrogen. Pharmacologically administered estrogens are found in the urine in either a free or conjugated state. When administered orally, substantial amounts enter the entero-hepatic circulation and are excreted via the feces.

Mechanism of Action and Biochemical Events

The molecular events surrounding the initial actions of female sex hormones on their target organs are not completely understood. Once estrogens are assimilated by a particular target organ, many subsequent biochemical changes occur rapidly within the gland. It has been suggested that estrogens act to derepress genetic materials found in the nuclei of the target cell resulting in stimulation of several metabolic events including ribonucleic acid (RNA) synthesis and protein anabolism. Lipid and carbohydrate metabolism are likewise enhanced.

The uterus, vagina, mammary glands, anterior pituitary gland and areas of the hypothalamus possess an avidity for estrogen. Once estrogen is assimilated in these anatomic areas, it is bound to proteins, specific macromolecules, located both in the cytoplasm and nucleus of the cells of the target organ. These are thought to be estrogen receptors. Whereas estrogens may exert some biochemical changes in their target organ cells before they attach themselves to these specific macromolecules, it is presumed that their major actions occur only after binding. Only a small portion of the estrogen localized within the target organ cell remains free or unbound.

The concept of estrogen receptors is rather complex in light of the diverse actions of these hormones. Although specific macromolecules can be extracted from estrogen target organs, this does not explain how this same hormone can produce behavioral changes as well as both stimulatory and inhibitory actions upon certain physiologic events.

The uterus and vagina are particularly sensitive to estrogens and very small amounts produce rather dramatic increases in several biochemical events within minutes. The growth and secretory activity of these tissues is increased markedly by estrogens. The vaginal mucosa proliferates and thickens, and the epithelial cells undergo cornification. The appearance of cornified epithelium in the vaginal fluid is a reliable index of estrogenic stimulation and is often used to determine female sex hormone activity. This is a very sensitive bioassay for estrogens. Estrogens increase the tone and excitability of uterine musculature. They produce changes in the water content of the uterus and the vagina. Estrogen administration leads to an imbibition of water by these tissues and hence an increased weight.

Estrogens produce many changes in intermediary metabolism within the uterus or vagina. DNA levels and the number of cellular mitoses increase quite early following the injection of female sex hormone. Ribosomal, messenger and transfer RNA rise. While some of the earliest changes induced by estrogens are related to nucleic acid synthesis, these hormones also produce stimulatory effects upon protein and carbohydrate metabolism.

Like the uterus and vagina, the mammary glands are particularly sensitive to estrogenic stimulation. The growth promoting effects of the estrogens on mammary tissues are evident at about the time of puberty. They cause a proliferation of the mammary ductile system. Physiologic and pharmacologic amounts of estrogens can lead to a retention of fluids within the breasts. This fluid retention may be seen just before menstruation when endogenous levels of estrogens are elevated. Pharmacologic amounts of estrogens, or the estrogen component present in certain oral contraceptive preparations, can often result in a sensation of increased fullness of the breasts.

The hypothalamus and the anterior pituitary gland play an important role in the regulation of female sex hormones (Chs. 42, 43). Physiologically speaking, estrogens can exert either a negative or a positive feedback effect upon pituitary gonadotropins. Pharmacologic amounts of estrogens almost always lead to an inhibition of the secretion of FSH and LH. The estrogen receptors located in the hypothalamus appear to be more sensitive to estrogens than similar areas in the anterior pituitary. The actions of estrogens upon the hypothalamus are mediated through specific releasing hormones (Ch. 42).

Therapeutic Uses of Estrogens

There are many indications for the pharmacologic use of estrogens (Table 47–4). Estrogens may be used briefly for a period of 2 or 3 days immediately following rape to prevent conception. Replacement regimens involve months or even years of treatment. Ovarian dysgenesis often requires very long term estrogen administration since the therapeutic rationale involves the complete replacement of female sex hormone. Female sex hormone therapy may be in-

dicated in the management of pathologic states, e.g., certain neoplasms. Estrogens alone can interfere with a variety of physiologic processes including ovulation. Estrogens are used in combination with progestational agents as in certain oral contraceptive preparations. (Ch. 48)

Dysmenorrhea is often alleviated by inhibiting ovulation with chronic estrogen therapy. More often, dysmenorrhea is treated with a combination of estrogens and progestational agents. Such a regimen allows the use of a lower dose of estrogen and thereby minimizes the incidence of undesirable adverse effects.

Estrogen administration can effectively prevent or reduce postpartum breast engorgement. In suppressing postpartum breast engorgement, it is important that the suckling stimuli not be initiated since it will enhance the milk-let-down process. Pharmacologic amounts of estrogen must be administered for a period of about a week immediately following parturition. They probably exert this action by inhibiting pituitary prolactin release and/or by directly reducing alveolar secretion in the mammary gland.

Estrogen replacement has been advocated in women suffering from the signs and symptoms of the menopause. Some of the symptoms may be psychologic whereas still others may be more closely associated with a deficit in physiologic levels of female sex hormones. Some women ex-

TABLE 47–4. Pharmacologic Uses of Estrogens

Indications	Comments on suggested therapy *
Dysmenorrhea	Diethylstilbestrol (up to 1 mg/day) for 21 days beginning on 4th day of cycle. Alternate cycles may be treated
Postpartum breast engorgement	Diethylstilbestrol (3 mg/day for first 3 days; 2 mg/day for next 3 days and 1 mg/day for 3 additional days)
Prostatic cancer	Diethylstilbestrol (2–10 mg/day)
Adjunct in prevention of habitual abortions	Variable dosages depending on duration of gestation
Menopause	Diethylstilbestrol (0.1–0.25 mg/day) or ethynyl estradiol (0.02–0.05 mg/day)
Certain breast cancers	Diethylstilbestrol (2.5–5 mg/t.i.d.) (Variable dose schedules)
Inhibition of blastocyst implantation	Diethylstilbestrol (25–50 mg/day x 5) or ethynyl estradiol (2–5 mg/day x 5) initiated immediately after suspected fertilization
Acne	Variable dose schedules
Endometriosis	Estrogen-progestin combination preparation. Therapy may be prolonged (e.g., 6–12 mo)
Functional uterine bleeding	Estrogen-progestin combination preparation. Dosage is variable. Large doses of conjugated estrogens recommended postovulation
Hirsuitism	Estrogen-progestin combination or sequential preparation
Prevention of ovulation	Wide choice of sequential and combination oral contraceptives

*Dosages are guidelines and may vary depending upon the specific circumstances of the endocrine disorder. Diethylstilbestrol is frequently recommended since it is an orally effective agent and relatively inexpensive compared to some of the steroid estrogens.

periencing the onset of menopause respond better to treatment with barbiturates or minor tranquilizers. While the therapy of postmenopausal osteoporosis is a controversial subject, recent experimental evidence suggests that it is best treated by a combination of supplemental calcium and vitamin D and small doses of fluoride rather than by estrogens.

Many etiologies may be involved in the failure of the ovaries to develop normally. Regardless of the etiology, estrogens can be used in an attempt to induce sexual maturation. Under such conditions, estrogen replacement will maintain the size and sometimes the function of reproductive structures. Secondary sex characteristics may develop following this type of estrogen therapy.

Estrogens, alone or in combination with progestational agents, may be of value in the management of functional uterine bleeding. Such bleeding is frequently associated with abnormally low levels of endogenous female sex hormones.

Hirsuitism may be related to increased endogenous secretion of androgens or androgen-like steroids. Because most masculinizing hormones are of ovarian origin, pharmacologic amounts of estrogen are generally capable of ameliorating this pathologic state. Estrogens act by suppressing pituitary secretion of gonadotropins thereby indirectly inhibiting ovarian steroidogenesis.

Estrogens can effectively block ovulation via an action on the hypothalamus and/or pituitary gland. Estrogens, alone or in combination with progestational agents, can effectively produce anovulatory cycles. This is the basis for their use as antifertility agents (Ch. 48).

Although estrogen deficiency may be a factor in women with a history of threatened or habitual abortion, female sex hormone therapy has not been particularly effective in increasing the incidence of live births. Estrogens are used in this condition because they increase endometrial development and proliferation, thereby affording a more optimal environment for implantation.

The growth of breast cancers can sometimes be suppressed in postmenopausal women with estrogen. Estrogens, however, may accelerate the growth of mammary tumors in premenopausal women as they are sometimes estrogen dependent. Accordingly, mammary carcinomas in premenopausal women are treated surgically or with chemotherapeutic agents and not with female sex hormones. Sometimes androgens are also used since they can inhibit some of the actions of endogenous female sex hormone.

Estrogens are often used in the treatment of prostatic carcinoma. Generally, estrogen therapy is initiated in the latter stages of this disease in an effort to induce a regression of the tumor and its possible metastases. The rationale for such therapy is based upon the antiandrogenic properties of the estrogens. Estrogen therapy not only directly inhibits the prostate gland, but suppresses pituitary gonadotropins leading to a reduction in testicular androgen production. Cyproterone is an antiandrogen but without significant estrogenic properties. It will inhibit prostatic function in experimental animals, but its therapeutic efficacy in man has not been impressive.

Estrogens have been used topically in males to alleviate acne, probably by antagonizing the stimulatory effect of androgens upon sebaceous glands. Estrogens seem to play a physiologic role in maintaining the texture of the skin.

Adverse Effects of Estrogens

In general, the estrogens have a fairly wide margin of safety. Fewer adverse effects would be expected in the management of ovarian dysgenesis where the therapeutic goal is simply a hormonal replacement. During such a therapeutic regimen, dosage would be chosen to provide physiologic levels. The same would apply to management of postmenopausal symptoms. In contrast, superimposing pharmacologic amounts of estrogens upon an already normal level of endogenous female sex hormones usually generates an increased incidence in the number of adverse effects.

The long term use of pharmacologic amounts of estrogens is not without its hazards (Table 47–5). Prolonged estrogenic therapy has been linked to an increased incidence of thromboembolic disorders. It is not clear just how female sex hormones alter the clotting of blood. Men treated with estrogens for prostatic carcinoma exhibit a higher than normal incidence of cardiovascular disorders. Likewise the estrogenic component of oral contraceptive combination preparations has been related to an increased incidence of thromboembolic disorders. Despite early suggestions it seems reasonably certain that estrogens do not increase the incidence of cervical carcinoma in humans. Women receiving estrogens for the abatement of menopausal symptoms may actually show a decreased incidence of cervical and mammary cancers.

TABLE 47–5. Adverse Effects of Pharmacologic Amounts of Estrogens

Nausea, vomiting, anorexia
Water retention and weight gain
Dizziness
Breast engorgement
Thrombophlebitis (and other blood clotting disorders)
Hepatic dysfunction
Hypertension

TABLE 47–6. Classification of Certain Estrogens

Chemical classification	Example	Common route of administration	Common dose range
Naturally occurring estrogen	Estradiol-17-β		
Semisynthetic steroid estrogens	Ethynylestradiol (Esteed, Estinyl)	Oral	0.05—0.1 mg
	Mestranol	Oral	0.1 —0.2 mg
	Quinestrol (Estrovis)	Oral	0.05—0.1 mg
	Estradiol valerate (Delestrogen)	IM	10—20 mg
	Estradiol cypionate	IM	5—10 mg
Nonsteroidal estrogens	Diethylstilbestrol (Stilbitin)	Oral	0.2 —1 mg
	Benzestrol (Chemestrogen)	Oral	3—6 mg
	Hexestrol	Oral	3—6 mg
	Methallenestril (Vallestril)	Oral	3—6 mg
	Chlorotrianisene (Tace)	Oral	10—20 mg
Polymeric estrogen	Polyestradiol phosphate (Estradurin)	IM	40 mg
Conjugated estrogen	Estrone sulfonate (Premarin)	Oral	1.0 —2.0 mg

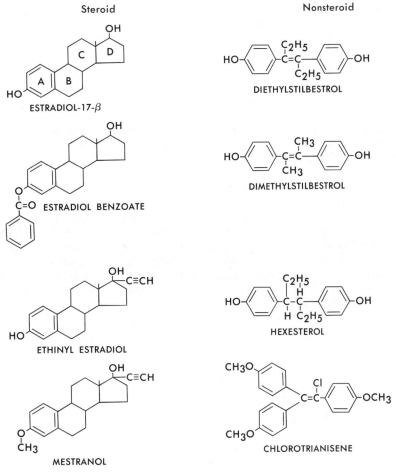

FIG. 47–2. Chemical structures of various estrogens.

Pharmacologic amounts of estrogen administered to immature or young girls can lead to precocious puberty. Premature development of secondary sex characteristics such as growth and proliferation of mammary gland tissue may occur. More seriously, estrogen administration in immature girls may stunt the growth of the long bones by accelerating the closure of the epiphyseal plate.

Certain of the side effects of estrogen therapy amount to nothing more than annoying actions. Nausea appears to be troublesome in many patients regardless of whether the estrogen is administered orally or parenterally. Stimulatory effects of the CNS may also be involved in the production of dizziness and vomiting. The nighttime administration of nonconjugated estrogen reduces the incidence of nausea.

Estrogens frequently lead to a retention of both salt and water and such retention may lead to an increase in body weight. It may be responsible for the increased tenderness of the breasts. This accumulation of fluids will usually recede after the early phases of estrogen treatment.

Estrogens may produce hypertension by activating the renin-angiotensin system and increase hormone transporting substances in the blood.

Pharmacologic Preparations of Estrogens

There are numerous preparations of estrogens or estrogen-containing combinations. Frequently, steroid estrogens can be chemically modified to increase their biologic activity. A chemical classification of estrogens may be seen on Table 47–6. **Estradiol,** estrone and estriol are all important physiologic female sex hormones (Figure 47–2), but estradiol is the only one of these three steroids that is used pharmacologically.

The majority of steroid estrogens are very poorly absorbed from the gastrointestinal tract. They are generally insoluble in water and consequently are usually suspended in either alcohol or oil vehicles. To be therapeutically effective, they must be administered parenterally or otherwise modified to render them orally active. Semisynthetic estrogens, such as ethynylestra-diol are orally effective steroid estrogens. Esterification will delay their absorption and prolong their biologic half-life.

Nonsteroidal estrogens are orally active and do not have to be chemically modified to achieve satisfactory pharmacologic activity. Nonsteroidal estrogens can also be administered parenterally and are usually quite soluble in water. These compounds are not altered as readily by hepatic metabolism nor are they bound as readily to plasma proteins as are the steroidal estrogens.

Estradiol-17-β, a naturally occurring estrogen, is not very orally active and must be administered parenterally. **Ethynylestradiol** is a very potent semisynthetic preparation. The ethynyl addition increases its effectiveness, renders it orally active and extends its biologic half-life. **Mestranol** is the 3-methyl ether of ethynylestradiol and is the most common estrogenic component of oral contraceptive combination preparations. The 3-cyclopentyl ether of ethynylestradiol is called **quinestrol.** Quinestrol is a long acting estrogen and a constituent of certain experimental preparations referred to as the-once-a-month-pill. There are other semisynthetic estrogens that have an equally long biologic half-life. **Estradiol valerate, estradiol dipropionate, estradiol benzoate** and **estradiol cypionate** all possess extended biologic activity related mainly to their slower rates of biotransformation by the liver.

The nonsteroidal estrogens, **diethylstilbestrol, dimethylstilbestrol, hexestrol, benzestriol** and **methallenestril** are orally active agents and are generally much cheaper than the steroid estrogens. Diethylstilbestrol is perhaps the most widely used.

Conjugated estrogens may be obtained from the urine of pregnant mares. Often these conjugated preparations contain sodium estrone sulfonate and equine estrogens. Synthetic conjugated estrogens also are available in the form of **piperazine estrone sulfate.**

Polymeric estrogens such as **polyestradiol phosphate** have been used in the hormonal treatment of prostatic cancer. It is doubtful that this polymeric form of estradiol is any more effective than estradiol itself.

FURTHER READING

ANDROGENS:

Longson D (1972): Androgen therapy. Practitioner 208:338

O'Malley BW (1971): Mechanism of action of steroid hormones. N Engl J Med 284:370

Shahidi NT (1973): Androgens and erythropoiesis. N Engl J Med 289:72

Walsh PC, Korenman SG (1971): Mechanism of androgenic action: effect of specific intracellular inhibitors. J Urol 105:850

Williams-Ashman HG, Reddi AH (1971): Actions of vertebrate sex hormones. Annu Rev Physiol 33:31

ESTROGENS:

Jensen EV, Mohla S, Gorell TA, DeSombre ER (1974): The role of estrophilin in estrogen action. Vitam & Horm 32:89

Kellie AE (1971): The pharmacology of estrogens. Annu Rev Pharmacol 11:97

Means AR, O'Malley BW (1972): Mechanism of estrogen action: early transcriptional and translational events. Metabolism 21:357

JOHN A. THOMAS

JOHN E. JONES

48. ORAL CONTRACEPTIVES

PHYSIOLOGIC CONSIDERATIONS

Progesterone, a precursor of many steroid hormones including the glucocorticoids, mineralocorticoids, androgens and estrogens, has inherent physiologic activity. It is secreted by several tissues, but physiologically significant amounts are only derived from the corpus luteum and the placenta.

The corpus luteum is formed shortly after ovulation from the remnants of the ruptured follicle. Progesterone secretion is initiated at the time, or even slightly before ovulation and is enhanced by LH (Fig. 48–1). Elevations in both FSH and LH occur prior to any demonstrable secretion of progesterone into the blood. If the ovum is not fertilized, progesterone secretion from the corpus luteum continues until the end of the cycle and gradually diminishes. During this luteal phase of the cycle, progesterone acts on the estrogen-primed uterus to stimulate glandular growth and development of the endometrium. The physiologic function of such actions is to prepare the endometrium for implantation of the fertilized ovum. The actions of progesterone, including biochemical effects, on the nonpregnant uterus are manifest only after priming by estrogens; it transforms a proliferating endometrium into a secretory type of endometrial growth. Thus the actions of estrogen and progesterone on the uterus are synergistic.

The actions of progesterone on the uterus render the uterine endometrium capable of accepting and supporting the growth of the fertilized ovum. If fertilization does not occur, the uterine endometrium is sloughed and menstruation occurs. Menstruation is characterized by extensive regression of the endometrium and by a loss of some stromal tissue of the uterus. If fertilization occurs, the life span of the corpus luteum is maintained by the hormone chorionic gonadotropin (HCG) and secreted by the placenta. When conception occurs, the corpus luteum continues to secrete progesterone for approximately a month and the uterine lining continues to grow and proliferate. Such growth and development is important in maintaining the pregnancy to full term. Occasionally, if endogenous progesterone secretion is not adequate, then pharmacologic supplementation may insure a successful full term pregnancy.

Progesterone depresses the contractility of the uterine myometrium. When the uterus shifts from a progesterone to an estrogen dominated state in late pregnancy, uterine excitability is increased. This increased excitability facilitates the expulsion of the fetus at parturition. Pharmacologic amounts of progesterone used in an estrogen primed animal can cause a regression of the endometrium but an increased growth of the myometrium.

Progesterone has little stimulatory effect upon the growth of the vagina, but can antagonize the actions of estrogens on the vagina, namely mitosis and the cornification of vaginal epithelium.

Progesterone transforms the estrogen dominated cervical secretions from a thin watery type to one that is thick and mucoid. Various oral contraceptive preparations exert similar actions. The increased viscosity of these secretions may act to impede the migration of spermatozoa in the female genital tract.

Estrogens will stimulate the ductal development of the mammary glands whereas progesterone will induce the alveolar proliferation of the ductal system. Growth hormone, prolactin (Ch. 43) and even the adrenocortical steroids (Ch. 46) also appear to be necessary for the optimal development of the mammary gland for lactation.

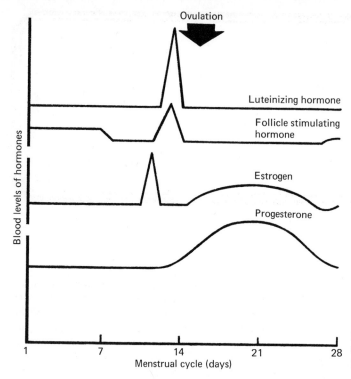

Blood levels of hormones

Ovulation

Luteinizing hormone

Follicle stimulating hormone

Estrogen

Progesterone

1   7   14   21   28

Menstrual cycle (days)

FIG. 48–1. Relationship between the pituitary follicle stimulating hormone and luteinizing hormone and the ovarian secretion of steroid.

Progesterone exerts actions upon the pituitary gland and/or the hypothalamus. In pregnancy, high doses of progesterone secreted by the placenta are sufficient to cause an inhibition of FSH and LH. This inhibition suppresses ovulation during the 9 month period of gestation. This suppression of pituitary gonadotropins is exploited pharmacologically and is the principal mechanism of action of the synthetic oral progestational contraceptives.

Progesterone possesses a thermogenic property which results in a slight elevation in body temperature shortly after ovulation. This elevation in basal body temperature sometimes is used to detect ovulation in women and is the basis of the rhythm method of birth control. The elevation is not a reliable index of ovulation.

SYNTHESIS, METABOLISM AND EXCRETION

The biosynthesis of progesterone occurs principally in the corpus luteum and the placenta. Small amounts of progesterone can be synthesized in other organs such as the testes and the adrenal cortex.

The synthesis of progesterone by the corpus luteum is stimulated by LH. How this pituitary hormone enhances steroidogenesis is unknown. LH reportedly increases cAMP formation and protein synthesis in the corpus luteum. Whereas no specific enzyme involved in the biosynthesis of progesterone seems to be particularly sensitive to the action of LH, some of the early steps in the

metabolic pathway of this steroid do appear to be influenced.

Progesterone itself is not a very effective pharmacologic agent since it has a relatively short biologic half-life. When ingested, it is readily inactivated by the liver. If it escapes inactivation by the liver, it can be stored in adipose tissue.

Chemical modifications of the progesterone structure render it pharmacologically useful, orally active, and prolonging its biologic half-life. Some chemical modifications result in derivatives that are more water soluble and that are bound more tightly to plasma proteins.

Two chemical classes of progestins are in current clinical use: **progesterone derivatives** e.g., hydroxyprogesterone, and steroids related to **testosterone** including the **19-norsteroids,** e.g., norethynodrel. The progestins resembling the 19-norsteroids are more apt to produce virilizing adverse effects. In general, the progesterone derivatives are more widely used for various gynecologic disorders whereas the 19-norsteroids seem to be used principally as constituents in oral contraceptive preparations.

Progesterone is metabolized primarily in the liver. Even though all of the metabolites of progesterone are not known, pregnanediol is found in the urine. These metabolites may be conjugated with glucuronides. A large portion of exogenous progesterone is excreted by the bile into the feces.

Little is known about the metabolism of the various synthetic progestational agents. Radioactive norethynodrel can be traced to the bile, urine and feces. Medroxyprogesterone acetate can be detected in the urine of women. Amounts of this synthetic progestin are conjugated as either glucosiduronates or sulfates. Certain of the synthetic progestins undoubtedly undergo some degree of biotransformation before being excreted by the kidneys.

MECHANISM OF ACTION AND BIOCHEMICAL EFFECTS

Recent reports indicate that a specific progesterone receptor exists in several tissues. Like other sex steroids, progesterone binds rather selectively to macromolecules in the cytoplasm and the nucleus of its target organs. There is undoubtedly some type(s) of progesterone receptors located in the hypothalamus and/or the anterior pituitary. Unfortunately, little progress has been made in elucidating CNS receptors for progesterone.

Once progesterone is secreted, it presumably enters its target cells and binds with either cytoplasmic or nuclear receptors. Like the estrogens or the androgens, the cytoplasmic binding is a necessary prerequisite for subsequent nuclear binding. In the nucleus, progesterone is bound to acidic proteins associated with chromatin.

Progesterone enhances the metabolic activity of several female reproductive organs. While progesterone (and close chemical derivatives) ordinarily enhances the growth and proliferation of the uterus, fallopian tubes, mammary glands etc., it is partially responsible for inhibiting the release of pituitary gonadotropins.

THERAPEUTIC USES

The development of new orally active derivatives made it more convenient to treat many gynecologic disorders with progestational agents (Table 48–1). Orally effective estrogens have been available for much longer periods of time; they share many of the same therapeutic indications as the progestational agents. However, the estrogens possess a higher incidence of undesirable and serious adverse effects (Ch. 47).

TABLE 48–1. Some Pharmacologic Uses of Progestational Agents

Prevention of ovulation (i.e., contraception)
Dysmenorrhea
Endometriosis
Functional uterine bleeding
Prevention of threatened or habitual abortion
Relief of premenstrual tension
Diagnosis of pregnancy

TABLE 48–2. Types of Oral Contraceptive Formulations

The combination pill (estrogen-progestin combination)
The sequential pill
Continuous progestin administration
Long acting pill (one-pill-a-month)
Long acting injectable preparations
Implants
Postcoital contraceptive and nonsteroidal antifertility agents

The discovery of the orally effective progestational agents has provided further impetus for studying the mechanism of ovulation. Undoubtedly, their main use is in the prevention of ovulation and they are utilized for this purpose by millions of women throughout the world. Oral contraceptives can be used in several specific circumstances: where pregnancy might be harmful to the health of the mother; for family planning; and for regulating the growth of the population. Further, the oral contraceptives may rarely be prescribed for young girls to control and regulate their menstrual cycles until sufficient endogenous steroid levels can be achieved. Frequently, the initiation of menstrual cycles in young girls is quite irregular, and this can sometimes be normalized by the administration of progestational agents. The doses used are different from those required for preventing ovulation.

There are several formulations of the oral contraceptives including the so-called combinations, sequentials and continuous types of preparations (Table 48–2). The combination type is most frequently prescribed. The oral contraceptives are ordinarily used for a period of 20–21 days during the menstrual cycle. Assuming a normal 28 day cycle, the oral contraceptive is administered on about the 5th day of the cycle and ingested every 24 hours until about the 25th day of the cycle (Fig. 48–2). To be effective, the oral contraceptive must be used daily for a period of approximately 20–21 days during the menstrual cycle. Menstruation usually occurs 40–72 hr after the final or 20th daily pill. Pills are not ingested during menstruation.

The blood levels of synthetic steroid must be sufficiently elevated to prevent midcycle ovulation. The progestational agent, if present in high amounts in the blood, will inhibit gonadotropin release by an action on pituitary and hypothalamic receptors. LH is believed to be the pituitary hormone responsible for causing ovulation. The oral contraceptives merely inhibit LH secretion resulting in an anovulatory cycle.

Forgetting to ingest a single pill during the 20 day regimen rarely leads to ovulation. A pill missed early in the normal cycle is more apt to result in an accidental pregnancy than a pill

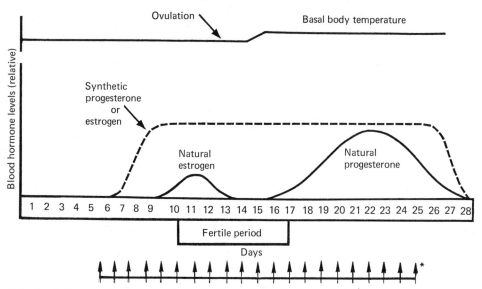

FIG. 48–2. Hormonal sequences during a normal menstrual cycle and the effect of an oral contraceptive. * Arrows indicate the daily ingestion of an oral contraceptive.

missed later on in the cycle. Needless to say, the dosage form must be adjusted to insure sufficient levels of synthetic steroid to suppress ovulation.

Progestational agents can be used for a variety of gynecologic disorders (Table 48–1). Several gynecologic disorders seem to stem from a lack or a deficiency of progesterone and/or estrogens. Functional uterine bleeding is often treated with progestational agents. While the exact etiology remains in question, there are abnormalities in the blood levels of estrogens and progesterone resulting in insufficient endometrial development in the latter stages of the menstrual cycle. When therapy is indicated, it is withdrawn near the end of the cycle to allow menstruation to take place. Frequently, combined therapy using both progestin and estrogen is more effective.

Dysmenorrhea or painful menses can frequently be relieved by progestational agents. Ovulation is often inhibited during therapy for dysmenorrhea. Many of the oral contraceptive preparations can be used in the management of this gynecologic disorder. Progestational agents may be indicated in endometriosis, a condition in which uterine mucosa is located in extrauterine sites. It is often characterized by severe dysmenorrhea.

Progestational steroids have been used to prevent threatened or habitual abortions. Unfortunately, women with histories of aborting seldom respond very well to this therapy. Progesterone deficiency appears to be only partly involved. Nevertheless, progestins are sometimes administered in an effort to carry the pregnancy to full term. A progestational agent with minimal an-

drogenic or virilizing properties should be selected to reduce masculinizing characteristics in the fetus.

If a reasonably normal menstrual cycle is interrupted by a missed period, a progestin can be used as an adjunct in the diagnosis of pregnancy. A short acting progestin-estrogen combination is administered. If withdrawal bleeding occurs within 4–9 days, the patient is not pregnant.

ADVERSE EFFECTS

These range from only mild annoying actions to more severe toxicity (Table 48–3). Some are

TABLE 48–3. Some Adverse Effects of Oral Contraceptives

Progestin related effects

   Fatigue, mental depression and lack of motivation
   Decreased menstrual flow
   Changes in liver function (17-α substitued steroids)
   Acne
   Weight gain
   Hirsuitism (17-α substituted steroids)

Estrogen related effects

   Nausea, dizziness and vomiting
   Fluid retention or edema formation
   Painful breast engorgement
   Hypertension
   Mild to severe headache
   Blood clotting disorders; thrombophlebitis and
     embolisms
   Alteration in liver function tests and jaundice
   Changes in blood glucose levels
   Increases in hormone binding proteins in the blood

merely subjective symptoms, while others are more objective and can be clearly associated with the use of these agents.

Perhaps most of the adverse effects of oral contraceptive preparations, in particular the combination type pill, are due to the estrogen—not the progestational component. Unfortunately, the estrogen component is regarded as a necessary constituent since it provides a better suppression of pituitary gonadotropin than progesterone. Efforts should be made to reduce the estrogen component to its lowest possible effective dose in the oral contraceptive formulation.

The milder adverse effects occur primarily during the initial cycles and tend to disappear with adjustments in dosage or simply with extended usage. Edema, nausea, vomiting, dizziness and headaches have been attributed to the estrogen component. Fluid retention can lead to painful breast engorgement. These steroids can precipitate hypertension. The estrogen component is believed to be responsible for alterations in blood clotting mechanisms. The mechanism whereby the oral contraceptives produce thromboembolic disease is still a matter of conjecture. There is, however, little doubt that some relationship exists between the use of oral contraceptives and venous thrombophlebitis and pulmonary embolism. For all the concern about the relationship between oral contraceptives and the incidence of fatal clotting disorders, it should be noted that pregnancy itself is associated with a higher incidence of mortality.

The reported fatigue, mental depression and lack of motivation are believed to be due to the progestational component. These effects are annoying and often will disappear with continued therapy. The 17-α alkyl side chain on the progestational molecule, while rendering it orally effective, can cause reversible liver damage. Some, but not all, oral contraceptives possess virilizing actions. Those progestational agents more closely related to 19-nortestosterone may cause acne, hirsuitism and some gain in body weight. An increased pigmentation of the skin (chloasma) has also been reported following the use of the oral contraceptives.

The oral contraceptives may be contraindicated in certain disease states, e.g., mammary carcinoma. In other conditions they may have to be prescribed with more discrimination, e.g., in diabetes. The following are generally accepted contraindications for the oral contraceptives; a medical history of thromboembolic disease, cervical or mammary carcinomas and liver disease. There are other conditions where the use of oral contraceptives are questionable and where mechanical forms of contraception should be encouraged: idiopathic visual disturbances; severe diabetes mellitus; hypertension; recurrent headaches—migraine; and during the growth of the long bones or in critical phases of skeletal growth.

Although the oral contraceptives possess certain conveniences and desirable attributes, certain women simply may not be able to tolerate their undesirable side effects. Aside from the rhythm method of birth control, other mechanical and chemical methods of contraception can be practiced including the intrauterine device (IUD), diaphragm or cervical cap and spermicidal agents (vaginal foams or jellies). In the male, the condom or vasectomy provide additional contraceptive methods.

It is generally agreed that the pregnancy or failure rate is lowest in those women practicing birth control using the oral contraceptives. The only other method of birth control which begins to approach the efficacy of the oral contraceptives is the IUD. If well intended or motivated women are faithful in the use of a properly fitted diaphragm, the pregnancy rate of this mechanical method begins to approach the efficacy of the oral contraceptives. The key to the success of such mechanical devices, however, lies in the motivation of the user.

PHARMACOLOGIC PREPARATIONS

The absorption of these steroids either parenterally or orally is quite rapid. Progesterone is bound to blood proteins, whereas many of the synthetic derivatives remain in a free or unbound state in the circulation. Progesterone is very soluble in lipids and hence tends to be stored in body fat depots. Similarly, **hydroxyprogesterone caproate** is very lipid soluble. Such a long acting derivative can be injected into subcutaneous fat, thereby affording a slow absorption into the circulation.

The chemical structures of some of the oral progestins may be seen in Figure 48–3. All of the steroids shown, except progesterone, possess a side-chain addition, 17-α alkyl group, which renders them more orally effective. **Norethindrone** and **norethynodrel** are considered 19-norsteroids. Norethynodrel is the first such steroid to have been referred to as "the pill."

The most widely used type of oral contraceptive, and probably the most effective, is the combination type formulation (Table 48–4). **Mestranol** is perhaps one of the most common estrogens found in oral contraceptive combination type preparations. It is an esterified derivative of ethynyl estradiol. There are approximately two dozen commercially available oral contraceptive preparations, each one existing in different dosage formulations. Usually it is the estrogen com-

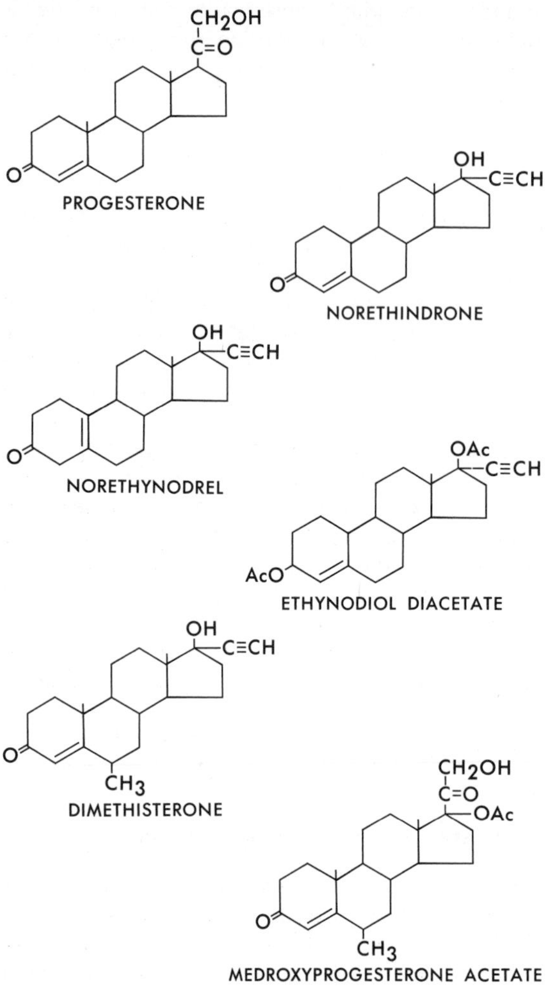

FIG. 48–3. Chemical structures of some of the more common progestins.

ponent that is found in different concentrations. Some women may not tolerate the higher dose increments of estrogen while in others the estrogen component may be too low leading to breakthrough or midcycle bleeding. The estrogen containing combination type pill must be titrated against its adverse effects and therapeutic effectiveness.

There are several other effective formulations (Table 48–2). The sequential type of pill is not as effective as the combination type in suppressing ovulation. The latter is used for 20 or 21 days during the menstrual cycle beginning on day 5 and ending on day 25. With the sequential formulation estrogen is initiated on day 5 and continues to day 25; progestin is included only from day 20 to day 25. Although the sequential type of oral contraceptive preparation more nearly approximates the normal cycle (i.e., estrogen priming followed by progesterone) its use results in a somewhat higher failure or pregnancy rate.

Potent progestins used alone and continuously throughout the cycle are capable of suppressing ovulation. Sometimes small amounts of estrogen are included in these so-called continuous preparations.

Long acting pills have been designed to suppress ovulation. Most of these are estrogens such as **quinestrol** (3-cyclopentyl ether of ethynylestradiol). This is orally active, but seems to have a great affinity for body fat where it is temporarily stored and slowly released.

Long acting injectable preparations such as **estradiol valerate** have undergone clinical trials and have been shown to suppress ovulation, but are not as popular as orally effective agents. These same estrogenic preparations can be implanted into subcutaneous fat. Sometimes these implants or steroid pellets are encapsulated in silastic to afford a more uniform and slow release of the drug. Implant preparations have not been too well received since termination of drug action involves surgical removal of the capsule or implant.

Estrogens are being used as the so-called "morning-after pill." If high doses of estrogen are administered for a few days following fertilization in the ovum, they prevent pregnancy by interfering with implantation of the egg. Either steroidal or nonsteroidal estrogens are capable of causing postcoital contraception. **Diethylstilbestrol** is frequently used in high doses immediately following cases of rape. The high doses necessary to interfere with implantation of the

TABLE 48–4. Steroid Components of Some Oral Contraceptive Preparations

Progestin	Estrogen	Trade name
Combination type		
Norethynodrel (5 mg)	Mestranol (0.075 mg)	Enovid
Norethindrone (10 mg)	Mestranol (0.06 mg)	Ortho-Novum
Norethindrone (1 mg)	Mestranol (0.08 mg)	Norinyl
Ethynodiol diacetate (1 mg)	Mestranol (0.1 mg)	Ovulen
Medroxyprogesterone acetate (10 mg)	Ethinylestradiol (0.05 mg)	Provest
Norgestrel (0.5 mg)	Ethinylestradiol (0.05 mg)	Ovral
Sequential type		
Dimethisterone (25 mg)	Ethinylestradiol (0.1 mg)	Oracon
Northindrone (2 mg)	Mestranol (0.08 mg)	Norquen

ovum are accompanied with rather severe nausea and vomiting. There are several non-steroidal antifertility agents that are being examined for their possible clinical use. Most of these nonsteroidal drugs such as **cyanoketone** act by interfering with enzymes involved in the synthesis of progesterone. Unfortunately, most of these nonsteroidal antifertility agents possess considerable degrees of teratogenicity.

FURTHER READING

Bingel AS, Benoit PS (1973): Oral contraceptives: therapeutics versus adverse reactions, with an outlook for the future. J Pharm Sci 62:179

Dickey RP, Dorr CH (1969): Oral contraceptives: selection of the proper pill. Obstet Gynecol 33:273

Diczfalusy E (1968): Mode of action of contraceptive drugs. Am J Obstet Gynecol 100:136

Drill VA (1975): Oral contraceptives: relation to mammary cancer, benign breast cancer and cervical cancer. Ann Rev Pharmacol 15:367

Emmens CW (1970): Antifertility agents. Annu Rev Pharmacol 10:237

Harris GW (1969): Ovulation. Am J Obstet Gynecol 105:659

Odell WD, Molitch ME (1974): The pharmacology of the oral contraceptives. Ann Rev Pharmacol 14:413

Simpson WM (1971): Oral contraceptives and untoward effects coincident with their use: a review. South Med J 64:1184

Warren MP (1973): Metabolic effects of contraceptive steroids. Am J Med Sci 265:4

JEREMY H. THOMPSON

49. HISTAMINE AND ANTIHISTAMINES

HISTAMINE

Histamine (Hist = tissue), is a **biogenic amine,** an organic base produced by living cells. Histamine, as its name implies, occurs in many tissues in nearly all forms of life. It occurs naturally in an inactive form, but is released in a free active state in response to injury or to antigen/antibody reactions. Histamine was first detected as a uterine stimulant in extracts of ergot (Ch. 19). The ubiquity of histamine, plus its potency, and, as originally described by Sir Henry Dale (1910–11), the similarity of many of its effects to anaphylactic shock and other allergic phenomena, suggests a fundamental role in biologic function. However, with few exceptions, there is widespread controversy concerning the role it plays in physiologic and pathologic functions.

Even though histamine and its analogs have *limited* therapeutic and diagnostic application, their study is of considerable pharmacologic interest and importance; histamine is intimately involved in a number of pathologic processes and therefore represents at least a potential site of pharmacologic attack; a large group of drugs known as the antihistamines is capable of antagonizing many of the effects of histamine, and certain chemical agents and drugs are capable of liberating histamine into the circulation from tissue storage sites, producing specific symptomatology.

Synthesis Distribution and Storage

Histamine [1-methyl-4-(β-amino-ethyl)-imidazole], is predominently synthesized from histidine by histidine decarboxylase, pyridoxal-5-phosphate being required as cofactor (Fig. 49–1). Rarely histidine may also be decarboxylated to histamine by nonspecific aromatic L-aminoacid decarboxylase (Dopa-decarboxylase). In man, using ^{14}C-L-histidine, it can be shown that about 5 mg of histamine are formed daily. It is unlikely that dietary histamine, or histamine synthesized in the gut lumen by bacteria, contributes significantly to the endogenous tissue histamine pool in spite of the fact that exogenously administered histamine can be taken up by a variety of different cell types. First, intralumenal histamine may be completely inactivated to N-acetyl-histamine by intestinal bacteria, and second, like serotonin, histamine is readily metabolized by enzymes in the gastrointestinal mucosa, liver and lungs, and excreted in the urine.

Histamine occurs in varying amounts in almost all tissues of almost all mammals. In man, the concentration is particularly high in the skin, the gastrointestinal mucosa (except the pyloric gland area of the stomach), the lungs and the bone marrow. In the brain, histamine has a pattern of distribution similar to that of serotonin, namely a high concentration in the hypothalamus, and a low concentration in the white matter and cerebral cortex. Additionally, although brain tissue contains histidine decarboxylase and N-methyl transferase, diamine oxidase (see below) is lacking. The histamine content of any tissue is no indication of the rapidity with which the amine is turning over, and there is only partial correlation between the histamine content, and the "histamine-forming capacity" (histidine decarboxylase activity), of tissues.

Histamine is stored through electrostatic forces in storage granules in several cell types. Mast cells universally contain high concentrations (e.g., rat mast cells contain about 10–15 mg histamine/10^6 cells) where it is bound along with heparin and serotonin. Gastrointestinal histamine occurs in at least three cell types; mast cells, cells of the APUD (amine precursor uptake

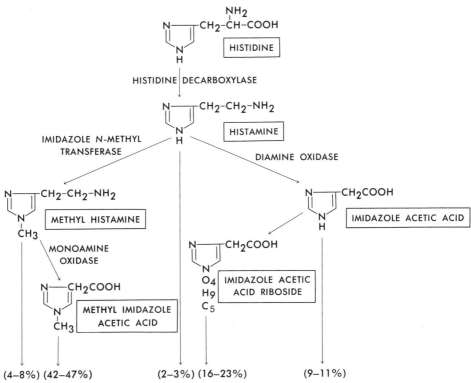

FIG. 49–1. Major routes of formation and metabolic disposition of histamine. The values in parentheses refer to percent recovery of histamine and its metabolites in the urine in 6 hr following intradermal (approximately 1 μg/kg) ^{14}C-histamine in 3 normal human males; percent of total radioactivity collected ranged from 81–84 (Schayer RW, Cooper JAD (1956): Metabolism of C^{14}Histamine. J Appl Physiol 4:481–483).

and decarboxylation) system, and a nonmast cell nonAPUD cell system. Histamine is also present in the polymorphonuclear basophil, in some nerves, nerve endings and synaptic vesicles.

Histamine binding probably occurs at the primary amino group that is protonated at physiologic pH allowing reaction with anionic groups.

Nonmast cell histamine has a more rapid turnover than mast cell histamine, and is probably of greater physiologic importance, since the associated histidine decarboxylase is "inducible," being subject to activation by such stimuli as gastrin, insulin hypoglycemia and nicotine. In animals, different histamine containing cell systems can be separated out by their susceptibility or resistance to depletion by compound 48/80 (a mixture of p-methoxy-N-methylphenyl ethylamines).

Metabolism

Histamine metabolism is indicated in Figure 49–1. Chlorpromazine (Ch. 25) depresses imidazole N-methyl transferase activity thereby augmenting tissue levels of histamine. With the exception of N-methylhistamine and N-dimethylhistamine which are potent gastric secretagogues, the various metabolites of hista-

mine possess little or no pharmacologic activity, and are excreted in the urine. The histaminase activity of plasma rises sharply during pregnancy but the reason for this is not clear.

PHARMACOLOGIC ACTIONS

The principal actions of histamine are exerted on the cardiovascular system, smooth muscles, exocrine glands and nerve endings. With a few exceptions, the **degree,** and even the **direction** of some of these actions differ markedly between species. The actions in man are discussed below.

Cardiovascular System

The most important effect of histamine in most species, including man, is hypotension. This is attributed primarily to dilatation of the small terminal arterioles (due to a direct effect on the smooth muscle), with subsequent passive post-capilliary venular dilatation, and to constriction in the larger veins. All of the small vessels in the body are involved, but the response following IV injection in man is most obvious over the face and upper trunk ("blushing area").

Histamine induced dilatation of the cerebral

vessels in man produces a severe, throbbing headache, due to stretching of dural pain sensors (Ch. 35).

Histamine has no significant direct effect on the heart, although reflex tachycardia and an increased cardiac output may occur as a response to the generalized vasodilatation. The systemic hypotension produced by histamine recovers rapidly as compensatory reflexes are activated, and the amine is destroyed. If given in large doses, histamine causes a profound progressive fall in blood pressure and histamine "shock," due to an exaggerated effect of the amine on the minute blood vessels causing increased pooling of blood, and tissue edema.

Histamine increases the permeability of the capilliary and the postcapilliary beds by causing "contraction" of endothelial cells and increasing the size of their gap junctions. This permits transudation of plasma proteins, with development of tissue edema.

When histamine is injected into the skin (or when the skin is scratched liberating endogenous histamine), the **triple response** of Sir Thomas Lewis is seen. This comprises: a **circumscribed erythematous zone** extending for several millimeters around the injection or scratch site due to terminal arteriolar dilatation. It develops within seconds, and after about a minute or so it becomes bluish, due to relative deoxygenation; a wider, **irregular area of erythema,** or "flare," developing over several minutes due to local arteriolar dilatation mediated by axon reflexes; and **localized edema** at the same site as the initial erythema due to increased permeability of the postcapilliary bed.

Smooth Muscle

Histamine is a powerful, direct stimulant of a variety of smooth muscles in laboratory animals, particularly uterine and bronchial smooth muscle. Bronchoconstriction is most obvious in guinea pigs in that it usually produces death. In normal man, histamine has little effect on extravascular smooth muscles, but in asthmatics it may precipitate an acute attack. Stimulation of the pregnant human uterus by histamine is insignificant.

Exocrine Glands

Although histamine has some stimulant effect on lachyrimal, salivary, bronchial and pancreatic exocrine gland function, its most important secretory effect is exerted on the parietal cells of the oxyntic gland area of the stomach. Doses of histamine less than those required to cause a sustained fall in arterial blood pressure, produce a copious secretion of gastric juice rich in both acid and pepsin. Following vagotomy in man the maximal secretory response to histamine may fall by about two-thirds. This permissive role of the parasympathetic nervous system may account in part for the partial antagonism of antimuscarinic agents for the secretory effects of histamine. Histamine antagonists (with three exceptions, burimamide, metiamide and cimetidine) do not antagonize the stimulant effect of histamine on gastric secretion (see below). Evidence suggests that histamine may be the "final common path" in stimulation of the parietal cells.

Nerve Endings

Histamine acts on various nerves. The "flare" of Lewis' triple response (see above) is ascribed to excitation by histamine of cutaneous sensory nerves eliciting an axon reflex, and afferent discharges evoked by the autacoid have been recorded in cutaneous nerves. When histamine is introduced into the superficial layers of the skin it induces pruritis. If the autacoid is administered more deeply it tends to evoke pain, often accompanied by pruritis. The pain and pruritis associated with various stings and venoms may, in part, be due to endogenous histamine release.

Various smooth muscles and exocrine glands are stimulated by histamine both directly, and indirectly by way of their motor nerves. Adrenal medullary chromaffin cells, for example, are stimulated by histamine directly, and indirectly through the splanchnic nerves, to secrete epinephrine and norepinephrine. In normal subjects catechol secretion in response to histamine is insignificant, but in patients with a phaeochromocytoma, sufficient amines may be released to raise the blood pressure (see below).

Mode of Action

Histamine receptors are distinct from those receptors stimulated by serotonin, acetylcholine and the catechols. It is well accepted that sympathomimetic amines can act on two separate adrenergic receptors (Chs. 14, 18), but although two histamine receptors, namely H_1- **and** H_2-receptors** have also been delineated in animal work, little is really known about their occurrence or specificity. Classification of adrenergic receptors was facilitated by the availability of appropriate, specific antagonists (Ch. 18) but with several exceptions, this has not been true of the histamine saga.

H_1-receptors are those involved in histamine stimulation of smooth muscle contraction in the gut, and bronchi, and which are blocked by classic antihistamines such as pyrilamine or triprolidine (see below). H_2-receptors are those involved in other actions of histamine such as stimulation of gastric acid secretion in animals and man, increase in the contraction frequency of cardiac muscle, e.g., in guinea pigs, increase in the mast and basophil cell stores of cyclic AMP and histamine in animals and man, and inhibition of contraction in the rat uterus. Actions of histamine on H_2-receptors are not blocked by classic antihistamines such as pyrilamine or triprolidine, but can be successfully reduced by burimamide, metiamide and cimetidine, recently introduced histamine antagonists.

Endogenous Histamine: Role in Physiologic and Pathologic Processes

The role of histamine in gastric secretion has been considered above under pharmacologic actions.

Anaphylactic Shock

The similarity between anaphylactic shock and the pharmacologic effects of histamine, led Dale and Laidlaw in 1910 to suggest that histamine may serve as a mediator of anaphylactic shock. It is now well established that histamine is released during antigen/antibody reactions, and that the intensity of many hypersensitivity phenomena may be considerably reduced by histamine antagonists. However, other autacoids are also liberated to varying degrees, in particular, bradykinin and other vasoactive kinins, prostaglandins, 5-hydroxytryptamine (serotonin), and an unsaturated fatty acid known as "slow reacting substance of anaphylaxis" (SRS-A). Their relative importance is in dispute. The limited effectiveness of antihistamines in some cases of "allergy" may be due, at least in part, to the mediation of other autacoids. For example, SRS-A may be important in human asthma.

As a result of antigen reacting with mast cell membrane-bound antibody, histamine containing storage granules undergo exocytosis. Histamine is then liberated from its weak ionic binding in exchange for extracellular cations, particularly calcium.

Other Physiologic and Pathologic Processes

It has been suggested that histamine plays a role in the **inflammatory reaction,** in the regulation of the **microcirculation,** in **tissue repair** and **growth,** and as a **neuroeffector transmitter** at certain synapses.

In patients with **hepatic cirrhosis** absorbed histidine and histamine bypass the liver, and may produce hypersecretion of gastric acid leading to peptic ulcer disease. Some patients with **gastric carcinoid tumors** (Ch. 50) secrete excessive quantities of histamine, and in **urticaria pigmentosa** and **systemic mastocytosis,** release of mast cell histamine may produce specific symptomatology. Patients with **chronic myelogenous leukemia** have high blood histamine levels, but surprisingly few symptoms, since the histamine is tightly bound in the basophils.

Histamine Release by Drugs and Physical Agents

Endogenous histamine may be released by a variety of physical agents and chemical substances (Table 49–1), and in sufficient magnitude to produce specific symptomatology ranging from pruritis or mild arterial hypotension, to a full-scale anaphylactic reaction. Rapid IV administration favors histamine release. The principal, and perhaps the only source of histamine liberated by these chemicals and physical agents are the mast cells, from which heparin, SRS-A, and vasoactive kinins, etc. are also released in varying amounts. Animal experiments have shown that drugs particularly likely to initiate histamine release possess two or more basic groups separated by, and carried on, an aliphatic, or aromatic moiety. Release with such agents may simply depend upon displacement of histamine, itself a base, from appropriate storage sites.

USES

Histamine, or one of its analogs, usually betazole (see below), are sometimes used as a test for gastric acid secretion. In the "augmented" (maximal histamine) test, 0.04 mg histamine/kg is given subcutaneously 30 min after 100 mg IM of the potent antihistamine pyrilamine that mini-

TABLE 49–1. Chemical and Physical Agents Releasing Histamine

Chemical agents	Physical agents
Antihistamines	Mechanical trauma
Chymotrypsin	Radiant energy
Compound 48/80	Thermal energy
Detergents	
Dextran	
Morphine	
Polymyxin B	
Polyvinylpyrrolidine	
Propamidine	
Reserpine	
Surface active agents	
Stilbamidine	
Toxins	
Tubocararine	
Venoms	

mizes the systemic but not the gastric secretory effects of histamine. This test gives a measure of the total number of functional parietal cells (parietal cell "mass") present, and is useful in identifying patients with true achlorhydria, defined as the failure to lower the gastric pH below 6 in response to maximal histamine stimulation. True achlorhydria is the hallmark of pernicious anemia.

Histamine (3 μg/kg, IV), **tyramine** (1.0 mg, IV) **glucagon** 0.5–1.0 mg, IV and **phentolamine** (Ch. 19) can be used as provocative tests for **phaeochromocytoma,** but false positive and negative responses occur in about 30% of patients. These tests should be done only when the laboratory data are equivocal and where the blood pressure is normal or only slightly elevated. Following the normal drop in blood pressure, a secondary rise greater than that resulting from a control cold pressor test, is a positive response. Since fatalities due to hypertensive crises and cerebrovascular accidents have been reported using these tests, they should be performed only in patients with an IV running and an α-adrenergic blocking agent (Ch. 19) available.

The use of histamine to treat peripheral artery disease, Ménières' syndrome and allergic diseases is obsolete.

PREPARATIONS

Histamine phosphate, *U.S.P.* is available as a solution for injection in concentrations of 100 μg, 200 μg and 1000 μg/ml. Doses of histamine are classically expressed in terms of the base, 2.75 mg of the phosphate salt are equivalent to 1 mg of histamine base.

BETAZOLE AND BETAHISTINE

Betazole, an isomer of histamine, possesses potent gastric secretagogue activity, but little or no

$$\text{CH}_2\text{-CH}_2\text{-NH}_2$$

BETAZOLE

systemic activity. Thus it is a convenient alternative to histamine in gastric secretory function tests since premedication with a systemic antihistamine is not required. Betazole hydrochloride *U.S.P.* (Histalog) is given in a dose of 0.5 mg/kg SC. Like histamine, betazole is being replaced by gastrin and congeners. **Betahistine hydrochloride** *N.F.* may possess some value in treating patients with Ménières' disease.

ANTIHISTAMINES

The pharmacologic actions of histamine can be countered in four ways. 1) By preventing or reducing histamine release, e.g., glucocorticoid-type agents can suppress the effects on the tissues of antigen/antibody reactions (Ch. 46), and cromolyn sodium (see below) stabilizes mast cell membranes. 2) By receptor antagonism, e.g., the antihistamines. 3) By increasing the rate of histamine catabolism using histaminase; this approach has not been valuable. 4) By using physiologic antagonists, drugs with opposite effects to those produced by histamine, e.g., epinephrine (see below and Ch. 18).

Antihistamine drugs can be divided into two groups depending upon whether they antagonise the effect of histamine on H_1- or H_2-receptors. Since only a few H_2-receptor antagonists are known, namely burimamide, metiamide and cimetidine the unified description that follows covers primarily the large group of classic antihistamines, those blocking the H_1-receptor. Properties of burimamide, metiamide and cimetidine will be indicated where known.

Subsequent to the synthesis of the first compound with significant antihistaminic activity by Bovet and Straub in 1937, dozens of powerful histamine antagonists have been made available for clinical use. These agents differ from each other primarily in **antihistamine potency, duration of action, adverse effects, cost** and in the possession of certain additional pharmacologic coincidentally associated properties such as **sedation.**

Structure Activity Relationships

Most of the important antihistamines contain a substituted ethylamine $-\text{CH}-\text{CH}-\text{N}=$ which is also present in histamine. However, this sequence is present in many compounds which possess no histamine antagonism. This moiety may present as a straight chain (e.g., diphenhydramine) or as part of a ring structure (e.g., chlorcyclizine); structural formulae of some representative antihistamines are shown in Figure 49–2.

Histamine Antagonism

Both H_1- and H_2-receptor antihistamines do not influence the formation or release* of histamine,

---

* When given rapidly by the IV route, some antihistamines may liberate histamine from storage sites (Table 49–1).

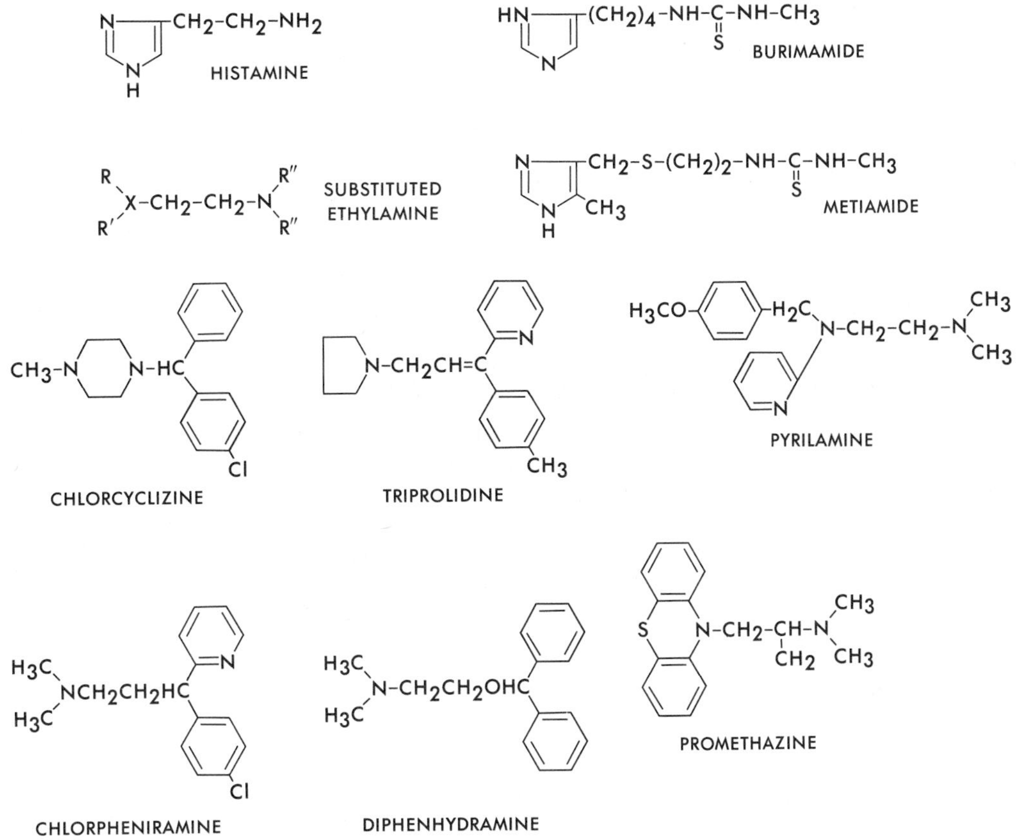

FIG. 49-2. Histamine and some representative histamine antagonists.

but selectively and competitively antagonize its actions presumably at specific receptor sites, without initiating a response. There is considerable variation in their efficacy for the different pharmacologic actions of histamine.

The effectiveness of antihistamines in blocking the actions of administered histamine is greater than in combating the various manifestations of anaphylaxis and allergy. This may be due to the concomitant liberation of other autacoids such as SRS-A, against which antihistamines are ineffective; the appropriate histamine receptor may be inaccessible to the antihistamine in sufficient concentration; and antigen/antibody reactions may under certain circumstances directly evoke a response without intervention of a humoral mediator.

ANTIHISTAMINES AND EXOGENOUSLY ADMINISTERED HISTAMINE. Antihistamines effectively block all the pharmacologic actions (see above) of exogenously administered histamine in animals and man. (However, effects mediated through H_2-receptors are only antagonized by burimamide and its analogs.) A dramatic example occurs in guinea pigs, where death by asphyxia following severe bronchospasm occurs with quite small doses of histamine (see above), yet, a hundred lethal doses of histamine may be given with impunity, if the animal is protected by an antihistamine.

ANTIHISTAMINES AND ENDOGENOUSLY RELEASED HISTAMINE. Antihistamines are only variably effective against the symptomatology of anaphylaxis and allergy, or following histamine release by histamine-releasing chemicals. Generally speaking, urticaria and pruritis are well antagonized by the antihistamines, but bronchoconstriction and hypotension are less well controlled. The effects on gastric hypersecretion are unaffected by H_1-antagonists.

Miscellaneous Actions

Some antihistamines possess a number of other pharmacologic properties that are probably dependent upon parasympatholytic activity rather than histamine antagonism and the magnitude of their occurrence varies widely with different agents. From the standpoint of their clinical use as antihistamines, these miscellaneous pharmacologic actions represent "adverse effects," but they are frequently exploited clinically, and form the basis of specific treatments.

CENTRAL NERVOUS SYSTEM. Some antihistamines produce drowsiness so consistently that they are used as sedatives, and occasionally in the treatment of petit mal. Rarely restlessness, nervousness and insomnia may occur, and in some patients with focal lesions of the cerebral cortex, antihistamines may initiate EEG activation and epileptiform seizures.

Some weak antihistamines possess the unique ability of suppressing motion sickness and the nausea and vomiting resulting from labyrinthine disturbance, without producing sedation. Other antihistamines lessen rigidity, and improve spontaneous movement and speech in Parkinson's disease and related drug induced extrapyramidal disorders.

PERIPHERAL NERVOUS SYSTEM. Most of the antihistamines possess local anesthetic actions, a property that may contribute to the relief of pruritis after topical application. Some antihistamines, when given IV in sufficiently high dosage may produce quinidine-like effects on myocardial conduction, a response consistent with their local anesthetic properties.

Absorption, Metabolism, Excretion

The antihistamines are readily absorbed following oral or parenteral administration. Pharmacologic effects are usually manifest within about 30 min, but the duration of action varies with different agents (Table 49–2). Little information is available on the metabolic fate or excretion of the different antihistamine preparations.

Adverse Effects

In therapeutic doses all antihistamines to varying degree elicit adverse effects that are rarely serious, but may in susceptable individuals necessitate discontinuence of therapy. Importantly,

TABLE 49–2. Major Groups of Official Antihistamine Preparations

Group and non proprietary name	Formulary	Trade name	Single adult dose (mg)	Duration of action (hr)	Comment
Alkylamines					
Chlorpheniramine maleate	U.S.P.	Chlor-Trimeton maleate, Histaspar Teldrin	4	4–6	Slightly sedative, but may cause excitement
Triprolidine		Actidil	2–5	8–12	Weak sedative, prolonged action
Ethanolamines					
Dimenhydrinate	U.S.P.	Dramamine	50	4–6	Similar actions to diphenyhydramine since it is the 8-chlorotheophyllinate salt of that compound
Diphenylhydramine hydrochloride	U.S.P.	Benadryl hydrochloride	50	4–6	Marked sedative, parasympatholytic, local anesthetic, useful in parkinsonism, and drug-induced extrapyramidal disorders. IV injection must be given very slowly
Ethylenediamines					
Pyrilamine maleate	N.F.	Neo-Antergan maleate, Para-minyl maleate, Pyramal maleate, Stamine, etc.	25–50	4–6	One of the most specific histamine antagonists known. Possesses no significant atropinic activity
Tripelennamine hydrochloride	U.S.P.	Pyribenzamine hydrochloride	50	4–6	Moderately sedative, local anesthetic, sometimes causes excitement and gastric irritation
Phenothiazines					
Promethazine hydrochloride	U.S.P.	Phenergan hydrochloride	25–50	4–6	Marked sedative, some atropinic action, effective against motion sickness. Prototype phenothiazine which led to development of tranquilizers (Ch. 25)
Piperazines					
Chlorcyclizine hydrochloride	N.F.	Di-Paralene hydrochloride	50	8–12	Slightly sedative, little atropinic activity
Cyclizine hydrochloride	U.S.P.	Marezine hydrochloride	50–100	6–8	Little sedative or atropinic activity, used primarily for motion sickness
Meclizine hydrochloride	U.S.P.	Bonine hydrochloride	25–50	8–16	Used mainly for motion sickness. Prolonged action

there is marked patient variation in predisposition to adverse effects.

Depression of the CNS with sedation, dizziness, tinnitus, incoordination, diplopia, amblopia and fatigue may develop. Very rarely central excitement may occur with development of euphoria, insomnia, nervousness and tremor. Sedation is by far the most common adverse effect, and some agents such as diphenhydramine produce drowsiness so frequently that they are used as sedatives. Sedation during antihistamine therapy may be a desirable phenomenon in overanxious patients, or those about to retire for the night, but occurring during the day it may interfere sufficiently with normal activities so that accidents occur (Ch. 7).

Some antihistamines possess antimuscarinic properties producing xerostomia, dysuria, blurring of vision, impotence and gastrointestinal symptoms. Anorexia, nausea and vomiting and alteration in bowel habit are not unusual, and can usually be controlled by administering the drug with meals. Depression of the bone marrow with development of leukopenia or agranulocytosis is rare. Since some antihistamines are teratogenic in animals, the use of these agents is contraindicated during pregnancy. The topical administration of antihistamines may result in hypersensitivity.

Because of the ease with which antihistamines are available, accidental acute poisoning is not uncommon, particularly in children. In general, 2-3 dozen capsules or tablets of most commercially available antihistamines constitutes a near-lethal or fatal dose in children. Whereas central depression with sedation usually accompanies therapeutic doses of antihistamines, toxic doses tend to produce stimulation with hallucinations, excitement, involuntary movements, convulsions, fixed dilated pupils and fever. Terminally, deepening cardiorespiratory collapse develops. Treatment is symptomatic and supportive. Mechanical support of ventilation and a short acting barbiturate to control convulsions are important adjuncts in therapy.

A few side effects (importantly, renal damage and leukopenia) have been reported with burimamide and metiamide, and possibly with cimetidine.

Preparations and Dosage

There are numerous antihistamines available, either singly, or in combination with other antihistamines, analgesics, decongestants or antibiotics, and "new" antihistamines are constantly being introduced into clinical practice often to the tune of exaggerated therapeutic claims.

The antihistamines fall into five chemical groups (Table 49–2); thus, it is not surprising that they vary in potency, duration of action and relative incidence of adverse effects. Variability in cost is usually not a problem, since chronic therapy is rarely undertaken with these agents.

Burimamide and its derivatives are thiourea analogs of histamine. Metiamide and cimetidine, the newer agents are about 5–10 times more potent than burimamide. These drugs are available in the United Kingdom and the United States for limited clinical study.

Uses

The antihistamines have achieved widespread popularity in the symptomatic treatment of many hypersensitivity states, and in the treatment of parkinsonism, insomnia and motion sickness.

HYPERSENSITIVITY STATES

The antihistamines are principally used in the symptomatic treatment of acute and chronic urticaria and pruritis where they serve as adjuncts to removal of the allergen(s), specific desensitization or suppression of the antigen/antibody reaction with glucocorticoids. Antihistamines may be given either systemically or topically. Topical administration may have the additional advantage of producing some relief from pruritis by a local anesthetic action, but *topical administration is often followed by hypersensitivity to the antihistamine.*

Specifically, antihistamines are of value in hay fever, vasomotor rhinitis, acute and chronic urticaria and in conditions where pruritis and/or urticaria are prominent; e.g., atopic and contact dermatitis, allergic drug reactions, insect bites and plant stings such as poison ivy or poison oak. In serum sickness, antihistamines reduce the pruritis and urticaria, but have no effect on the fever or arthalgia.

The antihistamines play a secondary role in therapy of anaphylactic shock, angioneurotic edema and bronchial asthma. Of prime importance in these conditions is the use of physiologic antagonists to histamine, namely **epinephrine,** in the treatment of **anaphylactic shock and angioneurotic edema,** and **epinephrine, theophyline** and **isoproterenol** in the treatment of **bronchial asthma.** Physiologic antagonists are desirable over antihistamines since these agents are more rapidly active than antihistamines and moreover produce an opposing effect rather than agonist blockade, and since autacoids other than histamine may be contributing to symptoms. Epinephrine, e.g., produces vasoconstriction in the presence of histamine, but in a similar situation antihistamines just antagonize the vasodilatation produced by histamine, but do not in themselves produce vasoconstriction.

MOTION SICKNESS, NAUSEA AND VOMITING

Piperazine class antihistamines and promethazine and diphenhydramine, are particularly useful in the symptomatic treatment of motion sickness, or the nausea and vomiting occurring postoperatively or following radiation exposure. Antihistamines have been used to treat nausea and vomiting of pregnancy, but it is preferable to avoid all unnecessary drugs under these circumstances.

Some antihistamines have been used in the treatment of parkinsonism and drug-induced extrapyramidal reactions, and may be of particular value by the IV route in treating an incapacitating disorder.

In spite of extravagant advertising claims, there is no evidence that antihistamines influence the course of the common cold, although some symptomatic benefit may be obtained, particularly if there is a superimposed allergic component.

Metiamide and cimetidine may become useful agents in the treatment of peptic ulcer disease and gastric acid hypersecretory states.

CROMOLYN SODIUM

Cromolyn sodium has been available in Europe and Canada since 1968, but has only recently been approved by the FDA as an adjunct for the management of patients with severe perennial bronchial asthma. It is available as a dry powder for inhalation by means of an oral inhaler.

Chemistry

Cromolyn sodium is a highly water soluble synthetic analog of khellin, the active spasmolytic ingredient extracted from the seeds of *Ammi visnaga,* a herb long used in eastern Mediterranean areas to prepare a tea found effective in treating colic in children. Chemically, cromolyn sodium is the disodium salt of 1, 3-bis (2-carboxychromon-5-yloxy)-2-hydroxypropane.

CROMOLYN   SODIUM

Mode of Action

Cromolyn sodium appears to "stabilize" the membrane of sensitized animal mast cells, preventing the release of histamine, serotonin, bradykinin, SRS-A, acetylcholine and other substances that mediate hypersensitivity reactions. It is ineffective once these substances have been released. Cromolyn sodium is not a smooth muscle relaxant, and it possesses no antiinflammatory activity.

Absorption, Metabolism, and Excretion

Since cromolyn sodium is poorly absorbed following oral administration, it should be inhaled by means of a special device known as the spinhaler. About 10% of the total dose administered is absorbed and rapidly excreted unchanged in the bile and urine, with a half-life of about 80 min. That portion of the inhaled dose which is not absorbed is either exhaled or cleared eventually through the gastrointestinal tract.

Adverse Effects

Adverse effects are not common. Maculopapular and urticarial skin rashes may be seen, but these usually clear on cessation of therapy. Occasionally patients may experience cough and or bronchospasm following inhalation of cromolyn sodium, and rarely an eosinophilic pneumonia has been reported.

In toxicity studies in macaque monkeys, cromolyn sodium was shown to be possibly associated with the development of proliferative arterial lesions in the kidneys and other organs. The relevance of these findings to man is as yet unknown, but it may assume importance in patients treated chronically with this agent. The safety of cromolyn sodium in pregnancy has not been determined.

Preparations and Dosage

Cromolyn sodium (Aarane, Intal) is available in capsules containing 20 mg of the drug in micronized form, together with 20 mg lactose powder to improve the flow properties of the material. The usual dose for adults and children 5 years or older, is one capsule inhaled 4 times daily for at least 2–4 weeks; some patients may require a longer period of exposure.

Cromolyn sodium appears to be most useful in the control or prevention of exercise-induced, and "extrinsic" asthma compared to "intrinsic" asthma. In "extrinsic" asthma patients have positive skin tests to at least one inhaled allergen, and develop symptoms of asthma when exposed to that allergen. In "intrinsic" asthma patients have negative skin tests, and symptoms are often associated with respiratory tract infections. Cromolyn sodium is not effective in the treatment of an acute attack of asthma or in the treatment of status asthmaticus. Children respond better to cromolyn sodium than do adults, and patients treated prophylactically may need lesser amounts of bronchodilators and steroid drugs.

Cromolyn sodium is worth trying in patients who cannot be managed without glucocorticosteroids.

FURTHER READING

Agents and Actions (1973): October, Vol 3, No 3

Eichler O, Farah A (ed) (1966): Histamine and Antihistamines, Handbook of Experimental Pharmacology. New York, Springer-Verlag Vol XVIII, Part 1

Wood CJ, Simkins MA (ed) (1973): International Symposium on Histamine H_2-receptor Antagonist. London, Deltakos (UK) Ltd

JEREMY H. THOMPSON

50. SEROTONIN AND SEROTONIN ANTAGONISTS

SEROTONIN

The discovery of serotonin as a naturally occurring amine resulted from independent investigations on two substances: *enteramine,* present in the enterochromaffin (argentaffin) cells of the gastrointestinal tract, and *vasotonin,* a vasoconstrictor present in serum. Both of these substances have been shown to be *serotonin* (5-hydroxytryptamine), which was first synthesized in 1951. Like histamine, serotonin is ubiquitous in nature, being found in almost all vertebrates and invertebrates and in many fruits (avocados, bananas, eggplant, passion fruit, pineapples, plantain, plums, tomatoes), nuts (walnuts), stings (cowhage, the source of "itching powder," nettle) and venoms (bee, scorpion and wasp).

The wide distribution of serotonin and its potent pharmacologic actions have prompted generous speculation on the functions of the amine in health and disease. However, in spite of an enormous quantity of research, the precise role of serotonin in the mammalian organism is far from clear.

CHEMISTRY AND BIOCHEMISTRY

Serotonin (Fig. 50–1) is 3(β-aminoethyl)-5-hydroxyindole and is usually prepared as the creatinine sulfate salt.

Synthesis, Distribution and Storage

The major pathway of serotonin synthesis is from dietary tryptophan (Fig. 50–1). Tryptophan is first hydroxylated to 5-hydroxytryptophan and then decarboxylated to serotonin. Local synthesis accounts for the serotonin content of mammalian tissues with the exception of the platelets that are devoid of 5-hydroxytryptophan decarboxylase. During passage through the splanchnic

area, platelets avidly take up the amine released from enterochromaffin cells and store it in an inactive form. Greater that 99% of the serotonin released from the gastrointestinal tract and not taken up by platelets is inactivated by uptake or catabolic processes in the hepatic and pulmonary vascular beds, thus "protecting" the systemic circulation. Many central neurons which normally synthesize and store serotonin also have the capacity to take up preformed serotonin from the cerebrospinal fluid; little serotonin passes the blood-brain barrier.

Approximately 1–2% of dietary tryptophan is converted into serotonin in normal subjects, but greater than 60% may be converted in patients with the carcinoid syndrome (see below).

The distribution and content of serotonin within the body vary widely in different species. The amount in man is about 10 mg, of which approximately 90% is present in the gastrointestinal tract. Of the remainder, the majority is present in platelets, lungs, bone marrow and brain, although most tissues can be shown to contain some serotonin. It should be stressed that quantitative data on the serotonin concentration within any given tissue is only of limited value, since the single measurement gives no indication of the rapidity of turnover, i.e., the degree of amine synthesis and storage, or of release and metabolism. For example, the gastrointestinal tract contains about 90% of the total body serotonin, whereas the brain contains about 3%; yet, the turnover times for gastrointestinal serotonin and brain serotonin are about 12–16 hr and 1 hr, respectively. In platelets, serotonin is strongly bound but liberated on platelet destruction.

Gastrointestinal serotonin is present in the enterochromaffin (argentaffin) cells, cells of the

APUD (Amine Precursor Uptake and Decarboxylation) series and in the myenteric plexus. Mast cells of many species, particularly rodents, contain serotonin, but the amine has only been identified in human mast cells from patients with the carcinoid syndrome. In studies on animals (particularly rodents), serotonin containing neurones have been found in the raphe nucleus of the lower brain stem, from which tracts innervate many diverse areas of the CNS.

The mechanisms of serotonin uptake and storage have been mainly studied using platelets. Serotonin is taken up by an active process into the cytoplasm, and from there it is incorporated by an energy dependent process into storage granules. Within the storage granules, serotonin is complexed with ATP and possibly other substances. Reserpine has similar actions on the storage of catecholamines and serotonin (Ch. 20). Reserpine blocks the energy dependent uptake of serotonin and promotes its release. Storage of serotonin in enterochromaffin granules and neuronal vesicles probably involves a similar energy-dependent storage process.

Metabolism

The metabolism of serotonin is subject to wide species variation, but in man two metabolites predominate (Fig. 50–1). In these two pathways, serotonin is initially oxidatively deaminated by nonspecific monoamine oxidase to 5-hydroxyindoleacetaldehyde, which is then further oxidized to predominately 5-hydroxyindoleacetic acid (5-HIAA), or reduced to the corresponding alcohol, 5-hydroxytryptophol (5-HTOL). Both 5-HIAA and 5-HTOL, mainly as glucuronides or sulfates, are excreted in the urine. About 5–10 mg 5-HIAA are excreted daily, but higher values are found in some patients with the carcinoid syndrome or in those eating serotonin containing foods. Ethyl alcohol ingestion greatly increases 5-HTOL excretion at the expense of 5-HIAA. Several other minor pathways of serotonin metabolism have been described, particularly oxygenation, conjugation, O-methylation, N-methylation and N-acetylation. These may assume importance when monoamine oxidase inhibitors are used.

PHARMACOLOGIC ACTIONS

Serotonin has numerous pharmacologic effects on various types of smooth muscle, nerves and exocrine glands in animals and man. Since serotonin causes direct, as well as indirect, and reflex effects, and since tachyphylaxis is common, the ultimate pharmacologic responses are invariably complex. Effects of serotonin show not only wide

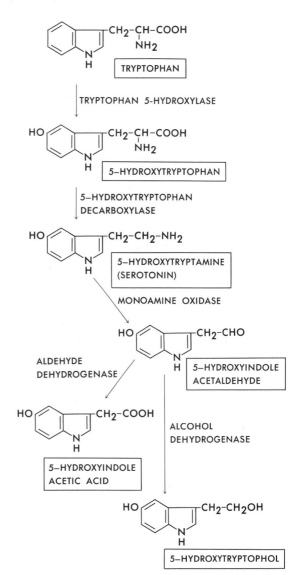

FIG. 50–1. Major pathways of serotonin synthesis and degradation in man.

species variation but also wide variation within a given species, and even variation between consecutive experiments in the same animal. The following description in general applies to man. Responses characteristic of a given animal species will be identified.

Cardiovascular System

Constriction or dilation of the arterial tree may be produced, depending upon the dose of serotonin administered and the vascular bed under study. Direct vasoconstriction is the classical response to 5-hydroxytryptamine and is the effect responsible for its names *vasotonin* and *serotonin*. Vasodilation occurs in skeletal muscles and cutaneous vessels, and in the latter bed it is responsible for the "flush" of the carcinoid syndrome. The flush, initially red, become bluish owing to stagnation (probably as a result of distal venoconstriction) and subsequent deoxygenation.

In rodents, serotonin is more potent than histamine in producing increased capillary permeability and edema, but these effects are not prominent in man. Serotonin causes positive inotropic and chronotropic responses on the myocardium, but these may be overshadowed by actions of the amine on afferent nerve endings initiating reflex cardiorespiratory changes (Bezold-like reflex). Most veins are strongly constricted by serotonin.

Extravascular Smooth Muscle

Low doses of serotonin (insufficient to alter arterial blood pressure) produce small intestinal motility and colonic relaxation. Responses in animals are exceedingly complex due to the variety of elements, both neuronal and muscular, responding to the amine. Serotonin produces bronchoconstriction in patients with bronchial asthma, but rarely in normal subjects. The human pregnant uterus is relatively insensitive to serotonin.

Exocrine Glands

Serotonin is generally inhibitory towards most exocrine glands. The amine depresses gastric acid and pepsin secretion, but it increases the output of mucosubstances by the gastric mucosa.

Miscellaneous Actions

Serotonin is capable of stimulating a variety of nerve endings, and many of its actions on the cardiovascular, respiratory and gastrointestinal systems are mediated by local nerve reflexes. The injection of serotonin into human skin is associated with pain and pruritis.

Serotonin increases the ventilatory minute volume, probably due to stimulation of aortic and carotid chemoreceptors. In animals, a variety of other actions can be demonstrated, particularly those associated with stimulation of various autonomic ganglia. In man, insulin hypoglycemia is followed by a rise in the serotonin levels of the hypothalamus and by growth hormone secretion. Cyproheptadine and methysergide (see below) prevent insulin hypoglycemia induced growth hormone secretion.

MODE OF ACTION

There is some evidence from animal experiments that there are two types of serotonin receptors, M-receptors (blocked by morphine, Ch. 29) in nerve elements and D-receptors (blocked by phenoxybenazmine, Ch. 20) in smooth muscle; however, the complexity of the pharmacologic responses to serotonin and the unavailability of potent and specific serotonin antagonists have made receptor characterization difficult. Serotonin receptors probably reside in the cell membrane.

ENDOGENOUS SEROTONIN: ROLE IN PHYSIOLOGY AND PATHOLOGY

The wide distribution of serotonin, its potent pharmacologic actions and its rapid turnover, particularly in the CNS, have generated numerous hypotheses concerning the possible role(s) of this autacoid in physiology and pathologic states. A few of the more probable hypotheses will be briefly mentioned.

Central Nervous System

Much evidence has been accumulated in recent years using animal experiments to suggest that serotonin is involved as a neurotransmitter at various synapses, but what role it serves is far from clear. Participation of serotonin in thought, perception and mood has been suggested, since many hallucinogens (Fig. 50–2) are chemically similar to serotonin, and drugs such as morphine, reserpine, phenothiazines, imipramine and monoamine oxidase inhibitors, interfere with serotonin (and catecholamine) metabolism and may induce psychoses. Alterations in serotonin metabolism have been identified in patients with schizophrenia and endogenous depression, but at present it is impossible to separate "cause from effect." Serotonin may be involved in sleep and thermoregulatory mechanisms, and low levels of the amine have been reported in patients with phenylketonuria, In rats, a brisk circadian rhythm in pineal gland serotonin is present, where the amine is precursor for melatonin (5-methoxy, N-acetyltryptamine).

Peripheral Nervous System

Again, based upon experiments in animals, there is evidence for the presence of "serotonin" transmission in the peripheral nervous system. Serotonin appears to be involved as a neurotransmitter in various cardiovascular and gastrointestinal reflexes.

Gastrointestinal Tract

In spite of the fact that about 90% of the total body serotonin is present in the gastrointestinal tract, its role in that tissue is not understood.

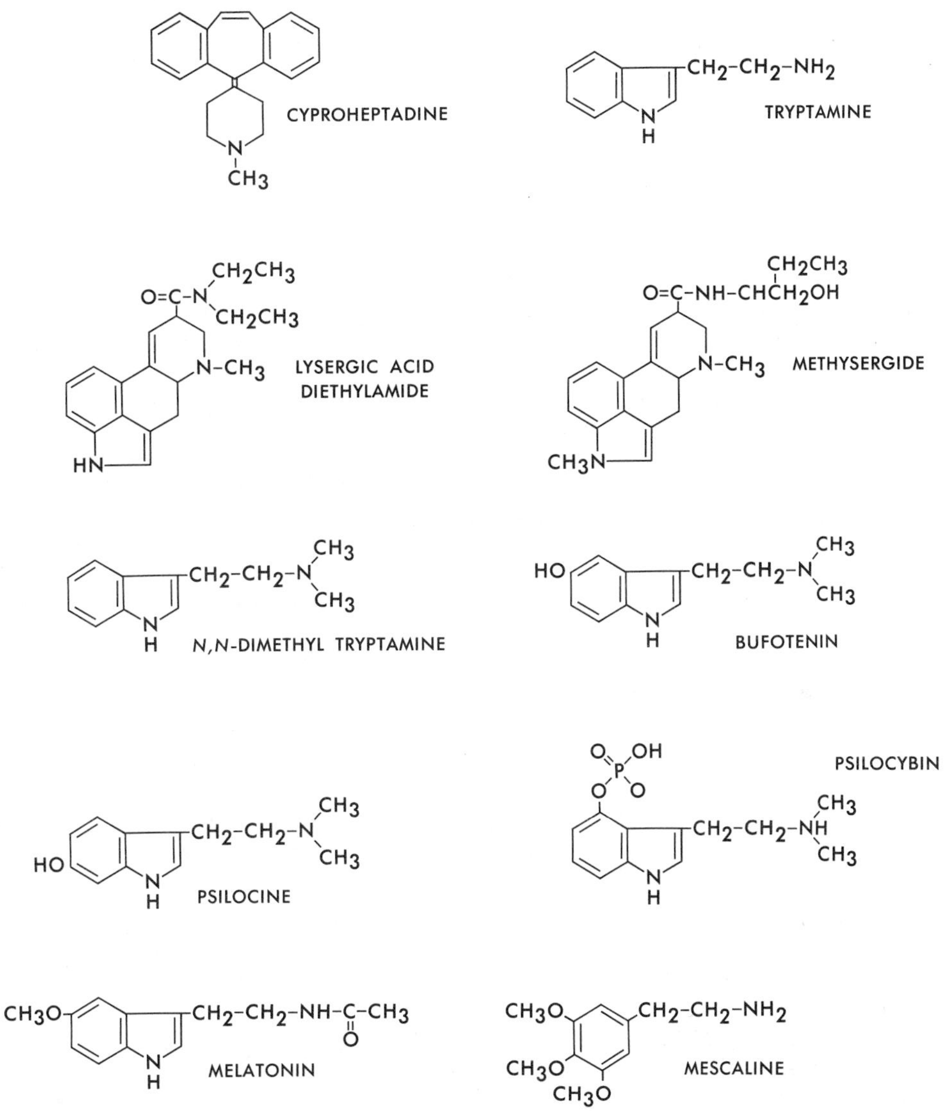

FIG. 50-2. Some potent serotonin antagonists and serotonin-like drugs.

Bowel serotonin may be involved in peristalsis, control of gastric secretion, intestinal absorption, epithelial cell renewal or release of polypeptide hormones. There is little doubt that platelet serotonin stores derive from the gut, but the role of platelet serotonin is also unknown; it may be involved in hemostasis and/or blood coagulation.

THE DUMPING SYNDROME. The dumping syndrome occurs in 5–10% of patients following operations that alter the normal gastroduodenal emptying mechanisms. Typically, there is a variable combination of intestinal (epigastric discomfort, fullness, cramps, hyperperistalsis, diarrhea) and vasomotor (weakness, dizziness, palor, palpitations, sweating, tachycardia) symptoms. Both components may be reproduced by the intravenous administration of serotonin. Since

blood levels of serotonin have been shown to be elevated during a glucose test meal in most patients with established dumping syndrome, this autacoid may be involved in its etiology.

If serotonin is in fact the humoral agent responsible for many of the symptoms of dumping, the question still remains as to how the amine reaches the peripheral circulation in view of the avid catabolic activity of the liver and lung. It may well be that serotonin is not directly involved in the symptomatology of the dumping syndrome but is released incidently by the "dumping" stimulus from APUD cells in conjunction with polypeptide hormones or other humoral agents.

THE CARCINOID SYNDROME. The important manifestations of the carcinoid syndrome are cutaneous flushing, bronchospasm, diarrhea, malabsorption, swings in blood pressure and occasionally mental symptoms. In chronic cases, a pellagra-like skin rash and right sided heart lesions of endocardial fibrosis with valvular incompetence may also be seen. The carcinoid syndrome was originally believed to occur only as a result of serotonin overproduction by malignant carcinoid tumors of the bowel with hepatic metastases, but it is now clear that the spectrum of symptoms produced by a carcinoid tumor depends upon many factors including the *cell of origin* (enterochromaffin, APUD, etc.), the *site of origin* (deriviation from fore, mid or hind gut), the *size of the tumor* and the *presence or absence of hepatic metastases* and the *mediator(s) produced.*

Apart from serotonin, 5-hydroxytryptophan, histamine, kallikrein and bradykinin have been implicated as mediators in some cases, but the role of prostaglandins, thyrocalcitonin and other substances normally associated with APUD cells is not clear.

Inappropriate hormone secretion from a variety of tumors has been recognized in recent years, indicating the varying hormonal potential of such lesions. In view of the origin of carcinoid tumors, it is not unreasonable to assume that they fall into a similar category, and that different carcinoids may be either occasionally or continually unihormonal or multihormonal with regard to their "endocrine secretion." Thus, because of the wide variations in symptomatology, the term **carcinoid spectrum** is preferred by some for this condition(s).

The *cutaneous flush* is typically a bright red, irregular flush that generally becomes bluish due to relative deoxygenation. Serotonin, histamine and kallikrein may all produce this lesion. Ethanol and catecholamines may precipitate flushing in patients with carcinoid tumors and are the basis of diagnostic tests. *Bronchospasm* in the carcinoid syndrome may depend upon serotonin or histamine release, but it does not respond well to either serotonin or histamine antagonists. The precise cause of the *malabsorption* seen in patients with the carcinoid syndrome is not well known, but no doubt diarrhea exacerbates the defect(s). The *swings in blood pressure* are unpredictable and probably depend upon the proportion of autacoids produced and upon the tone of the different vascular beds. The excessive diversion of tryptophan by the tumor leaves less available for the synthesis of protein and niacin. Consequently, *protein deficiency* and a *pellagra-like state* may develop in severe cases. One of the more intriguing manifestations of the carcinoid syndrome is the occurrence of *fibrotic lesions.* These take the form of fibrotic deposits in many parts of the body, particularly the endocardium and cardiac valves, but also in the pericardium, lungs, pleura, retroperitoneal area and skin. A related phenomenon may be the fibrosis which develops with methysergide therapy and in patients with endomyocardial fibrosis and schistosomiasis. In vitro, serotonin increases the growth of fibroblasts by shortening their lag phase, but it is not clear if this effect can be extrapolated to the genesis of fibrotic lesions in man. In the carcinoid syndrome, significantly more serotonin is contained in the platelets that show a dilated cannalicular system, bizarre shapes and exhibit unusual serotonin containing hyaloplasmic organelles not seen in normal platelets. There appears to be two separate absorption mechanisms for serotonin in platelets from patients with the carcinoid syndrome, and altered platelet and/or pulmonary function may encourage cardiac fibrosis.

Migraine

Some forms of migraine appear to be associated with altered serotonin metabolism. Attacks are frequently shown to be associated with a rapid release of bound serotonin in blood. Serotonin antagonists are not uniformly successful in treatment. For further discussion of migraine see Chapter 15.

SEROTONIN ANTAGONISTS

Antiserotonin drugs are either *direct,* or *indirect* or *physiologic antagonists.* Direct antagonists block the effects of serotonin on the end organ involved, indirect antagonists interrupt serotonin induced ganglionic transmission and physiologic antagonists exert balancing counteractions. Only the directly acting antagonists are considered here.

ERGOT ALKALOID DERIVATIVES

LYSERGIC ACID DIETHYLAMIDE (LSD). LSD was first shown by Gaddum to be a competitive antagonist of serotonin on uterine smooth muscle. It is more widely known as an hallucinogen (Chs. 9, 15, 14).

2-BROMOLYSERGIC ACID DIETHYLAMIDE (BOL). BOL has no hallucinatory properties but retains the antagonism of LSD for serotonin on smooth muscle. It has been mainly used in animals.

1-METHYL-D-LYSERGIC ACID BUTANOLAMIDE (METHYSERGIDE, Ch. 15).

Methysergide (Fig. 50–2) inhibits the effects of serotonin on smooth muscle and possesses only minimal ergot-like direct spasmogenic activity. Adverse reactions comprise gastrointestinal irritation (heartburn, anorexia, dyspepsia, cramps and diarrhea) and central nervous effects (insomnia, restlessness, nervousness, euphoria and unsteadiness). Retroperitoneal, pleuropulmonary or endocardial fibrosis may occasionally be seen in patients taking methysergide chronically. The fibrosis may regress on cessation of drug therapy but this is not always so. The occurrence of fibrosis is intriguing because of the structural similarities of methysergide to serotonin and the development of fibrotic lesions in the carcinoid syndrome.

Methysergide is of some value in the prophylaxis of migraine and in "cluster headaches." The beneficial effect of methysergide takes 1 or 2 days to develop, and "rebound" headaches may occur on cessation of therapy. Methysergide is of no benefit when given during an acute attack. Methysergide is also of occassional benefit in reducing diarrhea and malabsorption of the carcinoid syndrome, and in reducing symptoms in the postgastrectomy dumping syndrome. Contraindications to its use are pregnancy, thromboembolic disease, peripheral vascular disease, renal disease or coronary artery disease.

Methysergide bimaleate (Sansert) and methysergide base (Deseril) are available as tablets of 2 and 4 mg. The usual dose is 2–4 mg 2 or 3 times daily.

CYPROHEPTADINE

Cyproheptadine is related to the phenothiazine antihistamines, Like ergot derivatives, it possesses an N-substituted heterocyclic ring. Cyproheptadine is unique in that it is a potent antagonist of many of the peripheral actions of both serotonin and histamine in addition of possessing some parasympatholytic activity.

Adverse reactions are usually minimal. Drowsiness and dry mouth are most common and may disappear on chronic therapy. Skin rashes, dizziness, ataxia, anorexia and gastrointestinal irritation may also develop.

Cyproheptadine is mainly used in the treatment of pruritic dermatoses. It may be of some value in the postgastrectomy dumping syndrome and the carcinoid syndrome.

Cyproheptadine hydrochloride (Periactin) is available as 4 mg tablets and as a syrup containing 0.4 mg/ml. The usual dose is 4 mg 3 times daily.

PARACHLOROPHENYLALANINE (PCPA)

This experimental agent depresses tryptophan hydroxylase. Following the administration of 3–4 gm daily in man, the urinary excretion of 5-HIAA falls rapidly. In a few patients with the carcinoid syndrome, PCPA improved the intestinal symptoms but had no effect on flushing. Mild gastrointestinal irritation, ataxia and dyskinesia occasionally develop. In some animal species, PCPA has been shown to increase sexual behavior.

FURTHER READING

Erspamer V (ed) (1966): 5-Hydroxytryptamine and Related Indolealkylamines Handbook of Experimental Pharmacology. XIX Berlin, Springer

Gaddum, JH, Picarelli ZP (1957): Two kinds of tryptamine receptor. Br J Pharmacol 12:323–328

Garattini S, Valzelli L (eds) (1965): Serotonin. Amsterdam, Elsevier

Gyermek L (1961): 5-Hydroxytryptamine antagonists. Pharmacol Rev 13:339–439

Thompson JH (1971): Serotonin and the alimentary tract. Res Comm Chem Path Pharm 2:687–781

Thompson JH (1976): Serotonin in the regulation of gastrointestinal functions, in Serotonin in Health and Disease. Essman WB (ed) New York, Spectrum Publications, Ch 20

51. PROSTAGLANDINS

Few substances other than the prostaglandins have aroused so much pharmacologic interest in recent years. This is due largely to their ubiquitous occurrence in the body, diverse activities and numerous pathologic and therapeutic implications.

In the 1930s a pharmacologically active material was found in the human seminal fluid. Von Euler coined the term "prostaglandin" for this material, implicating the prostate gland as its source, although the seminal vesicles were later found to be more important. The prostaglandins (PGs) are now known to be present or formed in most if not all human secretions and organs.

Chemistry

PGs are a family of 20-carbon lipid acid containing a 5-membered ring, named prostanoic acid. They are grouped into the A, E, F, B and C types, the first three being the common natural products. Subdivision is made into mono-, bis- and trisunsaturated classes, according to the number of carbon-carbon double bonds in the parent E type PG, and designated by a subscript in the names of PGs. Over a dozen naturally occurring varieties have been identified. For example, PGE_1 is 9-oxo-11α-15(s)-dihydroxy-13-transprostanoic acid, or 11α-15-dihydroxy-9-ketoprost-13-enoic acid (Fig. 51–1).

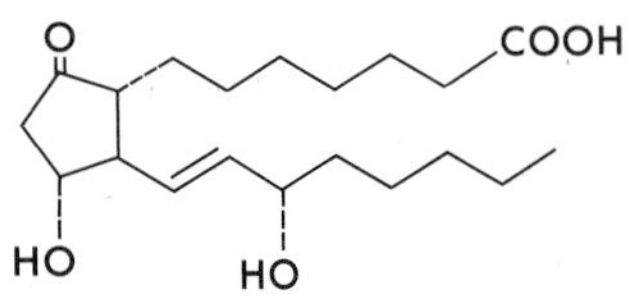

PGs are formed from polyunsaturated essential fatty acids in a great variety of tissues by a multienzyme complex referred to as "prostaglandin synthetase." While the stores of free PGs are rather limited, they are biosynthesized and released in response to stimuli. Once released, PGs, with the exception of the A series, are rapidly metabolized locally or in the general circulation, especially by the lungs, primarily by prostaglandin 15-hydroxydehydrogenase. Acting only close to their origin, PGE and F compounds may serve as local hormones or autacoids.

Pharmacology

Members of the PG family vary widely in their pharmacologic activities. The following description applies in broad outline to those of the E and A series. The F series frequently have different or opposite activities. Their actions on smooth muscle and adrenergic nerve function allow generalization regarding their overall effect in many organs. Formation of cyclic AMP (Ch. 18) is reported to be stimulated or inhibited by PGs, but it is premature to generalize concerning the significance of this phenomenon.

REPRODUCTIVE SYSTEM. PGs are best known for their action on the uterus. Both the E and F series cause contraction of the human uterus. They may stimulate pituitary gonadotrophin secretion and play a role in the ovulatory process and luteolysis.

NERVOUS SYSTEM. E, PGs are believed to be released at adrenergic neuroeffector synapses and reduce the release of adrenergic transmitter by a negative feedback mechanism. PGs may function as modulators or mediators of neurotransmission in the CNS.

CARDIOVASCULAR SYSTEM. E and A, PGs decrease the total peripheral resistance, plasma volume, cardiac output and arterial pressure. Renal blood flow is increased and water and sodium diuresis promoted. The F series is pressor. The systemic effects of the E and F members are curtailed by their rapid pulmonary metabolism.

GASTROINTESTINAL TRACT. Gastric acid secretion is inhibited by PGs, while intestinal motility is both stimulated and inhibited, depending on the compound and animal species. In general the E, PGs stimulate the longitudinal intestinal muscle and relax the circular muscle *in vitro;* F, PGs inhibit both.

RESPIRATORY SYSTEM. PGE compounds are potent bronchodilators, whereas $PGF_{2\alpha}$ is a bronchoconstrictor. In addition, PGE_2 prevents bronchoconstriction induced by histamine, serotonin, acetylcholine or bradykinin.

Pathophysiologic Roles

Many lines of evidence suggest that PGs play critical roles in normal function and in the pathophysiology of disease states. In no instance is the part played by the PGs established.

REPRODUCTION. As PGs are found in menstrual fluid, they have been implicated in the painful spasms of dysmenorrhea. PGs which occur in high concentrations in human semen may be absorbed from the vagina and affect motility of the uterus and Fallopian tubes and assist in fertilization. However, the seminal fluids of certain species are devoid of PGs. As $PGF_{2\alpha}$ appears in human blood during labor in waves that parallel the uterine contractions, it may be involved in parturition.

INFLAMMATION. Intradermal injection of PGE_1, e.g., induces wheal, flare, heat and pain in man. PGs are found in the inflammation exudates. Furthermore, the nonsteroidal antiinflammatory drugs, aspirin and indomethacin (Ch. 28), inhibit the biosynthesis of PGs. PGs may therefore play a role in inflammatory processes.

OTHER ROLES. Renal PGs may play a part in the regulation of arterial pressure. The circulating plasma PGA levels have been found to be lower in hypertensive compared to normotensive man. Carcinoid tumors contain a large quantity of PGs which may be responsible for diarrhea. PGE compounds induce fever when injected into cerebral ventricles of laboratory animals and occasionally during IV infusion in man. PGs may thus be responsible for hyperthermia. The antipyretic action of aspirin-like drugs has been thought to result from inhibition of PG synthesis.

Clinical Uses

FERTILITY CONTROL. Extensive clinical research is being made into the value of PGs for abortion. The initial approach favoring IV infusion has been discarded due to the high failure rates and frequent untoward effects, including hypotension, nausea, vomiting and diarrhea. Intravaginal PG administration which depends mainly on systemic absorption is associated with similar adverse effects. Intraamniotic instillation of PGs for the induction of midtrimester abortion is reported to be advantageous because the PGs are better localized and adverse effects are less frequent.

PGs used within several weeks of fertilization for contraceptive purposes owe their effect to the induction of early abortion. The success rate has been low and incidence of adverse effects high. Experiments in progress may improve the prospects of this application. PGs given IV induce labor as effectively as oxytocin and may be accepted for some specific indications.

OTHER USES. Because PGE_1 inhibits platelet aggregation, it has been used in the harvesting and preparation of platelests for therapeutic transfusion. In view of their bronchodilator and antiallergic activity, PGEs may prove useful in treatment of asthma. Other possible uses include that of PGA_1 for vasodilation, antihypertension, diuresis and inhibition of gastric secretion.

The major drawbacks to the clinical application of PGs have been their short duration of action, lack of effect given orally and systemic side effects. Synthetic analogs devoid of these drawbacks are actively being sought.

PROSTAGLANDIN INHIBITORS

An extensive search is being carried out for substances that prevent the effects of PGs. Such inhibitors may be useful in the treatment of such conditions as habitual abortion, premature labor, dysmenorrhea, diarrhea and inflammation. The compounds under study, although most are not available for general clinical use, have already substantially helped to elucidate the participation of PGs in the complex biologic events.

The inhibitors either prevent PG biosynthesis or PG actions at their receptor sites. The better known synthesis inhibitors include indomethacin, phenylbutazone and aspirin. A few other compounds, including a prostaglandin analog, specifically and competitively antagonize the smooth muscle contractile action of PGE_1 and E_2 or diminishes the PG induced formation of cyclic AMP in several tissues tested.

None of the compounds so far reported inhibit

all the actions of PGs. On the other hand, it would be desirable to develop compounds that discretely inhibit selected PG actions so as to achieve specific therapeutic results.

FURTHER READING

Kahn RH, Lands WEM (ed) (1973): Prostaglandins and Cyclic AMP—Biological Actions and Clinical Applications. New York, Academic Press

Karim SMM, Hiller K (1974): Prostaglandins: pharmacology and clinical application. Drugs 8:176–207

Ramwell PW (ed) (1973): The Prostaglandins. New York, Plenum Press

Wilson ED (ed) (1974): Symposium on prostaglandins. Arch Intern Med 133:29–146

CHEMOTHERAPY OF INFECTIONS AND NEOPLASIA

JEREMY H. THOMPSON

52. INTRODUCTION TO ANTIMICROBIAL AGENTS

Drugs used in the treatment of infectious diseases are either **antibiotics** or **chemotherapeutic agents.** Antibiotics, from **antibiosis,** are antiinfective substances of natural origin metabolically produced by, e.g., **fungi** (penicillin, griseofulvin), **bacteria** (bacitracin, colistin, polymyxin B), **streptomyces** (streptomycin, tetracyclines) and **micromonospora** (gentamicin), whereas chemotherapeutic agents are synthetic antimicrobial drugs (isoniazid, sulfonamides, etc.). The terms antibiotic, chemotherapeutic agent and antimicrobial agent are often used interchangeably to refer to either natural or synthetic drugs. Addi-

tionally, the term chemotherapeutic agent is often used to describe individual **anticancer drugs.** Paul Ehrlich coined the word "chemotherapy" in 1913 as "the injury of an invading organism without injury to the host."

Though nearly all antibiotics, at least initially, were obtained from living organisms, there are certain disadvantages in relying entirely upon natural sources for commercial purposes, and synthetic (e.g., chloramphenicol) or semisynthetic (e.g., the newer penicillins) production is becoming more common.

HISTORY OF ANTIMICROBIAL THERAPY

Ehrlich stressed that drugs should be sought which demonstrate greater effects on the pathogen than on the host. This concept which crystallized as the chemotherapeutic index is an attempt to relate drug potency and toxicity and to measure antimicrobial effectiveness. As defined by Ehrlich, the chemotherapeutic index Is:

$$\frac{\text{maximal tolerated dose}}{\text{minimum curative dose}}$$

Thus, no real therapeutic advantage is gained if a new drug is half as toxic as an old one and not more than half as active.

The unwitting application of "antibacterial" therapy is very old. Medical lore abounds with tales of the use of soil, plants and moldy ferments for the treatment of various skin lesions, the reported beneficial effects undoubtedly resulting from antibiotics produced by associated bacteria, fungi and actinomycetes. Several antiinfective drugs were available before Ehrlich's time. For example, malaria and dysentery were widely treated with the alkaloids of cinchona and ipecacuanha, mercury had been used in treating syphilis and carbolic acid had been introduced

as an antiseptic by 1865. Moreover, that bacteria could produce substances antagonistic to other bacterial species had been noted by Pasteur in 1877, while working with *Bacillus anthracis.* Ehrlich, however, established the major principles governing the investigation of experimental infections and pioneered the idea (in 1906) of *therapia sterilisans magna,* the total control of pathogenic bacteria with a single dose of a nontoxic chemical (a magic bullet).

Prior to the development of sulfonamides, several antiseptic and disinfectant arsenic, antimony, bismuth and dye compounds were introduced into therapy. Because of their systemic toxicity, they were used mainly topically. Some antimony compounds are still used (Ch. 63). The overwhelming therapeutic success of the sulfonamides and penicillin (introduced into therapy in 1935 and 1941, respectively) initiated systematic investigations into distribution of antibacterial drugs in nature. Over the past 30–35 years, thousands of new antimicrobial agents have been discovered and tested. Most of these drugs have proved too toxic for human use, but a sizable number have been retained. In spite of the introduction of many potent drugs, our hope for the elimination of all infections has not been realized, nor is it likely to be. Indeed, the indiscriminate use of antibiotics has frequently resulted in the development of a more serious infection than might otherwise have occurred. Many of the antimicrobial drugs have found other uses as tools in the investigation of cellular biochemistry and in laboratory bacteriology.

Antibiotics are widely used (15–20% of all prescriptions) and account for about 70–80% of hospital drug costs. Epidemiologic studies have shown that greater than 50% of antibiotics used are not needed, that an inappropriate agent is often chosen or that the dose used is incorrect. To facilitate an understanding of the correct use of antibacterial drugs, some of the basic principles governing their action are presented.

BASIC PRINCIPLES OF ANTIMICROBIAL CHEMOTHERAPY

Bactericidal and Bacteriostatic Drugs

On the basis of in vitro testing, antimicrobial drugs are classified as either **bactericidal** or **bacteriostatic.** Bactericidal drugs kill organisms and are more effective during logarithmic growth, since the increased metabolic activity provides maximum susceptibility. Bacteriostatic antimicrobial agents only prevent bacterial growth and clinically are less desirable; the terms *fungistatic, fungicidal, amebistatic, amebicidal,* etc., are self-explanatory. The classification into bactericidal and bacteriostatic drugs has some clinical usefulness, but the differences between the two groups of agents in vivo are to some extent dose dependent. Thus, bactericidal drugs usually exhibit a bacteriostatic effect if present in suboptimum concentrations, and bacteriostatic agents,

e.g., erythromycin, may be bactericidal at high drug concentrations.

If the body defense mechanisms are impaired (Table 52–1) the antibiotic may be unable to do more than slow the spread of infection, and a relapse occurs upon discontinuation of therapy. Although bactericidal drugs, in theory are capable of erradicating an infection without the help of host defense mechanisms, even the most potent bactericidal agents rarely eliminate the infection by a direct killing effect, and **intact host defense mechanisms and anatomical barriers are usually needed for full recovery.**

Antimicrobial Synergism and Antagonism

When used together in vitro, antimicrobial drugs can exhibit **additive, synergistic** or **antagonistic**

TABLE 52–1. Major Factors Predisposing to Local or Systemic Infections

Level of defense	Defense altering situations
Anatomic barriers and secretions	Foreign body (e.g., calculus, sequestrum)
	Congenital anomaly (e.g., ectopic ureter)
	Burns, local trauma or surgery
	Catheters (e.g., urinary, IV, intraarterial, tracheal)
	Diagnostic and therapeutic procedure (e.g., dental prophylaxis, ultrasonic nebulizers, IPPB apparatuses, cardiac prostheses)
	Bacterial proliferation in IV fluids stored at room temperature
	Increased secretions (e.g., pulmonary edema reduces the activity of alveolar macrophages)
	Reduced secretions (e.g., achlorhydria, Sjoegrens syndrome)
	Reduced blood flow
	Poor diet, alcoholism, major systemic metabolic disease
	Estrogens in oral contraceptives (produce dilatation of the upper urinary tract)
Normal bacterial flora	Contact with medical personnel (cross infection with drug resistant pathogens)
	Drug therapy (superinfections)
	Systemic metabolic disease (e.g., diabetes mellitus, sarcoidosis, uremia)
White blood cells	Disorders of granulocyte production (e.g., neutropenia, agranulocytosis, aplastic anemia)
	Depression of chemotaxis (e.g., glucocorticosteroids and ethyl alcohol)
	Depression of opsonization (e.g., glucocorticosteroids and tetracyclines)
	Depression of intracellular bacterial killing (e.g., glucocorticoids stabilize lysosomal membranes, and colchicine and vinblastine inhibit microtubule formation and stabilize lysosomal membranes)
Immunologic mechanisms	Antibody immunodeficiencies
	Cellular immunodeficiencies
	Combined immunodeficiencies
	Defects of the phagocytic system
	Defects of complement
	Immunodeficiencies associated with specific clinical conditions

effects. In vivo however, an additive effect is the usual response; synergism and antagonism may rarely occur, e.g., with penicillin plus streptomycin in the treatment of enterococcal endocarditis, or with penicillin plus tetracyclines in the treatment of pneumococcal meningitis, respectively. Since most bactericidal drugs act maximally on multiplying bacteria, and since bacteriostatic drugs depress bacterial cell multiplication and growth, a mixture of the two types may result in antagonism.

Antibacterial Spectrum

Antibiotics are often classified as **broad** or **narrow spectrum,** depending upon the range of organisms they affect. Thus, penicillin G has a **narrow spectrum** since it primarily affects only gram-positive organisms and neisseria, whereas, the tetracyclines have a **broad antibacterial spectrum** since they depress not only gram-positive and gram-negative bacteria but also the rickettsiae and the chlamydiae. Separation into broad and narrow spectrum antibiotics is often blurred, since overuse of "broad spectrum" agents (particularly ampicillin and the tetracyclines) has resulted in the emergence of many resistant strains. Thus, the *effective* spectrum of "broad spectrum" antibiotics may be narrower than that of some narrow spectrum antibiotics. Broad spectrum antibiotics should be restricted for the treatment of specific infections caused by a few organisms or even a single species of organism. *The property of "broad spectrum" should not be confused with a license for broad nonspecific use.*

Determination of Bacterial Sensitivity In Vitro

Two microbiologic methods are used to determine bacterial sensitivity to antibiotics. In the first method the isolated organism is inoculated into tubes, or onto plates of culture medium containing sequentially diminishing drug concentrations. Following suitable incubation, the lowest concentration of the drug inhibiting bacterial growth (the minimum inhibitory concentration: MIC) can be determined. Bactericidal activity usually occurs at drug concentrations 2–10 times greater than the MIC. Reported levels of antibacterial potency vary depending upon the test organism used and the size of the inoculum and upon the conditions, such as pH, temperature, presence or absence of oxygen, tissue fluid, pus, etc., of the in vitro test system.

The second method, which is more rapid but less precise, consists of application of standardized antibacterial, drug-impregnated, filter paper disks onto the surface of a uniformly seeded agar plate. A good indication of bacterial sensitivity may be obtained by measuring the zone of inhibition of bacterial colony growth; the size of the zone is related to all the conditions mentioned above (pH, temperature, etc.) plus the accuracy of the stated quantity of antibiotic present in the disk and the drugs diffusibility in agar. Because of the speed with which results may be obtained and because numerous antibiotics may be tested on the same agar plate, antibiotic disk testing is widely used in clinical microbiologic laboratories to give an indication of which antibiotic to use and the approximate level of dosage required to produce a therapeutic effect.

Two specific infections in which routine sensitivity testing may be misleading are subacute bacterial endocarditis and urinary tract infections. Subacute bacterial endocarditis has only rarely (if ever) been cured with bacteriostatic antibacterial drugs. Therefore, irrespective of the demonstration of sensitivity to bacteriostatic drugs on in vitro testing, bactericidal agents should be used in preference.

Two important considerations apply to urinary tract infections. First, some antibacterial agents excreted in the urine achieve higher concentrations there than those obtained in the blood and thus may be useful in treatment even though in vitro sensitivity testing (performed with antibiotic containing disks relating to commonly achieved blood levels) indicates that the organism is "resistant." Second, in vitro sensitivity testing is usually performed at pH 7.2–7.4, whereas urine is usually more acid at pH 5–6. Thus, antibiotics like streptomycin that possess greater antibacterial activity at an alkaline pH will appear more effective in vitro than they will be in vivo unless the urine is concomitantly alkalinized. On the other hand, antibacterial agents such as the tetracyclines or nalidixic acid which are more effective at an acid pH may appear to be ineffective when studied in vitro, whereas in acid urine in vivo, they might be clinically valuable. The rate of drug excretion may be influenced by the urine pH (Ch. 2). For example, the tetracycline antibiotics are more effective at an acid pH, but are also more slowly excreted.

Antibiotic Levels in Tissue Fluid

The distribution of antibiotics is an important factor in therapy. Distribution is usually equated in terms of "blood" or "serum levels," but, except in cases of septicemia, the blood antimicrobial concentration is not directly important. What is important is the concentration *achieved* and *maintained* in the infected tissue(s). This will depend upon many factors, such as the location of the infection, the causative organism, the presence of tissue fluid or an abscess cavity and the dose, route of administration and protein binding of the antimicrobial agent. For example, penicillin G, which produces an effective blood level for 2–4 hr following IM therapy, may persist in pus for 8–12 hr. Little is known about tissue levels of antimicrobial agents. Experimental work however has shown that the blood peak gives little indication of the tissue peak and that despite a high blood peak, some tissues may never be exposed to an adequate antimicrobial drug concentration. On the other hand, antimicrobial agents with a prolonged low peak may achieve satisfactory tissue distribution. In order to achieve and maintain adequate tissue levels of antimicrobial agents, rapidly excreted drugs should be given frequently, and in sufficiently high dosage, to ensure blood and tissue equilibration. Many drugs used in the treatment of urinary tract infections are effective in spite of low plasma levels, since they are concentrated in the urine.

BACTERIAL RESISTANCE TO ANTIMICROBIAL DRUGS

Considered by species, bacteria are susceptible to some antibacterial drugs and resistant to others (see above), but strains may develop that are resistant to drugs normally effective against that species. This is particularly true of staphylococci, gram-negative bacilli and *M. tuberculosis* but may occur with any organism; bacterial strains are known which are resistant to every antibiotic in current use. Bacterial resistance is a major medical problem because it severely limits the usefulness of many antibiotics and often necessitates the substitution of toxic and less potent drugs where the more acceptable agents are found to be ineffective.

Development of bacterial resistance makes it essential to revise periodically the drugs of choice for different bacterial infections and to determine the antibacterial sensitivity of the invading organism in all infections whenever possible. Failure to do this wastes time, money and needlessly exposes the patient to potentially harmful drugs. However, if antibiotics have to be administered before results of sensitivity testing are available, it is useful to know the probable sensitivity pattern (antibiogram) of a given bacterial species based upon the recent experience of the individual clinical laboratory.

Patterns of drug resistance may abruptly change when new antibiotics are introduced, or when there are changes in the customary usage of antibiotics within a hospital community. Thus, considerable variation in patterns of drug resistance may exist from hospital to hospital. Organisms that become resistant to one antibacterial drug usually exhibit **cross resistance** to related drugs. For example, bacteria developing resistance to sulfadiazine are resistant to equipotent concentrations of all other sulfonamides. Occasionally cross resistance may appear between two chemically dissimilar antibiotics, such as erythromycin and lincomycin.

Types of Bacterial Resistance

Bacterial resistance to antimicrobial drugs is either **natural** or **acquired; dependence,** a related phenomenon, is rare. The development of bacterial resistance is simply an expression of bacterial evolution, with survival of the fittest. Bacterial multiplication is so rapid that within $3\frac{1}{2}$ years an average strain of organism can have passed through as many generations as man has gone through in one million years.

NATURAL RESISTANCE. Natural resistance is genetically determined and depends upon the absence of a metabolic process affected by the antibiotic in question. Naturally resistant organisms proliferate as their sensitive brethren are killed. Natural resistance may be characteristic of an entire species, but sometimes as in the case of penicillin resistant staphylococci, is confined to particular strains within that species.

ACQUIRED RESISTANCE. Acquired resistance refers to resistance developing in a previously sensitive bacterial species. It can arise through **mutation** (spontaneous, induced), **adaptation** or through development of **infectious (multiple) drug resistance.**

By **spontaneous mutation** (about once per 10^5–10^{10} cells) a bacterial species produces de novo some members which differ from the parent strain. If the mutation is favorable, the bacteria will survive. If susceptible bacteria are exposed to subinhibitory concentrations of antibacterial drugs, drug resistant mutants may develop (**induced mutation**) either in one step (streptomycin type) or in a series of steps (penicillin type). Stepwise increase in resistance is probably due to mutations occurring in a number of different genes, each of which is responsible for a slight increase in resistance. One step increase in bacterial resistance is due to mutations occurring in more powerful genes which confer a considerable degree of resistance.

Adaptation presupposes that organisms contain low concentrations of antibacterial destructive enzymes, or the potential for synthesizing such enzymes, and that lethal enzyme concentrations are "triggered" through enzyme induction following antibiotic exposure, e.g., penicillinase induction following semisynthetic penicillin exposure in some strains of staphylococci (Ch. 55).

Infectious (multiple) drug resistance is the transfer in vivo or in vitro of genetic material (R factors) coding for resistance (e.g., β-lactamase production) from a resistant to a sensitive bacterium. Their presence was first reported in Japan in 1959–60 during an epidemic of Shigella dysentery; subsequently they have been identified all over the world. The origin of R factors remains unknown, but their development, as distinct from their spread, is probably not directly related to antibacterial chemotherapy. It is unclear why they have not spread throughout the entire bacterial population.

Genes for drug resistance may be associated with either **chromosomal** or **plasmid** DNA. Additionally, plasmids may affect bacteria in a variety of ways (phage typing, toxin production, fermentation reactions, etc.) confusing their identification. All plasmids contain genes (R factors) coding for resistance, but gram-negative bacteria possess in addition an RTF (resistance transfer factor:sex factor) that determines replication and transfer (see below). R factors transfer in one of three ways.

Transformation refers to the incorporation by a sensitive bacterium of free (naked) genes from a drug resistant cell. It occurs rarely (about $1/10^8$ cells) and is of little clinical importance. **Transduction** refers to the transfer of an R factor carrying plasmid by a temperate bacterial virus (bacteriophage) vector along with its own genes. It occurs mainly in gram-positive cocci, rarely in gram-negative bacilli, and usually resistance to one or two antibiotics only is transferred. Transduction occurs approximately once for every 10^3–10^6 exposed cells and is more readily accomplished if both the donor and recipient strains belong to the same group than if they belong to different groups. **Conjugation** depends upon a plasmid-containing, drug resistant "male" type bacterial cell passing R factor(s) and RTF to a drug sensitive "female" cell via a "sex pilus," the formation of which is induced by RTF. The infected "female" cell then becomes a "male" cell. Transfer factors have so far been determined in *E. coli*, *Shigella* spp., *Salmonella typhimurium*, *Klebsiella-Enterobacter* spp., *Vibrio cholerae*, *Pasturella* spp., *Proteus* spp., *Serratia marcessens* and *Pseudomonas aeruginosa*.

R-factor transfer is usually multiple, and resistance transfer to as few as one or as many as seven drugs at one time has been identified (chloramphenicol, erythromycin, penicillin, tetracycline, aminoglycosides, sulfonamides and fusidic acid). Donor and recipient strains may belong to different species, or even to different genera, and, more importantly, transfer can develop between pathogenic and nonpathogenic organisms indiscriminately.

DEPENDENCE. Organisms can become dependent on an antibacterial drug. Clinically, this may be seen occasionally in the treatment of tuberculosis with streptomycin (Ch. 56).

Clinical Implications of Drug Resistance

The spectrum of resistance conveyed by R-factors drastically curtails the antibacterial spectrum of many drugs. Thus, each hospital should develop an antibiotic policy, where certain drugs are reserved for specific use in critically ill patients infected with dangerous pathogenic organisms, e.g., *Staph. aureus* and *P. aeruginosa*. In addition, cross infection within the hospital environment should be controlled by careful attention to environmental hygiene, the treatment of carriers and the strict use of isolation procedures. It has long been held that clinical and veterinary use of antibiotics leads inexorably to an increase in bacterial resistance. However, this may not be true, since the frequency of resistance to some antibiotics falls if the use of those agents is abandoned or at least greatly curtailed. Tetracycline resistance is exceptional, since the gene determining resistance is closely linked to, or possibly part of, the genes involving transfer. Thus, selection for tetracycline resistance automatically selects for ability to transfer resistance from strain to strain, a situation deserving special consideration when tetracyclines are contemplated for prophylactic purposes, or for non-human use, e.g., in subtherapeutic doses in agriculture to increase the rate of weight gain in livestock.

Mechanisms of Resistance to Antimicrobial Drugs

When an organism has developed means for counteracting the antiinfective drug, it is said to be resistant; several mechanisms are known (Table 52–2). Resistance arising through alteration of the organism such that the drug either does not reach or does not interact normally with its bacterial target site generally occurs through mutational alteration of the cellular components. Resistance arising through enzymatic destruction of the antibiotic generally is associated with plasmids.

Factors Influencing Development of Bacterial Resistance

Bacterial resistance to antibiotics is a major therapeutic problem, as many pathogenic species

TABLE 52—2. Mechanisms of Resistance to Some Antimicrobial Agents

Antimicrobial drug	Mechanism(s) of resistance
Cephalosporins	Cleavage (hydrolysis) of the cephalosporin β-lactam ring by bacterial β-lactamases (cephalosporinases) (Ch. 55)
Chloramphenicol	Acetylation of the antibiotic by bacterial chloramphenicol acetyltransferases. Bacterial cells impermeable to chloramphenicol
Cycloserine	Increased production of alanine racemase and D-alanyl: D-alanine synthetase by bacteria. Increased production of D-alanine by bacteria (Ch. 53)
Erythromycin	Methylation of the 30S subunit of the bacterial ribosome by a plasmid-coded RNA methylase, resulting in failure of antibiotic binding
Fusidic acid	Presence of altered bacterial G factor resulting in failure of antibiotic binding (Ch. 53)
Gentamicin	Acetylation of amino groups, or phosphorylation or adenylation of hydroxyl groups by appropriate bacterial enzymes
Kanamycin	As for gentamicin
Lincomycin	As for erythromycin. Bacterial walls impermeable to the drug
Methicillin	Bacterial cells impermeable to the drug. Methicillin binds to penicillinases but is not destroyed by the enzyme.
Neomycin	As for gentamicin
Penicillin G, and other penicillinase sensitive penicillins	Cleavage (hydrolysis) of the penicillin β-lactam ring by bacterial β-lactamase (penicillinases) (Ch. 55)
Rifampin	Bacterial RNA polymerase possesses an altered β^1-subunit resulting in failure of antibiotic binding
Streptomycin	As for gentamicin
Sulfonamides	Bacterial production of para-amino benzoic acid, a direct sulfonamide antagonist. Development of alternate pathway of folic acid synthesis. Bacterial cells impermeable to the drug
Tetracyclines	Bacterial cells do not bind the antibiotic and may produce an inhibitor of tetracycline transport

which used to be highly sensitive are now resistant to the formerly effective drugs. Precautions to decrease the rate of emergence of resistant strains are avoiding unnecessary, promiscuous use of antibiotics and selection of antibiotics on the basis of in vitro bacteriologic investigation when possible. Additionally, antibiotics that usually demonstrate a wide spectrum of cross resistance, or that are likely to induce resistance should be avoided if possible. The combination of two or more antibacterial drugs reduces the development of resistance only in the treatment of tuberculosis (Ch. 56).

ANTIBACTERIAL DRUG COMBINATIONS

ANTIBIOTIC COMBINATIONS. The use of antibiotics in fixed dosage combinations is to be deprecated (Ch. 12). However, the simultaneous administration of two or more antibiotics, although not as fixed dosage preparations, may be justified under certain circumstances, e.g., in mixed bacterial populations (gram-positive and gram-negative pathogens) such as occur in bronchiectasis, otitis media, urinary tract infections and peritonitis; in gram-negative bacteremic shock (gentamicin plus a cephalosporin); in severe infections of doubtful etiology ("blunderbuss" therapy) until results of culture and sensitivity testing are known; to produce synergism (penicillin plus streptomycin) in *Strep. viridans* and *Strep. faecalis* subacute bacterial endocarditis (Ch. 56); to delay the emergence of resistant strains in tuberculosis and in severe *Ps. aeruginosa* infections (carbenicillin plus gentamicin). Some antibiotics with similar modes of action may antagonize each other and therefore should not be used; e.g., erythromycin and lincomycin may antagonize each other and chloramphenicol. Bactericidal and bacteriostatic drugs may show antagonism when combined.

CHEMOTHERAPEUTIC DRUG COMBINATIONS. There is ample justification for combining several sulfonamides to reduce renal toxicity (Ch. 60) or for combining antitubercular drugs (Ch. 56).

ANTIBIOTIC AND CHEMOTHERAPEUTIC DRUG COMBINATIONS WITH NONANTIBACTERIAL SUBSTANCES. Many fixed dosage preparations of antibiotics and chemotherapeutic agents plus analgesics, antihistamines, antipyretics, etc., are on the market. The physician is advised against using these.

In the clinical management of parasitic disease, the selection of the most suitable drug is only one aspect of therapy; adequate supporting measures must also be undertaken as *final recovery is dependent upon the host.*

Bacteriologic Diagnosis

In general, the selection of an antibiotic should be based upon an etiologic diagnosis. Culture of infected material (pus, etc.) will in most instances enable the pathogen(s) to be isolated and identified, with subsequent determination of its sensitivity (or resistance) to antimicrobial drugs. Although sensitivity determinations are desirable, particularly in infections caused by *E. coli, Proteus* spp., *Ps. aeruginosa* and *Staphylococcus* spp., they are not absolutely necessary in infections caused by some organisms (*T. pallidum,* pneumococci, gonococci, β-haemolytic streptococci), that are usually sensitive to drugs like penicillin.

Because many common pathogenic microorganisms show varying antibacterial resistance, a hit or miss philosophy in treatment is reprehensible; it can lead to a delay in administration of the correct drug and to diagnostic confusion. In some instances bacteriologic diagnosis and sensitivity determination are difficult. For example, in the acutely ill patient delay before instituting therapy may not be justified clinically, and treatment can be started after appropriate culture material has been taken. Additionally, appropriate material may not be readily available for culturing, and in these instances a Gram stain may be invaluable. The occasional necessity for administering a combination of antibiotics to febrile patients who are seriously ill and who are suspected of having an unknown overwhelming bacterial infection cannot be denied. However, the initiation of an antibiotic program should not commit the physician to its continuance if a change is suggested by the culture and sensitivity report. Thus, as soon as the pathogen is isolated, an antibiotic should be selected that has the most narrow spectrum against that organism in order to avoid superinfection (see below).

Major factors influencing the choice of an antibacterial drug in the absence of sensitivity testing are the location of the infection, a "statistical" guess as to the causative organisms, the presence of concomitant illness, knowledge of previous drug therapy and a history of drug reactions (Ch. 7).

Drug Response and Dosage

An antibacterial drug usually causes significant clinical improvement within 12–24 hr. If no clinical improvement is obvious after 48–72 hr of full therapy, it can usually be concluded that the organisms are resistant to that drug, or that some other problem such as an undrained abscess is preventing a favorable response. However, a knowledge of the natural history of a particular infection is exceedingly helpful. For example, the patient with pneumococcal pneumonia usually shows prompt improvement, whereas the patient with typhoid fever typically remains ill for several days after initiation of optimal antibiotic treatment. Antibacterial therapy should not be discontinued prematurely, and ample time should be available for full mobilization of host defenses. If symptoms and fever redevelop after a period of amelioration, *superinfection* with resistant organisms, *abscess formation* or an *adverse drug reaction* may be responsible.

Prophylactic Use of Antibacterial Drugs

Antimicrobial drugs have drastically altered the natural history of bacterial disease by reducing

TABLE 52–3. Some Indications for Prophylactic Antibiotics

Drug	Indication
Ampicillin	Used in prophylaxis of respiratory tract infections during the winter months in patients with chronic bronchitis
Ampicillin	Children with cystic fibrosis
Penicillin G	Used before oral surgery or other surgical manipulations to prevent the development of subacute bacterial endocarditis in patients with rheumatic endocarditis, congenital heart disease or a valvular prosthesis
Penicillin G	Used to prevent infections with group A streptococci in patients with rheumatic fever
Silver nitrate	Ophthalmia neonatorum
Sulfonamides	Used to prevent infections with group A streptococci in patients with rheumatic fever
Sulfonamides	Occasionally of value in prophylaxis of bacillary dysentery and meningococcal infections
Tetracyclines	Prophylaxis of household contacts of patients with cholera
Tetracyclines	Used in prophylaxis of respiratory tract infections during the winter months in patients with chronic bronchitis
Tetracyclines	Children with cystic fibrosis

Patients undergoing surgery, as a routine pre- or postoperative procedure
Patients with recurring ulcers of the mouth or lips due to *Herpes simplex*
Patients with nonspecific or virus infections, to prevent secondary bacterial infection
Patients with long-term indwelling urethral catheters
Patients taking corticosteroid or anticancer drugs
Patients in coma or with a tracheostomy

the morbidity and mortality from infections. Thus, it is not surprising that these same antimicrobial agents have been used in vain attempts to prevent rather than to treat infections. In general, there is no place for prophylactic antimicrobial therapy *unless prophylaxis is directed against one particular microorganism, or a small group of microorganisms.* Clinical situations in which antibacterial prophylaxis is indicated or probably ineffective and hazardous are listed in Tables 52–3 and 52–4, respectively.

Concomitant Drug Therapy

Gamma globulin and **antitoxic sera** are required as adjunct agents in specific circumstances. Glucocorticosteroids produce both beneficial and deleterious effects, but it is often not possible to predict which effect will be dominant. Glucocorticosteroids mask the symptoms of infection and alter the host-parasite relationship in favor of the parasite by inhibiting the inflammatory response, by enhancing tissue invasion and dissemination of pathogens, by depressing polymorphonuclear production, migration, phagocytosis and intracellular digestive mechanisms and by reducing interferon production. On the other hand, they possess beneficial antitoxic, antiallergic and antiinflammatory effects.

Their antitoxic property may be life saving in patients with septic shock caused by, e.g., gram-negative bacilli, where the steroid restores endotoxin-damaged vessel sensitivity to sympathomimetic amines, and in Herxheimer reactions (typhoid fever, leprosy, syphilis and filariasis) and viral hepatitis. Their "antiallergic" and antiinflammatory properties are of value, respectively, in counteracting severe or life threatening hypersensitivity reactions to an antibiotic (e.g., penicillin) which must be used, or as an adjunct agent in treating tuberculous meningitis (Ch. 56). Glucocorticosteroid therapy is mandatory in the Waterhouse-Friderichsen syndrome, and *additional* glucocorticosteroids are mandatory in patients on long-term steroid therapy who develop infections. With the exception of isoniazid therapy (Ch. 56), prophylactic antibiotics need not be given to patients on long term glucocorticosteroid therapy.

Conditions of the Host Which Modify the Response to Antimicrobial Drugs

Although the causative organism and the site of infection determine to a large extent the antibiotic(s) to be used, consideration of host factors is also of importance (Ch. 7). In particular, the state of gastrointestinal, renal and hepatic function are important determinants of antibiotic selection, since impairment usually alters drug pharmacokinetics (Ch. 77).

Failure of Antibacterial Therapy

The important reasons for difficulty and failure with antibacterial therapy are listed in Table 52–5. **Fever** may be caused by many factors other than infection. For example, mild temperature elevations may be seen in patients taking antihistamines or atropine and in certain disease states such as congestive heart failure. Additionally, patients with extensive skin disease, dysautonomia or congenital absence of the sweat glands are unable to loose body heat. **Antibacterial drugs may mask abscess formation** by reducing the spread of microorganisms. Abcesses are not cured by antibiotics and should be drained, with or without antibiotic irrigation. Drainage reduces the number of bacteria, increases antibiotic penetration, removes drug antagonists and may reduce the development of bacterial resistance.

Adverse Drug Effects

No antibacterial drug is totally devoid of toxicity, and specific adverse effects are described in the following chapters. **Superinfection** and **hypersensitivity,** common reactions to many drugs, are mentioned briefly here.

SUPERINFECTION. Superinfection (replacement infection) is the appearance of both microbiologic and clinical evidence of a new infection with pathogenic microorganisms or fungi (either a new strain or a new species) during antimicrobial treatment of a primary disease. It occurs in 2–4% of patients and is more common when an inappropriate drug, or too low a dosage is employed or when host resistance is impaired. Not all superinfections are the result of antibiotic use. Other important factors are frequent or prolonged catheterization, intubation or instrumentation, which provide the proper local condition for entry and colonization (Table 52–1).

In addition to some fungi, over 60 different species of bacteria normally inhabit the skin and the genitourinary, gastrointestinal and respiratory tracts. They are varyingly depressed on exposure to antibacterial drugs, broad spectrum

TABLE 52—5. Reasons for Difficulty and Failure of Antimicrobial Drug Therapy

Incorrect clinical diagnosis or procedures

Failure to recognize mixed infections
Treatment of "fever" or an undiagnosed condition
Treatment of untreatable infections (e.g., measles, mumps, upper respiratory tract viral disease, etc.)
Valueless prophylaxis
Complete reliance on culture and sensitivity reports
Improper dose (too large, too small), duration (too long, too short) or route of antibiotic administration
Antibiotic administration started too late
Concomitant administration of other drugs which interfere with antibacterial drugs (e.g., aluminum hydroxide binds tetracy-
    clines in the gut lumen, Ch. 37; barbiturates prevent the absorption of griseofulvin, Ch. 65; local anesthetics containing para-
    amino benzoic acid antagonise sulfonamides, Ch. 60)
Failure to control urinary pH (e.g., aminoglycosides are more active at an alkaline pH)
Inappropriate combination of bacteriostatic and bactericidal drugs

Incorrect bacteriologic diagnosis

Failure to recognize mixed infections (frequently anaerobic bacteria are missed)
Incorrect determination of sensitivity
Organism tested at incorrect pH (pertains particularly to organisms causing urinary tract infections)
Transfer of (contamination by) R factors

Bacterial factors

Development of bacterial resistance
Organism present in host in altered metabolic state (e.g., protoplasts, sphereoplasts, L-forms)
Development of bacterial persisters (development of forms other than L-forms)

Host factors

Failure of host defense mechanisms due to debility (malnutrition), disease (e.g., agammaglobulinemia, lymphoma),
    administration of other drugs (e.g., anticancer agents, corticosteroids) or radiation therapy (Table 52-1)
Inaccessibility of infection to drug (e.g., in meninges, bone, skin or urinary tract in patient with renal insufficiency)
Abscess formation. Failure to perform surgical drainage or debridement
Incurability of infection owing to presence of foreign body, kidney stone, malignancy, congenital anomaly, bronchiectasis,
    abnormal mucus (cystic fibrosis)
Presence of inadequately controlled or undiagnosed systemic disease such as diabetes mellitus, sarcoidosis, hypoparathyrodism
Presence of pus ("neutralization" of sulfonamides)
Inactivation of antibiotic by nonpathogenic host flora (e.g., penicillinase production)
Presence of nonantibacterial drugs which possess antibacterial activity and which contaminate collection of pus, etc., for in
    vitro study (e.g., by damaging the cytoplasmic membrane, lidocaine and procaine and preservatives in normal saline may
    be bactericidal)

Drug effects

Drug overdosage (e.g., failure to decrease the dose in renal or hepatic disease)
Drug cost (patient may not comply with dosage regimen due to high cost)
Development of superinfections (replacement infections)
Development of menningococcal and pneumococcal meningitis in patients on cephalothin. (Patients with severe systemic
    disease may develop menningeal infections with susceptible bacteria during therapy with cephalosporins since these
    agents pass poorly to the CSF)
Development of drug allergy, drug fever or some drug reaction
Problems associated with generic inequivalency
Drug intoxication, death

antibiotics producing a greater depression because of their wider range of antimicrobial activity. With depression of the normal nonpathogenic
bacterial flora, noncommensal or commensal
pathogenic organisms or fungi can more easily
initiate a superinfection. Thus, superinfection is
caused by organisms usually resistant to most of
the commonly used antibiotics, so creating a
therapeutic problem. Superinfection may occur
anywhere in the body, but the gastrointestinal
tract is most commonly involved. Symptoms of
gastrointestinal superinfection usually include
oral burning, xerostomia, stomatitis, glossitis,
cheilosis, black hairy tongue (Fig. 7–1), diarrhea,
signs of intestinal infection (enteritis, colitis) and
pruritus ani. Infection or superinfection trans-

mitted from another patient or a doctor or a
nurse is called **cross infection. Nosocomial infections** refer to cross infections acquired in a
hospital environment.

The **compromised host,** a patient with impaired
cellular immune and phagocytic defense mechanisms due to disease and/or drugs (Table 52–1),
may suffer a specific type of superinfection, **opportunistic infection.** This term refers to diseases
produced by ubiquitous parasites (Table 52–6)
which in normal man either live symbiotically, or
else produce minimal illness, and which are kept
in check by cellular immune and phagocytic
systems rather than by immunoglobins. *Opportunistic pathogens are not in themselves rare,
but their pathogenicity in comprised hosts*

TABLE 52—6. Principal Opportunistic Pathogens and Their Treatment*

Organism	Drug	Status on availability
Bacteria		
Bacteriodes spp.	Clindamycin Chloramphenicol (see Table 54—1)	
Listeria monocytogenes†	See Table 54—1	
M. Tuberculosis†	See Table 54—1	
Pseudomonas aeruginosa	Carbenicillin, gentamicin	
Serratia marcessens	Carbenicillin, gentamicin	
Viruses (DNA)		
Cytomegalovirus	Cytosine arabinoside	Drugs classified as experimental for treating these viruses, but of doubtful value
Herpes simplex	Idoxuridine	Available only at specific authorized centers
Varicella-zoster	Zoster immuno-globulin	
Fungi		
Asperigillus fumigatus	Amphotericin B	
Candida albicans	Amphotericin B	5-fluorocytosine classified as experimental for treating these infections. Most effective in *C. albicans* infection of the urinary tract. Available only at specific authorized centers
Cryptococcus neoformans	5-fluorocytosine	
Mucor	Amphotericin B	
Protozoa		
Pneumocystis carinii	Pentamidine isethionate	Available only from Parasitic Disease Drug Service, National Center for Disease Control, Atlanta (Table 54—2)
	Sulfadiazine and pyrimethamine Sulfamethoxazole and trimethoprim	Useful if pentamidine isethionate unavailable
Toxoplasma gondii (obligate intercellular pathogen)	Sulfadizaine and pyrimethamine Sulfamethoxazole and trimethoprim	
Other		
Nocardia asteroides	Sulfonamides, ampicillin	

* Intracellular pathogen.
† See also Table 54—2.

usually takes a form far different from and far more serious than that usually encountered.

HYPERSENSITIVITY. Hypersensitivity reactions can develop to most antibacterial drugs, particularly in atopic individuals, and those who have had allergic drug reactions (Ch. 7). In general, allergy to an antibacterial drug precludes its future use or the use of related drugs. For example, patients developing a sulfonamide allergy should never be exposed to any sulfonamide or to the chemically related drugs, acetazolamide, sulfonylurea compounds or thiazide diuretics.

FURTHER READING

Benveniste R, Davies J (1973): Mechanisms of antibiotic resistance in bacteria. Annu Rev Biochem 42:471–506

Dale DC, Petersdorf RG (1973): Corticosteroids and infectious Disease. Med Clin North Am 57:1277–1287

Editorial (1974): Plasmids: Lancet 1:249–250

Garrod LP, O'Grady F (1971): Antibiotic and Chemotherapy. (3rd ed) London, ES Livingstone

Kunin CM, Tupasi T, Craig WA (1973): Use of antibiotics. A brief exposition of the problem and some tentative solutions. Ann Intern Med 79:555–560

Levine, AS, Graw RG, Young RC (1972): Management of infections in patients with leukemia and lymphoma: Current concepts in experimental approaches. Semin Hematol 9:141–179

Stiehm ER, Fulginiti VA (1973): Immunologic Disorders in Infants and Children. Philadelphia, London, Toronto, WB Saunders

Watanabe T (1971): The origin of R factors. Ann NY Acad Sci 182:126–140

Weinstein L, Dalton AD (1968): Host determinants of response to antimicrobial agents. N Engl J Med 279:467–473; 524–531; and 580–588

JEREMY H. THOMPSON

53. MODE OF ACTION OF ANTIBIOTIC AGENTS

Antibiotics exhibit selective toxicity since host and bacterial cells differ structurally and functionally in many ways. Antibiotics act directly on microorganisms and do not increase host defense mechanisms. However, sometimes the opposite is true, as in β-hemolytic streptococcal infections when large doses of penicillin given early, by killing off all the bacteria, prevent adequate antibody production. Drugs capable of bolstering host defense mechanisms, such as levamisole (Tramisol), a veterinary anthelmintic, and

BCG and *C. parvum* vaccines, will no doubt achieve considerable development in the future.

Antimicrobial drugs can be generally classified with respect to their mode of action (Fig. 53–1), but many of them (particularly those inhibiting protein and nucleic acid synthesis) have more than one site of action so that secondary effects often confuse the picture. Furthermore, drugs given in combination may possess different patterns of action than when given individually, e.g., erythromycin and chloramphenicol.

INHIBITORS OF BACTERIAL CELL WALL FORMATION

The unique, rigid bacterial cell wall, a 100–200 Å thick coat external to the cytoplasmic membrane (bacterial cell membrane: cell envelope), represents a logical target for therapeutic attack. The wall serves primarily to **maintain the organisms' characteristic shape** and to **prevent cell rupture,** since bacteria sustain a high internal osmotic pressure—about 5 and 20 atm, respectively, for gram-negative and gram-positive bacteria. During cell division and growth, enzymes (peptidoglycan hydrolases) must break open strategic peptide links in the wall to allow interpolation of new building units. If wall synthesis is blocked by antibiotics (Fig. 53–1), the bacterium grows with gaps in its coat through which the cell membrane extrudes (due to imbibement of water), forming a protoplast (spheroplast) which eventually lyses (bactericidal effect). To facilitate an understanding of the mode of action of antibiotics preventing cell wall formation, a brief note concerning the structure and biosynthesis of cell wall peptidoglycans (mucopeptide: murein) in *Staph. aureus* and *E. coli* is presented.

Intracellular Biosynthesis of Subunits

Peptidoglycan subunits are oligosaccharide chains of two alternating amino sugars, *N*-acetyl-

glucosamine (Glu-NAc) and its 3-O-D-lactic acid derivative, *N*-acetylmuramic acid (Mur-NAc) linked β-1,4 (Fig. 53–2). Attached to carboxyl groups of the lactic acid side chain of the Mur-NAc moiety is a species dependant pentapeptide chain which in *Staph. aureus* is *L*-ala-*D*-glu-*L*-lys-*D*-ala-*D*-ala.

Transport of Subunits

The highly polar nonnucleotide portions of the peptidoglycans are transported across the cell membrane by a lipid soluble carrier (C_{55} isoprenoid alcohol pyrophosphate) (Fig. 53–2). During transportation, modifications to the pentapeptide moiety may be made, as in *Staph. aureus,* where a pentaglycine chain is added to the R_3 amino acid *L*-lys. Finally, under the influence of peptidoglycan synthetase, the subunit transfers to an acceptor, that in vivo is the growing point of a backbone glycan chain, releasing the carrier which is dephosphorylated by lipid pyrophosphatase to complete the cycle.

Assembly of Subunits

After transportation, three dimensional cross-linkages occur between polypeptide chains of

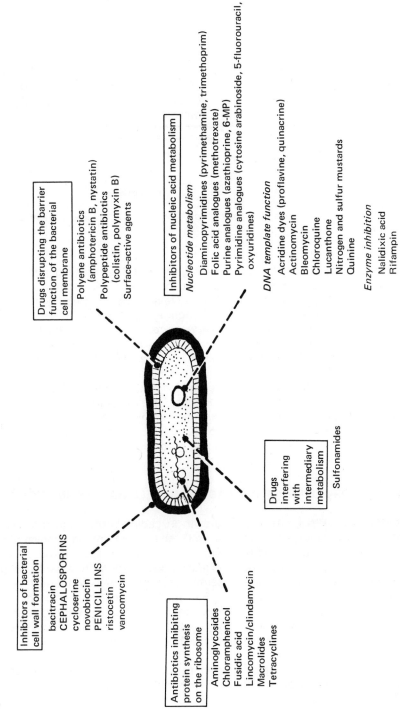

Inhibitors of bacterial
cell wall formation

bacitracin
CEPHALOSPORINS
cycloserine
novobiocin
PENICILLINS
ristocetin
vancomycin

Antibiotics inhibiting
protein synthesis
on the ribosome

Aminoglycosides
Chloramphenicol
Fusidic acid
Lincomycin/clindamycin
Macrolides
Tetracyclines

Drugs disrupting the barrier
function of the bacterial
cell membrane

Polyene antibiotics
  (amphotericin B, nystatin)
Polypeptide antibiotics
  (colistin, polymyxin B)
Surface-active agents

Inhibitors of nucleic acid metabolism

Nucleotide metabolism

Diaminopyrimidines (pyrimethamine, trimethoprim)
Folic acid analogues (methotrexate)
Purine analogues (azathioprine, 6-MP)
Pyrimidine analogues (cytosine arabinoside, 5-fluorouracil, oxyuridines)

DNA template function

Acridine dyes (proflavine, quinacrine)
Actinomycin
Bleomycin
Chloroquine
Lucanthone
Nitrogen and sulfur mustards
Quinine

Enzyme inhibition

Nalidixic acid
Rifampin

Drugs
interfering
with
intermediary
metabolism

Sulfonamides

FIG. 53-1. Mode of action of some antimicrobial and anticancer drugs.

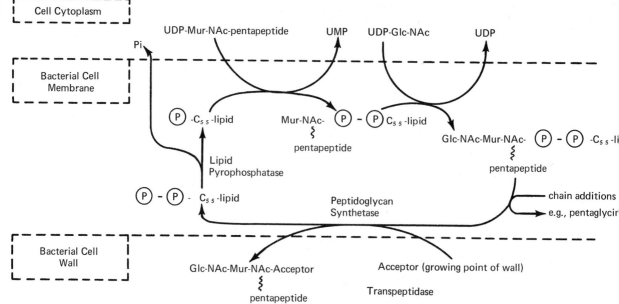

FIG. 53–2. Transport of peptidoglycan subunits in Staphylococcus aureus. The precise location of the enzymes within the membrane is not known.

adjacent peptidoglycans imparting stability to the wall. The pentapeptide of nascent peptidoglycans binds to a membrane bound transpeptidase forming an acyl-enzyme intermediate. The enzyme cleaves the terminal *D*-ala-*D*-ala bond, conserves the bond energy and utilizes it to form a new bond between the carboxyl group of the penultimate *D*-ala and the free amino group of either the diamino acid or the pentaglycine bridge in an adjacent peptidoglycan; the terminal *D*-ala is lost. In *E. coli,* the pentapeptide chains are joined together directly via peptide bonds, whereas in *Staph. aureus* cross-links are formed between the penultimate *D*-ala and an adjacent

pentaglycine bridge. Some peptide substituents do not form cross-links and have their terminal *D*-ala cleaved by a carboxypeptidase. Thus, although a *pentapeptide* is formed initially in *Staph. aureus* as part of the basic subunit, a *tetrapeptide* is the structure finally incorporated into the bacterial cell wall. Cross-linkage imparts unity and rigidity so that the final product resembles a wire netting fence. By virtue of the multiple cross-linkages, the bacterial cell wall can become one molecule composed of up to 12 or more peptidoglycan layers with, in some instances, a molecular weight of greater than 10^{12}.

ANTIMICROBIAL DRUGS INHIBITING BACTERIAL CELL WALL FORMATION

PENICILLIN AND CEPHALOSPORINS. As the first, and probably still the most clinically important antibiotic, penicillin G provided the impetus that led to our understanding of the reactions involving bacterial cell wall biosynthesis. All the other penicillins and all the cephalosporins probably act similarly to penicillin G.

Penicillin G can assume a structure similar to the acyl *D*-ala-*D*-ala end of the nascent peptidoglycan, probably binding covalently to the transpeptidase producing an inactive penicilloylated enzyme. This results in the accumulation of uncross-linked peptidoglycan chains and consequently the genesis of a "chain linked fence" without the links. In vitro, some subunits incorporated into nascent peptidoglycans during

growth in subinhibitory concentrations of penicillin G fail to cross-link on removal of the antibiotic. The reason for this is not clear, and its clinical importance with regards to premature termination of penicillin therapy is unknown.

Bacterial resistance to penicillins is achieved through modifications of the bacterium or the antibiotic; some resistant bacteria possess membrane lipopolysaccharides which prevent penicillin (methicillin) from reaching the appropriate transpeptidase (Table 52–2), whereas others destroy penicillin by penicillinases (β-lactamases) and amidase (Fig 55–1).

In vitro penicillin sensitive microorganisms grown in the presence of penicillin in a hypertonic (sucrose or sodium chloride) medium form protoplasts, which do not lyse; reconversion to normal shape and development occurs rapidly if the penicillin is washed out. This may have some clinical importance, as it is conceivable that bacteria might survive as viable protoplasts during therapy in sites where the medium is hypertonic, as in abscesses, osteomyelitis cavities or renal parenchyma. Thus, antibiotic inhibition of cell wall synthesis is not itself lethal but permits the growth of a defective-walled organism which ruptures under the force of its own osmotic pressure.

Bacterial persisters are cells which survive exposure to ostensibly lethal concentrations of bactericidal antibiotics, yet whose progeny remain fully sensitive to the agent; they occur about $1/10^6$ cells. The occurrence of persisters may explain recurrence of infection after "effective" antimicrobial therapy. Thus, if a small percentage of bacteria in a certain population are at a stage where their peptidoglycan coat is unbroken by peptidoglycan hydrolase, these cells cannot undergo growth and development until appropriate interpolation gaps are made. Penicillin and antibiotics depressing protein synthesis may inhibit hydrolase activity, thus selecting persisters.

CYCLOSERINE. By virtue of its similarity to *D*-ala (Ch. 55) cycloserine competitively inhibits alanine racemase and *D*-alanyl: *D*-alanine synthetase the enzymes required for the formation of the terminal *D*-ala-*D*-ala dipeptide of the peptidoglycan subunits. Since cycloserine acts through true competitive inhibition, its effect may be overcome by increasing the concentration of *D*-ala in the surrounding medium. Resistant mutants to cycloserine have been isolated that overcome inhibition through increased production of *D*-ala.

BACITRACIN, VANCOMYCIN, RISTOCETIN AND NOVOBIOCIN. Bacitracin is a specific inhibitor of membrane lipid pyrophosphatase (Fig. 53–2), probably by complexing with the lipid pyrophosphate portion of the peptidoglycan. It therefore deprives the growing cell of a necessary carrier, producing cessation of cell wall formation. Bacitracin also disrupts the bacterial cell membrane.

Vancomycin and **ristocetin** act similarly by inhibiting the action of the membrane polymerase, peptidoglycan synthetase (Fig. 53–2). They form stable 1:1 complexes with the moiety acyl-*D*-ala-*D*-ala presumably blocking peptidoglycan synthetase activity by altering the substrate. **Novobiocin** has been studied infrequently, but in vivo peptidoglycan residues accumulate in the presence of the drug, and it may also chelate magnesium cofactors.

ANTIBIOTICS AFFECTING THE BACTERIAL CELL MEMBRANE

The bacterial cell membrane (cytoplasmic membrane: cell envelope) is a semipermeable, triple layered, lipoprotein structure located between the cytoplasm and the cell wall. It is a dynamic structure, constantly undergoing modification, particularly during repair, growth and cell division, and possessing several vital functions. It poses an *osmotic barrier* between the interior and the exterior of the cell; it contains a *variety of enzymes* necessary for intermediary metabolism and cell wall formation and it contains various "binding proteins" and lipids responsible for the *transportation of amino acids and sugars,* etc., into the cell, and for transporting cell wall subunits out of the cell. Antibiotics may *disorganize membrane function, inhibit specific enzymes* involved in transport or growth or *alter ion permeability.*

Disorganization of Membrane Function

Drugs (surface active agents and polypeptide and polyene antibiotics) disorganizing membrane function are usually bactericidal. They possess well defined, but distinctly separated, hydrophobic and hydrophilic moieties which bind to complimentary portions in the membrane. Binding results in interference with the membranes' semipermeable properties, and essential substances such as purines, pyrimidines, sugars, amino acids and various ions are "leaked" (lost) from the cell.

Cationic surface active agents (e.g., CTAB, Ch. 62) possess a hydrophobic group such as a hydrocarbon chain or alkyl substituted benzene ring together with a positively charged hydrophilic moiety such as a quaternary ammonium group, etc. The activity of such agents increases with increasing pH, and substances of opposite charge may negate the effect. **Anionic surface active agents** (e.g., fatty acids, phenols) possess a hydrophobic group as described above in addition to a negatively charged hydrophilic group (carboxyl, sulfate, sulfonate, phosphate, etc.).

Polypeptide antibiotics (polymyxin B, colistin, tyrocidine) contain lipophilic and lipophobic groups and act like surface active agents. Sensitive bacteria bind and take up more antibiotic than resistant strains, and with polymyxin B there is a stoichiometric relationship between the quantity of drug present and the number of cells killed. Polymyxin B appears to bind to phosphate groups on the cell surface, and its activity can be reduced by soaps.

Polyene antibiotics contain a lactone ring (macrolides) which has a rigid hydrophobic polyene section and a flexible hydrophilic hydroxylated section. Polyenes complex with membrane sterols (primarily ergosterol) inducing breakdown of function; disorganization is proportional to the ratio of sterol : phospholipid, rather than to the presence of sterol per se. Polyenes may also produce specific blockade of nutrient uptake; e.g., nystatin blocks uptake of glycine at concentrations lower than those causing leakage of cell contents.

Inhibition of Specific Enzymes and Alteration in Permeability

Chlorhexidine, a potent inhibitor of bacterial cell membrane ATPase, inhibits growth, since ATPase is required for energy conversion and ion transport. Many other substances produce similar effects, but they are too toxic for human use. The gramicidins, along with several experimental antibiotics such as the macrotetralideactins, are cation conductors or "ionophores," consisting of cyclic molecules with lipophilic side chains oriented to the exterior of the molecule. Thus, by complexing cations in the center of the molecule they render them lipid soluble, enabling them to pass across membranes and be lost from the cell.

ANTIBIOTICS AFFECTING PROTEIN SYNTHESIS

Antibiotics affecting protein synthesis inhibit ribosomal function. However, little is known about the molecular basis of their action, since the structure, functions and interactions of ribosomes are still (often with the help of antibiotics) being elucidated. A brief review of protein synthesis (translation) will facilitate an appreciation of how important antibiotics may act (Fig. 53–3).

INITIATION. A 30S ribosomal subunit combines with mRNA and formylmethionyl-tRNA (f-met-tRNA), the latter at the A (amino acyl acceptor) site; a 50S subunit complexes to complete the 70S ribosome. The f-met-tRNA translocates to a second position, the P (peptidyl donor) site. Under some circumstances the f-met-tRNA may bind directly onto site P. At least three separate protein factors (F1, F2 and F3), not normally part of ribosomes, are necessary for initiation.

ELONGATION. The amino acyl-tRNA called for by the first mRNA codon binds to site A. Binding depends upon the formation of an amino acyl-tRNA-GTP complex with a "transfer factor" (TF 1). The complex delivers the amino-acyl-tRNA to site A with release of TF 1-GTP and Pi. Each binding step requires the splitting of one of GTP's high energy bonds. Then the f-met is transferred back to site A from site P under the influence of peptidyl transferase. Peptidyl transferase is a 50S ribosomal enzyme catalyzing peptide bond formation between the nascent peptide on site P to the amino acyl-tRNA on site A. This reaction results in polypeptide chain lengthening at its carboxy terminus by one amino acid residue. After peptide bond formation, the f-met-amino acyl-tRNA translocates to site P, displacing the discharged methionyl-tRNA and freeing site A for the next codon-directed amino acyl-tRNA. Translocation after peptide bond for-

mation requires the G(S_2) factor, and GTP is hydrolyzed to GDP and Pi in the process. *The puromycin reaction* (release of peptide from site A) is often referred to in analyzing drug effects on protein synthesis. Puromycin, an experimental anticancer drug, acts as an analog of amino acyl-tRNA. It binds to site A and takes part in peptide bond formation accepting the nascent polypeptide chain from site P, but since puromycin binds only weakly to ribosomes, the resultant peptidyl-puromycin moiety usually falls off the ribosome readily, and can be measured.

TERMINATION. Release of completed protein occurs when all the codons have been read; peptidyl transferase may be involved in the release mechanism. On termination, the 30S and 50S subunits dissociate, joining a pool of free subunits before combining with new mRNA.

Antibiotics Affecting Protein Synthesis

Chloramphenicol binds to the 50S subunit (approximately one molecule is bound per ribosome) inhibiting peptide bond formation. It may also inhibit mRNA : 30S ribosome attachment. The antibiotic blocks the puromycin reaction, possibly by inhibiting peptidyl transferase activity.

Streptomycin and other aminoglycosides interact with site A, causing instantaneous cessation of chain elongation by preventing adequate binding; additionally, they may prevent binding of amino acyl-tRNA to mRNA. Early studies suggested that the aminoglycosides caused misreading of the genetic code, but this is now considered artifactual.

Erythromycin and related macrolides bind to the 50S subunit inhibiting translocation between sites A and P. Additionally, they may block amino

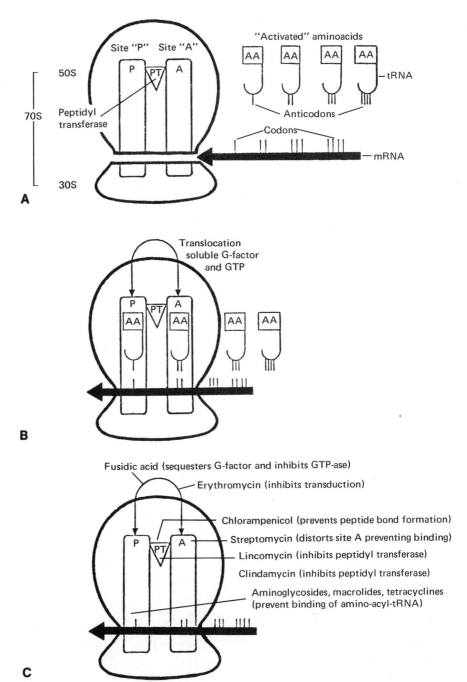

FIG. 53–3. Diagrammatic view of protein synthesis and mode of action of antibiotics interfering with protein synthesis. (A) Exploded diagrammatic view of the ribosomal components. (B) Diagrammatic view of an operational ribosome. (C) Antimicrobial drug targets.

acyl-tRNA binding to mRNA. In vitro, erythromycin prevents the attachment of chloramphenicol to the 50S subunit; the clinical importance of this interaction is unknown. **Lincomycin** and **clindamycin** inhibit peptidyl transferase activity and also prevent chloramphenicol binding.

The **tetracyclines** produce many effects, and it is impossible at present to separate out primary from secondary sites of action. They are excellent chelating agents (Ch. 57) and may bind necessary cofactors such as calcium, iron or magnesium. They also block binding of amino acyl-tRNA to mRNA and to site A.

Fusidic acid sequesters G factor and depresses GTPase activity, thus interfering with translocation.

Several antimicrobial and anticancer drugs interfere with nucleic acid synthesis in three general areas (Fig. 53–1 and 53–4).

Inhibition of Nucleotide Metabolism

INHIBITION OF DE NOVO PURINE AND PYRIMIDINE SYNTHESIS. Drugs inhibiting dihydrofolate reductase, an enzyme required for the synthesis of tetrahydrofolic acid, are of two classes: the anticancer folic acid analogs **methotrexate** and **aminopterin** (the "antifols"), and the antibacterial and antiprotozoal diaminopyrimines, **trimethoprim** and **pyrimethamine,** respectively. Tetrahydrofolic acid is required as a donor of one carbon units at several stages in purine, pyrimidine and methionine synthesis, and in the initiation of protein synthesis. Although the antifols inhibit dihydrofolate reductase from any source (mammalian or parasitic) in vitro, these agents possess no antibacterial or antiprotozoal properties in vivo. Conversely, the diaminopyrimidines possess no anticancer properties. There is a ready explanation for this apparent paradox.

Cells that require exogenous dihydrofolic acid (mammalian cells and most cancer cells) possess an active energy-requiring enzymic process for dihydrofolic acid uptake. The antifols, by virtue of their close structural similarity to the natural substrate, are readily taken up by the same system and inhibit dihydrofolate reductase intracellularly. The diaminopyrimidines, however, have no important inhibitory properties on mammalian dihydrofolate reductase since they penetrate poorly into mammalian and cancer cells, and their affinity for the enzyme is low. Bacteria

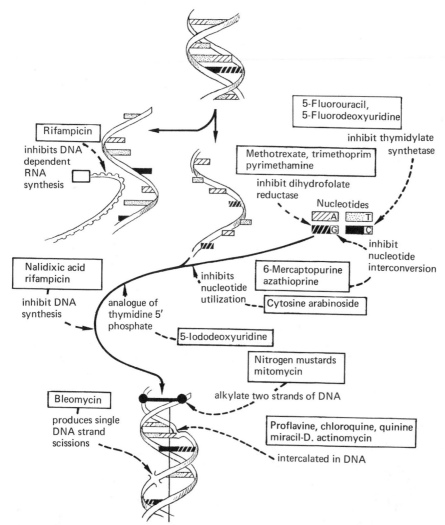

FIG. 53–4. Diagrammatic representation of the mode of action of drugs inhibiting nucleic acid metabolism.

and protozoa do not possess the active energy requiring process developed in mammalian cells for dihydrofolic acid uptake and must therefore synthesize their own de novo; thus, antifols have no significant antimicrobial properties. Trimethoprim and pyrimethamine, however, readily penetrate parasitic cells, and because of their higher affinity for parasitic dihydrofolate reductase than for the mammalian enzyme, they exhibit selective toxicity.

Pyrimethamine is primarily of value in the treatment of protozoal diseases such as malaria (Ch. 63), since the affinity of this agent is far greater for protozoal compared to bacterial dihydrofolate reductase. Conversely, trimethoprim possesses significant affinity for both bacterial and protozoal dihydrofolate reductase and thus is effective as an antibacterial (Ch. 60) and as an antiprotozoal agent (Ch. 63).

INHIBITORS OF NUCLEOTIDE INTERCONVERSION. 6-mercaptopurine (6-MP) and **azathioprine** (which converts in vivo to 6-MP by nonenzyme thiolysis) are metabolized to a nucleotide analog 6-thioinnosinic acid (Thio-IMP) that inhibits purine metabolism at a number of sites. **5-fluorouracil** and **5-fluorodeoxyuridine** are metabolized to 5-fluorodeoxy-UMP which inhibits thymidylate synthetase (Fig. 66–2), resulting in deprivation of thymine nucleotides and impairment of DNA synthesis.

INHIBITION OF NUCLEOTIDE UTILIZATION. Cytosine arabinoside (Ch. 66) inhibits nucleotide utilization, but its precise mode of action is not clear.

ANALOGS WHICH BECOME INCORPORATED INTO POLYNUCLEOTIDES. Many naturally occurring and synthetic analogs of nucleic acid components possess the normal sugars ribose and 2′-deoxyribose attached to purine and pyrimidine bases. These agents can become phosphorylated intercellulary to the triphosphate level and serve as unnatural substrates for DNA and RNA polymerization reactions, distorting the structure and properties of nucleic acid. For example, **5-bromodeoxyuridine** (BUdR) and **5-iododeoxyuridine** (IUdR) replace thymidine 5′ phosphate in DNA (Fig. 66–2), presumably leading to base-paring errors during replication

and transcription of viral DNA, with resulting impairment of the fidelity of gene expression.

Inhibition of DNA Template Function

Drugs may interfere nonspecifically with the role of DNA as a template in replication and transcription by reacting directly to form a complex, or by reacting indirectly to cause structural alterations. Such interference inhibits DNA and RNA polymerase activity.

DRUGS COMPLEXING WITH DNA. Drugs can complex covalently, noncovalently or through electrostatic binding (insertion—intercalation). For example, the **acridine dyes** (proflavine, quinacrine, neutral red), **chloroquine, quinine, lucanthone** (Miracil-D) and **actinomycin** intercalate between adjacent base pairs of the double helix.

DRUGS CAUSING STRUCTURAL ALTERATIONS IN DNA. **Mitomycin C** and the bifunctional **nitrogen** and **sulfur mustards** covalently bind as bifunctional alkylating agents to two sites of DNA (one on each strand) inhibiting its function as a template. Binding is accompanied by massive degradation of preexisting DNA but no alteration in RNA and protein synthesis. **Bleomycin** causes formation of single strand scissions (breaks) in the sugar phosphate backbone of DNA.

Inhibitors of Enzymic Processes in Nucleic Acid Synthesis

INHIBITORS OF RNA POLYMERASE. Rifampin is the most potent inhibitor known for DNA-dependent RNA polymerase in bacteria; DNA-dependent polymerase from eukaryotic cells, however, is not effected. Rifampin binds to RNA polymerase and blocks initiation of RNA synthesis. Rifampin-resistant bacteria produce DNA-dependent RNA polymerase which does not bind the antibiotic.

INHIBITORS OF DNA REPLICATION. Nalidixic acid inhibits DNA synthesis probably by interfering with specific enzymes. It is surprising that nalidixic acid possesses such activity, since it is a negatively charged compound and thus would not be expected to bind to the strongly negatively charged DNA.

DRUGS INTERFERING WITH INTERMEDIARY METABOLISM

Numerous drugs interfere with microbial intermediary metabolism, but little is known of their precise mode of action; only the sulfonamides are considered here.

Sulfonamides

All bacteria require dihydrofolic acid for the synthesis of folic acid cofactors. Sulfonamide-

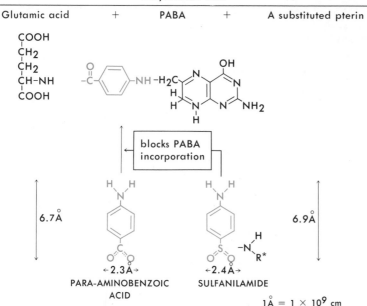

Dihydrofolic acid

| Glutamic acid | + | PABA | + | A substituted pterin |

PARA-AMINOBENZOIC ACID

SULFANILAMIDE

6.7Å

6.9Å

←2.3Å→

←2.4Å→

blocks PABA incorporation

$1\overset{\circ}{A} = 1 \times 10^9$ cm

FIG. 53–5. The dimensions of para-aminobenzoic acid and sulfanilamide and the mode of action of the sulfa drugs. **Asterisk** indicates the R in sulfanilamide, the site of N^1 substitutions, which is out of the plane of the main drug molecule and therefore does not prevent attachment of the sulfa onto the appropriate receptor. (Part of this figure is from Albert A (1960): Selective Toxicity. New York, Wiley p. 103.)

sensitive bacteria cannot assimilate performed dihydrofolic acid from the environment but must synthesize it de novo from precursors. Man requires preformed dihydrofolic acid. Dihydrofolic acid is synthesized in two steps. Under the influence of dihydrofolate synthetase, para-aminobenzoic acid and a substituted pterin form a dihydropteroate, which subsequently combines with glutamic acid forming dihydrofolic acid. Because of the close structural similarity between sulfonamides (as typified in Fig. 53–5 by sulfanilamide) and para-aminobenzoic acid (PABA), the sulfas reduce the synthesis of dihydrofolic acid either by *inhibiting dihydrofolate synthetase* or by, under certain circumstances, becoming incorporated by dihydrofolate synthetase into a *nonfunctional dihydropteroate.*

Although sulfonamides inhibit the synthesis of dihydrofolic acid in sensitive organisms immediately on exposure, there is a lag phase of several cell cycles during which growth continues normally. Presumably this growth is dependent upon stored cofactors. In vitro studies have shown that one molecule of PABA can competitively antagonize the bacteriostatic activity of 5,000–25,000 molecules of sulfanilamide, and in vivo bacteriosasis induced by sulfonamides is reversed by PABA and PABA-containing drugs, competitively.

Combination of a sulfonamide with trimethoprim or pyrimethamine (inhibitors of dihydrofolate reductase) results in a double sequential attack on folic acid metabolism (Ch. 60 sulfamethoxazole–trimethoprim).

Further Reading

Gale EF, Cundliffe E, Reynolds PE, Richmond MH, Waring MJ (1972): The Molecular Basis of Antibiotic Action. New York, Wiley and Sons

Hash JJ (1972): Antibiotic mechanisms. Annu Rev Pharmacol 12:35–56

JEREMY H. THOMPSON

54. DRUGS OF CHOICE FOR COMMON INFECTIONS

Chapters 55 through 66 describe the important antiparasitic agents. Since the classification and description of these drugs bear little relation to their current therapeutic usage, a summary table is presented here in an attempt to place each drug in the perspective of its clinical usefulness (Table 54–1). This table is only a *rough guide* to therapy based upon current opinions and should not be taken as absolute.

There are a number of drugs of proven therapeutic efficacy and safety used widely outside the United States but not available in this country through over-the-counter sales or through prescription. This unfortunate state of affairs exists since the demand for these drugs is small, and no American pharmaceutical firm has the time or money to spend in seeking FDA approval for these agents. These drugs are available, however, from the Center for Disease Control for use in specific disease states (Table 54–2).

The recommendation of a drug or drugs of choice for any specific infection is frequently debatable, since for some infections the physician may have available several drugs of approximately equal value. For the rational treatment of infections caused by bacterial species with variable antibiotic sensitivity patterns, e.g., enterobacter, bacteroides, *E. coli* proteus, pseudomonas and *Staph. spp.,* antibiotic susceptibility tests are mandatory. Furthermore, the selection of an antibiotic in other infections should also be based if at all possible, on the result of a culture and sensitivity determination. Sensitivity patterns of many bacteria vary between different hospitals reflecting primarily the degree of use of specific antibiotics. Other important factors determining antibiotic selection are the site and severity of infection, the presence of antibiotic allergy, the state of renal and hepatic function and other host factors (Ch. 52).

Drugs of choice for the following groups of diseases are listed elsewhere; for tuberculosis, Tables 56–3 and 56–4; for protozoal disease, Table 63–1; and mycotic infections, Tables 65–1, 65–2 and 65–3.

TABLE 54–1. Antimicrobial Drugs Commonly Used for Certain Infections (Drugs are listed Alphabetically in Each Category)

Organism	Clinical illness	Drugs of choice Primary	Drugs of choice Secondary (when indicated)
Alcaligenes faecalis	Various wound and urinary tract infections	Chloramphenicol, colistin, polymyxin B, sulfonamides	Gentamicin, kanamycin, neomycin, penicillin G, streptomycin, tetracyclines
Bacillus anthracis	Anthrax	Penicillin G	Cephalosporins, chloramphenicol, clindamycin, erythromycin, lincomycin penicillinase-resistant penicillins*, sulfonamides, tetracyclines
Bacteroides (various)	Bacteremia, various wound and urinary tract infections	Chloramphenicol Penicillin G	Ampicillin, carbenicillin, clindamycin, erythromycin, tetracyclines
Bartonella bacilliformis	Oroya fever	Chloramphenicol	Penicillin G, streptomycin, tetracyclines
Bordetella pertussis	Whooping cough	Erythromycin	Ampicillin, Chloramphenicol, tetracyclines
Brucella recurrentis (*Borrelia recurrentis*)	Relapsing fever	Tetracyclines	Chloramphenicol, penicillin G
Brucellae (various)	Brucellosis	Streptomycin plus tetracyclines, tetracyclines	Chloramphenicol plus streptomycin, erythromycin, kanamycin, streptomycin, sulfonamides
Calymmatobacterium granulomatis	Granuloma inguinale	Tetracyclines	Ampicillin and streptomycin
Clostridia (various)	Botulism, gas gangrene, tetanus	Antitoxin, penicillin G, tetracyclines	Erythromycin, Gentamicin
Corynebacterium diphtheriae	Diphtheria and the carrier state	Antitoxin, erythromycin penicillin G	Cephalosporins, clindamycin
Coxiella burnetii	Q fever	Tetracyclines	Chloramphenicol
Diplococcus pneumoniae	Arthritis, endocarditis, meningitis, otitis media, peritonitis, pharyngitis	Ampicillin, cephalosporins, penicillin G	Clindamycin, erythromycin, lincomycin, penicillinase-resistant penicillins,* tetracyclines
Enterobacter (aerobacter) spp.	Various wound and urinary tract infections	Gentamicin, carbenicillin, kanamycin	Ampicillin, cephalosporins colistin, nalidixic acid,† nitrofurantoin,† polymyxin B, sulfonamides, tetracyclines
Enterococci (streptococci of group D)	Bacteremia, bacterial endocarditis, various wound and urinary tract infections	Ampicillin plus streptomycin, penicillin G plus kanamycin, gentamicin, or streptomycin	Erythromycin plus streptomycin, tetracyclines, tetracyclines plus streptomycin, vancomycin
Erysipelothrix rhusiopathiae (*insidiosa*)	Erysipeloid	Penicillin G	Chloramphenicol, erythromycin, tetracyclines
Escherichia coli	Gastroenteritis	Ampicillin, carbenicillin, neomycin, polymyxin B, tetracyclines	Kanamycin
Escherichia coli	Urinary tract infections	Gentamicin,† nitrofurantoin,† sulfonamides†	Ampicillin,† cephalosporins,† chloramphenicol,† methenamine mandelate,† nalidixic acid†
Fusobacterium fusiformis (plus *Treponema vincentii*)	Vincent's angina	Penicillin G	Chloramphenicol, erythromycin, tetracyclines
Haemophilus ducreyi	Chancroid	Chloramphenicol, tetracyclines	Penicillin G, streptomycin, sulfonamides
Haemophilus influenzae	Bronchopneumonia, conjunctivitis, meningitis, otitis media	Ampicillin, chloramphenicol plus sulfonamides	Erythromycin, streptomycin plus sulfonamides, tetracyclines
Klebsiella spp	Osteomyelitis, pneumonia, urinary tract infections	Cephalosporins plus kanamycin, chloramphenicol plus streptomycin, gentamicin, or kanamycin, tetracyclines plus sulfonamides	Colistin, polymyxin B, sulfonamides
Large viruses (chlamydiae)	Ornithosis/psittacosis, trachoma, lymphogranuloma venereum, inclusion conjunctivitis	Chloramphenicol, tetracyclines	Erythromycin, sulfonamides
Leptospira canicola	Similar to Weil's disease	Penicillin G, tetracyclines	Clindamycin, lincomycin

TABLE 54—1. *(continued)*

Organism	Clinical illness	Drugs of choice	
		Primary	Secondary (when indicated)
Leptospira icterohae-morrhagiae	Weil's disease	Penicillin G, tetracyclines	Clindamycin, lincomycin
Listeria monocytogenes	Bacteremia, meningitis, Granulomata	Penicillin G	Ampicillin, chloramphenicol, erythromycin, kanamycin, tetracyclines
Mycobacteria (atypical)	Respiratory infections	Ethionamide, ethambutol	Erythromycin, streptomycin
Mycobacterium leprae	Leprosy	Sulfones	Cycloserine, thiosemicarbazones
Mycoplasma pneumoniae	"Atypical viral pneumonia"	Tetracyclines	Chloramphenicol, erythromycin, streptomycin
Neisseria gonorrhoeae	Gonorrhea: arthritis, endocarditis, genital infections	Penicillin G	Ampicillin, cephalosporins, clindamycin, erythromycin, kanamycin, lincomycin, penicillinase-resistant penicillins,* spiramycin, spectinomycin, sulfonamides, tetracyclines
Neisseria meningitidis	Bacteremia, meningitis	Penicillin G	Ampicillin, cephalosporins, chloramphenicol, erythromycin, sulfonamides, tetracyclines
Pasteurella pestis	Plague	Streptomycin, streptomycin plus sulfonamides, sulfonamides	Chloramphenicol, neomycin, penicillin G, polymyxin B, tetracyclines
Pasteurella (Francisella) tularensis	Tularemia	Streptomycin	Chloramphenicol, tetracyclines
Pasteurella multocida	Bacteremia, various infections	Penicillin G	Cephalosporins, erythromycin, tetracyclines
Pfeifferella (Actinobacillus) mallei	Glanders	Streptomycin plus sulfonamides, streptomycin plus tetracyclines	Chloramphenicol plus streptomycin
Pfeifferella whitmori	Melioidosis	Chloramphenicol plus streptomycin, tetracyclines	Kanamycin, streptomycin plus sulfonamides
Proteus (various)	Various urinary tract and wound infections	Gentamicin, kanamycin	Ampicillin, carbenicillin, cephalosporins, chloramphenicol, methenamine mandelate†, neomycin, nitrofurantoin†, streptomycin, sulfonamides, tetracyclines
Providencia	Various infections	Carbenicillin	Kanamycin, gentamicin
Pseudomonas aeruginosa	Various wound and urinary tract infections	Carbenicillin, Colistin, gentamicin, polymyxin B	Kanamycin, sulfonamides, tetracyclines
Rickettsiae (various)	Brills disease, Q fever, Rocky Mountain Spotted fever, typhus	Chloramphenicol, tetracyclines	Erythromycin, oleandomycin/troleandomycin
Salmonellae (various)	Typhoid and paratyphoid fevers	Ampicillin, chloramphenicol	Cephalosporins, colistin kanamycin, penicillin G, polymyxin B, trimethoprim plus sulfamethoxazole
Serratia marcessens	Various opportunistic infections	Gentamicin	Carbenicillin, chloramphenicol kanamycin
Shigellae (various)	Bacillary dysentery	Ampicillin, cephalosporins, sulfonamides	Chloramphenicol, colistin, kanamycin, polymyxin B, streptomycin, tetracyclines
Spirillum minus	Rat-bite fever	Penicillin G	Erythromycin, streptomycin, tetracyclines
Staphylococcus aureus (non-penicillinase-producing)	Various infections: abscesses, pneumonia, meningitis, osteomyelitis	Penicillin G	Bacitracin, cephalosporins, chloramphenicol, clindamycin erythromycin, gentamicin, kanamycin, lincomycin, nitrofurantoin†, oleandomycin/troleandomycin, spiramycin, streptomycin, tetracyclines, vancomycin
Staphylococcus aureus (penicillinase-producing)	Various infections: abscesses, bacteremia, endocarditis, acute pneumonia, meningitis, osteomyelitis	Cephalosporins, penicillinase-resistant penicillins*	Clindamycin, erythromycin, fucidin, gentamicin, kanamycin, lincomycin, oleandomycin/troleandomycin, spiramycin, vancomycin
Streptobacillus moniliformis	Rat-bite fever	Penicillin G	Erythromycin, streptomycin, tetracyclines

TABLE 54–1. *(continued)*

Organism	Clinical illness	Drugs of choice	
		Primary	Secondary (when indicated)
Streptococci (anaerobic)	Bacteremia, endocarditis, various wound infections	Penicillin G	Erythromycin, tetracyclines
Streptococcus pyogenes	Various infections: bacteremia, cellulitis erysipelas, otitis media, pharyngitis, pneumonia, scarlet fever	Penicillin G	Ampicillin, cephalosporins, clindamycin, erythromycin, lincomycin, penicillinase-resistant penicillins*
Streptococcus viridans	Oral infections, subacute bacterial endocarditis, urinary tract infections	Cephalosporins, penicillin G plus streptomycin, penicillin G	Ampicillin, cephalosporins, clindamycin, erythromycin, lincomycin, penicillinase-resistant penicillins,* vancomycin
Treponema duttoni	Trick-borne relapsing fever	Tetracyclines	Chloramphenicol, erythromycin, penicillin G
Treponema pallidum	Syphilis	Penicillin G	Arsenical salts, bismuth salts, cephalosporins, erythromycin, tetracyclines
Treponema pertenue	Yaws	Penicillin G	Bismuth salts, erythromycin, tetracyclines
Treponema recurrentis	Louse-borne relapsing fever	Tetracyclines	Chloramphenicol, penicillin G
Treponema vincentii (plus *Fusobacterium fusiformis*)	Vincent's angina	Penicillin G	Erythromycin, tetracyclines
Vibrio cholerae	Cholera	Tetracyclines	Chloramphenicol, erythromycin, streptomycin, sulfonamides

* Cloxacillin, dicloxacillin, methicillin, etc., Table 55–3
† Used for urinary tract infections only.

TABLE 54–2. Non FDA-Approved Drugs for Specific Disease Entities

Chemical name	Proprietary name	Indication
Bayer 2502	—	*Trypanosoma cruzi* infection (Chagas' disease)
Bithional *N.F.*	Lorothidol	Paragonimiasis
Dehydroemetine	—	Amebiasis
Melarsoprol	Arsobal, Mel B	*Trypanosoma gambiense* and *T. rhodesiense* infections of the CNS (African sleeping sickness)
Niclosamide	Yomesan	Various Helmintic infections (Table 64–1)
Niridazole	Ambilhar	Schistosomiasis, Dracunculiasis
Pentamidine	Lomidine	*Pneumocystis carinii* pneumonia, *Trypanosoma gambiense* infection
Sodium antimony dimercaptosuccinate	Astiban	Schistosomiasis
Sodium antimony gluconate	Pentostam	Leishmaniasis
Suramin (Bayer 205)	Antrypol	Early *Trypanosoma rhodesiense* infection

Drugs obtained from the Parasitic Disease Drug Service, Center for Disease Control, United States Public Health Service, Atlanta, Georgia

JEREMY H. THOMPSON

55. ANTIBIOTICS WHICH INTERFERE WITH THE BACTERIAL CELL WALL

Several important antimicrobial agents interfere with the biosynthesis of bacterial cell walls (Fig. 53–1). Of these, the most important are the **penicillins** and the **cephalosporins** and bacitracin, cycloserine and vancomycin (Table 55–1);

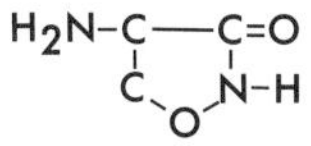

$$H_2N-C-C=O$$
$$C \quad N-H$$
$$O$$

CYCLOSERINE

ristocetin and novobiocin are not discussed since they are clinically obsolete. Most of the antibiotics described in this chapter act during the logarithmic phase of bacterial cell growth and have little or no effect on nongrowing organisms. The potential for antagonism of these drugs by bacteriostatic antibiotics is obvious and has been discussed above (Ch. 52).

THE PENICILLINS

HISTORY

At St. Mary's Hospital, London, in 1928, Alexander Fleming (later Sir Alexander Fleming) observed that a contaminating mold on one of his staphylococcal culture plates caused the adjacent bacterial colonies to undergo lysis. This mold, (*Penicillium notatum*), grown in broth culture was bactericidal in vitro against a variety of organisms; Fleming named the antibacterial principle **penicillin.** Desultory research continued on penicillin until 1939, when under the stimulus of World War II, Howard Walter Florey (later Sir Howard Florey) and Ernst Boris Chain, at the Sir William Dunn School of Pathology, Oxford University, England, began intensive work on this problem. Crude penicillin G became available for limited therapeutic trials in 1941; supplies were at first so scanty that the antibiotic was recovered from patients urine. In 1942 various centers in the United States undertook mass production of penicillin, since facilities were not available in England owing to the pressures of World War II. By 1943, sufficient quantities of the antibiotic were being produced to serve the allied forces, and in 1944 the antibiotic became available for limited civilian use.

The biosynthesis of penicillins up to 1958/9 depended upon the growth of *Penicillium notatum*

and *P. chrysogenum* in deep vat culture. It was fortuitously found that by adding various chemicals to this fermentation process a variety of new penicillins were produced by the mold (e.g., phenylacetic acid to induce penicillin G), and by international agreement these antibiotics were designated with letters of the alphabet; B, F, G, K, O, etc. However, the capacity of the molds to add new side chains was limited, and of all the early penicillins, only penicillin G has survived. Penicillin G (sodium penicillin G, sodium benzylpenicillinate, sodium benzylpenicillin) is the penicillin prototype, and **on a weight basis, provided an organism is susceptible, it is still the most potent.**

Unfortunately, penicillin G has several shortcomings. It is acid labile and therefore variably destroyed following oral administration; it is destroyed by bacterial β-lactamase(s) (penicillinase(s)); it has a relatively narrow antibacterial spectrum; it is rapidly excreted from the body; it penetrates poorly into tissue compartments, e.g., the cerebrospinal fluid and it is antigenic. When, in 1958, the basic penicillin nucleus, 6-aminopenicillanic acid (6-APA), was isolated, it became possible to add synthetically a multitude of side chains, producing a range of penicillins that collectively surmount the first four shortcomings of penicillin G. Although there are many differences

TABLE 55-1. Miscellaneous Bacterial Cell Wall Inhibitors

Drug	Source and properties	Adverse effects	Preparations, dosage and usage
Bacitracin	Bacitracin is the generic name for a group of at least four separate bactericidal polypeptide antibiotics, originally isolated from *Bacillus subtilis* contaminating a compound fracture in a young girl called Margaret Tracy; hence its name. About 80% of most commercial preparations is bacitracin A, a cyclic decapeptide with a molecular weight of about 1500 and containing a thiazolidine ring structure. Bacitracin has a gram-positive antibacterial spectrum resembling that of penicillin G and some activity against neisseriae and *H. influenzae*. Bacterial resistance is rare but may develop slowly. Antibacterial cross resistance has not been described Rapid absorption occurs following parenteral administration, drug clearance being by glomerular filtration. Bacitracin is given rarely for a local effect in the bowel lumen, since it is poorly absorbed. Some antibiotic inactivation may occur in the stomach from gastric acid	Bacitracin is safe when used topically, but following oral administration, superinfections and gastrointestinal upsets may occur. Parenteral administration is frequently followed by cutaneous hypersensitivity reactions, and renal toxicity, principally due to degeneration of the epithelium of the convoluted tubules. Renal toxicity results in proteinuria or hematuria in 30—70% of patients within the first week of therapy, but withdrawal of the antibiotic is required only if there is evidence of progressive renal impairment. Damage can be reduced by maintaining a high urinary output. In some individuals the cutaneous hypersensitivity reactions show cross reactivity to kanamycin and neomycin	Bacitracin, *U.S.P.* (Baciguent), is available in a wide range of topical preparations, usually in a concentration of 500 units/g; 1 unit is equivalent to the activity of 26 μg of the *U.S.P.* standard. Preparations for ophthalmic and dermatologic use usually contain in addition, neomycin, polymyxin B or tyrothricin; cutaneous hypersensitivity rarely results from continued topical use. The usual oral dose (rarely prescribed) of bacitracin is 20,000—30,000 units 3 times a day. Not more than 100,000 units a day should be injected IM, in divided doses; procaine hydrochloride should be added to reduce pain. Intrathecal bacitracin should never be more concentrated than 1000 units/ml, for a total of 5000 or 10,000 units
Cycloserine	A broad spectrum, bactericidal antibiotic, produced by *Streptomyces orchidaceus*. Its use should ordinarily be restricted to the treatment of tuberculosis. Mycobacterial resistance develops slowly and cross resistance has not been described Following oral administration rapid and almost total	Adverse reactions are dose-dependent and are more likely with blood levels greater than 50 μg/ml. With doses of 1 g or more daily, they can be expected in over 25% of patients, but this figure falls to about 2—5% with doses of 500 mg daily. Reactions may occur at any time, but most commonly appear within the	It is recommended that initial dosage of cycloserine (Oxamycin, Seromycin) be low (250 mg daily), and that this be increased over a 2 wk period to 250-500 mg twice daily

	absorption occurs, mainly from the stomach and upper small bowel. Cycloserine passes freely to most tissues and to the cerebrospinal fluid, and it is so diffusible that growth of bacilli inside macrophages may be inhibited. After conventional dosage, blood levels usually average 15—35 μg/ml. In prolonged therapy it is advisable periodically to check plasma drug levels, because cumulation may occur Cycloserine is partially degraded in the body, but 60—70% of an oral dose is excreted unchanged in the urine by glomerular filtration. Because the drug reaches high concentrations in the urine and is more effective at an acid pH, cycloserine is of special value in the treatment of renal tuberculosis. Cycloserine inhibits the metabolism of diphenylhydantoin	first 2 or 3 wk of therapy. Headaches, tremors, hyperreflexia, dysarthria, petit or grand mal (in 5—10%), vertigo, sleepiness or excitement, acute psychotic episodes (in 2 or 3%), and allergic dermatitis are not unusual. Seizures and psychotic episodes are more likely in those with a history of epilepsy and mood disturbances, such as depression or anxiety, and in those taking alcohol. Pyridoxine (100 mg daily), sedatives, tranquilizers or anticonvulsants may be administered with cycloserine in an attempt to reduce the CNS symptoms	
Vancomycin	A bactericidal antibiotic obtained from *Streptomyces orientalis*, primarily effective against gram-positive organisms; bacterial resistance is rare Minimal absorption follows oral administration, and since IM administration is painful, the antibiotic is usually given IV. The distribution and metabolic fate of vancomycin are unknown, but therapeutically effective cerebrospinal fluid levels do not occur in spite of the fact that only about 10% of the antibiotic is protein bound. Excreted by the kidney, 80% of an IV dose being cleared within 12—16 hr. Thus, patients with poor renal function rapidly achieve seriously high serum drug levels with conventional therapy	A relatively dangerous drug, chills, fever, allergic skin rashes, thrombophlebitis and anaphylactoid reactions occur, and superinfections with gram-negative bacteria and fungi may appear during long-term therapy. The most serious reactions are those involving the kidney and the eighth cranial nerve (cochlea). In both these instances lesions may progress despite drug withdrawal if renal function is inadequate impairing excretion	Sterile Vancomycin Hydrochloride, *U.S.P.* (Vancocin), in doses of 1 g IV, is given to adults twice daily, The usual dose for children is 44 mg/kg daily. Oral vancomycin 3—4 g daily, may be of value (with or without systemic administration) in the treatment of staphylococcal enterocolitis Vancomycin should not be used indiscriminately. It should be reserved for the treatment of seriously ill patients with gram-positive (particularly staphylococcal) infections resistant to less toxic antibiotics. It is widely used in hemodialysis patients to suppress staphylococcal shunt infections since it is not dialysable

among the various types of penicillin, a single and unified description of these drugs is presented. This is followed by a description of the more important penicillins and their properties; the generic term **penicillin** is used throughout to include the natural, the synthetic and the semisynthetic penicillins. New penicillins are being continually introduced, necessitating a full understanding of the properties of the older agents.

SOURCE

Commercial penicillin has been prepared from *P. notatum* and *P. chrysogenum.* Current production utilizes the 6-APA nucleus [obtained through the action of bacterial amidases (Fig. 55–1) on regular penicillin], with subsequent chemical manipulations. The 6-APA nucleus is also produced by *P. notatum* if no amino acids are available in deep vat culture, but the yield is small and the method complex and impractical. Total in vitro chemical synthesis of penicillin has been achieved, but the process has no commercial usefulness.

Natural penicillin is probably synthesized by fungi from residues of valine, cysteine and *L*-aminoadipic acid.

CHEMISTRY

The basic structure of all penicillins (Figure 55–1) is a sulfur containing thiazolidine ring (1), fused to a β-lactam ring, (2) upon which antibacterial activity depends, and a side chain (R″) which determines the individual penicillin characteristics (Table 55–4) the moiety R′ is the site of salt formation. Bacterial β-lactamase (penicillinase) and acids, such as gastric acid, and dilute bases, and primary or secondary amines, hydrolyze penicillin to pencilloic acid by breaking the β-lactam ring (3). Penicilloic acid has no antibacterial activity but is allergenic.

Penicillin salts, usually those of sodium and potassium, are stable for many months in the powder form, but they rapidly decompose to penicilloic acid and other metabolites following reconstitution with various solutions. Thus, solutions must be freshly prepared to ensure adequate antibacterial therapy and to minimize the infusion of potentially allergenic compounds.

Penicillin G and other acid labile penicillins are rapidly inactivated at an acid pH. Additionally, all penicillins are rapidly inactivated at an alkaline pH in the presence of carbohydrate; the mechanism of this inactivation is not known. Aqueous suspensions of procaine and benzathine penicillin G are stable for many months.

Measurement

The early natural penicillins were impure substances, and consequently measurement in international units by microbiologic assay (Ch. 5) was required. **The international unit of penicillin** is the specific penicillin activity contained in $0.6\mu g$ of the International Penicillin Master Standard, a sample of crystalline sodium penicillin G. The semisynthetic penicillins derived from 6-APA are

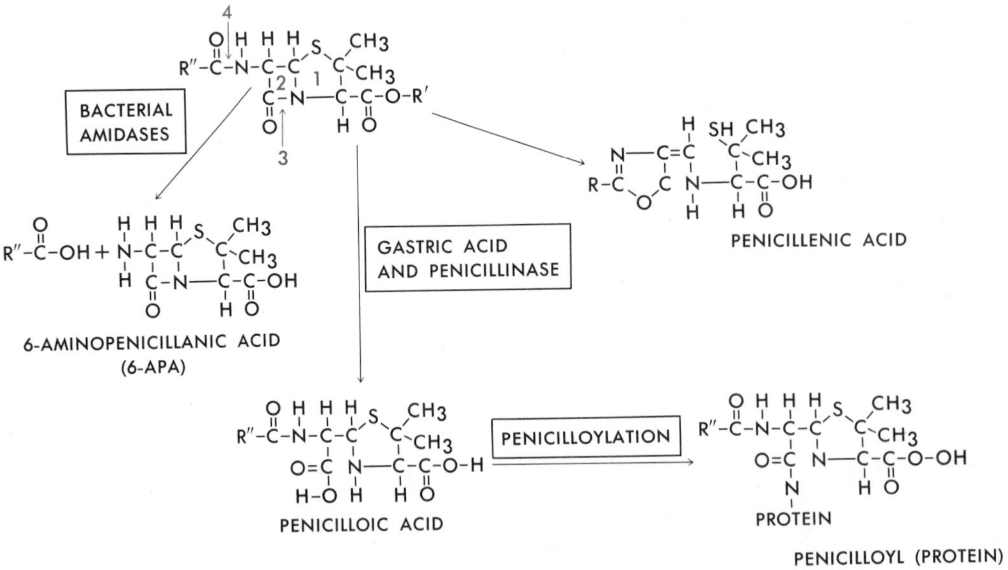

FIG. 55–1. **Penicillin, and various derivatives.** (1) thiazolidine ring; (2) β-lactam ring; (3) site of cleavage of the β-lactam ring by acid, penicillinase, etc: (4) site of cleavage by bacterial amidases; R′, site of salt formation; R″, site of side chain conferring individual penicillin characteristics.

measured in milligrams, and 1 mg of crystalline sodium penicillin G equals 1667 units. Because of the difference in atomic weight among sodium, potassium, calcium, etc., the equivalent penicillin salts have slightly different unit values. In clinical practice penicillin is usually measured either in milligrams or in megaunits (1,000,000 international units).

Antibacterial Spectrum

Apart from the recent "broad spectrum" penicillins, penicillin has a relatively narrow range of activity (Table 55–2). It is highly effective against most cocci, both gram-positive and gram-negative, although many strains of the staphylococcus are now resistant.

Mode of Action

Penicillin prevents the normal synthesis of bacterial cell walls (Ch. 53). It is a bactericidal antibi-

TABLE 55–2. Common Organisms Affected by Penicillin G

Organism	Sensitivity
Actinomyces israelii	++
Alcaligenes faecalis	+
Bacillus anthracis	++R
Bacillus subtilis	++R
Bacteroides spp	++
Bordetella pertussis	++
Borrelia	++
Clostridia	++
Corynebacterium diphtheriae	++R
Diplococcus pneumoniae	+++
Enterobacter aerogenes	+R
Erysipelothrix rhusiopathiae	+++
Escherichia coli	++R
Haemophilus ducreyi	++
Haemophilus influenzae	++
Klebsiella pneumoniae	+R
Leptospira icterohaemorrhagiae	++
Listeria monocytogenes	++
Neisseria gonorrhoeae	+++
Neisseria meningitidis	+++
Pasturella multocida	++
Pasturella pestis	+
Proteus mirabilis	++
Oroteus vulgaris	R
Salmonellae	++R
Shigellae	++R
Spirillum minor	++
Staphlococci	+++R
Streptobacillus moniliformis	++
Streptococci (groups A, C, G, H, L)	+++
Streptococci (groups B, E, F, K, N)	++R
Streptococci (group D)	+R
Treponema pallidum	+++
Treponema pertenue	++

R	In vitro testing essential, as many strains are penicillin-resistant
+++	High sensitivity
++	Moderate sensitivity
+	Some sensitivity (penicillin G not recommended for therapy)

otic, acting maximally during the logarithmic phase of cell growth. In some gram-negative bacteria penicillin may be more effective near the stationary growth phase rather than during logarithmic growth.

BACTERIAL RESISTANCE

Bacterial resistance to the penicillins is generally due to the elaboration of β-lactamases (penicillinases) which split the β-lactam ring (Figure 55–1); with the penicillinase-resistant penicillins, bacterial resistance is due to failure of antibiotic penetration (Table 52–2). Bacterial resistance is a major therapeutic problem, especially with staphylococci carried by medical and paramedical personnel in hospital environments. For example, during 1944/46, 10–20% of isolates of *Staph, aureus* were resistant to penicillin G, but by 1950 and 1960, the resistance rates were 50% and 80%, respectively.

Organisms developing resistance in vivo seldom revert to a sensitive strain, though their pathogenic and antigenic activity usually remain unimpaired. *Acquired penicillin resistance develops in a stepwise manner and may be delayed by a dose sufficiently large to overcome the emergence of first step mutants.* Some strains of microorganisms, e.g., pneumococci and *Strep. pyogenes,* rarely develop penicillin resistance in spite of the frequency with which infections caused by these organisms have been treated with the antibiotic.

Resistance to penicillinase in penicillinase resistant penicillins depends upon side chain R'' additions (Table 55–4) which diminish greatly the affinity between β-lactamase and the antibiotic at therapeutic concentrations. For example, the K_m for methicillin (concentration at $1/2$ V_{max}) is about 7000 μg/ml, and yet therapeutic drug levels are about 10 μg/ml at which point the degree of penicillinase activity is diminished about 1000-fold. Bacterial resistance to methicillin has become a severe therapeutic problem since about 50% of the strains are also resistant to cephalosporins.

β-LACTAMASES. Several β-lactamases are known, none being exclusively a penicillinase or a cephalosporinase (see below). Some microorganisms produce more than one type. Typically, β-lactamases from different microorganisms possess varying activities against the different β-lactam antibiotics. Penicillinase can be either exocellular or endocellular and may be constitutive or inducible, e.g., by methicillin, oxacillin and nafcillin. Penicillinase produced by host flora in the gut lumen is not absorbed into the general circulation to inactivate systemically administered penicillin.

Adverse Reactions

The incidence of adverse penicillin reactions is about 10–15% and of these about 10–15% are serious. Adverse penicillin reactions are divided into **sensitivity** (immediate, accelerated and delayed) reactions and **toxic** reactions.

Sensitivity Reactions

Hypersensitivity to the penicillins is of considerable practical and theoretical significance. Its practical significance is that it causes potentially fatal reactions and thus limits the use of these antibiotics; its theoretical significance is that it indicates how a simple nontoxic molecule can be altered into an extremely powerful immunizing and sensitizing antigen(s) (Ch. 7).

The penicillins are the most common drug causes of allergy, and reactions ranging from mild to fatal have been reported at one time or another to follow the administration of nearly all pencillins by almost all routes of administration. Although the incidence of allergic reactions is difficult to assess, there seems to be a greater risk with the use of procaine and benzathine penicillin G than with other preparations. This difference may be part due to occurrence of allergy to procaine or benzathine, or to the fact that these preparations may act as adjuvants (Ch. 7) and as depôts of antigen.

The incidence of penicillin sensitivity increases with prolonged therapy and high total dosage. *Topical application is most likely to produce sensitization;* oral administration is the least hazardous. Many individuals who manifest penicillin hypersensitivity have no history of prior penicillin exposure. They may, however, have been exposed unknowingly to the antibiotic in milk, food, drugs (ointments, vaccines) or from skin fungi.

PENICILLIN ANTIGENS. Since penicillin (as normally used) contains no free groups to covalently link with carrier proteins, the antigens must be degradation products. Major and minor antigenic determinants are responsible; these terms are somewhat confusing since they refer to the *frequency of their formation*, rather than to the *severity of reactions* they produce. Thus, when penicillin G breaks down in vitro and combines with protein, about 95% forms the penicilloyl group; this then constitutes the major antigenic determinant. The remaining 5% of penicillin G and its metabolites, such as penicillenic acid, penicillamine, penaldate, penicoyl conjugates, etc., constitute the minor antigenic determinants, but in many instances the exact chemical nature of the minor determinants is not known. Other antigens probably include fermen-

tation contaminants such as mycelial fragments or moieties derived from bacterial amidases linked with penicillin or its degradation products and nonprotein polymers of penicillin or its degradation products. Thus, the antigens formed by the penicillins are highly variable in origin, in structure, in conjugation patterns and in reactivity. Clinically they usually act together to produce complex patterns of hypersensitivity. *Antibodies to the minor antigenic determinants are more serious since they mediate the majority of anaphylactic reactions.* Synthesis of antibodies to both major and minor determinants may be linked. Characteristically, cross reactivity is the rule; hence a subject sensitized to one form of penicillin reacts with varying severity to other penicillins.

ANTIBODIES PRODUCED. The types of antibody produced are indicated in Table 55–3. Atopic individuals have a three-to four-fold increased risk of developing IgE antibodies compared to normal subjects. Between 60–100% of patients who have received penicillin, and many individuals who have never knowingly received the antibiotic, possess hemaglutinating IgG antibodies to the major determinant. Low titers of IgA and IgD may also develop. The concentration of antibodies is higher in those patients who have experienced some reaction to penicillin, and titers tend to be higher just after reactions and fall with time.

Penicillin Reactions

The *outstanding clinical feature of penicillin hypersensitivity is its unpredictability.* Severe allergic reactions can develop in subjects with no prior history of atopic disease, in patients who have never knowingly received the antibiotic before or in patients who have received penicillins without incident for days, months or years. Furthermore, having occurred once, a reaction may recur and persist for variable periods of time, or it may never reappear. Clinically, reactions are either **immediate, accelerated** or **delayed,** and they may be of varying severity (Table 55–3).

AMPICILLIN SKIN RASH. Ampicillin therapy (rarely with other penicillins) is associated in 7–8% of cases with an erythematous, maculopapular (exanthematous, morbilliform) lesion over the exterior aspects of the extremities and trunk developing within 5–8 days of commencing therapy; it is three times more common in women than men and is particularly associated with acute viral infections, especially those of the respiratory tract. In patients with infectious mononucleosis, cytomegalovirus infections and lym-

TABLE 55—3. Some Important Sensitivity Reactions to Penicillin

Type	Incidence	Time after penicillin exposure	Type of antibody	Antigenic determinants	Reactions and comments
Immediate	0.02—0.2% of patients attending venereal disease clinics	0—30 min	IgE	Minor (?major)	Angioedema, rhinitis, urticaria, bronchospasm, hypotension, anaphylactic shock. Cardiac arrhythmias and conduction defects may be contributory factors to sudden death in anaphylaxis
Acelerated	1—3%	30 min to 72 hr on	IgE (?IgM)	Major (?minor)	Urticaria, angioedema, serum sickness
Delayed	?		IgE (?IgM, IgG) may mediate "Arthus"-like or Serum Sickness reactions, or may modify other reactions by acting as blocking antibodies (Cell mediated)	Major (?minor)	Drug fever, eosinophilia, skin rashes (bullous, vesicular, maculopapular, scarlatiniform), contact dermatitis, erythema multiforme, Stevens-Johnson syndrome, exfoliative dermatitis, toxic epidermal necrolysis (Fig. 7—1), serum sickness, lymphadenopathy, purpura, recurrent arthralgia, neutropenia and thrombocytopenia. Combs positive hemolytic anemia. (Due to IgG directed against red cell — penicillin complex, and usually seen in patients receiving 80—100 mega units IV, daily.) Azotemia, proteinuria, and hematuria and hepatitis (particularly with methicillin, nafcillin and oxacillin). Collagen disease. (Rare. May develop in patients receiving numerous courses of penicillin who have had a series of reactions.)

phatic leukemia, the incidence rate approaches 90%. The rash is dose related, unaffected by corticosteroids and IgE antibodies are not present. It may be a "toxic" effect of ampicillin associated with the presence of abnormal lymphocytes or due to the presence of impurities. Patients may not respond similarly when challenged with the drug a second time. Of therapeutic importance, *the occurrence of the rash is not in itself a contraindication to future treatment with any penicillin, but it would be prudent to skin test such individuals beforehand.*

DIAGNOSIS OF HYPERSENSITIVITY. A history of a previous severe reaction to penicillin or a personal or family history of atopic disease should indicate caution before prescribing any penicillin. No really safe and reliable diagnostic test for penicillin sensitivity is yet available, and some of those in common use may be dangerous. Skin testing procedures have been widely used, since serologic tests have little or no predictive value. Skin scratch and intradermal testing with dilute penicillin G, a mixture of major and minor determinants or the major antigenic determinant penicilloyl reacted with polylysine (PPL) have been used.

Results of skin testing are not clear cut. All tests are associated with false negative reactions; however, negative skin tests to minor determinants suggest that immediate reactions are unlikely to occur and that the likelihood of accelerated reactions is also slight. *A positive reaction to the minor determinants carries a very high risk for the occurrence of immediate reactions, and a positive reaction to PPL only is associated with a higher incidence of accelerated reactions. Late reactions are exceedingly difficult to predict, since patients may become sensitized during penicillin therapy.* Several tests have been suggested for determination of penicillin hypersensitivity, namely, the basophil degranulation test, passive transfer of antibodies to guinea pigs, primates and humans and the lymphocyte transformation test; these have not proven highly satisfactory and are still under study.

TREATMENT OF HYPERSENSITIVITY. Oxygen, epinephrine and antihistamines serve as adjuncts to full supportive therapy in anaphylactic shock and other less serious immediate reactions; accelerated and late reactions are essentially self-limiting, and spontaneous resolution occurs on supportive therapy with antihistamines when penicillin is discontinued; corticosteroids are recommended by some authorities.

The use of penicillinase has no rational basis, since it degrades penicillin to penicillenic acid, an antigen, and furthermore is antigenic itself. In sensitive patients, milk, chocolate and other substances which might contain penicillin should be assiduously avoided. Penicillin O, once considered safe in penicillin sensitive individuals, is not safe.

Toxic Reactions

Penicillin G is remarkably nontoxic provided renal function is normal, and doses of up to 200 mega units/day IV have been tolerated without the appearance of toxic effects. In the case of the semisynthetic penicillins, however, particularly methicillin, bone marrow depression (neutropenia, elevation of the serum iron and saturation of the iron binding capacity) and renal damage may appear with excessive dosage.

When renal tubular function is impaired or in the presence of hyponatremia, penicillin may induce cerebral irritation with hyperreflexia and myotonic seizures. Penicillin produces partial depolarization and increased excitability of neural cells in tissue culture, suggesting that this may be the mechanism of penicillin-induced seizures in man. In addition, encephalopathy will follow conventional penicillin therapy in patients with renal failure if cerebrospinal fluid drug levels rise above 10 units/ml. Similarly, too concentrated intrathecal penicillin injections may result in chemical meningitis or transverse myelitis. It is well known that a breakdown (as yet unexplained) of the blood brain barrier occurs during cardiopulmonary bypass operations, and penicillin therapy in such individuals is very likely to be followed by CNS toxicity. Injection in the vicinity of a large mixed nerve, such as the sciatic, may be followed by severe and persistent pain in the peripheral nerve distribution and some residual loss of function, both motor and sensory. Procaine penicillin should be injected with extreme care, as pulmonary embolism and acute psychotic episodes have followed accidental intravascular injection.

Superinfection occurs in about 1% of patients. Oral therapy is frequently followed by intestinal upsets, nausea and vomiting. Local oral penicillin (lozenges or aerosol) is prone to produce cheilosis, buccal ulceration, black hairy tongue and glossitis—symptoms that are not necessarily due to superinfection. Patients with diminished renal reserve who are being given large doses of penicillin should be carefully checked for the development of cation intoxication: 3 megaunits of potassium penicillin G contains approximately 5 mEq of ionic potassium, and 4 g of sodium methicillin contains approximately 10 mEq of ionic sodium. Cardiac arrest due to transient hyperkalemia has been reported following the too rapid IV administration of potassium penicillins. Methicillin, oxacillin, nafcillin, cloxacillin and carbenicillin have been reported occasionally to cause evidence or liver damage (increase of serum glutamic oxaloacetic transaminase, alkaline phosphatase, lactic acid dehydrogenase and sulfobromophthalein retention). Carbenicillin therapy, particularly in patients with renal impairment, has been associated with a bleeding diathesis; it may produce thrombocytopenia, inhibit platelet aggregation and prolong the bleeding time.

Jarisch-Herxheimer reactions may develop within a few hours of primary penicillin exposure in the majority of patients with secondary syphilis, the syphilitic lesions becoming edematous and hyperemic. Serious symptoms occur if the granulomata are present at the coronary artery ostia or larynx.

PHARMACOLOGY OF PENICILLIN G

Absorption

ORAL. Penicillin G is erratically absorbed (usually 15–20%) from the gastrointestinal tract, primarily the duodenum, and no reliance should be placed on this form of therapy in severe infections. Nonabsorbed penicillin is variably destroyed by gastric acid or by colonic flora. Since absorption is influenced by the degree of gastric acidity, greater absorption is seen in neonates, elderly patients and those taking antacids due to the presence of relative achlorhydria. To minimize inactivation by gastric acid and food, penicillin G should be given no later than ½ hr before meals, or no earlier than 3 hr after meals.

PARENTERAL. Parenteral administration by either SC or preferably IM injection is the route of choice for serious infections; IV injection may occasionally be required. Following IM injection, peak serum levels develop within about 20 min but fall rapidly to therapeutically ineffective concentrations over the ensuing 3–4 hr due to renal excretion. Blood antibiotic levels in ambulatory patients 2 hr after IM penicillin administration are about twice as high as those occurring in patients confined to bed. Absorption of penicillin following IM administration may be reduced in patients with diabetes mellitus.

Several procedures can be adopted to prolong blood penicillin levels; the renal tubular excretion of penicillin can be blocked through the concomitant administration of probenecid, and repository preparations of procaine or benzathine penicillin may be used. Recent controlled studies, however, suggest that for many infections in man it is not mandatory to maintain a plateau of penicillin activity in the blood, but that peak levels for 6–8 hr/24 hr will suffice.

INTRATHECAL. Penicillin G passes slowly and erratically into the cerebrospinal fluid under normal circumstances. When the meninges are inflamed, antibiotic levels are higher but are still inconstant and unreliable. Intrathecal penicillin as an adjunct to systemic therapy is recommended by some authorities for pneumococcal meningitis or sensitive gram-negative meningitis in neonates. *Intrathecal penicillin administration is dangerous.* The maximal dose should be 5000 units administered in a concentration of not more than 1000 units/ml.

TOPICAL. Although penicillin G is available in creams and ointments for skin application, these preparations should never be used. They are very likely to induce hypersensitivity, an occurrence which precludes the future use of any penicillin by any route.

LOCAL. Penicillin G is available in suppository form, as an aerosol or for local instillation. into the pleural, peritoneal or joint cavities. There is rarely any justification for their use.

DISTRIBUTION, METABOLISM AND EXCRETION

Penicillin G is distributed widely in the body, tissue concentrations usually being about 20% of simultaneous plasma levels. The antibiotic concentrations in the kidney and urinary tract are high. Cerebrospinal fluid passage is discussed above. Penetration of penicillin G into joint fluid is usually excellent.

Penicillin G is partially broken down in the body by unknown mechanisms. About 90% of the drug is excreted unchanged by the kidney; some is excreted in the bile from where it may undergo an enterohepatic recirculation, and in the milk. Urinary excretion of penicillin is rapid and approximates total renal plasma flow. Thus, following the IM administration of aqueous penicillin G, 90% can be recovered from the urine after 2 hr. Excretion is by both glomerular filtration (10–15%) and tubular secretion (85–90%). The tubular secretion of penicillin is reduced by the excretion of other natural organic acids (pantothenic acid, uric acid, etc.) and by certain drugs e.g., probenecid (see below), acetyl salicylic acid, indomethacin, phenylbutazone and some sulfonamides. Penicillin clearance is diminished in the elderly patient and is relatively slow in the infant (Ch. 7).

Renal insufficiency may increase the plasma half-life from about 30 min to 10–15 hr. Under these circumstances, biliary excretion of the antibiotic increases. Patients with renal failure can be treated with penicillin G with reasonable safety as long as dosage is reduced; following a loading dose, maintenance doses can be given 10–12 hourly, but cation intoxication may be a problem in these circumstances.

Preparations

Three main types of penicillin G are available: penicillin G for **oral** use, aqueous penicillin G for **parenteral use** and **depôt** (repository, "slow release") **preparations** for parenteral use.

Sodium penicillin G, *N.F.,* and Potassium penicillin G, *U.S.P.,* are available as tablets. Penicillin G is available as a sterile powder for SC, IV or intrathecal administration; the calcium, aluminum and sodium salts are not as effective as the potassium salts. It should be reconstituted with sterile distilled water or normal saline; 5% dextrose is not recommended, since it has a pH of 4.5–5.5, that destroys the antibiotic. Potassium penicillin G, *U.S.P.,* is a popular preparation. The usual IM dose is 500,000 units every 6 hr; IV doses may be considerably higher.

Depôt penicillin G was developed for deep IM injection to provide a prolonged release of the active drug over a period of hours or days. Slow release from a muscle depôt avoids the wide fluctuations in plasma drug concentrations seen with multiple injections of aqueous penicillin G. *These preparations should never be injected IV, SC or intrathecally.* Commonly used preparations are Sterile Procaine Penicillin G. Suspension, *U.S.P.,* and Sterile Benzathine penicillin G Suspension, *U.S.P.* Following 600,000 units of procaine penicillin G IM, peak serum levels are achieved by about 2–4 hr, and measurable blood levels may persist for up to a week. This dose of procaine penicillin contains about 240 mg of procaine. Usually no adverse effects are seen due to the procaine, and it may, by virtue of its local anesthetic action, reduce the pain of the IM injection. Some patients, however, may develop a hypersensitivity reaction to the local anesthetic, and severe toxic reactions, e.g., cardiac arrhythmias and psychotic behavior frequently develop if the preparation is accidently injected intravascularly. In order to minimize rapid intravascular passage of procaine, subjects receiving procaine penicillin should not engage in any strenuous physical activity for several hours after receiving an injection. Benzathine penicillin G is even more slowly absorbed following IM administration than are procaine preparations. Following an injection of 600,000 units of benzathine penicillin G, therapeutic serum levels may persist for 10–20 days. This preparation should be used only for prophylaxis, e.g., against streptococcal throat infections in patients who have previously had an episode of rheumatic fever.

Use of Probenecid

Probenecid was specifically developed to block the renal tubular secretion of penicillin. It also blocks the renal tubular transport of other

CH₃–CH₂–H₂C,
CH₃–CH₂–H₂C / N–SO₂–⟨benzene⟩–COOH
PROBENECID

$CH_3\text{–}CH_2\text{–}H_2C$ and $CH_3\text{–}CH_2\text{–}H_2C$ attached to $N\text{–}SO_2$—〔ring〕—$COOH$
PROBENECID

organic acids (uric acid, pathothenic acid, the cephalosporins, etc.) and reduces organic acid transport into the cerebrospinal fluid. When used concomitantly with penicillin, plasma levels of the antibiotic are increased about two-fold and maintained for about twice as long as when penicillin is given alone.

Probenecid is almost totally absorbed following oral administration. Peak levels develop within 2–4 hr. The drug is bound to plasma proteins about 80–90%, and its half-life is between 6–12 hr.

Probenecid *U.S.P.* (Benemid) is costly. It causes gastrointestinal upsets and thus should be used with care in patients with peptic ulcer disease. Rarely hypersensitivity skin rashes may develop. The usual dose to augment serum penicillin levels is 0.5 g 6 hourly. Since probenecid is costly, and potentially toxic, it is rarely used in the conventional patient, since it is considered easier, safer and cheaper merely to give larger and more frequent doses of penicillin. Probenecid is of value, however, in single dose treatment of gonorrhea and in the rare patient who refuses parenteral therapy or in whom you cannot find veins. Probenecid is also used in the treatment of gout; uricosuric activity is due to blockade of renal tubular reabsorption of uric acid.

PHARMACOLOGY OF SOME PENICILLIN PREPARATIONS

There are well over 100 penicillin preparations on the market. Some of these are combinations of penicillin with other antimicrobial drugs or with probenecid, and they often carry misleading proprietory names. Thus, confusion is often apparent concerning the relative merits of any particular compound. In selecting a penicillin, the physician should base his choice on its potency and antibacterial spectrum, its optimum route of administration and protein binding, its susceptibility or resistance to penicillinase and its cost and intended use (therapeutic or prophylactic). The clinically useful penicillins can be readily classified into natural penicillin G preparations and the semisynthetic penicillins (Table 55–4).

been developed, but only a handful are important therapeutically (Table 55–4): acid resistant but penicillinase susceptible (penicillin V, phenethicillin); acid labile and penicillinase resistant (methicillin); acid and penicillinase resistant (nafcillin, oxacillin, cloxacilin, dicloxacillin, flucloxacillin); acid and penicillinase labile but broad spectrum (carbencillin), and acid stable, penicillinase labile and broad spectrum (ampicillin, indanyl carbenicillin). A few additional agents are undergoing clinical trial in the United Kingdom or the United States; their ultimate place in therapy remains to be seen. **Hetacillin,** derived from a condensation process during the synthesis of ampicillin, is hydrolyzed in vivo to ampicillin and acetone. **Amoxicillin** possesses a broad ampicillin-like spectrum; it may be of some value in the treatment of ampicillin-resistant typhoid fever. **Quinacillin, epicillin, azidocillin, ancillin, cyclacillin** and **ticarcillin** need to be evaluated but in all probability will not replace any of the current penicillins.

SEMISYNTHETIC PENICILLINS

The semisynthetic penicillins have been developed to overcome the shortcomings of penicillin G (see above). Almost 3000 different drugs have

THE CEPHALOSPORINS

Three major "cephalosporins," P, N and C, were isolated from the fungus *Cephalosporium acremonium,* obtained by Guiseppe Brotzu in 1945 from a sewage outlet off the coast of Sardinia. "Cephalosporin P" is a steroid antibiotic related to fusidic acid, possessing some activity against gram-positive organisms. "Cephalosporin N" is in reality a penicillin (penicillin N), since it possesses the 6-APA nucleus with a *D-α*-aminoadipic acid-derived side chain; it exhibits weak gram-positive and gram-negative activity. Cephalosporin C is the most important and has generated

a host of new and promising antibiotics. Cephalosporin C possesses a *D-α*-aminoadipic acid-derived side chain attached to 7-aminocephalosporanic acid (7-ACA), the cephalosporin building block.

7-ACA (Figure 55–2) is composed of a β-lactam ring (2) which is essential for antibacterial activity, fused to a dihydrothiazine ring (1) (in place of the thiazolidine ring of the penicillins). 7-ACA was readily isolated by dilute acid hydrolysis of cephalosporin C and can be considered in the same manner as the 6-APA ring system of the penicillins

TABLE 55–4. Some of the Major Penicillins

$$R'' - C - N - C - C - C - N - C - C - O - R'$$

(structure: $O=C-N-C-C-C-S-C(CH_3)(CH_3)$ with H, H, H substituents and $C=O$, $C-O-H$)

Drug Name		R'' Substitutions	Properties					Preparations and dosage
Chemical	Nonproprietary or generic		General	Penicillinase resistance	Broad spectrum	Route of administration	Plasma protein binding	
Benzyl	Penicillin G	CH_2- (phenyl)	See text	No	No	Parenteral (oral)	35–65%	See text
Phenoxymethyl	Penicillin V	$-OCH_2-$ (phenyl)	Similar to penicillin G but less potent. Following equivalent doses blood levels are 3–5 times higher than with penicillin G but sericidal activity is similar. The potassium salt is better absorbed than the free acid	No	No	Oral	55–88%	Potassium Phenoxymethyl Penicillin U.S.P. 250–500 mg, 8 hourly. Should be taken not earlier than 3 hr after food
Phenoxyethyl	Phenethicillin	$-OC_2H_4-$ (phenyl)	Similar to penicillin V	No	No	Oral	50–60%	Potassium Phenethicillin N.F. 250–500 mg, 8 hourly
Dimethoxy-phenyl	Methicillin	(phenyl with OCH_3, CH_3, OCH_3)	The first penicillinase resistant penicillin. Resistance due to the R''-substituted-CH_3 group that blocks hydrolysis by β-lactamase but not by acids. Antibacterial spectrum about equal to that of penicillin G, but *much less potent against nonpenicillinase producers*. Following IM injection plasma levels peak at about 40 min. Excreted rapidly in bile and urine. Methicillin resistance probably due to failure of antibiotic uptake by bacteria. May produce hepatic or renal damage	Yes, but variable	No	Parenteral	20–50%	Sodium methicillin U.S.P., 3–6 g 4–6 hourly because of its acid lability should not be dissolved in large volumes of acidic IV fluids, e.g., 5% dextrose. Methicillin and other penicillinase-resistant penicillins or a cephalosporin should be reserved for the treatment of infections due to penicillin G-resistant staphylococci and for initial treatment of all new staphylococcal infections until their sensitivity is determined

TABLE 55-4. *(continued)*

R'' Substitutions	Drug Name — Chemical	Drug Name — Nonproprietary or generic	General	Penicillinase resistance	Broad spectrum	Route of administration	Plasma protein binding	Preparations and dosage
(naphthalene with OC_2H_5 and CH_3)	6-(2-ethoxy-1) naphthamido	Nafcillin	Partially acid stable, but absorption following oral administration erratic and unreliable. Longer half-life than many other semisynthetic penicillins due to an enterohepatic recirculation. Highly irritating on parenteral administration	Yes	No	Parenteral (oral)	70–90%	Sodium Nafcillin, *U.S.P.* 0.5–1.0 g, 4–6 hourly
(phenyl isoxazolyl structure)	5-methyl-3 phenyl-4-isoxazolyl	Oxacillin	The first isoxazole penicillin to be developed. Less potent than penicillin G, but 6 times more potent than methicillin. About 60% of an oral dose is absorbed. Cleared in urine and bile	Yes	No	Oral parenteral	80%	Sodium Oxacillin *U.S.P.*, 250 mg–1 g, 4–6 hourly
(chloro-phenyl isoxazolyl structure)	5-methyl-3-0-chloro-phenyl-4-isoxazolyl	Cloxacillin	Similar to Oxacillin, but more readily absorbed after oral administration. Following IM administration blood levels are about twice those following oral administration	Yes	No	Oral parenteral	80–85%	Sodium Cloxacillin *U.S.P.*, 250–500 mg, 4–6 hourly
(dichloro-phenyl isoxazolyl structure)	5-methyl-2, 6-Dichloro-phenyl-4-isoxazolyl	Dicloxacillin	More potent than oxacillin or cloxacillin against penicillinase-producing staphylococci. Rapid absorption following oral administration with blood levels being about twice those seen with cloxacillin. Half-life longer than most other penicillins due to high plasma protein binding	Yes	No	Oral	80–95%	Dicloxacillin sodium 250–500 mg, 4–6 hourly
(fluoro-phenyl isoxazolyl structure)	5-methyl-2,	Flucloxacillin	Similar to dicloxacillin except less protein bound. Available only in England	Yes	No	Oral	60–80%	Flucloxacillin, 250–500 mg, 4–6 hourly
(phenyl with CH–NH_2)	α-aminobenzyl	Ampicillin	Gram-positive spectrum similar to that of penicillin G. Gram-negative spectrum against many strains of *E. coli, H. influenzae, Enterobacter aerogenes, Klebsiella, Proteus mirabilis, Salmonella, Shigella* and *Enterococci* Readily absorbed following oral and IM administration. Cleared in urine and bile. Biliary levels	No	Yes	Oral parenteral	15–25%	Sodium ampicillin *U.S.P., 500* mg orally, 6 hourly. In severe infections, 3–5 g, 6 hourly

α-carboxy benzyl	Carbenicillin	may reach 20—40 times simultaneous plasma levels and can be increased still further by probenacid, Sometimes useful in the treatment of biliary tract disease including the typhoid carrier state Similar antibacterial spectrum to ampicillin plus activity against *Ps. aeruginosa* and indole positive Proteus. Very high serum levels (40–200 $\mu g/ml$) are required to treat susceptible gram-negative organisms, levels only obtainable with parenteral therapy. CSF passage is poor and the drug cleared 80—100% in 4 hr by the kidney	No	Yes	Parenteral	50%	Carbenicillin sodium. Additive effects or synergism produced against *Ps. aeuruginosa* with concomitant gentamicin therapy. These antibiotics should not be mixed in the same container since gentamicin is rapidly inactivated
α-carboxy benzyl: indanyl	Indanyl carbenicillin	Only about 40% absorbed. Converted by plasma and tissue esterases to carbenicillin. The indanyl moiety excreted as glucuronide conjugates or sulfate esters in the urine. *Very low plasma levels are produced with this preparation,* and it should be reserved for treating mild urinary tract infections due to *Ps. aeruginosa* or indole positive proteus	No	Yes	Oral	50%	Indanyl carbenicillin

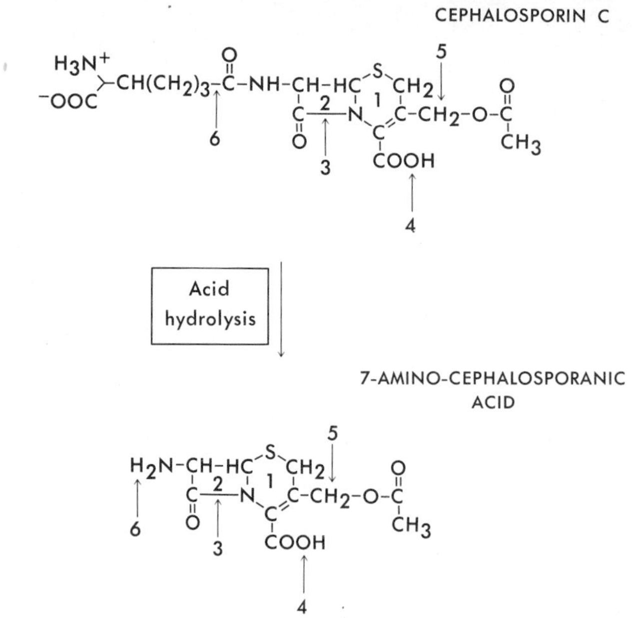

FIG. 55–2. Cephalosporin C and 7-amino-cephalosporinic acid. (1) dihydro-thiazine ring; (2) β-lactam ring; (3) site of action of cephalosporinase; (4) site of salt formation; (5) site for deacetylation and subsequent substitutions (Table 55–6); (6) site of acetylation and substitutions (Table 55–6).

(see above). The basic cephalosporin structure differs from that of the penicillins in that it possesses only two asymetric points compared to the three in 6-APA, and in that it has three instead of two sites at which chemical modifications may be made. Several semisynthetic cephalosporins have been produced from 7-ACA which possess greater antibacterial activity than the original cephalosporin C (Table 55–6).

TABLE 55–5. Common Microorganisms Affected by the Cephalosporins

Organism	Sensitivity
Actinomyces israelii	+++
Bacillus subtilis	+++
Diplococcus pneumoniae	+++
E. coli	++R
Haemophilus influenzae	++R
Cl. welchii	+++
Enterobacter aerogenes	R
Corynebacterium diphtheriae	+++
Listeria monocytogenase	+++
Klebsiella	+++
Neisseria gonorrhoeae	++R
Neisseria meningitidis	+++R
Proteus mirabilis	++
Salmonella	++R
Shigella	++R
Staph. aureus	+++R
Staph. epidermidis	+++
Strep. faecalis	+R
Strep. pyogens	+++
Strep. viridans	+++

R	In vitro testing essential, as many strains are resistant
+++	Highly sensitive
++	Moderate sensitivity
+	Some sensitivity

Antibacterial Spectrum

The cephalosporins have a relatively broad anti-bacterial spectrum (Table 55–5). In general, they are effective against all common gram-positive cocci except enterococci and methicillin-resistant staphylococci. They are somewhat more active against gram-negative bacilli than the penicillins, with the exception of carbenicillin which is the drug of choice for indole positive proteus, enterobacter and *Pseudomonas aeruginosa* infections.

Mode of Action and Bacterial Resistance

The cephalosporins probably act similarly to the pencillins (Ch. 53). Bacterial resistance may be due to failure of antibiotic penetration, or to production of β-lactamase (cephalosporinase); cephalosporins are not destroyed by penicillinase and may actually absorb it. Like penicillinase, cephalosporinase may be mediated by R factors (Ch. 52) and can be either exocellular or endocellular and constitutive or inducible.

Clinical Pharmacology

The cephalosporins released to date or under clinical evaluation can be divided into parenteral antibiotics rapidly excreted (cephalothin) parenteral antibiotics more slowly excreted (cephaloridine, cephazolin) and orally absorbed antibiotics

SODIUM CEPHALOTHIN

(cephaloglycine, cephalexin, cephradine). The drugs are variable excreted by both glomerular filtration and a renal tubular secretory mechanism similar to that for the penicillins. Details of absorption, metabolism and excretion are given for each agent (Table 55–6). Several newer agents under evaluation are **cephacetrile, cephapirin, cephramycin** and **cephamandole.**

ADVERSE REACTIONS

Similar adverse reactions may develop with all the cephalosporins, but some members of the group are particularly prone to produce specific lesions, e.g., renal damage with cephaloridine. More is known about cephalothin and cephaloridine, since these drugs have been more widely used than the newer agents.

The most important point regarding adverse reactions to the cephalosporins is the question of possible *cross sensitization between these antibiotics and the penicillins.* To date, the balance of clinical experience suggests that *clinically significant cross-sensitivity* is uncommon. This is not surprising since, unlike the penicillins, hydrolysis of the β-lactam ring of the cephalosporins is unusual, and when it does occur, the resulting compounds are highly unstable and do not readily form haptenes. However, several instances of cross sensitivity have been reported.

Hypersensitivity reactions (fever, eosinophilia, various skin rashes, urticaria, serum sickness and anaphylaxis) have been reported in 3–7% of patients. Neutropenia and thrombocytopenia may appear after 2–3 weeks of therapy, but agranulocytosis is rare. Superinfection with gram-negative microorganisms may appear, and with the presence of impaired renal function cation (sodium) loading is possible. A positive Coomb's test has been reported in some patients treated with doses of cephalothin greater than 10–12 g/day, particularly in the presence of hypoalbuminemia and impaired renal function. The reaction is not immunologic in nature but is the result of coating of the erythrocytes nonspecifically by a cephalothin/globulin complex that reacts with Coomb's serum in vitro. Rarely, cephalothin produces a hemolytic anemia. Cephalothin may produce renal toxicity in patients with preexisting renal disease, or when given in conjunction with gentamicin. A positive reaction for urinary sugar may occur with the "Clinitest" tablets, or with Benedict and Fehlings reagents, but not with specific tests for glucose such as "TesTape," which utilizes glucose oxidase. Thrombophlebitis may occur following IV administration. Elevation of serum glutamic oxaloacetic transaminase activity has been reported occasionally in children following IM administration, but this may reflect injection damage to muscles rather than hepatic damage.

Cephaloridine possessess many of the undesirable adverse effects of cephalothin. In addition, it is highly nephrotoxic, producing acute proximal tubular necrosis particularly in patients receiving 6–8 g or more/day. Acute renal damage is more common in patients with preexisting renal disease and in those taking other nephrotoxic drugs concomitantly. In order to minimize the occurrence of tubular necrosis, therapy with cephaloridine should be limited to 4 g/day in adults and 30–50 mg/kg/day in children. Probenecid may reduce the incidence of nephrotoxicity. Cephaloridine produces less pain following IM injection than cephalothin. Nail shedding has been reported following high doses of cephalosporins in patients with renal failure.

USES

The cephalosporins are of value in treating many gram-positive and gram-negative infections resistant to other antibiotics. Of particular importance is their action against *Staphylococcus aureus, Clostridium welchii,* most streptococcal and pneumococcal infections and some strains of *Klebsiella, Proteus* and *E. coli.* Cephalothin and cephaloridine have been used prophylactically to prevent infection in patients undergoing peritoneal dialysis, vaginal hysterectomy, cardiac and arterial graft surgery and major orthopedic surgery.

Cephaloridine and cephalexin may be used to treat syphilis and gonorrhea in a patient allergic to penicillins.

Since the cephalosporins pass poorly into cerebrospinal fluid, their use in treatment of bacterial meningitis is unreliable. In fact, cephalosporin sensitive bacteria have been known to initiate meningitis during treatment of systemic infections with the antibiotic. The cephalosporins are less effective than other antibiotic against *H. influenza* infections.

R'–C–HN–CH–CH–HC $\overset{S}{\underset{}{\diagdown}}$ CH$_2$
‖
O

$\overset{}{\underset{}{|}}$ C–N $\overset{}{\underset{}{\diagdown}}$ C–CH$_2$–R''
‖
O

COOH

TABLE 55–6. Some of the Major Cephalosporins

Drug name		Properties				Preparations and dosage	R' Substitutions	R'' substitutions
Chemical	Nonproprietary or generic	General	Route of administration	Half-life (min)	Plasma protein binding			
7-thiophene-2-acetamido-cephalosporanic acid	Cephalothin	Not measurably destroyed by gastric acid but absorption following oral administration poor. Best given IV since IM painful. Widely distributed except to the CSF; fetal blood levels usually reach 20% of maternal levels. About 30% converted in the liver to the weakly active O-desacetyl metabolite. About 60–90% excreted unchanged by the renal tubules producing with conventional therapy urinary levels of 800–3000 μg/ml. Probenecid delays tubular secretion. Almost completely removed during hemo- and peritoneal dialysis	IM IV	30	50–80	Sodium cephalothin available as 1 or 4 g powder in sterile ampules for reconstitution with normal saline or 5% dextrose. Usual adult dose is 1 g, 6 hourly. In serious infections or life-threatening infections 1 g, 3 hourly, or 1 g, 2 hourly IV, is recommended. The usual dose in children is 40–80 mg/kg/day in divided doses	S CH$_2$– (thiophene ring)	–O–C $\overset{O}{\underset{}{\|}}$ –CH$_3$
7-(2-thienyl-acetamido-3-pyridyl) methyl cephalosporanic acid	Cephaloridine	Possesses a similar antibacterial spectrum to cephalothin but has greater activity against some staphylococci, pneumococci and hemolytic streptococci and less activity against the neisseriae and *H. influenzae*. Following IM injection peak blood levels develop within 0.5 hr and are twice those produced by an equivalent dose of cephalothin. Passage into CSF is poor. Cephaloridine is a zwitterion and relatively nonpolar, and clearance is equivalent to the glomerular filtration rate. Thus, probenecid has little effect on its excretion	IM IV	60–90	20–30	Cephaloridine is available as 1 g dry powder for reconstitution, and as a solution of 500 mg/ml. The usual dose is 0.5–1 g, 6 hourly. A total daily dose of 4 g and 50 mg/kg should not be exceeded in adults and children, respectively	S CH$_2$ (thiophene ring)	$\overset{+}{N}$ (pyridinium ring)
7-(D-α-amino-α-phenylace-tamido-3-methyl-3-cephem-5-)carboxylic acid	Cephalexin	Acid stable. Less potent than cephalothin or cephaloridine. About 80% absorbed following oral administration. Rapidly cleared by glomerular filtration and tubular secretion	Oral IM IV	50–60	15–40	Under active study	–CH– NH$_2$ (phenyl ring)	–H

	Drug	Chemical name	Properties	Route			Dosage	R
$-CH-NH_2$ (phenyl)	Cephaloglycine	7-D-α-amino-phenyl-aceta-mido cephalo-sporanic acid	Hydrolysed to cephalothin in vivo. Slowly and incompletely (30%) absorbed following oral administra-tion resulting in low plasma levels. Partially metabolised to an O-desacetyl metabolite. Because of good renal clearance of free drug cephaloglycine has some place in treating urinary tract infections. Usually produces diarrhea	Oral	120	15–20	Cephaloglycine, 250–500 mg. 6 hourly. Should only be used for treatment of urinary tract infections	$-O-C{=}O$ / CH_3
$\begin{array}{c}N{=}N\\ \quad\ \ N{-}CH_2-\\N{=}H\end{array}$	Cephazolin	7-[1(1H)-tetrazolyl-acetamido]-3-[2-(5-methyl-1,3,4-thiadia-zolyl) thio-methyl]-Δ³-cephem-4-carboxylic acid	Less painful and possesses greater activity against enterobacter species than cephalothin. Follow-ing IM injections blood levels are 2–4 times higher than those achieved with similar doses of cephaloridine and cephalothin, respectively. Not removed by hemodialysis	IM / IV	120	70–90	Under active study	$\begin{array}{c}N{-}N\\ \quad\ \ C{-}CH_3\\-S\diagup\ \diagdown S\end{array}$
$-CH-NH$ (cyclohexadienyl)	Cephradine	7-amino-cyclo-hexadienyl-acetamido-cephalosporanic acid	Chemically similar to cephalexin but may be more potent against enterococci	Oral	40–60	15–20	Under active study	–H

FURTHER READING

Abraham EP (1962): The cephalosporins. Pharmacol Rev 14:473–500

Flynn EH (ed) (1972): Cephalosporins and Penicillins. Chemistry and Biology. New York, Academic Press

Kaye D (1973): Changes in the spectrum, diagnosis and management of bacterial endocarditis. Med Clin North Am 57:941–957

Parker CW (1975): Drug allergy. N Engl J Med 292:511–514; 732–736; 957–960

Simberkoff MS, Thomas L, McGregor D, Shenkein I, Levine BB, (1970): Inactivation of penicillins by carbohydrate solutions at alkaline pH. N Engl J Med 283:116–119

Stewart GT (1973): Allergy to penicillin and related antibiotics: antigenic and immunochemical mechanism. Annu Rev Pharmacol 13:309–324

Van Dellen RG, Gleich GJ (1970): Penicillin skin tests as predictive and diagnostic aids in penicillin allergy. Med Clin North Am 54:997–1007

Weinstein L, Kaplan K (1970): The cephalosporins, microbiological, chemical, and pharmacological properties and use in chemotherapy of infection. Ann Intern Med 72:729–739

JEREMY H. THOMPSON

56. ANTIBIOTICS WHICH INTERFERE WITH PROTEIN SYNTHESIS: I

The antibiotics discussed here and in Chapter 57 depress bacterial protein synthesis. Because they are so heterogenous, each group is described separately.

THE AMINOGLYCOSIDE ANTIBIOTICS

The aminoglycoside antibiotics comprise **streptomycin, dihydrostreptomycin, kanamycin, neomycin, gentamicin, viomycin** and **paromomycin** (Ch. 63); several promising aminoglycosides are currently under evaluation, namely, tobramycin, sisomycin, butirosin and BBK8. Some properties common to the group are discussed first.

Antibacterial Spectrum and Resistance

The aminoglycosides are broad spectrum antibiotics (Table 56–1), but the use of some agents should be restricted in therapy. Bacteria frequently develop permanent resistance to aminoglycosides. In any large population of microorganisms, naturally occurring, single step, high level resistant mutants appear and are rapidly selected. Resistance is more common with multiple exposure or prolonged therapy and is one of the most common reasons for therapeutic failure.

Cross resistance is usually complete within the group, but some exceptions are given in the text.

Mode of Action

Aminoglycosides inhibit protein synthesis, and by virtue of their strong cationic charges they damage bacterial cell membranes by combining with anionic membrane groups (Ch. 53); additionally, they may block energy production at the pyruvate-oxaloacetic acid step of the Krebs cycle. In vitro there is approximately (depending upon the antibiotic) a 10- to 80-fold increase in potency in going from pH 5.5–8.0; consequently, in the treatment of urinary tract infections the concomitant administration of urinary alkalinizers is advised. Aminoglycosides may be either bacteriostatic or bactericidal, depending upon the concentration achieved and the susceptibility of the organism. Low (subinhibitory) concentrations of streptomycin may produce dependence.

Absorption and Excretion

Since absorption following oral administration is poor (3–5%), and since little is destroyed in the gut lumen, the aminoglycosides (streptomycin, neomycin, kanamycin, paromomycin) may be given orally for a local effect in the gastrointestinal tract. If systemic activity is required, the drug (streptomycin, kanamycin, gentamicin, rarely neomycin) must be given either intramuscularly or intravenously. Topically, neomycin and gentamicin are exceptionally safe, but streptomycin may induce hypersensitivity reactions.

The aminoglycosides are primarily excreted in the urine. Thus, in the presence of renal insufficiency they must be given in reduced dosage to avoid toxicity. Sufficient antibiotic is absorbed following oral administration to produce toxicity in patients with renal insufficiency.

Adverse Effects

One of the major limiting factors in the use of the aminoglycosides is their propensity to damage either the labyrinthine and/or the auditory portions of the eighth cranial nerve. Other adverse effects, e.g., albuminuria and renal damage, may lead to irreversible damage if therapy is not discontinued at the first sign of toxicity. Most of the

TABLE 56–1. Some of the Organisms Affected by Streptomycin

Bacteroides fragilis	N. gonorrhea
Brucellae spp	P. pestis
Diplococcus pneumoniae	P. tularensis
Erysipelothrix	Proteus spp
E. coli	P. aeruginosa
H. ducreyi	Salmonellae spp
H. influenzae	Shigellae spp
L. monocytogenase	Staphylococci spp
K. granulomatis	Strep. faecalis
K. pneumoniae	Strep. pyogenes
M. tuberculosis	Strep. viridans

adverse effects, apart from hypersensitivity reactions, are dose dependent.

Risk factors for eighth cranial nerve damage with all the aminoglycosides are: increasing dose (particularly greater than 2 g/day) and duration of treatment, intrathecal administration (rare today), increasing age, renal insufficiency, prior or concomitant exposure to other ototoxic drugs, presence of CNS or eighth cranial nerve disease and dehydration. Whereas all the aminoglycoside antibiotics may damage the eighth cranial nerve, preferential damage to either the vestibular or the auditory divisions is characteristic of individual agents.

STREPTOMYCIN

Streptomycin was the first aminoglycoside to be isolated (Table 56–2). It is almost unique in that it is highly effective against most strains of human and bovine *M. tuberculosis* as well as possessing a broad antibacterial spectrum (Table 56–1).

STREPTOMYCIN

Bacterial Resistance and Dependence

Resistance may develop so explosively that within two or three generations organisms are over 1000 times less sensitive to the antibiotic. Development of mycobacterial resistance is delayed by the simultaneous use of one or more other antitubercular agents, but this is not necessarily true for other organisms.

On exposure of sensitive bacteria to subinhibitory concentrations of streptomycin in vitro, a paradoxical stimulation of bacterial cell growth may be seen. Additionally, a state of dependance may develop with bacteria *requiring* the antibiotic for growth (Ch. 52). Dependence is usually not permanent, since growth of organisms in subdependence inducing concentrations usually results in a reversion to sensitive or resistant bacteria. The clinical importance of dependence is not clear.

Adverse Effects

NERVOUS SYSTEM DAMAGE. In daily doses of 2 g or more, symptoms indicative of acute labyrinthine dysfunction develop in nearly all patients within a month. Even if therapy is stopped at this time, the condition may progress. About 10% of patients show some impairment of hearing after a week of 1 g of streptomycin daily, but whether the lesion is in the end organ, or centrally, is not known. High frequency sounds (outside the conversation range) are lost first, and with continuing therapy lower frequency sounds are gradually affected. High frequency sound loss is detected only by careful audiometric examination.

Streptomycin may rarely cause peripheral neuritis, facial and peripheral paresthesia and optic neuritis with scotomas. Excessive intrathecal streptomycin may be followed by chemical meningitis, radiculitis, transverse or patchy myelitis, convulsive seizures and encephalopathy.

NEUROMUSCULAR BLOCK. Streptomycin may induce a curare-like neuromuscular block, particularly when given intraperitoneally in large doses postoperatively to patients who have received neuromuscular blocking agents. The paralysis is partially reversed by neostigmine, but death may result from ventilatory paralysis. In patients with myasthenia gravis, streptomycin may induce a dramatic increase in skeletal muscle weakness.

HYPERSENSITIVITY. The most important hypersensitivity reactions are various skin rashes (in about 7% of patients), particularly maculopapular, erythematous and urticarial lesions; contact dermatitis in pharmacists, nurses and physicians who handle the drug frequently; exfoliative dermatitis; stomatitis; drug fever; eosinophilia; angioneurotic edema; serum sickness; lymphadenopathy and anaphylactic shock. Granulocytopenia may progress to agranulocytosis; aplastic anemia, thrombocytopenic purpura and hypoprothrombinemia occur rarely. Hypersensitivity reactions usually occur together but may appear as isolated reactions.

RENAL DAMAGE. Albuminuria is commonly seen with prolonged therapy; it is usually reversible. Reduced urine output may also be seen, a situation that potentiates systemic streptomycin toxicity.

MISCELLANEOUS EFFECTS. IV administration of streptomycin (not recommended) may produce transient hypotension. Pain occurs on IM injection, and injection sites should be alternated to avoid the development of sterile abscesses. Headaches occur commonly and may indicate the development of eighth cranial nerve damage. Gastrointestinal irritation usually follows oral therapy. Superinfection, primarily due to staphylococci and fungi may occur in about 5% cases.

Preparations, Dosage and Uses

Streptomycin sulfate is available in many preparations. Dosage is indicated in Table 56–2.

Limitations to the use of streptomycin are the risk of inducing bacterial resistance and eighth cranial nerve damage and the preferred mode of administration (IM). However, streptomycin is still one of the most important drugs for treating tuberculosis and for treating infections in patients hypersensitive to other drugs. With the introduction of new antibiotics, the need for streptomycin in other infections has decreased, but it is highly effective in tularemia, plague, severe brucellosis and, combined with penicillin, in group *D*-streptococcal endocarditis.

If streptomycin has to be given intrathecally, e.g., in treatment of *H. influenzae* meningitis, the total daily dosage should not exceed the following: in infants less than 12 months of age 10 mg, children 1–3 years of age 20 mg, children 4–10 years of age 40 mg and adults 60–100 mg. The antibiotic should be dissolved in normal saline from fresh powder. Commercial solutions should not be used, since they may contain a variety of irritating additives.

COMBINATION WITH OTHER ANTIMICROBIAL DRUGS.

In patients with *Haemophilus influenzae* infections who are allergic to a penicillin (ampicillin), use of streptomycin is an acceptable regimen providing it is given both intramuscularly and intrathecally in the presence of meningitis. Chloramphenicol or tetracyclines may be preferred in penicillin allergic individuals, particularly in treating meningitis. Synergism is frequently seen when penicillin and streptomycin are used against enterococci. In mixed urinary tract infections, streptomycin may be combined to advantage with nitrofurantoin or penicillin. Chloramphenicol may be combined with streptomycin (but preferably with kanamycin) in the treatment of serious *Klebsiella pneumoniae* infections. The many proprietary preparations containing fixed dosage ratios of penicillin and streptomycin should not be used (Ch. 12).

NEOMYCIN

Neomycin (Table 56–2) is primarily used orally for a local effect within the gastrointestinal tract and topically where susceptible organisms are inhibited by concentrations of about 10 μg/ml. Important organisms susceptible to neomycin are *E. coli, Proteus, Shigellae* and *Klebsiella* spp., and various gram-positive cocci. Variably resistant are *Pseudomonas aeruginosa* and *B. fragilis.*

Adverse Effects

When applied topically, neomycin is exceptionally safe, unless applied extensively to large, granulating surfaces from which appreciable absorption may occur to produce systemic toxicity. Topical use only occasionally produces sensitivity reactions, and under these circumstances cross sensitivity can be shown with other aminoglycosides. Oral neomycin commonly produces gastrointestinal upsets and superinfections with staphylococcal enterocolitis or fungus infections. Rarely, a patchy or generalized malabsorption syndrome resembling nontropical sprue may develop; normal bowel function appears on cessation of therapy, but a gluten free diet or glucocorticosteroids have no effect. Neomycin therapy is also associated with depression of intestinal disaccharidase activity caused by direct damage to the small intestinal brush border. Neomycin precipitates bile acids and may produce temporary hypocholesterolemia due to decreased sterol absorption. In sensitized patients, sufficient antibiotic will be absorbed to precipitate hypersensitivity reactions.

Parenteral neomycin is dangerous, and 500 mg daily in divided doses should not be exceeded. Neomycin is directly toxic to the sensory cells of the organ of Corti, and varying degrees of deafness may develop even several weeks *after the drug has been discontinued.* Similarly, neomycin is highly nephrotoxic, albuminuria developing in about 20% of patients. Hypersensitivity reactions may occur, such as various skin rashes, fever, paresthesias and headaches. Paradoxically, the incidence of hypersensitivity skin rashes is greater following parenteral than topical use. The incidence of renal damage and ototoxicity is greatly increased in patients with diminished renal function. Large doses of neomycin given by any route (particularly intraperitoneally) may induce ventilatory paralysis similar to that seen with streptomycin.

TABLE 56–2. Some Important Aminoglycoside Antibiotics

Drug	Source and chemistry	Properties	Preparations
Streptomycin	Isolated in 1944 from *Streptomyces gresius* following a carefully planned screening of soil Actinomycetes. A highly polar and complex glycosidic base usually prepared as the freely water soluble sulfate or hydrochloride	Only about 5% absorbed following oral administration necessitating SC or IM injection for systemic therapy. Streptomycin may rarely be given by intrathecal or intrapleural injection, but absorption following aerosol inhalation is very poor. *Topical preparations commonly induce hypersensitivity and should not be used* Streptomycin distribution is extracellular, but it is doubtful, even with large doses and with meningeal inflammation, whether satisfactory cerebrospinal fluid levels are obtainable. About 80% of the antibiotic is protein bound. Approximately 20% of administered streptomycin is degraded by unknown pathways. The remainder is excreted unchanged by glomerular filtration (70%) and by biliary excretion (10%) with a half-life of about 3 hr. In premature babies, the half-life is about 6–8 hr due to immature renal function	Streptomycin Sulfate *U.S.P.* is available for use by a variety of routes, the most important being IM. Dosage depends on the infection, but it is seldom desirable (except in the treatment of tuberculosis or subacute bacterial endocarditis) to exceed the average adult dose of 0.5–1.0 g twice daily for 7–14 days, best given by deep IM injection. Sufficiently large doses must be given in an attempt to prevent the development of bacterial resistance. Intravenous, intrapleural and intrathecal (25–100 mg/day in 10 ml of CSF) administration is rarely indicated. Many oral preparations for the treatment of diarrheal diseases (some of which may be of viral origin) contain streptomycin, but the efficacy of this antibiotic for this purpose is unproved and may even be dangerous because of the generation of multiple antibiotic resistance
Dihydrostreptomycin	Produced in 1947 by catalytic hydrogenation of of streptomycin	Not as potent as streptomycin while producing greater damage to the cochlear division of the eighth cranial nerve	Should not be used
Neomycin	Neomycins A, B and C are three closely related water soluble polybasic antibiotics obtained from *Streptomyces fradiae*. Neomycins B and C are isomers. Commercial preparations contain about 90% of neomycin B, the remainder being neomycin C	Only about 3% absorbed following oral administration. Only rarely given parenterally because of renal and eighth cranial nerve toxicity but rapidly absorbed following intramuscular injection with passage to most tissue compartments	Neomycin Sulfate, *U.S.P.* (Mycifradin), is available for topical, oral and parenteral administration. Topical preparations are often combined with other antibiotics, sulfonamides, cortisone, etc. The usual doses are: orally, 2–4 g 3 times daily; topically, 0.5% creams or ointments applied three times daily; IM, 250 mg twice daily
Kanamycin	A polybasic water soluble antibiotic obtained from *Streptomyces kanamyceticus*	Poorly absorbed following oral administration but readily distributed to most tissues and tissue fluid compartments with the exception of the CSF following parenteral injection. The half-life in normal adults is about 3 hr, and in premature babies about 18–20 hr. Excretion is primarily by way of renal glomerular filtration, but some kanamycin is secreted by the renal tubules. A single dose is essentially cleared in 24–48 hr if renal function is normal	Kanamycin Sulfate, *U.S.P.* (Kantrex) is available for oral, IM and IV use. For dosage see text

Gentamicin	A broad spectrum, bactericidal antibiotic, obtained from *Micromonospora purpurea* composed of three closely related fractions, gentamicins C_1, C_2 and C_{1a}. All fractions have similar molecular weights and are highly water soluble and stable in solution. Commercial preparations contain varying mixtures of the 3 fractions	Since absorption is poor following oral administration, the antibiotic is primarily given either topically or parenterally. Following IM administration, peak serum levels are achieved after about 1 hr, but absorption can be variable, necessitating the determination of serum levels to monitor therapy in severe infections. Gentamicin is bound about 30% to plasma proteins and in normal individuals has a half-life of 2–4 hr, with an apparent volume of distribution of 25–30% of the body weight. Gentamicin is primarily excreted unchanged by glomerular filtration, and in patients with uremia it may have a half-life of 40–50 hr or longer	Gentamicin Sulfate *U.S.P.* (Garamycin Sulfate) is available in 2 ml vials of 40 mg/ml and as a 0.1% ointment and cream. The usual dose for parenteral administration is 5–7 mg/kg in 3 divided doses on day 1 followed by 3 mg/kg from the 2nd day. For severe infections 2 mg/kg/8 hr may be given the 1st day irrespective of renal function. Thereafter, therapy should preferably be monitored by serum assays, attempting to maintain serum levels between 4–8 μg/ml. For severe bacterial meningitis, intrathecal gentamicin (4 mg/kg) should be combined with IM therapy. Dosage must be drastically reduced in patients with renal insufficiency
Viomycin	A highly water, soluble, strongly basic cyclic polypeptide produced by *Streptomyces puniceus*	Viomycin is not absorbed following oral administration, and must be given IM. Adverse reactions are more common with viomycin than with streptomycin. Hypersensitivity reactions (drug fever, eosinophilia and erythematous, maculopapular and pruritic skin rashes), and renal and eighth cranial nerve damage are common. Renal damage develops in over 50% of patients treated and may lead to edema with hypokalemia and hypocalcemia. These altered serum electrolyte patterns often produce electrocardiographic abnormalities suggesting direct myocardial damage. Skeletal muscle weakness and tetany may follow hypokalemia and hypocalcemia	Viomycin Sulfate *U.S.P.* (Viocin Sulfate) is usually given in doses of 1 g twice a day every 3 days. More frequent therapy increases the incidence of renal damage and ototoxicity. Viomycin should not be used to treat primary tuberculosis unless the causative organism is resistant to more potent chemotherapeutic agents, or where patients cannot tolerate these more potent drugs. When viomycin is used in the treatment of renal tuberculosis, concomitant urinary alkalinization potentiates its antitubercular effect

Uses

Neomycin is mainly used to reduce urease and ammonia producing organisms such as *Proteus* and Klebsiella spp. in patients with hepatic cirrhosis and in *E. coli* gastroenteritis in children. Additionally, neomycin with or without other drugs, such as erythromycin or tetracyclines, is advocated for preoperative bowel "preparation," since there is some evidence that its use is associated with a reduced incidence of septic complications following colon surgery.

Neomycin is highly effective topically for a variety of skin, external ear and conjunctival infections and for bladder irrigation. Commercial topical preparations frequently combine other antibiotics or glucocorticosteroids.

Parenteral neomycin is highly dangerous and is justified only as a life saving measure for infections due to bacteria demonstrated to be resistant to other similar less toxic agents such as gentamicin, the administration of which is more clearly defined.

KANAMYCIN

Kanamycin (Table 56–2) has an antibacterial spectrum very similar to that of neomycin and is effective against most strains of *Escherichia coli*, *Enterobacter*, *Proteus*, *Neisseria*, *Salomonella*, *Shigella*, *Staphylococcus* and *Klebsiella*. It is also weakly active against *Mycobacterium tuberculo-*

KANAMYCIN

sis. Most strains of *Pseudomonas aeruginosa* are resistant. Some bacteria resistant to kanamycin also show streptomycin resistance, but not all organisms resistant to streptomycin are kanamycin resistant.

Adverse Effects

Hypersensitivity maculopapular skin rashes, eosinophilia, drug fever, pruritis, headaches and various paresthesias may occur. Anaphylactic shock is rare. Like other aminoglycoside antibiotics, kanamycin tends to increase muscle weakness in patients with myasthenia gravis. Repeated kanamycin injections into the same muscle area may be followed by sterile abscess formation. Oral therapy may result in severe superinfection, diarrhea, cheilosis and proctocolitis. Like streptomycin and neomycin, kanamycin

may produce renal tubular damage and auditory and vestibular nerve injury. These are more common following IV administration of the antibiotic. Unlike deafness associated with neomycin, the auditory deficit does not progress on cessation of therapy. Kanamycin may induce a postoperative curare-like paralysis similar to that produced by streptomycin.

Uses and Dosage

Kanamycin is most often used in treating infections due to *E. coli, Klebsiella* spp., *Enterobacter*, and *Proteus* spp. It is a toxic drug which should be reserved for infections resistant to less dangerous antibiotics or for use in patients allergic to other drugs.

Orally it is of use in the treatment of hepatic coma (1–2 g three times daily for 5–10 days) and in preoperative bowel "sterilization."

Intramuscular therapy (10–15 mg/kg daily in two divided doses for 7–14 days) should be carefully monitored by frequent determinations of the state of renal function. A total daily dose of 1.5 g should not be exceeded irrespective of patient age, and a total dose of 15 g should not be exceeded for a single course of therapy. Optimum blood levels are probably in the range 20–30 μg/ml. If tinnitus, ataxia, dizziness or deafness occurs, kanamycin should be discontinued immediately.

Intravenous kanamycin should be reserved for the critically ill patient with a life threatening infection. *It should be given in reduced dosage in the presence of renal failure.* The usual dose is 10–15 mg/kg daily in divided increments, given by slow infusion as a 0.25% solution.

GENTAMICIN

Gentamicin (Table 56–2) possesses a broad antibacterial spectrum and is in general more potent than other aminoglycosides. It is effective against most strains of *Pseudomonas aeruginosa* which are inhibited by blood levels of about 10 μg/ml. It is also effective against many strains of *E. coli*, *Klebsiella*, *Enterobacter*, *Providencia*, *Serratia*, *Indole negative* proteus, *Shigella*, *Salmonella*, *Haemophilus influenzae*, *Mycoplasma*, *Neisseria*, *Staph. aureus*, group A streptococci and *D. pneumonia*. Indole positive proteus is variably sensitive. Either the tube dilution or agar diffusion tests are satisfactory for evaluating in vitro sensitivity to gentamicin. The Kirby/Bauer disk method yields irregular results.

Slow stepwise resistance has been demonstrated in vitro for a variety of organisms. Explosive resistance as seen with streptomycin therapy apparently does not occur. Gentamicin may be active against bacteria resistant to streptomycin, kanamycin and neomycin, but if organisms are resistant to gentamicin, cross resistance is invariably shown towards the other aminoglycosides except possibly BBK8.

Adverse Reactions

Adverse reactions to topical therapy are minimal. Following parenteral administration, maculopapular skin rashes, nausea, vomiting, headaches and signs of renal and hepatic damage (elevated blood urea nitrogen and serum glutamic oxaloacetic transaminase and alkaline phosphatase activity) may occur. By far the most serious toxicity is directed towards the eighth cranial nerve, with the vestibular division being more sensitive to damage. Vestibular damage tends to be irreversible. It is dose dependent and more likely to develop if peak gentamicin plasma levels exceed 10 μg/ml. Renal toxicity is not as common as vestibular damage but may develop when large doses of gentamicin are given, or in patients who have preexisting renal disease. In patients with preexisting renal disease, uncontrolled therapy may rapidly be followed by progressive renal failure. Neuromuscular block has not yet been reported to occur with gentamicin therapy. Following oral administration of gentamicin (rarely prescribed), gastrointestinal superinfections may develop.

Patients on gentamicin therapy should be monitored with respect to their plasma drug levels and to their renal and eighth cranial nerve functions.

Gentamicin is used locally in primary skin infections (e.g., impetigo, ecthyma, pyoderma gangrenosum, sycosis barbae) and secondary skin infections (e.g., pustular acne, pustular psoriasis). It has no antifungal activity but is occasionally useful in treating the secondary bacterial infections superimposed on such conditions (Ch. 65). The cream is preferable for moist areas and the ointment for dry locations. Topical gentamicin should be reserved for use in burn units and only be used in critically ill patients with *Pseudomonas, E. coli,* or *Klebsiella/Enterobacter* infections. It may on occasions be combined with success with mafenide (Ch. 60) or with silver nitrate (Ch. 62).

Parenteral gentamicin may be life saving in patients with serious infections due to gram-negative bacilli such as *Pseudomonas aeruginosa, E. coli* and *Klebsiella/Aerobacter* spp., resistant to less dangerous antibiotics. Carbenicillin may be given concomitantly in the treatment of Pseudomonas infections; however, care must be taken not to mix the two antibiotics in the same syringe since they interact and mutually destroy one another. When gram-negative

meningeal infections resistant to chloramphenicol are suspected, e.g., in the neonate, the subject with meningomyelocoel or in postoperative neurosurgical patients, intrathecal gentamicin may be life saving.

VIOMYCIN

Viomycin (Table 56–2) is a second line drug in the treatment of tuberculosis. It is weakly tuberculostatic, and mycobacterial resistance develops rapidly. Like other antitubercular drugs, the emergence of resistant strains can be delayed by the addition of one or more tuberculostatic drugs.

TREATMENT OF TUBERCULOSIS

Treatment of tuberculosis is a complex, long term procedure. This is primarily because of the characteristics of the causative organism, the nature and course of the disease process and because of the unpredictableness of host defense mechanisms. Drug treatment is the cornerstone of therapy, surgical intervention being required only rarely, but there are many factors to be considered in treatment as the disease is frequently associated with poverty, malnutrition, inadequate housing or a variety of other disease states.

Drug treatment of tuberculosis is twofold: therapy of active disease and prophylaxis.

TREATMENT OF ACTIVE DISEASE

Antitubercular drugs effectively treat active disease and control infectiousness. They are clinically divided into first line (primary) and second line (secondary) drugs (Table 56–3), depending upon their efficacy and degree of toxicity.

Between 5–10% of patients with primary tuberculosis yield cultures resistant to one first line drug. Therefore, it may be best to initiate therapy with three primary drugs, thus insuring that at least two drugs to which the mycobacteria are susceptible are given. However, the use of three or two first line drugs is controversial. Initial therapy should be continued in the dosage given in

TABLE 56–3. First and Second Line Antitubercular Drugs

First line	Second line
Isoniazid	Pyrazinamide
Streptomycin	Ethionamide
Para-aminosalicylic acid (PAS)	Cycloserine
Ethambutol	Kanamycin
Rifampicin (rifampin)	Viomycin
	Capreomycin
	Thiacetazone
	Streptovaricin
	Oxytetracycline
	Erythromycin

TABLE 56–4. Dosage of Antitubercular Drugs

Drug	Total dose	Details of administration
Streptomycin	1 g	Patients $<$40 yr, daily for 1st mo then 3/wk
	0.75 g	Patients $>$40 yr, daily for 1st mo then 3/wk
	1 g	2 or 3/wk with high dose isoniazid
Sodium PAS	12–16 g	In 2–4 divided doses daily
Isoniazid	300 mg	In 1 or 3 divided doses daily
	15 mg/kg	2 or 3/wk with streptomycin
Thiacetazone	150 mg	Single dose daily
Ethambutol	25 mg/kg	Single dose daily for first 2 mo
	15 mg/kg	Single dose daily after 2 mo
Rifampicin	450–600 mg	Single dose daily

Modified from Citron KM (1973): Tuberculosis. Br Med J 2:296–298

Table 56–4 for between 6 weeks to 6 months, depending upon the location and severity of the disease. Long term continuation therapy can then be initiated for 1–2 years, again depending upon the location and severity of the infection.

The use of two or three **first line drugs** in the treatment of active disease is of paramount importance, first to reduce the development of mycobacterial resistance and second to produce a potentiated tuberculostatic effect. Mycobacterial sensitivity should be determined in fresh cases, and periodically in chronic cases, but results of testing are often unreliable, and greater weight should be placed on clinical response and radiological findings.

The simultaneous use of the three primary drugs is justified in severe overwhelming infections and in new cases of active disease prior to the results of sensitivity tests, or when there is some indication that resistance to one of the primary drugs may be present.

Isoniazid, streptomycin and PAS are time honored first line drugs, but because of the difficulties of administering streptomycin and the problems associated with the use of PAS (Ch. 61), these latter two agents are being replaced by rifampin and ethambutol. Although rifampin and ethambutol are potent antitubercular agents producing fewer side effects than streptomycin and PAS, they are expensive, and only limited clinical experience has been accumulated on their use as first line drugs.

Secondary drugs are used in the face of mycobacterial resistance to the primary drugs or in the presence of allergy to the primary drugs. All secondary drugs exhibit low potency, and most are considerably more toxic than the primary ones and must be discontinued after several months. It is usually considered advantageous to combine three secondary drugs; however, various combinations of primary or secondary drugs are employed. Secondary drugs may be of real value in giving short term chemotherapeutic cover during the surgical removal of tubercular tissue.

DRUG RESISTANCE. Resistance to antitubercular drugs is a major therapeutic problem. Patterns of drug resistance show striking differences in different populations. For example, the higher incidence of drug resistance in India and the near East may reflect the added hazards of poor housing and nutrition as well as (presumably) irregular and inconstant self-medication. In the United States, resistant organisms have been reported to be more common in the Black subject than in the Caucasian. As indicated above, the use of a second drug tends only to reduce the likelihood of emergence of drug resistance; *it will not prevent its occurrence.* Mycobacteria resistant to isoniazid may be less pathogenic than isoniazid susceptible organisms. *Uncontrolled intermittant therapy or failure to take both or all antitubercular drugs favors the development of resistant strains and are the principle causes of therapeutic failure.*

USE OF CORTICOSTEROID DRUGS. Adrenocorticosteroid drugs are frequently advocated as adjunctive agents in the treatment of tuberculosis, to reduce symptoms and inflammatory adhesions and to facilitate healing of caseous foci. Apart from their indispensability in adrenal insufficiency, their value is debatable. Many authorities believe that if the mycobacteria are highly sensitive to the primary drugs, a short concomitant course of corticosteroids is of value in tuberculous meningitis with intraspinal or intracisternal block, in tuberculous pneumonia or in miliary tuberculosis. Corticosteroids depress the tuberculin reaction.

If glucocorticosteroids are required for nontuberculous disease in a patient with either inactive tuberculosis, or a positive skin test, they need not be withheld provided adequate prophylactic therapy with isoniazid (300 mg/day for the duration of steroid therapy and continued for an additional 6 months) is undertaken. Glucocorticosteroids may be of symptomatic benefit in the treatment of allergies to antitubercular drugs.

Prophylaxis

Prophylaxis with isoniazid or isoniazid plus PAS is often undertaken to prevent the development of active tuberculosis in persons at high risk. Prophylaxis can either be **primary** (prevention of infection) or **secondary** (prevention of disease in an infected patient) and should usually be continued for at least 1 year. There is some debate as to whom should receive prophylactic therapy and as to the dosage and time sequence of therapy.

A strong case can be made for prophylaxis in the following situations: recent skin test converters; contacts, especially young children, and all subjects with positive skin tests in the following categories: adolescent females, pregnant women (treatment is started in the last trimester and continued for 1 year), patients with silicosis, lymphoma or unstable diabetes mellitus and in postgastrectomy patients or in those taking glucocorticosteroids.

Conventionally, isoniazid alone, 100 mg 8 hourly is used; PAS 4 g 8 hourly is added by some authorities. However, since patient compliance on daily therapy is far from 100%, it has been suggested that large doses of two antitubercular drugs should be given twice or three times a week (preferably supervised by a physician or a Public Health employee) in order to minimize the development of mycobacterial resistance. Recommended twice weekly therapy has been either isoniazid 15 mg/kg plus PAS 12 g, or isoniazid 15 mg/kg plus streptomycin 1 g (Table 56–4). The intermittant nature of twice weekly therapy is apparently not followed by a higher incidence of drug resistance as one might expect, since there is a delay of several days in the establishment of logarithmic growth in mycobacteria following clearance of antitubercular drugs.

TREATMENT OF ATYPICAL MYCOBACTERIA

Atypical mycobacterial infections are difficult to treat. There is frequently a poor correlation between in vitro testing and clinical effectiveness, particularly with infections caused by the Battey strain. The five primary drugs are usually administered concomitantly. Pyrazinamide or cycloserine may replace PAS. Treatment is complicated by the high degree of mycobacterial resistance, the necessity for surgical intervention in localized disease and even with sensitive strains the need for a prolonged course of drug exposure.

FURTHER READING

Citron, KM (1973): Tuberculosis. Br Med J 2:296–298

Faloon, WW (1970): Metabolic effects of nonabsorbable antibacterial agents. Am J Clin Nut 23:645–651

Fox, W (1971): General considerations in intermittent drug therapy of pulmonary tuberculosis. Postgrad Med J 47:729–736

JEREMY H. THOMPSON

57. ANTIBIOTICS WHICH INTERFERE WITH PROTEIN SYNTHESIS: II

Several important antibiotics inhibiting protein synthesis are presented in this chapter.

THE TETRACYCLINES

Tetracyclines were originally isolated from various species of *Streptomyces* (Fig. 57–1). Recently, however, several semisynthetic derivatives have been introduced into therapy, some of which have subsequently been found in nature. The generic term **tetracycline** is used to describe the whole group. Some physicians claim that one tetracycline is clinically superior to another, but the major compounds are essentially similar, showing only slight differences in acid stability, amount or rapidity of absorption, height of tissue level, rate of clearance or degree of toxicity (Fig. 57–1; Table 57–2). This allows a single and unified description of this class of compounds. Important differences among the various members are indicated in the text.

Chemistry

Tetracycline crystalline bases are yellowish, odorless and slightly bitter compounds. They are poorly water soluble but readily form highly soluble sodium and hydrochloride salts. Dry powders are highly stable, but aqueous solutions usually show appreciable loss of activity within 24–48 hr, particularly at an elevated pH. Rolitetracycline is buffered to neutral pH but is the least stable of the tetracyclines; demeclocycline is the most stable.

Antibacterial Spectrum and Resistance

The tetracyclines are *broad spectrum antibiotics* with an antibacterial spectrum overlapping those of the penicillins and cephalosporins, the aminoglycosides, and chloramphenicol (Table 57–1).

Gram-positive bacteria are usually affected by lower concentrations of the antibiotics than are gram-negative species. *Broad spectrum* must not be confused with *license for broad nonspecific use* (Ch. 52).

Bacterial resistance develops in a slow, stepwise manner, as with penicillin, and mechanisms of resistance are discussed above (Ch. 52). Organisms resistant to one tetracycline are almost invariably resistant to equipotent concentrations of all other tetracyclines. Rarely, organisms *dependent* upon chlortetracycline have been isolated from man. Bacteria may show varying susceptibility to the different tetracyclines on in vitro testing, but it is not certain how important these differences are in clinical infections. Antibacterial cross resistance for gram-negative organisms is common with chloramphenicol.

Mode of Action

The tetracyclines depress protein synthesis (Ch. 53) and may additionally disrupt the bacterial cell membrane by complexing essential divalent metals. They are usually bacteriostatic, but under exceptional circumstances they may be bactericidal.

Absorption and Metabolism

In general, the tetracyclines are incompletely and irregularly absorbed following oral administration, with as much as 30% being excreted unchanged. Absorption, however, is usually adequate to treat most infections. Absorption is depressed by food (except for doxycyline), calcium, magnesium, iron and aluminum salts, and slightly by milk, since the tetracyclines form nonabsorbable chelates with heavy metals. The addition of phosphate (as in tetracycline phosphate complex) may partially neutralize the chelating

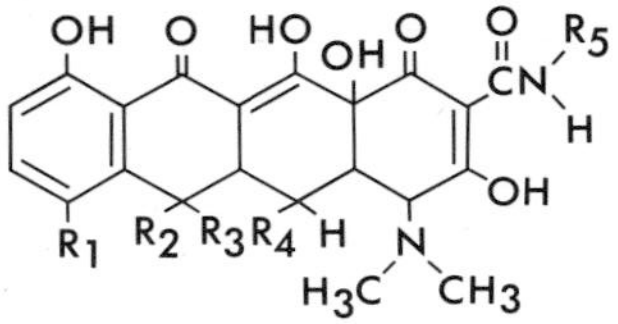

Drug	Source	Plasma protein binding (%)	Renal clearance (ml/min)	Half-life (hr)	SUBSTITUTIONS				
					R$_1$	R$_2$	R$_3$	R$_4$	R$_5$
Chlortetracycline (1948)	*Streptomyces aureofaciens*	40–70	30	4–6	Cl	CH$_3$	OH	H	H
Oxytetracycline (1950)	*Streptomyces rimosus*	20–35	85	8–10	H	CH$_3$	OH	OH	H
Tetracycline (1952)	Semisynthetically derived from chlor-tetracycline	25–60	60	8–9	H	CH$_3$	OH	H	H
Demeclocycline (1959)	*Streptomyces aureofaciens*	40–90	25–35	10–17	Cl	H	OH	H	H
Rolitetracycline (1960)	Synthetically derived from tetra-cycline	?	?	?	H	CH$_3$	OH	H	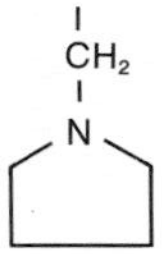 –CH$_2$–N (pyrrolidinyl)
Methacycline (1961)	Semisynthetically derived from oxytetracycline	75–90	30	10–16	H	CH$_2$	H	OH	H
Doxycycline (1966)	Hydrogenation of methacycline	25–90	20–30	12–20	H	CH$_3$	H	OH	H
Minocycline (1970)	Semisynthetically derived from tetracycline	70–75	10	12–19	N (CH$_3$)$_2$	H	H	H	H

FIG. 57–1. **The major tetracycline antibiotics.** The year of introduction into therapeutics is indicated in parenthesis.

TABLE 57-1. Common Organisms Affected by the Tetracyclines

Organism	Sensitivity	Organism	Sensitivity
Actinobacillus malleii	++	*Klebsiella pneumoniae*	++R
Actinomyces israelii	+++	*Leptospira icterohemorrhagiae*	++
Enterobacter aerogenes	++R	*Listeria monocytogenes*	++
Bacillus anthracis	++	*Mycoplasma pneumoniae*	+++
Bacteroides spp	++R	*Neisseria gonorrhoeae*	++
Balantidium coli	++	*Neisseria meningitidis*	++
Borrelia recurrentis	+++	*Pasturella pestis*	++
Brucellae spp	+++R	*Francisella (Pasturella)*	
Chlamydia (Bedsonia)	+++	*tularensis*	++
Cholera vibrio	+++	*Pseudomonas pseudomalleii*	++
Calymmatobacterium granulomatis	+++	*Rickettsiae*	+++
Clostridium perfringens	++	*Salmonellae*	++R
Clostridium tetani	++	*Shigellae*	++R
E. Coli	++R	*Staphylococcus aureus*	+R
Entameba histolytica	++	*Streptococci*	++R
Haemophilus duceyi	+++	*Treponema pallidum*	+
Haemophilus influenzae	+++R	*Treponema pertenue*	+

R In vitro testing essential, as many strains are resistant
+++ High sensitivity
++ moderate sensitivity
+ Some sensitivity but tetracyclines not recommended for therapy

effect of calcium. In order of decreasing absorbability are doxycycline, minocycline, methacycline, demeclocycline, tetracycline, chlortetracycline and oxytetracycline; the rate of absorption has little influence on their half-lives (Fig. 57–1).

A single oral dose of 100 mg doxycycline produces plasma levels similar to 300 mg twice daily of demeclocycline and 250 mg four times daily of chlortetracycline, tetracycline and oxytetracycline. The prolonged plasma levels seen with doxycycline and demeclocycline are primarily due to slow renal excretion (Fig. 57–1), making these agents effective for outpatient use. Methacycline has a long half-life resulting from high plasma protein binding.

For IV administration the tetracycline solution should be less than 5 mg/ml to minimize thrombophlebitis. Intramuscular tetracycline is effective but painful; the antibiotic can be detected in plasma within about 15 min and peak levels develop within 60 min. Chlortetracycline is poorly absorbed from IM sites.

The tetracyclines have a volume of distribution a little larger than that of total body water, and since they are cleared by the liver, high antibiotic

TABLE 57-2. Some Popular Oral and Parenteral Tetracycline Preparations

Drug	Doses for oral administration (mg)		Doses for parenteral administration (mg)*	
	Loading	Maintenance	IV	IM
Chlortetracycline hydrochloride, *N.F.*	500	250–500, 6 hourly	Must be freshly prepared since relatively unstable. 250–500, 12 hourly	100, 8 hourly
Demeclocycline hydrochloride, *N.F.*	600	150–300, 6–12 hourly	—	—
Doxycycline	100–200	100 mg, 12–24 hourly	—	—
Methacycline hydrochloride, *N.F.*	300	150, 6 hourly	—	—
Minocycline	200	100 mg, 12 hourly	—	—
Oxytetracycline hydrochloride *U.S.P.*	500	250–500, 6 hourly	250–500, 12 hourly	100, 8 hourly
Rolitetracycline *N.F.*			Reserved for management of severe infections where oral administration is impossible. 150–300, 12 hourly	Reserved for management of severe infections where oral administration is impossible. 150–300, 12 hourly
Tetracycline hydrochloride, *U.S.P.*	500	250–500, 6 hourly	250–500, 12 hourly	100, 8 hourly
Tetracycline phosphate complex	500	250–500, 6 hourly	—	—

* Do not give more than 2 g tetracycline/day parenterally, since this is likely to produce hepatic damage

concentrations occur in both hepatic parenchyma and in the bile, reaching 10–30 times simultaneous plasma levels. Biliary excretion results in a diminishing enterohepatic recirculation. Tetracycline levels in the cerebrospinal fluid are primarily dependent on duration of therapy rather than on actual dosages and usually average about one-fifth of simultaneous plasma levels. Tetracycline passes most readily into the cerebrospinal fluid and demeclocycline least readily. Tetracycline and oxytetracycline readily cross the placenta (demeclocycline and chlortetracycline do so poorly) to the fetus, and antibiotic concentrations in milk during lactation may be one-third to one-half simultaneous plasma levels (see below).

Excretion

Tetracyclines are excreted primarily in the urine by glomerular filtration (Fig. 57–1), and to a lesser extent in the bile, and in the milk during lactation (see below). Oxytetracycline is preferentially excreted in the urine and chlortetracycline in the bile.

Adverse Effects

Adverse reactions to the tetracyclines are classified as **hypersensitivity reactions** and **biologic and toxic reactions.**

HYPERSENSITIVITY REACTIONS. Gastrointestinal disturbances including cheilosis, black hairy tongue (Fig. 7–1), glossitis and anogenital pruritus, burning, pain or tenesmus occur in about 20–30% of patients. These may be partly hypersensitivity or toxic reactions and partly due to superinfection; vitamin deficiencies are probably not involved. Skin rashes of all types may occur, particularly morbiliform rashes and urticaria, and in severe cases, exfoliative dermatitis. Skin rashes may be accompanied by fever, eosinophilia, angioedema or anaphylactic shock, which is supposedly more common after demeclocycline. Lightheadedness, Jarisch-Herxheimer-like reactions, pancreatitis, burning of the eyes and periorbital areas and blood dyscrasias (thrombocytopenia, lymphocytosis and "toxic" granulation of the leukocytes) are rare.

Demeclocycline and doxycycline may cause phototoxic dermatitis; other tetracyclines produce the reaction rarely. The reaction is more common with doses of demeclocycline exceeding 100 mg/day. Usually phototoxicity is accompanied by high fever, eosinophilia and, in severe cases, shedding of the hair and nails and residual nail pigmentation.

BIOLOGIC AND TOXIC REACTIONS: TISSUE IRRITATION. When taken orally, the tetracyclines (particularly oxytetracycline) produce dose dependant gastrointestinal irritation, particularly nausea, vomiting, anorexia and diarrhea. Consequently, they should be given with care to patients with peptic ulcer disease. The diarrhea of irritation must be differentiated from the diarrhea of superinfection (see below), since the latter demands prompt cessation of tetracycline therapy, the institution of supportive measures and a new antibiotic. Milk and calcium and aluminum antacids reduce the gastrointestinal symptoms of oral tetracycline therapy but also depress its absorption. Intramuscular administration of tetracyclines is painful. Injection sites should be alternated. Intravenous therapy can induce thrombophlebitis, a reaction which is minimized by keeping the tetracycline concentration less than 0.5%.

SUPERINFECTION. The broad spectrum tetracyclines rapidly depress the normal body flora, particularly that of the gastrointestinal tract, and after a couple of days of therapy, the feces become soft, unformed and odorless, and superinfection (Ch. 52) is likely. Usual superinfecting organisms are penicillinase producing staphylococci, various strains of *Proteus* and *Pseudomonas* and *Candida albicans.* Necrotizing (pseudomembranous) enterocolitis may also develop.

DAMAGE TO TEETH, BONES AND NAILS. Tetracyclines readily bind to unerupted teeth at the time of their development and calcification, with the formation of tetracycline-calcium orthophosphate complexes. Antibiotic binding depends upon the individual tetracycline and the total dose given, but not upon duration of therapy; oxytetracycline and doxycycline appear to be the least likely to bind to teeth and bones. Antibiotic binding results in **tooth staining** and with high exposure partial or complete **enamel hypoplasia** (Fig. 7–1) probably due to interference with the presecretory and secretory ameloblasts. Tooth staining is seen shortly after eruption as yellowish bands which fluoresce under ultraviolet light. Fluorescence is gradually lost as the tetracycline is oxidized to gray-brown metabolites. Stained and hypoplastic teeth may be more inclined to carious degeneration than are normal teeth, and furthermore they pose a cosmetic problem.

Damage to deciduous and or permanent teeth occurs, depending upon the time and duration of exposure in relationship to tooth development. Exposure of the fetus from about the third month of gestation, or of the neonate and baby up to about 12 months of age, can result in staining and enamel hypoplasia of the deciduous teeth. Similar effects may be seen in the permanent dentition if antibiotic exposure occurs from about 6 months of gestation up to 8–10 years of age.

Osseous deposition of tetracyclines can cause a reversible depression of linear bone growth in premature infants. Yellow, brown or gray discoloration and pitting of the nails can also appear following tetracycline therapy in any age group.

METABOLIC EFFECTS. The tetracyclines may depress liver function, particularly when given parenterally in doses of 2 g or more per day. Oxytetracycline and tetracycline are the least hepatotoxic of the tetracyclines, but they still may produce this condition. Histologically, hepatocytes show vacuolation and fatty infiltration, and progression to massive hepatic necrosis may occur. Contributing factors to necrosis are renal insufficiency (resulting in higher plasma levels) and pregnancy; the increased demand for protein anabolism during pregnancy may make the liver more susceptible to drugs, such as the tetracyclines, which depress this function. Tetracyclines produce weight loss and a negative nitrogen balance, presumably due to a direct depression of host protein synthesis.

Tetracyclines may prolong blood coagulation either indirectly by depressing prothrombin synthesis (depression of colonic bacterial flora) or directly by chelating serum calcium and/or interfering with plasma lipoproteins. An increase in the quantity of urinary bilirubin, and a decrease in the urobillinogen, may result from depression of the colonic flora. Tetracyclines increase the urinary excretion of folic acid and riboflavin and may produce increased intracranial pressure (pseudotumor cerebrii) in children. In advanced renal failure, if the dose of tetracycline is not adjusted downwards, progressive azotemia, acidosis, hyperphosphatemia, negative nitrogen balance, potassium loss in the urine, anorexia and nausea and vomiting will develop.

RENAL DAMAGE. Tetracyclines were originally buffered with citric acid, which used to lose its buffering capacity under extremes of temperature and humidity with the production of (among others) anhydrotetracycline and 4-epianhydrotetracycline. These compounds could produce in a few days reversible facial lesions resembling systemic lupus erythematosus and a Fanconi-like syndrome (nausea, vomiting, glycosuria, polyuria, polydipsia, aminoaciduria, proteinuria and acidosis). Parenteral tetracyclines are currently buffered with lactose, which is more stable than citric acid. However, lactose buffered tetracyclines usually contain small quantities of anhydrotetracycline and 4-epianhydrotetracline, and although these levels increase only slightly during conditions of proper storage, they increase rapidly under extremes of storage.

Demeclocycline may induce nephrogenic diabetes insipidus, and tetracyclines when given in association with methoxyfluorane anesthesia may produce acute renal tubular necrosis.

Preparations and Dosage

Many preparations (Table 57–2) are available for oral, parenteral and topical administration either singly, in combinations or with other drugs such as antifungal agents. Tetracyclines with antifungal agents have been suggested for use in patients with malignant or metabolic disease to prevent *C. albicans* superinfection (Ch. 52); their value is questionable.

Oral administration of tetracyclines is safest. Parenteral administration seldom needs to be continued more than a few days, but more prolonged treatment may be required for the unconscious patient and for those who do not respond promptly or who cannot ingest or absorb oral preparations. Slow IV infusion (5 mg/ml or less) is preferred to IM injection which should be combined with a local anesthetic. Tetracyclines should *never* be given intrathecally, and apart from the conjunctival sac in solutions or ointments of 0.5–1.0%, topical application is not recommended. In general, the newer tetracyclines offer no advantage over the older preparations, whereas they tend to be considerably more expensive.

Uses

ANTIBACTERIAL USES. Tetracyclines are usually contraindicated during pregnancy, lactation, peptic ulcer disease and hepatic disease; in the last instance, administration is especially dangerous. Doses larger than 1 g/day are seldom required and *doses greater than 2 g/day parenterally should not be given.*

Because of their broad antibacterial spectrum, the tetracyclines enjoy wide popularity, but other drugs may be more potent and desirable, particularly if a bactericidal effect is required. The tetracyclines are effective in the treatment of many infections, notably those due to the rickettsiae, the Chlamydia, Mycoplasmae (PPLO), bacterioides, hemolytic streptococci and staphylococci. They are also effective in cholera, relapsing fever, tularemia, chancroid, granuloma inguinale, syphilis, yaws, gonorrhea, leptospirosis, actinomycosis and nocardiosis. In the treatment of melioidosis, brucellosis and glanders, streptomycin may be added to tetracycline with advantage. Some gram-negative urinary tract infections may be susceptible. The mode of action of tetracyclines in the treatment of *Balantidium coli* and *Entamoeba histolytica* infections is probably indirect (Ch. 63). Tetracyclines are the drugs of choice for Whipple's disease, the "Blind Loop" syndromes and Tropical sprue. In the penicillin allergic patient, the tetracyclines or chloramphenicol are the agents of choice for *H. influenzae*, pneumococcal and meningococcal meningitis. Doxycycline and minocycline may possess greater activity against some anaerobic bacteria and some staphylococci, respectively, than other tetracyclines. In addition, minocycline may be superior to other related agents and the sulfonamides in the prophylaxis of meningococcal infections, and in meningococcal carriers.

Chronic tetracycline therapy with topical desquamating agents is used for severe inflammatory, recalcitrant acne; noninflammatory acne (comedones) does not respond to antibacterial

TABLE 57—3. Some Antibiotics Inhibiting Protein Synthesis

Drug	Properties	Preparations
Chloramphenicol	Chloramphenicol is unique in that it contains a nitrobenzene radicle. Only the *L*-form is biologically active. Rapidly absorbed after oral administration with peak plasma levels of 30 μg/ml developing within 2 hr following a 2 g dose. Poorly absorbed following IM administration. Highly diffusable, and appears in most body tissues and secretions and in the fetus. Bound about 40—50% to plasma proteins and has a half-life of 2–3 hr. Degraded by glucuronyl transferase. Free chloramphenicol is cleared by glomerular filtration and the glucuronated metabolite by tubular secretion	Oral: Chloramphenicol *U.S.P.* (Chloromycetin), capsules and Chloramphenicol Palmitate Oral Suspension *U.S.P.* which is hydrolyzed in the bowel lumen to chloramphenicol Parenteral: Sterile Chloramphenicol for Suspension *N.F.* is for IV or IM use. Sterile Chloramphenicol Sodium Succinate *U.S.P.,* is a water soluble preparation for IV use only Topical: Chloramphenicol Ophthalmic Ointment *U.S.P.* contains 1% of the antibiotic
Erythromycin	Erythromycin base is partially destroyed by gastric acid but sufficiently absorbed to treat most infections; food, by delaying gastric emptying, reduces its absorption. Erythromycin stearate, erythromycin base in enteric-coated capsules or erythromycin estolate are not acid labile, and thus higher blood levels are achieved with these preparations. Following 500 mg of the stearate, e.g., peak blood levels of 5—15 μg/ml develop in 1—4 hr Erythromycin diffuses well into most tissue compartments except the CSF. It is concentrated in the liver and bile, and concentrations there may reach 20—50 times simultaneous plasma levels. Following a single oral or IV dose only about 5–15% of the antibiotic appears, respectively, as active drug in the urine	Oral: Erythromycin Base *U.S.P.* (Ilotycin) and Erythromycin Sterate *U.S.P.* are available in tablets and enteric-coated tablets of 100 and 250 mg. Erythromycin Estolate *N.F.* (the lauryl sulfate salt of the propionic acid ester of erythromycin) is available as capsules of 125 and 250 mg and as a liquid of 25 mg/ml. Erythromycin Stearate and Erythromycin Ethyl Carbonate *U.S.P.* are available as dry powders for reconstitution or as oral suspensions Parenteral: Erythromycin Ethylsuccinate (50 mg/ml) contains the local anesthetic 2% butyl amino benzoate for IM administration. Erythromycin Lactobionate *U.S.P.* and Erythromycin Gluceptate *U.S.P.* are available in doses of 0.25, 0.50 and 1.0 g for IV administration Topical: Erythromycin Base *U.S.P.* is available as a 0.5 or 1.0% ointment
Oleandomycin	A weak basic macrolide antibiotic isolated from *Streptomyces antibioticus.* Primarily bacteriostatic but may assume bactericidal properties. Similar to erythromycin in antibacterial spectrum, mode of action and adverse effects. Bacterial resistance develops rapidly. Acid stable and well absorbed following oral administration. Very poorly absorbed following IM injection. Well distributed except to the CSF. Excreted by the kidneys and in the bile	Oleandomycin Phosphate *N.F.* is given orally in doses of 250–500 mg 6–8 hourly. The total daily dose should not exceed 3 g. Oleandomycin Phosphate for Injection *N.F.* is usually given in doses of 500 mg 8 hourly
Troleandomycin	Synthetic triacetyl derivative of oleandomycin, but not as potent. Troleandomycin administered orally is detected as oleandomycin in the plasma. About 30% of patients taking troleandomycin for greater than 10 days develop intrahepatic cholestasis (see erythromycin, adverse effects)	Troleandomycin *N.F.* is given orally in doses of 250–500 mg 6–8 hourly. The total daily dose should not exceed 3 g
Spiramycin	Resembles erythromycin in most of its properties but is less potent, and bacterial resistance is only of limited importance. Not acid labile and absorbed rapidly following oral administration. Available only in Canada and France	Spiramycin Base (Rovamycin) is usually given orally in doses of 0.5—1.0 g 6 hourly

therapy. The lesions in inflammatory acne result from a disorganization of follicular epithelium with subsequent blockade of the sebum gland duct. This leads to rupture of the follicular contents into the dermis, where free fatty acids liberated from sebum triglycerides by lipases from *Propionibacterium acnes* and other organisms cause inflammation. Antibiotics benefit the acne lesions by killing the microorganisms that produce the lipases. Tetracycline dosage is empirical; 500–1000 mg/day and adjusted downwards to about 250 mg every 2 days. Full antilipolytic effect may not be seen for several weeks. Tetracyclines are also effective in the long term treatment of chronic bronchitis and cystic fibrosis (Table 52–3).

Because the bacterial flora in the colon is depressed by the tetracyclines, 5 mg of vitamin K orally is a useful adjunct to therapy. Riboflavin and folic acid deficiency are thereoretically possible, and with chronic tetracycline therapy a multivitamin preparation is desirable.

NONANTIBACTERIAL USES. All tetracyclines (particularly demeclocycline) have the property of binding to some cancerous tissues and exhibiting a golden yellow fluorescence when exposed to ultraviolet light. This property has been used as the basis of several diagnostic tests for gastric and colonic cancer. Tetracyclines have also been used to determine the rate of bone turnover.

CHLORAMPHENICOL

Chloramphenicol is a broad spectrum bacteriostatic antibiotic originally isolated from *Streptomyces venezuelae* but now produced synthetically. Its clinical use should be restricted due to the dangers of bone marrow toxicity.

CHLORAMPHENICOL

Antibacterial Spectrum and Resistance

Chloramphenicol has a broad spectrum of activity, almost equivalent to that of the tetracyclines. It is effective against many gram-positive and gram-negative organisms and demonstrates activity against the Chlamydiae and rickettsiae. Because of its toxicity, chloramphenicol should be restricted to the treatment of salmonelloses and infections due to rickettsiae, *Haemophilus influenzae,* gram-positive organisms resistant to less toxic antibiotics, the Chlamydiae, and anaerobic infections, particularly with *Bacteroides fragilis.* R factor mediated bacterial resistance is of increasing clinical consequence, but it develops slowly. Resistance is not seen in rickettsial organisms nor in *Bacteroides fragilis.* Para-aminosalicylic acid therapy favors the resistance of *Escherichia coli* to chloramphenicol, and some enteric bacteria may demonstrate cross resistance with the tetracyclines or erythromycin.

Mode of Action and Properties

Chloramphenicol inhibits protein syntheses (Ch. 53). It is primarily bacteriostatic, but with some organisms under certain conditions it may be bactericidal. Its important properties are indicated in Table 57–3.

Adverse Effects

HEMATOPOIETIC TOXICITY. Chloramphenicol is directly hematotoxic. In every patient, if the antibiotic is given for long enough and in high enough dosage (particularly blood levels of greater than 25 μg/ml), bone marrow depression can be seen. Marrow depression (reticulocytopenia, an elevated serum iron, prolonged plasma iron clearance, evidence of vacuolation of both the red and white cell series on marrow examination) in this instance is dose dependent, reversible and not an indication to stop therapy. These changes usually revert promptly to normal on cessation of therapy, but rarely they may persist for several months.

Chloramphenicol may rarely (1:2,000–1:50,000) cause aplastic anemia as an idiosyncratic or hypersensitivity response. Since white cells turn over more rapidly than red cells, aplasia usually appears as neutropenia rather than anemia. *Danger signs necessitating immediate cessation of chloramphenicol therapy are neutropenia below 4000/cu mm or less than 40%* polymorphonuclear leukocytes in a peripheral differential white cell count. Aplastic anemia with pancytopenia has accounted for about 75% of all blood dyscrasias reported following chloramphenicol therapy. Other rare dyscrasias include selective depression of each cellular component (thrombocytopenia, erythroid hypoplasia, leukopenia, agranulocytosis) and various combinations. Aplastic anemia is three times more common in females compared to males and more common in adults compared to children; it has been reported in twins but not in children less than 2–3 years of age. It may be more common after repeated courses of the antibiotic, particularly following oral therapy for viral infections, but it may not appear until several weeks after therapy has been discontinued. Phenylalanine does not protect against aplastic anemia.

HYPERSENSITIVITY REACTIONS. Apart from blood dyscrasias, fever, various skin rashes (macular, papular, vesicular), angioedema and Jarisch-Herxheimer reactions in the treatment of brucellosis and typhoid fever may develop. Glossitis, stomatitis, cheilosis and pruritis ani may be due not only to hypersensitivity but also to superinfection.

NONHYPERSENSITIVITY REACTIONS. Chloramphenicol has a bitter taste, and oral therapy may induce nausea, vomiting, gastric irritation, pruritis ani and diarrhea, which may be associated with the low salt syndrome. Therapy may be followed by superinfection with a wide range of organisms, in particular, *Staph. aureus, Pseudomonas, Proteus* and *Candida;* necrotizing (pseudomembranous) entercolitis may also be seen. Purpura, excessive bleeding from mucosal surfaces (accentuated by reduced prothrombin levels, see below), hemolytic anemia in patients with glucose-6-phosphate dehydrogenase deficiency, optic and peripheral neuritis, "glove and stocking" paresthesias, headaches, mood disturbances, myalgia, renal glomerular and tubular damage and chromosomal breakages may also be seen. Chloramphenicol therapy may reduce plasma prothrombin levels, due to a sterilizing effect on the colonic microflora and possibly also to a reduction in hepatic prothrombin synthesis. Chloramphenicol interferes with other aspects of protein synthesis, namely, histocompatibility antigen formation in lymphocytes and antibody production, and prevention of the response to hematinics such as vitamin B_{12} or iron. Depression of the colonic microflora is associated with a lower urine urobilinogen excretion. In man, the biotransformation of tolbutamide, diphenylhydantoin and dicourmarol is retarded, leading to prolonged plasma half-lives with resulting toxicity (Ch. 4).

ADVERSE EFFECTS IN THE NEONATE. Additionally, the neonate readily develops the gray (blue) baby syndrome, characterized by progressive abdominal distension, vomiting, refusal to suck, dyspnea, cyanosis and loose greenish stools. Within a day or so the baby develops a grayish color, and peripheral vascular collapse; death occurs in about 50% of cases within 4–5 days. The syndrome results from immaturity of glucuronyl transferase activity (so that chloramphenicol is not detoxitified), accentuated by immaturity of renal clearing mechanisms (Ch. 7). If chloramphenicol is needed in a neonate, the dose should not exceed 25mg/kg/day.

Preparations, Uses and Dosage

Chloramphenicol preparations are available for oral, IV topical and IM (not recommended) administration (Table 57–3).

Chloramphenicol should be reserved for the treatment of typhoid fever and other salmonelloses, meliodosis, some rickettsial diseases, *Haemophilus influenzae* meningitis, staphylococcal infections resistant to the semisynthetic penicillins or cephalosporins, anaerobic infections, particularly with *Bacteroides fragilis,* and urinary tract infections resistant to other antibiotics. It is mandatory that therapy be monitored with hemoglobin determinations and a white cell count and differential every 24–48 hr.

There are several dosage regimens for typhoid fever. One popular regime is 1 g every 6 hr for 1 week followed by 1 g every 8 hr for 1–3 weeks. Parenteral administration is preferable. It is probably wise not to give a loading dose, as Jarisch-Herxheimer-like reactions can be serious in a debilitated patient. Some physicians add corticosteroids in serious cases. Ampicillin is a valuable alternative.

For rickettsial disease and melioidosis, the usual dose is 50–75 mg/kg of body weight in 4 divided doses daily until 48 hr *after* the temperature has returned to normal. Tetracyclines may be preferable. For *H. influenzae* meningitis the usual dose is 50–75 mg/kg daily in 4 divided doses for 2 weeks.

THE MACROLIDE ANTIBIOTICS

The macrolide antibiotics (lactone ring containing), comprise **erythromycin, oleandomycin, troleandomycin, spiramycin** and **carbomycin** (Table 57–3). Carbomycin is no longer available because of its high toxicity.

ERYTHROMYCIN

Erythromycin, isolated in 1952 from *Streptomyces erythreus,* enjoyed wide popularity for several years in the treatment of many common pathogenic organisms. Its clinical effectiveness has somewhat diminished owing to the development of bacterial resistance. Erythromycin depresses protein synthesis (Ch. 53) and, depending upon the organism and the duration of exposure, it is bacteriostatic or bactericidal.

Antibacterial Spectrum, Bacterial Resistance and Properties

Erythromycin has an antibacterial spectrum between that of penicillin G and the tetracyclines. It is primarily effective against some gram-positive cocci (staphylococci, streptococci, enterococci and pneumococci), neisseriae, listeriae, *Bacteroides fragilis, Corynebacterium diptheriae, Haemophilus influenzae,* brucellae, some rickettsiae, the large viruses, spirochetes and *Entamoeba histolytica.* It is also highly effective against *Mycoplasma pneumoniae* but not against yeasts and fungi. Antibacterial resistance develops fairly rapidly and is becoming more widespread. Cross resistance is usually complete between the macrolides. Cross resistance rarely develops with penicillin. A variety of erythromycin preparations is available (Table 57–3).

Adverse Effects

Erythromycin has low toxicity. With oral therapy, nausea, anorexia, diarrhea, glossitis, stomatitis, cheilosis and superinfection are common. Erythromycin is rarely given IM or IV, since severe pain with local induration and thrombophlebitis, respectively, usually develop. Hypersensitivity reactions with fever, eosinophilia, lymphocytosis, headaches and a variety of skin rashes are sometimes seen and are more common in those patients who have received the drug on repeated occasions. Erythromycin estolate may produce either silent elevation of liver function tests particularly the transaminases, or a syndrome of acute intrahepatic cholestasis resembling viral hepatitis or acute cholecystitis; abdominal pain is usually severe. The syndrome which is more common in atopic individuals usually develops 10–20 days after starting therapy and may be accompanied by fever and eosinophilia; it usually regresses rapidly on cessation of therapy. The offending agent may not be erythromycin but the associated lauryl sulfate salt. However, whether or not erythromycin base is safe in these individuals is not clear.

Preparations and Dosage

There is a variety of oral, parenteral and topical preparations of erythromycin available (Table 57–3).

The usual oral dose of erythromycin is 500 mg 4–6 times daily for 10 days. The base must be taken on an empty stomach, while the other preparations are not influenced by food or gastric acid. Intramuscular injections should never be more concentrated than 50 mg/ml and are often impractical because of excessive pain. The usual IV dose is 1.0–1.5 g four times daily.

Uses

Erythromycin is of limited value in the treatment of penicillin resistant gram-positive infections and in the treatment of infections such as syphilis in patients allergic to penicillin. However, the gradual emergence of erythromycin-resistant strains is becoming a problem. If both penicillin and the sulfonamides are contraindicated, erythromycin may be used in the prophylactic treatment of rheumatic fever. Erythromycin is effective in the diphtheria carrier state and in mycoplasma pneumonia and in amebiasis (Ch. 63).

Use of the Oleandomycins

The clinical usefulness of oleandomycin and troleandomycin is limited to the treatment of severe infections resistant to other more potent antibiotics or for the treatment of severe infections in patients hypersensitive to less toxic drugs. Since the oleandomycins are excreted in an active form both in bile and urine, they are of particular use in gram positive infections of these fluids. If tetracyclines and chloramphenicol are contraindicated, some rickettsial diseases may respond dramatically to oleandomycin. Liver function should be monitored if the patient requires troleandomycin for longer than 10 days.

Use of Spiramycin

Spiramycin is effective in most gram-positive infections resistant to penicillin. If used for renal infections, concomitant urinary alkalinization is desirable. It has been reported to be highly effective in some cases of gonorrhea resistant to penicillin.

FURTHER READING

Gorbach, SL, and Bartlett JG (1974): Anaerboic infections. N Engl J Med 290:1177–1184; 1237–1245; 1289–1294.

Scott, JL, Finegold SM, Belkin GA, Lawrence JS (1965): A controlled double-blind study of the hematologic toxicity of chloramphenicol. N Engl J Med 272:1137.

Suhrland LG, Weisberger AS (1969): Delayed clearance of chloramphenicol from serum in patients with hemotologic toxicity. Blood 34:466–471

Wallerstein RO, Condit PK, Kasper CK, Brown JW, Morrison FR (1969): Statewide study of chloramphenicol therapy and fatal aplastic anemia. JAMA, 208:2045–2050

JEREMY H. THOMPSON

58. ANTIBIOTICS WHICH INTERFERE WITH THE BACTERIAL CELL MEMBRANE

The bacterial cytoplasmic membrane is the site of cell wall synthesis in many organisms. Furthermore, it serves as an osmotic barrier and as an organ for the selective intracellular transport and concentration of essential cell nutrients. The "surface active" antibiotics described in this chapter, and some antifungal drugs (Ch. 65), all damage bacterial cell membranes by increasing their permeability (Ch. 53). The antibiotics described in this chapter are polypeptides derived from species of the *Bacillus* genus; they have poor sensitizing capacity following topical application but are highly nephrotoxic when administered systemically. Nephrotoxicity is usually dose dependent and is increased in the presence of underlying renal disease.

TYROTHRICIN

Tyrothricin is mainly of historical interest, since chronologically it was the first antibiotic to be introduced into therapeutics. Dubos, who isolated tyrothricin from the gram-positive, aerobic, spore bearing soil microbe, *Bacillus brevis,* was impressed by the fact that soil contains very few viable bacteria in spite of the numbers added to it each day. He proposed that chemicals like tyrothricin cleared the soil by the phenomenon of *antibiosis* (Ch. 52).

Commercial tyrothricin is a mixture by weight of approximately 80% **tyrocidine,** a basic, cyclic polypeptide, and 20% **gramicidin,** a neutral, cyclic polypeptide. It is bactericidal primarily against gram-positive bacteria; its gram-negative spectrum is of little or no clinical use. The activity of tyrothricin is not decreased by the usual proteolytic enzymes or tissue breakdown products, and it acts as a cationic surface active detergent or disinfectant (Ch. 53). Gramicidin, which is more potent than tyrocidine, acts by selectively depressing intracellular oxidative phos-

phorylation. The development of bacterial resistance is rare.

Tyrothricin should only be applied topically or by local instillation into a closed cavity. Tyrothricin solutions used in the mouth, nose or paranasal sinuses should not have access to the subarachnoid space, as anosmia or chemical meningitis may ensue. Hypersensitivity reactions are almost nonexistent, but bleeding may be profuse from fresh skin wounds and pain develops occasionally.

Tyrothricin, *N.F.* (Soluthricin), is available in a multitude of ointments, sprays and alcoholic solutions, usually in a concentration of 0.5 mg/ml. It is used for the local treatment of gram-positive skin infections. Many proprietary preparations have been used as throat lozenges.

POLYMYXIN B

Polymyxin is a generic name for half a dozen strongly basic cyclic polypeptides (polymyxins A,B,C,D,E and M), all differing in amino acid content and elaborated by various strains of *Bacillus polymyxa,* an aerobic spore forming bacillus found in soil. Polymyxin E is the same as colistin (see below). Polymyxin B is the only other antibiotic of this group with therapeutic usefulness; the remainder are more toxic and less potent. Polymyxin B has a molecular weight of about 1000 and readily forms water soluble salts with mineral acids. The usual preparation is polymyxin B sulfate, which is unstable in alkaline solutions.

Antibacterial Spectrum

Polymyxin B has a gram-negative spectrum. Microorganisms generally susceptible are *Enterobacter aerogenes, E. coli, Haemophilus influenzae, Bordetella pertussis, Klebsiella pneu-*

moniae, Pseudomonas aeruginosa, salmonella, and shigellae. Proteus spp. are highly resistant to this antibiotic and often produce superinfections during therapy.

Mode of Action and Bacterial Resistance

Polymyxin B is bactericidal even in hypertonic media, and sensitive organisms bind the drug. It complexes with phospholipid components of the cell membrane and, by virtue of its lipophilic and lipophobic groups, becomes oriented between lipid and protein membrane components, impairing their functions (Ch. 53). *The bactericidal effect of polymyxin B is reduced by serum and tissue fluid and by soaps and other substances that antagonize surface active agents.* Bacterial resistance develops slowly and is rare. Cross resistance is demonstrated with colistin. Some bacteria resistant to the tetracyclines and chloramphenicol show cross resistance to polymyxin B, although the reverse is uncommon.

Absorption, Metabolism and Excretion

Polymyxin B is usually administered topically with almost none being systemically absorbed from this site. Rarely oral, IV or intrathecal administration is warranted. Intestinal absorption in children reaches significant proportions but is absent in the adult. Following parenteral administration, peak blood levels develop within about 1 hr. Polymyxin B does not reach the cerebrospinal fluid and intrathecal administration is occasionally necessary in patients with CNS infections. Little is known about the metabolism or excretion of polymyxin B, but the drug is primarily cleared through the kidneys. There is a slight delay in the commencement of renal excretion, and elimination persists for up to 3 days or so following cessation of therapy. In the presence of renal insufficiency, toxic plasma levels of polymyxin B develop rapidly with conventional doses.

Adverse Effects

Adverse effects are minimal after topical application, since the drug is not absorbed. Nausea, vomiting and diarrhea, and the development of superinfections with gram-positive bacteria, proteus spp. or fungi, may follow oral therapy. Serious adverse effects are seen following parenteral therapy. Pain at the injection site is common. Facial flushing, paranasal, circumoral, lingual and "glove and stocking" paresthesiae may occur, as can drug fever and various skin rashes including urticaria. General skeletal muscle weakness, vertigo, ataxia, diplopia, ptosis and a depression of reflexes are less common.

Neuromuscular paralysis unaffected by neostigmine or calcium gluconate may rarely develop. Skeletal muscle weakness in patients with myasthenia gravis may get worse.

Kidney damage, with the development of proteinuria and hematuria, is the most important adverse reaction that can develop, and patients receiving the drug systemically should be hospitalized for this reason. Kidney damage is dose dependent and easily induced in those patients already suffering from diminished renal function; it is usually reversible in the early stages. Chemical meningitis often follows intrathecal therapy. Acute overdosage may occur in children. Polymyxin B lyses mast cells releasing histamine. Symptoms attributable to acute histamine release may develop.

Preparations and Dosage

Polymyxin B Sulfate, *U.S.P.* (Aerosporin), is available in many preparations for local, oral and systemic administration. It is frequently combined with other antibiotics (bacitracin and neomycin) and with hydrocortisone for topical application only.

The average oral dose of polymyxin B is 4.0 mg/kg daily. Intramuscularly or preferably, IV, the daily dose is 1.5–2.5 mg/kg in 3 or 4 divided doses. A daily dose of 200 mg should not be exceeded in parenteral administration. Procaine hydrochloride is often added to the IM preparation. Intrathecally, a dose of 5 mg/day with a concentration of 0.5 mg/ml should not be exceeded. Procaine hydrochloride should *never* be given intrathecally. Topical polymyxin B is usually a 0.25% cream or ointment.

Uses

Polymyxin B is of value in the treatment of *Pseudomonas aeruginosa* infections, particularly those of the urinary tract, skin, external ear, conjunctiva and meninges, and in septicemia when other drugs such as carbenicillin and gentamicin are ineffective. Other gram-negative skin infections are usually highly susceptible to therapy. Oral therapy may rarely be advisable in the treatment of salmonella carrier states.

COLISTIN

Colistin, a bactericidal polypeptide antibiotic obtained from *Bacillus colistinus,* is identical with polymyxin E. It is available as colistin sulfate for oral administration and sodium colistimethate, the methanesulfonate derivative, for IM administration.

Antibacterial Spectrum and Resistance

Colistin has an antibacterial spectrum and mode of action similar to that of polymyxin B but is less potent. It is not antagonized by serum. Resistance develops rarely. Cross resistance is present with polymyxin B.

Absorption, Metabolism and Excretion

In children under 5 years of age colistin sulfate is absorbed following oral administration. No absorption occurs in the adult. Sodium colistimethate releases colistin slowly by hydrolysis from the IM injection site, and after an injection of 150 mg peak plasma levels of about 10–20 μg/ml develop within 2 hr. Release of colistin from the muscle site maintains fairly uniform blood and urinary drug levels. Colistin is excreted by glomerular filtration, and dangerous serum drug levels rapidly develop in the patient with diminished renal function. Colistin passes readily across the placenta but not into the cerebrospinal fluid.

Adverse Effects

Colistin demonstrates a pattern of toxicity similar to that of polymyxin B. In addition, peripheral neuritis, amblyopia, nystagmus, transient deafness and leukopenia may occur. In general, less side effects are seen with parenteral colistin compared to parenteral polymyxin B.

Preparations and Dosage

Colistin Sulfate, *N.F.* (Coly-Mycin Oral Suspension), is suspended in distilled water (5 mg/ml) immediately prior to use. The usual dose for children is 3–5 mg/kg daily in divided doses. Colistin sulfate is present in some topical preparations containing neomycin and hydrocortisone.

Sodium Colistimethate, *U.S.P.* (Coly-Mycin Injectable), is available for IM administration in doses of 150 mg, with the local anesthetic dibucaine, 8 mg; the IV and intrathecal preparations do not contain the dibucaine. The usual IM dose is 2.5–5.0 mg/kg daily in divided doses. A total daily dose of 10 mg/kg may rarely be given for severe infections but should not be exceeded. For IV therapy the drug should be diluted with dextrose or sodium chloride solution and injected over a 30 min period, twice daily. The maximum intrathecal dose per day in children and adults is 5 and 20 mg, respectively. Parenteral therapy must be drastically reduced in the presence of renal insufficiency.

Uses

Colistin has therapeutic applications similar to those of polymyxin B. It has been suggested that colistin and polymyxin B be reserved for the treatment of systemic *Pseudomonas aeruginosa* infections in those patients in whom other more potent but less toxic antibiotics such as gentamicin and carbenicillin are ineffective.

JEREMY H. THOMPSON

59. MISCELLANEOUS ANTIBIOTICS

There are several antibiotics whose precise classification is unclear. For convenience, they are grouped together and considered in this chapter.

LINCOMYCIN AND CLINDAMYCIN

Lincomycin is a water soluble, acid stable, bactericidal antibiotic produced by *Streptomyces lincolnensis,* unrelated chemically to any known antibacterial agent. Clindamycin is 7-chloro-deoxylincomycin. Compared to lincomycin, clindamycin is more potent and bactericidal for more strains, and more readily absorbed following oral administration.

ANTIBACTERIAL SPECTRUM

LINCOMYCIN HYDROCHLORIDE MONOHYDRATE

Lincomycin possesses a gram-positive antibacterial spectrum. In particular, it is effective against most pathogenic streptococci (not *Strep. faecalis),* staphylococci, pneumococci, corynebacteria and most if not all anaerobes except *Bacteroides fragilis.* Clindamycin possesses a similar antibacterial spectrum to that of lincomycin, but it inhibits sensitive bacteria in considerably lower concentrations. Furthermore, it is highly effective against *Bacteroides fragilis.*

MODE OF ACTION

Both lincomycin and clindamycin act similarly by inhibiting protein synthesis (Ch. 53). Erythromycin may block lincomycin and clindamycin induced inhibition of protein synthesis by preventing antibiotic binding to or displacement from the ribosome. Thus, in bacteria that bind macrolide antibiotics but are resistant to them, the activity of lincomycin and clindamycin may be blocked even though the organism(s) are highly sensitive to these agents.

Bacterial resistance is of slow, stepwise onset, and clinically it is of limited importance. Cross resistance has been shown in vitro with erythromycin, but this may not occur in vivo.

ABSORPTION, METABOLISM AND EXCRETION

Only about 20–30% of an oral dose of lincomycin is absorbed, and food measureably decreases absorption still further. With doses of 500 mg, peak plasma levels of 2–5 μg/ml are seen within 1–3 hr, and the antibiotic has a biologic half-life of 5–6 hr. Following IM administration, peak levels are seen within 30 min.

Clindamycin hydrochloride is rapidly and almost completely absorbed following oral administration, doses of 300 mg yielding plasma levels of 3 μg/ml within 1–2 hr; the presence of food has no measurable influence on absorption. For any given dose, peak serum levels are about twice as high with clindamycin compared to lincomycin, but clindamycin has a shorter half-life of about 3 hr. Clindamycin phosphate is well absorbed following parenteral administration, blood levels of 12 μg/ml being achieved with doses of 300 mg.

Lincomycin and clindamycin pass readily into most tissues and tissue fluids, including saliva, but poorly into cerebrospinal fluid even in the

CLINDAMYCIN PHOSPHATE

presence of meningitis. The metabolism of clindamycin is complex. It is partially metabolized in the liver to the antibacterially active N-demethylated and sulfated metabolites. The parent antibiotics, as well as their metabolites, are excreted in the free form and as their glucuronides in the urine and bile.

Lincomycin is present in umbilical cord blood in concentrations approaching 25% of simultaneous maternal blood levels; no significant accumulation is seen in the fetus with repeated dosage.

ADVERSE EFFECTS

Adverse reactions to lincomycin are primarily related to the gastrointestinal tract. Crampy abdominal pains, nausea, vomiting, diarrhea, proctocolitis and bleeding may occur. These symptoms may rapidly progress with the development of a "toxic megacolon." The pathogenesis of this reaction is not known, but it may develop following both oral or parenteral drug administration. Furthermore, it is more likely to develop in the elderly, in those with a compromised blood supply to the bowel and in those concomitantly taking antidiarrheal medications. Pruritis ani, vulvovaginitis, hypersensitivity skin rashes, generalized pruritis, photosensitivity, headaches, myalgia, dizziness and urticaria have developed rarely. A few cases of mild granulocytopenia, thrombocytopenia and jaundice have been reported, and in some individuals, liver function tests have been abnormal; superinfections with gram-negative bacilli and Candida albicans may be a problem. True generalized hypersensitivity with angioedema, serum sickness and anaphylactic shock is rare. Cardiovascular collapse can follow a too rapid IV administration of lincomycin. Post-operative neuromuscular block has been reported rarely.

Adverse effects to clindamycin appear to be similar to those seen with lincomycin. However, clindamycin appears to produce a picture of "toxic megacolon" and pseudomembranous colitis more frequently than does lincomycin. It must be stressed that clindamycin is a new antibiotic, and almost certainly a broader spectrum of adverse reactions will be reported subsequent to its wider use.

PREPARATIONS AND DOSAGE

Lincomycin hydrochloride U.S.P. (Lincocin) is available in tablets and capsules of 250 mg, as a sterile solution of 300 mg/ml for injection and as a syrup containing 50 mg/ml.

Usual adult doses are 500 mg orally, 3–4 times daily, 600 mg IM 2–4 times daily and 600 mg IV 2–3 times daily. In children equivalent doses are 50 mg/kg daily orally and 10 mg/kg daily parenterally in divided doses.

Clindamycin is available for oral (Cleocin hydrochloride) and parenteral (Cleocin phosphate) administration. Usual adult doses are 150–450 mg 3–4 times daily orally and 300–600 mg 3–4 times a day parenterally.

USES

Lincomycin is useful primarily for mild or moderately severe infections in patients who are allergic to the penicillins. It may be effective in some gram-positive infections (Staphylococcus aureus, group A streptococci and pneumococci) resistant to the penicillins, cephalosporins or erythromycin. Lincomycin has been claimed to be more effective in osseous infections, but this is probably not true. It may be of value both in acute diphtheria and in the carrier state.

The precise role of clindamycin in therapy is uncertain. There is no doubt that it is more potent than lincomycin and that it is effective against some organisms such as Bacteroides fragilis which are resistant to lincomycin. However, the incidence of adverse reactions to this antibiotic, particularly those involving the liver and the gastrointestinal tract, may limit its general acceptance.

SPECTINOMYCIN

Spectinomycin dihydrochloride is obtained from Streptomyces spectabilis. It is used to treat acute genital and rectal gonorrhea, but it has no activity against extragenital or extrarectal gonorrhea or against syphilitic infections. Cross resistance of gonococci between penicillin and spectino-mycin has not been reported. Spectinomycin inhibits protein synthesis at the level of the 30s subunit of the ribosome, but its exact mode of action is unknown.

Spectinomycin is given by IM injection. Absorption is rapid, with peak serum levels of

100 μg/ml developing within an hour following the administration of 2 g. Protein binding of spectinomycin is low, but little is known about its metabolism and excretion.

Spectinomycin may cause pain following injection, and drug fever, various skin rashes including urticaria, nausea, insomnia and dizziness have been reported. Rarely, evidence of hematologic, renal and hepatic damage may appear, with falls in the hemoglobin and hematocrit, elevation of the BUN, and decreased creatinine clearance or elevation of liver function tests be-

coming manifest. Penicillin-sensitive patients appear to tolerate spectinomycin readily.

Spectinomycin (Trobicin) is indicated only in the treatment of acute gonococcal urethritis, proctitis and cervicitis when due to susceptible strains of *Neisseria gonorrhoea*. It is ineffective in extragenital and extrarectal gonorrhea and in syphilis. The value of spectinomycin has not yet been established in children or in pregnant women. The usual dose in man is 2 g/day and in women 4 g/day.

FUSIDIC ACID

Fucidin is the sodium salt of fusidic acid, a steroid antibiotic obtained from *Fusidium coccineum* and related structurally to cephalosporin P. Fusidic acid contains the steroid cyclopentenoperhydrophenanthrene ring system (Ch. 46) but is essentially devoid of any steroid biologic activity. It is only available in Europe.

FUCIDIN

Fucidin has a gram-positive spectrum similar to that of penicillin G and when combined with that antibiotic demonstrates an additive bactericidal effect. Its mode of action has been discussed in Chapter 53. Fucidin is absorbed following oral administration and passes to most tissue compartments except the cerebrospinal fluid. Protein

binding is high. Renal excretion amounts to less than 5% of the administered dose, elimination being primarily by way of the bile. Thus, an enterohepatic circulation may develop. Fucidin should not be given IM, since it may cause necrosis; IV administration may lead to hypotension, hemolysis or thrombophlebitis.

Apart from minor gastrointestinal upsets, dizziness and mild skin rashes, fucidin has been shown to be relatively nontoxic. It should be stressed that the antibiotic has not been in use for a long enough time to permit a definite evaluation of its long range toxicity.

Fucidin has been mainly used in the treatment of *Staphylococcus aureus* infections resistant to penicillin, since it is not destroyed by penicillinase. In general, staphylococci are inhibited by concentrations of about 0.01 μg/ml, levels readily achieved by conventional therapy. Resistance may develop rapidly, and cross resistance is observed with cephalosporin P. There is some evidence that fucidin resistance develops less rapidly with concomitant penicillin, erythromycin or novobiocin therapy. The suggested dose is 500 mg 3 or 4 times daily.

RIFAMPIN (RIFAMPICIN)

Rifampin (rifampicin) is a semisynthetic derivative of rifamycin B, one of a group of complex macrocyclic antibiotics produced by *Streptomyces mediterranei*. It is a zwitterion and is soluble in water at an acid pH. Rifampin inhibits DNA dependent RNA polymerase by forming a very stable complex with the enzyme in a well-defined stoichiometric ratio; the macrocyclic ring is the portion of the molecule responsible for enzyme binding (Ch. 53). Bacterial species resistant to rifampin contain an RNA polymerase which does not form a complex with the antibiotic and thus is not inhibited. RNA polymerase from mammalian cells does not bind to rifampin.

Rifampin is a broad spectrum antibiotic possessing inhibitory properties against many gram-positive cocci (e.g., gonococci and meningo-

RIFAMPIN

cocci) and gram-negative bacteria (e.g., some strains of *E. coli, Pseudomonas aeruginosa,* indole positive and negative proteus and anaerobes such as *Bacteroides fragilis*). It is also highly effective against most strains of *Mycobacterium tuberculosis* and many atypical mycobacteria. Its potency against gram-positive bacteria lies between penicillin G, which is more potent, and the cephalosporins, erythromycin and lincomycin/clindamycin, whereas it is far less potent than the aminoglycosides, colistin or the tetracyclines against gram-negative bacteria such as *E. coli, Pseudomonas aeruginosa* and indole positive and negative proteus. As indicated above, rifampin is highly effective against *Mycobacteirum tuberculosis,* and the minimum inhibitory concentration for this organism is between 0.01–0.1 μg/ml, levels which are easily achievable in man following oral therapy.

Bacterial resistance develops rapidly in one or two steps (streptomycin type), an occurrence that reduces the potential usefulness of rifampin. Thus, in the treatment of tuberculosis, the addition of a second drug is essential (Ch. 56). However, most wild strains of *Mycobacterium tuberculosis* have a remarkably small proportion of rifampin-resistant mutants, about one-tenth that encountered with isoniazid. An unsettled question is: What is the potential danger of using rifampin alone in the treatment of gram-positive infections insofar as this may lead to the development of resistance in mycobacteria present in concomitant but unrecognized tuberculosis infections? Acid fast and nonacid fast organisms resistant to other antibiotics are usually sensitive to rifampin.

Rifampin is well absorbed in the fasting state following oral administration, but the presence of food reduces absorption. Peak serum levels develop within 2–4 hr, and measurable antitubercular activity persists for 12–18 hr. Rifampin diffuses well into most body tissues and has a half-life of 3–5 hr. The antibiotic is primarily concentrated in the liver and then excreted in the bile as the free drug and as a desacetylated metabolite which possesses some antitubercular activity. Free rifampin undergoes an enterohepatic circulation, but the desacetylated metabolite is poorly absorbed. About 30% of any given dose is excreted in the urine; about half of this is free rifampin, the remainder being the desacetylated metabolite. Probenecid depresses the hepatic uptake of rifampin, thus prolonging its half-life.

ADVERSE EFFECTS

Apart from the occurrence of liver toxicity, rifampin has proved relatively nontoxic to date. However, with increased usage a broader range of adverse effects will almost certainly be reported. Central nervous system side effects of headache, drowsiness, fatigue, blurred vision and dizziness are fairly frequent, and rifampin may also cause a Coombs positive hemolytic anemia, leukopenia, thrombocytopenia, eosinophilia, drug fever, an elevated BUN and hyperuri-

cemia. Body secretions, such as sweat, tears, saliva, urine, etc., may be colored red. Various skin rashes including urticaria may be seen, but generalized hypersensitivity is rare. Rifampin most commonly produces side effects and toxicity in the gastrointestinal tract. Most often encountered are epigastric distress, nausea, vomiting and diarrhea, and more rarely liver toxicity, which can be fatal. Liver toxicity may be more common in alcoholics, in those with cirrhosis or in patients on oral contraceptive steroids or taking the antibiotic intermittently. Increased BSP retention can occur during rifampin therapy, but this may not reflect the development of liver damage since the antibiotic competes with BSP at its site of excretion.

Rifampin and various orally administered x-ray contrast media interact in the bowel lumen resulting in reduced rifampin absorption. Similarly, PAS can delay the absorption of rifampin when both agents are administered simultaneously. Thus, in the treatment of tuberculosis with PAS and rifampin, there should be at least an 8–12 hr interval between the single daily dosage of each agent. Rifampin may decrease the prothrombin time, the effect becoming manifest about 1 week after the start of therapy.

Rifampin has been reported to be teratogenic and immunosuppressive in experimental animals.

Rifampin (Rifadin, Rimactane) is available as capsules of 300 mg. The usual dose is 600–900 mg/day on an empty stomach since food reduces absorption. In children, the dosage is 10–20 mg/kg/day, not to exceed 600 mg/day. PAS reduces the absorption or rifampin (see above) following concomitant oral administration. The drug is expensive.

USES

Rifampin plus at least one other antitubercular drug has shown great promise in the treatment of tuberculosis, and the antibiotic may approach or even surpass isoniazid both in its efficasy and in its freedom from toxicity (Ch. 56). However, the reliability and efficacy of rifampin has not yet been widely accepted. Because of the prolonged blood levels obtained with rifampin, the possibility and efficacy of intermittent therapy has been studied, but no fixed guidelines are as yet available (Ch. 56). Rifampin should not be used for single drug therapy for tuberculosis, or for long term prophylaxis.

A 4–7 day course of treatment has been recommended for the meningococcal carrier state. Rifampin *should not* be used, however, to treat meningococcal meningitis. Rifampin plus clindamycin has shown some promise in the treatment of nocardiosis.

CAPREOMYCIN

Capreomycin is a recently introduced, water soluble cyclic peptide bacteriostatic antibiotic isolated from *Streptomyces capreolus*. It is used as a second line drug in the treatment of tuberculosis. Capreomycin consists of four active components, capreomycins IA, IIA, IB and IIB. The commercial preparation contains about 80% capreomycin IA and IB with the remainder being a mixture of capreomycins IIA and IIB. Mycobacterial resistance is of the streptomycin type. Occasionally, antibacterial cross resistance is shown with viomycin and kanamycin. One strange phenomenon reported with capreomycin is that mycobacteria resistant to streptomycin and PAS may be more susceptible to capreomycin than are normal strains. Capreomycin has produced eosinophilia, some degree of deafness and tinnitus and, rarely, elevation of the blood nonprotein nitrogen levels and proteinuria. It is given by IM injection in doses of 1 g daily. Excretion is by way of the urine. The precise clinical usefulness of this antibiotic has not yet been determined, but it must be given with at least one other antitubercular drug (Ch. 56). It is relatively expensive.

FURTHER READING

Mattson K (1973): Side effects of rifampin. A clinical study. Scand J Resp Dis [Supp] No. 82

Radner DB (1973): Toxicologic and pharmacologic aspects of rifampin. Chest 64:213–216.

JEREMY H. THOMPSON

60. CHEMOTHERAPEUTIC AGENTS: I

THE SULFONAMIDES

History

In 1908, Gelmo synthesized the intermediary dye chemical sulfanilamide for use in the dye industry. Subsequently, sulfanilamide and a variety of other diazo dyes were used as urinary antiseptics following the demonstration that these chemicals had some in vitro antimicrobial activity. However, it was not until 1932–1935 that Domagk reported the in vivo effectiveness of Prontosil in preventing hemolytic streptococcal infections in mice, a discovery for which he was awarded the Nobel Prize in Medicine in 1938. Soon after the introduction of Prontosil, it was shown that its action depended on rupture of the azo (-N = N-) linkage in the host, with the production (Fig. 60–1) of the active sulfonamide, sulfanilamide (para-aminobenzenesulfonamide). The term **sulfonamide (sulfa drug)** is commonly used as a generic name for all derivatives of sulfanilamide.

Thousands of sulfonamides have been developed, but few have been found to possess sufficient advantages to render them effective therapeutic agents. Although there are many differences among the individual sulfa drugs, they have sufficient in common to warrant a single and unified description. Individual therapeutically useful antibacterial sulfonamides are evaluated later in this chapter. Antidiabetic ''sulfonamides'' and diuretic ''sulfonamides'' are discussed in Chapters 45 and 38, respectively.

Chemistry

The sulfonamides can be considered as substituted derivatives of sulfanilamide. They are all white crystalline powders, mostly poorly soluble in water. Soluble sodium salts are easily pre-pared. The minimal basic chemical requirements for sulfa antibacterial action are contained in sulfanilamide (Fig. 60–1). The para-NH_2 group is essential for maximal antibacterial activity and can only be replaced by chemical groupings that are converted to a free amino group in the host, as in Prontosil. Ortho- and meta-NH_2 substitutions are almost devoid of antibacterial activity. The sulfamyl ($-SO_2NH_2$) group is not essential for antibacterial activity as such, but the sulfur atom is, and should be linked directly to the benzene ring. Because the sulfamyl group is the most important moiety of sulfanilamide, the N of its amide NH_2 is designated N^1; the N of the para-NH_2 is then designated N^4. The majority of effective substituted sulfonamides are N^1 sulfanilamide derivatives (Fig. 60–2). Of these, sulfas with an additional heterocyclic ring are the most potent. Sulfonamides containing a single benzene ring are considerably more toxic than heterocyclic ring N^1 substitutions. Direct benzene ring substitution yields totally inactive compounds.

Antibacterial Spectrum

The antibacterial spectrum of the old sulfa drugs is not as wide as that of most of the newer agents. Most of the currently popular sulfonamides have approximately equal spectra. Highly sensitive in vitro are the majority of the group A streptococci, *Haemophilus influenzae*, *Haemophilus ducreyi*, pneumococci, *Escherichia coli*, *Brucellae*, *Pasteurella pestis*, *Bacillus anthracis*, *Corynebacterium diptheriae*, *Cholera vibrio*, nocardiae, actinomycetes and the large viruses (agents producing inclusion conjunctivitis, psittacosis/ornithosis, lymphogranuloma inguinale and trachoma). Gonococci, meningococci and shigellae are variably sensitive, while some

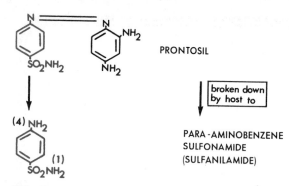

PRONTOSIL

broken down
by host to

PARA-AMINOBENZENE
SULFONAMIDE
(SULFANILAMIDE)

FIG. 60–1. The N of the amide NH$_2$ in all sulfonamides is designated as N^1, and the N of the para NH$_2$ as N^4.

strains of *Klebsiella, Enterobacter* and *Proteus* may be sensitive only to very high concentrations, such as might be obtained in the urine. Many staphylococci, enterococci, clostridia and pseudomonas spp. are highly resistant.

Mode of Action

Sulfa drugs are primarily bacteriostatic agents (Ch. 53), and intact host cellular and humoral defense mechanisms are essential requirements for satisfactory clinical improvement. Exceptionally, some sulfonamides may reach bactericidal concentrations in vivo, as in the urinary tract following therapy with soluble sulfa drugs, and in the ocular tissues following topical application of sulfacetamide.

Interference with Action of Sulfonamides

Weight for weight, the sulfonamides are less potent than the majority of antibiotics because their activity is reduced by pus, tissue fluids and some drugs, all of which contain para-amino benzoic acid (PABA). In vitro studies have shown that one molecule of PABA can competitively antagonize the bacteriostatic activity of 5,000–25,000 molecules of sulfanilamide. Sulfonamide-antibiotic combinations are discussed at the end of this chapter.

Bacterial Resistance

Acquired bacterial resistance to sulfa drugs, first seen in gonococcal infections, has subsequently developed in a variety of meningococci, staphylococci, hemolytic streptococci, pneumococci and shigellae. Almost certainly, resistance develops by random mutation both in vivo and in vitro. In vitro, resistant organisms may reconvert to sensitive bacteria on repeated subculture, while in vivo, acquired resistance is usually permanent. Bacteria resistant to one sulfonamide are resistant to equipotent concentrations of all

other sulfonamides. In the majority of cases the mechanism(s) of acquired resistance is unknown. However, some organisms may produce excessive quantities of para-aminobenzoic acid, while others adapt to utilize the drug.

Acquired bacterial resistance is one of the most important causes of sulfonamide therapeutic failure. It may be prevented by avoiding promiscuous use of sulfonamides, by using sulfonamides only if they are the most satisfactory agents available, by commencing adequate therapy promptly and by giving an adequate dose for sufficient time to eradicate the infection (Ch. 52).

Administration

ORAL ADMINISTRATION. This is the easiest, safest and most economical method of sulfonamide therapy. Systemic sulfonamides (see below) are rapidly and almost totally absorbed, with peak blood levels developing within 2–4 hr. Oral administration of the poorly absorbed sulfonamides allows these drugs to act locally in the intestinal lumen.

PARENTERAL ADMINISTRATION. If oral administration is impossible or impractical, the soluble sodium sulfonamide salts may be injected parenterally.

Slow IV infusion (taking up to 10 min) is preferable to either SC or IM injection because sodium sulfonamides are intensely irritating to the tissues. Intravenous administration is rarely necessary for longer than 36–48 hr, and it should be stressed that renal complications (see below) are approximately doubled with this route of therapy. Because of their irritating properties, sulfa drugs should *never* be injected intrathecally.

TOPICAL APPLICATION. Local application of sulfa creams and ointments, etc., should be used only in the conjunctival sac, the otic canal and the vagina. Topical application of the drugs elsewhere should be avoided, since their use entails considerable risk of generating sensitivity (allergic) reactions, and antibacterially, they are inefficient. One exception, however, appears to be mafenide (see below).

Absorption

Except for the sulfonamides designed to be used for their antibacterial effects in the bowel lumen, sulfa drugs as a class are rapidly absorbed from the gastrointestinal tract, principally the small bowel. Sodium bicarbonate may increase the rate, but not the total amount, of sulfonamide absorbed.

Blood Levels

There is poor agreement between serum sulfonamide levels and clinical response, but generally speaking, therapeutically effective levels lie between 5 and 15 mg/100 ml. These are easily obtained with standard loading and maintenance doses.

PROTEIN BINDING. The protein binding of all sulfonamides is almost directly proportional to the plasma albumin concentration and varies considerably among members of the class. In general, acetylated sulfonamide metabolites are more highly bound than the parent drug.

Sulfonamides and unconjugated bilirubin occupy similar receptor areas on plasma proteins, but sulfonamides are preferentially carried. Hence, sulfonamides displace unconjugated bilirubin from plasma albumin, and may produce kernicterus (see below) in the neonate (Ch. 11). Similarly, sulfonamides may displace acidic drugs such as methotrexate, the coumarins, phenylbutazone, aspirin, etc., producing an immediate increase in the plasma concentration of free drug. This may be followed by an enhanced therapeutic or toxic effect of the displaced agent (Ch. 4).

Distribution

Sulfa drugs are widely distributed throughout the body and readily pass the placental barrier. Equilibrium with most tissues occurs usually within 2–4 hr. With usual systemic dosage, the drugs cross the blood-brain barrier to varying degrees. Cerebrospinal fluid levels of sulfadiazine, e.g., may reach up to 80% of simultaneous plasma levels. Drug levels are even greater in pleural, peritoneal and articular fluids, and since these fluids usually contain minimal protein concentrations most of the drug in the free active form.

Metabolism

Sulfonamides vary as to the degree to which they are metabolized. They are mainly degraded in the liver by N^4 acetylation and oxidation. A small percentage may be conjugated with glucuronic acid, and some may be sulfated or sulfamated. The percentage of sulfonamide acetylated is proportional to the duration of time the sulfa remains in the body. Acetylsulfonamides have no antibacterial activity, are potentially toxic and are usually less soluble than the parent drug.

Most sulfonamides are acetylated polymorphically, while others, such as salicylazosulfapyridine are acetylated monomorphically as are hydralazine, phenelyzine and isoniazid (Ch. 61). Thus, patients with a slow acetylator phenotype tend to suffer a higher incidence of adverse reactions to many sulfonamides compared to patients with a rapid acetylator phenotype.

Excretion

Sulfa drugs are excreted in both free and inactive forms and circadian variations have been described. Elimination is principally in the urine, but some loss in the sweat, tears, saliva, milk and feces occurs and can be therapeutically important. The sulfas are handled by the kidney like urea. Free drug is filtered by the glomerulus and may be partially reabsorbed. Sulfacetamide, however, is not absorbed to any significant extent. Some tubular secretion of sulfa drugs may also occur. Acetylated derivatives are filtered through the glomerulus, and since there is no tubular reabsorption, a greater concentration of acetylated drug compared with free drug develops. Free sulfa drug levels in the renal tubules may be 15–25 times simultaneous plasma levels, explaining the effectiveness of sulfa drugs in some urinary tract infections.

Adverse Effects

In spite of their simple chemical structure, the sulfonamides are potentially dangerous drugs. The overall incidence of their varied adverse effects, that may involve almost every body system, is probably about 5–10%. Many adverse reactions are of a minor nature, yet if they remain unrecognized and untreated, they may progress to potentially lethal disturbances. It should be stressed that if a patient has had a hypersensitivity reaction to any sulfonamide subsequent exposure to sulfa drugs, including the related thiazide diuretics (Ch. 38) and the oral hypoglycemic agents (Ch. 45), may be hazardous. The incidence of hypersensitivity reactions depends on the sulfonamide used, the dose and duration of exposure, and the route of administration. Cross-sensitivity even between systemic and topically applied sulfonamides occurs. Although they are described separately, it should be stressed that hypersensitivity reactions often occur together. Repeated exposure to sulfa drugs increases the likelihood of sensitization.

KIDNEY DAMAGE. Sulfonamide crystals may precipitate in the renal tubules, renal pelvis or ureter resulting in crystalluria. Depending upon their size, crystals may cause epithelial irritation, with bleeding or complete obstruction. Tissue damage produced by crystal formation may act as a site for infection. The development of crystalluria is dependent on the concentration and the solubility properties of the individual sulfonamide and its metabolites in the urine, and is more common following parenteral than oral administration. Urinary solubility of the sulfa drugs and their acetylated metabolites varies widely, but with few exceptions it is increased by urinary alkalinization. The measures taken to reduce crystalluria are described below under Triple Sulfonamide Preparations. Toxic nephrosis and focal or generalized nephritis may rarely be seen. They are probably hypersensitivity reactions. The nephritis may be either an isolated local reaction or part of a general hypersensitivity response.

BLOOD DISORDERS. Blood dyscrasias are rare, but are potentially fatal. Hemolytic anemia may be either acute or chronic. In some cases, the anemia is a hypersensitivity reaction. Anemia can also develop rapidly in red blood cells deficient in glucose-6-phosphate dehydrogenase (Ch. 7). Acute hemolytic anemia usually develops within the first 2–7 days of drug exposure and is commonly associated with fever. Acute renal tubular necrosis may follow the associated hemoglobinuria. Mild chronic hemolytic anemia may occur in patients exposed to prolonged low dosage therapy.

Agranulocytosis (0.1%) usually appears between the 2nd and 6th week of therapy. Bone marrow examination frequently shows maturation arrest at the myeloblastic stage. Agranulocytosis is almost certainly a sensitization phenomenon. Its incidence seems to be independent of either total drug dosage or duration of exposure. It usually develops abruptly, but may be preceded by progressive neutropenia. *All patients taking sulfonamides should be instructed to watch for symptoms of early agranulocytosis and, if these develop, to stop all drugs immediately and consult their physician.* Periodic blood counts, particularly during the first 2 months of therapy, may detect the development of neutropenia.

Thrombocytopenic purpura, eosinophillia and aplastic anemia are all encountered rarely. They probably have an allergic basis, although marrow aplasia may result from a myelotoxic effect of the drugs.

HYPERSENSITIVITY REACTIONS. A variety of hypersensitivity reactions may be seen; some have already been mentioned above under kidney damage and blood disorders.

Numerous reactions in the skin and mucous membranes may develop. Commonly seen within 10–12 days of commencing therapy are generalized skin rashes (morbilliform, purpuric, papular, vesicular, petechial, scarlatiniform), urticaria and photodermatitis (Ch. 7). In patients with a history of sulfonamide sensitivity, the rashes develop in a matter of hours and may rapidly progress to exfoliative dermatitis. Contact dermatitis is becoming less common owing to the reduced use of topical sulfonamide drugs. Behçets syndrome, erythema nodosum, erythema multiforme, the Stevens-Johnson syndrome and epidermolysis bullosa may rarely be seen. The Stevens-Johnson syndrome may be more common following the use of long acting sulfonamides (see below).

Drug fever (3%) is almost certainly a hypersensitivity reaction. It usually develops within 10 days of commencing therapy and is often accompanied by systemic features, thus resembling serum sickness. Drug fever must be distinguished from fever due to a recurrence of the original infection, or fever associated with the onset of acute hemolytic anemia or agranulocytosis. In previously nonsensitive individuals a typical serum sickness syndrome may appear within 10–20 days. In previously sensitized patients a syndrome of anaphylactic shock may develop abruptly. Lesions similar to local or generalized polyarteritis nodosa, to temporal arteritis or to lupus erythematosus are rare adverse reactions (0.1%).

Patients with lupus erythematosus should avoid sulfonamides, and the chemically related drugs acetazolamide (Ch. 38), the sulfonylureas (Ch. 45), and the thiazides (Ch. 38).

GASTROINTESTINAL DISTURBANCES. About 2% of patients taking sulfa drugs experience nausea, anorexia and vomiting. These symptoms are probably of CNS origin since they may also occur with parenteral therapy. Superinfection and diarrhea do not often occur.

MISCELLANEOUS EFFECTS. Other rare adverse reactions include peripheral neuritis, changes in mood (fatigue, depression, anxiety, drowsiness, insomnia, nightmares and psychotic episodes), ataxia, vertigo, tinnitus, hepatitis, goiter with or without hypothroidism, arthralgia, conjunctivitis, hypersensitivity myocarditis, pulmonary infiltration, porphyria and "cyanosis" (from methemoglobinemia and sulfonamide oxidation products). Sulfacetamide may produce systemic acidosis with a lowered carbon dioxide combining power of the blood. Sulfonamides may depress the rate of metabolism of some drugs such as phenytoin.

EFFECTS IN THE FETUS AND NEONATE. In addition to the adverse reactions described above, sulfonamides may produce kernicterus in the fetus and neonate (Ch. 11). Sulfonamides are teratogenic in some laboratory animals, but so far they have not been shown to cause such lesions in man. However, because of this potential risk it seems prudent to avoid their use during pregnancy.

PHARMACOLOGY OF COMMON SULFONAMIDES

The sulfa drugs may be classified into four groups (Fig. 60-2 and Table 60-1). Sulfonamides of **group 1 are used topically.** Because of the risk of inducing sensitization, the only apparently safe products for use on the skin are mafenide and silver sulfadiazine; other products may be introduced with safety into the conjunctival sac, the otic canal and the vagina. **Group 2 (short acting sulfonamides)** comprises the vast majority of all sulfa drugs. These are rapidly absorbed after oral or parenteral administration, and are rapidly metabolized and excreted. **Sulfonamides of group 3 (long acting sulfonamides)** are absorbed rapidly following oral or parenteral administration, but are excreted slowly. Sulfonamides in **group 4 are poorly absorbed** after oral administration and are used only for their local effect in the bowel lumen in the treatment of spe-

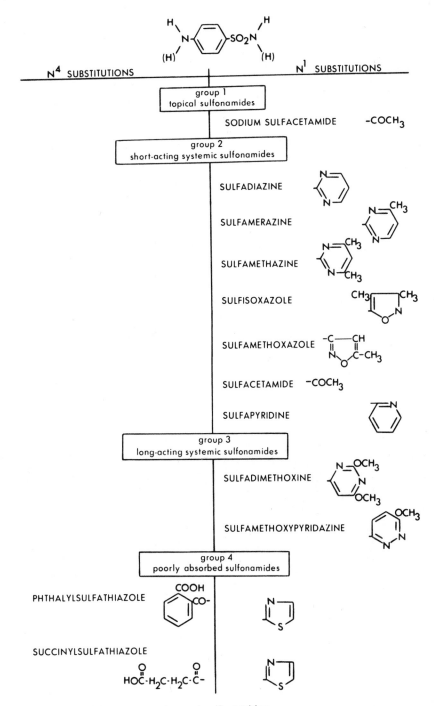

FIG. 60-2. Some commonly used sulfonamides.

TABLE 60–1. Some Popular Sulfonamides

Drug	Properties	Preparations and dose
Group 1. Sulfas for topical use		
Sodium sulfacetamide	Highly water soluble (100 times that of sulfadiazine). A 30% solution has a pH of 7.5 that is nonirritating. Bacteriostatic or bactericidal concentrations rapidly develop in ocular tissues following conjunctival application. Sulfa of choice for infections of the conjunctival sac. Should not be applied if an open wound is present	Sodium sulfacetamide U.S.P. Sodium sulamyd) as an ophthalmic ointment (10%) and as an ophthalmic solution (30%). Applied 2–8 hourly
Mafenide (α-amino-para-toluenesulfonamide)	Differs from other sulfas in that it may not act by PABA inhibition. Contains a methyl group between the amino radical and the benzine ring. Used topically, particularly on burns, to prevent *Pseudomonas* infections. Inhibits carbonic anhydrase resulting in an alkaline urine. Rarely produces a maculo-papular eruption and local pain and burning due to hypertonicity. Mafenide hydrochloride may produce hyperchloremic acidosis in patients with reduced pulmonary function	Mafenide acetate (Sulfamylon) available as a 5% solution and a 10% cream. The burned surface should be carefully cleaned prior to application. Adequate bacteriostatic concentrations usually maintained for 12 hr with use of nonocclusive dressings. The cream is more effective and therapy should be continued for 2–3 wk
Silver sulfadiazine	Equal antibacterial spectrum to mafenide. It is painless on topical administration, does not produce hyperchloremic acidosis and is less rapidly metabolised than mafenide	Silver sulfadiazine U.S.P.
Sulfisoxazole	Primarily a group 2 sulfa, but used topically in the eye, nose, ear and vagina.	Sulfisoxazole diethanolamine, 4% for general application. Sulfisoxazole U.S.P. (Gantrisin), 10% cream, for vaginal application
Group 2. Short acting systemic sulfas		
Sulfadiazine	Rapidly and almost completely absorbed following oral or parenteral administration with peak serum levels obtained between 2–4 hr. At serum levels of 10 mg/100 ml the drug is 50% bound to plasma proteins. About 30% acetylated, and acetyl sulfadiazine *more* soluble than the parent drug. About 200 mg/100 ml and 20 mg/100 ml of free sulfa are soluble in urine at pH 7.0 and 5.5, respectively. Free sulfa is absorbed about 70% by renal tubules	Sulfadiazine, U.S.P., 2–4 g initially followed by 1 g 4–6 hourly for systemic infections. For urinary tract infections 1 g 4–6 hourly Sodium Sulfadiazine Injection U.S.P., 25–50 mg/kg 8 hourly diluted in normal sodium chloride, 1/6 molar sodium lactate, or Ringers solution. Concentrations should not exceed 2.5–5.0% for SC and IV administration, respectively, to minimize sloughing or thrombophlebitis
Sulfamerazine	Similar to sulfadiazine. About 50% acetylated and about 80% reabsorbed by the renal tubules	Usually used as a component of triple sulfonamides. See text
Sulfamethazine	Similar to sulfadizine. About 70% acetylated and about 85% absorbed by the renal tubules	Usually used as a component of triple sulfonamides. See text
Double or Triple Sulfas	See text	Trisulfa pyrimidines U.S.P. (sulfadiazine, sulfamerazine, sulfamethazine) Sulfadiazine and sulfamerazine N.F. Sulfacetamide, sulfadiazine and sulfamerazine N.F.
Sulfisoxazole	Following comparable dosage, blood levels are twice those of sulfadiazine. About 30% is acetylated and urinary solubility of both free and acetylated sulfisoxazole is greater than that of sulfadizine. The incidence of adverse reactions is about 0.1–0.2%	The loading dose for each preparation is 2–4 g followed by 1 g 6–8 hourly Sulfisoxazole U.S.P. (Gantrisin) is available in tablets of 500 mg. The initial oral dose of 2–4 g is followed by 1–2 g 4–6 hourly See above for topical preparations
Sulfamethoxazole	Closely related to sulfisoxazole, but more slowly absorbed and less rapidly excreted than that compound permitting twice daily administration. See text under Trimethoprim: Sulfamethoxazole	Sulfamethoxazole U.S.P. (Gantanol), 1–2 g initially, followed by 1 g 8–12 hourly

Drug	Description
Sulfacetamide	High urine solubility (2%) and rapid renal excretion permit treatment of urinary tract infections. Adverse reactions other than crystalluria develop in about 2% of patients. "Cyanosis" due to production of methemoglobin and oxidation products appears in about 5% of patients
Sulfapyridine	An early sulfa. Far more toxic than newer agents, but is the drug of choice for dermatitis herpetiformis

Group 3. Long acting systemic sulfas

Drug	Description
Sulfadimethoxine	Rapidly absorbed, and excreted mainly (80%) as the glucuronide. Free drug absorbed by the renal tubules about 95%. Following an oral dose of 2 g, peak plasma levels of 10–20 mg% develop within 4–6 hr, and 24 hr later are still 5–15 mg%
Sulfamethoxypyridazine	Rapidly absorbed but poorly excreted due to 80–90% plasma protein binding and avid renal tubular reabsorption of free sulfa. Following an oral dose of 2 g peak plasma levels of 10–20 mg% develop within 3–5 hr, and after 4 days are still in the range of 1–3 mg%. About 10% is acetylated

Group 4. Poorly absorbed sulfas

Drug	Description
Succinylsulfathiazole	Hydrolysed in the bowel with release of the active principle sulfathiazole. The small quantity of sulfa absorbed (3–5%) can initiate hypersensitivity in sensitized individuals. Not effective in diarrhea
Phthalylsulfathiazole	Superior to succinylsulfathiazole in that it is effective in the presence of diarrhea. Absorbed about 3–5%
Salicylazosulfapyridine	Insoluble derivative of sulfapyridine used in ulcerative colitis

Sulfacetamide N.F. (Sulamyd) 1–3 g initially followed by 1 g 8 hourly

Sulfapyridine U.S.P., is given in doses of 500 mg 4–12 hourly

Sulfadimethoxine, N.F. (Madribon), 1–2 g initially followed by 0.5–1 g daily

Sulfamethoxypyridazine U.S.P. (Kynex, Midicel), 1 g initially followed by 0.5–1 g daily

Succinylsulfathiazole U.S.P. (Sulfasuxidine), 250 mg/kg/day in 4–6 divided doses

Phthalylsulfathiazole N.F. (Sulfathalidine), 50–125 mg/kg/day in 3–4 divided doses

Salicylazosulfapyridine U.S.P. (Azulfidine), 4–8 g daily in 4–8 divided doses

cific intestinal diseases such as Shigellae infections, and occasionally in reducing the lumenal bacterial population prior to bowel surgery. Their value in preoperative patients is being questioned, and their place in the treatment of bacillary dysentry is gradually becoming obsolete due to emergence of resistant organisms and to the introduction of the more potent antibiotics. Because they suppress the normal bacterial flora, the synthesis of vitamin K may be depressed below that required to maintain adequate host synthesis of prothrombin. Consequently, patients taking the poorly absorbed sulfa drugs over prolonged periods should receive vitamin K.

Double and Triple Sulfonamide Preparations

One of the common and yet avoidable adverse effects of the sulfonamides is crystalluria. Crystals are primarily composed of acetylsulfonamide metabolites, but may contain free drug. The more effective sulfonamides unfortunately are usually less soluble in acidic urine, and thus crystalluria may readily result. Measures taken to reduce crystal formation (adequate hydration and urinary alkalizers) are not always practical or desirable. For example, an adequate fluid intake may be impossible in a dehydrated patient who also has diarrhea and vomiting. Alkalinizing drugs (sodium bicarbonate, lactate, acetate or citrate), although they raise urinary pH, also lower blood sulfa drug levels by enhancing renal excretion. Furthermore, large doses of alkali may be contraindicated in patients with renal failure, and soluble sodium sulfonamides may be contraindicated in patients with edema and congestive heart failure.

The solubility of most free and acetylated sulfonamides is not interfered with by addition of a second or a third sulfonamide to the solution. By using a double or triple sulfonamide mixture, additive antibacterial activity is produced with the retention of independent solubility. Thus, a higher total concentration of sulfonamide can be obtained in the urine (without the likelihood of drug precipitation) than would be possible if a single sulfa was used.

Triple sulfa prepartions do not have a broader antibacterial spectrum, nor is the overall incidence of adverse reactions (with the exception of crystalluria) less than that of single drugs. The reduction in crystalluria is greater with a triple sulfa mixture than with full dosage of sulfadiazine plus an alkali. Combination of a triple sulfonamide and an alkali is even safer.

Adverse Effects of Long Acting Sulfas

The clinical usage of long acting sulfas should be limited to prophylactic (*E. coli* urinary tract infections) or suppressive therapy (malaria). They should not be given to patients with renal failure or to neonates.

The incidence of adverse reactions to the long acting sulfonamides is about 10–20%. Hypersensitivity skin rashes are more common with these sulfonamides than with other members of the class, particularly the Stevens-Johnson syndrome. In the neonate, severe kernicterus may be induced (Ch. 11). Adverse drug reactions developing in a patient receiving long acting sulfonamides are more serious because of delayed drug excretion and a number of deaths have followed their use.

USE OF SULFONAMIDES

The indications for the use of sulfonamides become fewer as the more potent antibiotics are made available. However, sulfas are easy to administer, relatively cheap and rarely followed by superinfection. Sulfonamides should be given only if there is a reasonable chance of their being effective and then only under careful supervision. All pateints should be instructed to watch for signs and symptoms of toxicity (in particular, fever, headaches, sore throat, diarrhea, jaundice, hematuria, loin pain) and to contact their physician immediately and discontinue all drugs at the first suspicious sign. It should be remembered that many of the severe adverse reactions develop within a few days to weeks of commencing treatment, and careful monitoring of the peripheral blood count should be considered. With systemic sulfonamide therapy, an adequate fluid intake (sufficient to produce at least 2.0 liters of urine per day) is of paramount impor-

tance. Urinary alkalinizing agents may also be prescribed.

Determination of bacterial sensitivity to the sulfas in vitro is desirable, but the tests are frequently misleading. Measurement of blood levels of the sulfonamides may be valuable in monitoring treatment in patients with renal insufficiency who must be given sulfonamides. In general, the choice of a sulfonamide is based primarily on pharmacologic and toxicologic factors since in vivo comparisons are unreliable.

TOPICAL SULFONAMIDES

Sodium sulfacetamide is a valuable preparation for some cases of blepharitis and conjunctivitis, as prophylaxis against infection following penetrating eye injuries in the newborn and in the treatment of trachoma and inclusion conjunctivitis. Probably the 30% solution is more useful than the 10% cream. For the treatment of trachoma and inclusion conjunctivitis, topical therapy should be combined with full doses of a short acting sulfonamide by mouth.

Mafenide is finding wide favor in the treatment of burns, particularly those infected with *Pseudomonas aeruginosa*; silver sulfadiazine is probably equally effective.

$$H_2NCH_2 - \bigcirc - SO_2NH_2$$

MAFENIDE

Sulfisoxazole preparations may be used as is sulfacetamide, and are also of value in treating some vaginal infections, and infections in the nose and otic canal.

SHORT ACTING SYSTEMIC SULFONAMIDES

The short acting systemic sulfonamides are bacteriostatic for a wide variety of organisms. However, antibiotics are nowadays preferred in the majority of instances, although the low cost of sulfonamides is an important advantage.

Bacterial Infections

Many organisms causing acute or chronic pyelonephritis and/or acute cystitis, such as *E. coli,* proteus spp. and Klebsiella spp. may still be sensitive to sulfonamides. However, in many instances the responsible organism shows multiple drug resistance. (Ch. 52).

Sulfonamides are the drugs of choice for chancroid and nocardiosis. In the latter condition, high doses of 4–6 g/day are required and ampicillin or a tetracycline may be added with advantage. Sulfonamides plus streptomycin or chloramphenicol used to be the agents of choice for *Haemophilus influenzae* meningitis, but they have been replaced in this disease by ampicillin, except in those patients allergic to the penicillins. Sulfonamides have also been replaced in the treatment of most cases of shigellosis where ampicillin, tetracyclines or chloramphenicol may be more active. The problem of multiple drug resistance (Ch. 52) applies particularly with this species. However, the sulfonamides may be of some value for prophylactic treatment in epidemics of shigellosis caused by sensitive strains. In the case of meningococcal meningitis, ampicillin, penicillin G or chloramphenicol are probably the agents of choice, since many strains of *Neisseria menningitidis* are sulfonamide resistant; a sulfonamide plus trimethoprim may prove to be of value in treating the carrier state although either rifampin, or minocycline are probably more effective. Most strains of gonococci are now resistant to sulfonamides but recent clinical experience has suggested that a sulfonamide plus trimethoprim is highly effective in many newly acquired infections. Several studies have shown the value of sulfonamides in the long term prophylaxis of group A β-hemolytic streptococcal infections in patients allergic to the penicillins or the cephalosporins.

Protozoal Infections

Sulfonamides are of value in chloroquine-resistant malaria (Ch. 63), and in combination with pyrimethamine, they are of value in toxoplasmosis and *Pneumocytis carinii* infection. In the latter condition pentamadine isethionate is also of value.

Large Viruses (Chlamydia) Infections

Sulfonamides are the drugs of choice for many infections caused by the large viruses. Tetracyclines are valuable alternative agents. In trachoma and inclusion conjunctivitis both topical and oral sulfonamide therapy is desirable.

Fungus Infections

Sulfonamides are the drugs of choice combined with penicillin in the treatment of some cases of actinomycosis. South American blastomycosis, histoplasmosis and maduromycosis may also respond to sulfa therapy, although amphotericin B is more desirable.

Other Uses

Sulfapyridine is the sulfa of choice for dermatitis herpetiformis.

LONG ACTING SYSTEMIC SULFONAMIDES

The only theoretical advantage of the long acting sulfonamides is in prophylactic or suppressive therapy. However, most physicians now agree that it is safer to give a shorter acting sulfa drug more frequently than to rely on a small dose of a long acting preparation. Recently the use of the long acting sulfa drugs has achieved some success in the treatment of chloroquine-resistant malaria infections (Ch. 63).

POORLY ABSORBED SULFONAMIDES

Phthalysulfathiazole is the sulfonamide of choice for reducing the bowel flora prior to colonic surgery. It is of no value in bacillary dysentery. Succinylsulfathiazole is as effective as the systemic sulfonamides in the treatment of acute bacillary dysentery, but its use may reduce the incidence of the carrier state. Salicylazosulfapyridine may be useful in the long term management of

HOOC

HO

N=N

SO₂NH

SALICYLAZOSULFAPYRIDINE

ulcerative colitis, and is sometimes helpful in regional enteritis. Although the poorly absorbed sulfonamides diminish the colonic fecal flora, there is little clinical evidence to show that such an effect yields a lower incidence of postoperative infections than no prophylactic treatment. On the contrary, preoperative bowel "sterilization" may be followed by *a higher* incidence of postoperative infections.

SULFONAMIDE-ANTIBIOTIC MIXTURES

An additive effect may be produced when sulfonamides are combined with bacteriostatic antibi-

otics, e.g., with chloramphenicol or streptomycin in the treatment of *Haemophilus influenzae* meningitis and *Klebsiella pneumoniae* infections, or with tetracyclines for nocardiosis. However, there is a theoretical objection to combining a bactericidal antibiotic with the bacteriostatic sulfonamides (Ch. 52). There have been few investigations comparing possible sulfonamide antibiotic combinations, and until any combination has been conclusively shown to be superior to either agent used separately, these mixtures should be avoided. Exceptions to this categorical statement are the combinations of sulfadiazine and streptomycin or chloramphenicol in the treatment of *Haemophilus influenzae* and the combination of sulfadiazine and penicillin in actinomycosis and anthrax. However, in the latter diseases penicillin alone may be preferable. The concomitant use of sulfonamides and inhibitors of folic acid cofactor synthesis is discussed below.

SULFAMETHOXAZOLE: TRIMETHOPRIM

Trimethoprim, an antimalarial agent, has recently achieved popularity in fixed dosage combination with sulfamethoxazole. The mixture possesses a wider antibacterial spectrum and potentiated antibacterial effects than observed with the use of either agent alone, and produces a double sequential attack on bacterial metabolism (Ch. 53). Sulfonamides other than sulfamethoxazole have been combined, but not as fixed dosage preparations with trimethoprim and related drugs in the treatment of malaria (Ch. 63), but sulfamethoxazole was selected over other short acting sulfonamides for combination with trimethoprim since both agents are absorbed and excreted at about the same rate.

Some important properties of the combination are discussed here; the other pharmacologic properties of sulfamethoxazole and trimethoprim are discussed above, and in chapter 63, respectively.

Bacterial resistance to trimethoprim is retarded by the addition of sulfamethoxazole. Transfer of trimethoprim resistance by conjugation (Ch. 52) is rare.

Absorption, Metabolism, and Excretion

Alone or in combination, trimethoprim and sulfamethoxazole are well absorbed after oral administration. Following a single dose of 160 mg trimethoprim plus 800 mg sulfamethoxazole, plasma levels peak between 1–2 μg/ml and 40–60 μg/ml, respectively, within 2–4 hr; equivalent

steady state plasma levels are achieved after 2–3 days of similar doses twice a day. Sulfamethoxazole and trimethoprim are bound about 70 and 40% respectively to plasma proteins; the binding of sulfamethoxazole to plasma proteins is reduced in uremic plasma.

Trimethoprim has a volume of distribution of 100 liter and its concentration in tissues exceeds that of plasma; the opposite is true of sulfamethoxazole. Trimethoprim and sulfamethoxazole have half-lives of 8–17 and 8–12 hr respectively. After a single maternal dose, peak amniotic fluid levels develop at 10 hr and 14 hr respectively for sulfamethoxazole and trimethoprim.

Both agents are principally excreted in the urine both in the free and metabolized form. With normal renal function, urine levels are approximately 3-fold and 100-fold higher than in plasma for sulfamethoxazole and trimethoprim, respectively. Sulfamethoxazole clearance is increased by a high urine flow rate and urinary alkalization; trimethoprim clearance is increased only in acid urine. The clearance of both agents falls rapidly in renal insufficiency.

Adverse Reactions

The adverse reactions of the sulfamethoxazole and trimethoprim mixture are the reactions seen with either compound individually. There is some evidence that trimethoprim may increase the gastrointestinal and hematologic toxicity of sulfamethoxazole. Some clinical evidence suggests that the acute toxicity of the mixture may be significantly increased by the concurrent administration of D-amphetamine sulfate, or chlorpheniramine maleate.

Preparations and Dosage

Sulfamethoxazole 400 mg and trimethoprim 80 mg are available in a fixed dosage preparation (Bactrim, Septra). A ratio of 5 parts sulfa to 1 part trimethoprim appears satisfactory, since this yields on absorption a blood ratio of about 1:2, a ratio that appears optional on in vitro testing.

Uses

Sulfamethoxazole and trimethoprim have a potentiated antibacterial effect against many organisms causing urinary and respiratory tract infections, and against gonococci and salmonellae. The combination is not recommended for use in children under 12 years of age or during pregnancy.

FURTHER READING

Bushby SRM, Hitchings GH (1968): Trimethoprim, a sulfonamide protector. Br J Pharmcol 33:72–90

Craig WA, Kunin CM (1973): Trimethoprim—Sulfamethoxazole: pharmacodynamic effects of urinary pH and impaired renal function. Ann Intern Med 78:491–497

Finland M, Kass EH (1973): Trimethoprim—Sulfamethoxazole. J Infect Dis [Suppl] Nov 128:5433–5816

Shuck JM, Moncrief JA (1969): Safeguards in the use of topical mafenide (sulfamylon) in burned patients. Am J Surg 118:864–870

Woods DD (1962): The biochemical mode of action of the sulfonamide drugs. J Gen Microbiol 29:687–702

JEREMY H. THOMPSON

61. CHEMOTHERAPEUTIC AGENTS: II

Apart from the sulfonamides (Ch. 60) and the antiseptics (Ch. 62), there are many valuable antimicrobial chemotherapeutic agents. Some of the more important ones are discussed below under drugs for **tuberculosis** (Isoniazid, the amino-salicylates, ethambutol, pyrazinamide and ethionamide), **leprosy** (the thiosemicarbazones and the sulfones) and **urinary tract infections** (methenamine mandelate, nalidixic acid and the nitrofurans).

DRUGS FOR TUBERCULOSIS

ISONICOTINIC ACID HYDRAZIDE (ISONIAZID)

Isoniazid (INAH, INH), the official name for isonicotinic acid hydrazide, has been the mainstay in antitubercular treatment. It is widely used in the treatment of all types of tuberculosis and occasionally in atypical mycobacterial infections. Isoniazid is related to the thiosemicarbazones (see below), the monoamine oxidase inhibitor iproniazid (Marsilid) (Ch. 24) that is no longer available, and the vitamin, nicotinic acid (Ch. 72). Its numerous derivatives are either less active or more toxic.

ISONIAZID

Bacterial Resistance and Mode of Action

Isoniazid resistance develops rapidly and is a function of the size of the bacterial population present in the lesion(s). It is relevant that isoniazid mutants are often deficient in catalases and peroxidases (see below) and have diminished virulence for guinea pigs. The clinical significance of isoniazid resistance depends on the type of tuberculous disease. It is significant if there are large foci of persistent infection, but less significant if there is minimal disease. The addition of a second or a third antitubercular drug retards the onset of resistance (Ch. 56). Cross resistance with other antitubercular drugs occurs rarely.

Isoniazid is tuberculocidal or tuberculostatic in vitro, depending upon various factors including the number of organisms present and the drug concentration. The minimum tuberculostatic concentration of isoniazid for most strains appears to be about 0.05 μg/ml.

There is a relation between mycobacterial drug binding and tuberculocidal and tuberculostatic activity. Isoniazid is probably catabolized in the host to a more active compound by catalases and peroxidases produced by the mycobacteria. Many resistant bacteria have been shown deficient in these enzymes. In vitro, sensitive mycobacteria lose their acid fastness and may show a disruption of porphyrin metabolism, or depression of protein synthesis on isoniazid exposure.

The precise mode of action of isoniazid is unknown, but it may depress DNA synthesis. Isoniazid acts more effectively against dividing organisms and there is a lag phase of up to several days after exposure to the drug during which time sensitive mycobacteria do not reenter logarithmic growth. This phenomenon has been one main argument for *intermittant,* rather than *daily* therapy in the treatment of tuberculosis.

Absorption, Metabolism and Excretion

Isoniazid is rapidly absorbed following oral administration and diffuses freely to most tissues and tissue fluids. Active therapeutic levels may still be present in slow inactivators (see below) 24 hr later. Cerebrospinal fluid concentrations are usually at least half simultaneous blood levels, and bacteriostatic levels may be achieved in caseous foci and inside macrophages. IM, IV or intrarectal (suppository) administration is possible, but rarely used.

Isoniazid is primarily metabolized by acetylation to acetylisoniazid, which is therapeutically inactive and almost devoid of central and peripheral nervous system toxicity; other inactive metabolites are isonicotinic acid, isonicotinyl glycine, isonicotinyl hydrazone and N-methyl isoniazid. Isoniazid and its metabolites are excreted in the urine.

Acetylation of isoniazid occurs mainly in the liver, bowel mucosa and kidney, and depends upon the transfer of acetyl groups from coenzyme A. The rate of acetylation is under genetic control and may be "slow" or "rapid" (Ch. 8). Family studies have demonstrated that following a standard dose of isoniazid (9.8 mg/kg) blood levels six hr later show a bimodal distribution with the antimode at 2.5 μg/ml. Thus, "slow" inactivators have plasma levels greater than 2.5 μg/ml and "rapid" inactivators have levels less than this figure. The slow inactivator is an autosomal homozygous recessive, whereas "rapid" inactivators are either homozygous dominants, or heterozygotes; known heterozygotes have slightly higher blood levels than homozygous dominants, but only in the Japanese population, and using low testing doses of isoniazid can these two groups of "rapid" inactivators be separated. The major gene controlling isoniazid metabolism operates against a background provided by a variety of other genes.

The distribution of phenotypes varies in different populations. Among Europeans and black and white Americans about 50% of the population are "slow" inactivators. On the contrary, about 80–90% of Eskimos and most Orientals are "rapid" inactivators.

BIOCHEMICAL BASIS FOR ISONIAZID POLYMORPHISM. The difference between slow and rapid inactivators is due to the quantity of acetylase present and not to its quality. No differences in the rate of absorption, or in the rate of renal excretion of isoniazid are demonstrable between "slow" and "rapid" inactivators.

OTHER DRUGS METABOLIZED BY ACETYLATION. Hydrazine and some sulfonamides may also be acetylated polymorphically, but the majority of the sulfonamides, PAS and ethionamide are acetylated monomorphically. Steric factors probably determine by which system drugs are acetylated. PAS and ethionamide delay the acetylation of isoniazid even though they are metabolized by a different enzyme, since these two agents preferentially combine and utilize coenzyme A.

CLINICAL SIGNIFICANCE OF ISONIAZID POLYMORPHISM. "Slow" inactivators have more prolonged plasma levels of isoniazid following a standard dose than do "rapid" inactivators, and are more likely to develop adverse reactions such as peripheral neuropathy. There is no relationship between the rate of isoniazid inactivation and the development of mycobacterial resistance, but there may be a poorer clinical response in "rapid" inactivators. "Rapid" inactivators should not be treated with twice weekly dosage regimens (Ch. 56).

Adverse Reactions

Adverse reactions developing with conventional isoniazid therapy occur in 1–5% of patients, but with daily doses above 10 mg/kg the incidence of reactions increases to 15–20%. Following oral therapy, xerostomia, headaches and mild gastrointestinal upsets with nausea and vomiting are common. Superinfection does not occur. Peripheral neuritis occurs in up to 25% of patients taking 6 mg/kg/day. It may be the consequence of the drug competing with vitamin B_6 for the enzyme apotryptophanase. Other nervous system reactions are vertigo, ataxia, tinnitus, monoamine oxidase inhibitor-like mood changes (euphoria; depression, drowsiness, restlessness), hallucinations, psychotic episodes, optic neuritis, optic nerve atrophy, hyperreflexia, muscle twitching, paresthesiae, increased appetite, hesitancy of micturition and increased libido. Convulsive episodes may be produced, particularly in epileptic patients. Such patients usually require increased anticonvulsant drug coverage during isoniazid therapy. With massive doses of isoniazid, toxic encephalopathy and coma (with EEG changes) and severe metabolic acidosis may appear. Neurologic toxicity is more common in "slow" inactivators of the drug as well as in patients who are malnourished.

Isoniazid hypersensitivity produces fever, various pruritic skin rashes, eosinophilia, agranulocytosis, proteinuria and, rarely, polyarteritis nodosa. With high doses of the drug, hypotension, mild bronchoconstriction, methemoglobinemia and hyperglycemia may occur. Diabetic patients may require more insulin during high dosage therapy, since the drug is diabetogenic, and pellagra can be precipitated in malnourished patients. It has been suggested that isoniazid is carcinogenic if taken for a long time, but this appears unlikely. Hepatic necrosis may develop as late as after 8 months of therapy. It tends to be preceded by a prodromal period of fatigue, malaise, weakness, anorexia, fever and arthralgias; it may be more common in rapid inactivators, particularly after ingesting ethanol, or some other enzyme inducer. Various arthrithides, such as low back pain, shoulder-hand syndrome and nonspecific arthralgias and sideroblastic anemia may rarely develop.

Peripheral neuropathy is rarely seen in association with dosage schedules of less than 3–5 mg/kg daily. Peripheral neuropathy and some of the adverse effects of isoniazid on the central nervous system are usually preventable by the concomitant administration of 100 mg of vitamin B_6 daily. Pyridoxine has no antagonistic effect on the tuberculocidal action of isoniazid, and does not influence plasma levels of the drug.

Preparation and Use

Isoniazid *U.S.P.,* is available in many proprietary preparations (Table 61–1). The usual dose is 3–5 mg/kg/day, in 3 divided doses. In severe life-threatening disease (miliary tuberculosis, tubercular meningitis, severe tubercular pneumonia) doses as high as 30 mg/kg/day may be given for a short period of time. The incidence of serious adverse reactions however, increases rapidly with increasing dose.

Recently, some authorities have recommended that isoniazid be given in one dose per day rather than in three divided doses. This is controversial however, since the incidence of drug toxicity is higher with single dose therapy, in spite of the concomitant administration of pyridoxine. In the treatment of mild tuberculosis in slow inactivators, isoniazid may be given twice weekly instead of daily.

Isoniazid is highly effective against mycobacteria, is distributed widely in the body, is active inside macrophages, is easy to take, is cheap and may have a potentiated antimycobacterial effect in the presence of fever. Isoniazid given in high dosage can also be used to treat some infections caused by atypical mycobacteria.

THE AMINOSALICYLATES

The aminosalicylates, used only in the treatment of tuberculosis, include para-aminosalicylic acid (PAS); its sodium potassium, and calcium salts; the phenyl ester; and calcium benzoylpas. When given in equivalent amounts, all these agents are therapeutically similar. The salts are more stable, are less irritating to the gastrointestinal mucosa and have higher urinary solubilities than the free acid. The aminosalicylates possess to a slight degree some of the classical pharmacodynamic actions of the salicylates (Ch. 28), such as analgesic and antipyretic activity.

The following description applies to PAS. PAS has a sour taste and a bitter aftertaste. Its weak bacteriostatic activity against human and bovine

PAS

Mycobacterium tuberculosis is potentiated by isoniazid or streptomycin. Although mycobac-

TABLE 61–1. Some Chemotherapeutic Drugs Used in Tuberculosis

Drug	Preparations and dosage
Isoniazid	Isoniazid *U.S.P.* available in many proprietary preparations, usually tablets of 50–100 mg, and injectable preparation of 100 mg/ml and a flavoured syrup of 10 mg/ml. Dosage — see text and Ch. 56
The amino-salicylates	Aminosalicylic acid *U.S.P.* (para-aminosalicylic acid) and its salts are available in numerous dosage forms in uncoated, enteric-coated and powder form. Many fixed dosage preparations with other antitubercular drugs, antacids, etc., are available, but the physician is advised against using these preparations (Ch. 77). The usual dose of PAS is 8-20 g daily in divided doses
Ethambutol	Ethambutol (Myambutol) is available in tablets of 100 mg and 400 mg of the *d*-isomer which is about 200 times more active than the *l*-form. The usual dose is 15 mg/kg/day in a single dose
Pyrazinamide	Pyrazinamide *U.S.P.* (Aldinamide) is available in tablets of 500 mg. The usual dose is 20–25 mg/kg in divided doses; a daily dose of 3 g should not be exceeded
Ethionamide	Ethionamide, *U.S.P.* (Trecator) is available in tablets of 125 mg and 250 mg with or without enteric-coating. Suppository preparations are available for children. The usual adult dose is 250 mg twice daily increased by 125 mg/wk to a maximum dose of 500 mg twice daily
Thiacetazone	Thiacetazone (Tibione) is given in doses of 200 mg/day

terial resistance is of slow onset, not appearing until after 3–4 months of therapy, PAS should only be given in combination with other antitubercular drugs in an attempt to delay resistance further. Cross resistance has not been described.

Mode of Action

PAS is bacteriostatic, but its exact mode of action is unknown. The closely related compound, para-aminobenzoic acid, can antagonize the effect of PAS in vitro, but appears to block a different receptor site from that involved in sulfonamide antagonism. (Ch. 53). Large doses of PAS are required for the treatment of disease; high, continuous blood levels are probably essential.

Absorption, Metabolism and Excretion

The absorption of PAS following oral administration is rapid and almost complete, the sodium salt being absorbed more rapidly than the free acid. After a 4 g dose, peak blood levels of about 6–8 mg/ml develop with 1–2 hr. The drug is distributed in total body water, passing easily into most tissue compartments with the exception of the cerebrospinal fluid, where drug concentrations are only one-tenth simultaneous plasma levels. Penetration into caseous material is usually satisfactory.

PAS is degraded by acetylation and competes successfully with isoniazid for cofactors (see above). This competition assumes some clinical importance because, of the two drugs, PAS is preferentially acetylated, allowing isoniazid to persist longer in an active form. Both free PAS and its acetylated derivative are promptly excreted (over 90% in 12 hr) by renal glomerular filtration and tubular secretion. Probenecid prevents the tubular secretion of the drug and may be combined with advantage in PAS therapy (Ch. 55). Free PAS is poorly soluble in acid urine, and the acetylated derivative is even less soluble. As with the sulfonamides, urinary drug precipitation (crystalluria) may develop (Ch. 60). Crystalluria can be minimized by urinary alkalinization. The various salts of PAS and their acetylated metabolites, have higher solubilities in urine than PAS itself.

Adverse Reactions

Gastrointestinal symptoms and various manifestations of hypersensitivity are seen in about 5% of patients; other reactions are rare. Gastrointestinal irritation is manifest in a variety of symptoms including nausea, epigastric distress with pain or heartburn, anorexia and diarrhea. Gastric bleeding may develop, and the drug should be given with caution to patients with peptic ulcer disease. Gastrointestinal symptoms may be lessened by giving the drug with meals, with an antacid or through the use of the less irritating preparations such as the various salts or enteric-coated tablets. Abdominal distress is also minimized by starting therapy with low doses of PAS, such as 2–3 g/day, and gradually increasing the dose to optimum levels.

Hypersensitivity reactions usually develop between the 2nd and 8th week of therapy. Fever, headache, general malaise, a variety of skin rashes which may rarely progress to exfoliative dermatitis, photosensitivity reactions, myalgias, arthralgias and eosinophilia may be seen. Chemical and clinical evidence of pancreatitis, hepatitis or nephritis may be seen less commonly. Agranulocytosis, lymphocytosis, thrombocytopenia, progressive mental deterioration, eosinophilic pneumonitis and coma may also develop. Anaphylactic shock, meningitis, radiculitis and neuronitis are rare. A clinical picture similar to that of infectious mononucleosis may appear, but without the presence of heterophil antibodies.

PAS may depress the hepatic synthesis of prothrombin and factor VII (proconvertin), depress serum cholesterol levels and cause mild hyperglycemia. It reduces bronchial secretions and may produce goiter with hypothyroidism. Hemolytic anemia can occur in patients with glucose-6-phosphate dehydrogenase deficiency. Since PAS is a strong organic acid, acidosis may develop, particularly in children. Crystalluria has been mentioned. With large doses of the sodium, potassium or calcium salts, cation intoxication may be a problem in the face of diminished renal function. PAS delays the absorption of rifampin.

Preparations, Dosage and Uses

Amino salicylic acid, *U.S.P.* (Para-aminosalicylic acid), the sodium, potassium and calcium salts of PAS and calcium benzoylpas are available in many preparations (Table 61–1). The various salts of PAS and calcium benzoylpas cause less gastrointestinal irritation, are more stable and are more soluble in acid urine than PAS itself. Administration of PAS with antacids and after meals may reduce the intolerable nausea.

PAS is used exclusively as a first line drug in the initial treatment of tuberculosis (Ch. 56). *It is of great clinical importance and cannot be stressed too strongly that because of its sour taste and irritant properties, patients often do not take PAS as prescribed. If a patient is prescribed PAS and a second antitubercular agent, such as isoniazid, but does not take the PAS, mycobacterial resistance develops more rapidly than otherwise to isoniazid.*

ETHAMBUTOL

Ethambutol (ethylene diamino-di-l-butanol dihydrochloride) an odorless, white crystalline compound, is used as a first line drug in the treatment of tuberculosis. It is a bacteriostatic agent, depressing RNA synthesis, and about 70–80% of strains of human *Mycobacterium tuberculosis* are sensitive to 1 μg/ml. Mycobacterial resistance develops slowly, and no antibacterial cross resistance has been described to date.

Ethambutol (Table 60–1) is almost completely absorbed following oral administration, with peak plasma levels developing within 2–4 hr. In general, it passes poorly into the various body compartments with the exception of the cerebrospinal fluid and red blood cells. About 90% of the parent drug is excreted unchanged in the urine. The remaining 10% is composed of a ter-

$$CH_2OH \qquad\qquad C_2H_5$$
$$H\text{-}C\text{-}NH\text{-}CH_2\text{-}CH_2\text{-}HN\text{-}C\text{-}H$$
$$C_2H_5 \qquad\qquad CH_2OH$$

ETHAMBUTOL

minal butyric acid metabolite and an intermediary aldehyde.

Adverse reactions are very uncommon with doses less than 20 mg/kg/day, but fairly common with doses greater than 50 mg/kg/day. Manifestations of anaphylactic shock, and leukopenia and thrombocytopenia may occur. The most serious side effects are ataxia, a decrease in visual acuity with scotomata and enlargement of the blind spot with a concomitant loss in ability to perceive the color green. The dosage of ethambutol must be drastically reduced in the presence of renal insufficiency.

PYRAZINAMIDE

Pyrazinamide is used only in the treatment of tuberculosis. It is related to nicotinamide, and may depress protein synthesis. In experimental infections in animals, pyrazinamide is more tuberculostatic than PAS, viomycin or cycloserine, but less active than isoniazid or streptomycin. If given alone in vivo, mycobacterial resistance develops within 6–8 weeks. However, the onset of resistance can be delayed by combining a second or third antitubercular drug. Cross resistance may rarely occur with isoniazid. Pyrazinamide is readily absorbed after oral administration and is widely distributed in the body. A dose of 1 g produces peak plasma levels of 40–50 μg/ml in 2 hr. Tuberculostatic levels occur both in caseous foci and in macrophages. Pyrazinamide is excreted by glomerular filtration and tubular secretion.

Adverse Reactions

Pyrazinamide toxicity is dose-dependent. Biochemical evidence of hepatic damage develops in 5–15% of patients. These effects are usually reversible by reducing the dosage or temporarily discontinuing the agent, but death from hepatic necrosis can occur. All patients receiving pyra-

PYRAZINAMIDE

zinamide should be hospitalized and have careful and continued evaluation of liver function during therapy. Gastrointestinal upsets, with nausea and vomiting, arthralgia, spiking temperature, general malaise, lymphadenopathy, anemia and dysuria may occur. Because pyrazinamide decreases the renal tubular excretion of urate, hyperuricemia may complicate therapy, and precipitate acute gouty arthritis in susceptible patients; thiazide diuretics and furosemide may potentiate this response. Diabetic patients may be difficult to control since their insulin requirements may change.

Uses

Because of its toxicity, pyrazinamide is usually reserved for the treatment of tuberculosis resistant to the primary drugs (Ch. 56). It is particularly valuable in short courses as an adjunct to minimize the local spread of infection.

ETHIONAMIDE

Ethionamide is related to nicotinic acid and is a second line drug for the treatment of tuberculosis (Ch. 56). In vitro, its tuberculostatic activity is 3–5 times as effective as that of streptomycin. Sensi-

tive mycobacteria lose their acid fastness on exposure to ethionamide, but its mode of action is not known. It is more effective against human than against bovine strains and may be converted in vivo into a more active form. Mycobacterial resistance develops rapidly when ethionamide is given alone, but can be delayed by the addition of other drugs; tetracyclines, kanamycin and cycloserine are less effective than other second line drugs in this regard. Cross resistance occurs with the thiosemicarbazones, but not with streptomycin, PAS, isoniazid, viomycin and cycloserine.

Ethionamide (Table 61–1) is usually given orally in enteric-coated capsules to minimize mucosal irritation, but may rarely be given in suppository form or IV. Absorption following the use of suppositories or enteric-coated capsules is slower and more irregular than that following oral administration of the uncoated tablets, but blood levels persist for longer periods of time.

ETHIONAMIDE

Ethionamide is widely distributed, tuberculostatic concentrations developing in most tissues and tissue fluids, including the cerebrospinal fluid. It has a shorter half-life than isoniazid.

Ethionamide has been shown to be as effective as PAS in reducing the acetylation of isoniazid in vitro. Ethionamide is cleared primarily in the urine. However, only about 1–5% of free drug is excreted, the balance being made up with numerous metabolites.

Adverse Reactions

Numerous adverse reactions may develop with ethionamide therapy. These may be minimized by careful adjustment of dosage. Gastrointestinal irritation with nausea and vomiting, stomatitis, sialorrhea and a metallic after-taste develop in most patients. These may be minimized by using enteric-coated tablets or by taking the uncoated tablets after meals. Headaches, mental depression, convulsions, sleepiness, postural hypotension, allergic skin rashes, acne, purpura, menorrhagia, gynecomastia, impotence, peripheral neuritis, hyperuricemia and hepatitis occur rarely with prolonged therapy. Fetal abnormalities have been described, and some diabetic patients have increased insulin requirements.

DRUGS FOR LEPROSY

THIOSEMICARBAZONES

Most of the thiosemicarbazones are no longer used therapeutically. The exceptions are methisazone, used in the chemoprophylaxis of smallpox (Ch. 66), and thiacetazone, used occasionally in the treatment of pulmonary tuberculosis and tuberculoid leprosy. Thiacetazone is less tuberculostatic than PAS and its mode of action is unknown. *Mycobacterium leprae* becomes resistant more readily than *M. tuberculosis*.

Thiacetazone (Table 61–1) is well absorbed following oral administration with excretion occurring primarily in the urine. Anorexia, nausea and vomiting and various skin rashes are common with thiacetazone. More serious reactions which may develop are blood dyscrasias with leukopenia, hemolytic anemia and thrombocytopenia. If the drug is not discontinued promptly at the first sign of a falling white blood cell count, agranulocytosis may develop. Thiacetazone may also produce hepatic and renal damage.

TABLE 61–2. Some Chemotherapeutic Sulfones Used in Leprosy

Drug	Properties, preparations and dosage
Dapsone (4,4'-diamino-diphenyl sulfone)	Dapsone *U.S.P.* (Avlosulfon) is available in tablets of 10, 25, 50 and 100 mg. Initial dosage is 25 mg twice weekly. At intervals of 4–6 wk the dose is increased to 50, 100, 200 and 300 mg twice weekly
4,4'-diacetyl-diamino-diphenyl sulfone	Long acting, experimental sulfone under clinical trial in Africa. Releases dapsone or its monoacetylated derivative through action of tissue enzymes. The dose is 225 mg IM every 11 wk
Glucosulfone sodium (Promin)	A highly toxic agent of mainly historical interest since it was the first sulfone used in therapy. Highly water soluble. Administered IV to minimize toxicity; oral and topical preparations also available
Sulfoxone sodium (Diasone sodium)	A water soluble derivative of dapsone for oral use
Thiazolsulfone (Promizole)	A poorly water soluble for oral use
Sulfetrone sodium (Cimedone)	A complex diamino substituted derivative of dapsone for oral administration

SULFONES

There are several sulfones (Table 61–2), all of which are derived from 4,4'-diamino-diphenyl sulfone (dapsone, DADPS, DDS) and are related to the sulfonamides. Many of the sulfones break down to dapsone in vivo, but it is still not clear in which form these agents exert their antibacterial effects; it may be dapsone itself, or one of its mono-substituted derivatives. The following description applies to dapsone, the drug of choice for the treatment of leprosy. Important pharmacologic properties of other sulfones occasionally used in the treatment of leprosy, will be discussed below.

DAPSONE

Dapsone is used for the treatment of leprosy, in which it is primarily bacteriostatic. Its mechanism of action is not known, but some antagonism is produced by para-aminobenzoic acid (Ch. 53). Dapsone has a weak antitubercular effect, but is too toxic to be used for this purpose.

DIAMINODIPHENYL SULFONE
(DAPSONE)

Dapsone is slowly but completely absorbed following oral administration. It is about 50% bound to plasma proteins, and is distributed in total body water. Dapsone is concentrated in the liver, muscles, kidney and skin, but passage into the cerebrospinal fluid is poor. Concentration in the skin may be 10–15 times greater in inflamed than in normal skin. Dapsone is conjugated in the liver with glucuronic acid and excreted in the urine and in the milk. Free drug is also excreted in the urine and bile. Because an enterohepatic circulation follows biliary excretion of the free drug, a single dose of dapsone may be detected in the plasma for up to 12 days. Thus, in long term therapy, it is advisable to discontinue medication every few months to allow drug excretion to "catch up" with drug administration.

Adverse Reactions

Adverse reactions developing with sulfone therapy are nearly all dose-dependent. Gastrointestinal upsets (nausea, vomiting, anorexia, abdominal pains and diarrhea) occur in about 10% of patients. Headaches, excitement, nervousness, insomnia, cholestatic jaundice, amblyopia, psychotic episodes, a variety of skin rashes particularly erythema nodosum and erythema multiforme, paresthesias, pruritis, drug fever, goiter and hematuria and severe renal failure develop occasionally. Use of dapsone in high doses (200–300 mg/day) may be associated with methemoglobinemia and Heinz-body formation. Dapsone is a potent electron donor and may produce hemolysis in both normal and glucose-6-phosphate dehydrogenase-deficient red cells. Hemolytic anemia is unusual unless there is an associated defect of red cell formation. Dapsone may occasionally produce the "Sulfone-syndrome". This is a Jarisch-Herxheimer-like reaction of fever, exfoliative dermatitis, hepatitis, methemoglobinemia, progressive anemia and lymphadenopathy, seen after about 4–6 weeks of therapy in the occasional patient with lepromatous leprosy. Dapsone may rarely be associated with an infectious mononucleosis-like syndrome, which can be fatal.

Uses

Dapsone (Table 61–2) is the drug of choice for leprosy and some cases of dermatitis herpetiformis. It also may be of value in some cases of recalcitrant eczematous dermatitis and in malaria. In the treatment of leprosy, long courses of therapy (up to 5 years) may be required, and therapy should be carefully tailored to each individual patient. The incidence of adverse reactions is greatly diminished if therapy is commenced slowly and excessive drug cumulation prevented by periodic cessation of therapy. Adjunct therapy with corticosteroids, aminoglycosides or "antimalarial" agents may be helpful. Thalidomide, now withdrawn from the market (Ch. 7), in doses of 100–400 mg/day was highly effective in many cases of leprosy.

DRUGS FOR URINARY TRACT INFECTIONS

METHENAMINE MANDELATE

Menthenamine mandelate is the salt of methenamine and mandelic acid (Fig. 61–1), two old urinary antiseptic agents that today are rarely given individually.

Methenamine is a condensation of formaldehyde and ammonia from which at a pH of 5.5 or lower the active bactericidal principle, formaldehyde, is liberated:

$$(H^+)$$

$$N_4(CH_2)_6 + 6H_2O \rightarrow 4\ NH_3 + 6HCHO$$

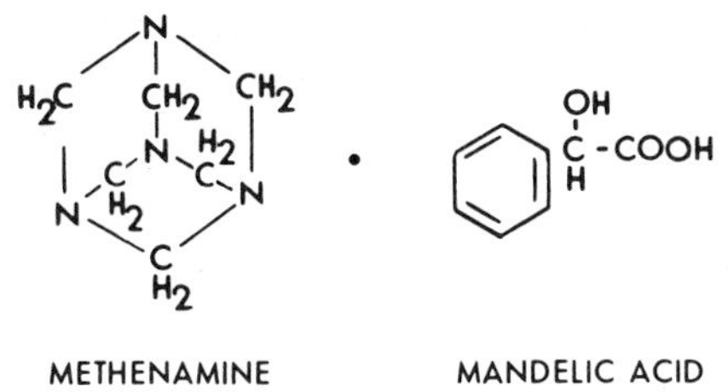

METHENAMINE   MANDELIC ACID

FIG. 61–1. Methenamine mandelate.

Mandelic acid is a simple aromatic acid which is weakly bactericidal in an acid medium. Methenamine mandelate is primarily effective against gram-negative bacteria, especially important, is *E. coli*. Bacterial resistance and antibacterial cross resistance do not develop. Following oral administration, methenamine mandelate is rapidly absorbed and concentrated in the urine; almost no drug can be detected in the serum. Since as much as 20–30% of any given dose may be prematurely converted to formaldehyde in the stomach by gastric acid, the drug is often given in enteric-coated capsules to prevent inactivation.

Even though the compound itself acidifies the urine, the concomitant administration of some urinary acidifying agent such as ammonium chloride or sodium acid phosphate, is recommended. The antibacterial effect of methenamine mandelate decreases markedly as the urinary pH increases above 4.5., as, e.g., during and following meals when the urinary pH may rapidly become alkaline. Urine acidifying drugs are mandatory in treating infections caused by ammonia-producing organisms such as *Proteus vulgaris.*

Adverse reactions developing with therapy are minimal. Skin rashes are unusual. Occasionally excessive formaldehyde liberated by gastric acid can produce unpleasant intestinal symptoms. Similarly, bladder irritation (urinary frequency, burning pain) from formaldehyde can be troublesome, and with large doses mild proteinuria or hematuria may develop. The drug is contraindicated in patients with renal insufficiency. Sulfonamides should not be given simultaneously, as they precipitate out in acid urine. Furthermore, some sulfonamides are directly precipitated by formaldehyde. Infrequently, reversible eighth cranial nerve damage has been reported. Much more common than reactions to methenamine mandelate are episodes of systemic acidosis due to large doses of acidifying drugs in patients who have renal failure and who are unable to excrete an exogenous acid load.

Methenamine mandelate (Mandelamine) is available in two preparations: Methenamine Mandelate Tablets, *U.S.P.*, and Methenamine Mandelate Oral Suspension, *U.S.P.* The usual dose for adults is 3–6 g in divided doses daily. Mandel-amine usually clears the urine within a week if the organisms are susceptible and if strict attention is paid to maintaining an acid urinary pH. This drug enjoys wide popularity because of its lack of systemic toxicity and because bacterial resistance does not develop. Methenamine hippurate (Hiprex) is also popular.

NALIDIXIC ACID

Nalidixic acid is 1-ethyl-7-methyl-4-oxo-1, 8-naphthyridine-3-carboxylic acid. It is an expensive urinary antiseptic agent, being particularly valuable against some strains of *E. coli, Enterobacter aerogenes, Klebsiella* spp., and *Proteus* spp. In general, *Pseudomonas aeruginosa* is highly resistant. Nalidixic acid also possesses a gram-positive antibacterial spectrum, but this is of little clinical importance. Although nalidixic acid is a bactericidal agent, its activity is reduced by tissue fluid.

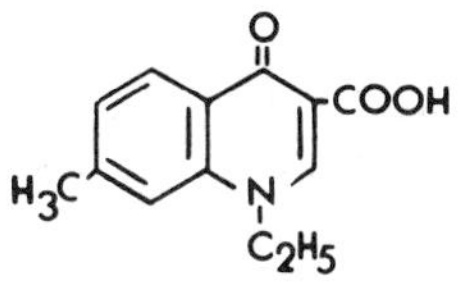

NALIDIXIC ACID

Nalidixic acid depresses protein synthesis (Ch. 53). Bacterial resistance develops rapidly, but so far no cross resistance has been described. The drug may possess some mild antipyretic activity.

Nalidixic acid is rapidly and well absorbed following oral administration. It is only rarely given parenterally. It is rapidly concentrated in the urine both as free drug (20%) and as glucuronated metabolites (80%). There is no likelihood of urinary drug precipitation (crystalluria).

Adverse reactions are common and may be serious. Gastrointestinal upsets can be controlled by administering the drug after meals. Transient fever, myalgia, polyarthritis, headaches, eosinophilia, sleepiness, vertigo and amblyopia may develop. Allergic skin rashes, including urticaria, photodermatitis and pruritus, may be troublesome. Convulsions have been precipitated in susceptible individuals, and occasionally abnormal liver function tests (elevated serum glutamic oxaloacetic transaminase levels and increased thymol turbidity) and blood dyscrasias occur. Superinfection is rare. Administration during pregnancy should be avoided, and in young children nalidixic acid may produce an increased intracranial pressure. The glucuronide conjugate of nalidixic acid may give rise to a false-positive glucose reaction with Benedict's reagent or Clinitest.

Nalidixic Acid Tablets *N.F.* (NegGram) are available in tablets of 250 and 500 mg. The usual adult dose is 1 g 4 times daily for 2 weeks, followed by 1 g twice daily for a further 2 weeks. The usual dose for children is 55 mg/kg daily.

Nalidixic acid is occasionally used in the treatment of acute and chronic urinary tract infections, for long term suppressive therapy or for prophylaxis following genitourinary manipulations. In the latter instance, therapy can be either systemic or by instillation into the bladder. No control of urinary pH is required, but because of the rapidity with which bacterial resistance develops, bacterial culture and sensitivity tests are essential before commencing therapy.

THE 5-NITROFURANS

Several chemotherapeutic agents derived from 5-nitro-2-furaldehyde (Table 61–3) exhibit mild antibacterial, anticandida or antiprotozoal activity, probably by depressing the formation of acetyl coenzyme A. The presence of the nitrogroup in the 5 position of the furan ring is essential for antibacterial activity. The development of antibacterial resistance is of limited therapeutic importance. Cross resistance is complete within the group.

The nitrofurans may produce hemolytic anemia in patients with glucose-6-phosphate dehydrogenase deficiency. In several strains of animals,

5-NITRO-2-FURALDEHYDE

NITROFURANTOIN

high doses of nitrofurazone and furazolidone have produced a depression of spermatogenesis by a direct action on the seminiferous tubules. No such effect has been reported in man with normal testicular function or in those with testicular tumors.

NITROFURANTOIN

Nitrofurantoin, (1-(5-Nitrofurfurylideneamino)-hydantoin) is a urinary antiseptic. It is effective against many gram-positive and gram-negative bacteria, but many strains of *Proteus, Escherichia coli, Enterobacter aerogenes,* neisseriae, staphylococci, streptococci and *Pseudomonas aeruginosa* may exhibit resistance. It is primarily a bacteriostatic agent and blood plasma reduces its activity.

Nitrofurantoin is usually given orally. Very rarely may it be given IV as the highly soluble sodium salt. Following oral administration, absorption of nitrofurantoin is rapid and almost complete. The antiseptic is poorly bound to plasma proteins and plasma levels rarely achieve bacteriostatic concentrations due partly to rapid renal excretion, and partly to breakdown of the drug by tissue enzymes. Nitrofurantoin readily passes the placental barrier but the concentration achieved is too low to be either toxic or antibacterially effective. Between 30–50% of a dose is cleared by the kidney within 6 hr; most of the remainder is excreted in the urine as inactive brown metabolites. There is some tubular reabsorption of nitrofurantoin that helps to concentrate the drug locally in the renal parenchyma. Nitrofurantoin is more soluble at an alkaline pH, but crystalluria (Ch. 60) is not a problem. Nitrofurantoin exhibits a bright yellow fluoresence in urine.

TABLE 61–3. Some 5-Nitrofurans

Drug	Properties, preparations and dosage
Nitrofurantoin (Furadantin)	Nitrofurantoin Oral Suspension *U.S.P.,* 0.5%, and Nitrofurantoin Tablets *U.S.P.* are the official preparations. The usual adult dose is 5–10 mg/kg/day in divided doses for 2 wk. If a further course of treatment is necessary, a 1–2 wk rest period should be observed. Not more than 360 mg of the soluble sodium salt should be injected IV per day
Nitrofurazone	Used primarily for the topical treatment of mixed bacterial skin infections, and rarely in the treatment of *T. gambiense* sleeping sickness (Ch. 63). Its antibacterial activity not reduced by pus, blood or tissue fluids, and it does not depress wound healing. Topically it induces hypersensitivity in about 5% of patients In a 0.2% concentration it is available in many proprietary dressings, suppositories and powders as Nitrofurazone Solution *N.F.,* Nitrofurazone Ointment *N.F.,* and Nitrofurazone Cream *N.F.*
Nifuroxime	Occasionally effective in the topical treatment of vaginal candidiasis (Ch 63). Often combined with furazolidone (see below)
Furazolidone (Furoxone)	Furazolidone is usually available in combination with nifuroxime (see above) as a powder (Furazolidone and Nifuroxime Powder *N.F.*), or as suppositories (Furazolidine and Nifuroxime Suppositories *N.F.*). The usual adult dose is 100 mg 4 times daily

Adverse Reactions

Apart from "hypersensitivity" reactions including polyneuropathy and allergic pneumonitis, the adverse reactions occuring with nitrofurantoin are probably dose dependent.

Gastrointestinal upsets are common, but may be reduced by taking the drug with meals, antacids or milk. Jaundice and hallucinations may rarely occur. Hemolytic anemia may be produced in patients with glucose-6-phosphate dehydrogenase deficiency, and a folic acid-dependent megaloblastic anemia may develop in patients receiving several courses of therapy. This anemia may depend upon the "hydantoin" moiety of the drug and be akin to the folic acid-dependent anemia occasionally seen with diphenylhydantoin therapy.

Allergic reactions are rare, but transient myalgia, fever, a variety of skin rashes including urticaria and anaphylactic shock, may occur. An allergic infiltrative pneumonitis resembling either multiple pulmonary emboli, or pneumonic consolidation, associated with fever, cough, dyspnea and eosinophilia may develop, but usually resolves rapidly on cessation of therapy.

Nitrofurantoin may cause an ascending sensorimotor polyneuropathy which does not appear to be dose related. This begins within 45 days of commencing therapy, and is far more likely to occur in the presence of renal insufficiency. In about 20% of patients there is an accompanying increase in cerebrospinal fluid protein. Recovery from the neuropathy tends to be inversely related to the severity of symptoms, but the lesion may progress even after cessation of therapy. It is not clear if the neuropathy is a toxic effect of the drug or a metabolite, or whether it results from a specific interference with intermediary metabolism. In a high percentage of normal volunteers, nitrofurantoin produces changes in sensory and motor nerve conduction velocity and electromyographic changes in muscle function.

FURAZOLIDONE

This derivative is an antibacterial and antiprotozoal drug. In vitro, it is effective against some species of *Salmonella, Shigella, Vibrio cholera, Proteus, Streptococcus, Staphylococcus,* and *Escherichia coli.* Furthermore, it demonstrates some antiprotozoal activity against *Giardia lamblia* and *Trichomonas vaginalis.* Furazolidone is administered orally, but poor absorption restricts its antibacterial and antiprotozoal effects to the intestinal lumen. The agent is also used topically in the vagina.

Gastrointestinal upsets are common, but may be reduced by careful spacing of the drug doses with meals. Fever, arthralgia, various skin rashes, pruritis, angioneurotic edema, deafness, dizziness and anaphylactic shock are rare. Patients taking furazolidone should not imbile alcohol, since a serious Antabuse-like reaction may develop (Ch. 10). Furazolidone inhibits monoamine oxidase activity and thus sensitizes the patient to sympathomimetic amines.

Furazolidone has been used for the treatment of bacterial diarrheas and intestinal giardiasis (Ch. 63). The combination of Furazolidone and Nifuroxime is effective in treating vaginal trichomoniasis and candidiasis (Ch. 63,65).

FURTHER READING

De Gowin RR (1967): A review of therapeutic and hemolytic effects of dapsone. Arch Intern Med 120:242–248

Maddrey, WC, Boitnott JK (1973): Isoniazid hepatitis. Ann Intern Med 79:1–12

Shepard CC (1969): Chemotherapy of leprosy. Annu Rev Pharmacol 9:37–50

Youatt J (1969): A review of the action of isoniazid. Am Rev Resp Dis 99:729–749

PETER LOMAX

62. ANTISEPTICS AND DISINFECTANTS

Antiseptics and disinfectants are probably the most widely used group of drugs. Although the concept that all infectious diseases are the result of the spread of microorganisms was accepted only slowly by the medical profession at the turn of the last century, the layman, aided and abetted by all the forces of the mass advertising media of the present day, grasped the idea with alacrity and enthusiasm. Antiseptics are now freely applied to almost all the tissues of the body—by eye and mouth washes, throat and nasal sprays, vaginal douches, antiseptic deodorants and soaps, etc. Apart from the phobia they induce in some people, these are actually harmful to the tissues in many instances.

Although the importance of antiseptics in clinical practice has declined somewhat since the introduction of antibiotics, the former agents still have an important place in the treatment of local infections. Disinfectants are widely used for home and hospital sanitation.

The current terminology is rather imprecise, and common usage does not entirely reflect the original derivations. While both antiseptics and disinfectants kill or prevent the growth of microorganisms, the terms have become more restricted in medical parlance. Nowadays **antiseptic** is used in reference to substances applied to the tissues, while **disinfectant** connotes a chemical applied to inanimate objects. The term **germicide** is frequently used to cover both antiseptics and disinfectants.

An ideal germicide would have high efficacy and a wide antimicrobial spectrum. It should be lethal to bacteria, bacterial spores, fungi, viruses and protozoa. In the case of an antiseptic, the compound should not be damaging to the tissues; it should be active in the presence of body fluids, yet not discolor the tissues unduly or have an offensive odor. Disinfectants should penetrate into organic matter and into nooks and crannies, retain activity in the presence of organic matter (blood, sputum, feces, etc.) and be compatible with soaps. Additionally, disinfectants should be stable in solution and not be corrosive to surgical instruments and other materials.

MECHANISMS OF ACTION

Germicidal activity depends on three basic mechanisms of action. Coagulation of protein is frequently adduced as the means by which microorganisms are destroyed, and this may be the major effect of moist-heat sterilization. Many of the new agents, the surfactants, act by destroying the normal permeability characteristics of the cell membrane. It is probable, however, that most germicides act directly by poisoning the enzyme systems in the bacterial cells. For many germicides, however, it is not possible to state precisely their mechanism of action.

The classification of such a varied group of compounds as the antiseptics and disinfectants is difficult, since too rigid a regimen is liable to confuse rather than elucidate. Apart from physical agents, it is generally found most useful (or least objectionable) to discuss the germicides according to their chemical structure.

PHYSICAL AGENTS

HEAT

Saturated steam at 2 atmospheres pressure (120° C) is the most important single method of destroying microorganisms in general clinical use. Both the vegetative and spore forms of most bacteria are killed after exposure for 20 min. Dry heat is much less efficacious: 3 hr at 140° C may be needed. Simple boiling at normal atmospheric pressure may be inadequate to destroy organisms such as those of infectious hepatitis, and in office practice it is advisable to use disposable syringes and needles.

ULTRAVIOLET LIGHT

The maximum antibacterial effect of light energy is manifest around a wave length of 2700 Å. Organisms vary considerably in resistance to ultraviolet light, gram-negative, nonsporing organisms being most susceptible. Staphylococci, streptococci and viruses are resistant. Although not convenient and too expensive for general use, light sterilization is being employed to prevent airborne cross infection in burns units by creating a light screen between patients. Such techniques find greatest applicability in special hospital units such as burn wards and premature baby units.

CHEMICAL AGENTS

ACIDS

BORIC ACID. Boric acid forms a 5% solution at room temperature. Only mildly antiseptic, it does not irritate the skin or delicate surfaces (e.g., the cornea), and this may account for its wide usage. Also available is an ointment containing 10% boric acid.

BENZOIC ACID. This is a weak, tasteless, nontoxic bacteriostatic agent used extensively as a preservative in food and drink in a concentration of 0.1%. High concentrations can be applied to the skin. It is used in the treatment of ringworm and other skin infections (Ch. 65).

MANDELIC ACID. This agent is used for urinary tract infections (Ch. 61). For maximum effect the urine pH should be maintained at less than 5.5 by the coadministration of ammonium chloride. The oral dose of mandelic acid as the sodium salt is 8–12 g daily.

SALICYLIC ACID. This weak antiseptic and fungicidal agent is also used as a keratolytic (loosens the horny layer epidermis).

ALKALIES

Strong alkalies (e.g., sodium hydroxide, potassium hydroxide) are occasionally used for disinfecting excreta, particularly from patients with virus infections such as poliomyelitis. Sodium borate solution is sometimes employed as a skin antiseptic.

SURFACE-ACTIVE AGENTS (SURFACTANTS)

In recent years a large number of these agents have been synthesized. They all act, as does soap, by lowering the surface tension of solutions. Surfactants can be classified according to the nature of the ionic charge on the hydrophobic group.

ANIONIC SURFACTANTS. These include the common soaps. Soaps are active against grampositive, but not gram-negative, organisms. However, it is probable that the soaps owe their antiseptic action primarily to the dislodging, during the physical process of scrubbing, of bacteria embedded in the skin. Sometimes other antiseptics, such as mercuric iodide and phenols, are incorporated in the soap. Of the new anionic surfactants, octylphenoxyethoxyethyl ether sulfonate (pHisoderm) has been most widely used. When combined with hexachlorophene (see below), the mixture is named pHisoHex. This latter preparation has replaced soap for preoperative scrubbing in many hospitals since the mechanical effect of handwashing is augmented by the additional action of the surfactant and the antibacterial properties of hexachlorophene.

CATIONIC SURFACTANTS. These have positively charged hydrophobic groups. Many are dimethyl ammonium compounds of the general structure shown in Figure 62-1. These agents are generally more effective than the anionic compounds; they can be used in more dilute solutions (1:20,000 range); and their activity covers a wider range of organisms. In dilute solutions (0.1–1.0%) they are used for preoperative skin preparation. Common preparations include Benzalkonium Chloride, *U.S.P.* (Zephiran); Benzethonium Chloride, *U.S.P.* (Phemerol); and Cetylpyridinium Chloride, *U.S.P.* (Ceepryn). These are usually used as 10% solutions or as 0.1% tinctures.

PHENOLIC COMPOUNDS

The introduction of phenol by Lister in the 1860s marked the beginning of modern antiseptic tech-

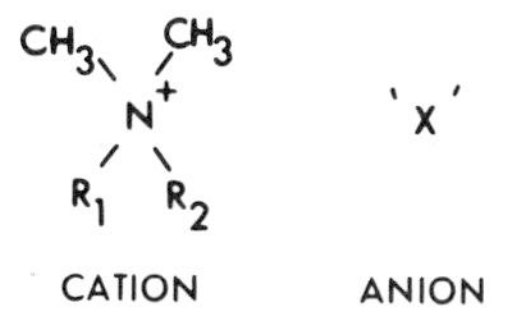

FIG. 62–1. The dimethyl ammonium cationic surfactants.

niques. Subsequently phenol became the standard against which other compounds were measured, hence the term "phenol coefficient." Such comparisons are now rarely made. A large number of phenolic derivatives have been prepared and used as germicides. These are all effective against nonsporing pathogens but are inactive against bacterial spores.

PHENOL. This agent exhibits relatively weak activity and high tissue toxicity.

CRESOL. This compound is about 10 times more active than phenol with about the same toxicity. It is not too soluble in water and is used as a soapy emulsion referred to as Lysol.

THYMOL. This has been used as an anthelmintic agent. A mixture of the iodides of thymol (mainly consisting of thymol diiodide) has been employed as a dusting powder.

HEXYLRESORCINOL. Its broad anthelmintic spectrum renders hexylresorcinol a useful agent in helmintic infestations when administered orally. It is frequently used in throat lozenges on account of its spreading and penetrating properties.

HEXACHLOROPHENE. This new phenolic derivative is active against gram-positive and some gram-negative organisms in a concentration of 2–5%. It is incorporated in a variety of soaps for scrubbing-up, including Dial and pHisoHex. Hexachlorophene has an affinity for the skin and becomes incorporated in the deeper layers so that scrubbing time may be reduced following repeated use. Sensitivity occurs in some individuals and keratitis can follow introduction into the eye.

ALCOHOLS

ETHYL ALCOHOL. This is extensively used for cleaning the skin prior to parenteral injections. It is most effective in a concentration of 70% by weight (78% by volume). Solutions of greater or lesser dilutions are reputed to have less antiseptic action.

ISOPROPYL ALCOHOL. Rubbing alcohol has a lower volatility and higher activity than ethyl alcohol. It is active in solutions ranging from 30–90%, and the effectiveness is not so sensitive to dilution as is the case with ethyl alcohol.

HALOGENS

IODINE. This agent is effective in the elemental form only. It possesses high fungicidal, virucidal and bactericidal activity. Iodine stains and is locally toxic to the tissues. Severe idiosyncrasy can occur. The 2% aqueous solution, stabilized with sodium iodide, appears to be the best preparation. Tinctures in ethyl alcohol are common.

IODOPHORES. These are large organic molecules carrying loosely bound iodine which is liberated slowly. They are expensive and little more effective than elemental iodine solutions.

CHLORINE. Chlorine is an effective germicide at very low concentrations (2:1,000,000) owing to its action in suppressing enzymes associated with glucose metabolism. Hypochlorous acid is formed on reaction with water, and this is the basis for the use of chlorine in the sterilization of drinking water and swimming pools. A 5% sodium hypochlorite solution. (Dakin's solution) is used for cleaning wounds, since the liberated chlorine sterilizes the tissue and dissolves fibrinous tissues. There are several organic chlorides (chloramines) which release chlorine, but these are not much used. Examples are chloramine-T, halazone and chloroazodin.

OXIDIZING AGENTS

HYDROGEN PEROXIDE. As a 3% solution, this agent has been extensively used for cleaning wounds. The compound is unstable and nascent oxygen is released, particularly on contact with organic matter. The evolution of oxygen mechanically loosens pus and tissue debris as well as killing bacteria.

POTASSIUM PERMANGANATE. This acts in the same way as hydrogen peroxide. It has the disadvantage of staining skin and clothing and is irritating to mucous membranes. Strong solutions such as Condy's fluid have been used for sterilizing feces.

SODIUM PERBORATE. This agent releases oxygen on contact with tissues. As a 2% solution, it is used as a mouthwash. Chronic changes in the oral mucous membranes may follow prolonged use of strong pastes.

HEAVY METALS*

MERCURIC CHLORIDE. Although highly toxic, mercuric chloride is used as a hand sterilizing agent on the unbroken skin as a 1:2000 solution.

THIMEROSAL (MERTHIOLATE). This is an

---

* Dyes and vital stains used in the treatment of superficial mycoses are discussed in Chapter 65.

organic complex containing about 50% mercury. Solutions of 1:1000 are used for sterilizing the skin and mucous membranes but may lead to sensitivity reactions.

SILVER NITRATE. This is extensively used as a 1% solution for instilling into the conjunctival sac of infants as prophylaxis against gonorrheal ophthalmia neonatorum.

FURTHER READING

Reddish GF (ed) (1957): Antiseptics, Disinfectants, Fungicides, and Chemical and Physical Sterilization. Philadelphia, Lea & Febiger

JEREMY H. THOMPSON

63. DRUGS USED IN THE TREATMENT OF
PROTOZOAL DISEASES

The protozoa that commonly cause infections in man are listed in Table 63–1. The drugs used to treat these infections are discussed separately under each disease state.

MALARIA

Malaria is a parasitic disease endemic in territory occupied by some 1000 million people, nearly one-third of the world's population. It has been estimated that several hundred million persons suffer from the disease, and that between two and three million die annually from either malaria or its complications. Malaria is caused by infection with one or more of the parasites of the genus *Plasmodium. P. falciparum,* causing falciparum malaria (malignant tertian, MT), and *P. vivax,* causing vivax malaria (benign tertian, BT), are the parasites most commonly responsible for human infection. *P. malariae,* causing quartan malaria (Q), is not uncommon, whereas *P. ovale,* causing ovale malaria (ovale tertian, OT), is rare. Several other strains are responsible for disease in animals. *P. falciparum* produces a more serious disease than the others; however, paradoxically, it is theoretically easier to treat (see below, under Life Cycle of the Malaria Parasite).

Malaria is usually transmitted to man by the bite of a female *Anopheles* mosquito (inoculation of sporozoites) or rarely, through inoculation of trophozoites and/or merozoites via a blood transfusion, or by syringes and needles contaminated with parasite-containing blood. Malaria is becoming more common in the United States owing to present day jet travel and should be considered in all cases of obscure fever. Military and paramilitary personnel returning from Asia may be infected with parasites showing resistance to the usually effective drugs.

LIFE CYCLE OF THE MALARIA PARASITE

Knowledge of the life cycle (Fig. 63–1) of the malaria parasite facilitates an understanding of the mode of action of the drugs used in the prevention and treatment of this condition. In the mosquito, there is one partial cycle (completion of gametogony) and one complete cycle (sporogony), whereas in man there are two complete cycles (exoerythrocytic schizogony and erythrocytic schizogony) and one partial cycle (gametogony).

SEXUAL CYCLE IN THE MOSQUITO. Macrogametes (female) and microgametes (male) ingested by the female *Anopheles* fuse in her bowel lumen, forming sequentally a zygote, an oöcyst, and sporozoites. Sporozoites pass to the mosquito salivary glands and are ready to infect man.

ASEXUAL CYCLES IN MAN. Exoerythrocytic (preerythrocytic) schizogony develops following inoculation of sporozoites by the mosquito. The sporozoites rapidly leave the circulation, and mature in the liver parenchymal and possibly other tissues cells, for about 7–10 days. Merozoites are then produced that, when liberated, initiate the phase of erythrocytic schizogony. In BT, OT and Q malaria, the exoerythrocytic phase may persist in some form or other, causing the relapses so characteristic of the disease. The exoerythrocytic phase of MT malaria does not persist, and therefore the infection cannot initiate a relapse if the erythrocytic phase has been completely destroyed. The persistance of the exoerythrocytic stage in BT, OT and Q malaria is almost certainly not due to reinfection with merozoites, since in blood transfusion-induced malaria (see above) an exoerythrocytic stage of the disease suppos-

TABLE 63–1. Cause and Treatment of Some Protozoal Diseases of Man

Disease	Protozoan	Effective drugs
Amebiasis	*Entamoeba histolytica*	See Figure 63—2
Ciliate dysentery	*Balantidium coli*	Oxytetracycline
Giardiasis	*Giardia lamblia*	Quinacrine, Chloroquine, Metronidazole
Leishmaniasis	*Leishmania donovani, L. tropica, L. braziliensis*	Antimony compounds, aromatic diamidines
Malaria	*Plasmodium falciparum, P. vivax, P. malariae, P. ovale*	See Figure 63—1
Pneumocystis carinii pneumonia	*Pneumocystis carinii**	Pentamidine isethionate
Toxoplasmosis	*Toxoplasma gondii*	Pyrimethamine plus sulfadizaine or a triple sulfonamide Trimethoprim plus sulfamethoxazole
Trichomoniasis	*Trichomonas vaginalis*	Metronidazole
Trypanosomiasis	*Trypanosoma gambiense, T. rhodesiense, T. cruzi*	Suramin, pentavalent arsenicals Bayer 2502 *(T. cruzi)*

* Sometimes classified as a fungus

edly never develops; this point, however, is disputed.

Erythrocytic asexual schizogony results from red cell parasitization by merozoites with the subsequent formation of trophozoites. These trophozoites divide and grow, eventually rupturing the red cell with the release of further merozoites, which initiate a new red cell cycle. Some merozoites do not develop asexually, but initiate the third phase of development, gametogony. Of clinical importance is the fact that *gamete production is more active in recent cases of infection and in the early stages of relapses.* Gametocytes cause no symptoms and remain dormant until they are ingested by the mosquito.

PATHOGENIC EFFECTS OF MALARIA.
The pathogenic effects of plasmodial infection are all related to the asexual erythrocytic stages of the disease. It is the periodic red cell rupture with release of cell products and foreign proteins (merozoites), that causes the fever and chills of the malaria attack, and eventually contributes to the anemia. In addition, massive hemolysis can produce hemoglobinemia (blackwater fever). Indirect effects due to various "toxic" factors produced by the asexual erythrocytic parasites may also be seen, i.e., increased capillary permeability, release of pharmacologically active peptides, disseminated intravascular coagulation and adherence of parasitized red cells to capillary endothelia. In the latter situation, interference with the microcirculation in the brain can lead to the grave condition, cerebral malaria.

PRINCIPLES OF TREATMENT OF MALARIA

The attack on malaria is twofold: measures taken against the mosquito vector and treatment of the disease in man.

CONTROL OF THE VECTOR. Eradication of the vector mosquito is an important Public Health measure, and has been effective in controlling malaria in some communities. Swamp and marsh drainage and chemical sprays (DDT, DDVP and organophosphates) are of most importance; many strains of *Anopheles* are now resistant to chemical sprays.

TREATMENT OF THE DISEASE IN MAN. It has not been possible to induce artificial immunity through the use of vaccines; however, patients with malaria develop a gradual immunity which is of considerable importance in their recovery. For clinical purposes, malaria patients may be divided into nonimmune and semiimmune subjects. The aims of treatment in the two groups are different. In the nonimmune patient, the object is complete eradication of the parasites whereas in the semiimmune, it is the control of the attack. Treatment for the semiimmune is predicted upon a high risk of reinfection, otherwise radical cure would be attempted. Drug therapy can best be considered with reference to that stage of the plasmodial life cycle that is to be depressed. Some strains of plasmodia, particularly *P. falciparum*, now exhibit resistance to the commonly used antimalarial agents.

Causal Prophylaxis

True causal prophylaxis is not yet available, since no drug selectively kills the inoculated sporozoites **before** they initiate the exoerythrocytic phase of development. **Causal prophylactics** are drugs that kill the exoerythrocytic parasites. Obviously, they must be taken for as long as the individual remains in a malarious region. The 8-aminoquinolines, chloroguanide and pyrimethamine are causal prophylactics for MT ma-

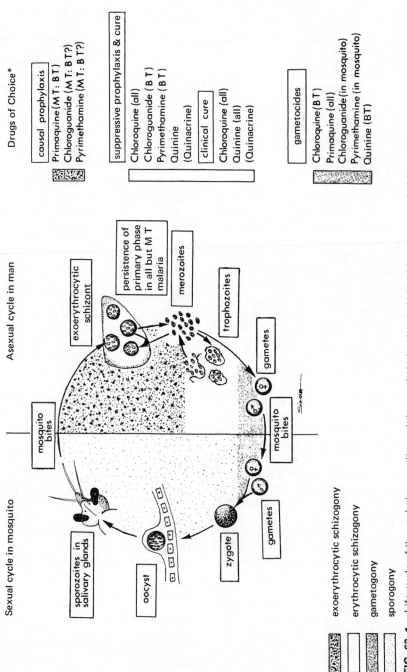

FIG. 63-1. Life cycle of the malaria parasite and drugs of choice for malaria.* Many strains of plasmodia are resistant to the commonly used drugs, and sulfonamides or sulfones may be added with advantage to pyrimethamine or chloroguanide regimens (see text).

laria, but are only weakly active against BT, OT and Q malaria.

Suppressive Prophylaxis (Suppressive Treatment)

Since a true causal prophylactic is unavailable, particularly for BT malaria, suppressive prophylaxis is the method of choice. Any of the drugs acting on the asexual erythrocytic stage will either prevent its development or keep it at such a low level that clinical disease is not produced. *Suppressive prophylaxis is not curative,* except if carried out for many years when the patient may outlive the parasites (see below, under Suppressive Cure), and fullblown attacks of malaria may develop after drug therapy is discontinued. This is particularly true in the case of BT malaria. The 4-aminoquinolines, chloroguanide and pyrimethamine are effective suppressive prophylactic agents. They should be taken during periods of exposure and for several weeks after leaving a malarious zone. Short term suppressive prophylaxis may be of value in patients with a history of malaria who are undergoing severe stress (e.g., travel, infection or surgery).

Suppressive Cure

As indicated above, suppressive prophylaxis is usually not curative. However, under certain circumstances, if carried out for many years, it may lead to suppressive cure because the patient outlives the parasites.

Clinical Cure

Drugs that interfere with erythrocytic schizogony (schizonticides) suppress the symptoms of the acute attack. The 4-aminoquinolines and quinine are the drugs of choice. However, in certain circumstances, depending on the drug susceptibility of some strains, chloroguanide may be required.

Complete Cure (Radical Cure)

Complete cure is usually possible in patients who have attacks of malaria after leaving a malarious area. It comprises eradication of both exoerythrocytic and erythrocytic phases of infection. In the case of MT infection, adequate treatment of the clinical attack will result in complete cure, since the exoerythrocytic stage of the disease does not persist with this strain (see above). The 8-aminoquinolines in combination with chloroquine are the drugs of choice for radical cure of BT, OT and Q malaria.

Gametocidal Drugs

Several drugs are actively gametocidal both in man and possibly also in the mosquito. The 8-aminoquinolines for example, are active against the gametes of all types of malaria, and quinine and chloroquine are gametocidal for BT malaria. Chloroguanide and pyrimethamine may prevent gametocyte maturation in the mosquito rendering them noninfective. It is not clear, however, if this is due to irreversible damage produced by the drugs in man, or to a specific effect of these agents following their ingestion incidentally by the mosquito. The efficient application of drugs in producing causal or suppressive prophylaxis and clinical cure prevents the development of gametes.

CINCHONA ALKALOIDS: QUININE

There are about two dozen alkaloids in the bark of the cinchona tree, the most important being quinine (Table 63–2) and its *d*-isomer, quinidine (Ch. 34). The pharmacologic properties of cinchona bark are due almost entirely to quinine, which is discussed here. Quinine has had a long and romantic history in the treatment of "fevers" and "agues." Commercially, it is produced from natural sources. For the most part, quinine has been replaced by less toxic, more effective antimalarials, but it still is a useful agent against plasmodia resistant to other drugs. *These are becoming more common.* Quinine has the great advantage of being cheap, and thus more readily available for widespread use in poor countries. Numerous congeners of quinine have been developed, but none are as potent as the parent drug.

Antimalarial Actions

Quinine has been used for suppressive prophylaxis and clinical cure in all types of malaria since it is actively schizoticidal. It is also weakly gametocidal for BT, OT and Q malaria. It may act by interfering with the cellular oxidation of glucose.

Nonantimalarial Actions

Quinine has actions on many organ systems, some of which are of therapeutic importance. It has no effect on cardiac muscle in therapeutic doses, but with overdosage, or in idiosyncratic subjects, a quinidine-like effect may be apparent (Ch. 34). In skeletal muscle, quinine increases the refractory period and decreases the excitability of the motor-end-plate, (curare-like effect), making it useful in some types of muscle disease (Table 63–2). The smooth muscle stimulating

TABLE 63—2. Preparations, Dosage and Uses of Some Antimalarial Drugs

Drug	Preparations	Uses and dosage
Quinine	Quinine Sulfate *U.S.P.* is formulated in gelatin capsules due to its bitter taste Totaquine (about 10% quinine) is used in poor countries for the treatment of malaria where quinine sulfate is too expensive. Quinine dihydrochloride, *N.F.* Quinine and Urea Hydrochloride, *U.S.P.*	Uses in malaria: In the acute attack, 600—650 mg, 8 hourly after meals, for 7 days, Given with quinine it may produce radical cure in BT malaria Nonmalaria uses: nocturnal muscle cramps, myokymia, myotonia congenita (Thomsen's disease), dystrophia mytonia and torsion spasm Drug of choice for cerebral malaria in presence of chloroquine resistance. Infused IV under electrocardiographic monitoring. The usual dose is 500—600 mg in normal saline or glucose. Can be repeated at 8 hourly intervals, but oral therapy should be initiated as soon as possible Sclerosing agent for varicose veins
Quinacrine	Quinacrine hydrochloride *U.S.P.* (Mepacrine, atabrine)	Uses in malaria: Used like quinine for suppressive prophylaxis and clinical cure in malaria if quinine or chloroquine are contraindicated. In the acute attack a loading dose of 200 mg plus 1 g of sodium bicarbonate (to reduce nausea) in a suitable flavored liquid medium, is followed by 200 mg 6 hourly for the 1st day, and then by 100 mg 3 times daily for 1 wk. Suppressive prophylaxis is accomplished by 100 mg daily, commencing 2 wk before entering an area where the disease is endemic, and continuing for 1 mo after leaving the area Nonmalaria uses: Occasionally of value in worm infections (Ch. 64), giardiasis, leishmaniasis, amebiasis and trichomoniasis
Chloroquine	Chloroquine phosphate *U.S.P.* (Aralen phosphate), and chloroquine hydrochloride *U.S.P.* (Aralen hydrochloride) are available for oral and parenteral administration, respectively	Uses in malaria: Chloroquine is the drug of choice for treating an acute attack of malaria (clinical cure) and for suppressive prophylaxis. BT, OT and Q malaria tend to relapse on cessation of therapy, but in MT malaria chloroquine may produce complete cure. Unfortunately, many strains of plasmodia causing MT and BT malaria are now chloroquine-resistant In the acute attack, 1 g chloroquine phosphate is followed by 250—500 mg in 6—8 hr, and then by 2 daily doses of 250—500 mg. This is usually sufficient to cure malaria, but BT malaria may relapse. IM (200 mg base 6 hourly) or slow IV infusion (400 mg base 8 hourly) are required in the severe

	attack; oral therapy should be undertaken as soon as possible. Suppressive prophylaxis is accomplished with 250–500 mg/wk, and continued for 4–6 wk after leaving the malaria area
Hydroxychloroquine	Hydroxychloroquine sulfate *U.S.P.* (Plaquenil) Nonmalaria uses occasionally are: amebiasis, giardiasis, porphyria cutanea tarda, discoid lupus erythematosus, rheumatoid arthritis and certain other collagen diseases such as systemic lupus erythematosus and pulmonary sarcoidosis. Chloroquine may reduce the symptoms of infectious mononucleosis, but it has no effect on the heterophil antibody titer or the lymphocytosis. Dosage is usually about 250 mg daily. In the treatment of an acute attack of malaria, an 800 mg loading dose is followed by 400 mg in 6–8 hr and then 400 mg daily for 2 days. Suppressive prophylaxis is accomplished with 400 mg weekly. In the collagen diseases and rheumatoid arthritis the usual dose is 200–800 mg daily. Giardiasis is usually cleared by 200 mg 3 times daily for 1 wk
Primaquine	Primaquine phosphate *U.S.P.* Radical cure of BT malaria may be expected in over 95% of patients given primaquine 15 mg base daily for 2 wk, plus chloroquine. Rarely doses as high as 45 mg base/day may be tolerated, but frequent blood examinations should be performed during therapy. Chloroquine can be given concomitantly, since it may reduce the development of plasmodial resistance; furthermore, it eliminates the erythrocytic stage of the disease. Quinacrine should never be used in association with primaquine, as the toxicity of the latter is greatly increased. Primaquine is the only really effective drug available for causal prophylaxis of BT malaria, and patients taking it should be instructed to watch for signs of hemolysis or agranulocytosis
Chloroguanide	Chloroguanide hydrochloride (Proguanil hydrochloride) The usual dose for causal prophylaxis of malaria in nonimmune patients is 100 mg daily for 1 wk before entering and for 4 wk after leaving, a malaria area. In the treatment of an acute attack (rarely used) of BT malaria, 600 mg should be followed by 300 mg daily for 10–14 days
Pyrimethamine	Pyrimethamine, *U.S.P.* (Daraprim) Uses in malaria: Pyrimethamine is useful in both nonimmune and semiimmune subjects as a prophylactic and suppressant in a dose of 25 mg/wk. It should be taken regularly on the same day each wk in order to minimize the development of resistance. Therapy should commence 1 wk before entering, and continue for 3 mo after leaving a malarial area. Pyrimethamine is of no use in the treatment of an acute attack since it acts too slowly, but in prophylactic and suppressive treatment it effectively prevents the development of gametes. Pyrimethamine may produce suppressive cure of some strains of BT malaria if continued for 12–15 mo Nonmalaria uses: Toxoplasmosis, and rarely in the treatment of polycythemia rubra vera. It is under investigation in the treatment of *Pneumocystis carinii* infection in combination with a sulfonamide

properties of quinine are poorly understood, but are of some therapeutic importance since bronchoconstriction may be severe in asthmatic subjects, and oxytocic effects may be seen that become stronger as pregnancy advances; quinine used to be employed to induce labor, and toxic doses may produce abortion.

Absorption, Metabolism and Excretion

Following oral administration, quinine is rapidly and effectively absorbed, mainly from the upper small bowel, with peak plasma levels developing within 1–3 hr; about 70–80% is protein bound. Quinine is degraded in the liver, only about 5–10% of the active drug being recoverable in the urine. Quinine base is avidly reabsorbed from the renal tubules in alkaline urine, but in spite of this, significant cumulation usually does not occur. Subcutaneous and IM administration are not advisable, since intense pain, sloughing of the skin, and sterile abscess formation may develop.

Adverse Effects

Quinine can produce a variety of adverse effects, often collectively termed **cinchonism** (Ch. 34). Idiosyncrasy is common, and symptoms of cinchonism are rapidly produced in such individuals by therapeutic doses. Quinine should not be used in patients who show idiosyncrasy to either it or quinidine, and because of its oxytocic properties it should not be used in pregnant patients. The fatal oral dose of quinine is in the order of 8g. Quinine should be given cautiously to patients with myasthenia gravis, since its neuromuscular blocking action may lead to death; small doses of quinine may be used diagnostically in this disease. In the treatment of a patient with MT malaria, quinine may induce blackwater fever. Other adverse effects of quinine are similar to those of quinidine (Ch. 34).

ACRIDINE DYES: QUINACRINE

Quinacrine is the only acridine dye still used in malaria. It is a yellow crystalline light-sensitive drug related to methylene blue. For uses of other acridine derivatives see Chapters 62 and 66.

Mode of Action

Quinacrine is readily intercalated into DNA thus effectively blocking DNA and RNA polymerase activity (Ch. 53). Additionally, quinacrine depresses cholinesterase activity, and interferes with lactate production from glucose through depression of 6-phosphofructokinase. Plasmodial resistance is rare. Cross resistance may appear with chloroquine.

Antimalarial Actions

Quinacrine produces the same effect as quinine and chloroquine by destroying the asexual erythrocytic parasites in all types of malaria (Table 63–2). Thus it produces effective clinical cure and suppressive prophylaxis and cure; in some cases of MT malaria quinacrine may be curative. Quinacrine is less toxic and more active than quinine, but less active and more toxic than chloroquine.

Absorption, Metabolism and Excretion

Quinacrine is readily absorbed from the gastrointestinal tract, widely distributed in the body and bound by many tissues, particularly the liver, spleen, lungs, kidneys, nails and hair. Thus cumulation regularly occurs, and quinacrine has

QUINACRINE

been found in skin and nails 2 years after cessation of therapy. Quinacrine is slowly excreted by the kidney, clearance being more rapid in acid urine. Acid urine is colored a deep yellow by quinacrine and its metabolites. Quinacrine prevents the degradation of 8-aminoquinolines (see below).

Adverse Effects

Quinacrine is moderately well tolerated, and only a small proportion (probably 2%) of patients develop serious adverse reactions. Gastrointestinal upsets (nausea, vomiting, diarrhea), headaches, mild fever, sweating, myalagia, arthralgia, vertigo, insomnia, pruritus and a variety of skin rashes are common and rapidly disappear on cessation of therapy. Yellowing of the skin, nails and sclerae (owing to local tissue drug binding) occurs in most patients. This may be of cosmetic inconvenience or may be confused with jaundice. Under ultraviolet light nails and blond hair exhibit a yellowish-green fluorescence. Very rarely quinacrine produces corneal edema, bone marrow depression and violent psychotic reactions (mepacrine madness) usually with hallucinations, excitement, restlessness or a Korsakoff-like state. With large doses or in patients hypersensitive to its action, cardiac arrhythmias may occur. Quinacrine should be given with extreme caution to patients with psoriasis, since the latter condition may deteriorate rapidly. Quinacrine potentiates the toxicity of the 8-aminoquinolines through retarding their metabolism.

4-AMINOQUINOLINES: CHLOROQUINE

Of the several hundred 4-aminoquinolines developed, only chloroquine, hydroxychloroquine, amodiaquine (camoquin), amopyroquine and cycloquine have been retained in therapy. The 4-aminoquinolines all contain the same alkyl side chain present in quinacrine. Chloroquine and hydroxychloroquine are the most widely used (Table 63–2).

Mode of Action

The exact mechanism of plasmodicidal action of chloroquine is not known, but the drug intercalates with DNA (Ch. 53). Intercalation may partially explain chloroquine tissue binding, and its antimalarial properties; parasitized erythrocytes selectively accumulate chloroquine over nonparasitized erythrocytes and plasma.

Chloroquine has a number of other actions which cannot be related; stabilization of lysosomes, some antiinflammatory and antihistaminic activity, and increase in the prostaglandin

CHLOROQUINE

content of some tissues. It also binds to melanin which accounts for its deposition and adverse effects on the retina (see below).

Antimalarial Actions

Chloroquine is highly effective against the asexual erythrocytic parasites of MT, BT and Q malaria, and is gametocidal against most strains of *P. vivax*. Because of its rapid action, chloroquine is the drug of choice for the acute attack. It is usually curative of MT malaria, but only suppressive of other forms. Chloroquine does not prevent infection when given prophylactically; neither does it prevent recurrence of BT malaria after suppression of an acute attack. However, in the latter case it significantly prolongs the intervals between relapses.

Several strains of *P. falciparum* and *P. vivax* have been reported resistant to chloroquine; in some of these instances quinine and pyrimethamine plus a sulfonamide (see below) have been effective. Cross resistance may occur with quinacrine.

Absorption, Metabolism, and Excretion

Chloroquine is rapidly and almost completely absorbed following oral administration. It is con-centrated in several tissues, particularly red and white blood cells, liver, spleen, skin, kidney, lung and retina. In the liver, chloroquine levels may be up to 600 times the plasma concentration, a discovery that suggested its use in amebiasis (see below). Chloroquine is primarily degraded by the liver, and numerous metabolites have been identified, some of which possess antimalarial properties. Chloroquine is excreted slowly in the urine; excretion is increased with urinary acidification and following the use of dimercaprol (Ch. 9). Other 4-aminoquinolines and pamaquine may delay its degradation.

Because of its tissue binding, clinically significant cumulation may develop with long term therapy. For example, following prolonged treatment for a collagen disease, the drug may be detected in some tissues up to 5 years after the last dose.

Adverse Effects

Short term administration of chloroquine may rarely produce mild gastrointestinal irritation (nausea, anorexia, and vomiting), headaches, a variety of skin rashes, transient amblyopia due to difficulty in accommodation and pruritis. Acute accidental overdosage in children may cause hypotension, convulsions, cardioventilatory depression and coma, and is often fatal; it should be treated vigorously with demercaprol and acid diuresis.

When chloroquine is administered over a long period of time in low doses for malaria suppression the drug is relatively safe, but when used chronically in high doses in the treatment of diseases such as collagen disorders, it may produce serious adverse effects. Drug deposition in the cornea, ocular muscles and retina can lead to corneal opacities, muscle palsies and retinal damage. The early lesion of chloroquine retinopathy is a mottling of the macula with loss of the foveal reflex. Later, areas of depigmentation and hyperpigmentation can be seen in the macula, eventually leading to the classic "bulls-eye" appearance (Fig. 7–1); at this stage generalized areas of depigmentation and hyperpigmentation may be seen over the entire retina. Retinal damage leads to partial or total loss of vision. It may progress after all therapy has been discontinued. In addition to ocular toxicity, chronic chloroquine therapy may produce transient attacks of dizziness, insomnia, psychoses, leukopenia, porphyria and peripheral neuritis. Furthermore, deposition in the skin and nails may produce pigment changes or a chronic pruritic eruption similar to lichen planus, and bleaching of cranial hair and eyelashes and alopecia may be minor cosmetic inconveniences. Chloroquine may produce T wave changes in the electrocardiograph, but without any other evidence of cardiotoxicity. Patients with psoriasis may suffer a serious relapse, and the drug may be teratogenic.

4-AMINOQUINOLINES: HYDROXY-CHLOROQUINE AND AMODIAQUINE

Hydroxychloroquine and amodiaquine are similar to chloroquine in pharmacology, clinical usefulness and adverse effects. Some physicians claim that they are safer.

8-AMINOQUINOLINES: PRIMAQUINE

Primaquine has the greatest therapeutic index of all the 8-aminoquinolines and is the only one now used (Table 63–2). It has replaced pamaquine, pentaquine and isopentaquine.

Mode of Action and Resistance

The mode of action of primaquine is unknown, but it may breakdown in vivo to a more active 5, 6-quinolinequinone metabolite. Primaquine suppresses the mitochondrial functions of plasmodia in the exoerythrocytic stages and possibly also the activity of structures equivalent to mitochondria in the erythrocytic forms. It may also intercalate into DNA (Ch. 53). Some cases of plasmodial resistance to primaquine have been reported in animals and man.

Antimalarial Actions

Primaquine is highly active against the exoerythrocytic phase of MT malaria, but less active against BT malaria. It also exhibits a weak action against the asexual erythrocytic forms of

$$CH_3$$
$$NH-CH-CH_2-CH_2-CH_2-NH_2$$

$$H_3CO$$

PRIMAQUINE

BT malaria, but the effect is so erratic that it is of little clinical consequence. Primaquine is gametocidal for MT, BT, Q and OT malaria.

Absorption, Metabolism and Excretion

Primaquine is slowly but almost completely absorbed following oral administration. The drug is rapidly excreted, over 90% of a single oral dose being cleared within 24 hr. Quinacrine and the biguanides delay the metabolism of primaquine by an unknown mechanism, a phenomenon which is not therapeutically desirable since toxicity of the 8-aminoquinolines is also increased about tenfold. Since quinacrine is slowly excreted, interference may still be demonstrable 12–15 weeks or more after cessation of therapy.

Adverse Effects

Crampy abdominal pains and gastrointestinal upsets occur in many patients. Headaches, leukocytosis and leukopenia are less common; rarely leukopenia will rapidly progress to agranulocytosis. Primaquine was one of the first drugs to be incriminated in the production of hemolytic anemia in patients with glucose-6-phosphate dehydrogenase deficiency (Ch. 7; Table 75–23). Methemoglobinemia is provoked in patients with NADH methemoglobin reductase deficiency. Quinacrine, by retarding its catabolism, potentiates the adverse effects of the primaquine.

BIGUANIDES AND DIAMINOPYRIMIDINES: CHLOROGUANIDE

A series of biguanide and diaminopyrimidine compounds was developed during World War II. Both groups are closely related, since the pyrimidine ring of the diaminopyrimidines can be opened producing a biguanide. The biguanides in active use, **cholorguanide, chloroproguanil** and **cycloguanil pamoate,** and the **diaminopyrimidines** are discussed below and in Table 63–2.

Mode of Action

Chloroguanide is converted in vivo to a triazine ring compound that competitively inhibits dihydrofolate reductase (Ch. 53).

$$HN$$
$$Cl \qquad NH \qquad =NH$$
$$H_3C \quad CH_3$$

CHLOROGUANIDE

Antimalarial Actions

In moderately severe MT and BT malaria, chloroguanide can suppress the acute attack; it acts more slowly than chloroquine and should not be used in severe MT infection, particularly in a nonimmune subject. Chloroguanide is a causal prophylactic for MT malaria and a suppressant prophylactic for BT malaria; it is not curative in BT malaria since the exoerythrocytic stage of the parasite is not killed. Chloroguanide is not gametocidal in man, but prevents gametocyte and zygote maturation in the mosquito gut. Resistance (particularly in *P. falciparum* malaria) develops rapidly, tends to be of a high order and survives mosquito passage. Cross resistance occurs with chloroproguanil and pyrimethamine. Combination of a sulfonamide or a sulfone with chloroguanide may delay the emergence of resistant strains and potentiate its effect (see below: diaminopyrimidines).

Absorption, Metabolism and Excretion

Chloroguanide is slowly absorbed following oral administration and is concentrated in red blood cells. Metabolism and excretion are rapid. Chloroguanide delays the degradation of primaquine.

Adverse Effects

Adverse reactions to chloroguanide are few and generally not serious. Minor gastrointestinal upsets, headaches and occasionally hematuria and proteinuria with epithelial casts may appear, and the drug depresses gastric secretion. With long term therapy, an increase in the peripheral blood myelocyte count may be observed. Of clinical importance is the fact that malarial resistance develops rapidly to chloroguanide.

CHLORPROGUANIL

Chlorproguanil is a chloroguanide analog with essentially similar pharmacology and degree of antiprotozoal activity, but with a longer duration of action. Antimalarial resistance develops rapidly, and cross resistance is demonstrated with chloroguanide.

CYCLOGUANIL PAMOATE

The recently introduced cycloguanil pamoate (chloroguanide triazine pamoate) is a poorly soluble chloroguanide salt which is given parenterally as a repository preparation. Absorption from the injection site is a first order process, influenced by the particle size of the preparation. One injection of 2–5 mg/kg IM maintains suppressive blood levels for several months, but the exact value of this drug in long term therapy is not yet certain since its use may encourage the emergence of resistant strains. Use of cycloguanil pamoate combined with a depot sulfone which slowly releases diaminodiphenyl sulfone (Ch. 61), may be superior.

DIAMINOPYRIMIDINES

Many diaminopyrimidines have been tested for antimalarial activity, but only two, **pyrimethamine** and **trimethoprim** are of any value. They all inhibit the conversion of dihydrofolic acid to tetrahydrofolic acid by selectively inhibiting dihydrofolate reductase (Ch. 53).

Since protozoa synthesize their own dihydrofolic acid from precursors, they are open to "sequential blockade" by both the sulfonamides or the sulfones in addition to the diaminopyrimidines. This concept of sequential blockade has been a major advance in chemotherapy. There are two main advantages of sequential blockade. First, combined therapy reduces the rate of emergence of resistant strains and second, plasmodia resistant to either the sulfonamides or sulfones, or the diaminopyrimidines, may still be sensitive to a combination of a diaminopyrimidine (pyrimethamine or trimethoprim) plus a sulfonamide (sulfadiazine, triple sulfonamide, sulfamethoxazole) or a sulfone (diaminodiphenyl sulfone).

PYRIMETHAMINE

Antimalarial Actions

The antimalarial actions of pyrimethamine are similar to those of chloroguanide, but pyrimethamine is more potent since it acts directly and has a longer half-life. Because pyrimethamine acts on late stage trophozoites and because it takes a finite time to exhaust parasitic stores of tetrahydrofolic acid, its effect in an acute attack of malaria is of slow onset. The effect on gamete development is probably weaker than that of chloroguanide. Plasmodial resistance develops rapidly, and cross resistance is usually complete with chloroguanide. Pyrimethamine-resistant strains of plasmodia have an altered dihydrofolate reductase to which the drug does not readily bind. Furthermore, the mutant enzyme is produced in larger quantity than the normal enzyme, compensating for the presence of the inhibitory drug.

Absorption, Metabolism, and Excretion

Pyrimethamine is well absorbed following oral administration. Little is known about its metabolism or excretion.

Adverse Effects

Minor gastrointestinal upsets, a variety of skin rashes and megaloblastic anemia (reversed by folinic acid administration) are rarely produced.

TRIMETHOPRIM

Trimethoprim is principally used as an antibacterial agent (Ch. 60). It is under investigation in

TRIMETHOPRIM

combination with a sulfonamide in the treatment of multiresistant (particularly to chloroquine) strains of plasmodia.

General Usage of Antimalarial Drugs

The following summary is only a brief guide to the usage of the antimalarial drugs. *Susceptibility or resistance of local strains should be checked.* Many strains of MT malaria, particularly those in Asia, are now resistant to chloroquine. In the treatment of resistant strains, adjunct therapy with the sulfonamides, the sulfones or the tetracyclines may be of value. Doses are listed in Table 63–2.

Treatment of Acute Attack

Chloroquine phosphate is the drug of choice. **Amodiaquine** and **hydroxychloroquine** may replace chloroquine, but are usually considered inferior. **Quinine sulfate,** and **quinacrine** may be used in place of 4-aminoquinolines if resistance is suspected.

The above drugs will lead to cure in nearly all cases of MT malaria; however, in BT, Q and OT malaria the addition of a second drug active against the exoerythrocytic phase of the infection is necessary. **Primaquine** is the agent of choice.

Treatment of the Serious Attack

In the treatment of the grave attack of malaria, when heavily parasitized red blood cells are clogging arteries, speed is essential. The drugs of choice are either **chloroquine hydrochloride** or **quinine dihydrochloride,** depending upon the level of plasmodial resistance.

The defibrination syndrome (disseminated intravascular coagulation) may develop rapidly in falciparum malaria and heparinization is urgently needed. However, great care must be exercised since its use may be followed by cerebral hemorrhage. Dexamethazone is of value in cerebral edema. IV infusion of low molecular weight dextran may reduce red cell "stickiness" and improve flow through small spastic vessels. Inhalation of 5% carbon dioxide for 5–10 min every hour may improve cerebral blood flow.

Prophylaxis and Suppression

In the abscence of resistance, **chloroguanide hydrochloride,** 100 mg daily, and **pyrimethamine,** 25 mg weekly, commencing 1 week before entering, and continuing for 4 weeks after leaving, a malarious area, are the drugs of choice for MT prophylaxis. **Chloroquine phosphate,** 500 mg weekly, and **quinacrine,** 100 mg daily, commencing 2 weeks before entering, and for 4 weeks after leaving, a malarious zone, are alternative regimens.

Experimental investigation of malaria. Until about 10 years ago antimalarial compounds were tested against the avian parasite P. gallinaceum in the chick. Two new and useful laboratory models have now replaced this unsatisfactory test system, i.e., rodent malaria P. berghei infection in mice, and P. falciparum infection in the South African monkey Aotus trivirgatus. This latter is the only simian species in which human malaria parasites will readily develop.

New antimalarial drugs are urgently needed principally to combat multiple resistant strains of P. falciparum, but also to provide radical cure of B.T. malaria. In recent years more than 250,000 compounds have been screened for antimalarial activity and some promising leads, (phenanthrene methanols, 4-quinoline methanols, diaminoquinazolines and diaminohydrothiazines) are being followed.

AMEBIASIS

Amebiasis is caused by invasion of the gastrointestinal mucosa, liver and other tissues by trophozoite (vegetative) forms of the protozoal organism *Entamoeba histolytica.* Amebiasis is widespread in many parts of the world. In the United States, as many as 5% of the people in the southern states may be carriers. It is fairly common in southern California, Arizona and New Mexico owing to the proximity of ubiquitous infection in Mexico. Pathogenic amebas are differentiated microscopically on the basis of morphology. The protozoan must be identified to prove etiology, since pathogenic and nonpathogenic amebas look alike. Usually clinical infection is present as either acute or chronic colitis or as extraintestinal infection, most frequently liver abscess. However, the parasite may remain as a commensal in the lumen of the bowel producing cysts but without serious mucosal invasion.

The life cycle of E. histolytica is indicated in Figure 63–2. The basis of drug therapy is to kill the trophozoite forms of the parasite in the bowel, as cystic amebas cease to be produced when all trophozoites are killed. Most drugs are directly amebicidal; broad spectrum antibiotics are indirectly amebicidal by eliminating the colonic bacterial flora required by E. histolytica for normal growth and maturation; some drugs may be cystocidal. The occurrence of natural or ac-

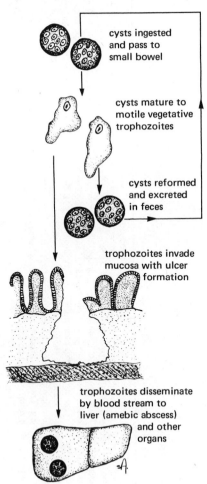

cysts ingested
and pass to
small bowel

cysts mature to
motile vegetative
trophozoites

cysts reformed
and excreted
in feces

trophozoites invade
mucosa with ulcer
formation

trophozoites disseminate
by blood stream to
liver (amebic abscess)
and other
organs

Carbarsone
(Diloxanide furoate)
Glycobiarsol
8-Hydroxyquinolines
(metronidazole)

Carbarsone
(Diloxanide furoate)
Glycobiarsol
8-Hydroxyquinolines
(metronidazole)

Antibiotics
Carbarsone
(Diloxanide furoate)
Emetine
Glycobiarsol
8-Hydroxquinolines
(Metronidazole)

Antibiotics (Erythromycin)
Chloroquine
Emetine
(Metronidazole)

FIG. 63–2. Life cycle of *Entamoeba histolytica* and drugs of choice for amebiasis.

quired resistance of E. histolytica to amebicides is controversial.

IPECACUANHA ALKALOIDS: EMETINE

Ipecacuanha is obtained from the dried rhizomes or roots of *Cephaelis ipecacuanha* and *C. acuminata*. Its amebicidal activity is due entirely to its alkaloid content, mainly emetine and cephaeline. Emetine is the only ipecacuanha alkaloid in

EMETINE

current use (Table 63–3). It's name derives from its propensity to produce vomiting. It is occasionally used today and is an important drug for histortial reasons.

Adverse Effects

Emetine mainly affects the cardiac and skeletal muscles and the gastrointestinal tract.

CARDIOVASCULAR SYSTEM. Tachycardia from stimulation of the S.A. node, precordial pain, dyspnea and systemic hypotension may develop. Electrocardiographically, T-wave flattening and inversion, and a gradual widening of the PR and QRS intervals are characteristic; all types of cardiac irregularities may appear and acute cardiac failure and death may supervene rapidly.

SKELETAL MUSCLE. Emetine may partially block transmission at the myoneural junction. Commonly it produces localized (at the site of injection) and generalised myositis, with weakness, aching pain and tenderness. Myositis most commonly affects the muscles of the neck and the distal muscles of the extremities. The incidence of cardiac and skeletal muscle damage is dramatically increased if the patient is ambulatory.

TABLE 63–3. Some Antiamebic Drugs

Drug	Properties	Preparations and dose
Emetine	Emetine depresses protein synthesis probably by preventing the attachment of aminoacyl tRNA onto the ribosome, and depresses aerobic glycolysis. It is amebicidal for trophozoite forms of the parasite in the bowel wall, liver or other tissues, but has no effect on trophozoites in the bowel lumen or on cysts since a sufficiently high concentration does not develop there. Thus the use of emetine alone in an acute attack of dysentery may initiate a chronic carrier state. Emetine is an intense irritant when taken orally and thus must be given parenterally. Absorption is rapid from both SC and IM sites, but the former is preferred since it is less painful. The drug is excreted slowly by the kidney, and because of cumulation a single course of injections should not last longer than 10 days	The usual daily dose of Emetine hydrochloride, *U.S.P.* in adults is 1.0 mg/kg of body weight, not to exceed 60 mg. This is given SC in either 1 or 2 doses. Therapy should be monitored clinically by pulse rate, blood pressure and electrocardiographically, and must be discontinued if evidence of cardiac toxicity appears. If no symptoms or signs of toxicity develop, a 10 day, 600 mg course of emetine should not be exceeded. At least 2 mo should elapse before a repeat course is given. The patient should remain in bed for the duration of emetine therapy and for at least 1 wk afterwards, and remain sedentary for a further 3–6 wk. The drug should be used with extreme caution, if at all, in children, and in patients with impaired renal or cardiac function
8-hydroxyquinolines	The halogenated hydroxyquinolines are directly amebicidal for vegetative forms of the parasite in the bowel lumen and bowel wall, probably by blocking essential enzyme systems. Due to their poor absorption, they have no effect on systemic disease. They may be cystocidal Minimal absorption occurs following oral administration, their antiamebic effects being due to a local action in the bowel lumen. Little is known about the distribution, metabolism and excretion of the absorbed hydroxyquinolines.	Many preparations are available, either singly or in combination. **Chiniofon** (Yatren) is usually prescribed in a dose of 500 mg—1 g 3 times daily for 10 days. It is wise to commence with 250 mg 3 times daily and gradually increase the dosage to minimize gastrointestinal irritation. **Iodochlorhydroxyquin** (Clioquinol, Vioform) is available in a variety of official *U.S.P.* and *N.F.* preparations for use in amebiasis and skin infections. Enteric-coated tablets are used in the treatment of amebiasis, the oral dose being 250–500 mg 3 times daily for 10 days. A repeat course should only be given after a 2–3 wk rest period. Retention enemas of 2 g/200 ml water are rarely used. Topical preparations are usually 3% powders, creams and ointments after combined with glucocorticosteroids. They are usually applied 3 times daily

Drug		
	Plasma iodine levels do not effectively measure the degree of drug absorption	**Diiodohydroxyquin,** *U.S.P.* (Diodoquin), is usually given orally in a dose of 650 mg 3 times daily for 7–20 days. A repeat course should only be given after a 3–4 wk rest period. The drug is too insoluble for administration in an enema
Chloroquine	See text	The recommended dose in extraintestinal infection is 250 mg 6 hourly for 3 days, followed by 250 mg twice daily for 14–21 days. If the patient has hepatic amebiasis, symptoms will usually start to abate within 48 hr of commencing therapy. Chloroquine is about equipotent with emetine but considerably less toxic
Metronidazole	The mode of action of metronidazole is not known. The drug is well absorbed following oral administration and passes successfully to most organs including the liver, the gastrointestinal tract and most genitourinary tissues and fluids. It is excreted unchanged and as various unknown metabolites	Metronidazole, *U.S.P.* (Flagyl) is available for oral administration. The optimum dosage for amebiasis has not yet been decided, but 300–800 mg 3 times a day for 5–10 days has been shown highly effective in several trials. It may also be effective in prophylaxis. In trichomoniasis the usual oral dose in females is 250 mg 3 times daily for 7–10 days, and concurrent vaginal therapy may also be advisable; local vaginal therapy may be ineffective by itself. It is essential to treat sexual partners concurrently if they are infected; the dose for males is 250 mg twice a day for 7–10 days. If a repeat course is needed in either sex it is wise to wait for 4–6 wk. With repeated courses carefully monitoring of the blood count is advisable
Carbarsone	Carbarsone probably acts by -SH group inactivation. It is absorbed after oral administration, but excretion, both in the urine and bile, is slow, and cumulation may develop rapidly, particularly in patients with renal and hepatic disease	Carbarsone is available in capsules (Carbarsone Capsules, *N.F.*), tablets (Carbarsone Tablets, *U.S.P.*), and as suppositories (Carbarsone suppository, *N.F.*). The usual dose for acute or chronic amebic colitis is 250 mg 3 times daily for 7–10 days. If a second course is required, a 2 wk rest period should be observed. Carbarsone suppositories are of use in some cases of trichomoniasis
Glycobiarsol	Poorly absorbed, and acts locally in the intestinal lumen	The usual oral dose of glycobiarsol, *N.F.* (Milibis), in amebiasis is 500 mg 3 times daily for 7–12 days. It may be more active in the subacute or carrier state than in acute colitis. Suppositories of 250 mg 3 times daily for 7–12 days are also used in the treatment of vaginal candidiasis or trichomoniasis
Paromomycin	Paromomycin is poorly absorbed from the gastrointestinal tract, but exhibits a local action in the bowel lumen. It is too toxic to be given systemically, producing severe renal damage	Paromomycin sulfate *N.F.* (Humatin) is usually prescribed as 10–25 mg/kg/day in divided doses for 5 days. A repeat course of therapy can follow a 10–15 day rest period

GASTROINTESTINAL TRACT. Nausea, vomiting and bloody diarrhea develop from both central and peripheral nervous system stimulation, and may be confused with a relapse of the infection.

MISCELLANEOUS EFFECTS. Emetine frequently produces headaches, dizziness and faintness (systemic hypotention) and a variety of skin rashes, and urticaria and purpura are common.

Uses

USE IN AMEBIASIS. Emetine is effective in acute amebic colitis, acute relapses of chronic amebic colitis and in amebic abscesses. It is of no use in the treatment of the asymptomatic carrier since the drug does not achieve satisfactory amebicidal levels in the bowel lumen. Emetine is a highly toxic drug, and the dosage and duration of therapy outlined (Table 63–3) should not be exceeded. In colitis, emetine is usually given until the acute symptoms have abated (2–5 days) and then its administration is stopped. Another drug active against the intralumenal vegetative amebas should also be given to avoid induction of the carrier state. For amebic abscesses, a 10 day course of emetine in combination with chloroquine is recommended. Chloroquine and metronidazole are gradually replacing emetine in therapy.

OTHER USES. Emetine is of limited value in the treatment of balantidiasis (see below) and some helmintic infections (Ch. 64).

DEHYDROEMETINE AND EMETINE BISMUTH IODIDE

Racemic **2-dehydroemetine** is a simple congener of emetine. The drug is excreted more rapidly and has been shown experimentally to be concentrated more in the liver and less in the heart than natural emetine. The side effects of 2-dehydroemetine are similar to those of emetine.

Emetine bismuth iodide contains about 25% emetine and about 20% bismuth. It is an orally administered compound releasing emetine slowly in the bowel lumen. Side effects are similar to emetine.

8-HYDROXYQUINOLINES

There are three 8-hydroxyquinolines (Table 63–3) of use in the treatment of amebiasis. Because of their similarity they can be considered together. They are all tasteless yellow powders: **chiniofon** is moderately water soluble, whereas **iodochlorhydroxyquin** and **diiodohydroxyquin** are poorly water soluble.

Adverse Effects

In the absence of hypersensitivity to iodine, adverse reactions are usually minimal. Recently, however, use of these agents (particularly iodochlorhydroxyquin) has been associated with the development of severe subacute myelo-optic neuropathy. Diarrhea and pruritis ani are produced frequently, but clear when the drugs are discontinued. Headaches, gastric irritation with nausea and vomiting, and hepatic damage are less common. Iodine released from the 8-hydroxyquinolines augments the plasma protein-bound iodine level and may alter thyroid function tests and rarely produce iodism. Patients sensitive to iodine and patients with hepatic, renal or thyroid disease should not be exposed to these agents without extreme caution.

Uses

USE IN AMEBIASIS. All the 8-hydroxyquinolines are effective in the treatment of acute or chronic amebiasis and in treatment of the carrier state but *they should not be used alone.* Clinically there is little to choose among them. If repeated courses of antiamebic therapy are required, a 2–3 weeks rest period between individual programs is advisable. These drugs are cheap compounds that are valuable in the treatment of large populations. Furthermore, no restriction of activity is required. The single major hazard to therapy is the development of optic neuritis. Metronidazole may eventually replace the 8-hydroxyquinolines.

OTHER USES. Iodochlorhydroxyquin is of value in some cases of superficial fungal disease (Ch. 65), trichomonal vaginitis (see below), and various skin disorders, such as acrodermatitis enterohepatica, where it may be used in combination with hydrocortisone. Diiodohydroxyquin is occasionally used in the treatment of giardiasis and ciliate dysentery (see below).

4-AMINOQUINOLINES: CHLOROQUINE

Chloroquine (Tables 63–2 and 63–3), the most popular 4-aminoquinoline used in amebiasis, is discussed above. The effectiveness of chloroquine and the 8-hydroxyquinolines in amebiasis is almost certainly due to their quinoline nucleus. Chloroquine is actively amebicidal for extraintestinal parasites, particularly hepatic and pulmonary infection, but it has no effect on the bowel forms of the disease. The absence of effect on the intestinal parasites may result from its rapid and almost complete absorption in the upper bowel and its storage in the liver. Chloroquine should always be combined with an amebicide active against intestinal parasites.

Metronidazole

Metronidazole (2-methyl-5-nitroimidazole) has been in use for many years in the treatment of urogenital trichomoniasis and ulcerative gingivitis. Recently however, it was found to offer great promise in the treatment of amebiasis and giardiasis. In amebiasis it is unique in that it exhibits antiprotozoal activity against both bowel

METRONIDAZOLE

and tissue forms of the disease. In general, however, higher doses are required to eradicate amebic infection from the gastrointestinal tract than from the liver.

Adverse Effects

Superinfections (particularly with *Candida albicans*), xerostomia, stomatitis, nausea, vomiting, abdominal pain, diarrhea, dysgeusia, headaches, flushing, a variety of skin rashes, pruritis, urethral and vaginal burning pain, leukopenia and in rare instances, dizziness, vertigo, ataxia and paresthesias of the arms and legs may appear. Agranulocytosis has not yet been reported; however, metronidazole should be given with caution to patients with hepatic or hematologic pathology. Until more experience has been gained with this drug, its use during pregnancy should be avoided. Following high doses, unknown drug metabolites can cause a reddish-brown discoloration of the urine. Patients taking metronidazole may rarely experience a disulfiram-like (an Antabuse-like) reaction on taking alcohol (Ch. 10).

Uses

Metronidazole may become the drug of choice for both intestinal and extra intestinal amebiasis and for prophylaxis. Additionally, it is a highly specific local and systemic trichomonacidal drug, effective in treating trichomoniasis in men and women. It is trichomonacidal in serum, urine, semen and all genitourinary tissues, so that eradication of deep seated infection is possible. Metronidazole may also be of some value in the treatment of giardiasis (lambliasis), particularly if quinacrine is contraindicated, and in Vincent's Angina. Metronidazole has been used experimentally in the treatment of alcoholism. Its use may be associated with "Antabuse-like"

reactions and it may also suppress the desire for alcohol and alter its positive hedonic effect.

ARSENIC PREPARATIONS

Several arsenical and bismuth preparations have been advocated for the treatment of amebiasis. *N*-**carbamoylarsanilic acid** (Carbarsone) and **glycobiarsol** (Milibis) are the most commonly used (Table 63–3). Acetarsol, diphetarsone and several thioarsenites are rarely used.

Carbarsone

Carbarsone contains about 29% arsenic. It is amebicidal for intestinal amebas and may exhibit some cystocidal activity. It has no value in the treatment of extraintestinal amebiasis. Carbarsone is about as active as the 8-hydroxyquinolines but it is considerably more toxic.

Adverse reactions are rare and primarily those of arsenical poisoning. Gastrointestinal upsets, skin rashes (particularly exfoliative dermatitis),

CARBARSONE   GLYCOBIARSOL

polyneuritis, optic neuritis, encephalopathy, psychotic reactions and renal and bone marrow damage are typical. The drug is contraindicated in patients with renal or hepatic disease.

Glycobiarsol

Glycobiarsol contains about 42% bismuth and 15% pentavalent arsenic. It is of value in the treatment of intestinal amebiasis only, being primarily amebicidal; it may also have some direct cystocidal activity. Adverse reactions are similar to those occurring with carbarsone. In addition, the bismuth colors feces black.

DILOXANIDE FUROATE

Diloxanide furoate, the 2-furoic acid ester of diloxanide (dichloracet-4-hydroxy-N-methylanilide), is a recently introduced directly acting amebicide at present under clinical trial. It acts primarily against trophozoite forms in the bowel lumen possessing no significant activity against extraintestinal parasites. Toxicity to date has been that of gastrointestinal upsets but with greater use a wider spectrum of adverse effects will undoubtedly appear. Diloxanide furoate is available in tablets of 500 mg. The usual dose is 500 mg 3 times a day for 10 days. It has been used successfully in the treatment of acute, subacute and chronic amebic colitis, and particularly in the treatment of the asymptomatic cyst excretor. It is available for clinical trial purposes only.

ANTIBIOTICS

Chlortetracycline, oxytetracycline, erythromycin (Ch. 57), neomycin (Ch. 56), bacitracin (Ch. 55), and paromomycin (see below) all demonstrate some antiamebic activity. However, it is not certain whether this is a direct amebicidal effect, an indirect action due to the suppression of the colonic flora, or both. Irrespective of their antiamebic activity, these antibiotics are of value in reducing the secondary bacterial infection of the ulcerated mucosa.

Paromomycin

Paromomycin is a broad spectrum antibiotic obtained from *Streptomyces rimosus,* closely related to the aminoglycoside antibiotics (Ch. 56).

PAROMOMYCIN

It is effective against vegetative intestinal amebas, some gram-negative organisms, *Trichomonas vaginalis* and some helminths. Adverse reactions are gastrointestinal upsets, skin rashes, vertigo and headaches. Diarrhea commencing early in therapy may regress in spite of continuing treatment. Superinfection is common.

Paromomycin has been used in the treatment of intestinal amebiasis, trichomoniasis, some types of bacterial dysentery, preoperatively to suppress the colonic flora and in hepatic coma and precoma and in some cases of taeniasis. In amebiasis it is of particular value in patients hypersensitive to the 8-hydroxyquinolines.

PRINCIPLES OF TREATMENT OF AMEBIASIS

A correct diagnosis is essential, and prior use of antibiotics or barium enemas may temporarily depress the excretion of amebic cysts and vegetative forms. None of the drugs presently available has been proved effective in treating both intestinal and extraintestinal amebiasis, and successful therapy depends upon concomitant or sequential treatment with at least two drugs. Metronidazole (see above) and niridazole (Ch. 64) may prove effective against both intestinal and extraintestinal amebiasis.

Treatment of Acute Amebic Colitis

This is best treated with 5–7 days of **tetracyclines,** 3 weeks of an **8-hydroxyquinoline,** and 2 weeks of **chloroquine,** all drugs started simultaneously. If this regimen fails, emetine is the drug of choice. Usually a 3–5 day course is sufficient to produce clinical arrest of the attack. There is no point in continuing emetine any longer than necessary. If therapy commences with emetine, sequential adjunct therapy with either the 8-hydroxyquinolines, the arsenicals, or the antibiotics is essential in order to prevent a carrier state. If antibiotics are given alone relapses are common. Metronidazole may become the drug of choice.

Treatment of Chronic Amebic Colitis

Chronic amebic colitis is best treated with a 3 week course of **8-hydroxyquinolines** or the **arsenicals,** plus **cholorquine.** Several courses may be required. Emetine and antibiotics may be necessary in treating acute flareups. Emetine should be given as described above in treatment of the acute attack.

Treatment of the Asymptomatic Carrier State

The asymptomatic carrier is usually best treated with the **8-hydroxyquinolines,** the **antibiotics** (preferably paromomycin), or **carbarsone** or **glycobiarsol.** Several courses of treatment may be required. A course of chloroquine should also be given to eradicate any asymptomatic extraintestinal infection. Metronidazole is probably less effective than diiodohydroxyquin.

Prophylaxis

Subacute myeloneuropathy is a grave risk of prophylaxis with the 8-hydroxyquinolines, and thus these agents once widely used are becoming less popular. Metronidazole may become the drug of choice.

Treatment of Extraintestinal Amebiasis

Chloroquine and **emetine** are the drugs of choice for either acute or chronic extraintestinal amebiasis. Usually the liver is the site of infection, but many other tissues can be involved. Open surgical drainage or needle aspiration of abscesses may be required (Ch. 52). Some authorities recommend erythromycin as an adjunct agent in the treatment of hepatic amebiasis since this antibiotic is selectively concentrated in the liver. Metronidazole may become the drug of choice for extraintestinal amebiasis in so far as it possesses activity against both intestinal and extraintestinal infection.

Extraintestinal disease is always secondary to intestinal infection even though the intestinal phase may have remained asymptomatic. Thus, after successful therapy of extraintestinal amebiasis eradication of symptomatic or asymptomatic colonic infection should be undertaken to prevent the recurrence of extraintestinal infection.

LEISHMANIASIS

Leishmaniasis is a term applied to several diseases caused by protozoal organisms of the genus *Leishmania*. Kala-azar is caused by *L. donovani,* oriental sore by *L. tropica,* and mucocutaneous leishmaniasis (South American leishmaniasis) by *L. braziliensis.* In all instances, a *Phlebotomus* sandfly vector hosts part of the protozoal life cycle. The treatment of leishmaniasis is twofold: treatment of the disease itself and measures taken against the vector. In this chapter only a brief mention of the available drugs is made.

ANTIMONY COMPOUNDS

Antimony is used only in the form of its organic preparations, and these are either trivalent or pentavalent compounds. Trivalent antimony readily forms thio antimonites with –SH groups of cellular constituents, but this may not be true in vivo with pentavalent antimony compounds. Many of the antimony preparations are obsolete.

Trivalent Antimony Compounds

Tartar emetic (Antimony Potassium Tartrate, *U.S.P.*) has been replaced by the pentavalent arsenical compounds in the treatment of leishmaniasis. It is of limited use in *Schistosoma japonicum* infections and in chlonorchiasis and filariasis (Ch. 64), and in mycosis fungoides and granuloma inguinale. Its one advantage is its cheapness.

Antimony sodium tartrate is similar to tartar emetic. **Antimony thioglycollamide** and **antimony sodium thioglycollate** are claimed to be less toxic and more potent than tartar emetic. They may be given IM or IV. **Stibophen (Fuadin) and antimony dimercaptosuccinate** are trivalent antimony compounds of some use in schistosomiasis.

Pentavalent Antimony Compounds

The pentavalent antimony compounds are more active, less toxic and more parasiticidal in leishmaniasis but more expensive than the trivalent compounds. **Stibamine glucoside** (Neostam) is a 4% solution that is injected IV in doses of 2.2 mg/kg. **Ethylstibamine** (Neostibosan) is usually given IM or IV in doses of 200–300 mg every 2nd day. **Sodium stibogluconate** (Pentostam) which contains 100 mg of pentavalent antimony/ml is the antimony compound of choice. It is usually given IM or IV in daily doses of 600 mg for 6–10 days.

Adverse effects caused by these compounds include nausea, vomiting, diarrhea, perspiration, headaches, dizziness, arthralgia, purpura, proteinuria, skin rashes, bradycardia, coughing and respiratory arrest. Reactions may develop during or immediately after drug injection, and antimony compounds should be given with caution to patients with hepatic or renal disease.

Aromatic Diamidines

There are several aromatic diamidines, but only **hydroxystilbamidine isethionate,** *U.S.P.* and **pentamidine isethionate** (Lomidine) are used clinically. These drugs are injected IM or IV, and may be followed by the rapid development of headache, palpitations, dyspnea, dizziness, sweating, tachycardia, nausea, vomiting, diarrhea or abdominal pain. These symptoms are partly due to histamine release (Ch. 49) and peripheral adrenergic blockade. The original aromatic diamidine, stilbamidine, was discarded because of the frequency with which it produced acute yellow atrophy of the liver and fifth cranial nerve nuclear degeneration. Neither of these reactions has been reported with hydroxystilbamidine nor pentamidine.

These drugs are probably inferior to antimony compounds in the treatment of leishmaniasis primarily because of their toxicity, but they may be used with success in antimony resistant cases.

Hydroxystilbamidine is occasionally of benefit in the treatment of North American blastomycosis, and pentamidine isethionate in a dose of 4 mg/kg/day for 2 weeks is of dramatic benefit in some cases of *Pneumocystis carinii* pneumonia.

Principles of Treatment of Leishmaniasis

TREATMENT OF KALA-AZAR. Stibamine glucoside, ethylstibamine and sodium stibogluconate are more popular than the trivalent antimony compounds. Pentamidine (4 mg/kg IM for

10 days) and hydroxystilbamidine (5 mg/kg IV for 10 days) are often dramatically successful in cases that do not respond to antimony compounds.

TREATMENT OF ORIENTAL SORE. Local measures are more important than antimony compounds. Probably local intralesion injection of quinacrine, or cautery, x-irradiation and carbon dioxide snow are of more value. Pentavalent arsenicals or tartar emetic can be given for widespread lesions.

TREATMENT OF MUCOCUTANEOUS DISEASE. Treatment of mucocutaneous leishmaniasis is a chronic therapeutic problem. Intravenous sodium antimony gluconate, trivalent antimony compounds, arsenicals, chloroquine, amphotericin B, cycloguanil pamoate and the aromatic diamidines have all been used.

TRYPANOSOMIASIS

Trypanosomiasis is a term applied to diseases caused by protozoal organisms of the genus *Trypanosoma*. African sleeping sickness is caused by *T. gambiense* or *T. rhodesiense,* and South American sleeping sickness (Chagas' disease) by *T. cruzi.* In this chapter only a brief mention of the available drugs is made.

SURAMIN

Suramin, a benzidine derivative, has been used in the treatment and prophylaxis of trypanosomiasis and in the treatment of pemphigus and onchocerciasis. Synergistic activity may be demonstrated between it and the pentavalent arsenicals or the aromatic diamidines. The mechanism of action of suramin is unknown. However, it does inhibit a variety of enzyme systems. Suramin is not absorbed following oral administration but must be given IV. Little is known about its metabolism, but the drug is excreted very slowly due to poor glomerular filtration (it is highly bound to plasma proteins) and avid tubular reabsorption. Following a single dose, the drug may be detected in the plasma for up to 3 months.

Adverse reactions are serious. Violent gastrointestinal upsets, hypotension and loss of consciousness may follow too rapid IV injection. A variety of skin rashes, paresthesias, photophobia, sweating and renal damage may appear rapidly, particularly in malnourished patients. Agranulocytosis and hemolytic anemia are rare.

Suramin is of use in *T. gambiense* and *T. rhodesiense* infections, when it is given IV in a 10% aqueous solution. The initial test dose of 200 mg should not be exceeded. This is followed by 1 gm of suramin on days 6, 14 and 16; 1 g of tryparsamide on days 21, 26, 31 and 36; and 2 g of tryparasamide on day 41. Suramin (Bayer 205) is available in 1 g ampoules.

Tryparsamide

Tryparsamide *U.S.P.* contains 25% pentavalent arsenic. It is highly effective in some cases of trypanosomiasis, particularly if combined with suramin. It is given IV in the dosage described above, under Suramin. Tryparsamide passes readily into the CSF, a property of extreme value in treating late stage trypanosomiasis. The overall incidence of adverse reactions may reach 25%, while ocular symptoms usually develop in at least 10% of patients treated. Ocular symptoms may be minimal (e.g., hemeralopia, fortification phenomena, transient amblyopia) but may progress to total blindness. Hepatitis, skin rashes and gastrointestinal upsets are also common adverse reactions.

MELARSOPROL

Melarsoprol (Mel B) is a dimercaprol derivative of melarsen oxide, and probably acts by –SH group inhibition. Small but therapeutically significant trypanocidal CSF levels develop following conventional therapy, a factor of some importance in the treatment of severe, advanced sleeping sickness and *T. rhodesiense* infection.

Mel B produces a variety of adverse reactions, particularly a toxic encephalopathy, and renal and hepatic damage. It may induce erythema nodosum in patients with leprosy.

Mel B is given by slow IV infusion in propylene glycol. Since it is highly irritating to vascular endothelium it may produce thrombophlebitis. Patients receiving this drug should be hospitalized so that appropriate adjunct therapy with glucocorticosteroids or dimercaprol may be given. Dosage should be based not upon body weight, but upon severity of disease. Melarsoprol has three advantages over tryparsamide: it is rapidly acting; it possesses no ocular toxicity; and trypanosomes resistant to tryparsamide usually retain their sensitivity to melarsoprol.

MELARSONYL (MEL W)

Melarsonyl is a water soluble derivative of Mel B; it resembles the latter pharmacologically. It is given IM.

PRINCIPLES OF TREATMENT OF TRYPANOSOMIASIS

The object in the treatment of trypanosomiasis is to clear the blood, tissues and CSF of parasites. In *T. gambiense* infection, either suramin and tryparsamide or pentamidine and tryparsamide may be effective. If CNS involvement has developed, melarsoprol is the drug of choice. Melarsoprol is also the drug of choice for most cases of *T. rho-* *desiense* infections. Early infections with *T. cruzi* may respond to the 8-aminoquinolines (see above, under Malaria). Nitrofurazone (Ch. 61), 10 mg/kg 3 times daily for 10 days, may be effective if given early in the course of infection.

The prophylaxis of trypanosomiasis is best accomplished by a single IM injection of 250 mg of pentamidine. This will afford adequate protection for 4–6 months.

TRICHOMONIASIS

Trichomoniasis is a veneral disease caused by the protozoan *Trichomonas vaginalis.* Of the many drugs available for the topical treatment of this disease, the pentavalent arsenicals, the 8-hydroxyquinolines, hexetidine, hydrogen peroxide, silver nitrate and furazolidone are popular. However, these drugs, although eradicating the infection in many women, often fail when the infection is chronic. **Metronidazole,** a trichomonacidal drug in males and females (see above), represents an important step forward in drug therapy since infection in males (which cannot be treated with topical preparations) is often the source of female reinfection through sexual contact.

TOXOPLASMOSIS

Toxoplasmosis is caused by congential or acquired infection with the protozoan *Toxoplasma gondii.* Treatment depends upon the type and extent of the infection. However, drugs effective in the treatment of experimental toxoplasmosis are not always equally useful in human infection.

Pyrimethamine (see above, under Malaria) and sulfadiazine, or trimethoprim and sulfamethoxazole (Ch. 60) are the most important drugs in use. In patients with severe chorioretinitis, it is advisable to add a glucocorticosteroid to the antiprotozoal regimen. Folinic acid should also be added to prevent the development of megaloblastic anemia.

GIARDIASIS

Giardiasis (lambliasis) is caused by *Giardia lamblia,* a protozoan that may occur in the gastrointestinal tract. Quinacrine hydrochloride, diiodohydroxyquin, chloroquine, hydroxychloro- quine and metronidazole (see above) have all been used with success in treatment. Probably **quinacrine** is the drug of choice. It is given in doses of 100 mg 3 times for 7–10 days.

BALANTIDIASIS (CILIATE DYSENTERY)

Balantidiasis is caused by the protozoan *Balantidium coli* (not to be confused with *Bacterium* [*Escherichia*]*coli*). The tetracyclines, pentavalent arsenicals, diiodohydroxyquin, emetine and silver nitrate have been used with varying success.

Probably the **tetracyclines,** particularly oxytetracycline and chlortetracycline, are the drugs of choice. They are given in doses of 500 mg 3 times daily for 10 days.

FURTHER READING

Most H (1972): Treatment of common parasitic infections of man encountered in the United States. N Engl J Med 287:495–498; 698–702

Ross Institute (1972): Antimalarial drugs, Bulletin No. 2 (rewritten). London, London School of Hygiene and Tropical Medicine

Rozman RS (1973): Chemotherapy of malaria. Pharmacol Rev 13:127–152

WHO Technical Report (1973); Malaria. Report Series No. 529. Geneva, WHO

JEREMY H. THOMPSON

64. DRUGS USED IN THE TREATMENT OF HELMINTHIASIS

Worm infection (helminthiasis) includes parasitization with cestodes (tapeworms), nematodes (roundworms) and trematodes (flukes) (Table 64–1). Helminthiasis is present in approximately half the world's population and is not limited to tropical or subtropical countries, but is endemic in many areas because of poor sanitation, poor family hygiene, malnutrition, disease and crowded living conditions. The anthelmintic drugs are toxic compounds acting directly on the parasite. In the case of anthelmintic agents acting against intestinal helminths (vermifuges), they kill or sterilize the worms, or paralyze them so that they lose hold of the intestinal mucosa and are expelled. Host immunity seems unimportant for recovery. Treatment is frequently complicated by drug toxicity, mixed infections, "Jarisch-Herxheimer-like" reactions to liberated helmintic protein, coincident disease, malnutrition, anemia or dehydration. Improvement of the patient's general condition as regards nutrition, and correction of anemia, electrolyte imbalance, etc., are important aspects of therapy.

When treating intestinal parasitism, a 24 hr fast prior to drug administration may be advisable. It is suggested that the drug package insert be consulted for special precautions regarding dosage or administration, since in this chapter only principal adverse effects are given for each agent and no attempt is made to list all precautions and contraindications to therapy. Infection with more than one type of worm is common. Thus drug therapy must take into account a possible effect on a second parasite. When selecting a drug, the cost should be considered, since many patients requiring these agents are financially destitute. The drugs are discussed alphabetically (Table 64–2).

TABLE 64–1. Cause and Treatment of Helmintic Infections of Man

Disease	Helminth	Drugs used in treatment
Cestode (tapeworm) infections		
Intestinal taeniasis	*Diphyllobothrium latum*	*Quinacrine,* Aspidium, (Dichlorophen, Niclosamide)
	Hymenolepsis nana	*(Dichlorophen, Niclosamide)* Aspidium,* Hexylresorcinol,* Mebendazole, Quinacrine*
	Taenia saginata, T. solium	*Quinacrine,* Aspidium, Mebendazole, (Dichlorophen, Niclosamide)
Somatic taeniasis (cysticercosis)	*T. solium*	None
Nematode (roundworm) infections		
Ancylostomiasis	*Ancylostoma duodenale*	*Bephenium,* Hexylresorcinol, Mebendazole, Tetrachloroethylene,* Thiabendazole
	Necator americanus	*Bephenium,* Hexylresorcinol, Tetrachloroethylene,* Thiabendazole
Ascariasis	*Ascaris lumbricoides*	*Piperazine, Pyrantel,* Bephenium, Diethylcarbamazine, Hexylresorcinol,* Mebandazole, Thiabendazole
Enterobiasis	*Enterobius vermicularis*	*Piperazine, Pyrantel, Pyrvinium,* Gentian violet,* Hexylresorcinol,* Mebendazole, Niclosamide,* Oxytetracycline, Thiabendazole
Filariasis	*Wuchereria bancrofti*	*Diethylcarbamazine,* Mebendazole, Merarsonyl
	B. malayi	*Diethylcarbamazine,* Mebendazole, Merarsonyl
	Loa loa	*Diethylcarbamazine,* Mebendazole, Merarsonyl
Onchocerciasis	*Onchocerca volvulus*	*Diethylcarbamazine* plus suramin, Mebendazole, Merarsonyl, (Niridazole)
Strongyloidiasis	*Strongyloides stercoralis*	*Thiabendazole,* Gentian violet,* Pyrvinium
Trichiniasis	*Trichinella spiralis*	Corticosteroids, Thiabendazole
Trichuriasis	*Trichuris trichiura*	*Hexylresorcinol,* Mebendazole, *Thiabendazole,* Bephenium
Trematode (fluke) infections		
Clonorchiasis	*Clonorchis sinensis*	*Chloroquine,* Antimony Sodium Tartrate, Bithionol, Emetine, Gentian violet
Fascioliasis	*Fasciola hepatica*	*Emetine plus Sulfonamides,* Bithionol, Chloroquine
	Fasciolopsis buski	*Hexylresorcinol,* Tetrachloroethylene
Heterophyiasis	*Heterophyes heterophyes*	*Tetrachloroethylene,* Hexylresorcinol
Paragonimiasis	*Paragonimus westermani*	*Bithionol,* Chloroquine, Emetine plus Sulfonamides*
	P. kellicotti	Bithionol, Chloroquine, Emetine plus Sulfonamides*
Schistosomiasis (bilharziasis)	*Schistosoma haematobium*	*Stibophen, Lucanthone, Niridazole,* Sodium Antimony Dimercaptosuccinate
	S. mansoni	*Stibophen,* lucanthone, *niridazole,* Sodium Antimony Dimercaptosuccinate
	S. japonicum	*Potassium Antimony Tartrate,* Niridazole, Stibophen

Italics indicate current drugs of choice.
Parentheses drugs available for limited use only.
Asterisks drugs rarely used.

TABLE 64–2. Some Anthelmintic Drugs

Drug	Properties	Adverse effects	Preparations, dosage and usage
Antimony compounds	Potassium and sodium antimony tartrate, stibophen and antimony dimercaptosuccinate may all be used. Properties are discussed in Ch. 63. They selectively inhibit schistosomal phosphofructokinase, which catalyses the conversion of fructose-6-phosphate to fructose-1-6-diphosphate	See Ch. 63	Potassium and sodium antimony tartrate are given IV in increasing doses from 60-120 mg every 2nd day. Used in some cases of schistosomiasis, clonorchiasis and filariasis. Stibophen is given IM in doses of 100 mg every 2nd day for 1-3 wk
Aspidium	Aspidium is a dark green evil smelling oil (oleoresin) extracted from the rhizome and stipes of the male fern *Dryopteris filix mas*. The active principal filixic acid, is rarely used in resistant cases of taeniasis when quinacrine has failed. Aspidium depresses most cestodes (except *Hymenolepsis nana*) and is highly irritating to the intestinal mucosa if given undiluted. It is poorly absorbed, but even so absorption should be reduced by giving a saline cathartic 4-6 hr after the last dose	Abdominal pain, nausea, vomiting and diarrhea are common. Excessive absorption occurs if the bowel contains a fatty meal, castor oil or dioctyl sodium sulfosuccinate (Ch. 37) or if the mucosa is extensively ulcerated. Systemic intoxication produces progressive amblyopia, xanthopsia, deepening coma with convulsions, ventilatory depression and death; jaundice and albuminuria may develop terminally. The drug should not be given during pregnancy since it may induce abortion, nor should it be given to debilitated patients or those with cardiac, renal or severe intestinal ulceration	The usual adult dose is 4-6 g by duodenal tube with about 30 ml of mucilage acacia, 30 ml of sodium sulfate, and 30-50 ml of water. This is divided into 3 or 4 parts and injected every 10-15 min. If one administration of the drug has failed to evacuate the parasite, re-exposure should not be attempted for at least 2 wk
Bephenium hydroxynaphthoate	A quaternary ammonium compound, the drug of choice for treating infections with hookworms in man since it is less toxic than tetrachloroethylene. It is more active against *Ancylostoma duodenale* than against *Necator americanus*. Several related drugs are used as anthelmintics in veterinary practice. A single oral dose is often effective, but since the drug is relatively nontoxic, little is lost by continuing therapy for 3-7 days	Bephenium has a bitter taste and may produce nausea, vomiting, diarrhea and abdominal pain	Bephenium (Alcopar) is given orally in 5 g doses for 3-7 days. Special attention to diet is not required and no sequential catharsis is necessary. It can be used safely if concomitant ascariasis is present since it does not stimulate *A. lumbricoides*
Bithionol	A phenolic compound developed in Japan. The drug of choice for paragonimiasis and occasionally in fascioliasis		The usual oral dose is 50 mg/kg every 2nd day for 10 doses
Carbon tetrachloride	A halogenated hydrocarbon obsolete in the treatment of helminthiasis but still frequently used in the dry cleaning industry (as a cleaner) and as a solvent in rubber and paint industries. Thus accidental and occupational exposure are important toxicologically (Ch. 13)	Highly hepatotoxic, and fatalities have resulted from occupational exposure	None
Chloroquine	Chloroquine has been used in clonorchiasis, but most cases do not require therapy. It may depress ova output, but it does not kill the worms. See Ch. 63	See Ch. 63	See Ch. 63
Dichlorophen	A new taeniacide whose mode of action is unknown. It detaches the scolex from the bowel wall so that the worm dies and is rapidly digested. Thus fecal examination is valueles in determining success of treatment	Gastrointestinal irritation, urticarial skin rashes, lassitude and depression may develop. Since the worm is digested intraluminally, cysticercosis may result from autoinfection by ova liberated from *T. solium*	Dichlorophen (Anthiphen) is available only in Europe. The usual dose is 6 g, orally, repeated twice. No bowel preparation required, but a saline cathartic should be given 2-4 hr after the drug to minimize the danger of cycticercosis

Drug	Activity	Adverse reactions	Dosage
Diethylcarbamazine	A piperazine ring-containing phenothiazine effective against several species of filarial parasite. It is inactive in vitro but highly active in vivo, probably sensitizing the microfilaria so that they become phagocytosed by fixed tissue macrophages. No phagocytosis occurs in the blood stream. The drug kills adult *Brugia malayi* and *Loa loa*, and most adult *Wuchereria bancrofti*; it has minimal activity against adult *Onchocerca volvulus* Rapidly absorbed following oral administration with diffusion throughout most tissues and tissue compartments. It is excreted as the free drug and as a mixture of four metabolites, all of which contain a piperazine ring but are therapeutically inactive	Adverse reactions usually minimal and rarely necessitate discontinuance of therapy. Commonly seen are headaches, arthralgia, lymphadenopathy, gastrointestinal upsets, a general feeling of weakness, dermatitis, and fever. Transient leukocytosis and eosinophilia may appear. In initial therapy for onchocerciasis or filariasis, severe allergic or febrile reactions may occur due to release of helminthic protein on worm disintegration; corticosteroids or antihistamines may be useful in controlling these reactions	Diethylcarbamazine citrate, *U.S.P.* (Banocide, Hetrazan), is highly stable under extremes of heat and humidity. The usual dose is 2 mg/kg 3 times daily for 1-3 wk, depending on the type of infection. *W. bancrofti and B. malayi* are usually cured by one course of therapy. Loaiasis may require several spaced courses for complete cure; in onchocerciasis repeated courses, usually combined with suramin (Ch. 63), are required to keep the disease in check. Diethylcarbamazine is also of value in ascariasis, larva migrans and tropical pulmonary eosinophilia
Emetine	See Ch. 63	See Ch. 63	Rarely used in facioliasis. See Ch. 63
Gentian violet	See Ch. 62	See Ch. 62	Rarely used in clonorchiasis, strongyloidiasis and enterobiasis resistant to more potent drugs
Hexylresorcinol	Introduced originally as a urinary antiseptic, but subsequently found to paralyze various worms, in particular *Ascaris lumbricoides, Ancylostoma duodenale, Taenia saginata, Hymenolepsis nana, Trichuris trichiura,* and *Fasciolopsis buski.* Many of the newer drugs are more effective anthelmintics, but hexylresorcinol has the advantage of a wide spectrum of activity and low toxicity. Thus it may rarely be used in cases of mixed infection where the use of a more potent drug acting against a single parasite might be dangerous. About 30% of an oral dose is absorbed	Glossal and buccal ulceration may develop if the tablets are chewed and not swallowed whole or are held in the mouth. Gastrointestinal irritation is common, and the drug should not be used in patients with ulcerative or obstructive conditions of the intestine. Coating of the buttocks with petroleum jelly prior to the use of hexylresorcinol enemas may prevent perianal irritation and ulceration	Hexylresorcinol, *N.F.* (Caprokol) is available as 100 and 200 mg gelatin-coated tablets. The usual dose for adults, 1 g, should be followed 2-4 hours later by a saline cathartic. It should be given after an overnight fast since fatty food depresses intraluminal activity. Hexylresorcinol can be administered as an enema (1:100) in water. Used occasionally to treat *Trichuris trichiura, Fasciolopsis buski,* and *H. nana,* and rarely in patients with enterobiasis, and piperazine- and pyrantel-resistant ascariasis
Hycanthone	The hydroxymethabolite of Lucanthone possessing marked schistosomicidal activity. It may replace lucanthone	Gastrointestinal upsets, headache, myalgia, dizziness and altered liver function	Hycanthone (Etrenol) used in treating *S. mansoni* and *S. haematobium* infections
Lucanthone	Effective against adult *Schistosoma haematobium* and *S. mansoni,* but only weakly, if at all, effective against *S. japonicum.* It prevents helmintic ova production or release and subsequently destroys the parasite. Fully absorbed following oral administration passing into most tissue spaces. Only about 10-15% is excreted unchanged into the urine	Children tolerate lucanthone better than adults, and tolerance is poor among Egyptians and Latin Americans. Gastrointestinal irritation develops in 15-20% of patients. The drug has a bitter taste. Vertigo, tinnitus, convulsions, acute psychoses and circulatory failure are rare. Antihistaminics or atropine may protect against the development of some of these adverse effects. The skin and sclerae may turn yellow or orange (drug pigment) during therapy; this usually requires 4-6 wk to regress. The drug should be used with caution if severe renal or hepatic disease is present	Lucanthone Hydrochloride *U.S.P.* (Miracil D), is given in doses of 5 mg/kg 2 or 3 times a day for 5-10 days. It is of use only in schistosomiasis
Mebendazole	A new broad spectrum anthelmintic showing activity in ascariasis, ankylostomiasis, trichuriasis, enterobiasis, filariasis, taeniasis and strongyloidiasis		Mebendazole (Vermox) is usually given in doses of 100 mg twice a day for 1-5 days

(continued)

TABLE 64–2. *(continued)*

Drug	Properties	Adverse effects	Preparations, dosage and usage
Niclosamide	Taeniacidal in man and effective against *Echinococcus granulosus* in dogs. Poorly absorbed following oral administration. Mode of action not known, but it detaches the scolex from the mucosa permitting worm digestion	Gastrointestinal irritation. May initiate cysticerosis (see above dichlorophen)	Niclosamide (Cestocide, Yomesan) is available only in Europe; it is used in the U.S. on an investigational basis, but its use is prohibited for treating *T. solium* infections. The usual dose is 2 g (four tablets) in the morning after an overnight fast. In the U.S. niclosamide is under investigation for treatment of beef and fish tapeworm infection, and infection with *H. nana*
Niridazole	A relatively new drug related to the Nitrofurans and metronidazole which has mainly been used in Africa. In schistosomes it prevents maturation of the egg and shell in females, and produces degeneration of the testes in males. Niridazole is well absorbed following oral administration but largely metabolized by the liver on its first passage. The parent drug and its metabolites are avidly protein bound; excretion is by kidney and liver	Gastrointestinal upsets (nausea, anorexia, vomiting, abdominal pains, diarrhea), various skin rashes and paresthesias are common. Flattening and inversion of T waves may appear on electrocardiographic examination without any other evidence of myocardial toxicity. Rarely, central effects of insomnia, aggitation, visual and auditory hallucinations, confusion and epileptiform convulsions may develop. Hemolytic anemia occurs in subjects with glucose 6-phosphate dehydrogenase deficiency. Patients may complain of an objectional body odor and the urine may be colored dark	Niridazole (Ambilhar) is not available in the U.S. The usual dose is 25 mg/kg/day for 5-10 days. It is schistosomicidal in *S. haematobium* and *S. mansoni* infections, but a poor response other than a decreased cell count is seen in *S. japonicum* parasitization. Niridazole is of some value in guinea worm infection, cutaneous leishmaniasis, and possibly intestinal and extraintestinal amebiasis and onchoceriasis
Piperazine	Highly effective against *Ascaris lumbricoides* and *Enterobius vermicularis*. In *A. lumbricoides*, it blocks the effect of acetylcholine at the myoneural junction causing relaxation of the worm's hold on the mucosa with subsequent expulsion by normal peristaltic activity or cathartics. Its mode of action in enterobiasis is not known. Readily absorbed following oral administration, but still highly effective against *A. lumbricoides* in the small bowel and *E. vermicularis* in the colon. The majority is excreted unchanged	Gastrointestinal irritation and headaches are common. Urticaria, skin rashes, amblyopia and transient muscle weakness may develop, but are rare. Cerebellar ataxia ("worm wobble") is a rare but serious adverse effect and is more likely to develop if other phenothiazine compounds are administered concomitantly	Piperazine citrate, *U.S.P.* (Antepar), and piperazine adipate (Entacyl) are popular amongst the many available preparations. In enterobiasis the usual dose is 65 mg/kg. Two short courses of therapy lasting 7 days, with a week's rest in between, are probably sufficient. Simultaneous treatment of the entire family is desirable. In ascariasis, 3-5 mg daily for 1-3 days for adults usually results in complete cure. The usual dose for children is 50-75 mg/kg daily for 1-3 days
Pyrvinium	A poorly absorbed red cyanine dye which selectively depresses essential anaerobic metabolic reactions in *Trichuris trichiura*, *Strongyloides stercoralis*, *Ascaris lumbricoides*, and *Enterobius vermicularis*. The pamoate is more effective and less irritating than the chloride. One dose cures 80-95% of cases of enterobiasis for a 2-3 wk period	Gastrointestinal irritation and photodermatitis may occur. Feces are colored red. Underclothes may also become heavily stained	Pyrvinium Pamoate, *U.S.P.* (Povan), is available as a 50 mg tablet and as a suspension of 10 mg/ml. For enterobiasis the drug is given orally in doses of 5 mg/kg (maximum 300 mg) every 2 wk. Attempts to prevent reinfection with pinworms by simultaneous treatment of the whole family is often undertaken, but is rarely successful. It is also used occasionally in strongylyoidiasis
Pyrantel	A new drug for the treatment of enterobiasis and ascariasis probably acting by producing neuromuscular blockade in the worms permitting their expulsion. It is poorly absorbed following oral administration	Gastrointestinal upsets, headache, lassitude, elevation of liver function tests and a variety of skin rashes may develop	Pyrantel pamoate (Antiminth) is given in a single dose of 11 mg/kg with a maximum dose of 1.0 g. Many physicians consider it to be the drug of choice for enterobiasis and ascariasis

Drug	Pharmacology / Properties	Toxicity	Administration and Uses
Quinacrine	only about 10% of any given dose being excreted in the urine as free drug or metabolites Rarely used for cestode infections. The worm is stained yellow and identification of the scolex is relatively easy. Properties are covered in Ch. 63	See Ch. 63	A semisolid diet is eaten for a couple of days and a saline cathartic or enema given the night before. Quinacrine is administered in 4 doses of 200 mg, 10-15 min apart. It may be necessary to give 400-600 mg of sodium bicarbonate with each dose to prevent nausea and vomiting. Increased efficacy is seen if the drug is administered intraduodenally in solution. A saline cathartic or enema should be given 1-2 hr later.
Sulfonamides	See Ch. 60	See Ch. 60	The sulfonamides, Ch. 60, are occasionally combined with emetine in the treatment of fascioliasis and paragonimiasis
Suramin	See Ch. 63	See Ch. 63	Suramin, Ch. 63, can be combined with diethylcarbamazine in the treatment of onchocerciasis. The recommended dose is 1.0 g/wk for 5-10 wk after a 200 mg test dose
Tetrachloroethylene	An unsaturated chlorinated hydrocarbon chemically related to carbon tetrachloride and chloroform but of no value as an anesthetic because of its low vaporization and high boiling point. It is more effective against *Necator americanus* than against *Ancylostoma duodenale*, and it probably paralyzes the worms so that they lose their attachment to the mucosa and are evacuated by normal peristaltic activity. Intestinal absorption is minimal in the absence of fat or alcohol	Gastrointestinal irritation (burning pain, nausea, vomiting and diarrhea) is common. Rarely excessive absorption occurs producing chloroform-like central nervous system effects (giddiness, drowsiness, vertigo, progressive coma)	Tetrachloroethylene, *U.S.P.* is available in gelatin capsules which are heat and light labile. The usual dose is 0.12 ml/kg (maximum 5 ml) orally. The capsules should be emulsified and given orally or by duodenal tube since if swallowed whole, they may dissolve caudal to the worm; subsequent catharsis is probably not necessary. The patient should be on an alcohol and fat free diet for at least 36 hr before and after therapy. In cases of mixed infection with both *Ascaris lumbricoides* and hookworms, it is advisable to reduce the ascaris infection first with piperazine or pyrantel, or some other drug prior to the administration of tetrachloroethylene, since the latter may excite *A. lumbricoides* and stimulate migration or induce intestinal obstruction. Some authorities prefer to use bephenium instead, since this drug is active in both ascariasis and ancylostomiasis
Thiabendazole	A potent anthelmintic in vitro, possessing marked activity against *Strongyloides stercoralis* and *Trichinella spiralis;* in animal muscle in vivo, it kills *Trichinella spiralis* larvae. Thiabendazole is rapidly absorbed following oral administration with peak serum levels developing within 1 hr. About 90% of the drug is excreted in the urine in the free form or as glucuronide and sulfate conjugates	Adverse effects are frequent and often severe. Gastrointestinal upsets (nausea, anorexia, vomiting, crampy abdominal pain, diarrhea), lassitude, headache, dizziness, tinnitus, paresthesias and sleepiness may develop. A variety of hypersensitivity phenomena may appear due to allergy to either the drug or to parasitic protein: skin lesions (urticaria, maculopapular rashes), fever and lymphadenopathy. Rarely hypotension, altered liver function tests, hyperglycemia and xanthopsia may develop	Thiabendazole *U.S.P.* (Mintezol) is available as a suspension of 100 mg/ml. The usual dose is 25 mg/kg/day with 3.0 g maximum daily dose. It is of value in the treatment of multiple parasitic infections, particularly strongyloidiasis, enterobiasis, ancylostomiasis, cutaneous larva migrans, trichinosis and trichuriasis. It also may be of some benefit in visceral larva migrans

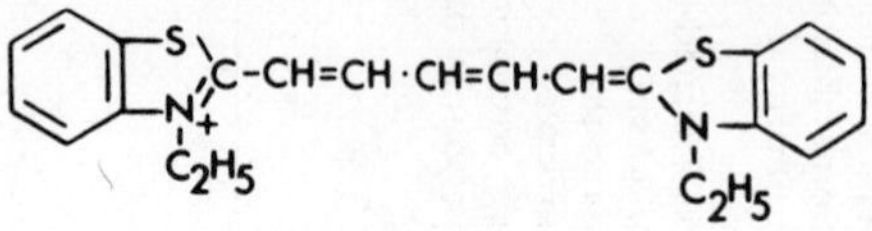

DITHIAZANINE IODIDE

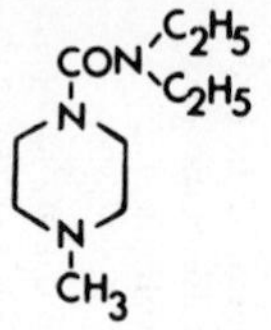

DIETHYLCARBAMAZINE

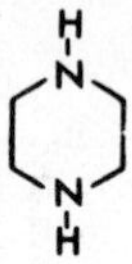

PIPERAZINE

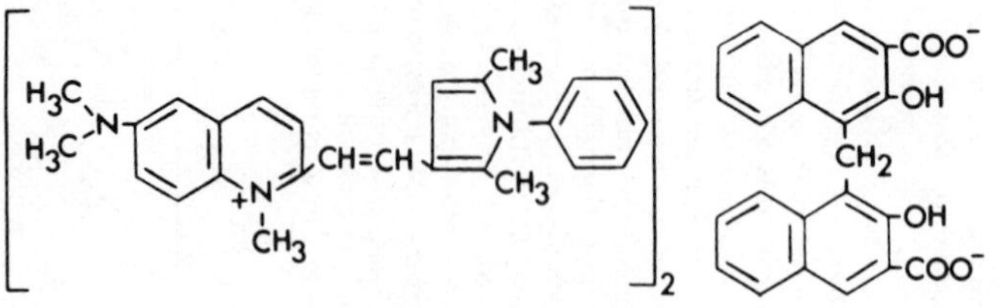

PYRVINIUM PAMOATE

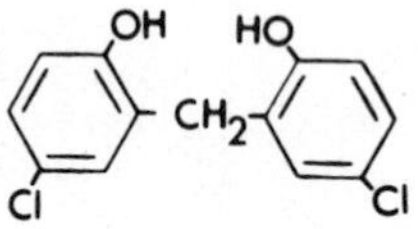

DICHLOROPHEN

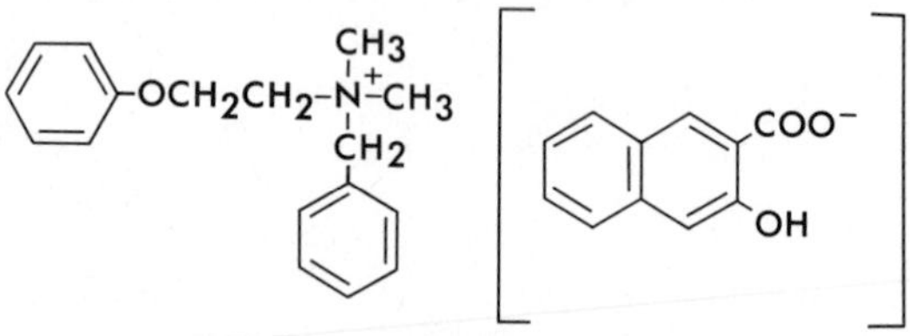

BEPHENIUM HYDROXYNAPHTHOATE

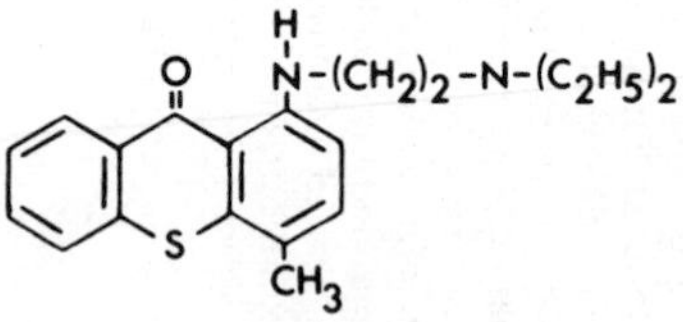

LUCANTHONE

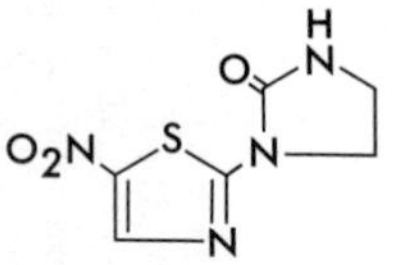

NIRIDAZOLE

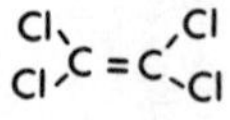

TETRACHLOROETHYLENE

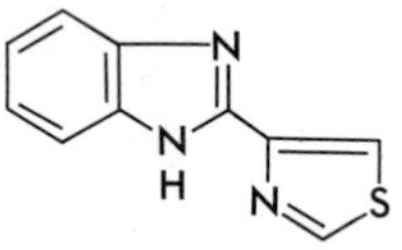

THIABENDAZOLE

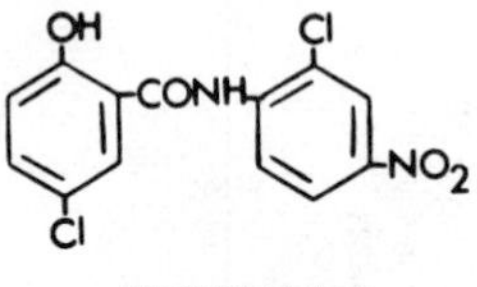

NICLOSAMIDE

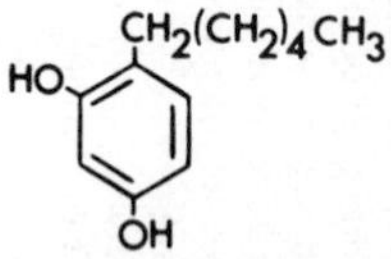

HEXYLRESORCINOL

FURTHER READING

Desowitz RS (1971): Antiparasite chemotherapy. Annu Rev Pharmacol 11:351–368

Goble, FC (ed) (1969): The pharmacological and chemotherapeutic properties of niridazole and other antischistosomal compounds. Ann NY Acad Sci 160:423–946

Most H (1972): Treatment of common parasitic infections of man encountered in the United States. N Engl J Med 287:495–498; 698–702

Turner JA (1973): Enterobiasis. Hagerstown, Harper and Row, Pract Med Vol 4, Ch 51

JEREMY H. THOMPSON

65. DRUGS USED IN THE TREATMENT OF MYCOTIC DISEASES

The fungi that may infect man can be divided into two groups depending upon whether they produce **superficial** or **deep infections. Superficial infections** are confined to the epidermis, the hair and the nails, whereas **deep infections** involve the dermis, bones, viscera, etc. Fungi that produce lesions in the skin or its appendages do so by their ability to penetrate the horny layer and proliferate within it. In hair and nails, where keratin is more compact, infection tends to occur at the zone where new keratin is being formed in the hair follicle and in the nail bed, respectively. But some involvement may only occur at the distal portion of the nail.

Superficial fungal disease is caused by a variety of fungi. Ringworm (e.g., tinea capitis, tinea corporis, tinea cruris, tinea unguium) is caused by various strains of *Microsporum, Trichophyton,* and *Epidermophyton;* tinea versicolor, by *Malassezia furfur;* candidiasis, by *Candida albicans;* and tinea nigra, by *Cladosporium werneckii* and *C. mansoni.*

The most frequent organisms causing deep fungal diseases are listed in Table 65–3.

Both superficial and deep mycotic infections are commonly precipitated by an easily recognizable cause. Predisposing local factors for superficial disease are skin maceration, chafing and occlusive shoes. Predisposing factors for deep fungal disease are malignancy, uremia, tuberculosis, sarcoidosis, diabetes mellitus, hypoparathyroidism, therapy with broad spectrum antibiotics, glucocorticosteroids or antineoplastic drugs, malnutrition, burns, debilitation, or radiation exposure (Ch. 52). The control or elimination of predisposing factors is often of more importance than the antifungal therapy itself (Fig. 65–1).

CHEMOTHERAPY OF SUPERFICIAL MYCOSES

There are many preparations available for topical use in the treatment of superficial fungal disease (Table 65–1). Most of these have become obsolete with the introduction of **griseofulvin,** but some, along with several recently introduced preparations retain limited therapeutic usefulness.

Based on in vitro testing, antifungal drugs can be either *fungistatic* or *fungicidal* (Ch. 52). There usually is poor correlation between in vitro activity and in vivo effectiveness since the drug may not be able to reach the site of fungal infection deep in the nails, hyperkeratotic epidermis or hair follicles. Cure is thus difficult because of a high rate of relapse, and to a lesser extent, to reinfection.

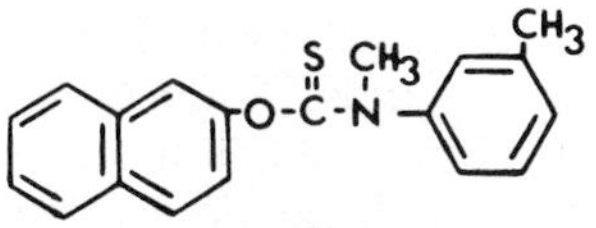

Keratolytic agents, e.g., salicylic acid, are often used concomitantly to increase drug penetration and hasten the shedding of heavily infected stratum corneum. Similarly, drugs that reduce hyperhidrosis may be valuable adjunct agents. Superficial mycoses, particularly if they are untreated or overtreated, often give rise to second-

SALICYLANILIDE

TOLNAFTATE

ary skin eruptions or mycides (dermatophytides). Furthermore, bacterial superinfection is common and demands prompt treatment. Superinfection

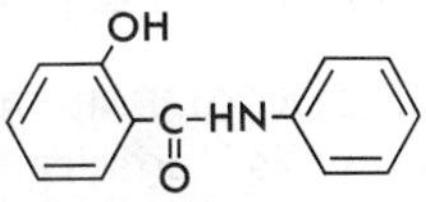

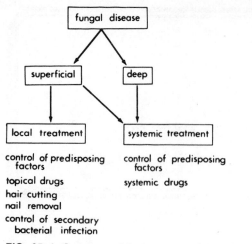

FIG. 65–1. Summary of the treatment of superficial and deep fungal disease.

superficial → local treatment

control of predisposing factors

topical drugs

hair cutting

nail removal

control of secondary bacterial infection

systemic treatment

control of predisposing factors

systemic drugs

can often be controlled by soaks or compresses of Burow's solution or warm potassium permanganate solution (1 : 10,000), or by adequate removal (debridement) of heavily infected stratum corneum. Some authorities have recommended a short course of antibiotic therapy, but the wisdom of this is doubtful, since antibiotics may initiate further superinfection, and may cross react with fungal products, producing "id" reactions. Preliminary corticosteroid therapy has been suggested for progressive eczematous lesions and to control dermatophytides and allergic phenomena. Systemic corticosteroids (plus antifungal therapy) may be of special value in human cases of animal ringworm, since by virtue of their antiinflammatory activity steroids minimize the degree of final scarring.

SYSTEMIC DRUGS FOR TINEA INFECTIONS

Griseofulvin

Griseofulvin is obtained from *Penicillium griseofulvum dierckx* and *P. janczewski*. It is the only available systemic agent for treating superficial mycoses due to most strains of *Microsporum, Trichophyton,* and *Epidermophyton*. It is ineffective against the deep mycoses. Griseofulvin is fungicidal for growing cells and fungistatic for resting cells.

GRISEOFULVIN

MODE OF ACTION. Griseofulvin may act by depressing nucleic acid synthesis. It rapidly binds to keratin precursor cells and makes them resistant to fungal infection. Thus new skin, hair and nails are the first to become free of fungal elements, and therapy must be continued until the infected keratin has been replaced by keratin containing griseofulvin. This usually takes 3–10 weeks for skin and hair mycoses and up to 18 months for nail disease. Infection of the soles of the feet is rarely cured by griseofulvin alone. Mycotic resistance to griseofulvin is rare.

ABSORPTION, METABOLISM, AND EXCRETION. Griseofulvin is erratically absorbed, mainly because of its poor solubility. Small-sized particles ($<3.0~\mu$ in diameter; microcrystalline form) are absorbed 2–3 times as rapidly as large particles ($<10.0~\mu$). Fatty meals increase absorption. Griseofulvin is metabolized in the liver to the inactive metabolite, 6-demethylgriseofulvin and excreted in the urine. Loss also occurs in the feces. Barbiturates and primidone may accelerate the hepatic microsomal catabolism of griseofulvin through enzyme induction and phenobarbital reduces the gastrointestinal absorption of griseofulvin.

ADVERSE EFFECTS. Gastrointestinal upsets, fever, thirst (xerostomia), frequency of micturition, chest pain, dyspnea, a variety of skin lesions (including lupus erythematosus-like eruptions, urticaria, lichen planus, erythema multiforme and photodermatitis), headache and serum sickness are among the most common adverse reactions, and may develop in up to 5% of patients. The headaches tend to be severe during early therapy, but usually diminish in frequency and severity with continued exposure. Griseofulvin has a structural similarity to colchicine, and although it depresses spermatogenesis in mice, it has not been shown to do so in man. Cross sensitivity has not been described in patients sensitive to penicillin. Griseofulvin may precipitate symptoms of porphyria in patients with this disease or with advanced liver disease, and recently it has been incriminated in producing forgetfulness, apathy, amblyopia, vertigo and disorientation—symptoms that may be potentiated by concomitant alcohol ingestion. Temporary leukopenia, granulocytopenia, punctate basophilia and monocytosis are rare. Because of the occurrence of white cell depression, periodic blood counts during long term therapy are advisable. Griseofulvin may also produce peripheral neuritis, albuminuria, stomatitis and dysgeusia. Some children have developed gynecomastia and hyperpigmentation of the nipples, areolas and external genitalia. Superin-

TABLE 65–1. Some Topical Drugs for Tinea Infections

Drug	Properties	Adverse effects	Preparations
Heavy metals	Penetrate fungal cytoplasm and oxidize enzyme sulfhydryl groups (Ch. 62)		Ionic copper, thiomerosal, bismuth
Iodine	Used in tinea corporis. Do not use on toes or groin since severe blistering may develop	Iodine should never be mixed with a mercuric salt, as the highly irritating red iodide of mercury is formed	Alcoholic iodine, 2%
Detergents (surface active agents)	Polar compounds possessing hydrophobic and hydrophilic groups which disturb osmotic functions of cell membrane (Ch. 53)		Benzalkonium chloride and cetyltrimethylammonium bromide (Ch. 62)
Selenium	Used in the control of dandruff and nonspecific dermatoses	Poisonous if ingested	Selenium sulfide *U.S.P.*
Castellani's paint	Mixture of 0.3% basic fuchsin, 1.0% boric acid, 10% resorcinol, and 4.5% phenol. Of some use in tinea pedis, cruris and axillaris, and in nonspecific dermatoses	Stains clothes deeply	Carbol-fuchsin Solution *N.F.*
Fatty acids	Fungistatic activity increases with an increase in the number of carbon atoms up to 11. Straight chains are more active than branched chains. The antifungal activity of sebum due to propionic and caprylic acids. Used in tinea pedis and corporis (Undecylenic and caprylic acids) or in bakery products (propionates)	Possesses unpleasant, rancid, sweat-like odor. Rarely produce sensitization	Undecylenic acid *N.F.*, zinc undecylenate *N.F.*, caprylic acid, caprylic compounds (10% sodium caprylate plus 5% zinc caprylate). Sodium and calcium propionates
Whitfield's ointment	Fungistatic (benzoic acid 6%) and keratolytic (salicylic acid 3%) agent used in tinea versicolor and ringworm		
Salicylanilide	Salicylic acid derivative of aniline. Weak fungistatic agent often combined with undecylenic acid	Photosensitivity reactions	Salicylanilide *N.F.*, 5% ointment. Present in many soaps
Glyceryl triacetate	Releases acetic acid locally under influence of host and mycotic esterases. Weakly active against ringworm fungi but not *C. albicans*		Triacetin ointment, 25%. Triacetin powder, 33%
Tolnaftate	Effective against most dermatophytoses and erythrasma. No effect on tinea of the hair or nails, or on *C. albicans*. Should be combined with keratolytics in treatment of tinea of palms and soles		Tolnaftate *U.S.P.*, 1% solution
Haloprogin	Used in tinea infections		Haloprogin, 1% cream or solution
Acrisorcin	Used in tinea versicolor. Antifungal activity reduced by soaps. Should be applied twice daily for at least 1 mo after the infection has cleared	Sensitivity reactions	Acrisorcin, 2% cream
Thymol	Used in many dermatophytoses. Often added to Whitfield's ointment		Thymol, *U.S.P.*, 1% alcoholic solution, or 2% powder
Miconazole nitrate	Used in tinea infections		Miconazole nitrate, 2% cream

fection with *Canadian albicans* has been reported occasionally.

PREPARATIONS AND DOSAGE. Griseofulvin, *U.S.P.*, is the official form; there are many proprietary preparations. Because of irregular gastrointestinal absorption, the total daily dose should be divided into three or four portions and administered after meals. Duration of therapy varies depending on the location of the fungus. The usual daily doses for adults and children are 0.5–1.0 g and 10 mg/kg, respectively.

USES. Griseofulvin is highly effective in the treatment of fungal infections of the skin, hair and nails caused by *Microsporum, Tricophyton* and *Epidermophyton* species. Pruritus and burning are usually relieved within 1–3 days, which coincides with the time griseofulvin appears within the basal layers of the stratum corneum.

Treatment should be continued for about 3–4 weeks if the nails, palms and soles are not involved. Infection of the highly keratotic palms and soles, and of the nails, requires therapy for 4–12 weeks and 4–12 months, respectively. Griseofulvin should not be used if the tinea will respond to topical agents (Table 65–1), since there is little justification for the use of a potentially toxic drug when less dangerous chemicals will suffice. A definite mycologic diagnosis should always be required prior to commencing therapy, as treatment is often prolonged and costly.

Griseofulvin in doses of 0.5g–1.0 g may be of symptomatic benefit in Raynaud's disease.

BASIC PRINCIPLES OF TREATMENT OF TINEA

Griseofulvin is the drug of choice for uncomplicated tinea capitis, for favus and for kerions. Some authorities recommend an initial trial of topical drug therapy in tinea barbae, corporis, cruris and manuum, with the addition of griseofulvin if local therapy fails, but for severe tinea the concomitant use of both topical and systemic drugs is justified. Other adjunctive procedures are hair clipping or shaving plus warm compresses and debridement in tinea barbae, and application of mild keratolytic agents in tinea corporis. Tinea pedis is a chronic therapeutic problem, the infection persisting because of the thick stratum corneum present. Apart from griseofulvin and tolnaftate, haloprogin, miconazole and Whitfield's ointment are of most value; undecylenic acid and zinc undecylenate are not as effective. Strict attention to foot hygiene, avoidance of reinfection from communal shower rooms, etc., and avoidance of wool and synthetic fiber socks is of greater importance. Dusting powders can also be valuable. Tinea unguium is difficult to cure. Griseofulvin is the drug of choice, combined in selected cases with nail avulsion. Tinea versicolor tends to recur, but Whitfield's ointment and acrisorcin are of some value. Tinea nigra may respond to Whitfield's ointment.

TOPICAL DRUGS FOR SUPERFICIAL CANDIDIASIS

Candida albicans can cause superficial infection, deep infection, or both. Several drugs are available for topical therapy, some of which may also be given systemically. Nystatin is the most important, other agents are indicated in Table 65–2.

Nystatin

Nystatin, so named because it was located in the New York State Department of Health (1951), is a polyene antibiotic obtained from *Streptomyces noursei*. Polyenes are complex molecules with a large conjugated double bond system (–CH=CH–) in a lactone ring linked to an amino sugar. Nystatin is a conjugated tetraene linked to the amino sugar mycosamine. Nystatin exhibits both fungistatic and fungicidal activity, depending on the drug concentration; the presence of blood, pus or tissue fluid that reduce activity; and the susceptibility of the fungus. It is measured in milligrams or units (1 mg = 3500 units).

Nystatin may act by altering fungal cell membrane permeability, probably by complexing with membrane sterols (Ch. 53). Its lack of antibacterial activity may be related to the relative absence of sterols in bacterial cell membranes. Fungal resistance develops rarely. Cross resistance occurs with amphotericin B (see below).

Nystatin is usually applied topically or given orally for its local effect in the bowel lumen. Parenteral administration is undertaken rarely.

ADVERSE EFFECTS. Even in large doses, nystatin is relatively innocuous when applied topically, but cutaneous irritation may develop following repeated exposure. Contact sensitivity is very rare. Minor gastrointestinal symptoms follow oral administration. Superinfection is never a problem. Administration of nystatin IM is painful and rarely may produce hemolytic anemia through complexing with red blood cell sterols.

PREPARATION AND DOSAGE. Nystatin, *U.S.P.* (Mycostatin), is present in a variety of topical preparations, often combined with gentian violet, procaine hydrochloride, antibiotics or hydrocortisone. The oral dose is 0.5–1 million units 3 times daily. Topical powders, ointments, creams and suppositories are applied three times daily.

USES. The main use of nystatin is in the treatment of candidiasis of the skin, mouth, intestine and vagina. Nystatin can be given parenterally for the rare systemic cases of candidiasis. Several preparations of broad-spectrum antibiotics (tetracyclines, neomycin, etc.) are available with nystatin (Ch. 57) for the purpose of reducing Candida superinfections which occasionally develop. The effectiveness of these combinations has not been proved.

TABLE 65–2. Some Drugs Used for the Treatment of Candidiasis

Drug	Properties	Adverse effects	Preparations
Nystatin	See text		Ointment or cream 3-5%
Chloroquinaldol (Sterosan)	Has mild gram-positive antibacterial, anticandida and keratoplastic activity		
Hexetidine (Sterisil)	Used in treatment of vulvovaginal candidiasis and trichomoniasis (Ch. 63). Detergents reduce its antifungal activity	Vulval or vaginal irritation	Hexetidine gel, 0.1% for vaginal use only. The usual dose is 7 ml of the gel inserted high in the vaginal vault daily for 1 wk
Gentian Violet, *U.S.P.*	Effective in some cases of oral, vaginal or cutaneous candidiasis	Stains deeply. Rarely sensitizing	Available as a 2% solution, and for vaginal infections as a 1% solution in glycerine
Chlordantoin	A derivative of an agricultural fungicide. Used in cutaneous, paronychial and vaginal candidiasis	Cutaneous irritation	Combined with benzalkonium chloride (Sporostacin)
Candicidin (Candeptin)	A heptaene fungistatic and fungicidal antibiotic obtained from *Streptomyces greseus* with an antifungal spectrum similar to that of amphotericin B and nystatin. It is 15-30 times more active, however, than either of these agents against *C. albicans* in vitro. Probably acts by complexing with cell membrane sterols (Ch. 53). Not absorbed after topical, vaginal or oral administration	Cutaneous sensitivity rare. Vulvovaginitis following local therapy. Cross sensitivity not reported	Available as an ointment (0.06%) and as tablets (0.30 mg)
Miconizole nitrate (Monistat)	Used in vulvovaginal candidiasis	Vulvovaginal irritation	Cream, 2%
Amphotericin B	See text		
Clotrimazole	See text		
Natamycin	See text		
Iodochlorhydroxyquin	Weak, anticandida activity. See Ch. 63		

CHEMOTHERAPY OF DEEP MYCOSES

Chemotherapy of deep fungus disease is unsatisfactory since there are only a limited number of drugs available whose use is associated with severe toxicity, and since the patients concerned are usually seriously ill with a variety of disease states (see above). The drugs of choice for most of the deep fungal diseases are indicated in Table 65–3. Apart from potassium iodide and amphotericin B, these are discussed in detail elsewhere. The control of predisposing factors (see above), and continuance of drug therapy long enough to reduce the likelihood of relapse, are of prime importance in the treatment of deep mycotic disease (Fig. 65–1).

Sulfonamides

Sulfonamides are the drugs of choice for nocardiosis. They may have to be given IV, since plasma levels of 10 mg/100 ml or greater, are desirable. Erythromycin, ampicillin, streptomycin, tetracyclines or capreomycin may be given in place of sulfonamides if these agents cannot be used.

Penicillin

The penicillin of choice for actinomycosis is benzyl penicillin G. It should be given IV in doses of 10–20 mega units per day. In patients hypersensitive to penicillin, erythromycin, a cephalosporin, clindamycin, streptomycin or a tetracycline may be used instead.

Hydroxystilbamidine

Hydroxystilbamidine is a valuable drug for many deep fungal diseases. There is some evidence that it should be combined with amphotericin B in the treatment of North American blastomycosis. IV infusions of hydroxystilbamidine should not be more concentrated than 1 mg/10 ml.

Potassium Iodide

Potassium iodide, *U.S.P.* possesses a limited ability to resolve chronic granulomas, a property that has been of therapeutic usefulness in the treatment of syphilis and some deep fungal dis-

TABLE 65—3. Cause and Treatment of Deep Mycoses

Disease	Fungus	Drugs used in treatment
Actinomycosis	*Actinomyces israeli**	Penicillin, erythromycin, sulfonamides, cephaloridine, cephalothin, tetracyclines
Aspergillosis	*Aspergillus fumigatus, A. niger*	Amphotericin B, nystatin
Blastomycosis (North American)	*Blastomyces dermatitidis*	Amphotericin B, hydroxystilbamidine
Blastomycosis (South American)	*Blastomyces brasiliensis*	Amphotericin B, sulfonamides
Candidiasis (moniliasis)	*Candida albicans*	Nystatin (superficial); amphotericin B, flucytosine (deep)
Chromoblastomycosis	*Fonsecaea, Phialophora, Cladosporium*	Potassium iodide, amphotericin B
Coccidioidomycosis	*Coccidioides immitis*	Amphotericin B, hydroxystilbamidine
Cryptococcosis (torulosis)	*Cryptococcus neoformans*	Potassium iodide, amphotericin B, flucytosine
Geotrichosis	*Geotrichum candidum, etc.*	Potassium iodide, nystatin, amphotericin B
Histoplasmosis	*Histoplasma capsulatum*	Potassium iodide, amphotericin B, hydroxystilbamidine, sulfonamides
Maduromycosis	*Madurella mycetomi, Madurella grisea, Allescheria boydii*	Sulfonamides, tetracyclines, amphotericin B
Phycomycosis	*Mucor spp.*	Amphotericin B, hydroxystilbamidine
Nocardiosis	*Nocardia asteroides**	Sulfonamides, tetracyclines, erythromycin
Penicilliosis	*Penicillium spp.*	Amphotericin B
Rhinosporidiosis	*Rhinosporidium seeberi*	Amphotericin B
Sporotricosis	*Sporotrichum schenckii*	Potassium iodide, amphotericin B

* Not a true fungus

eases. It is available as a saturated solution of 1 g/ml. The starting dose is 1 g 3 times daily; this may be gradually increased to 12 g daily in severe cases. Some authorities recommend commencing with the full dosage. Therapy should be continued for 4–6 weeks after all lesions appear to have healed. It is of particular value in cutaneous and lymphatic sporotricosis, but should be used with caution in pulmonary or disseminated disease. Use of potassium iodide interferes with thyroid function tests (Ch. 76), and iodism may develop. Prominent symptoms of iodism are a metallic taste in the mouth, parotitis, acneiform skin rashes and coryza. If iodism develops, therapy should be discontinued for several days and resumed at a lower dosage.

Amphotericin B

Of the two amphotericins, A and B, isolated in 1958 from *Streptomyces nodosus,* only the conjugated heptaene amphotericin B is used in therapeutics. It is a heat-labile and light-sensitive fungistatic antibiotic with a wide spectrum of activity (Table 65–3) and some effect in American leishmaniasis (Ch. 63). The antifungal effects are maximal between pH 6.0–7.5. Resistance in vivo is rare. Cross resistance occurs with nystatin, but is uncommon. The drug may act by depressing phosphate uptake, and by complexing with cell membrane sterols (Ch. 53).

ABSORPTION, METABOLISM, AND EXCRETION. Amphotericin B is poorly absorbed after oral administration and is usually given IV, intrathecally or topically. After IV injection, the drug passes poorly into the cerebrospinal fluid, levels normally reaching only one-thirtieth to one-fiftieth simultaneous plasma levels. The drug is excreted by the kidney over 24–36 hr.

ADVERSE EFFECTS. Amphotericin B is a toxic drug, and with systemic therapy, adverse reactions develop in almost all patients. In general, the crystalline preparations are less toxic than the solubilized preparations. Adverse effects include fever, general malaise, chills, myalgia, arthralgia, gastrointestinal upsets with bleeding, headaches, vertigo, hypotension and sweating. Thrombophlebitis is common and may be reduced by adequate drug dilution and slow infusion. Ventricular fibrillation and cardiac arrest rarely may follow too rapid infusion. Hypersensitivity maculopapular skin rashes, anaphylactic shock, leukopenia, thrombocytopenia, hypochromic anemia, peripheral neuritis, amblyopia, diplopia, convulsions and acute hepatic failure are less common.

Over 80% of patients develop some impairment of renal function as indicated by proteinuria, microscopic or macroscopic hematuria, hypokalemia, hypomagnesemia and elevated blood urea nitrogen or creatinine levels. The renal lesions are usually reversible, but may progress to tubular acidosis and nephrocalcinosis. Renal damage is due to a direct toxic effect of the antibiotic on the renal tubules and to renal vasoconstriction. Intrathecal administration of amphotericin B may be followed by lumbar pain, amblyopia, diplopia, chemical meningitis, nerve palsies, urinary retention and severe headaches. Death has occurred. Concomitant therapy with cortisone, antipyretics, antihistamines and antiemetics may counteract some of these adverse reactions. Heparin may delay the onset of thrombophlebitis, but should be used sparingly.

PREPARATIONS AND DOSAGE. Amphotericin B, is available as a microcrystalline suspension and an aqueous colloid suspension. The microcrystalline preparation is available either as a 3% amphotericin preparation for topical application in candidiasis (see above) or as an oral preparation combined with neomycin or tetracycline. The colloidal preparation, amphotericin B. *U.S.P.* (Fungizone), contains about 0.8% sodium desoxycholate per milligram plus a phosphate buffer and sodium chloride. It is the only preparation available for IV or intrathecal therapy.

Colloidal amphotericin B for IV or intrathecal use should be freshly prepared and protected from light even during infusion. It may be stored for several hours in the cold after reconstitution. A trial dose should always be given. The drug should be reconstituted with 5% dextrose. Normal saline must not be used, as the drug may precipitate. The IV infusion should be run in slowly and should never be more concentrated than 0.1 mg/ml. The usual dose is 0.25–1.0 mg/kg, not to exceed 1.5 mg/kg. Renal toxicity is reduced by keeping the patient hydrated, prolonging the infusion time, giving the drug on alternate days and alkalinizing the urine.

For intrathecal use 0.5 mg amphotericin B should be diluted in distilled water or cerebrospinal fluid to a concentration of between 0.1–0.25 mg/ml and slowly injected with hydrocortisone 2 or 3 times a week for several months. It may be advisable to alternate between lumbar and cisternal injection sites. Duration of therapy depends on the severity of the infection and the occurrence of side effects, which may necessitate temporary cessation of treatment. For chromoblastomycosis, injection of amphotericin B *into* the lesion is often the treatment of choice.

USES. In spite of its toxicity, amphotericin B represents an important therapeutic advance, since it is the only currently available drug for treating the progressive systematic mycoses. Amphotericin B should be reserved for severe infections. Adjunctive surgical resection of localized chronic granulomas may be clinically desirable. The duration of amphotericin B treatment varies with the severity of the disease and with the occurrence of adverse effects such as severe renal damage that may necessitate interruption of therapy. All patients receiving amphotericin B must be hospitalized and their renal function and serum electrolytes carefully monitored. The minimal duration of treatment is 4–6 weeks, but severe deep fungal disease may require 4–6 months of therapy.

5-Fluorocytosine (Flucytosine)

Flucytosine is unlike other fluorinated compounds such as 5-fluorouracil, the riboside and deoxyriboside of fluorocytosine, in that it lacks significant cytotoxic properties in man.

5-FLUOROCYTOSINE

MODE OF ACTION. Flucytosine is readily taken up into fungal cells and is converted through various steps into an uridine triphosphate intermediary, that blocks thymidylate synthetase. Synergism may be observed when flucytosine is combined with amphotericin B since the polyene antibiotic by disrupting the fungal cell membrane (Ch. 53) permits greater uptake of the more potent agent.

ANTIFUNGAL SPECTRUM. Flucytosine is effective against a variety of fungi, in particular, *Candida albicans, Cryptococcus neoformans, Torulopsis glabrata,* and *Sporotrichum schenckii,* and some species of *Aspergilli* and *Chromoblastomyces.* It is inactive against *Blastomyces dermatitidis, Coccidiodes immitis,* and *Histoplasma capsulatum.* Resistance has been reported. Care should be observed when testing for sensitivity to flucytosine in vitro, since commonly used culture media contain beef and yeast extracts and peptones, which effectively compete with the antifungal agent for incorporation into the cultured fungus.

ABSORPTION, METABOLISM AND EXCRETION. Flucytosine is well absorbed following oral administration with peak levels developing within 4–6 hr. It is widely distributed within the body and cerebrospinal fluid levels are 60–100% of plasma levels. Flucytosine is metabolized to about 10% and excreted by the kidney. It has a half-life of 5–8 hr.

ADVERSE EFFECTS. Flucytosine produces gastrointestinal irritation with nausea, anorexia, crampy abdominal pains and vomiting; occasionally it will produce a malabsorption syndrome with steatorrhea. Reversible liver dysfunction, with elevation of serum glutamic oxaloacetic transaminase and alkaline phosphatase activity develops in about 10% of patients. Rarely flucytosine has been associated with progressive leukopenia, thrombocytopenia, confusional states, hallucinations, severe headache and vertigo. Hematologic damage is more likely in those patients concomitantly receiving cytotoxic drugs or x-irradiation, or who have some hematologic disease. Blood counts should be performed twice weekly during therapy.

In rodents, which metabolize flucytosine to 5-fluorouracil, the drug is teratogenic; the human organism does not metabolize flucytosine to 5-fluorouracil.

PREPARATIONS AND DOSAGE. Flucytosine (Ancobon) is available in capsules of 250 and 500 mg. It has been given in a variety of dosages between 5–200 mg/kg/day. It has been particularly valuable in the treatment of *Candida albicans* endocarditis, and cryptococcal meningitis and cryptococcal pulmonary disease. However, resistant organisms frequently emerge during treatment. Patients with septicemia due to *T. glabrata* and with various infections caused by *Aspergilli* have responded to therapy with flucytosine, but in general, experience with the drug has been meager. Synergistic activity may be seen in combination with amphotericin B. The main advantages of flucytosine are its rapid absorption following oral administration, its wide tissue distribution, and its relative lack of serious adverse effects. The effectiveness of the drug is limited by the development of resistance during therapy in cryptococcal disease, and by the high incidence (50%) of resistance in initial isolates of *Candida albicans.*

Clotrimazole

Clotrimazole is a recently introduced imidazole possessing fungistatic activity. It is presently available on an experimental basis in Europe. In vitro, clotrimazole inhibits *Histoplasma capsulatum, Cryptococcus neoformans, Coccidioides immitis, Aspergillus fumigatus, Blastomyces dermatitidis, Candida albicans, Microsporum* spp., *Epidermophyton floccosum* and *Trichophyton tonsurans.* In vitro effectiveness has not been fully evaluated, but clotrimazole has proved valuable in some cases of septicemia, pneumonia, renal disease and endocarditis due to candida, and in pulmonary aspergillosis. Clotrimazole is heat and light resistant, and is rapidly absorbed following oral administration. There have been few adverse effects reported to date with doses of 60 mg/kg/day.

Clotrimazole is available for oral and topical use. The 1% solution for topical application is nonsensitizing and has been used successfully in the treatment of various dermatophytes.

Hamycin

Hamycin is an experimental polyene antibiotic obtained from *Streptomyces pimprima* and related to amphotericin B. The drug is well absorbed following oral administration and possesses activity against a variety of fungi, particularly *Blastomyces dermatitidis, Histoplasma capsulatum, Aspergillus fumigatus, Cryptococcus neoformans,* and *Candida albicans.* Adverse reactions reported to date have been limited to the gastrointestinal tract.

Hamycin (Primamycin) is available on an experimental basis for oral and topical use. Relapses are common, particularly in the treatment of deep fungal infections. Hamycin may be applied topically in the treatment of vaginal candidiasis.

Natamycin

Natamycin is a tetraene antifungal antibiotic obtained from *Streptomyces natalensis.* It possesses a wide antifungal spectrum against common dermatophytes. It is also active against *Trichomonas vaginalis,* but it possesses no antibacterial activity. Natamycin is applied topically and vaginally; it is not absorbed following oral administration, but is occasionally given by this route in the treatment of intestinal candidiasis. Adverse reactions have not been described following topical or vaginal application, but minor symptoms of gastrointestinal irritation may follow oral administration.

Natamycin is available in a variety of preparations in a strength of 2% (pimafucin, pimaricin). It is effective in the treatment of chronic candidal paronychia and vulvovaginitis. It may also be used for tinea versicolor.

X-5079C

X-5079C (RO-2-7758: Saramycetin) is a sulfur (13%)-containing fungistatic polypeptide antibiotic, derived from a strain of streptomyces. It has been found effective in the treatment of some deep mycoses, particularly, *Blastomyces dermatitidis, Histoplasma capsulatum,* and *Sporotrichum schenckii.* It has no activity against *Cryptococcus neoformans.* The potential of this agent has not yet been fully explored due to its relative unavailability. Side effects reported with X-5079C have been various skin rashes, particularly urticaria and liver damage. It is usually given in doses of 3–5 mg/kg for 4–6 weeks. X-5079C is still investigational.

FURTHER READING

Hamilton-Miller JMT (1973): Chemistry and biology of the polyene macrolide antibiotics. Bacteriol Rev 37:166–196

JEREMY H. THOMPSON

66. DRUGS USED IN THE TREATMENT OF VIRAL DISEASES

Viruses can be divided into the "**large viruses**" (chlamydia) responsible for molluscum contagiosa, psittacosis/ornithosis, trachoma, inclusion conjunctivitis, lymphogranuloma venereum and the rickettsial infections, and the **true (small) viruses** (the poxviruses, herpesviruses, adenoviruses, piconaviruses, etc.). The "large viruses" possess both DNA and RNA and differ from the true viruses both in morphology and in mode of multiplication. They also show varying susceptibility to the penicillins, the tetracyclines, chloramphenicol and the sulfonamides. They are not considered in this chapter.

The true viruses contain a core of either DNA (smallpox, chickenpox, herpes simplex, herpes zoster) or RNA (poliomyelitis, mumps, measles, rabies), but not both, and can replicate only inside host cells through the use of host enzyme systems (see below). Thus, there are two major obstacles to effective antiviral therapy. First, since viral replication is intracellular, antiviral drugs must be highly selective and not seriously interfere with normal cellular functions of the host. Second, most viral diseases are of short duration, and the prodromal phase of rapid virus growth is usually asymptomatic. Two additional pertinent problems to the successful development of potent, selective antiviral agents are: the relative lack of intrinsic virus enzyme systems that may serve as specific targets for drugs; and,

the poor correlation between in vitro activity and in vivo response. For these reasons most of the major advances in the treatment of viral diseases have been in the area of **prevention,** e.g., by the control of the vectors. Some success has been achieved by **active immunization** with either attenuated or killed virus vaccines (Ch. 73) and by **passive immunization.** Passive immunization involves the use of antibodies. Antibodies can be prepared in animals (high titer hyperimmune gamma globulin) but are rarely used in the treatment of human viral diseases since they may induce allergic reactions. Human gamma globulin is prepared from pooled blood of healthy donors or from convalescent patients. Antibodies are most effective when used prophylactically in persons who have been exposed to such viral diseases as measles, rubella (particularly pregnant women), rabies, infectious hepatitis, mumps and occasionally varicella. Antivaccinia gamma globulin is of prophylactic value in patients with defective immune mechanisms who require smallpox vaccination, and in the treatment of eczema vaccinatum and vaccinia gangrenosa.

Neither active nor passive immunization is of value once the disease has appeared, and, with few exceptions, the treatment of viral disease consists of alleviating symptoms rather than attacking the causative organism.

BIOLOGY OF VIRUSES

A knowledge of the biology and reproduction of the true viruses facilitates understanding of the action of the antiviral drugs.

Viral Structure

Viruses contain a core or genome of nucleic acid (either RNA or DNA, but not both) surrounded by a coating of protein subunits or capsomers, the

viral antigens. The capsomeres protect the nucleic acid and may be responsible for the attachment (adsorption) of viruses onto host cells.

Viral Specificity

Like the more complicated bacteria, viruses demonstrate a wide range of host and tissue specificity. Thus, mumps virus is pathogenic for man only, and polio-virus has a marked affinity for anterior horn cells. This implies that the virus protein coat is not merely a protective envelope but has configurations that lead to discriminatory cell attachment and possibly enzymes important in the process of penetration (see below).

Viral Reproduction (Fig. 66–1)

Since viruses contain no intracytoplasmic enzymes capable of reproducing viral nucleoprotein, the virus must invade a host cell and instruct its synthesizing mechanisms to produce viral rather than cellular components. The cycle of viral reproduction is readily divided into the phases described below.

FREE VIRAL PARTICLE. At present no major drugs are active against the free virus particle, but it can be destroyed in vitro by heat, ultraviolet light, x-irradiation and β propiolactone.

VIREMIA. After the free virus particles have entered the host, a viremia occurs and the particles localize in their preferred tissue(s). While the particles are in this extracellular environment, they may be inactivated by endogenous or exogenous (gamma globulin) antibodies. For example, poliomyelitis antibody attacks viral intercapsomeric junctions. No drugs other than antibody are known that act at this stage.

ADSORPTION. Before a virus can penetrate a cell, it must become absorbed onto the cell's surface, presumably at specialized receptor areas.

PENETRATION. Cellular penetration may depend on a process analogous to phagocytosis (pinocytosis). Viruses may penetrate in toto, or leave behind some of their outer coat proteins. One drug, amantadine (see below), may interfere with the penetration of, but not absorption onto, host cells by some myxoviruses (particularly influenza A_2 virus).

ECLIPSE. Following penetration, the virus particle becomes uncoated with separation of the genome and the covering protein. Virus messenger RNA then harnesses the host cell nutrients and protein-synthesizing machinery and produces inhibitors of host cell macromolecular synthesis, new viral nucleic acid, protein and lipids and "repressors," which control virus synthesis. The length of the eclipse phase may be as short as 10 min for some bacteriophages or as long as 9 hr for herpesviruses.

In general, DNA viruses first code for mRNA (transcription) which then attaches to host cell ribosomes initiating protein synthesis (translation). The nucleic acid of RNA viruses may serve indirectly as mRNA, or the RNA can be transcribed to a complementary messenger.

Because of its complexity, the eclipse phase offers the most likely target site for the development of antiviral drugs possessing selective toxicity. The **deoxyuridines** act during the eclipse

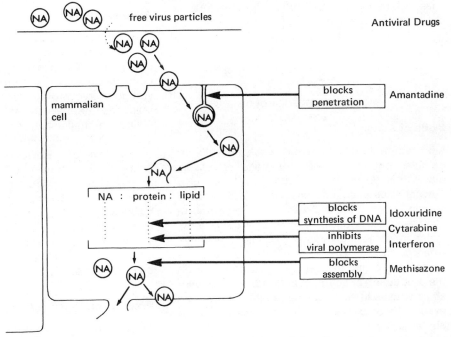

FIG. 66–1. Proposed mechanism of virus synthesis and the site of action of antiviral drugs.

phase (see below). Two other drugs, **2-(α-hydroxybenzyl)-benzimidazole** (HBB) and **guanidine,** are of some interest, not because they are highly effective in vivo, but because they have demonstrated that the selective inhibition of viral protein synthesis is possible. Both these agents inhibit the synthesis of viral RNA polymerase.

ASSEMBLY.   Assembly, or aggregation of newly synthesized virus particles, occurs in the nucleus (adenoviruses), in the cytoplasm (poxviruses) or at the cell surface (influenza virus). One drug, **N-methylistatin β-thiosemicarbazone,** may block viral assembly.

RELEASE.   The release of new virus particles is usually associated with host cell death. The released virus is ready to reinfect new host cells.

Viral Interference

The ability of one virus to interfere with the development of a second virus in the same tissue or host is called viral interference. It was first observed by Jenner, who showed in 1804 that vaccinia reacted weakly on skin involved in an herpetic eruption. Isaacs and Lindenmann, in 1957, discovered a soluble mediator of viral interference which they called **interferon.** Interferon is a polypeptide with a molecular weight of about 30,000. Its production is induced in host cells by virus or viral compounds.

Interferon is thought to inhibit viral nucleic acid replication shortly after genome release, either by selective inhibition of viral polymerase, or by preventing the combination of viral mRNA and host ribosomes. Its production in vivo may play an important role in the recovery from some viral infections, but this is not true in every case. The fungal products helenine and statolon (an anionic polysaccharide produced by *Penicillium stoloniferum)* induce the formation of interferon. Recently, **enhancer agents** or **stimulon** have been found in virus-infected cells. These substances counteract the effectiveness of interferon.

ANTIVIRAL DRUGS*

1-ADAMANTANAMINE HYDROCHLORIDE (AMANTADINE HYDROCHLORIDE)

Amantadine is a symmetrical heterocyclic primary amine which inhibits the growth of several viruses (influenza A, A_1, A_2 and C viruses) in cultures of chick-embryo fibroblasts and may offer some protection against infection by some strains of the influenza viruses (particularly influenza A_2) in man. A congener **Rimantadine** is similar to amantadine.

AMANTADINE HYDROCHLORIDE

Mode of Action

Amantadine does not prevent absorption of viral particles onto host cells, but does selectively block their penetration. In addition, it may also prevent virus uncoating and virus release under certain circumstances. Amantadine has no curative properties and only acts as a partial prophylactic in some individuals. It is most effective when given within 24–48 hr of infection, and the earlier it is given, the better. It has no effect on the production or action of antibody. Among sensitive viruses in vitro, complete inhibition is rare even at the maximum nontoxic concentration of about 50 mg/ml.

* The use of antiviral drugs in relation to cancer is not discussed in this book.

Absorption, Metabolism and Excretion

Amantadine is well absorbed from the gastrointestinal tract and has a biologic half-life of about 20 hr. So far no patterns of drug metabolism have been identified; the drug is excreted in the urine, where as much as 90% may be present in unchanged form.

Adverse Effects

The major adverse effects of amantadine involve the central nervous system and tend to be dose related. Slurred speech, somnolence, inability to concentrate, ataxia, a drunken feeling, insomnia, vertigo, nervousness, tremor and some psychic reactions (depression, feelings of detachment, Lilliputian hallucinations and paranoia) may occur, particularly with drug doses of greater than 300 mg/day. However, they may develop in patients on conventional dose schedules. Blurred vision, epileptiform seizures, various skin rashes, urinary frequency, xerostomia and gastrointestinal upsets may also develop. In general, toxic doses of amantadine are very near therapeutic doses, and geriatric patients, or those with a history of psychic upsets or seizures should not be given the drug.

Preparation, Dosage, and Uses

Amantadine Hydrochloride (Symmetrel) may be of some use in the **prophylaxis** of influenza infection in man. Occasionally accelerated rather than reduced influenza infection has occurred in test animals. The reasons are not clear. Recently amantadine has achieved popularity as a psychedelic drug. The chemoprophylaxis of influenza has one theoretical advantage over active immunization. For vaccination to be successful, it must be administered 4–8 weeks *prior* to the expected time of infection, whereas chemoprophylaxis can be initiated immediately. However, since amantadine is not 100% effective, it still seems prudent for prophylaxis to use a vaccine containing a current strain of influenza virus rather than amantadine.

The usual adult dose of amantadine is 200 mg once per day for 10 days, or for as long as the local epidemic persists. In children 1–9 years of age, the daily dose is 4–8 mg/kg/day with a maximum of 150 mg/day. In the case of 9–12 year-olds, the dose of amantadine is 100 mg twice a day.

Amantadine has been used successfully in the treatment of Parkinson's disease (Ch. 32). It probably acts similarly to L-dopa, although the level of benefit may be less with amantadine. Amantadine has also been used with limited success in the treatment of subacute sclerosing panencephalitis and Creutzfeldt-Jakob disease.

5-IODO-2'-DEOXYURIDINE

Of the four halogenated pyrimidine deoxyribosides—iodo-, fluoro-, bromo-, and chlorodeoxyuridine, iododeoxyuridine is the most important and effective (Fig. 66–2).

5-Iodo-2'-deoxyuridine (2'-deoxy-5-iodouridine, IDU, IUDR, idoxuridine) inhibits the replication of DNA viruses (particularly *Herpes simplex* and *Vaccinia).* In general, RNA viruses, with one or two possible exceptions (e.g., Rous sarcoma virus), are not affected.

Mode of Action and Viral Resistance

Idoxuridine inhibits a variety of enzymes involved in DNA synthesis, including thymidylic synthetase, thymidylic phosphorylase, nucleoside diphophate reductase and DNA polymerase. However, its most important action is almost certainly that of competing with thymidine-5'-phosphate.

IDOXURIDINE

In vivo, idoxuridine is sequentially converted by kinases into mono-, di-, and triphosphate forms. The triphosphate competes with thymidine-5'-phosphate (Fig. 66–2) in the formation of DNA by DNA polymerase. DNA polymerase is unable to distinguish between idoxuridine and thymidine, because the van der Waals radius of iodine (2.15) is essentially similar to that of the methyl group of thymidine (2.0). It is generally understood that the idoxuridine DNA does not function properly, but leads to the production of defective nucleic acid (lethal viral synthesis). Resistance to idoxuridine has been described for some isolates of *Herpes simplex.*

Pharmacology

Because idoxuridine is rapidly incorporated into host DNA following systemic administration, the

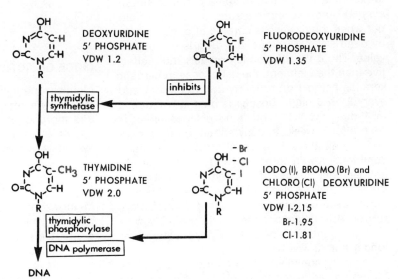

FIG. 66–2. Mode of action of the deoxyuridines (*VDW*, van der Waals radius).

present use of this drug is usually confined to local therapy in the conjunctival sac or on the skin. Small quantities may be absorbed but are rapidly excreted in the urine as iodine, ribose and uracil.

In rare circumstances idoxuridine may be given by IV infusion, e.g., in the treatment of herpes encephalitis.

Adverse Effects

Adverse effects resulting from topical conjunctival idoxuridine therapy are usually minimal. Periorbital burning, tingling pain or discomfort, lacrimation, edema and erythema accompanied by photophobia are common and may reflect irritation from the drug base and not the idoxuridine itself. There may be an increased occurrence of subepithelial opacities following its use, but this has not been proved. Care should be taken that the insoluble petrolatum base is not incorporated into deep corneal lesions. Adverse effects following IV therapy are severe, but the disease states so treated are potentially lethal. Stomatitis, marrow aplasia and hepatic degeneration have been described. The drug may be teratogenic and carcinogenic.

Preparations

Idoxuridine *U.S.P.* is available in a 0.1% solution (Dendrid, Herplex, Stoxil); in a 0.1% solution in polyvinyl alcohol (Herplex); and as a 0.5% ointment in a petrolatum base (Stoxil). The solution is heat and light sensitive and should be kept refrigerated. The ointment is heat stable.

Preparations, Dosage and Usage

Idoxuridine is effective in some cases of *herpes simplex* and vaccinia keratitis of recent origin, but when the disease is chronic or accompanied by deep stromal lesions, the drug is of doubtful value. The 0.1% solution is probably more effective than the ointment, the usual dose in herpetic keratitis being 1 drop hourly during the day and every 2 hr at night. Dosage is gradually reduced to 1 drop every 2–4 hr. If no obvious effect is seen after a week, therapy should be discontinued. When there is deep stromal involvement, combination with corticosteroids, cycloplegics or antibacterial drugs (if secondary infection is present) may be desirable, but boric acid must not be used concomitantly. Even if a satisfactory response is being obtained, it is probably wise not to continue idoxuridine application for longer than 3 weeks.

Topically administered, idoxuridine sensitizes herpesviruses to the lethal effects of irradiation, an effect that can be demonstrated in herpes keratitis. The clinical efficacy of a combination of idoxuridine plus irradiation is under investigation.

Idoxuridine has been used to treat other herpetic infections, and infections due to cytomegalovirus, but the results have not been impressive. In patients with potentially fatal herpesvirus encephalitis, idoxuridine has been administered by constant IV infusion in a dose of 80–100 mg/kg/day for 5 days; the concomitant administration of idoxuridine intrathecally appears to offer no additional advantage. Idoxuridine 40% in dimethylsulfoxide (DMSO) has been shown to be of some benefit in herpes zoster, reducing the duration of pain and accelerating healing, and in primary herpetic whitlow. Idoxuridine, 5% in DMSO has also been shown to shorten the course of some cutaneous herpetic lesions in man.

N-METHYLISATIN β-THIOSEMICARBAZONE (METHISAZONE)

Methisazone has a wide antiviral spectrum on in vitro study but activity in vivo is confined to treatment of infections caused by the pox viruses. Methisazone has been shown to protect against smallpox and alastrim (variola minor) and may be of some use in complications of primary vaccination. In one early series reported from Madras, India, 6 mild cases of smallpox with 2 deaths developed in 2297 patients treated with methisazone, in contrast to 114 cases of smallpox with 20 deaths in 2842 nontreated controls.

N-METHYLISATIN β-THIOSEMICARBAZONE

MODE OF ACTION

Methisazone may prevent the synthesis of a protein that is required for normal virus assembly and morphogenesis or maturation. Methisazone has no effect on viral DNA replication or on the synthesis of mRNA.

Pharmacology and Adverse Effects

Methisazone is absorbed after oral administration with peak plasma levels developing within 4–7 hr. Little is known about its metabolism. In limited clinical usage, the only adverse effects noted have been nausea and vomiting, some impairment of mentation, dermatitis and jaundice.

Methisazone prevents the conjugation of bilirubin with glucuronic acid.

Uses

Methisazone (Marboran) is an approved drug in Great Britian, and in doses of 1.5–3.0 g daily, has been shown to be effective in the prophylaxis of smallpox when given *before* the 8th or 9th day of the incubation period. It also effectively prevents the development of variola minor in contacts of the disease. In some instances methisazone prophylaxis has been more effective than revaccination, but it is unlikely that this agent will replace conventional primary immunization.

Even though methisazone has no effect in smallpox once the disease has developed, there is some evidence that the drug combined with antivaccinal gamma globulin is of therapeutic value in patients with complications of vaccination, particularly in the modification of primary vaccination in a patient who *must* be vaccinated in the presence of some contradiction (eczema, myeloproliferative disease, etc.).

CYTOSINE ARABINOSIDE

Cytosine arabinoside (1-β-D-arabinofuranosylcytosine:ARAC:Cytarabine) was originally developed as an antileukemia drug. It is now available on an experimental basis for topical and parenteral administration in some virus diseases. Cytarabine possesses a similar antiviral spectrum to that of idoxuridine, but antiviral resistance has been reported only rarely. The drug inhibits

CYTARABINE

nucleoside reductase and DNA polymerase and depresses the reduction of cytidilic acid to deoxycytidilic acid thus depleting the pool of deoxycytidine triphosphate available for DNA synthesis. However, its primary site of action is not clear.

Absorption, Metabolism, and Excretion

Following IV administration, cytarabin is rapidly inactivated by deamination, primarily in the liver and kidney. However, the drug persists for longer periods of time following intrathecal administration, since specific deaminases are absent in brain tissue. Cytarabine is widely distributed following IV injection but is rarely, if at all, incorporated into DNA.

Adverse Effects

Adverse effects following topical administration have been minimal, but following IV injection severe dose-dependent reactions may be seen; typically produced are hepatic damage, bone marrow depression, gastrointestinal disturbances and supression of immunity.

Uses

Cytarbine has been used successfully in the conjuntival sac in the treatment of herpetic keratitis. It has also been used with some success in the treatment of other localized and generalized infections caused by *herpes simplex,* and *herpes zoster varicella* viruses, but convincing proof of clinical efficacy is lacking. Results in the treatment of cytomegalovirus infections have not been encouraging, but cytarabine has been used successfully in the treatment of smallpox.

Cytarabine has been given in doses of 20–200 mg/sq m/day for 1–7 days.

Cytarabine possesses several advantages over idoxuridine. First, herpesviruses, particularly type 2-herpesviruses, are generally more sensitive to cytarabine than to idoxuridine. Second, cytarabine is rarely if ever incorporated into host DNA, whereas idoxuridine is readily incorporated, an occurrence which makes this agent a potential carcinogen and teratogen. Third, resistance develops rapidly to idoxuridine, but has not been a problem with cytarabine.

PHOTODYNAMIC INACTIVATION OF HERPESVIRUSES

Photodynamic inactivation of viruses is a new, but simple approach to virus chemotherapy, which is still under study.

Exposure of viruses to a variety of congeners of the heterocyclic dye acridine orange, namely neutral red, toluidine blue and proflavine, results in a complex formation between the dye and viral nucleic acid presumably through intercalation (Ch. 53). Minimal or no change in viral infectiousness occurs in the dark, but upon exposure to light, the guanine moiety of nucleic acid is rapidly deleted with resulting loss of infectivity.

Although many viruses are susceptible to photodynamic inactivation in vitro, only herpesvirus has been shown to be affected in vivo. Resistance to photodynamic inactivation has been described.

The dyes are avidly taken up by normal cells, but adverse reactions other than mucosal irritation and contact dermatitis have not been described.

Herpetic infection of the skin, recurrent herpes labialis and herpes progenitalis have been successfully treated by the topical application of 0.1% neutral red followed by light exposure.

MISCELLANEOUS ANTIVIRAL DRUGS UNDER INVESTIGATION

6-azaruridine inhibits orotidylic acid decarboxylase, and has been shown to inhibit several DNA and RNA viruses in vitro. It is on trial for the treatment of measles and subacute sclerosing panencephalitis. **Vidarabine** is a congener of idoxuridine and cytarabine, and has a similar antiviral spectrum. It may possess some advantages over the older drugs. **5-Trifluoromethyl-2'-deoxyuridine** and **5-ethyl-2'-deoxyuridine** are congeners of idoxuridine. They show certain promise in DNA virus infections. **Adenine arabinoside (Ara A)** is a purine that possess potent antiviral properties against DNA viruses in vitro and in vivo.

VIDARABINE

Rifampin (Ch. 59) inhibits the replication of poxviruses and adenoviruses in vitro, but in vivo trials have been disappointing. It probably interferes with the assembly of virus DNA and protein when the virus envelope is formed. **Isoprinosine** is a congener of inosine that may prove effective in vivo. **Quinacrine** (Ch. 63) has been used experimentally against arbor viruses. **Flumidin** (N'N'-anhydrobis [β-hydroxyethyl] biguanide hydrochloride, ABOB) has been reported in early studies to have some prophylactic activity against influenza. **Xenalamine** may have some prophylactic and therapeutic activity in influenza and chickenpox. **Phagicin,** a polypeptide produced by bacteriophage-infected *Escherichia coli,* may be of use in systemic viral disease.

INTERFERON. Therapy with exogenous interferon has not yet shown significant results, primarily because of its short half-life (about 10 min), and because human cells must be used to produce interferons for the treatment of viral infections in man. Interferon exhibits greatest protective activity in vitro if added at least 24 hr prior to virus inoculation. Limited clinical use has indicated that it may be of some value in *herpes simplex* and vaccina keratitis. However, interferon has been found to be antigenic on repeated administration. There is some hope the induction of endogenous interferon in man may become therapeutically practicable, either by the use of attenuated viruses or specific inducers of nonviral origin.

FURTHER READING

Adamson RH, Levy HB, Baron S (1972): The interferon system in Search for New Drugs. In Rubin AA (ed): Medicinal Research Series. N 6. New York, Dekker, pp 291–316

Bauer DJ (1973): Antiviral chemotherapy: the first decade. Br Med J 2:275–279

Prusoff WH, Goz B (1973): Potential mechanisms of action of antiviral agents. Fed Proc 32:1679–1687

Weinstein L, Chang T-W (1973): The chemotherapy of viral infections. N Engl J Med 289:725–730

CHARLES M. HASKELL

MARTIN J. CLINE

67. ANTICANCER DRUGS

The treatment of cancer with drugs was initiated in 1941 by Huggins, with the discovery that estrogens palliate prostatic cancer, and subsequently by the development of the polyfunctional alkylating agents as a result of experimental work performed during World War II. Since then there has been a tremendous increase in the number of chemotherapeutic agents available. The purpose of this chapter is to provide an introduction to the anticancer drugs and to summarize the factors that influence their usefulness in treating human malignant diseases.

SELECTIVE TOXICITY

The clinically useful anticancer agents have a greater cytotoxicity for malignant tissues than for normal cells of the tumor-bearing host. They are therefore said to exhibit selective toxicity. Selective toxicity is possible because of metabolic differences between malignant and normal cells. Unfortunately, these differences are generally quantitative rather than qualitative, leading to at least some degree of toxicity to normal tissues during the treatment of cancer with drugs. Most of the quantitative differences between normal and cancer cells relate to biochemical pathways, transport processes and DNA-repair mechanisms. For example, the synthesis of major macromolecules, including DNA and RNA, are more easily damaged by some anticancer drugs in certain cells than in normal cells. In addition, there may be differences in the ability of normal cells and cancer cells to repair damage to these critical molecules.

The target of therapy in malignant disease is the cancer cell. It is a variable and fluctuating target. One of the major factors influencing the response of a cancer to drug therapy is the fraction of the tumor cells that are in the replicative cycle. Thus the cell cycle of an individual tumor cell and the kinetics of growth of a tumor cell population must be considered in the evaluation of selective toxicity. Specifically, the activity of drugs during different phases of the cell life cycle must be noted. Drugs that kill cells only during specific phases of the cycle (phase specific), must be differentiated from drugs which kill cells during all or most phases of the cell cycle (phase nonspecific). The phases of the cell cycle are illustrated in Figure 67–1.

Although both normal cells and cancer cells which divide go through these same phases, differences exist between populations of normal cells and populations of cancer cells in the number and distribution of cells in cycle. Both normal and neoplastic cells may be influenced by certain growth factors and both appear to divide more rapidly when the population size is small, and more slowly when it is large. Recently, the quantitative rates of growth of both experimental tumors and human tumors have been measured. When the size is small and growing rapidly, a relatively high proportion of its cells are synthesizing DNA (in S-phase) at any given time. At this point in the life history of the cancer one should logically use cycle-active drugs effective against rapidly dividing cells. In contrast, an advanced tumor with a very low growth fraction and a slow increase in size may respond better to a phase nonspecific drug.

It is important to reemphasize that the differences between normal tissues and a malignant tissue may be slight. Many normal tissues have a high proliferative capacity rivaling and in some instances exceeding that of malignant tissues. Such normal tissues, including bone marrow elements, gastrointestinal epithelium and hair follicles bear the brunt of the toxic effects of certain anticancer drugs. Fortunately, the rapidly proliferating normal and cancer cells are not always equally vulnerable, and the principle

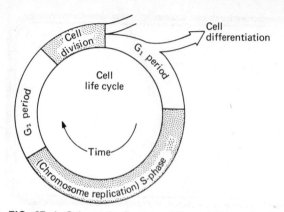

FIG. 67–1. Schematic diagram of the cell life cycle. G_1 is the first "gap" period and G_2 is the second "gap" period. (From Morton DL (1972): Ann Intern Med 77:443.)

of selective toxicity can still be utilized. It is apparent, however, that the margin of safety is often a very narrow one.

MECHANISM OF ACTION OF ANTICANCER DRUGS

The majority of antineoplastic drugs appear to act by effecting either enzymes, or substrates acted upon by enzymes systems (Fig. 67–2). Usually, the effects on enzymes or substrates relate to DNA synthesis or function, and consequently these drugs appear to exert their major toxic and antitumor effects by inhibiting cells that undergo DNA synthesis at some time in their life cycle. Drugs which act primarily by inhibiting the enzymes of nucleic acids synthesis are called

antimetabolites. Methotrexate, a structural analog of folinic acid, acts as a nearly irreversible inhibitor of the active site of the enzyme dihydrofolate reductase. Another commonly used antimetabolite is **5-fluorouracil,** which appears to act as a reversible inhibitor of the enzyme thymidylate synthetase. The antimetabolites act directly on enzymes as either reversible or irreversible inhibitors, leading either to disruption of DNA synthesis due to the lack of an essential building block or to the synthesis of abnormal DNA due to the incorporation of an abnormal building block.

A variety of major drugs appear to work primarily by effecting substrates. The usual substrate effected is the DNA macromolecule, although some of these agents will interfere with other substrates such as proteins. At least five major chemical classes of drugs appear to act by effecting specific substrates. The **alkylating agents** are extremely reactive compounds which can substitute an alkyl group (e.g., $R-CH_2-CH_2^+$) for the hydrogen atoms of many organic compounds. The primary compounds effected by alkylation appear to be nucleic acids, primarily DNA. Such alkylation produces breaks in the DNA molecule and cross-linking of the twin strands of DNA, thus interfering with DNA replication and the transcription of RNA. These effects are somewhat similar to what is seen with ionizing radiation, and for that reason this class of compounds is sometimes called "radiomimetic."

A second group of compounds that work primarily on substrates are the **antibiotics.** These

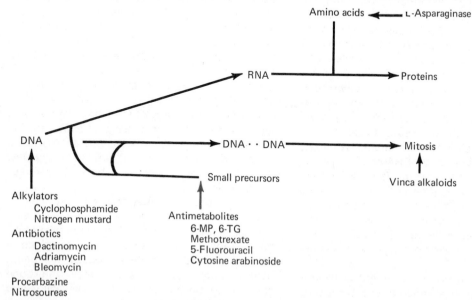

FIG. 67–2. Site of action of chemotherapeutic agents. The red arrow indicates drugs acting primarily as inhibitors of enzymes. Black arrows indicate specific substrates acted upon by drugs of that class. (Modified from Cline MJ, Haskell CM (1975): *Cancer Chemotherapy* (2nd ed). Philadelphia, WB Saunders, p. 3.)

are natural products derived from certain soil fungi. They produce their antineoplastic effect by forming relatively stable complexes with DNA, thereby inhibiting the synthesis of DNA and RNA.

A third class of drugs acting primarily on substrates are the **vinca alkaloids.** Although their total mechanism of action may not be completely defined, this class of drugs binds to microtubular proteins necessary for cell division. These proteins form the spindle apparatus which allows the chromosomes to separate to either end of the dividing cell. The vinca alkaloids appear to be able to dissolve this protein, leading to death of the cell during mitosis.

Other drugs which appear to work by specifically inhibiting substrates are **procarbazine** and the experimental enzyme L-**asparaginase.** Procarbazine interacts directly with DNA leading to depolymerization whereas L-asparaginase eliminates L-asparagine from extracellular fluids, leading to specific starvation of cells requiring this amino acid for protein synthesis.

Many drugs useful in the treatment of patients with cancer have not had their mechanisms of action completely defined. For example, the mode of action of many of the steroid hormones as anticancer agents is not certain. Some may have their primary effect on membrane transport processes of susceptible cells, and it is clear that they require binding to specific cytoplasmic receptors. Some drugs appear to act on both enzymes and substrates. An example of this group is the **nitrosoureas,** that have alkylating and antimetabolic activities.

The interested student is referred to the references given later for more detailed reading into the mechanisms of action of the useful anticancer drugs. The chemical structures of some of these drugs are illustrated in Figure 67–3 for the purpose of demonstrating the similarities of chemical structure within the classes of drugs.

THE LOG CELL KILL HYPOTHESIS

Anticancer drugs are thought to be incapable of killing all cancer cells at any given exposure. Rather they will kill a variable fraction of cells from a few percent up to a maximum of 99.999%. The observed fractional tumor cell kill can frequently be graphed as a line with a negative exponential slope, so experimental chemotherapeutic data is often expressed in logarithmic terms. Since the body burden of tumor cells in man with an advanced malignancy may be greater than 10^{12} cells (1 kg), and since the best one can hope for with a single maximal exposure of tumor cells to a drug is somewhere between 2 and 5 logs of cell kill, it is apparent that treatment must be repeated many times in order to

achieve even partial control. This hypothesis also suggests that chemotherapeutic drugs alone may not be capable of totally eradicating any given population of tumor cells. There is evidence that immunologic approaches to therapy may not face this restriction, since the immune system can totally eradicate small numbers of tumor cells; however, it may be ineffective against large tumor cell masses. The approximate order of magnitude for this latter effect is 10^5 cells.

PHARMACOLOGIC FACTORS

Factors altering the concentration of a drug at its primary site of action, or the period of time which that drug is available at the biologic receptor, must be considered in the use of cancer chemotherapeutic drugs. This relationship is sometimes expressed as the product of drug concentration multiplied by drug exposure time, or the $C \times T$ function. The important factors relating to this function are known for some drugs, and are being explored for others. These will be considered below (see Table 67–1).

Route of Administration and Absorption

A variety of routes of administration may be chosen to optimize availability. Drugs may be administered orally, IV, IM, intraarterially or instilled into a local site such as a malignant effusion in the pleural space or into the spinal fluid. By carefully selecting the route of administration the antitumor effect of a given drug may be improved by allowing it to reach high concentrations in the areas involved by a tumor. One very specialized example of this approach has been with isolation-perfusion of an extremity with high doses of alkylating agents for regional malignant melanoma.

Distribution and Transport

The distribution and transport of anticancer drugs may profoundly influence their effectiveness. After a drug is absorbed, it may enter or pass through various body compartments including the vascular spaces, extracellular spaces, and into cells. In some cases drugs may accumulate in certain areas as a result of binding, active transport or solubility in fat. The converse of this is that some drugs may be excluded from certain areas because of binding, solubility or transport phenomena. Since most anticancer drugs exert their effect directly on an intracellular target molecule, the ability of that drug to get to the cancer cell is of vital concern. If tumor cells are in an area of the body which is inaccessible to anticancer drugs, then the concentration

ALKYLATING AGENTS

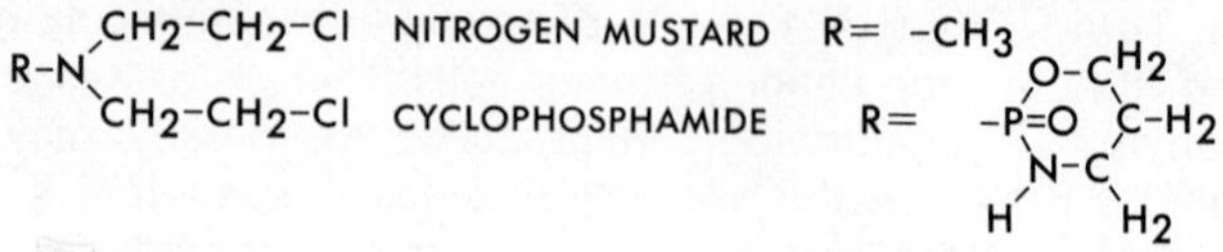

CH₂–CH₂–Cl NITROGEN MUSTARD R= –CH₃

R–N

CH₂–CH₂–Cl CYCLOPHOSPHAMIDE R= ...

ANTIMETABOLITES

NORMAL METABOLITE

STRUCTURAL ANALOG

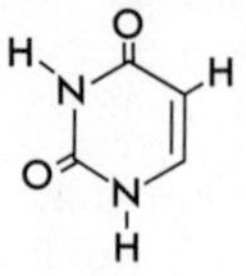

URACIL

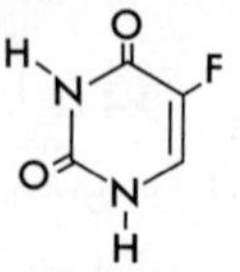

5-FLUOROURACIL

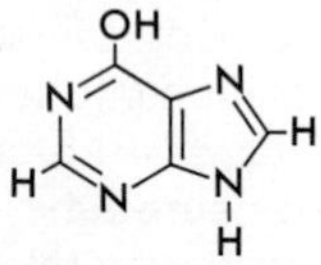

HYPOXANTHINE

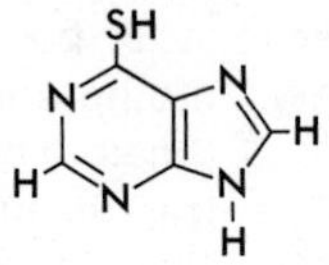

6-MERCAPTOPURINE

VINCA ALKALOIDS

VINCRISTINE
VINBLASTINE

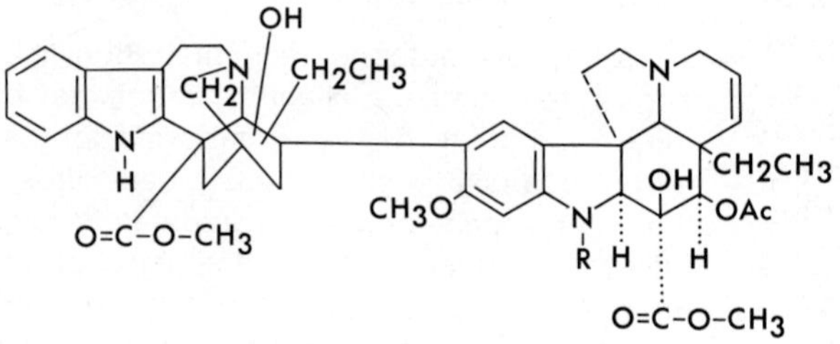

VINCRISTINE
R is O=C–H

VINBLASTINE
R is CH₃

ANTIBIOTICS

ACTINOMYCIN-D

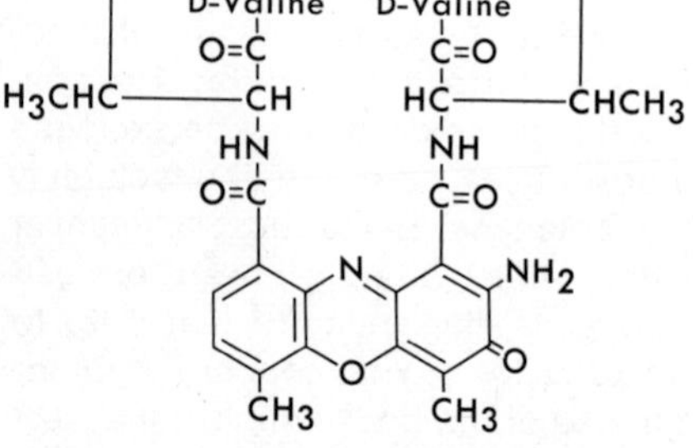

Sarcosine   Sarcosine

L-Proline   L-Proline

D-Valine   D-Valine

FIG. 67–3. Chemical structures of selected anticancer drugs.

TABLE 67–1. Pharmacologic Characteristics of Selected Anticancer Drugs

Drug	Cell cycle phase specificity	Plasma T 1/2	Plasma protein binding	Entry into CNS	Biotransformation Activation	Biotransformation Degradation	Main route of excretion	Major toxicities
Alkylating agent Cyclophosphamide	NS	6.5 hrs	10%	Moderate	Oxidized by hepatic microsomal enzymes to biologically active and inactive products		Renal	Myelosuppression; cystitis; alopecia
Antimetabolites Methotrexate	S	12 hrs	50%	Minimal	None	None	Renal	Myelosuppression; stomatitis; hepatic dysfunction
6-Mercaptopurine	S	90 min	10-20%	Moderate	To nucleotide	Oxidation to 6-thiouric acid via xanthine oxidase	Renal	Myelosuppression; stomatitis; hepatic dysfunction
Cytosine arabinoside	S	2 hrs	Negligible	Moderate	To nucleotide	Deamination to uracil arabinoside	Renal	Myelosuppression
5-Fluorouracil	NS	20 min	? negligible	Extensive	To nucleotide	Extensive	Lung and renal	Myelosuppression; gastrointestinal; integument
Vinca alkaloids Vincristine	S	A few min	? negligible	? negligible		? extensive	Bile	Neuropathy; alopecia
Antibiotics Dactinomycin	NS	A few min	? negligible	Low	None	None	Bile	Myelosuppression; gastrointestinal; integument
Adriamycin	NS	27 hrs	Extensive	? negligible	Extensive biotransformation to active and inactive metabolites		Bile	Myelosuppression; stomatitis; alopecia; cardiac damage
Hormones Prednisone	NS	24 hrs	90%	Low	——	Conjugation and reduction in liver	Renal	Peptic ulcer; psychosis; diabetes m.; electrolyte problem; myopathy

Abbreviations: S — phase specific   NS — phase nonspecific   CNS — central nervous system   ? — undetermined or estimated from known properties of the drug or a closely related drug

Cline MJ, Haskell CM (1975): *Cancer Chemotherapy* (2nd ed). Philadelphia, WB Saunders, p. 29

times time factor for those drugs will be negligible and the cancer cells will survive. This phenomenon is sometimes referred to as the "sanctuary" effect. An example of such a sanctuary is the brain, where tumor cells appear to be inaccessible to many anticancer drugs by virtue of the "blood-brain barrier." Most commonly used anticancer drugs are relatively lipid insoluble (Ch. 2). Access to the brain is restricted in large part to molecules which are highly fat soluble.

Biotransformation

The metabolism of an anticancer agent may be an important consideration. Some drugs are inactive before administration, requiring biotransformation to achieve their active form. One example of this is the alkylating agent, **cyclophosphamide,** which is metabolized in the liver from an inactive to an active form. A variety of other drugs can modify the activation process, including barbiturates and corticosteroids.

Excretion

The route of excretion of an anticancer drug may also be critical in clinical therapy. Methotrexate, a folic acid antagonist, is primarily excreted by the kidneys. Even a moderate elevation of blood urea nitrogen may be associated with major hematologic toxicity from the use of relatively low doses of methotrexate. Similarly, vincristine, a mitotically active plant alkaloid, which is excreted primarily by bile, may lead to severe neurotoxicity when administered to patients with liver disease.

Drug Interactions

Most patients with cancer receive a variety of potent noncancer drugs for the control of symptoms from their treatment of their neoplastic disease. Such drugs may include a barbiturate for sedation, a phenothiazine for nausea or mental symptoms, analgesics and allopurinol for the prevention of uric acid nephropathy. Indeed, it is not uncommon for a patient with cancer to be receiving as many as eight or more drugs at the same time. In recent years an extensive literature has developed concerning some of the interactions between drugs used in clinical medicine; however, there is a paucity of data concerning such interactions between drugs used in the treatment of human cancer. Drug interactions may occur by a variety of mechanisms. Interactions of anticancer agents and other drugs are as follows:

1. Direct chemical or physical interaction (e.g., nitrogen mustard and aqueous solutions)

2. Interaction during intestinal absorption (e.g., methotrexate-antibiotics)

3. Interaction at plasma or blood transport sites (e.g., methotrexate-aspirin)

4. Interaction at the cellular receptor site (e.g., methotrexate-folinic acid)

5. Interaction by accelerated or inhibited metabolism (e.g., cyclophosphamide and drugs influencing hepatic metabolism)

6. Altered acid-base balance leading to changes in drug distribution and renal clearance (e.g., theoretical—not established for anticancer drugs)

7. Alterations of renal function that influence rates of renal excretion (e.g., methotrexate excretion)

8. Alterations in cellular transport mechanisms (e.g., L-asparaginase-methotrexate)

9. Alterations in cellular biochemical pathways and drug resistance (e.g., 6-mercaptopurine-allopurinol)

Specific examples of some of these interactions, as they relate to cancer chemotherapy, may be cited. Nitrogen mustard and many of its derivatives are highly reactive compounds. Thus direct chemical inactivation in physical mixtures of drugs in infusion solutions is a likely problem. Methotrexate absorption may be profoundly altered by concomitant use of antibiotics which suppress gastrointestinal microbial flora. Methotrexate is transported by serum and both aspirin and sulfonamides are known to displace this drug and to thereby markedly alter free drug levels and drug toxicity. Cellular transport of specific drugs may be altered by other drugs; one recently described example of this is the inhibition of methotrexate transport across cell membranes by L-asparaginase. Finally, it is important to reemphasize the possibility that allopurinol, a potent xanthine oxidase inhibitor, can profoundly effect the metabolism of **6-mercaptopurine,** a purine analog. Clinically this effect results in markedly augmented toxicity when the two drugs are used in combination, and it is therefore necessary to appropriately decrease the dose of 6-mercaptopurine.

DRUG RESISTANCE

Another factor which often limits the clinical usefulness of a chemotherapeutic agent is the emergence of a line of malignant cells resistant to that drug. It is a common clinical experience to find that the first trial of a given drug with a cancer patient is successful and that subsequent trials are often progressively less successful until no apparent beneficial effect is achieved by administering the drug.

Probably a number of cellular mechanisms are involved in drug resistance: altered drug metabolism (increased deactivation, decrease or loss of the essential activation process), impermeability of the cell to the active compound, altered specificity of an inhibited enzyme, increased production of a target molecule, repair of cytotoxic lesions and in some cases alternative biochemical pathways may bypass an inhibited reaction. There is obviously an analogy between the development of resistance to drugs in cancer therapy and the appearance of antibiotic resistant strains of bacteria during the course of an infection. The approach of the clinician is often the same in both situations—change drugs or, less often, use larger doses of the same drug.

DRUG SCHEDULES AND COMBINATION CHEMOTHERAPY

Studies with experimental animal tumors have conclusively demonstrated the importance of drug scheduling in therapy. **Cytosine arabinoside,** an antimetabolite which kills cells only in S-phase, must be given frequently in order to assure contact with cancer cells during this critical period. When this drug is so employed, it is possible to cure some forms of murine leukemia, whereas maximally tolerated doses of the drug given at less frequent intervals fail to prolong survival. On the other hand cyclophosphamide, which is phase nonspecific, achieves optimal suppression of most experimental animal neoplasms when given on a high dose intermittent schedule.

A second factor related to drug scheduling is the growth status of any given tumor. In general, solid tumors with a large tumor mass will be growing slowly and will have a small growth fraction (less than 10%). Since relatively few of these cells will be dividing, it should not be surprising that the tumors are generally insensitive to phase specific drugs. Thus, the usual treatment for advanced nonhematologic tumors has been with phase nonspecific drugs such as alkylating agents. However, successful treatment with such phase nonspecific drugs may render the tumor more susceptible to phase specific drugs, by converting the tumor from one with a low growth fraction with few of the cells in S-phase, to a smaller tumor with a high growth fraction with many cells in S-phase.

In recent years it has become obvious that the optimal way of treating many kinds of tumors has been by combinations of drugs. The optimal combinations of drugs for the primary therapy of advanced neoplasms, and as early therapy in combination with surgery and radiation therapy are under active study. Several theoretical and practical advantages to combination therapy have emerged. At the risk of oversimplification, it is perhaps useful to amplify this principle by thinking of a population of malignant cells as resembling a culture of bacteria. In both, combinations of agents can delay or suppress the emergence of drug-resistant cells and can prolong the time necessary for the population of dividing cells to reach a density that produces clinically apparent disease. Addition of an anti-cancer drug to malignant cells results in the killing of the drug-sensitive cells, just as the addition of an antibiotic to bacteria results in the killing of the susceptible bacteria. If the drug is not completely effective, then a portion of the cancer (or bacterial population) survives. The surviving population contains drug-resistant cells. If the drug-resistant cells are capable of replication, they give rise to a drug-resistant tumor or bacterial population. The administered drug thus has a selective mode of action leading to the emergence of a resistant cell line. The frequency of emergence of an antibiotic-resistant bacterium can be determined precisely. It is less easy to determine the frequency of occurrence of drug-resistant cancer cells. It is obvious, however, that the chances for the development of a drug-resistant line will not be as good if two or more drugs of dissimilar modes of action are used in a treatment combination. This principle can be demonstrated by a simple example.

A patient with acute lymphocytic leukemia may have 10^{12} malignant cells in his body. If a single drug, e.g., **prednisone,** is 99.999% effective (i.e., if it kills 99,999 of every 100,000 tumor cells), then 10^7 malignant cells remain after prednisone therapy. If, in addition, a second agent with a different mode of action such as vincristine, is 99.9% effective, the population of malignant cells can be further reduced to 10^4 cells. If still more agents are used, it is theoretically possible to reduce the cell population to nearly zero. At present, this goal is not obtainable because of many factors: limitations imposed by toxicity to normal tissues are compounded by multiple agents; malignant cells are concentrated in sites not reached by the drug (i.e., the CNS); cells may be in a prolonged G_1 or G_0 phase and thus unaffected by cell cycle phase-specific drugs.

Several principles underlying combination chemotherapy warrant special emphasis. Since cancer chemotherapy generally involves the use of toxic drugs, programs of combination chemotherapy must be designed with care to minimize dangerous toxicity. In general, the successful programs of combination chemotherapy have been designed with the following criteria in mind: 1) only drugs active against the tumor in question are included in the combination:

TABLE 67–2. Clinical Characteristics of Selected Anticancer Drugs

Drug	Usual dosage	Toxicity Acute	Toxicity Delayed	Major indication for use
Alkylating agents:				
Cyclophosphamide (Cytoxan)	30–40 mg/kg IV every 3—4 wk 2—4 mg/kg/day PO	Nausea and vomiting	Myelosuppression; alopecia; cystitis	Hodgkin's and nonHodgkin's lymphomas; multiple myeloma; lymphocytic leukemia; many solid tumors
Melphalan (Alkeran)	0.25 mg/kg/day X 4 PO every 4–6 wk	None	Myelosuppression	Multiple myeloma; breast and ovarian cancer
Mechlorethamine (nitrogen mustard; Mustargen)	0.4 mg/kg IV or IP in single or divided doses	Nausea and vomiting; local irritant	Myelosuppression	Hodgkin's disease; locally for malignant effusions
Antimetabolites:				
Methotrexate (MTX)	0.4 mg/kg/day IV push X 4—5 or 0.4 mg/kg IV push 1 or 2 times/wk	Occasional diarrhea	Oral and GI ulcers; myelosuppression; hepatotoxicity	Choriocarcinoma; acute lymphocytic leukemia; carcinoma of cervix and head and neck
Fluorouracil (5-FU)	12.5 mg/kg/day IV X 3–5 d or 15 mg/kg/wk IV	Nausea	Myelosuppression; stomatitis; diarrhea	Carcinomas of breast, ovary and large bowel
Cytosine arabinoside (Cytarabine HCl; arabinosyl cytosine; ara-C; Cytosar)	2–3 mg/kg/day IV until response or toxicity	Nausea and vomiting	Bone marrow depression	Acute leukemia
6-Thioguanine (6-TG)	2 mg/kg/day PO	Occasional nausea and vomiting	Myelosuppression	Acute leukemia

Vinca alkaloids:			
Vincristine sulfate (Oncovin)	0.01–0.03 mg/kg/wk IV	Local irritant	Mild myelosuppression; neuropathy; constipation; alopecia	Acute leukemia; Hodgkin's disease; other lymphomas and solid tumors
Vinblastine sulfate (Velban)	0.1–0.2 mg/kg/wk IV	Nausea; local irritant	Alopecia; neuropathy; myelosuppression	Hodgkin's disease; miscellaneous solid tumors
Antibiotics			
Dactinomycin (actinomycin D; Cosmegen)	0.015–0.05 mg/kg/wk IV	Nausea; vomiting;	Myelosuppression; alopecia; GI ulcers	Wilms' tumor; sarcomas; testicular carcinomas
Mithramycin (Mithracin)	0.025–0.050 mg/kg IV every other day for up to 8 doses	Nausea and vomiting; hepatotoxicity	Myelosuppression; hypocalcemia	Embryonal carcinoma of testis
Adriamycin	60 mg/m² body surface area IV every 3–4 wk	Nausea and vomiting; local irritant	Myelosuppression; alopecia; cardiac damage; stomatitis	Sarcomas; lymphomas; breast cancer; thyroid cancer
Bleomycin	10–15 units/m² 1 or 2 times/wk	Nausea, vomiting; fever, anaphylaxis	Pulmonary fibrosis; alopecia; stomatitis; edema	Hodgkin's and nonHodgkin's lymphomas; cancer of head and neck
Hormones:			
Prednisone	10–100 mg/day PO	None	Hyperadrenocorticism	Leukemia; lymphoma; multiple myeloma; breast cancer
Diethylstilbestrol (DES)	1,5 or 15 mg/day PO (1 mg in prostate)	None	Hypercalcemia; fluid retention; feminization; uterine bleeding; may cause vaginal carcinoma of offspring when given during pregnancy	Breast and prostatic carcinoma
Calusterone (Methosarb)	200 mg/day PO	None	Hypercalcemia; fluid retention; virilization	Breast carcinoma
Medroxy progesterone acetate (Provera)	100–200 mg/day PO; 200–600 mg 2 times/wk	None	None	Endometrial carcinoma; renal cell carcinoma

2) drugs included must have different mechanisms of action, to minimize the possibility of drug resistance; and 3) drugs chosen have generally had different spectra of clinical toxicity, allowing the administration of full or nearly full doses of each of the active agents. A final factor is the preference of most investigators to utilize intermittent courses of intensive combination chemotherapy rather than continuous programs of drug administration. This approach tends to maximize tumor cell killing, to be better tolerated by patients and appears to cause less immuno-suppression (see below).

IMMUNOSUPPRESSION

Many of the commonly used anticancer drugs are capable of suppressing both cellular and humoral immunity. In view of the increasing evidence implicating host immunologic factors in the control of small numbers of tumor cells, the potential effect of cancer chemotherapeutic drugs on the immune system becomes of increasing importance. There is evidence in experimental tumor systems that the preservation and in some cases the augmentation of immunity is important to the antitumor effects of chemotherapy. Conversely, there is evidence in man that response to chemotherapy may be correlated with a patient's immune status prior to treatment.

A great deal has been learned about how drugs effect the immune system, and it is apparent that drugs can be distinguished which achieve immunosuppression primarily when administered prior to antigenic stimulation, coincident with antigenic stimulation, and/or following antigenic stimulation. This relates to the mechanisms of action of the immunosuppressive drugs, as well as to the specific sequence of cellular events associated with the immune response.

Immunosuppression may vary depending on the precise dose and schedule of the drug given, either by itself or in combination with other drugs. Intermittent, intensive courses of chemotherapy appear to suppress cellular immunity much less than continuous low dose chemotherapy. In general, the immunosuppressive effects of most of the anticancer drugs commonly used do not extend beyond the period of active drug administration. Indeed, in some patients an "immunologic overshoot" occurs after drug administration. Thus, when short courses of combination chemotherapy are given every 2–4 weeks, the patient's immunologic function may be normal most of the time.

CLINICAL USE OF ANTICANCER DRUGS

In Table 67–2 clinically useful examples of the classes of commonly used anticancer drugs are listed together with the usual dose, toxicity and responsive major tumor types. The information provided is meant to be illustrative rather than encyclopedic and the interested student should consult the references given below for the practical application of these agents to clinical problems.

FURTHER READING

Cline MJ, Haskell CM (1975): Cancer Chemotherapy. 2nd ed Philadelphia, Saunders

Holland JF, Frei E, III (1973): Cancer Medicine. Philadelphia, Lea and Febiger

Livingston RB, Carter SK (1970): Single Agents in Cancer Chemotherapy. New York, Plenum Publishing Corp

Zimmerman AM, Padilla GM, Cameron IL (eds) (1973): Drugs and the Cell Cycle. New York, Academic Press

PART III

MISCELLANEOUS TOPICS AND REFERENCE MATERIAL

JOSEPH H. BECKERMAN

68. COMMONLY USED DIAGNOSTIC DRUGS

The names, purposes, and doses of the drugs commonly used in diagnostic procedures are presented in Table 68-1.

Before using any drug in a test procedure, the practitioner should read and completely familiarize himself with the information contained in the package insert. In addition, he should remember that although commonly used, few of these diagnositic agents are without adverse effects, some of which may be serious. These should be borne in mind when the diagnostic drug is prescribed.

In particular, contrast media containing organic iodine compounds may produce serious adverse effects or even fatal anaphylactic reactions. Individuals with a history of allergy are more likely to have adverse reactions or exaggerated reactions to these compounds. Thyroid function tests may be affected by these agents.

TABLE 68—1. Commonly Used Diagnostic Drugs

Drug	Trade name	Method of administration	Usual dose
Contrast media for visualizing gastrointestinal tract			
Barium Sulfate, *U.S.P.*		Oral	300 g
		Rectal	400 g
Meglumine Diatrizoate, *U.S.P.*	Gastrografin	Oral	30-90 ml of 76% solution
		Rectal	240 ml of 76% solution diluted to 1000 ml with water
Sodium Diatrizoate, *U.S.P.*	Hypaque Sodium	Oral	90-180 ml of 25-40% solution
		Rectal	500-1000 ml of 15-25% solution
Contrast media for visualizing gallbladder and bile ducts			
Ipodate Calcium, *N.D.*	Oragrafin-Calcium	Oral	3 g
Ipodate Sodium, *N.D.*	Oragrafin-Sodium	Oral	3 g
Iopanoic acid, *U.S.P.*	Telepaque	Oral	3 g
Meglumin iodipamide, *U.S.P.*	Cholografin Meglumine	IV	20 ml of 52% solution
Sodium iodipamide, *U.S.P.*	Cholografin Sodium	IV	40 ml of 20% solution
Contrast media for outlining body cavities			
Iodized Oil, *N.F.*	Lipiodol	Intrathecal Intratracheal	For myelography, 3-5 ml; for bronchography, 10 ml per side
Iophendylate, *U.S.P.*	Pantopaque	Intrathecal	For myelography, 6 ml
Propyliodone, *U.S.P.*	Dionosil	Intratracheal	For bronchography, 10 ml
Contrast media for pyelography and angiography			
Iodopyracet, *N.F.*	Diodrast	IV	For excretory pyelography, 20 ml of 35% solution; for cardiopulmonary visualization, 40-45 ml of 70% solution

TABLE 68–1. *(continued)*

Drug	Trade name	Method of administration	Usual dose
Meglumine Diatrizoate *U.S.P.*	Renografin	IV	For excretory pyelography, 25 ml of 60% solution; for cerebral angiography, 10 ml of 60% solution
Meglumine Iothalamate, *U.S.P.*	Conray	IV	For excretory pyelography, 30 ml of 60% solution; for angiocardiography, 25-50 ml of 60% solution
Sodium Diatrizoate, *U.S.P.*	Hypaque Sodium	IV	For excretory pyelography, 30 ml of 50% solution; for angiocardiography, 50 ml of 75 or 90% solution (combination of sodium and meglumine salts)
Sodium Iothalamate, *U.S.P.*	Angio-Conray	IV	For excretory pyelography, 25 ml of 66.8% solution; for angiocardiography, 40-50 ml of 66.8 or 80% solution
Sodium Methiodal, *N.F.*	Skiodan	IV Retrograde	20 g in 50 ml of solution amount varies according to number of exposures and diagnosis; 2-3 g in 10-15 ml solution usually suffices

Drugs used to test gastric function

Drug	Trade name	Method of administration	Usual dose
Azuresin, *N.F.*	Diagnex Blue	Oral	2 g with 500 mg of caffeine and sodium benzoate
Betazole Hydrochloride, *U.S.P.*	Histalog	Subcutaneous	50 mg
Histamine Phosphate, *U.S.P.*		Subcutaneous	300 μg of base

Drugs used to test kidney function

Drug	Trade name	Method of administration	Usual dose
Inulin		IV	In 10% solution; dose depends on procedure
Mannitol, *N.F.*		IV	In 25% solution; dose depends on procedure
Phenolsulfonphthalein, *U.S.P.*	Phenol Red, P.S.P.	IV IM	6 mg 6 mg
Sodium Aminohippurate, *U.S.P.*		IV	2 g
Sodium indigotin disulfonate, *U.S.P.*	Indigo Carmine	IV	40 mg

Drugs used to test kidney function

Drug	Trade name	Method of administration	Usual dose
Galactose		Oral	40 g
Rose Bengal Sodium I^{131} Injection, *U.S.P.*	Robengatope	IV	150 μc
Sodium Sulfobromophthalein, *U.S.P.*	Bromsulphalein, B.S.P.	IV	5 mg/kg body weight

Drugs used for miscellaneous tests

Drug	Trade name	Method of administration	Usual dose
Evans Blue, *U.S.P.*		IV	For blood volume estimation, 25 mg
Metyrapone, *U.S.P.*	Metopirone	Oral	For pituitary function determination, 750 mg every 4 hr for six doses
		IV	30 mg/kg of body weight in 1000 ml sodium chloride injection over 4-hr period

PETER LOMAX

69. ENZYMES

Certain enzymes are used for topical application to tissues or for hypodermic injection. These actions are thus generally limited to the local site of application.

HYALURONIDASE

Hyaluronidase is prepared commercially from bovine testes and is available as a dry sterile, amorphous solid for injection.

Mechanism of Action

Hyaluronidase depolymerizes hyaluronic acid found in the interstitial substances of tissues, particularly in the skin and synovial fluid. Hyaluronic acid consists of a chain of glucuronido-N-acetylglucosamine units polymerized by stable glucosidic linkages. Hyaluronidase breaks down these latter linkages. The resultant reduction in viscosity facilitates the spreading of substances through the tissues.

Uses

Hyaluronidase can be added to parenteral fluids such as saline, dextrose, lactate and plasma to speed absorption and diminish local distention of the tissues. The drug is particularly useful in hypodermoclysis (the subcutaneous injection of a large quantity of saline solution) in infants.

A variety of agents, such as antibiotics, alkaloids, steroids and antisera, can be more rapidly absorbed if hyaluronidase is added to the injection solution. Used during infiltration anesthesia with local anesthetics, hyaluronidase increases the area of skin anesthesia.

The rate of absorption of regions of traumatic or postoperative edema or hematoma can be hastened by infiltration of hyaluronidase and the use of a pressure bandage. Similarly, the inflammation due to accidental extravasation of irritant solutions can be reduced.

Many other applications for hyaluronidase have been described.

Adverse Effects

Hyaluronidase, being a protein enzyme, may stimulate antibody formation and cause allergic reactions when large repeated injections are used.

Dose

During hypodermoclysis, 150 *N.F.* units are injected either into the infusion area immediately prior to commencing infusion or into the tubing of the infusion equipment, or they are mixed with the infusion fluid. For local anesthesia 150 units of hyaluronidase are added to each 25–50 ml of local anesthetic solution. To hasten absorption of hematomata and other exudates, up to 3000 units may be used according to the size of the area involved.

STREPTOKINASE AND STREPTODORNASE

Streptokinase and streptodornase are enzymes derived from the growth of a strain of hemolytic streptococcus.

Mechanism of Action

Streptokinase activates plasminogen present in fibrin deposits. The activated plasminogen catalyzes the fibronolytic process which leads to the rapid dissolution of fibrinous exudates, the fibrin being broken down to large polypeptides.

The streptodornase group of enzymes are desoxyribonucleases and lead to depolymerization of desoxyribonucleoprotein and desoxyribonucleic acid, which make up the major portion of purulent exudates. The splitting of the nucleoprotein into purine bases and pyrimidine nucleosides markedly reduces the viscosity of the pus and aids dissolution. The enzymes have no effect on the nuclei or nucleoprotein of living cells.

Uses

A mixture of streptokinase and streptodornase is used to facilitate the removal of clotted blood or fibrinous or purulent material so that the action of antibiotics and the process of tissue repair are facilitated. This therapy may be beneficial in conditions, such as empyema, hemothorax, chronic pleural adhesions and hematoma, where local drainage is employed. The drugs are injected directly into the affected parts. Oral administration has been used in these conditions and in acute thrombophlebitis, bronchiectasis and bronchitis.

Adverse Effects

The injection of the enzymes may cause local pain. Transient rashes, urticaria and a febrile reaction have been reported and ulceration of the mucosa can follow buccal use. Nausea, vomiting and diarrhea may occur following oral administration.

Interference with normal clotting mechanisms precludes the use of these agents when there is active hemorrhage.

Dose

The enzymes are supplied in vials containing 100,000 units of streptokinase and 25,000 units of streptodornase; 10–20 ml of water are added before use. For empyema and hemothorax, up to two vials are injected. An initial dose of 10,000 units of streptokinase and 2500 units of streptodornase is recommended for maxillary sinus empyema. Similar doses are used for local application.

One tablet containing 10,000 units of streptokinase and 2500 units of streptodornase is given orally four times daily.

TRYPSIN

Trypsin is a proteolytic enzyme crystallized from ox pancreas. The enzyme acts directly to hydrolyze proteins, but does not affect living cells.

Uses

Trypsin is used in the same way as streptokinase and streptodornase in the debridement of ulcers, abscesses, necrotic wounds and empyemas. Intramuscular injection has been employed in the treatment of thrombophlebitis, inflammation of the eye, and varicose and diabetic ulcers.

Adverse Effects

Adverse effects are negligible when trypsin is applied topically. Pain, induration and febrile reactions may follow IM injection. Trypsin should not be used in the patient with hepatic insufficiency, since severe liver damage may occur.

Dose

A dose of 2.5–5.0 mg is injected IM, and 5 mg tablets are given orally. The dry powder is applied directly to wounds.

CHYMOTRYPSIN

Chymotrypsin is a yellowish-white powder obtained from ox pancreas. In general, the actions, uses and doses of chymotrypsin are similar to those of trypsin.

FURTHER READING

Symposium (1950): Ground substances of mesenchyme and hyaluronidase. Ann NY Acad Sci 52:945

JOHN A. BEVAN

70. HYPERBARIC OXYGEN

Hyperbaric oxygen is usually administered to subjects at pressures between two and three, but never more than four, atmospheres. The patient is placed in either a small chamber in which the ambient gas is oxygen under pressure or a large chamber containing ambient air under a pressure similar to the oxygen inhaled from an appropriate apparatus. The resultant increased oxygen content of hemoglobin, plasma and tissues is not linearly related to pressure.

The duration of safe exposure is dependent on the oxygen pressure and is limited by the susceptibility of the retinal cells to oxygen toxicity. It has been shown that visual acuity and fields of vision are reduced after 2 hr exposure at 3 atmospheres. However, there is considerable evidence that the procedure relatively is free from danger if it is correctly carried out and its restrictions realized.

The value of hyperbaric oxygen in clinical practice is due to three biologic effects: the relief of hypoxia and anoxia, the potentiation of ionizing radiation (radiosensitizing effect), and the inhibition of bacterial growth and toxin production. Clinical areas in which hyperbaric oxygen is valuable are summarized in Table 70–1.

TABLE 70–1. Clinical Uses and Mechanism of Action of Hyperbaric Oxygen

Biologic effect	Clinical uses	Mechanism of action
Relief of hypoxia and anoxia	In cardiovascular surgery, especially prior to inflow occlusion and cardiotomy, and as an aid to anesthetic control	Increases oxygen content of hemoglobin, plasma, and tissues, with resultant increased margin of safety to ischemia
	For relief and prevention of traumatic ischemia, as after severance of main vessel(s) to a limb	
	In treatment of carbon monoxide and cyanide poisoning	
	In treatment of decompression shock in divers and aviators	
Potentiation of ionizing radiation	During radiotherapy, reducing total dose needed for therapeutic effect	Enhances production of active radicles in aqueous solution and increases oxygenation and threefore radiosensitivity of some cancer cells
Inhibition of bacterial growth and toxin production	In control and treatment of gas gangrene infection (*Clostridium welchii*)	Inhibits toxin production
	Possibly in management of large burned surfaces and in aiding wound healing	Exerts bacteriostatic and wound-drying effect

FURTHER READING

Behnke AR, Saltzman HA (1967): Hyperbaric oxygenation. N Engl J Med 276:1423, 1478

Fundamentals of Hyperbaric Medicine (1966): National Academy of Sciences, National Research Council, Pub. No. 1298 Washington, DC

JOHN A. BEVAN

71. VASOACTIVE POLYPEPTIDES

BRADYKININ, ANGIOTENSIN AND SUBSTANCE P

A number of pharmacologically active polypeptides have been extracted from tissues or prepared by the action of enzymes on plasma proteins. Three such polypeptides with dominant actions on smooth muscle are described in Table 71–1. Their physiologic role, if any, is not understood; they may be important in some disease states, but are not used therapeutically.

TABLE 71–1. Characteristics of Three Vasoactive Polypeptides: Biologic Pathways of Change Are Indicated by Arrows: Enzymes Effecting Change Are Italicized

Characteristic	Bradykinin (kallidin)	Angiotensin	Substance P
Precursor or source Activating enzymes	Bradykininogen (a-2-globulin) *Kallikrein (also trypsin, snake venom)*	Angiotensinogen (a-2-globulin) *Renin* Angiotensin I (inert, decapeptide) *Converting enzyme*	Brain, intestine (Extraction purification)
Active agent	Bradykinin (nonapeptide) Lysl-bradykinin Methionyl-lysl-bradykinin	Angiotensin II, (octapeptide)	Polypeptide (MW ~ 1700)
Fate	*Kininase* Inactive fragments	*Angiotensinase* Inactive fragments	Unknown; possibly inactive fragments
Pharmacologic actions	1. Vasodilation-hypotension	1. Vasoconstriction-hypertension by direct action on vascular smooth muscle and by facilitation of transmitter release	1. Vasodilation
	2. Action on nonvascular smooth muscle: a. Contraction of rat uterus and guinea pig ileum in vitro b. Bronchoconstriction in vivo	2. Contraction of nonvascular smooth muscle.	2. Increased intestinal motility
	3. Increased capillary permeability	3. Action on kidney a. Antidiuresis in man and due to vasoconstriction b. Mild antidiuresis followed by sodium diuresis in rodents	3. Sedation
	4. Mobilization of leukocytes	4. Stimulation of aldosterone secretion	
	5. Production of pain by stimulation of nerve endings		
Possible physiologic or pathologic significance	Possible involvement in inflammatory response	1. Possible role in certain hypertensive states 2. Regulation of aldosterone secretion	1. Possible role in regulation of peristaltic activity 2. Possible role in function of central nervous system
Clinical uses	None	Has been used to treat hypotensive conditions	

FURTHER READING

von Euler US, Eliasson R (1967): Prostaglandins. Med Chem 8:1

JOHN A. BEVAN

72. VITAMINS

This chapter contains a synopsis of our knowledge of vitamins, their sources and uses in the human being. A depressingly high percentage of the world's population is underfed and presumably exhibits vitamin deficiencies. Otherwise except in infants, some pregnant women and patients with some specific disorder (Ch. 8), it is hard to justify routine supplementation of the diet by vitamin preparations.

TABLE 72–1. Vitamins

VITAMIN A: Vitamin A_1 (retinol); vitamin A_2 (dehydroretinol). Precursor is β-carotene. All have vitamin A activity

Properties

Red or yellow crystals, fat-soluble, water-insoluble. Easily oxidized in presence of oxygen. Often used as yellow coloring for food (e.g., in oleomargarine)

Physiologic function

1. Prosthetic group for photosensitive pigments of retinal rods and cones
2. Essential to normal function of epithelial cells, osteoblasts and odontoblasts
3. Peripheral antagonist to estrogens
4. Essential to normal pregnancy and fetal development

Normal requirements

Recommended daily allowance (IU)

Infant	1500
Child (under 12)	2000–4500
Adult	5000
Pregnant woman	6000
Lactating woman	8000

Minimum daily requirement (U.S.P.U.)

Infant	1500
Child (under 12)	3000
Adult	4000

Food sources

Fish liver oils, liver, eggs, milk, butter, green leafy and yellow vegetables

Suggested clinical applications

Prophylactic in conditions impairing vitamin utilization
Curative in various optic and visual disorders, hyperkeratosis and various other skin disorders, hyperestrogenism

Therapeutic dosage

25,000–100,000 IU/day, orally.

Untoward effects

Hypervitaminosis with symptoms of hard tender lumps in extremities, cortical thickening of bones, affections of skin and mucosa, fatigue and possibly hepatomegaly or jaundice

VITAMIN B_1: Thiamine. Thiamine pyrophosphate-cocarboxylase is active form

Properties

Colorless crystals, water-soluble, fat-insoluble. Thermolabile except in acid solution. Stable to oxygen but not to oxidizing agents or ultraviolet light

Physiologic function

1. Prosthetic group in metabolism of α-keto acids
2. Essential in energy metabolism of neurons and cardiac muscle

(continued)

TABLE 72–1. *(continued)*

3. Essential to production of acetylcholine
4. Necessary in detoxification of pyruvate

Normal requirements

Recommended daily allowance (mg)

Infant	0.4
Child (under 12)	0.5–1.0
Adult	0.8–1.4
Pregnant woman	1.0
Lactating woman	1.2

Minimum daily requirement (mg)

Infant	0.25
Child (under 12)	0.5–0.75
Adult	1.0

Food sources

Yeast, whole grains, pork, liver, fresh green vegetables; much lost in cooking

Suggested clinical applications

Beriberi (three forms), polyneuritis, alcoholism, Wernicke's psychosis, cardiac disease, lead poisoning, other neuritides

Therapeutic dosage

5-30 mg/day

Untoward effects

May produce anaphylactic-type reaction when given IV

VITAMIN B$_2$: Riboflavin

Properties

Orange-yellow crystals. Water- and alcohol-soluble, fat-insoluble. Thermostable dry. Stable to oxygen. Unstable to light and alkali

Physiologic function

1. Prosthetic group of several coenzymes involved in many redox systems
2. Necessary to normal growth and development of fetus
3. Essential to health of tissues of ectodermal origin, including CNS
4. Has role in release of ACTH from pituitary
5. Shares with vitamin A and nicotinamide in visual process

Normal requirements

Recommended daily allowance (mg)

Infant	0.6
Child (under 12)	0.8–1.4
Adult	1.2–1.7
Pregnant woman	1.6
Lactating woman	1.0

Minimum daily requirement (mg)

Infant	0.6
Child (under 12)	0.9
Adult	1.2

Food sources

Yeast, liver, organ meats, milk, leafy vegetables, muscle meats, egg white

Suggested clinical applications

Deficiency characterized by seborrheic lesions, glossitis, ocular disorders, anogenital pruritus and exhaustion; may occur with pellagra

Therapeutic dosage

10 mg/day

Untoward effects

None known

NIACIN: Nicotinic acid. Nicotinamide is the naturally occurring form. Precursor is tryptophan

Properties

White crystals or powder. Soluble in water and alcohol; insoluble in fat solvents. Stable to heat and oxidizing agents

Physiologic function

1. Prosthetic group of coenzymes I and II, which have role in carbohydrate and protein metabolism and in cell respiration
2. Has role with B vitamins in maintaining healthy CNS, skin and GI tract

(continued)

TABLE 72—1. *(continued)*

Normal requirements

Recommended daily allowance (mg)

Infant	6
Child (under 12)	9—16
Adult	13—22
Pregnant woman	17
Lactating woman	21

Minimum daily requirement (mg)

Child under 6	5.0
Child over 6	7.5
Adult	10.0

Food sources

Yeast, liver, organ meats, milk, eggs

Suggested clinical applications

Nicotinamide: Pellagra, radiation sickness, sprue, dermatosis of alimentary or toxic origin, delirium tremens, scurvy (with vitamin C)

Therapeutic dosage

Niacinamide:	100—1000 mg/day
Nicotinic acid:	150— 450 mg/day

Untoward effects

Nicotinic acid: Oral administration may cause flushing, nausea, vomiting and vertigo. Parenteral administration may cause sudden fall in blood pressure or anaphylaxis

VITAMIN B_6: Pyridoxine, pyridoxol

Properties

Soluble in water, alcohol and acetone. Stable to heat, acid and alkali, but not to light

Physiologic function

1. Acts as coenzyme in many steps of amino acid metabolism
2. Has role in synthesis of unsaturated fatty acids from protein
3. Necessary to health of entire organism, especially CNS and skin

Normal requirements

Recommended daily allowance

Not established, but thought to be about 1.5—2.0 mg/day for adults (requirement increased with increased protein consumption)

Minimum daily requirement

Not established

Food sources

Yeast, liver, meats, fish, whole grains, corn, legumes

Suggested clinical applications

Idiopathic and metabolic neurologic disorders, certain dermatoses, hyperemesis gravidarum and other prolonged vomiting, radiation sickness. Supportively in other B-complex deficiencies and in prolonged isoniazid therapy

Therapeutic dosage

25—100 mg/day

Untoward effects

None known

VITAMIN B_{12}: Cyanocobalamin

Properties

Red crystals. Water soluble. Hygroscopic, stable at room temperature and to boiling in neutral aqueous solutions. Unstable in alkaline or heated acid solutions

Physiologic function

1. Essential to normal metabolism of carbohydrates, fats and protein
2. Important to maturation of erythrocytes, neural function and growth

Normal requirements

Recommended daily allowance

Not established, but estimated at 3—5 μg/day in diet (1—1.5 μg absorbed).

Minimum daily requirement

Not established

Food sources

Liver, organ meats, beef, pork, eggs, dairy products

Suggested clinical applications

Pernicious anemia; supportively in megaloblastic anemia caused by vitamin B_{12} deficiency and in various neuritides

(continued)

TABLE 72–1. *(continued)*

Therapeutic dosage

For pernicious anemia: 100–200 μg IM daily for a wk; then monthly for life

Untoward effects

None known

VITAMIN C: Ascorbic acid

Properties

White crystals. Water soluble. Unstable to oxidizing agents, alkalis, and certain metals

Physiologic function

1. Important in redox systems and certain other metabolic processes
2. Essential to normal growth, especially of bones and teeth
3. Role as antistress factor, including effect on adrenals and antiinfectious action
4. Antiscorbutic effect

Normal requirements

Recommended daily allowance (mg)

Infant	30	
Child (under 12)	40–80	Adult
Adult	70–80	
Pregnant woman	100	
Lactating woman	100	

Minimum daily requirement (mg)

Infant	10
Child (under 12)	20
Adult	30

Food sources

Citrus fruits, parsley, green peppers, vegetables of the cabbage family

Suggested clinical applications

Scurvy and other vitamin C deficiencies; supportive in infectious disease (especially tuberculosis); possible prevention of the common cold

Therapeutic dosage

100–120 mg/day

Untoward effects

None known

VITAMIN D: Ergocalciferol (vitamin D_2); cholecalciferol (vitamin D_3)

Properties

Odorless crystalline compounds. Soluble in fats and fat solvents, insoluble in water. Slightly sensitive to light

Physiologic function

Regulates calcium and phosphorus metabolism and is thus necessary to normal growth of bone and normal muscle function

Normal requirements

400 IU for all ages

Food sources

Fish liver oils, eggs, dairy products, sunlight

Suggested clinical applications

Rickets, osteomalacia, infantile tetany, acute lead poisoning, lupus vulgaris, hypoparathyroidism, adjunctively in disorders of renal function

Therapeutic dosage

400–4000 IU/day, orally

Untoward effects

Hypervitaminosis D may result in severe disturbances of calcium and phosphorus metabolism

FOLIC ACID: Pteroylmonoglutamic acid

Properties

Orange-yellow crystals, tasteless, odorless. Slightly soluble in water, insoluble in fat solvent. Thermostable in basic or neutral solutions, unstable to heat in acid solutions. Decomposed by light

(continued)

TABLE 72—1. *(continued)*

Physiologic function
1. Provitamin of citrovorum factor
2. Associated with vitamin B_{12} in nucleic acid synthesis and nucleoprotein function
3. Active in metabolism of amino acids, purines and pyrimidines
4. Necessary to utilization of pantothenic acid by organism
5. Essential to growth and reproduction
6. Important in erythropoiesis

Normal requirements
Recommended daily allowance
Not established; thought to be approximately 0.05 mg
Minimum daily requirement
Not established

Food sources
Leafy green vegetables, yeast, liver, kidney

Suggested clinical applications
Megaloblastic anemia; adjunctively in diseases with concomitant anemia, in acute leukemia of infancy and in certain complications of pregnancy

Therapeutic dosage
1—15 mg/day

Untoward effects
May mask pernicious anemia, leading to spinal cord damage

BIOTIN: α-Biotin; β-biotin

Properties
Soluble in water and alcohol. Stable to heat. Inactivated by acids, alkalies, rancid fats and choline

Physiologic function
1. Coenzyme for certain carboxylations
2. Necessary to utilization of pantothenic acid
3. Important in ectodermal metabolism
4. May be involved in biosynthesis of fatty acids, amino acids and proteins

Normal requirements
Recommended daily allowance
Not established; probably 150—300 μg
Minimum daily requirement
Not established

Food sources
Present in all foods and synthesized by intestinal flora

Suggested clinical applications
Dermatoses (acne, furunculosis, seborrhea of infancy)

Therapeutic dosage
Not established

Untoward effects
None known

PANTOTHENIC ACID: Usually prepared as the calcium salt or the alcohol-panthenol

Properties
Yellow, viscous oil. Soluble in water. Unstable to heat, acid and alkali. Calcium salt is thermostable and water-soluble

Physiologic function
1. Component of coenzyme A
2. Important to adrenal function, antibody production and epidermal growth

Normal requirements
Recommended daily allowance
Not established; estimated at 10 mg
Minimum daily requirement
Not established

Food sources
Yeast, organ meats, egg yolk, vegetables

(continued)

TABLE 72–1. *(continued)*

Suggested clinical applications

Adjunctively in pituitary adenoma, Addison's disease, cirrhosis, diabetes, postoperative intestinal atony, wound healing and poisoning due to isoniazid

Therapeutic dosage

50–500 mg/day

Untoward effects

None known

VITAMIN E: The tocopherols α, β, and γ are the most common of the seven forms; α is most active

Properties

α, β, and γ tocopherols are viscous oils, insoluble in water; stable to heat, light and acid in absence of oxygen. Unstable to ultraviolet light, alkali, oxidizing agent, rancid fats. Esters are more stable

Physiologic function

1. Protective effects against oxidation of fatty acids, certain types of liver degeneration, erythrocyte hemolysis, anoxia and hyperoxia of the lungs
2. Role in normal function of kidney, muscle, respiratory enzyme systems and pituitary
3. Role in formation of dental enamel and liver tissue

Normal requirements

Recommended daily allowance
Not established; thought to vary between 10-30 mg for adults; 0.5 mg/kg for infants
Minimum daily requirement
Not established

Food sources

Vegetable oils, cereals, eggs. Not destroyed by cooking

Suggested clinical applications

In acute carbon tetrachloride poisoning, as protective liver therapy; adjunctively in various degenerative diseases and anemias; may be useful as nonspecific antioxidant especially if body contains unsaturated lipids; may protect lipid constituents against formation of toxic peroxides

Therapeutic dosage

Not known; may be 50–300 mg

Untoward effects

None known

VITAMIN K: Menadione; phytonadione (vitamin K_1)

Properties

Menadione: Yellow crystals, insoluble in water, soluble in alcohol and vegetable oils. Stable in air; unstable to light, alkalis and reducing agents

Physiologic function

Essential to production of prothrombin and, thus, to normal blood clotting

Normal requirements

Not established

Food sources

Leafy green vegetables, tomatoes, liver

Suggested clinical applications

Prophylactic in hemorrhagic diathesis of newborn, prior to liver surgery, during prolonged antibiotic therapy
Curative in prothrombinopenia, overdosage of coumarol-type anticoagulants, bite of various pit vipers

Therapeutic dosage

Varies with K-analog used and indication

Untoward effects

May cause temporary refractoriness to anticoagulant. Overdosage in infants may result in hemolytic anemia or kernicterus

Modified from Pearson S (1968): **Table on Vitamins.** Roche Laboratories, Division of Hoffmann-La Roche, Inc., Nutley, NJ

JEREMY H. THOMPSON

73. IMMUNOBIOLOGIC AGENTS AND ACTIVE IMMUNIZATION

Active immunization is produced by stimulation of host defense mechanisms (antibody) by administered vaccines. The resulting immunity may last a lifetime or only a few months. Vaccines are prepared from microorganisms or their products (toxins) that have been changed so that they retain their antigenic potential but have lost their ability to produce disease. Reduction of pathogenicity may be produced by heat or formaldehyde inactivation (**killed vaccines**) or by the development of attenuated strains (**live vaccines**) of organisms. Usually artificially induced immunity is less satisfactory than that resulting from the corresponding natural infections. Furthermore, killed microorganisms are usually less effective than attenuated microorganisms. There are 20 active immunizing agents presently available (Table 73–1), the first 6 being recommended for all healthy infants. Table 73–2 gives the recommended schedule for active immunization and tuberculin testing of normal infants and children; it is based upon the recommendations on immunization policies and procedures formulated by the Advisory Committee on Immunization Practices (ACIP) of the United States Public Health Service, and the Committee of Infectious Diseases of the American Academy of Pediatrics.*

Smallpox

The United States Public Health Service and the Committee on Infectious Diseases of the American Academy of Pediatrics have recently revised

* A variety of immunobiologic agents and drugs is available from the USPHS, Center for Disease Control. These agents are listed in Tables 54-2, 73-3, 73-4, 73-5. They can be obtained by calling the Center for Disease Control, telephone, (8:00am–4:30pm), [404] 633-3311, or (4:30pm–8:00am), [404] 633-2176.

their recommendations concerning routine vaccination against smallpox.

The risk of contacting smallpox in the United States is so low that the routine, compulsory vaccination of infants and children should be abandoned; smallpox vaccination occasionally results in severe adverse reactions which may be fatal. Smallpox vaccination is still recommended for all medical and hospital personnel, and for all travelers to areas where smallpox is endemic or where vaccination is required. Individuals who require smallpox vaccination and who have a contraindication to its administration may be managed successfully with adjunct therapy with gamma globulin and methisazone (Ch. 66).

Gamma Globulin Therapy

Many antibody deficiencies can be treated successfully with repeated IM injections of human gamma globulin. Gamma globulin is of no value in pure cellular immuno deficiencies, but may be of limited value in those patients with combined antibody and cellular immunodeficiency.

Immune Serum Globulin (human) *U.S.P.,* is prepared by alcoholic fractionation of pooled human serum from about 500 donors. Fractionation removes most other serum proteins and the hepatitis virus. It is reconstituted as a sterile 16.5% solution, and it contains 95% IgG with trace quantities of IgA and IgM and other serum proteins. IgA and IgM globulins are therapeutically insignificant in view of their rapid half-life (about 7 days compared to about 25 days for IgG), and their low concentration.

Patients on long term gamma globulin therapy require more frequent injections during times of infection, since the rate of protein catabolism is increased.

Gamma globulin is given IM, and care should be taken in children not to give more than 5 ml

TABLE 73–1. Active Immunizing Agents

Diphtheria (toxoid)	Influenza
Tetanus (toxoid)	Mumps
Pertussis antigen	Tularemia
Poliomyelitis	Typhus
Measles	Rocky Mountain spotted fever
Rubella	Cholera
BCG	Plague
Yellow fever	Adenovirus
Rabies	Vaccinia
Typhoid	Anthrax

Krugman A, Ward R (1973): Active immunization for the prevention of infectious diseases in *Infectious Diseases of Children and Adults* (5th ed) Ch. 33. St. Louis, CV Mosby, and Immunobiologic agents and drugs. The Center for Disease Control, United States Public Health Service, Atlanta, Ga.

TABLE 73–2. Recommended Schedule for Active Immunization and Tuberculin Testing of Normal Infants and Children

2 mo	DTP, type 1 OPV, or trivalent OPV*
4 mo	DTP, type 3 OPV, or trivalent OPV
6 mo	DTP, type 2 OPV, or trivalent OPV
9-11 mo	Tuberculin test
12 mo	Measles vaccine, Rubella (mumps)
15-18 mo	DTP, trivalent OPV
2 yr	Tuberculin test
3 yr	DTP, tuberculin test
4 yr	Tuberculin test
6 yr	TD, tuberculin test,† trivalent OPV
8 yr	Tuberculin test†
10 yr	Tuberculin test†
12 yr	TD, tuberculin test‡
14 yr	Tuberculin test†
16 yr	Tuberculin test†

*OPV, oral polio vaccine. If trivalent OPV is used, interval should be 6 weeks or longer.

DPT, diphtheria and tetanus toxoids and pertussis vaccine combined.

TD, tetanus and diphtheria toxoids, adult type.

Immunization may be started at any age. The immune response is limited in a proportion of young infants, and the recommended booster doses are designed to ensure or maintain immunity. Protection of infants against pertussis should start early. The best protection of newborn infants against pertussis is avoidance of household contacts by adequate immunization of older siblings. This schedule is intended as a flexible guide that may be modified within certain limits to fit individual situations.

†Frequency of repeated tuberculin tests depends on the risk of exposure of children under care and the prevalence of tuberculosis in the population group.

‡After age 12 follow procedure recommended for adults, i.e., combined tetanus and diphtheria toxoid booster every 10 years as TD.

Krugman A, Ward R (1973): Active immunization for the prevention of infectious diseases, in *Infectious Diseases of Children and Adults* (5th ed) Ch. 33. St. Louis, CV Mosby.

in any one site. In adults, the maximum volume per injection site can be doubled. The usual dose in adults and children is 100 mg/kg/month (0.7ml/kg).

Adverse Reactions

Various manifestations of allergy may develop. Anaphylactic shock however, is rare, and following such an occurrence the subject should be tested for the presence or absence of hypersensitivity to gamma globulin from different manufacturers. Local muscle pain, sterile abcess formation and nerve damage may result from injection trauma.

In patients with isolated IgA deficiency, anaphylactic shock is particularly likely to occur to the trace quantities of IgA present in most gamma globulin preparations.

TABLE 73–3. Immunobiologic Agents and Drugs Procured, Distributed and Stored by Immunobiologics Activity, Center for Disease Control (CDC), with Information about their Source, Licensure and Investigational New Drug (IND) Application

Biologic	Source	Licensed or IND approved	Distributed to	Conditions for distribution	Storage
Antitoxins					
Botulinum Equine antitoxin (ABE)	Connaught Laboratories	Licensed	MD as required	Emergency	4° C
Diphtheria (Equine) antitoxin	Merrell-Nat'l Laboratories	Licensed	MD as required	Emergency	4° C
Antivenin					
North American coral snake *(Micrurus fulvius)* Antivenin (Equine)	Wyeth Laboratories	Licensed	MD as required	Emergency	4° C in *8 SE* states; Calif., Ill., Md., Nev., N.J., Ohio, Okla., Texas and Wisc.
Globulins and Plasmas					
Vaccinia immune globulin (VIG)	Hyland Laboratories	Licensed	MD as required	Emergency	4° C
Western Equine Encephalitis (WEE) immune globulin	CDC	IND approved	MD as required	Emergency	-20° C
Zoster Immune Globulin (ZIG)	CDC	IND approved	MD as required	Emergency	-20° C
Immune plasma:					
Calif. E.	CDC		MD as required	Emergency	-20° C
EEE	CDC		MD as required	Emergency	-20° C
Herpes simian B	CDC		MD as required	Emergency	-20° C
Junin	CDC		MD as required	Emergency	-20° C
Lassa fever	CDC		MD as required	Emergency	-20° C
Machupo	CDC		MD as required	Emergency	-20° C
RSSE	CDC		MD as required	Emergency	-20° C
SLE	CDC		MD as required	Emergency	-20° C
WEE	CDC		MD as required	Emergency	-20° C
Niclosamide (Yomesan)	Farbenfabriken, Germany	IND approved	MD as required	Emergency	Room temp.
Pentamidine isethionate (Lomidine)	May & Baker, Ltd., British Isles	IND approved	MD as required	Emergency	4° C
Skin test antigens					
Tularemia skin test antigen	CDC	IND approved	MD as required		4° C
Vaccines					
Anthrax vaccine, absorbed	Michigan State Health Laboratories	Licensed	MD as required	Prophylaxis	4° C
Botulinum toxoid, pentavalent (ABCDE)	Ft. Detrick (Parke, Davis)	IND approved	Investigators	Physician-to-physician basis	4° C
Eastern equine encephalitis (EEE) vaccine, inactivated, dried	Merrell-Nat'l Laboratories	IND approved	Investigators	Physician-to-physician basis	-20° C
Tularemia vaccine, live, attenuated	Merrell-Nat'l Laboratories	IND approved	Investigators	Physician-to-physician basis	-20° C
Venezuelan equine encephalitis (VEE) vaccine	Merrell-Nat'l Laboratories	IND approved	Investigators	Physician-to-physician basis	-20° C

TABLE 73—4. Recommended Treatment Dosages and Frequencies of Administration of Antitoxins and Antivenins Available from the Center for Disease Control

Clinical disease	Immunobiologic agent	Dosage	Interval
Botulism (types A,B,E)	Botulinum antitoxin, trivalent (Equine) types A, B and E	1 vial IV, 1 vial IM	Further similar dosages in 2—4 hr if signs or symptoms worsen
Diphtheria	Diphtheria antitoxin (purified, concentrated globulin, equine)	20,000—80,000 units or more IM or slow IV drip, depending upon site, severity, duration of infection	Additional similar dosages in 24 hr if local or general improvement is not apparent. Continue until symptoms controlled, or other etiologic agent identified
Coral snake envenomation	North American coral snake *(Micrurus fulvius)* antivenin (equine)	3—5 vials (30—50 ml) by slow IV injection or drip (in 250—500 ml to run in over 30 min)	Additional similar dosages as required. Response to treatment may be rapid and dramatic

TABLE 73—5. Recommended Prophylactic Dosages and Frequencies of Administration of Antitoxins and Globulins Available from the Center for Disease Control

Disease entity	Immunobiologic agent	Dosage	Interval
Botulism (types A,B,E)	Botulinum antitoxin trivalent (equine) types A, B and E	1/5 to 1 vial IM*. Details and precautions supplied with antitoxin	Single dosage; may repeat one dosage if signs or symptoms occur
Chickenpox, Herpes Zoster	Zoster immune globulin (ZIG) (human)	Details and precautions supplied with globulin	Single dosage
Complications of smallpox inoculation, etc.	Vaccinia immune globulin (VIG) (human)	0.3—0.6 ml/kg IM (never administer IV†)	Single dosage only; may be repeated at discretion of physician
Diphtheria	Diphtheria antitoxin (purified, concentrated globulin, equine)	1000—5000 units IM* Details and precautions supplied with antitoxin	Single dosage
Western equine encephalitis (WEE)	Western equine encephalitis (WEE) immune globulin (human)	5—10 ml IM (never administer IV†)	Single dosage

* Denotes intramuscular route of administration
† Denotes intravenous route of administration

FURTHER READING

Buescher EL (1967): Immunization for foreign travel. Med Clin North Am 51:843

Chanock RM (1970): Control of acute mycoplasmal and viral respiratory tract diseases. Science 169:248—256

Immunization information for international travel. United States Public Health Service Publications No. 384, Washington, DC, GPO, July 1967-1968.

Report of the Committee on the Control of Infectious Diseases (1966): 5th ed Evanston, American Academy of Pediatrics

Stiehm ER, Fulginiti VA (1973): Immunologic Diseases in Infants and Children. Philadelphia, London, Toronto, W.B. Sanders

JEREMY H. THOMPSON

74. DRUG INTERACTIONS AND INCOMPATIBILITY

Therapeutics is the pouring of drugs of which one knows nothing into a patient of whom one knows less.
Voltaire

The whole problem of drug incompatibility is changing as our knowledge of drug metabolism enlarges. The term "incompatibility" comes from the Latin *in* (not) and *compactilis* (to join together). Drug incompatibility exists if the therapeutic aim of the physician has been invalidated by the interaction of administered therapeutic agents. Incompatibility can either be physical, chemical or therapeutic.

Physical incompatibility occurs if the physical state of the individual drugs in a mixture changes when the drugs are blended. Amphotericin B, e.g., precipitates if it is mixed with normal saline instead of 5% dextrose (Ch. 65). **Chemical incompatibility** occurs when components of a drug mixture interact chemically. For example, IV methicillin should not be given in 5% dextrose solutions since the antibiotic is destroyed at an acid pH (Ch. 55).

Physical and chemical incompatibility are frequently produced by the careless mixing of drugs for parenteral administration (Table 74–1). In many instances there is observable evidence of incompatibility, such as color change, gas evolution or formed precipitate. However, a reduction of therapeutic potency can occur *without any observable signs.* While obvious evidence of incompatibility does not imply total loss of therapeutic potency, drug mixtures showing evidence of interactions should not be used. It should be stressed that our knowledge of physical and chemical drug incompatibilities is limited and that Table 74–1 represents only a partial list. Realistically, *data on compatibility of the majority of mixtures of specific agents are not known.*

Therapeutic incompatibility results when drugs interact in the patient (Ch. 4). Although "blunderbuss" therapy, with complex fixed-dosage preparations, is rare today, there is still a psychologic appeal in prescribing more than one drug. A recent study revealed that an average of 14 other drugs (range 6–32) were prescribed for each patient taking sodium methicillin. Another report indicated that of 138 randomly selected IV solutions, 24% contained 2 drugs and 14% contained five or more drugs. In many instances, this polypharmacy may lead to serious drug interactions. The problem is compounded when a patient is seen by several specialists, each of whom is ignorant of the others' therapy.

In Table 74–2 some common therapeutic drug incompatibilities are listed. Where known, the mechanism of the interaction is indicated as well.

TABLE 74–1. Some Important Physical and Chemical Drug Incompatibilities

	Aminophylline	Ammonium Chloride	Amobarbital Sodium	Ascorbic Acid	Benzyl Alcohol	Calcium Chloride	Calcium Gluconate - Glucoheptonate	Chloromycetin Succinate #	Chlorpheniramine Maleate	Chlortetracycline HCl	Chlorothiazide Na (Diuril Sodium)	Corticotrophin Aqueous	Dextran	Dextrose	Diphenhydramine HCl (Benadryl HCl)	Diphenylhydantoin Na (Dilantin Na)	Ephedrine Sulfate	Epinephrine HCl (Adrenalin HCl)
Aminophylline				I												I		
Ammonium Chloride																		
Amobarbital Sodium															I			
Benzyl Alcohol								I										
Blood (Whole)																		
Calcium Chloride									I	I								
Calcium Gluconate																		
Chlorpheniramine Maleate						I												
Chloromycetin Succinate #					I											I		
Chlortetracycline (Aureomycin)						I				H			I					
Corticotrophin Aqueous																		
Dexamethasone-21-Phosphate																		
Dextran				I						I								
Dextrose																		
Dihydromorphinone HCl																		
Dimenhydrinate (Dramamine)	I	I	I													I		
Diphenylhydantoin Sodium	I							I							I			
Ephedrine Sulfate																		
Epinephrine HCl (Adrenalin HCl)																		
Erythromycin Glucoheptonate #								I								I		
Heparin Sodium																		
Hyaluronidase (Wydase)																		I
Hydrocortisone Succinate			I														I	
Hydroxyzine HCl (Vistaril HCl)	I		I					I								I		
Insulin Aqueous			I								I					I		
Kanamycin Sulfate (Kantrex)														I		I		
Levarterenol Bitartrate (Levophed Bitartrate)			I						I		I					I		
Lincomycin HCl (Lincocin)																I		
Magnesium Sulfate							I											
Methicillin Sodium (Dimocillin)																		
Metarminol Bitartrate (Aramine)																I		
Morphine Sulfate	I		I								I					I		

	Erythromycin Glucoheptonate #	Heparin Sodium	Hyaluronidase (Wydase)	Hydrocortisone Succinate	Hydroxyzine HCl (Vistaril HCl)	Insulin, Aqueous	Kanamycin Sulfate	Levarterenol Bitartrate	Magnesium Sulfate	Meperidine HCl (Demerol HCl)	Metaraminol Bitartrate (Aramine)	Methicillin Sodium	Narcotic Salts +	Nitrofurantoin Na (Furadantin Na)	Novobiocin Sodium	Oxytetracycline HCl (Terramycin HCl)	Penicillin G, K or Na	Pentobarbital Na
Aminophylline					I					I			I			I		
Ammonium Chloride													I					
Amobarbital Sodium				I	I	I		I		I			I					
Benzyl Alcohol																		
Blood (Whole)								I			X							
Calcium Chloride																		
Calcium Gluconate									I						I			
Chlorpheniramine Maleate								I										I
Chloromycetin Succinate #	I				I										I	I		
Chlortetracycline (Aureomycin)																		
Corticotrophin Aqueous															I			
Dexamethasone-21-Phosphate																		
Dextran																		
Dextrose							I								I			
Dihydromorphinone HCl																		
Dimenhydrinate (Dramamine)		I		I	I													I
Diphenylhydantoin Sodium	I				I	I	I	I		I	I		I			I	I	I
Ephedrine Sulfate				I														I
Epinephrine HCl (Adrenalin HCl)			I												I			
Erythromycin Glucoheptonate #		I													I			I
Heparin Sodium	I		I	I	I		I			I			I		I			
Hyaluronidase (Wydase)		I																
Hydrocortisone Succinate		I					I				I	I			I	I		I
Hydroxyzine HCl (Vistaril HCl)		I															I	I
Insulin Aqueous														I	I			I
Kanamycin Sulfate (Kantrex)		I		I														
Levarterenol Bitartrate (Levophed Bitartrate)														I	I			I
Lincomycin HCl (Lincocin)																	I	
Magnesium Sulfate															I			
Methicillin Sodium (Dimocillin)				I						I	I		I					
Metarminol Bitartrate (Aramine)				I							X	I					I	
Morphine Sulfate		I								I		I		I	I			

	Phenobarbital Sodium	Procaine HCl	Prochlorperazine Maleate (Compazine)	Promazine HCl (Sparine HCl)	Protein Hydrolysate	Sodium Bicarbonate	Sodium Iodide	Streptomycin Sulfate	Succinylcholine Chloride	Sulfadiazine Sodium	Sulfisoxazole Diethanolamine (Gantrisin)	Tetracycline HCl	Thiopental Na (Pentothal Na)	Vancomycin HCl	Vitamin B-12	Vitamin B Complex with Ascorbic Acid	Vitamin K_1	Warfarin Na (Panwarfin Na)
Aminophylline		I	I											I		I		
Ammonium Chloride											I							
Amobarbital Sodium		I						I				I		I				
Benzyl Alcohol																		
Blood (Whole)																	X	
Calcium Chloride																		
Calcium Gluconate			I					I										
Chlorpheniramine Maleate																		
Chloromycetin Succinate #			I									I		I				
Chlortetracycline (Aureomycin)				*	I													
Corticotrophin Aqueous						I												
Dexamethasone-21-Phosphate			I											I				
Dextran																	I	
Dextrose															I			I
Dihydromorphinone HCl						I							I					
Dimenhydrinate (Dramamine)	I		I										I					
Diphenylhydantoin Sodium	I	I	I					I			I	I		I		I	I	
Ephedrine Sulfate	I												I					
Epinephrine HCl (Adrenalin HCl)																		*
Erythromycin Glucoheptonate #	I							I				I						
Heparin Sodium			I					I				I		I				
Hyaluronidase (Wydase)																		
Hydrocortisone Succinate	I		I									I		I		I		
Hydroxyzine HCl (Vistaril HCl)	I										I					I		
Insulin Aqueous	I					I				I	I		I					
Kanamycin Sulfate (Kantrex)	I										I							
Levarterenol Bitartrate (Levophed Bitartrate)	I					I	I	I		I	I		I					
Lincomycin HCl (Lincocin)																		
Magnesium Sulfate		I				I												
Methicillin Sodium (Dimocillin)			I			I								I				
Metarminol Bitartrate (Aramine)													*					*
Morphine Sulfate	I					I	I			I	I		I					

Row labels (drugs) for the compatibility matrix:

- Narcotic Salts +
- Nitrofurantoin Na (Furadantin Na)
- Novobiocin Sodium (Albamycin)
- Oxytetracycline HCl (Terramycin)
- Penicillin G, K or Na
- Pentobarbital Sodium
- Phenobarbital Sodium (Luminal Na)
- Phenylephrine HCl (Neo-Synephrine)
- Prednisolone-21-Phosphate
- Procaine HCl
- Prochlorperazine Maleate
- Promazine HCl (Sparine)
- Promethazine HCl (Phenergan HCl)
- Secobarbital Sodium (Seconal Na)
- Sodium Bicarbonate
- Sodium Cephalothin (Keflin)
- Sodium Iodide
- Streptomycin Sulfate
- Succinylcholine Chloride
- Sulfadiazine Sodium
- Sulfisoxazole Diethanolamine (Gantrisin)
- Tetracycline HCl (Achromycin HCl)
- Thiopental Sodium (Pentothal Na)
- Tripelennamine HCl (Pyribenzamine HCl)
- Vancomycin HCl (Vancocin)
- Vitamin B-12 (Rubramin)
- Vitamin B Complex with C (Folbesyn)
- Vitamin K₁ (Aqua-Mephyton)
- Warfarin Sodium (Panwarfin)

Patel JA: A guide to physical compatibility of intravenous drug admixtures. Amer J Hosp Pharm 23:409.

Legend:

I   Incompatible

*   Incompatible in 5% dextrose injection

Dissolve first in water for injection

X   Therapeutic dose must be diluted with large volume prior to infusion

A   Incompatible in dextrose 5% injection, fructose, invert sugar, lactated Ringer's, sodium lactate, ammonium chloride

B   Incompatible in lactated Ringer's, sodium lactate

C   Incompatible in dextrose 5% injection, fructose, invert sugar, lactated Ringer's, ammonium chloride

D   Incompatible in dextrose 10% with sodium chloride, lactated Ringer's

E   Incompatible in lactated Ringer's, sodium lactate, Ringer's solution

F   Incompatible in fructose, invert sugar, lactated Ringer's, sodium lactate, ammonium chloride

G   Incompatible in ammonium chloride

H   Incompatible in lactated Ringer's, ammonium chloride, Ringer's solution.

J   Incompatible in lactated Ringer's, ammonium chloride

+   Narcotic Salts: Codeine Phosphate, Leritine HCl, Levo-Dromoran Bitartrate, Methadon HCl

TABLE 74–2. Some Important Therapeutic Drug Incompatibilities

Primary drug	Known interactants	Result
Alcohol	Furazolidone, metronidazole, nitroglycerin, sulfonylureas, tetraethyl thiuram disulfide (Antabuse)	Hypotension, nausea, vomiting, diarrhea (Antabuse-like reaction)
Alcohol	CNS depressants, narcotics, tranquilizers	Alcohol potentiates effect of the other drugs
Alcohol	Griseofulvin	Apathy, forgetfulness, impaired cerebral function
Alcohol	Vancomycin	Convulsions
Anticoagulant	Aspirin	Patients controlled on anticoagulant therapy may bleed owing to added anticoagulant effect of aspirin
Anticoagulant	Phenyramidol	Hypoprothrombinemia
Chlorpromazine	Orphenadrine	Hypoglycemia
Chlorpromazine	Dextromoramide	Hallucinations
Chlorpromazine	Trifluoperazine	Hypoglycemia
Coumarin anticoagulants	Indomethacin, oxyphenbutazone, phenylbutazone	Patients well controlled on anticoagulant therapy may bleed owing to displacement of plasma-bound coumarin
Coumarin anticoagulants	Anabolic steroids, barbiturates, chloral hydrate, clofibrate, gluthethimide, griseofulvin, phenobarbitone, primidone, D-thyroxine	Patients well controlled on anticoagulant therapy *plus* one of these drugs may bleed if second drug is discontinued without reduction of anticoagulant dosage. These drugs probably stimulate hepatic microsomal enzymes responsible for coumarin metabolism
Digitalis	Diuretics	Digitalis intoxication due to diuretic-induced potassium loss
Digitalis	Calcium gluconate	Digitalized patients rapidly develop toxic reactions if given calcium gluconate intravenously; Ca^{++} synergizes the action of glycosides
Diphenhydramine	Thioridazine	Epistaxis, dry mouth, dizziness, disorientation
Guanethidine	Methylphenidate	Cardiac arrhythmia
Imipramine	Amitriptyline	Alternating drowsiness and agitation leading to convulsions and coma
Insulin	Indomethicin	Hypoglycemia; indomethicin may block catecholamine-induced glycogenolysis
Isoniazid	Para-aminosalicylic acid, ethionamide	Severe side effects may result from isoniazid in slow inactivators (Ch. 61).
Methandrostenolone	Coumarin	High prothrombin time resistant to vitamin K_1
Methotrexate	Aspirin, sulfonamides	Displacement of methotrexate from its plasma albumin binding
α-Methyldopa	Amitriptyline	Agitation, tremor
Monoamine oxidase inhibitors	Meperidine	Exaggeration of effects of meperidine
Monoamine oxidase inhibitors	*Drugs* Alcohol, amphetamines, anesthetics (some), antihistamines (some), hypotensives (some), imipramine, metaraminol, α-methyldopa, morphine, muscle relaxants (some), pethidine, pressor agents (some), reserpine, sympathomimetics (some) *Foods* * Beer, broad beans, cheese, chicken liver, chocolate, game, pickled herrings, wines, yeast extract	Hypertensive crises and visual hallucinations (Ch. 20) may occur following any one combination
Nondepolarizing muscle relaxants	Bacitracin, colistin, kanamycin, neomycin, polymyxin B, streptomycin	Prolonged neuromuscular block
Phenylbutazone	Acetohexamide	Potentiation of acetohexamide; phenylbutazone blocks renal excretion of chief metabolite of acetohexamide, hydroxyhexamide
Phenylbutazone	Phenobarbital, promethazine	Reduced half life of phenylbutazone
Phenylhydantoin	Coumarins	Prolonged action of phenylhydantoin
Phenylhydantoin	Phenylbutazone, phenyramidol, sulfaphenazole	Prolonged action of phenylhydantoin; possible inhibition of phenylhydantoin metabolism
Phenyramidol	Phenylhydantoin	Inhibition of phenylhydantoin metabolism
Probenecid	Salicylates	Hyperuricemia; transient gout
Quinidine	Nondepolarizing and depolarizing muscle relaxants	Prolonged muscle relaxation
Reserpine	General anesthetics	Profound fall in blood pressure due to failure of compensatory mechanisms

(continued)

TABLE 74-2. (continued)

Primary drug	Known interactants	Result
Sulfonamides	Para-aminobenzoic acid-containing local anesthetics	Inactivation of sulfonamide (Ch. 60)
Sulfonylurea	Monoamine oxidase inhibitors, oxyphenbutazone, probenecid, salicylates, sulfonamides	Potentiation of hypoglycemic effect of sulfonylurea
Sympathomimetics (direct acting)	Bethanidine, bretylium, guanethidine	Hypertension
Tetracyclines	Antacids, metals, milk	Decreased tetracycline absorption
Thiazide diuretics	Glucocorticosteroids	Hyperglycemia
Tolbutamide	Sulfonamides	Hypoglycemia due to displacement of tolbutamide from albumin fraction

* Foods containing tyramine or L-dopa.

FURTHER READING

Donn R (1967): Intravenous solution manual and incompatibility file. Am J Hosp Pharm 24:459

Edward M (1967): pH: An important factor in the compatibility of additives in intravenous therapy. Am J Hosp Pharm 24:440

Fowler TJ (1967): Some incompatibilities of intravenous admixtures. Am J Hosp Pharm 24:450

Garb S (1970): Clinical Guide to Undesirable Drug Interactions and Interferences. New York, Springer Publishing Co

Gallelli JF (1967): Stability studies of drugs used in intravenous solutions. Am J Hosp Pharm 24:425

Hansten PD (1973): Drug Interactions. 2nd ed Philadelphia, Lea and Febiger

King JC (1975): Guide to Parenteral Admixtures. Cutter Laboratories

Martin EW (1971): Hazards of Medication, Philadelphia, Toronto, Lippincott

Parker EA (1967): Solution additive chemical incompatibility study. Am J Hosp Pharm 24:434

Swindler G (1971): Handbook of Drug Interactions. New York, Wiley Interscience

JEREMY H. THOMPSON

75. DRUG-INDUCED DISEASE (TABLES)

No drug escapes the stigma of causing disease (Ch. 7). This section contains tables of drugs which have been associated with specific pathology. Diagnostic difficulties abound however since in many cases the pathogenesis is not clear. The references contain a more detailed presentation of this information.

TABLE 75–1. Drugs That May Produce an Alteration in Skin Pigmentation

ACTH	Gold salts
Arsenic	Lucanthone
Bismuth	Nitrofurantoin
Bromides	Novobiocin
Catecholamines	Phenolphthalein
Chloroquine	Potassium iodide
Chlorpromazine (the "Purple People")	Quinidine
Cytotoxic agents	Quinacrine
Diphenylhydantoin	Silver salts
Estrogen-containing oral contraceptives (stimulate melanocytes)	Sulfonamides
	Zinc oxide

TABLE 75–2. Drugs That May Produce an Exanthematic Rash

Anticonvulsants	Methaminodiazepoxide
Anticholinergics	Nitrofurantoin
Antihistamines	Novobiocin
Atropine	Organic extracts
Barbiturates	Para-aminosalicylic acid
Bromides	Penicillins
Chloral hydrate	Phenothiazines
Chlordiazepoxide	Phenylbutazone
Chloroquine	Primidone
Chlorothiazide	Quinacrine
Chlorpromazine	Quinine
Diethylstilbestrol	Reserpine
Diphenylhydantoin	Salicylates
Erythromycin	Serums
Gold salts	Streptomycin
Griseofulvin	Sulfonamides
Insulin	Sulfones
Meprobamate	Tetracyclines
Mercurials	Thiouracil

TABLE 75–3. Drugs That May Produce Contact Dermatitis

Acriflavine	Mepyramine
Amethocaine	Mercurials
Antazoline	Neomycin
Antihistamines	Nitrofurazone
Arsphenamine	Novobiocin
Bacitracin	Para-aminosalicyclic acid
Benzocaine	Parabens
Benzoyl peroxide	Penicillins
Cetrimide	Peru balsam
Chloramphenicol	Phenindamine
Chlorcyclizine	Phenol
Chlorhexidine	Potassium hydroxyquinoline sulfate
Chlorhydroxyquinoline	
Chloroxylenol	Procaine
Chlorphenesin	Promethazine
Chlorpromazine	Propamidine
Crotamiton	Pyribenazmine
Cyclomethycaine	Quinacrine
Diphenhydramine	Quinine
Domiphen bromide	Resorcin
Ephedrine	Salicylates
Formaldehyde	Selenium sulfide
Gold salts	Spiramycin
Halogenated phenolic compounds	Streptomycin
	Sulfonamides
Iodine and Iodides	Sulfur and salicylic acid ointment
Iodochlorhydroxyquinoline	
Isoniazid	Tetracyclines
Lanolin	Thiamine
Menthol	Thimerosal
Meprobamate	

TABLE 75-4. Drugs That May Produce an Acneiform Eruption

ACTH	Glucocortico steroids
Androgenic hormones	Iodides
Barbiturates	Methandrostenolone
Bromides	Oral contraceptives
Diphenylhydantoin	Vitamin B_{12}

TABLE 75-5. Drugs That May Cause A Fixed Drug Eruption

Acetanilid	Meprobamate
Acetarsone	Mercury salts
Acetophenetidin	Methenamine
Acetylsalicylic acid	Neoarsphenamine
Acriflavine	Opium alkaloids
Aminopyrine	Oxophenarsine
Amobarbital	Oxytetracycline
Amodiaquine	Para-aminosalicylic acid
Amphetamine sulfate	Penicillins
Anthralin	Phenacetin
Antimony potassium tartrate	Phenobarbital
Antipyrine	Phenolphthalein
Arsphenamine	Phenylbutazone
Barbital	Phenylhydantoin
Barbital sodium	Potassium chlorate
Belladonna	Pyrimidine derivatives
Bismuth salts	Quinacrine
Bromides	Quinidine
Chloral hydrate	Quinine
Chloroguanide	Reserpine
Chloroquine	Salicylates
Chlorothiazide	Santonin
Chlorpromazine	Saccharin
Chlortetracycline	Scopolamine
Cinchophen	Sodium salicylate
D-amphetamine	Streptomycin
Diallybarbituric acid	Strychnine
Diethylstibestrol	Sulfadiazine
Digilanid	Sulfaguanidine
Digitalis	Sulfamerazine
Dimenhydrinate	Sulfamethazine
Diphenhydramine	Sulfamethoxypyridazine
Diphenylhydantoin	Sulfapyridine
Disulfiram	Sulfarsphenamine
Ephedrine	Sulfathiazole
Epinephrine	Sulfisoxazole
Ergot alkaloids	Sulfobromophthelein sodium
Erythrosine	Tetracyclines
Eucalyptus oil	Thiambutosine
Formalin	Thonzylamine HCl
Frangula	Tripelennamine
Gold salts	Trisodium arsphenamine
Griseofulvin	sulfate
Iodine	Tryparsamide
Ipecac	Vaccines and immunizing
Karaya gum (Sterculia gum)	agents
Magnesium hydroxide	

TABLE 75-6. Drugs That May Cause Eczematous Dermatitis

Antibiotics	Mercurials
Antihistamines	PAS
Arsenicals	Penicillins
Bromides	Quinacrine
Chloral hydrate	Streptomycin
Iodides	Sulfonamides

TABLE 75-7. Drugs That May Cause Bullous Eruptions

Acetophenetidin	Ergot
Aminopyrine	Gold salts
Antipyrine	Griseofulvin
Arsenicals	Insulin
Atropine	Iodides
Barbiturates	Mercurial diuretics
Bismuth	Penicillins
Bromides	Phenolphthalein
Chloral hydrate	Phenothiazines
Cinchophen	Quinine
Digitalis	Salicylates
Diphenylhydantoin	Streptomycin
Diuretics	Sulfonamides

TABLE 75–8. Drugs That May Cause Photodermatitis

Acetohexamide	Coal tar	Methoxsalen	Reserpine
Acridine dyes	Cyclamates	5-Methoxypsoralen	Rose bengal perfume
Agave lechuguilla	Demeclocycline	8-Methoxypsoralen	Rue
(amaryllis)	Desipramine	Monoglycerol para-	Salicylanilides
Agrimony	Dibenzopyran derivatives	aminobenzoate	Salicylates
9-Aminoacridine	Dicyanine-A	Mustards	Sandalwood oil (perfume)
Aminobenzoic acid	Diethylstilbestrol	Nalidixic acid	Silver salts
Angelica	Digalloyl trioleate	Naphthalene	Stilbamidine isethionate
Anthracene	Dill	Nortriptyline	Substituted benzoic acids
Arsenicals	Diphenhydramine	Oral contraceptives	(sun screens)
Barbiturates	hydrochloride	Oxytetracycline	Sulfonamides
Bavachi (corylifolia)	Diphenylhydantoin	Para-dimethylaminoazobenzene	Sulfonylureas
Benzene	Doxycycline	Paraphenylenediamine	Tetrachlorsalicylanilide
Benzopyrine	Estrone	Perloline	Tetracyclines
Bergamot (perfume)	Fennel oil	Perphenazine	Thiazide diuretics
Bithionol	Fentichlor	Phenanthrene	Thiophenes
Blankophores (sulfa	Fluorescein dyes	Phenazine dyes	Thiopropazate dihydrochloride
derivatives)	5-Fluorouracil	Phenolic compounds	Tribromosalicylanilide
Bulosemide (Jadit)	Glyceryl p-aminobenzoate	Phenothiazine	Trichlormethiazide
Bromchlorsalicylanilid	Gold salts	Phenoxazines	Triethylene melamine
4-Butyl-4-chlorosalicy-	Griseofulvin	Phenylbutazone	Triflupromazine hydrochloride
lanilide	Hexachlorophene	Prochlorperazine	Trimeprazine tartrate
Carbamazepine	Imipramine	Promazine hydrochloride	Trimethadione
Carbinoxamine	Isothipendyl	Protriptyline	Trypaflavine
Carbutamide	Lantinin	Promethazine hydrochloride	Trypan blue
Cedar oil	Lavender oil	Psoralens	Vanillin oils
Chlordiazepoxide	Lime oil	Pyrathiazine hydrochloride	Water ash
Chlorpromazine	Meclothiazide	Pyridine	Xylene
Chlorpropamide	Mepazine	Quinethazone	Yarrow
Chlortetracycline	9-Mercaptopurine	Quinidine	
Citron oil	Methotrimeprazine	Quinine	

TABLE 75–9. Drugs That May Cause Exfoliative Dermatitis

Acetazolamide	Mesantoin
Allopurinol	Methotrimeprazine
Antimony compounds	Nitroglycerin
Arsenicals	PAS
Barbiturates	Penicillins
Bismuth	Phenacetamide
Carbamazepine	Phenindione
Chloroquine	Phenothiazines
Demeclocycline	Phenylbutazone
Diphenylhydantoin	Quinacrine
Furosemide	Quinidine
Gold salts	Streptomycin
Griseofulvin	Sulfonamides
Hydroflumethiazide	Sulfonylureas
Iodides	Tetracyclines
Isorbide	Thiazide diuretics
Measles virus vaccine	Vitamin A
Mercurials	

TABLE 75–11. Drugs That May Cause Stevens-Johnson Syndrome

Antipyrine	Phenylbutazone
Arsenicals	Quinine
Barbiturates	Salicylates
Belladonna	Smallpox vaccine
Carbamazepine	Sulfadimethoxine
Chloramphenicol	Sulfamethoxypyridazine
Chlorpropamide	Sulfisomidine
Codeine	Tetracyclines
Diphenylhydantoin	Thiacetazone
Hydralazine	Thiazides diuretics
Measles vaccine	Thiouracil
Mercurial diuretics	Trimethadione
Methylphenylethylhydantoin	Triple sulfonamides
Paramethadione	(sulfadiazine,
Penicillins	sulfamethazine,
Phenolphthalein	sulfamerazine)
Phensuximide	

TABLE 75–10. Drugs That May Cause Erythema Nodosum-Like Lesions

Bromides	Salicylates
Iodides	Sulfonamides
Penicillins	

TABLE 75–12. Drugs That May Cause Erythema Multiforme-Like Lesions

Acetophenetidin	Gold salts
Aminopyrine	Iodides
Antihistamines	Meprobamate
Antipyrine	Penicillins
Arsenicals	Phenolphthalein
Barbiturates	Phenothiazines
Bismuth	Phenylbutazone
Bromides	Salicylates
Chloramphenicol	Streptomycin
Cinchophen	Sulfonamides
Diphenylhydantoin	Sulfonylureas
Erythromycin	Thiazide diuretics

TABLE 75–13. Drugs That May Cause Toxic Epidermal Necrolysis

Acetazolamide	Methyl salicylate
Allopurinol	Neomycin sulfate
Aminopyrine	Nitrofurantoin
Antihistamines	Opium powder
Antipyrine	Penicillins
Barbiturates	Phenophthalein
Brompheniramine	Phenylbutazone
Chenopodium oil	Polio vaccine
Diphenylhydantoin	Sulfonamides
Ethylmorphine HCl	Sulfones
Gold salts	Tetanus antitoxin
Ipecac	Tetracyclines
Isoniazid	Tolbutamide

TABLE 75–14. Drugs That May Produce Lupus Erythematosus

Aminosalicylic acid	Para-aminosalicylic acid
Barbiturates (long term?)	Paramethadione
Chlorpromazine	Penicillamine
Chlortetracycline	Penicillins
Digitalis (long term)	Phenothiazines
Diphenylhydantoin	Phenylbutazone
Ethosuximide	Primidone
Gold compounds (long term)	Procainamide
Griseofulvin	Propranolol
Hydralazine	Propylthiouracil
Isoniazid	Quinidine
Mephenytoin	Reserpine (long term)
Methsuximide	Streptomycin
Methyldopa	Sulfadimethoxine
Methylthiouracil	Sulfamethoxypyridazine
Oral contraceptives (mestranol?)	Tetracycline (degraded)
	Thiazides (long term)
Oxyphenisatin	Trimethadione

TABLE 75–15. Drugs That May Cause "Collage" Disease

Busulfan	Mercurial diuretics
Chloramphenicol	Penicillins
Chlortetracycline	Phenylbutazone
Diphenylhydantoin	Pyromen
Iodides	Sulfonamides
Iproniazid	Thiouracil

TABLE 75–16. Drugs That May Induce Acute Porphyria (A) or Cutaneous Porphyria (C) in Man

Aminopyrine	A
Androgens	A, C
Barbiturates	A, C
Chlordiazepoxide	A
Chloroquine	C
Diphenylhydantoin	A
Estrogens	A, C
Ethyl alcohol	C
Griseofulvin	A
Hexachlorobenzene	C
Meprobamate	A
Oral contraceptives	A, C
Sulfonamides	A
Sulfonylureas	A, C

TABLE 75–17. Drugs That May Produce Purpura

Acetophenetidin	Diphenylhydantoin
ACTH	Ergot
Allopurinol	Fluoxymesterone
Anticoagulants	Gold salts
Antihistamines	Griseofulvin
Antipyrine	Heparin
Arsenicals	Insulin
Arsenobenzols	Iodides
Barbiturates	Isoniazid
Bismuth	Mepesulfate
Bromides	Meprobamate
Carbamides	Nirvanol
Cephalosporins	Penicillins
Chloral hydrate	Phenothiazines
Chloramphenicol	Phenylbutazone
Chlorothiazide	Quinidine
Chlorpromazine	Quinine
Chlorpropamide	Salicylates
Cinchophen	Sulfonamides
Corticosteroids	Thiazide diuretics
Digitalis	Thiouracils
Digitoxin	Trifluoperazine

TABLE 75–18. Drugs That May Cause Urticaria

ACTH	Mercurials
Barbiturates	Nitrofurantoin
Bromides	Novobiocin
Chloramphenicol	Opiates
Dextran	Penicillinase
Diphenylhydantoin	Penicillins
Enzymes	Phenolphthalein
Erythromycin	Phenothiazines
Glutethimide	Propoxyphene
Griseofulvin	Salicylates
Insulin	Sera
Iodides	Streptomycin
Iodopyracet	Sulfonamides
Liver extracts	Tetracyclines
Meprobamate	Thiouracil
Meperidine	

TABLE 75–19. Drugs That May Cause Lichenoid and Lichen Planus-Like Reactions

Amiphenazole	Propylthiouracil
Chloroquine	Quinacrine
Gold salts	Quinidine
Organic arsenicals	Thiazide diuretics
PAS	

TABLE 75–20. Drugs That May Cause Alopecia

Allopurinol	Methimazole
α-methyl dopa	Methotrexate
Anticoagulants	Norethindrone acetate
Arsenic	Oral contraceptives
Aspirin	Propylthiouracil
Amphetamines	Quinacrine
Clofibrate	Selenium sulfide
Cyclophosphamide	Sodium warfarin
Diphenylhydantoin	Thallium
5-Fluorouracil	Trimethadione
Gentamicin	Triparanol
Gold salts	Uracil mustard
Heparin	Vinblastine
Iodine	Vincristine
Mepesulfate	Vitamin A
Mephenytoin	

TABLE 75–21. Drugs That May Cause Gynecomastia

Adrenocortical hormones
Androgens
Busulfan
Chlortetracycline
Diethylstilbestrol
Digitalis
Digitoxin
Estrogens
Ethionamide
Griseofulvin
Haloperidol
HCG (human chorionic gonadotropin)
Heroin
Isoniazid
Methyldopa
Methyltestosterone
Oral contraceptives
Phenaglycodol
Phenelzine
Phenothiazines
Reserpine
Spironolactone
Stilbestrol
Vincristine
Vitamin D_2

TABLE 75–22. Drugs That May Produce Serum-Sickness

Antihistamines
Arsenicals
Barbiturates
Bismuth
Digitalis
Diphenylhydantoin
Heparin
Hydralazine
Insulin
Iodides
Mercurial diuretics
Penicillins
Phenylbutazone
Procainamide
Quinidine
Salicylates
Streptomycin
Sulfonamides
Thiouracils
Vaccines

TABLE 75–23. Compounds That May Produce Hemolysis of Glucose-6-Phosphate Dehydrogenase-Deficient Red Cells

Analgesics:
Acetanilid
Acetophenetidin (phenacetin)
Acetylsalicylic acid*
Antipyrine
Pyramidone

Sulfonamides and sulfones:
Dapsone
N_2-Acetylsufanilamide
Salicylazosulfapyridine
Sulfacetamide
Sulfanilamide
Sulfamethoxypyridazine
Sulfapyridine
Sulfisoxazole*
Sulfoxone*
Thiazolsulfone

Antimalarials:
Chloroquine
Primaquine
Pamaquine
Pentaquine
Quinocide
Quinacrine

Nonsulfonamide antibacterial agents:
Chloramphenicol‡
Furazolidone
Furmethonol
Neoarsphenamine
Nitrofurantoin
Nitrofurazone
Para-aminosalicylic acid

Miscellaneous:
α-Methyldopa
Dimercaprol*
Hydralazine
Mestranol
Methylene blue*
Nalidixic acid
Naphthalene
Niridazole
Phenylhydrazine
Probenecid
Pyridium
Quinine+
Trinitrotoluene
Vitamin K (water soluble)

* Slightly hemolytic in Blacks or only in very large doses
+ Hemolytic in Caucasians, but not in Blacks
‡ Possibly hemolytic in Caucasians but not in Blacks or Orientals
Taken in part from: Beutler E (1974): Glucose-6-phosphate dehydrogenase deficiency in *The Metabolic Basis of Inherited Disease*. 3rd ed. Stanbury JB, Wyngaarden JB, Frederickson DS (eds). New York, McGraw Hill

TABLE 75–24. Drugs That May Cause Blood Dyscrasias

Drug	Agranulocytosis (Leukopenia)	Aplastic anemia	Hemolytic anemia	Megaloblastic anemia	Pancytopenia	Thrombocytopenia
Acetanilid			*			
Acetazolamide	*	*			*	*
Acetophenetidin		*	*		*	*
Acetylphenylhydrazine			*			
Acetylsalicylic acid	*	*	*		*	*
Allyl-isopropyl-acetylcarbamide						*
Aminopyrine	*	*	*			
Antihistamines	*					
Antineoplastics	*	*			*	
Antipyrine			*			
Arsenicals	*					
Arsenobenzenes						*
Barbiturates		*		*	*	*
Busulfan					*	*
Carbamazepine	*	*				*
Cephalothin sodium			*			*
Chloramphenicol	*	*	*		*	*
Chloroquine	*		*			
Chlorothiazide	*	*			*	*
Chlorpromazine	*		*			
Chlorpropamide		*			*	*
Cinchophen	*					
Clofibrate	*					
Colchicine		*		*		
Corticotropin	*					
Cycloserine				*		
Cytarabine	*		*	*		*
Diaminodiphenylsulfone			*			
Digitalis glycosides	*	*			*	*
Dimercaprol			*			

(continued)

TABLE 75–24. *(continued)*

Drug	Agranulo-cytosis (Leukopenia)	Aplastic anemia	Hemolytic anemia	Megalo-blastic anemia	Pancyto-penia	Thrombo-cytopenia
Diphenylhydantoin	*			*		*
Dipyrone	*					
5-Fluorouracil				*		
Furazolidone			*			
Gamma benzene hexachloride	*					
Glutethimide				*		
Gold compounds	*	*			*	*
Hydralazine	*					
Hydrochlorothiazide						*
Imipramine	*					
Indomethacin		*				
Iothiouracil	*					
Irradiation (radioactive drugs)		*				
Isoniazid			*			
Mepazine	*	*			*	
Meprobamate	*	*			*	
6-Mercaptopurine	*	*		*	*	*
Methotrexate	*	*		*	*	*
Metformin				*		
Methiamazole	*	*			*	*
Methophenobarbital				*		
Methyldopa	*	*	*		*	*
Methylene blue			*			
Neomycin				*		
Nitrofurantoin			*	*		
Nitrofurazone			*			
Novobiocin	*					
Oral contraceptives				*		
Oxyphenbutazone	*					
Pamaquine			*	*		
Para-aminosalicylic acid			*	*		
Penicillin	*	*	*		*	*
Pentaquine			*			
Pentamidine isethionate				*		
Phenacetin	*					
Phenantoin		*	*		*	
Penindione	*					
Phenothiazines	*					
Phenylbutazone	*	*			*	*
Phenylhydrazine			*			
Phenytoin sodium	*	*		*		
Primaquine			*			
Primidone				*		
Probenecid			*			
Procainamide	*					
Prochlorperazine	*					
Promazine	*					
Propylthiouracil	*					
Pyrimethamine				*		
Quinacrine	*	*	*			*
Quinidine	*	*	*		*	*
Quinine			*			*
Rifampin						*
Salicylates	*					
Streptomycin	*	*		*		
Stibophen			*			
Sulfonamides	*	*	*		*	*
Sulfoxone			*			
Tetracyclines	*		*		*	*
Thiazides	*					
Thiazolsulfone			*			
Thioridazine	*					*
Thiouracil	*					*
Tolbutamide	*	*			*	
Triamterene				*		
Trimethadione	*	*			*	
Trimethoprim				*		
Tripelennamine	*					
Vitamin K water-soluble analogs			*			

TABLE 75—25. Drugs That Cross the Human Placental Barrier and That May Endanger the Fetus During Pregnancy or in the Prenatal Period

Drug	Adverse effect(s)
Acetophenetidin	Methemoglobinemia
Alphaprodine	Fetal respiratory depression
Aminopterin	Abortion, anomalies, cleft palate
Ammonium chloride	Acidosis
Anesthestics (volatile)	Depressed fetal respiration
Androgens	Advanced bone age; clitoral enlargement, labial fusion, masculinization
Barbiturates	Anomalies, depressed respiration
Bishydroxycoumarin	Fetal death and intrauterine hemorrhage
Bromides	Neonatal skin eruptions (bromoderma)
Busulfan	Cleft palate
Chloral hydrate (large doses)	Fetal death
Chlorambucil	Abortion, anomalies
Chloroquine	Thrombocytopenia
Chlorpromazine	Neonatal jaundice, prolonged extrapyramidal signs, neonatal goiter
Chlorpropamide	Prolonged neonatal hypoglycemia, neonatal goiter?
Cholinesterase inhibitors	Muscular weakness (transient)
Cortisone	Cleft palate
Cyclophosphamide	Defects of extremities, stunting, fetal death
Cyclopropane	Neonatal respiratory depression
D-amphetamine sulfate	Transposition of vessels?
Diphenylhydantoin	Anomalies
Estrogens	Advanced bone age, clitoral enlargement, labial fusion, masculinization, vaginal cancer (20 years later)
Ether	Neonatal apnea
Ethyl biscoumacetate	Fetal death, neonatal hemorrhage
Ganglionic blocking agents	Neonatal ileus
Heroin	Initial neonatal addiction, neonatal death, respiratory depression
Hexamethonium bromide	Neonatal ileus, death
Iodides	Goiter
Iophenoxic acid	Hypothyroidism, retardation
Iothiouracil	Neonatal goiter
Isoniazid	Retarded psychomotor activity
Levorphanol	Fetal respiratory depression
Lithium carbonate	Neonatal goiter
Lysergic acid diethylamide	Chromosomal damage, stunted offspring
Mecamylamine	Fatal neonatal ileus
Mepivacaine	Fetal bradycardia, neonatal depression
Methimazole	Neonatal goiter, hypothyroidism, mental retardation
Methadone	Fetal respiratory depression
Methotrexate	Abortion, anomalies, cleft palate
Morphine	Initial neonatal addiction, respiratory depression, neonatal death
Nicotine (smoking)	"Small for dates" neonates
Nitrofurantoin	Fetal hemolysis
Nitrous oxide	Respiratory depression
Novobiocin	Hyperbilirubinemia
Oral progestogens	Clitoral enlargement, labial fusion, masculinization
Paraldehyde	Respiratory depression
Phenmetrazine	Multiple skeletal and visceral anomalies
Phenobarbital	Respiratory depression, death
Phenylbutazone	Neonatal goiter
Podophyllum	Fetal resorption, deformities
Potassium iodide	Cyanosis, goiter, mental retardation, respiratory distress
Propylthiouracil	Neonatal goiter, hypothyroidism, mental retardation
Quinine	Deafness, thrombocytopenia
Radioactive iodine	Congenital goiter, mental retardation, hypothyroidism
Reserpine	Nasal block, respiratory obstruction
Salicylates	Anomalies, neonatal bleeding

(continued)

TABLE 75—25. *(continued)*

Drug	Adverse effect(s)
Smallpox vaccination	Fetal vaccinia
Sodium warfarin	Intrauterine hemorrhage, fetal death
Streptomycin	Hearing loss, eighth cranial nerve damage, micromelia, multiple skeletal anomalies
Sulfonamides (long acting)	Kernicterus, hyperbilirubinemia, acute liver atrophy, anemia, neonatal goiter
Sulfonylureas	Neonatal goiter, prolonged neonatal hypoglycemia
Tetracyclines	Discolored teeth, inhibits long bone growth, micromelia, syndactyly
Thalidomide	Phocomelia, hearing defects, fetal death
Thiazides	Neonatal death, thrombocytopenia
Thiouracil	Hypothyroidism, neonatal goiter, mental retardation
Tolbutamide	Congenital anomalies and prolonged neonatal hypoglycemia
Tribromoethanol	Depressed fetal respiration
Vitamin A (large doses)	Cleft palate, congenital anomalies, eye damage, syndactyly
Vitamin D (large doses)	Hypercalcemia, mental retardation
Vitamin K analogs (large doses)	Hyperbilirubinemia, kernicterus

TABLE 75–26. Some Drugs Excreted in Human Milk

Acetaminophen	Ether	Phenacetin
Alcohol	Ethinamate	Phenaglycodol
Allergens (egg, peanuts, etc.)	Ethyl biscoumacetate	Phenolphthalein
Ambenonium chloride	Folic acid	Phenylbutazone
Aminophylline	Heroin	Phenytoin
Amphetamines	Hexachlorobenzene	Potassium iodide
Anthraquinone cathartics	Hydroxypylcarbamate	Prochlorperazine
Antihistamines	Hydroxyzine	Propoxyphene
Arsenical salts	Iodine[131]	Propylthiouracil
Aspirin	Iopanoic acid	Pseudoephedrine
Atropine	Imipramine	Pyrimethamine
Barbiturates	Isoniazid	Quinidine
Bishydroxycoumarin	L-propoxyphene	Quinine sulfate
Bromides	Mandelic acid	Reserpine
Brompheniramine	Mefanamic acid	Rh antibodies
Caffeine	Meperidine	Rhubarb
Calomel	Metals	Riboflavin
Cascara	Methadone HCl	Salicylates
Chloral hydrate	Methdilazine	Scopolamine
Chloramphenicol	Methimazole	Senna
Chloroform	Methocarbomal	Sodium salicylate
Chlorpromazine	Metronidazole	Streptomycin
Codeine	Morphine	Sulfamethoxazole
Copper	Narcotics	Sulfadimethoxine
Cortisone	Neomycin sulfate	Sulfanilamide
Cyclophosphamide	Niacin	Sulfapyridine
Cyclopropane	Nicotine	Sulfathiazole
Cycloserine	Nitrofurantoin	Tetracyclines
Danthron	Novobiocin	Thiamine
DDT	Oral contraceptives	Thiazide diuretics
D-amphetamine	Oxacillin	Thiopental
Diazepam	Oxyphenbutazone	Thiouracil
Diphenhydramine	Pantothenic acid	Thyroid hormones
Diphenylhydantoin	Papaverine	Tolbutamide
Ephedrine	PAS	Trifluoperazine
Ergot alkaloids	Penethamate hydriodide	Vitamins A,B,B_{12},C,D,E,K
Erythromycin	Penicillin G	
Estrogens	Pentazocine	

TABLE 75–27. Drugs That May Cause Intestinal Malabsorption

Drug	Substance(s) involved
Alcohol (ethanol)	Folic acid, vitamin B_{12}, fat, D-xylose
Aluminum hydroxide	Tetracycline antibiotics
Bacitracin	As for neomycin
Bisacodyl	Fat, protein, potassium
Calcium carbonate	Fatty acids
Chlorothiazide diuretics	Water and sodium
Cholestyramine	Bile salts, digitalis, lincomycin, sterols, carbohydrates, iron, fat soluble vitamins, etc.
Clofibrate	As for cholestyramine
Colchicine	Vitamin B_{12}, cholesterol, fat, carotine, sodium, potassium, D-xylose
Contraceptives, oral	Folic acid
Diphenylhydantoin	Folic acid
Ethacrynic acid	Water and sodium
5-Fluorouracil	Severe general malabsorption
Kanamycin (oral)	As for neomycin
Methotrexate	Severe general malabsorption
Neomycin	Cholesterol, disaccharides, Vitamin B_{12}, carotine, iron, potassium, sodium, chloride, nitrogen
Paromomycin	As for neomycin
PAS	Folic acid, vitamin B_{12}, cholesterol, iron, D-xylose
Phenformin	Glucose
Phenolphthaline	Fat, vitamins A,D,E,K, calcium
Polymyxin B	As for neomycin
Potassium chloride	Vitamin B_{12}
Triparenol (MER-29)	Severe general malabsorption

FURTHER READING

Martin EW (1971): Hazards of Medications. Philadelphia, JB Lippincott

D'Arch PF, Griffin JP (1972): Iatrogenic Disease. New York, Oxford Medical Publications

Meyler L (1970): Side Effects of Drugs. 5th ed. Princeton, NJ, Excerpta Medica Foundation

JEREMY H. THOMPSON

76. INFLUENCE OF DRUGS ON LABORATORY TESTS

Drugs may interfere with the results of laboratory procedures in two main ways: by causing pharmacologic and toxicologic changes or by interfering with analytical procedures. Pharmacologic effects occur frequently and are usually dose dependent. For example, iodine containing substances (such as Metrecal, x-ray contrast media, potassium iodide, the halogenated hydroxyquinolines) elevate the protein bound iodine (PBI) level. This is a spurious elevation, since it does not represent the true concentration of hormone. Data indicating how drugs affect the PBI level have been presented in detail by Sisson.

Analytical interference occurs when the drug or its metabolites interferes with the test procedure. For example, mercurial diuretics inhibit the color reaction in the determination of PBI by the chloric acid technique, and reserpine and its metabolites inhibit the Porter-Silber color reaction of 17-hydroxycorticosteroid estimation.

The effect of the complex and potent drugs available today on laboratory procedures presents an increasingly difficult problem. A knowledge of these patterns of drug interference is the responsibility of the physician and frequently enables him to explain some puzzling and unexpected test results. Tables 76–1, 76–2 and 76–3 present some common patterns of drug interference which have been noted over several years; they do not pretend to be complete. Additions, deletions or corrections to this list will be gratefully received and acknowledged. In general, the drugs have been listed alphabetically by generic name. In order to keep the tables within manageable proportions, many drug groups have been used, e.g., anabolic steroids, barbiturates, oral contraceptives, tetracyclines and thiazide diuretics. Since analytical tests frequently differ between laboratories, the exact test has been specified where possible. Detailed effects of drugs on the red and white blood cell series (hemolytic anemia, aplastic anemia, leukocytosis, agranulocytosis) are not presented; the interested reader should consult the article by Best.

A list of selected references is given at the end of the chapter.

SYMBOLS USED IN TABLES

+ = False positive elevation due to possible pharmacologic or toxic effect
− = False negative depression due to possible pharmacologic or toxic effect
+ = False positive elevation due to interference with analytical procedure

− = False negative depression due to interference with analytical procedure
S = See Supplementary Information on Drug Effect, following each table
? = Effect reported but ambiguous

TABLE 76–1. Influence of Drugs on Tests of Blood, Serum and Plasma

Drug	Acid phosphatase	Albumin	Alkaline phosphatase	Amino acids	Ammonia	Amylase	Bicarbonate	Bilirubin	Blood urea nitrogen (BUN)	Bromsulphalein (BSP)	Calcium	Carbon dioxide combining power	Carbon dioxide content	Cephalin flocculation	Ceruloplasmin	Chloride	Cholesterol	Clotting time	Coagulation time	Coombs'	Copper
Acetaminophen								+													
Acetanilide																					
Acetazolamide					+											+					
Acetohexamide		+						+	+												
Alcohol (ethyl)						+															
Allopurinol		+																			
Aluminum antacids									+												
Amantadine																					
Aminocaproic acid																					
Aminophylline																					
Aminopyrine																				+S	
Aminosalicylic acid															−						
Amphotericin B								+	+												
Ampicillin		+												+							
Anabolic steroids		+S						+S		+S	+			+S			+				
Androgens	+S	+						+		+	+			+			± S				
Angiotensin amide																					
Anthraquinone derivatives															−						
Antipyrine																					
Arsenicals								+													
Aspidium oleoresin								+S		+S											
Avocado																					
Bacitracin									+												
Barbiturates		+				− S			+					+							
Biguanides						−															
Bilirubin																	+				
Bishydroxycoumarin												?									
Bismuth salts			+																		
Bromide									+							+	+S				
Bromsulphalein		+S							+	+S											
Caffeine						−															
Calcium antacids									+			+									
Carbamazepine		+								+S											
Cephaloridine		+							+											+S	
Cephalothin		+																		+S	
Chiniofon									+												
Chloral hydrate								+S													
Chloramphenicol		+																			
Chlordiazepoxide		+				+															
Chlorobutanol								S													

Cortiscosteroids	Creatinine	Creatinine phosphokinase	Eosinophil count	Factors VII, VIII	Factor IX	Glucose	Glucose tolerance	Iron	Lactic dehydrogenase	LE cells	Lipids (total)	Methemoglobin	Paper electrophoresis	pH	Phenylketonuria	Phosphorus (inorganic)	Platelet count	Potassium	Protein (total)	Prothrombin time	RBC sedimentation rate	Serotonin	SGOT, SGPT	Sodium	Thymol turbidity	Typing, crossmatching	Uric acid	WBC alkaline phosphatase	WBC count	Zinc
						−						+											+							
												+																		
																−	−										+			
						−																	+				+			
																							+				−			
								−S								−				−S										
																							+							
																	+													
																			+											
			+					+			+	+				−	−		+				+							
	+		+													−	−						+							
			+																				+							
																							+S	+	+S					
																							+	+	+					
																											+			
																	−			+					−					
																	−													
																						S								
	+		+								+										S	+			+					
								−								+														
															?			+							+					
																			+				+				?			
+																			+				+							
						+																								
																								−						
											+												+							
			+															+					+				+			
			+																				+		+					
			+																											
																				+S										
								+S								−				+										
																				+S				+						

(continued)

TABLE 76–1. (continued)

Drug	Acid phosphatase	Albumin	Alkaline phosphatase	Amino acids	Ammonia	Amylase	Bicarbonate	Bilirubin	Blood urea nitrogen (BUN)	Bromsulphalein (BSP)	Calcium	Carbon dioxide combining power	Carbon dioxide content	Cephalin flocculation	Ceruloplasmin	Chloride	Cholesterol	Clotting time	Coagulation time	Coombs'	Copper
Chloroquine																					
Chlorpropamide			+							+					+		−				
Chlorthalidone				+	+					+											
Cholestyramine							−										−				
Cinchophen																	−				
Clofibrate	+									+							−				
Clomiphene										+											
Cloxacillin			+																		
Codeine						+															
Colchicine			+																		
Colistin									+												
Copper											**+**										
Corticosteroids				+		+											−	+	−		
Corticotropin				+													−	+	−		
Cycloserine																					
Cyproheptadine						+															
Dehydrocholic acid										+							+				
Dextrans								?											+		
D-thyroxine																	−				
Diazoxide																					
Digitalis																					
Diiodohydroxyquin										+											
Diphenylhydantoin								+													
Dithiazanine iodide										+											
Epinephrine				+																−	
Erythromycin		+						+S		+				+			−				
Estrogens	+	+								+	+			+			−				
Ethacrynic acid						+			+							−					
Ethchlorvynol																					
Ethionamide																					
Ethoxazene								?		+											
Ethyl aminobenzoate																					
Ethylenediaminetetraacetic acid											−	−									
Florantyrone										+				+							
Fluoride			−							+											
Furazolidone																					
Furosemide			+			+			+							−					
Gentamicin									+												
Glucose (IV)				+S			−			−											
Glutethimide																					

Cortiscosteroids	Creatinine	Creatinine phosphokinase	Eosinophil count	Factors VII, VIII	Factor IX	Glucose	Glucose tolerance	Iron	Lactic dehydrogenase	LE cells	Lipids (total)	Methemoglobin	Paper electrophoresis	pH	Phenylketonuria	Phosphorus (inorganic)	Platelet count	Potassium	Protein (total)	Prothrombin time	RBC sedimentation rate	Serotonin	SGOT, SGPT	Sodium	Thymol turbidity	Typing, crossmatching	Uric acid	WBC alkaline phosphatase	WBC count	Zinc
																	−						+							
			+			−																			+					
						+											−	−									+			
											−									+										
																											−			
+	+								−										+	−S			+				−			
			+																				+							
																							+							
																	−						+							
+			+																											
																	+								+					
S	−					+	+	−		−S								−		−			+					±S	+	
	−					+	+	−										−					+				−			
																							+							
						−																								
																					+					+S				
																					S									
						+																			+					
			+							+																				
			+			+				+										+S										
			+			+								−			−										+			
			+																				+S		+					
					+S	+	+				−												+		+					
			+			+											−	−						−				±S		
																				−S										
																							+				+			
												+																		
														−S																
			+																						+					
						−		?																						
			+																											
						+													−				+	−			+			
																							+							
						+																								
												+								−S										

(continued)

TABLE 76-1. (continued)

Drug	Acid phosphatase	Albumin	Alkaline phosphatase	Amino acids	Ammonia	Amylase	Bicarbonate	Bilirubin	Blood urea nitrogen (BUN)	Bromsulphalein (BSP)	Calcium	Carbon dioxide combining power	Carbon dioxide content	Cephalin flocculation	Ceruloplasmin	Chloride	Cholesterol	Clotting time	Coagulation time	Coombs'	Copper
Gold salts			+																		
Griseofulvin										+											
Guanethidine									+												
Guanoxan										+											
Haloperidol																	=				
Heparin					+S					+	−						=			−S	
Histamine						+															
Hydralazine																					
Hydroxyzine																					
Indomethacin			+			+	+	+	+					+			+				
Inorganic iodides										+											
Insulin				+							−										
Iodine containing drugs										+S											
Iodochlorhydroxyquin										+											
Ion exchange resin					+											+					
Iothiouracil																					
Iron (oral)																					+
Iron sorbitol																					+
Isocarboxazid			+							+				+			+				
Isoniazid					+		+														
Kanamycin									+	?				?			−				
Lactobacillus acidophilus					−																
L-thyroxine																	−				
Lincomycin			+											+							
Lithium carbonate																					
Magnesium antacids									+		−										
Mannitol																−					
Mechlorethamine																					
Mefenamic acid																					
Meperidine			+							+				+			+				
Mephenytoin																					
Mercurial diuretics																−					
Metaxalone										+				+							
Methadone			+							+				+			+				
Methicillin					+				+		−	−									
Methocarbamol									+												
Methotrexate										+				+			+				
Methyldopa			+					+	+	+				+						+S	
Methylene blue																					
Methysergide																					

Cortiscosteroids	Creatinine	Creatinine phosphokinase	Eosinophil count	Factors VII, VIII	Factor IX	Glucose	Glucose tolerance	Iron	Lactic dehydrogenase	LE cells	Lipids (total)	Methemoglobin	Paper electrophoresis	pH	Phenylketonuria	Phosphorus (inorganic)	Platelet count	Potassium	Protein (total)	Prothrombin time	RBC sedimentation rate	Serotonin	SGOT, SGPT	Sodium	Thymol turbidity	Typing, crossmatching	Uric acid	WBC alkaline phosphatase	WBC count	Zinc
			+							+							−													
										+										−										
																								+						
										+														+						
																				−										
+S						+			− S							+				+				−	+					
			+							+																				
																				+										
						+														+				+	+					
			+							+			S																	
						−									−		−													
			+							+			S																	
			+							+			S	+																
										+																				
								+										+						+						
								+										+						+						
																							+	+						
			+					+		+		+					+						+							
	+		+																	+										
	S																													
																								+	+					
						+																								
																					− S									
	+															?	−								+					
																	−							+			+ S			
																	−													
																								+	+					
										+																				
																			−					−				+		
																								+	+					
	+		+													+	+							+	+		+			
																	−							+	+			−		
+S			+							+						−				?	+			+	+	S				
												−																		
			+																	+	−									

(continued)

TABLE 76–1. (continued)

Drug	Acid phosphatase	Albumin	Alkaline phosphatase	Amino acids	Ammonia	Amylase	Bicarbonate	Bilirubin	Blood urea nitrogen (BUN)	Bromsulphalein (BSP)	Calcium	Carbon dioxide combining power	Carbon dioxide content	Cephalin flocculation	Ceruloplasmin	Chloride	Cholesterol	Clotting time	Coagulation time	Coombs'	Copper
Monoamine oxidase inhibitors					−					+											
Morphine		+				+				+				+							
Nafcillin								+													
Nalidixic acid								+													
Neomycin					−			+												−	
Nicotinic acid								+	+					+						−	
Nitrofurantoin								+		?		?	?								
Novobiocin								+S		+											
Oral contraceptives		+								+	+			+	+		+				+
Oxacillin		+						+	+	+				+							
Pancreozymin						+															
Para-aminobenzoic acid																					
Paraldehyde																					
Para-thor-mone											+										
Pargyline		+						+	+	+				?							
Penacillamine		+												+							
Penicillin	+																			+S	
Pentazocine						+															
Phenacetin																					
Phenazopyridine								+		+											
Phenformin																	−				
Phenindione												?									
Phenolphthalein										+											
Phenolsulfonphthalein										+											
Phenothiazines		+						+	?	+				+			+				
Phenylbutazone																	+				
Phenyramidol																	−				
Physostigmine																					
Piperazine																					
Pitressin																					
Polymyxin B									+												
Potassium chloride																+					
Prilocaine																					
Primaquine																					
Primidone																					
Probenecid		+								+				+							
Procainamide		+																			
Procaine																					
Progesterones		+								+	+										

Cortiscosteroids	Creatinine	Creatinine phosphokinase	Eosinophil count	Factors VII, VIII	Factor IX	Glucose	Glucose tolerance	Iron	Lactic dehydrogenase	LE cells	Lipids (total)	Methemoglobin	Paper electrophoresis	pH	Phenylketonuria	Phosphorus (inorganic)	Platelet count	Potassium	Protein (total)	Prothrombin time	RBC sedimentation rate	Serotonin	SGOT, SGPT	Sodium	Thymol turbidity	Typing, crossmatching	Uric acid	WBC alkaline phosphatase	WBC count	Zinc
																							+		+					
			+																				+							
			+																				+		+					
																				+										
						+	+																+				+			
			+																				+							
			+																											
				+S		+	+			+										−			+	+	+					−
			+																				+							
						−																								
						−																								
															−															
						−																	+		+					
			+														−				+				+					
			+							+							−	+S						+S						
						−						+											+							
			+																											
																	−													
+																														
			+			+				+					?			−			+		+		+		−			
										+								−		+				+			+			S
																				+										
						+																								
																												+		
																+														
						−													+						+					
												+																		
												+																		
										+																				
			+																				+		+			−		
			+							+																				
			+																											

(continued)

TABLE 76–1. (continued)

Drug	Acid phosphatase	Albumin	Alkaline phosphatase	Amino acids	Ammonia	Amylase	Bicarbonate	Bilirubin	Blood urea nitrogen (BUN)	Bromsulphalein (BSP)	Calcium	Carbon dioxide combining power	Carbon dioxide content	Cephalin flocculation	Ceruloplasmin	Chloride	Cholesterol	Clotting time	Coagulation time	Coombs'	Copper
Propoxyphene																					
Propranolol								+													
Propylthiouracil																					
Pyrazinamide								+													
Pyrimethamine																					
Quinacrine																					
Quinethazone																					
Quinidine																				+S	
Quinine																				+S	
Reserpine																					
Salicylates	+					+						?					−				
Sodium bicarbonate				−							+										
Sodium chloride				−							+					+					
Spironolactone				+				+													
Stibophen								+												+S	
Streptokinase, ustreptodornase								+										+			
Streptomycin																					
Sulfinpyrazone																					
Sulfonamides			+				+	+	+				−S								
Tetracyclines						+		+	+									−	−	+S	
Thiabendazole														+							
Thiazide diuretics						+		+			+					−					
Thyroglobulin																	−				
Thyroid (desiccated)																	−				
Tolazamide		+																			
Tolbutamide	+	+								+			+								
Triacetyloleandomycin		+						+		+			+				+				
Triamterene							−		+						+						
Triiodothyronine																	−				
Trimethadione																					
Vancomycin								+													
Viomycin						+			−												
Vitamin A																	+				
Vitamin B₁₂																					+
Vitamin C																					
Vitamin D		−									+										
Vitamin E																					
Vitamin K							+S														
X-ray contrast media	+					+	+	+	+									−S	−S		

Influence of drugs on laboratory tests (continued)

Cortiscosteroids	Creatinine	Creatinine phosphokinase	Eosinophil count	Factors VII, VIII	Factor IX	Glucose	Glucose tolerance	Iron	Lactic dehydrogenase	LE cells	Lipids (total)	Methemoglobin	Paper electrophoresis	pH	Phenylketonuria	Phosphorus (inorganic)	Platelet count	Potassium	Protein (total)	Prothrombin time	RBC sedimentation rate	Serotonin	SGOT, SGPT	Sodium	Thymol turbidity	Typing, crossmatching	Uric acid	WBC alkaline phosphatase	WBC count	Zinc
						−																								
						−	−S																+							
									+											+										
																			−	−			+				+			
														−																
			+																								+			
						+																								
			+													−				+										
			+													−				+										
									+																+					
			+					−				+			?	−	−			−			+				+−S			
																									+					
																	+										−			
			+																											
	+		+																											
									+											+										
			+													−											−			
			+							+		+				−				−			+							
			+			−				+						+	+		−	−			+							
						+																	+							
						+	+			+							−	−									+			
+S																														
+S																														
						−																	+							
						−																			+		+			
																							+		+					
+	+					+											+							−			+			
										+										−										
	+																													
−	+																			−										
																				+	+									
+																											+			
																+														
																	+													
																				−										
													S																	

(continued)

Aluminum antacids	Chronic use may produce iron-deficiency anemia May retard absorption of bishydroxycoumarins
Aminopyrine	May produce false positive result in Coombs' test (direct)
Anabolic steroids	17-α-Alkylated steroids may produce intrahepatic cholestasis
Androgens	May elevate acid phosphatase level in female patients. Androsterone may lower serum cholesterol level
Aspidium oleoresin	If absorbed, may produce jaundice. If absorbed, may produce BSP retention
Avocado	Avocado, banana, blue plum, brinjal, eggplant, papaw, passion fruit, pineapple, plantain, red plum, tomato, and walnut may elevate blood serotonin levels owing to their high serotonin content
Barbiturates	Low amylase level may develop in poisoning. Reduce effectiveness of bishydroxycoumarins through enzyme induction
Bromide	May produce false elevation of cholesterol when this is estimated directly
Bromsulphalein	May directly interfere with estimation of alkaline phosphatase and calcium
Carbamazepine	May produce BSP retention through intrahepatic cholestasis
Cephaloridine	May produce false positive result in Coombs' test (direct)
Cephalothin	May produce false positive result in Coombs' test (direct)
Chloral hydrate	Produces interfering color with Nessler's reagent for BUN determination. Reduces effectiveness of bishydroxycoumarins through enzyme induction
Chloramphenicol	Elevates serum iron level as early sign of bone marrow toxicity
Chlordiazepoxide	May reduce effectiveness of bishydroxycoumarins through enzyme induction
Chlorobutanol	Produces interfering color with Nessler's reagent for BUN determination
Clofibrate	Reduces rate of bishydroxycoumarin metabolism
Corticosteroids	May interfere with creatinine clearance. May suppress LE cells in patient with systemic lupus erythematosus. In normal individuals, may produce fall in serum uric acid level; however, rapid elevation of serum uric acid level may follow treatment of patient with acute leukemia
Dextrans	Dextrans 110/150 prevent satisfactory red cell agglutination
D-thyroxine	Increases effect of bishydroxycoumarins by displacing protein-bound drug
Diphenylhydantoin	Increases effect of bishydroxycoumarins by displacing bound drug and reducing its metabolism
Erythromycin	Erythromycin estolate may produce syndrome of acute intrahepatic cholestasis resembling viral hepatitis or acute cholecystitis. Produces false positive elevation of SGOT level determined by azone-fast violet B and diphenylhydrazine collimetric methods
Estorgens	May increase Factor IX level in serum
Ethacrynic acid	May produce hyperuricemia following oral administration
Etchchlorvynol	May increase metabolism of bishydroxycoumarins by enzyme induction
Ethylenediaminetetraacetic acid	May lower pH slightly due to calcium chelation
Glucose (IV)	May elevate blood ammonia level in patient with portosystemic anastomoses
Glutethimide	May increase metabolism of bishydroxycoumarins by enzyme induction
Heparin	May elevate blood ammonia level. May alter positive Coombs' test (direct) to negative. Benzyl alcohol in heparin may interfere with spectrophotofluorometric estimation of corticosteroids. May suppress LE cells in patient with systemic lupus erythematosus
Inorganic iodides	May interfere with reading of many tests on paper electrophoresis
Iodine containing drugs	May elevate result of BSP or PSP tests due to chemical interference. May interfere with reading of many tests on paper electrophoresis
Iodochlorhydroxyquin	May interfere with reading of many tests on paper electrophoresis
L-thyroxine	May interfere with creatinine clearance
Magnesium antacids	Retard absorption of bishydroxycoumarins
Mechlorethamine	Causes hyperuricemia owing to cell destruction
α-Methyldopa	May produce false positive result in Coombs' test (direct). May interfere with creatinine estimation by alkaline picrate method. May interfere with determination of uric acid level by phosphotungstate method
Novobiocin	Retards conjugation of bilirubin. Produces a yellow color in serum which clinically can be confused with jaundice and which biochemically interferes with bilirubin estimation
Oral contraceptives	May stimulate synthesis of Factors VII and VIII by liver
Penicillin	May produce false positive result in Coombs' test (direct). In patient with renal failure, therapeutic doses of potassium or sodium penicillin salts may rapidly produce cation overload
Phenylbutazone	May induce glandular-fever-like cells
Propranolol	Prevents response of plasma glucose and free fatty acids in insulin tolerance test
Quinidine	May produce false positive result in Coombs' test (direct)
Quinine	May produce false positive result in Coombs' test (direct)
Salicylates	Small doses produce hyperuricemia
Stibophen	May produce false positive result in Coombs' test (direct)
Sulfonamides	Sulfacetamide may produce systemic acidosis
Tetracyclines	Increase coagulation time due to calcium chelation and/or interference with plasma lipoproteins
Thyroglobulin	Interferes with creatinine clearance
Thyroid (desiccated)	Interferes with creatinine clearance

Vitamin K	Large doses in the neonate may produce hyperbilirubinemia
X-ray contrast media	Diatrizoate sodium may lower clotting and coagulation times; several other agents have also been implicated. May interfere with reading of many tests on paper electrophoresis

TABLE 76–2. Influence of Drugs on Tests of Urine

Drug	Acetone	Albumin	Amino acids	Blood (benzidine, guaiac)	Calcium	Catecholamines	Color	Creatine, creatinine	Diacetic acid	Diagnex blue	Estrogens	Galactose	Glucose (Ames' method)	Glucose (Benedict's method)	5-HIAA	Phenolsulfonphthalein (PSP)	Porphyrins	Pregnanediol	Protein	Specific gravity	Uric acid	Urobilinogen	Vanillylmandelic acid (VMA)
Acetaminophen	+S																						
Acetanilide	+S													+	+S								
Acetazolamide															−							−	
Acriflavine							S										S						
Alcohol (ethyl)												+			−		S						+
Allopurinol																				−			
Aluminum antacids										+S													
Aminophylline																		+					
Aminopyrine														+									
Aminosalicylic acid							S							+			+S		+			+S	
Amitriptyline							S																
Amphotericin B																			+				
Ampicillin		+												+					+		+	−	
Anabolic steroids					+			+															
Androgens					+			+															
Anileridine																							+
Anthraquinone derivatives							S								+								
Antipyrine	+S							+						+								+	
Arsenicals																			+				
Aspidium oleoresin													+S										
Avocado															S								
Bacitracin																			+				
Barbiturates															−S		S						+
Barium sulfate										+S													
Biguanides	+																						
Bishydroxycoumarin							S														+		
Bismuth salts													+S	+S					+				
Bromide		+																					
Bromsulphalein	+															+						+	
Caffeine								−S															+
Calcium antacids										+S													
Cephaloridine														+S								−	
Cephalothin														+S								−	
Chiniofon		+	+																				
Chloral hydrate														+			+S						+
Chloramphenicol														+								−	
Chloroform														+									
Chloroquine							S										+S						
Chlorpropamide																	+S						

592   MISCELLANEOUS TOPICS AND REFERENCE MATERIAL

Drug	Acetone	Albumin	Amino acids	Blood (benzidine, guaiac)	Calcium	Catecholamines	Color	Creatine, creatinine	Diacetic acid	Diagnex blue	Estrogens	Galactose	Glucose (Ames' method)	Glucose (Benedict's method)	5-HIAA	Phenolsulfonphthalein (PSP)	Porphyrins	Pregnanediol	Protein	Specific gravity	Uric acid	Urobilinogen	Vanillylmandelic acid (VMA)
Chlorzoxazone							S																
Cholestyramine					+																		
Cinchophen														+									
Cloxacillin																							−
Colistin																			+				
Copper				+																			
Corticosteroids		+							+	+			+	+							+		
Corticotropin		+							+				+	+							+		
Cyproheptadine																−							
Dextrans																				+			
Diphenylhydantoin							S																
Dithiazanine iodide																			+	+			+
Epinephrine													+S	+S									+
Erythromycin						+																−	+
Ethacrynic acid														+		−						−S	
Ethoxazene							S								+	+S							
Furazolidone							S																
Gentamicin																			+			−	
Glucose (i.v.)													+	+									
Glutethimide																							+S
Glyceryl guaiacolate															+								
Gold salts																			+				
Griseofulvin																	+S		+				
Guanethidine																							−
Guanoxan																							+
Heparin														−S									
Hydralazine				+S																			
Indomethacin														+									
Inorganic iodides	+		+																				
Iodine-containing drugs	+		+													−							
Iodochlorhydroxyquin	+		+																				
Iodopyrine			+																				
Iron (oral)										+S													
Iron sorbitol							S												+				
Isoniazid													+S	+S					+				
Kanamycin																			+			−	
Kaolin										+S													
Lithium carbonate													+S	+S					+				
Magnesium antacids										+S													

(continued)

TABLE 76–2. (continued)

Drug	Acetone	Albumin	Amino acids	Blood (benzidine, guaiac)	Calcium	Catecholamines	Color	Creatine, creatinine	Diacetic acid	Diagnex blue	Estrogens	Galactose	Glucose (Ames' method)	Glucose (Benedict's method)	5-HIAA	Phenolsulfonphthalein (PSP)	Porphyrins	Pregnanediol	Protein	Specific gravity	Uric acid	Urobilinogen	Vanillylmandelic acid (VMA)
Mefenamic acid																			+				
Mephenesin														+S									+S
Mercurial diuretics														−		−							
Metaxalone														+					+				
Methenamine hippurate														+S	+S								
Methenamine mandelate				+		+								+S	−	+S			+S			?S	+
Methicillin																			+			−	
Methocarbamol							S								+S								+
Methyldopa						+	S														?S		
Methylene blue							S		+S														
Methysergide														−									
Metronidazole							S																
Morphine													+	+		+S							
Nafcillin																						−	
Nalidixic acid														+									
Neomycin																			+			−	
Nicotinic acid						+			+			+S	+S										
Nitrofurantoin							S																
Novobiocin																		?					
Oral contraceptives																		+					
Oxacillin																			+			−	
Paraldehyde																			+				
Para-thor-mone					+																		
Penacillamine																			+				
Penicillin		+												+		−			+				
Phenacetin	+S						S							+									
Phenazopyridine							S		+S							+	+S					+S	
Phenformin	+S																						
Phenindione																			+				
Phenolphthalein							S									+							
Phenolsulfonphthalein	+						S																
Phenothiazines						+	S	+S	+S							−S	+					+	
Phensuximide							S																
Phenylhydrazine																	+						
Pitressin																	+						
Polymyxin B																			+				
Primaquine							S																
Probenecid														+		+					+		
Procaine																	+S					+S	

Test

Drug	Acetone	Albumin	Amino acids	Blood (benzidine, guaiac)	Calcium	Catecholamines	Color	Creatine, creatinine	Diacetic acid	Diagnex blue	Estrogens	Galactose	Glucose (Ames' method)	Glucose (Benedict's method)	5-HIAA	Phenolsulfonphthalein (PSP)	Porphyrins	Pregnanediol	Protein	Specific gravity	Uric acid	Urobilinogen	Vanillylmandelic acid (VMA)
Progesterones																		+					
Quinacrine							S		+														
Quinidine						+	S		+														+
Quinine						+	S		+							+							−
Reserpine						+	S		+														
Riboflavin							+																+
Salicylates	S	+											+	+		−	+		+		+		+
Sodium bicarbonate				−S					+							−			+S				
Stibophen																			+				
Streptomycin												+		+								−	
Sulfinpyrazone														+		?					+		
Sulfonamides							S						+	+		−	+S		S			+S	
Tetracyclines			+S		+						+S		+S	+S								−	+
Thiazide diuretics					−			−					+	+		−						−	
Tolbutamide	+																						
Tolonium chloride							S																
Triamterene				−			S	−													+		
Trimethadione				−															+				
Viomycin				−																			+
Vitamin B complex																							+
Vitamin B12												+											
Vitamin C				−S									+	+							+		
Vitamin D					+							+							+				
Vitamin E																			+				
Wheat germ extracts																			+				
X-ray contrast media		+	+											+S					+S	+			

(continued)

Acetaminophen	Produces interfering color in ferric chloride test for acetone
Acetanilide	Produces interfering color in ferric chloride test for acetone
	Increases color reaction in 5-HIAA determination
Acriflavine	Colors urine greenish-yellow
	Produces interfering color in spectrophotofluorometric test for porphyrins
Alcohol (ethyl)	May induce acute intermittent porphyria
Aluminum antacids	May displace diagnex blue from its resin, producing false positive test result
Aminosalicylic acid	Colors urine yellow
	Produces interfering yellow color with Ehrlich's aldehyde reagent for urobilinogen and porpho-bilinogen determinations
Amitriptyline	Colors urine bluish-green
Anthraquinone-containing drugs	Color urine yellow or red, depending on pH
Antipyrine	Produces interfering color in ferric chloride test for acetone
Aspidium oleoresin	If absorbed, may produce false positive result in Benedict's test
Avocado	Avocado, banana, blue plum, brinjal, eggplant, papaw, passion fruit, pineapple, plantain, red plum, tomato, and walnut may elevate urinary 5-HIAA excretion owing to their high serotonin content
Barbiturates	Depress color reaction in 5-HIAA determination
	May induce acute intermittent porphyria, particularly when used as a general anesthetic
Barium sulfate	May displace Diagnex blue from its resin, producing false positive test result
Bishydroxycoumarin	Colors alkaline urine orange/red
Bismuth salts	May produce glycosuria
Caffeine	Produces more rapid excretion of resin in Diagnex blue test
Calcium antacids	May displace Diagnex blue from its resin, producing false positive test result
Cephaloridine	Produces interfering brown color in Benedict's test for glucose
Cephalothin	Produces interfering brown color in Benedict's test for glucose
Chloral hydrate	May induce attack of acute intermittent porphyria
Chloroquine	Colors urine yellowish-brown
	May induce attack of acute intermittent porphyria
Chlorpropamide	May induce attack of acute intermittent porphyria
Chlorzoxazone	Colors urine red/orange-purple/blue
Diphenylhydantoin	Colors alkaline urine red/brown
Epinephrine	Large doses may produce glycosuria
Ethacrynic acid	Produces uricosuria following intravenous administration
Ethoxazene	Colors urine orange/red
	Interferes with determination of porphyrins by spectrophotofluorometry
Furazolidone	Colors urine red/brown
Glutethimide	May produce color change which interferes with VMA measurement
Griseofulvin	May induce attack of acute intermittent porphyria
Heparin	May lower 5-HIAA excretion in patient with metastatic carcinoid disease
Hydralazine	Interferes with determination of catecholamines by spectrophotofluorometry
Iron (oral)	May displace Diagnex blue from its resin, producing false positive test result
Iron sorbitol (IM)	May produce dark brown color in urine on standing
Isoniazid	May produce glycosuria
	May produce false positive result in Benedict's test in absence of glycosuria
Kaolin	Kaopectate may split Diagnex blue from its resin, producing false positive test result
Lithium carbonate	May produce glycosuria
Magnesium antacids	May displace Diagnex blue from its resin, producing false positive test result
Mephenesin	Increases color reaction in 5-HIAA determination
	May produce interfering color in test for VMA
Methenamine hippurate	Hippuric acid liberation may produce false positive result in Benedict's test
	May alter PSP excretion
Methenamine mandelate	Formaldehyde liberation may produce false positive result in Benedict's test
	Large doses may liberate sufficient formaldehyde to produce renal damage
	Formaldehyde production may interfere with color test for urobilinogen
Methocarbamol	May produce dark brown, black, or greenish color in urine on standing
	Increases color reaction in 5-HIAA determination
α-Methyldopa	May produce darkening of urine on standing
	May interfere with determination of uric acid by phosphotungstate method
Methylene blue	Colors urine blue/greenish-yellow
	Blue color directly interferes with color determination of Diagnex blue test
Metronidazole	May produce dark brown color in urine on standing
Morphine	May induce acute intermittent porphyria
Nicotinic acid	May produce glycosuria
Nitrofurantoin	Colors urine yellow/brown
Phenacetin	Produces interfering color in ferric chloride test for acetone
	Acetophenetidin may color urine brown/wine red
Phenazopyridine	Colors urine orange/red
	May produce false positive result in Diagnex blue test by imparting additional color
	Interferes with spectrophotofluorometric determination of porphyrins

(continued)

Phenazopyridine *(continued)*	Produces interfering yellowish to pink color with Ehrlich's aldehyde reagent for urobilinogen determination
Phenformin	Induces false color in test for acetone
Phenolphthalein	May color alkaline urine pink/red
Phenolsulfonphthalein	Colors alkaline urine pink
Phenothiazines	May color urine reddish-brown
	May interfere with determination of diacetic acid level
	May interfere with urinary estrogen determination by Kober method
	Depress color reaction in 5-HIAA determination
Phensuximide	Colors urine red/brown
Primaquine	Colors urine red/brown
Procaine	Interferes with Ehrlich's aldehyde reagent for porphobilinogen and urobilinogen determinations
Quinacrine	Colors urine yellow
Quinidine	May color urine brown/black
Quinine	May color urine brown/black
Riboflavin	Colors urine yellow
Salicylates	Produce interfering color in ferric chloride test for acetone
Sodium bicarbonate	Reduces urinary calcium excretion in alkaline urine
	May produce false positive result in test for proteinuria by Albutest method
Sulfonamides	May color urine yellow/brown
	Interfere with Ehrlich's aldehyde reagent for porphobilinogen and urobilinogen determinations
	Crystalluria may produce proteinuria
	Sulfisoxazole may produce false positive result in test for proteinuria
Tetracyclines	Parenteral forms containing large quantities of vitamin C may produce false positive result in test for glycosuria
	Chlortetracycline may produce false positive result in Benedict's test
	May interfere with urinary estrogen determination by fluorometric method
	Degraded tetracyclines may induce reversible symptoms resembling De Toni-Fanconi syndrome
Tolbutamide	Metabolite produces false positive result in tests for proteinuria using acetic acid, sulfosalicylic acid, or heat
Tolonium chloride	May color urine blue/green
Triamterene	Produces blue fluorescence in urine
Vitamin C	May produce false negative result in guaiac test
X-ray contrast media	Diatrizoate sodium produces black color in Benedict's test
	Several agents produce false positive result in tests for proteinuria using nitric acid and sulfosalicylic acid

TABLE 76–3. Influence of Drugs on Endocrine and Miscellaneous Tests

Drug	Cerebrospinal fluid protein (CSP)	Electrocardiography	Fat	17-hydroxycorticosteroids	I^{131} uptake	17-ketogenic steroids	17-ketosteroids	Metyrapone response	Occult blood (benzidine, guaiac)	Pregnancy (immunologic)	Protein bound iodine (PBI)	Pseudolymphoma	Sarcoidosis	Schilling	Sex chromatin	Skin (intradermal)	Spermatozoa (postcoital)	Urobilinogen	T$_3$ uptake
Acetaminophen									+										
Acetanilide									+										
Acetazolamide				?															
Alcohol (ethyl)									+										
Aminosalicylic acid			+	−					+		−							+S	
Amphetamines				?															
Ampicillin																		−	
Anabolic steroids							+				−								+S
Androgens					−S		+				−S				S				
Antipyrine																		+	
Bacitracin			+																
Barbiturates					?	S													
Barium sulfate											+S								
Bishydroxycoumarin			+						+		−								+
Bromide									+		+S								
Bromsulphalein											+							+	
Caffeine				+															
Carisoprodol								−											
Cephaloridine									+									−	
Cephalothin									+									−	
Chiniofon					−						+								
Chloral hydrate				+							−								
Chloramphenicol									+									−	
Chlordiazepoxide				+S	−		?												
Chlorpropamide											−								
Cinchophen									+										
Cloxacillin																		−	
Colchicine			+	+					+		−								
Corticosteroids				+	−		−		+							S			
Corticotropin				+	−		−		+		−					S			
Dexamethasone				−			−		+										
D-thyroxine											+								
Diazepam					−														
Digitalis		S		?					+										
Diiodohydroxyquin					−				+		+								
Diphenylhydantoin					−		−	−			−S	S	S						+
Dithiazanine iodide											+								
Emetine		S							+										
Epinephrine											−								

TABLE 76–3. *(continued)*

Drug	Cerebrospinal fluid protein (CSP)	Electrocardiography	Fat	17-hydroxycorticosteroids	I¹³¹ uptake	17-ketogenic steroids	17-ketosteroids	Metyrapone response	Occult blood (benzidine, guaiac)	Pregnancy (immunologic)	Protein bound iodine (PBI)	Pseudolymphoma	Sarcoidosis	Schilling	Sex chromatin	Skin (intradermal)	Spermatozoa (postcoital)	Urobilinogen	T₃ uptake
Erythromycin										+									−
Estrogens				−			−				+S				S		S		−
Ethinamate							+S												
Fluoride											−								
Gentamicin																		−	
Glutethimide							+S												
Gold salts											−								
Heparin									+										
Histamine									+										
Hydroxyzine				+S															
Indomethacin									+										
Inorganic iodides				+	−				+		+								
Iodine-containing drugs				+	−				+		+								
Iodochlorhydroxyquin				+	−				+		+S								
Iodopyrine									+		+								
Iothiouracil											+								
Iron (oral)									+S										
Kanamycin	+																		−
L-thyroxine					−						+								
Lithium carbonate					−S						−S								
Mannitol	+																		
Mechlorethamine											+								
Meprobamate				+S	−		+S	−											
Mercurial diuretics											−S								
Methenamine mandelate				+S		+S	+S				+								
Methicillin																		−	
Methotrexate	+								+										
Metrecal											+S								
Monoamine oxidase inhibitors								−											
Morphine									+S										
Nafcillin																		−	
Nalidixic acid						+	+												
Neomycin	+																		
Nitrofurantoin				+															
Oral contraceptives				−S	−		−S	−			+S								−
Oxacillin																		−	
Paraaminobenzoic acid											−								
Paraldehyde				+			?												
Penicillin						+S	+S												

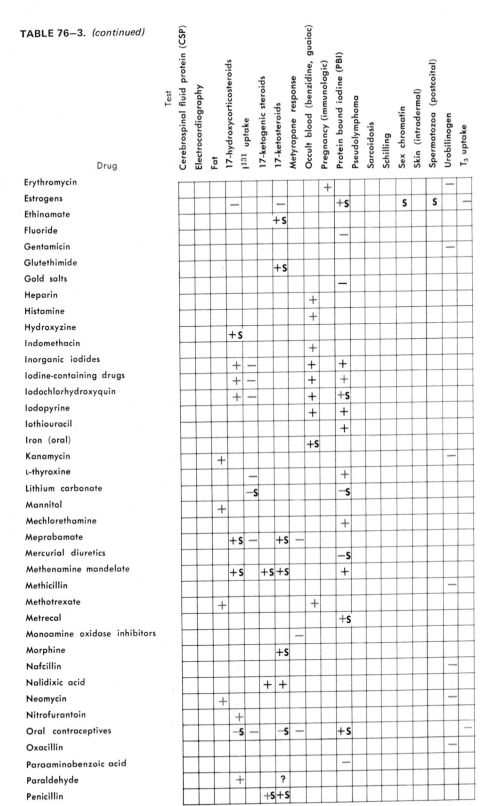

(continued)

TABLE 76–3. (continued)

Drug (Test →)	Cerebrospinal fluid protein (CSP)	Electrocardiography	Fat	17-hydroxycorticosteroids	I^{131} uptake	17-ketogenic steroids	17-ketosteroids	Metyrapone response	Occult blood (benzidine, guaiac)	Pregnancy (immunologic)	Protein bound iodine (PBI)	Pseudolymphoma	Sarcoidosis	Schilling	Sex chromatin	Skin (intradermal)	Spermatozoa (postcoital)	Urobilinogen	T_3 uptake
Perphenazine											+								−
Phenacetin	+S								+										
Phenaglycodol				+		+	+												
Phenazopyridine							?												
Phenindione									+										
Phenolphthalein			+																
Phenothiazines	+S	S		−S			+S	−		+S	+								
Phenylbutazone					−				+		−	S							+
Polymyxin B			+																
Potassium chloride									+S										
Probenecid									−										
Progesterones											+				S		S		
Propoxyphene				+															
Propylthiouracil											−								−
Pyrazinamide							−				+								
Quinidine		S																	
Quinine		S		+			?												
Reserpine				−S			−		+										
Resorcinol											−								
Salicylates	+S								+		−		S						+
Spironolactone				+			+												
Streptomycin	+S																−		
Sulfonamides	+S			+	−						−								
Tetracyclines			+														S	−	
Tetraiodofluorescein											+								
Thiazide diuretics				−	−		?				−								
Thyroglobulin					−						+								
Thyroid (desiccated)					−						+								
Tolbutamide											−								
Triacetyloleandomycin				+S			+S												
Triiodothyronine					−						+								
Vitamin A											+								
Vitamin B_{12}														+					
Vitamin C							+S	−											
Vitamin D											+								
X-ray contrast media					−						+								

Aminosalicylic acid	Interfering yellow color produced with Ehrlic's aldehyde reagent for urobilinogen and porphobilinogen determination
Anabolic steroids	Decrease thyroxine binding capacity of plasma proteins
Androgens	Testosterone may reduce ^{131}I uptake. Testosterone may displace protein-bound thyroxine. Testosterone may reduce number of Barr bodies
Barbiturates	May inhibit metyrapone response
Barium sulfate	Iodine contaminants may elevate PBI
Bromide	Iodine contaminants may elevate PBI
Chlordiazepoxide	May produce false positive increase in 17-hydroxycorticosteroid level determined by Glenn-Nelson method
Corticosteroids	Depress most intradermal skin tests, e.g., for tuberculosis
Corticotropin	Depresses most intradermal skin tests, e.g., for tuberculosis
Digitalis	All manifestations of digitalis on EKG must be interpreted in light of clinical diagnosis; for discussion of changes, see Chapter 33
Diphenylhydantoin	Displaces thyroxine from plasma protein-binding sites. May induce lymph node changes suggestive of lymphoma. May induce lymph node changes suggestive of sarcoidosis
Emetine	Produces typical EKG changes; prolongation of PR and QT intervals; flattening and inversion of T waves
Estrogens	Augment protein binding of thyroxine. May increase number of Barr bodies. Increase number and motility of spermatozoa
Ethinamate	Produces interfering color in Zimmermann test for 17-ketosteroids
Glutethimide	Increases color reaction in 17-ketosteroid determination
Hydroxyzine	Produces interfering substance in Glenn-Nelson technique for 17-hydroxycorticosteroid estimation
Iodochlorhydroxyquin	Augments protein binding of thyroxine
Iron (oral)	Ferrous fumarate may produce false positive result in orthotolidine test for occult blood
Lithium carbonate	May reduce thyroid function
Meprobamate	Interferes with Glenn-Nelson test for 17-hydroxycorticosteroids. Interferes with Zimmermann test for 17-ketosteroids
Mercurial diuretics	Produce false negative PBI level in tests using chloric acid and distillation
Methenamine mandelate	Interferes with phenylhydrazine tests for 17-hydroxycorticosteroids, 17-ketogenic steroids, and 17-ketosteroids
Metrecal	Increases PBI level due to high iodocasein content
Morphine	Increases color reaction in 17-ketosteroid determination
Oral contraceptives	Estrogen component may increase quantity of cortisone-binding plasma protein. It may also increase quantity of cortisone-binding, etc., with resultant decrease in urinary 17-hydroxycorticosteroid and 17-ketosteroid excretion
Penicillin	High doses intravenously may cause depression of 17-ketogenic steroid and 17-ketosteroid excretion. Increases color reaction in 17-ketosteroid determination
Perphenazine	Increases thyroxine binding capacity of plasma proteins
Phenacetin	Acetophenetidin may produce false positive result in test for cerebrospinal fluid protein by sulfosalicylic acid method
Phenothiazines	Prevent determination of cerebrospinal fluid protein; produce false positive result in test for CSF protein by Folin-Ciocalteu method. Produce typical EKG changes: sinus tachycardia, prolongation of QT interval, flattening of T wave. Depress or inhibit formation of corticosteroid bisphenylhydrazone in Porter-Silver test. May produce false positive increase in 17-ketosteroid estimation by Zimmermann test. Thorazine may produce false positive immunologic test for pregnancy
Phenylbutazone	May induce lymph node changes suggestive of lymphoma
Potassium chloride	May produce small bowel ulceration
Progesterones	May reduce number of Barr bodies. Decrease number and motility of spermatozoa
Quinidine	Produces typical EKG changes: sinus tachycardia, SA block, prolongation of QT interval, bizarre rhythm changes particularly after digitalis
Quinine	Rarely produces EKG changes
Reserpine	Produces interfering substance in Glenn-Nelson technique for 17-hydroxycorticosteroid estimation
Salicylates	May produce false positive result in test for cerebrospinal fluid protein by Folin-Ciocalteu method. May displace thyroxine from plasma protein-binding sites
Streptomycin	Prevents determination of cerebrospinal fluid protein
Sulfonamides	Prevent determination of cerebrospinal fluid protein; sulfanilamide may produce false positive result in test for cerebrospinal fluid protein by Folin-Ciocalteu method
Tetracyclines	Increase number and motility of spermatozoa
Triacetyloleandomycin	Interferes with Porter-Silber test for 17-hydroxycorticosteroids and with Drekter test for 17-ketosteroids
Vitamin C	Increases color reaction in 17-ketosteroid determination

FURTHER READING

Best LR (1963): Drug-associated blood dyscrasias. JAMA 185:286

Bohnen RF, Ultmann JE, Gorman JG, Farhangi M, Scudder J (1968): The direct Coombs' test: The clinical significance. Ann Intern Med 68:19

Hicks JT (1967): Drugs affecting laboratory values. Hosp Formulary Management 3:19

Martin EW (1971): Hazards of Medication. Philadelphia, Toronto, JB Lippincott

Sisson JC (1965): Principles of, and pitfalls in, thyroid function tests. J Nucl Med 6:853

Young DS, Thomas DW, Friedman RB, Pestaner LC (1972): Effects of drugs on clinical laboratory tests. Clin Chem 18:1041–1303

JEREMY H. THOMPSON

77. ANTIBIOTIC THERAPY IN RENAL FAILURE

Many antibiotics and their metabolites are eliminated from the body primarily by renal excretion, and compounds may reach the urine by either glomerular filtration and or tubular secretion. For example, the penicillins are cleared by both filtration and secretion, whereas vancomycin is removed by filtration only. Some of the filtered or secreted antibiotic may undergo tubular reabsorption into the renal parenchyma or bloodstream. Cephaloridine, for example, is partially reabsorbed by the renal tubules.

There are two risks faced by the patient with compromised renal function when he has to be treated with a drug which is mainly excreted by the kidney. First, there is the danger of toxicity due to high blood concentrations of the drug or metabolites resulting from impaired excretion, and, second, there is the danger that specific drugs will be withheld because of fear of inducing toxicity. Unfortunately, the pharmacokinetics of most antibiotics have not been well studied in renal impairment, and thus dosage guidelines are mostly empirical. A summary table is included here, based upon data in the literature, but it is far from being entirely satisfactory (Table 77–1). Selection of an appropriate dose is usually difficult, and when hemodialysis or peritoneal dialysis is being performed, further adjustment of antibiotic dosage is imperative if the drug is being lost in the dialysis fluid.

Because of the wide physiologic variability of patients with respect to drug responses in renal impairment, it is impossible to predict with certainty that any given dosage schedule will either be effective or produce toxicity, and thus, where possible, posology should be controlled by the determination of blood drug levels and through clinical judgment. Several formulas for calculating drug dosage in renal impairment have been proposed, but none are universally satisfactory.

TABLE 77-1. A Guide to the Dosage of Antibiotics in Renal Failure

Antibiotic	Serum half-life (h) Normal	Oliguria	Hepatic failure	Mechanism of removal (%)	Duration of effective serum level (h)	Major toxicity in uremia
Amphotericin B	18—24	?	No effect	Kidney	24	Anemia, renal tubular acidosis, K loss, nephrotoxicity
Ampicillin	0.5	8—15	Slight effect	Kidney-T	4	Epileptiform seizures
Bacitracin	1—2	?	?	Kidney (10—30)	?	Nephrotoxicity
Carbenicillin	IV 1	15	25	Kidney		Sodium lode, clotting abnormalities
Cefazolin	2.0	56	?	Kidney	8	Skin rashes, shedding of hair and nails
Cephalexin	PO 1	20	Slight effect	Kidney		Skin rashes, drug fever
Cephaloridine	0.5—1.5	20—24	No effect	Kidney-G (60—70)	8	Renal tubular damage
Cephalothin	0.5—1.0	6—18	No effect	Kidney (60—90)	4	Skin rashes, drug fever, GI upsets
Chloramphenicol	1.5—4.0	3—5	Moderate increase	Liver (90—95) Kidney-G (5—10)	8	Not increased unless hepatic failure present
Chlortetracycline	5—6	6—11	Marked increase	Kidney-G Liver	6	Hepatic failure
Clindamycin	2—3	10	Moderate increase			Skin rashes, GI upsets, altered liver function
Cloxacillin	0.5	0.8	?	Kidney (G:T)	4	Seizures
Colistimethate	1.5—3	48—72	No effect	Kidney-G (40—80)	12	Nephrotoxicity, peripheral neuritis, resp. paralysis
Demeclocycline	9—12	50	Marked increase	Kidney-G Liver	6	Hepatic failure
Dicloxacillin	0.7	1.0	?	Kidney (G:T)	8	Seizures
Doxycycline	17	Slight increase	Marked increase	Liver		Skin rashes, GI upsets
Erythromycin	1—1.5	4—6	Moderate increase	Liver (85), Kidney-G (15)	6	Usual reactions
Ethambutol	4—6	7—14	?	?	?	Altered perception, color green
Gentamicin	2—6	4—72	No effect	Kidney-G (80—100)		Nephrotoxicity, ototoxicity
Isoniazid	1—4	?	Moderate increase	Liver	8	Ataxia, peripheral neuritis
Kanamycin	2—4	72—96	No effect	Kidney-G:T (50—90)	12	Nephrotoxicity, ototoxicity
Lincomycin	4—5	10—15	Moderate increase	Liver (85—90) Kidney (10—15)	6	Skin rashes, GI upsets
Methacycline	14	?	?	Kidney Liver	20	Skin rashes, GI upsets, hepatic failure
Methicillin	0.5	4.0	No effect	Kidney-G:T	4	Epileptiform seizures, nephritis, hepatitis
Minocycline	10—15	35	Moderate increase			Skin rashes, hepatic failure
Nafcillin	1.0	?	?	Kidney (G:T)	9	Seizures
Nitrofurantoin	0.5	?	Moderate increase	Kidney-G:T (30—60)		
Novobiocin	2—3		Marked increase	Liver		
Oxacillin	0.5	2.0	Slight increase	Kidney-G:T	6	Skin rashes, epileptiform seizures
Oxytetracycline	8	66	?	Kidney Liver	12	Skin rashes, GI upsets, hepatic failure
Penicillin G	0.2—0.5	3.5—20	No effect	Kidney-G (10—30) -T (70—90)	4	Epileptiform seizures, hyperkalemia
Polymyxin B	6—7	48—72	No effect	Kidney-G	12	Nephrotoxicity, peripheral neuritis
Rifampin	1.5—5	Slight increase	10—15			Nephrotoxicity, hepatic failure
Streptomycin	2—4	48—96	No effect	Kidney-G (30—80)	12	Nephrotoxicity, ototoxicity
Tetracycline	IV 6 PO 8—9	48—108	Slight increase	Kidney-G (20—70) Liver	6	Hepatic failure
Vancomycin	4—6	216		Kidney-G (30—100		Nephrotoxicity, ototoxicity

G=glomerular filtration, T=tubular secretion, IV=intravenous, PO=per oral, U=unit, d=day, ?=data not available

Drug removal by dialysis		Dosage schedule			
		Renal failure		During dialysis	
Peritoneal	Hemodialysis	Moderate	Severe	Peritoneal	Hemodialysis
No	No	0.5 mg/kg/3 d	0.5 mg/kg/4–5 d	As for severe renal failure	As for severe renal failure
No	Slight	Normal	0.5–10 g/8–12 hr	As for severe renal failure	0.5 g/6 hr
?	?	100,000 U/d	?	?	?
Slight	Slight	2 g/8 hr	2 g/8–12 hr	2 g/6 hr	2 g/6 hr
?	?	0.4 g/d	0.25 g/d	?	?
Slight	Slight	250–500 mg/24 hr	250–500 mg/24 hr	250 mg/12 hr	250 mg/12 hr
Yes	Yes	Do not use	Do not use	Do not use	Do not use
Yes	Yes	Normal	1 g/8–12 hr	Add 20μg/ml	1 g/6 hr
No	No	Normal	10–25% reduction	As for severe renal failure	As for severe renal failure
Slight	Yes	Do not use	Do not use	Do not use	Do not use
No	No				
?	?	Normal	?	?	?
15%	No	150 mg/2–4 d	100 mg/2–4 d	As for severe renal failure	As for severe renal failure
Slight	No	Do not use	Do not use	Do not use	Do not use
?	?	Normal	?	?	?
No	No	Normal	25% reduction	As for severe renal failure	As for severe renal failure
No	No	Normal	Normal	Normal	Normal
Slight	Slight	10 mg/kg/d	5-10 mg/kg/d	?	?
Slight	Yes	25% reduction	80 mg/2 d		1.5 mg/kg
Yes	Yes	Normal			100 mg/d
40%	Yes	0.5 g/1.5d	0.5 g/3 d	250 mg	7.5 mg/kg
No	No	Normal			
?	?	0.3 g/1-3 d	0.3 g/3-4 d	?	?
No	Slight	Normal	1-2 g/8 hr	As in severe renal failure	1 g/6 hr
No	No	Do not use	Do not use	Do not use	Do not use
?	?	Normal	?	?	?
		Do not use	Do not use	Do not use	Do not use
		Normal	25% reduction	As in severe renal failure	As in severe renal failure
No	Slight	Normal	1–2 g/6 hr	1–2 g/6 hr	1–2 g/6 hr
?	?	0.25 g/8 hr	0.25 g/d	?	?
No	Slight	Normal	1.6×10⁶ U/6–12 hr	1.6×10⁶ U/6–12 hr	1.6×10⁶ U/6 hr
No	No	100 mg/2–4 d	50 mg/2–4 d	50 mg/2–4 d	50 mg/2–4 d
?	?		300 mg/kg/24 hr	?	?
Yes	Yes	0.5 g/1.5 d	0.5 g/3 d	0.5 g/3 d	0.5 g/3 d
Slight	No	Do not use	Do not use	Do not use	Do not use
?	?	0.5 g/216 hr	0.5 g/216 hr	0.5 g/216 hr	0.5 g/216 hr

FURTHER READING

Bennett WM, Singer I, Coggino CH (1973): Guide to drug usage in adult patients with impaired renal function: A supplement JAMA 223:991–997

Bulger RJ, Petersdorf RG (1970): Antimicrobial therapy in patients with renal insufficiency. Postgrad Med 47:160–165

Jackson EA, McLeod DC (1974): Pharmacokinetics and dosing of antimicrobial agents in renal impairment, Parts I and II. Am J Hosp Pharm 31:36–52; 137–148

Kovnat P, Labovitz E, Levinson SP (1973): Antibiotics and the kidney. Med Clin North Am 57:1045–1063

Mirkin BL (1970): Drug therapy in patients with impaired renal function. Postgrad Med 47:159–164

JOSEPH H. BECKERMAN

78. PROLONGED ACTION DOSAGE FORMS

Many medications have been specially formulated to produce prolonged therapeutic action after administration. The benefits of these dosage forms are a more uniform and therefore more effective blood level pattern, greater convenience in administration and an economy resultant upon the administration of fewer doses.

There are a number of ways to effect a prolonged or predetermined release of medication from its dosage form. The three methods most often used are addition of a second pharmacologically active substance, chemical modification of the drug and alteration of the physical properties of the drug or formulation.

PHARMACOLOGIC MEANS OF PROLONGING DRUG ACTION

The action of a drug may be prolonged by the addition of an active substance which decreases blood flow and slows absorption. The technique has been used effectively to prolong the action of local anesthetics. Vasoconstrictors, such as epinephrine, have been combined with procaine, lidocaine, mepivacaine and other similar agents (Ch. 22). A second substance may be selected for its ability to slow the excretion rate of a drug administered systematically. Probenecid is an excellent example of this method of pharmacologic prolongation of drug action. Probenecid, a substance which inhibits the renal tubular transport of organic acids, was developed specifically to raise and maintain the plasma level of penicillin (Ch. 58).

CHEMICAL MEANS OF PROLONGING DRUG ACTION

Chemical methods have been used to convert a drug into a less soluble form which may delay excretion or slow the rate of absorption. This method has been successfully applied to penicillin and insulin therapy. Procaine penicillin is prepared by reacting an aqueous solution of sodium or potassium penicillin G with an equimolar quantity of procaine hydrochloride. The resultant compound is used every 12–24 hr instead of every 3–6 hr to maintain effective levels.

Unmodified or soluble insulin is rapidly absorbed and has a duration of action of 12–16 hr. However, when insulin is modified by the addition of zinc chloride so that the solid phase of the suspension consists of a mixture of crystals and amorphous insulin in a ratio of approximately 7 parts of crystals to 3 parts of amorphous material, the duration of action is extended to 30 hr.

PHYSICAL MEANS OF PROLONGING DRUG ACTION

There are a great number of techniques used to modify the physical properties of drugs and their vehicles to induce slower absorption. Compression of a drug into a hard, sterile pellet is used for the administration of steroid hormones such as desoxycorticosterone acetate. Another commonly used method for prolonging activity is the use of gelatin solution as a vehicle for subcutaneous or intramuscular injections. An example of this physical modification is the use of this vehicle for the administration of sodium heparin.

Medication in oral dosage forms for prolonged action has been designated as delayed release, continuous action, sustained release, sustained action, timed release, and time disintegration medication. The majority of these preparations are designed to produce a continuous therapeutic effect for 8–12 hr.

One of the widely used dosage forms in the Spansule, a capsule containing many tiny pellets with varying disintegration times. These pellets are usually divided into four groups: uncoated beads, beads resistant to dissolution for 3 hr, beads resistant to dissolution for 6 hr and beads resistant for 9 hr. These beads are then encapsulated. A variation of this procedure (used in Spacetabs) is to include coated granules in the regular tablet granulation.

Another type of timed release formulation is the Timespan, a tablet with a slow release core. In this case the drug is mixed in a core such as carnauba wax. The core slowly dissolves and the drug leaches out. An outer core containing immediately available drug can be compressed onto the slow release core, as in Extentabs.

Repeat action tablets (Repetabs) are not truly sustained release preparations. They resemble enteric coated tablets except that an immediate release portion is applied outside the barrier coat. This allows a second dose 4–6 hr later, but not a continuous release.

Enteric coated tablets designed to disintegrate in basic pH never break up to release the drug, since the pH in the lower part of the small intestine is seldom higher than 7.0. However, some enteric coatings (e.g., Enseals) are designed to release the drug by simple erosion.

In the preparation of multiple layer tablets (e.g., Spantabs) the sustained release granulation is compressed into one layer, and the immediate release granulation is compressed into a second layer.

Cationic drugs can be complexed with polar cationic exchange resins (as in Ionamin), and release from this preparation is dependent upon pH and electrolyte content of the intestinal tract.

Drugs with amine groups (e.g., antihistamines and alkaloids) can be complexed with tannic acid to form slightly soluble salts. Release is dependent upon the pH of the stomach. An example of this is cryptenamine tannate, an alkaloidal fraction of veratrum (Ch. 20).

The prescriber should remember that while many of these dosage forms perform ideally in vitro, their action in the human organism is often far from suitable.

JOSEPH H. BECKERMAN

79. COMMONLY USED PARENTERAL SOLUTIONS

Intravenous fluid therapy plays an important role in the management of the sick. Diarrhea, burns, a draining fistula, the use of gastrointestinal suction or intubation, extensive trauma, hemorrhage, vomiting, large open wounds and even lactation may result in the loss of large amounts of water and electrolytes. Intravenous fluid may also serve as an important vehicle for the administration of drugs when a rapid response is desirable or when other routes are not available.

The prescriber should carefully select the proper fluid for the particular condition. Adverse reactions may occur if an infusion is given too rapidly or if too large a volume is given. This may result in acid base imbalance, circulatory overload or congestive heart failure, especially in patients with cardiorenal disease. Orders by prescriber should clearly indicate amount and flow rate of fluid therapy.

TABLE 79–1. Commonly Used Parenteral Solutions

Solution	Formula	Grams/liter	Milliequivalents per liter							
			Na^+	K^+	Ca^{++}	Mg^{++}	NH_4^+	Cl^-	Lactate	HPO_4^{--}
Ammonium Chloride 2.14%	Ammonium chloride	21.40					400	400		
Dextran 6% in sodium	Dextran	60.00	154					154		
Chloride 0.9%	Sodium chloride	9.00								
Dextrose in water 2.5%	Hydrous dextrose	25.00								
Dextrose in water 5%	Hydrous dextrose	50.00								
Dextrose in water 10%	Hydrous dextrose	100.00								
Dextrose in water 20%	Hydrous dextrose	200.00								
Dextrose 2.5% in sodium	Hydrose chloride	25.00	77					77		
Chloride 0.45%	Sodium chloride	4.50								
Dextrose 2.5% in sodium	Hydrous dextrose	25.00	154					154		
Chloride 0.9%	Sodium chloride	9.00								
Dextrose 5% in sodium	Hydrous dextrose	50.00	34					34		
Chloride 0.2%	Sodium chloride	2.00								
Dextrose 5% in sodium	Hydrous dextrose	50.00	77					77		
Chloride 0.45%	Sodium chloride	4.50								
Dextrose 5% in sodium	Hydrous dextrose	50.00								
Chloride 0.9%	Sodium chloride	9.00	154					154		
Dextrose 10% in sodium	Hydrous dextrose	100.00	154					154		
Chloride 0.9%	Sodium chloride	9.00								
Lactated Ringer's	Sodium lactate	3.10	130	4	3			109	28	
(Hartmann's) solution	Sodium chloride	6.00								
	Potassium chloride	0.30								
	Calcium chloride	0.20								
Mannitol 10% in sodium	Mannitol	100.00	77					77		
Chloride 0.45%	Sodium chloride	4.50								
Mannitol 20% in water	Mannitol	200.00								

Solution	Constituent	g							
Peritoneal dialysis with 1.5% dextrose	Hydrous dextrose	15.00	141		3.5	1.5	101	45	
	Sodium lactate	5.00							
	Sodium chloride	5.60							
	Calcium chloride	0.26							
	Magnesium chloride hexahydrate	0.15							
Peritoneal dialysis with 4.25% dextrose	Hydrous dextrose	42.50	141		3.5	1.5	101	45	
	Sodium lactate	5.00							
	Sodium chloride	5.60							
	Calcium chloride	0.26							
	Magnesium chloride hexahydrate	0.15							
Polyionic 48 in dextrose 5%	Hydrous dextrose	50.00	25	20		3	22	23	3
	Sodium lactate	2.60							
	Potassium chloride	1.30							
	Magnesium chloride hexahydrate	0.31							
	Dibasic potassium phosphate	0.26							
Polyionic 75 in dextrose 5%	Hydrous dextrose	50.00	40	35			40	20	15
	Sodium lactate	2.30							
	Potassium chloride	1.50							
	Dibasic potassium phosphate	0.26							
	Sodium chloride	0.91							
Ringer's	Sodium chloride	8.60	147	4	4		155		
	Potassium chloride	0.30							
	Calcium chloride	0.33							
Sodium chloride (normal saline)	Sodium chloride	9.00	154				154		
Sodium chloride 0.45% (half normal saline)	Sodium chloride	4.50	77				77		
Sodium chloride 5%	Sodium chloride	50.00	855				855		
Sodium lactate 1/6 molar	Sodium lactate	18.70	167					167	

JOHN A. BEVAN

80. SOURCES OF INFORMATION IN PHARMACOLOGY

DRUG REFERENCES

The Pharmacopeia of the United States of America (*The United States Pharmacopeia; U.S.P.*) (1975) New York

Conservative, official compendium of drugs of proved therapeutic value. Contains directions regarding sources, identification, assay, standards of purity, etc. Revised every 5 years by an independent committee of the Pharmacopeial Convention. Because of its conservative approach to selection, many recent widely used drugs are not included. Standards are recognized by the Food and Drug Administration.

The National Formulary (*N.F.*) (1975): Washington, DC, American Pharmaceutical Association

Conservative publication, revised every 5 years, complementary to the *U.S.P.* Criterion for inclusion is *now* only therapeutic value, not extent of use, as in older editions. Standards are recognized by the Food and Drug Administration.

The British Pharmacopoeia (*B.P.*) (1973): Published under the recommendation of the Medicines Commission for Her Majesty's Stationery Office, Cambridge, England, University Printer House

The British equivalent of the *U.S.P.*, revised every 5 years.

Physicians' Desk Reference. Oradell, New Jersey, Medical Economics

Compiled, organized information regarding major pharmaceutical specialties, biologicals, and antibiotics. Published annually. Information is based upon material supplied by the manufacturers whose products are included.

The Merck Index: An Enclyclopedia of Chemicals and Drugs (1968): Rahway, New Jersey, Merck

An encyclopedial reference to the chemistry and physical characteristics of drugs. Revised every 8 years.

The United States Dispensatory (1973). By Osol A, et al. Philadelphia, Lippincott

A collection, alphabetically arranged, of articles on individual drugs and of general articles on pharmacologic classes of drugs.

Pharmaceutical Compounds and Their Synonyms (1967): By Negwer M New York, Pergamon Press

A compendium of important tables introducing 3900 drugs and more than 26,000 synonyms in international use.

PHARMACOLOGY AND TOXICOLOGY REFERENCES

The Pharmacological Basis of Therapuetics (1970): Goodman LS, Gilman A (eds) New York, Macmillan

Drill's Pharmacology in Medicine (1971): DiPalma JR (ed) New York, McGraw-Hill

Clinical Toxicology of Commercial Products (1973): Gleason MN, Gosselin RE, Hodge HC, Smith RP (eds) 3rd ed. Baltimore, Williams & Wilkins

CLINICAL PHARMACOLOGY REFERENCES

Accepted Dental Remedies (1967): Chicago, American Dental Association

Drugs used in dental practice, including a list of brands accepted by the Council on Dental Therapeutics of the American Dental Association. A handbook of therapeutics, not a textbook of pharmacology.

Current Therapy (1974): Conn RB (ed) Philadelphia, Saunders

Current and authoritative information on the treatment of disease. Renewed annually.

Dilemmas in Drug Therapy (1967): Beckman H (ed) Philadelphia, Saunders

One author's opinion on the use and abuse of. drugs, common and uncommon, in certain clinical situations.

New Drugs: By the Council on Drugs of the American Medical Association. Chicago, The Association

A review, replacing *New and Nonofficial Drugs*, which provides information on single-entity drugs introduced during the past 10 years and a comparative review of older drugs in a particular therapeutic group. Not a comprehensive reference book of drug therapy or a textbook of pharmacology. Published annually.

Side Effects of Drugs as Reported in the Medical Literature of the World. Meyler L (ed): Amsterdam, Excerpta Medica Foundation

Presents information obtained through the abstracting services of *Excerpta Medica* and the *Index Medicus* of the United States National Library of Medicine. Published annually.

PUBLICATIONS OF THE AMERICAN SOCIETY FOR PHARMACOLOGY AND EXPERIMENTAL THERAPEUTICS

Journal of Pharmacology and Experimental Therapeutics. Baltimore, Williams & Wilkins

Molecular Pharmacology. New York, Academic Press

Pharmacological Reviews. Baltimore, Williams & Wilkins

OTHER JOURNALS

Agents and Actions. Basel, Switzerland, Birkhaüser Verlag

Annual Review of Pharmacology. Cutting WC, Dreisbach RH, Elliott HW (eds). Annual Reviews, California, Palo Alto

Archives Internationales de Pharmacodynamie et de Thérapie. Belgium, Ghent

Biochemical Pharmacology. New York, Pergamon Press

British Journal of Pharmacology and Chemotherapy. British Pharmacological Society, London, British Medical Association

Clinical Pharmacology and Therapeutics. St. Louis, CV Mosby

Drug Surveillance Information. The Boston Collaborative Drug Surveillance Program, Director Dr. H. Jick, Boston University Medical Center, pools data particularly on drug exposure and adverse events from 14 hospitals in the United States, Canada, New Zealand, Israel and Scotland. Its aim is to provide clear statistical data on drug hazards.

European Journal of Pharmacology. Amsterdam, North Holland Publishing Co

Journal of Pharmacy and Pharmacology. London, Pharmaceutical Society of Great Britian

Naunyn-Schmiedebergs Archiv für experimentelle Pathologie und Pharmakologie. Berlin, Springer

Pharmacology. Basel, Switzerland, Basel

Physiology and Pharmacology for Physicians. Washington, DC, American Physiological Society
Brief reviews of therapeutic usefulness of drugs. Designed for the practitioner of medicine.

Toxicology and Applied Pharmacology. Official Journal of the Society of Toxicology. New York, Academic Press

Toxicon. Oxford, Pergamon Press, Ltd
An international society devoted to the exchange of knowledge on the poisons derived for the tissues of plants and animals.

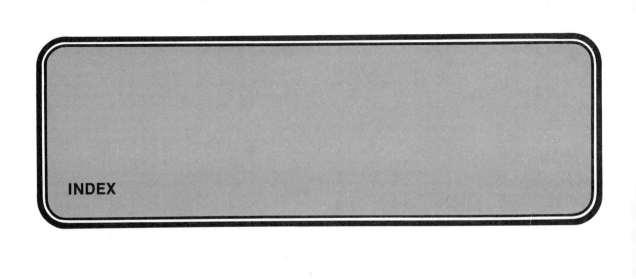

INDEX

A

Abortion
  prevention with progestational
    agents, 376
  prostaglandins for induction of,
    397
Abscesses, treatment of, 421
Absorption of drugs, 9—11
  in childhood, 82
  interactions during, 28—29
  malabsorption
    and adverse drug reactions, 55
    drugs causing, 577
  pH affecting, 9—10
  and routes of administration,
    10—11
Abuse of drugs, 66—74
  alcohol, 79—80
  amphetamines and stimulants,
    71—72
  barbiturates and other sedatives,
    70—71
  and dependence, 67—68
  hallucinogens, 72—73
  heroin and other opiates, 68—70
  marihuana, 73—74
  permissive drugs, 66
  prescriptive drugs, 67
  proscriptive drugs, 67
  and tolerance, 67
Acceptors
  binding with drugs, 4
  drug interactions at sites for, 30
Accessibility of drugs, barriers
    affecting, 6
Acetaminophen, 226
  affecting laboratory tests, 580—
    581, 592, 596, 598
  chemical structure of, 22
  excretion in milk, 576
Acetanilid
  adverse effects of, 569, 572
  affecting laboratory tests, 580—
    581, 592, 596, 598

Acetanilid *(continued)*
  blood dyscrasias from, 573
Acetarsone, adverse effects of, 569
Acetazolamide, 242, 246
  adverse effects of, 570, 571
  affecting laboratory tests, 580—
    581, 592, 598
  blood dyscrasias from, 573
  diuretic action of, 304, 307
Acetic acid, in alkali poisoning, 101
Acetohexamide, 353
  adverse effects of, 570
  interaction with other drugs, 32,
    566
Acetone in urine, drugs affecting
    tests for, 592—595
Acetophenetidin. *See* Phenacetin
Acetylation rate, genetic factors in,
    61—62
Acetylcholine, 116—117
  antagonism by antimuscarinic
    agents, 128
  chemistry of, 116
  depolarizing action of, 161—162
  mechanism of action, 117
  and neurohumoral transmission,
    111—112
  pharmacologic effects of, 116—
    117
  striatal, in parkinsonism, 248—
    249, 252
Acetylcholinesterase, 120, 161
Acetylphenylhydrazine, blood
    dyscrasias from, 573
Acetylsalicylic acid, 223—226
  adverse effects of, 569, 572
  blood dyscrasias from, 573
  excretion in milk, 576
  interaction with other drugs, 29,
    32, 566
Acetylsulfanilamide, adverse effects
    of, 572
Achlorhydria, histamine test in,
    384
Achromycin. *See* Tetracycline

Acid(s)
  corrosive, antidotes for, 101
  germicidal activity of, 489
Acidic drugs, interaction with other
    agents, 29, 32
Acidosis, renal tubular, diuretics in,
    311—313
Acne
  antibiotics in, 455—456
  estrogen therapy in, 369, 370
Acneiform eruption, drug-induced,
    569
Acoustic nerve, aminoglycosides
    affecting, 441—442
Acridine dyes
  adverse effects of, 570
  in malaria, 498
  mode of action, 417
Acriflavine
  adverse effects of, 568, 569
  affecting laboratory tests, 592,
    596
Acrisorcin, in tinea infections, 521
ACTH. *See* Corticotropin
Actidil, 386
Actinobacillus. See Pfeifferella
Actinomyces israelii, drugs affect-
    ing, 427, 436, 452
Actinomycin D
  in cancer, 539, 543
  mode of action, 417
  structure of, 538
Actinomycosis, 524
  penicillin in, 523
Active transport of drugs, 9
Activity of drugs
  selectivity of, 3
  structural factors in, 4
Adaptation, bacterial, and resis-
    tance to drugs, 403
Addiction to drugs, 68—71. *See*
    also Abuse of drugs
  antipsychotic drugs, 194
  narcotics, 233
Addison's disease, 356

Antihistamines *(continued)*
  therapeutic uses of, 387—388
  in vestibular disturbances, 132
Antihypertensive drugs, 150—159
  adrenergic neuron blocking
    agents, 155—157
  bretylium, 157
  ganglionic blocking agents, 154—
    155
  ganglionic stimulating agents, 154
  guanethidine, 155—157
  gyancydine, 153
  hydralazine, 153
  in hypertensive crises, 158
  α-methyldopa, 157—158
  minoxidil, 153
  monoamine oxidase inhibitors,
    158
  programs of therapy with, 159
  rationale of therapy with, 150—
    151
  reserpine, 152—153
  veratrum alkaloids, 151—152
Antiinflammatory agents, 223—229
  acetaminophen, 226
  adrenocorticoids, 358, 359—360
  colchicine, 228
  indomethacin, 227—228
  investigational, 229
  phenacetin, 226
  pyrazolon derivatives, 226—227
  salicylates, 223—226
Antimetabolites, 538, 539, 542
  mechanism of action, 536
Antimicrobial agents, 400. *See also*
    Antibiotics
Antiminth, 516
Antimony compounds
  adverse effects of, 570
  in helminthiasis, 514
  in leishmaniasis, 509
Antimony dimercaptosuccinate
    sodium, 422
Antimony gluconate sodium, 422
Antimony poisoning, antidote in,
    102
Antimony potassium tartrate
  adverse effects of, 569
  as anthelmintic, 514
  in leishmaniasis, 509
Antimuscarinic agents, 128—134
  absorption, excretion and
    metabolism of, 131
  adverse effects of, 133—134
  antipsychotic drugs, 195—196
  chemistry of, 128—129
  mechanism of action, 129
  pharmacologic effects of, 130—
    131
  poisoning from, 134
  therapeutic use of, 131—133
Antipsychotic drugs, 187—196
  addiction and tolerance to, 194
  adverse effects of, 194—196
  butyrophenones, 190—191
  choice of agent, 192
  contraindications to, 196
  dibenzodiazepines, 191
  dosage of, 193
  duration of treatment with, 192
  pharmacology of, 188—191

Antipsychotic drugs *(continued)*
  phenothiazines, 188—190
  rauwolfia alkaloids, 191
  therapeutic uses of, 191—192,
    193—194
  thioxanthenes, 190
Antipyretic agents, 224, 226, 227
Antipyrine, 226
  adverse effects of, 569, 570, 571,
    572
  affecting laboratory tests, 580—
    581, 592, 596, 598
  blood dyscrasias from, 573
  localization in organs, 13
Antiseptics and disinfectants, 488—
    491
  chemical agents, 489—491
  mechanisms of action, 488
  physical agents, 488—489
Antispasmodics, 132
Antitoxins, 561, 562
Antitussive agents, 233, 235, 238
Antivenins, 561, 562
Antodyne, 168—169
Anxiety, 206—210
  antipsychotic drugs in, 193
  benzodiazepines in, 207—210
  propanediols in, 207
Apoferritin, 314
Apomorphine, emetic effects of, 90
Appetite
  stimulants of, 288
  suppressants of, 142, 186, 288
Apresoline. *See* Hydralazine
Aralen. *See* Chloroquine
Aramine. *See* Metaraminol
Arfonad camphorsulfonate, 155
Arlidin. *See* Nylidrin hydrochloride
Arrhythmias, 266—275
  and action of antiarrhythmic
    drugs, 271
  digitalis in, 261—262
  from digitalis, 264
  diphenylhydantoin in, 274, 275
  EEG effects of drugs in, 274
  lidocaine in, 273—274, 275
  pathophysiology of, 266—267
  phenytoin, 274, 275
  procainamide in, 273, 275
  propranolol in, 148, 273, 275
  quinidine in, 271—272, 274—275
Arsenicals
  adverse effects of, 568, 569, 570,
    571, 572
  affecting laboratory tests, 580—
    581, 592
  in amebiasis, 507
  blood dyscrasias from, 573
  excretion in milk, 576
  poisoning from, antidote in, 102
Arsenobenzenes, blood dyscrasias
    from, 573
Arsenobenzols, adverse effects of,
    571
Arsphenamine, adverse effects of,
    568, 569
Artane, in parkinsonism, 252
Arteritis, necrotizing, from amphe-
    tamine abuse, 71
Arthritis
  gouty, allopurinol in, 230

Arthritis
  gouty *(continued)*
    colchicine in, 228
  rheumatoid, salicylates in, 224
  treatment of, 421
Arvin, 322—323
Ascariasis, 513
Ascorbic acid, 556. *See also* Vita-
    min C
L-Asparaginase, in cancer, 537
Aspergillosis, 524
Aspidium
  affecting laboratory tests, 580—
    581, 590, 592, 596
  in helminthiasis, 513, 514
Aspirin, 223—226. *See also* Acetyl-
    salicylic acid
Asthma
  adrenocorticoids in, 360
  cromolyn sodium in, 388—389
  ephedrine in, 141
  isoproterenol in, 140
  xanthines in, 255
Astrafer, 315
Atabrine. *See* Quinacrine
Atarax. *See* Hydroxyzine
Atria, digitalis affecting, 259
Atrioventricular node, digitalis
    affecting, 259
Atropine, 128—134
  absorption, excretion and meta-
    bolism of, 131
  adverse effects of, 568, 569
  chemistry of, 128—129
  excretion in milk, 576
  interaction with other drugs, 28
  mechanism of action, 129
  pharmacologic effects of, 130—
    131
  as poison antidote, 101, 125
  poisoning from, 134
    antidote in, 103
  preanesthetic medication with,
    220
  therapeutic uses of, 131—133
Auerbach plexus, 110
Aureomycin. *See* Chlortetracycline
Automaticity, cardiac, 266
Automatism, from barbiturates,
    202
Autonomic nervous system
  anatomy of, 108—110
  antipsychotic drugs affecting,
    195—196
  imipramine affecting, 182
  physiology of, 110
Aventyl. *See* Nortriptyline
Avertin. *See* Tribromoethanol
Avocado, affecting laboratory tests,
    580—581, 590, 592, 596
Azapetine, 145, 279
Azathioprine, mode of action of,
    417
Azuresin, 548
6-Azauridine, in virus infections,
    534

B

Bacillus
  anthracis, drugs affecting, 420, 427, 452, 467
  subtilis, drugs affecting, 427, 436
Bacitracin, 424
  adverse effects of, 568
  affecting laboratory tests, 580–581, 592, 598
  in amebiasis, 508
  interaction with other drugs, 566
  malabsorption from, 577
  mode of action, 413
  in renal failure, 604–605
Bacteremia, treatment of, 420, 421, 422
Bactericidal drugs, 401
Bacteriostatic drugs, 401
Bacteroides, drugs affecting, 420, 427, 442, 452, 457, 458, 462, 464
BAL therapy. See Dimercaprol
Balantidiasis, 452, 511
Banocide, 515
Barbital, 201
  adverse effects of, 569
Barbiturates, 201–203
  absorption, metabolism and excretion of, 201–202
  abuse of, 70–71
  addiction to, 202
  adverse effects of, 202, 568, 569, 570, 571, 572
  affecting laboratory tests, 580–581, 590, 592, 596, 598, 601
  as anticonvulsant agents, 201, 242, 244–245
  in anxiety, 210
  blood dyscrasias from, 573
  chemistry of, 201
  contraindications to, 202–203
  crossing placental barrier, 575
  excretion in milk, 576
  interaction with other drugs, 566
  overdose of, 202
  poisoning from, 99
    amphetamine in, 142
    diuretics in, 313
  porphyria from, 53
  therapeutic uses of, 202
  tolerance to, 31
Barium sulfate, 547
  affecting laboratory tests, 592, 596, 598, 601
Barriers in distribution of drugs
  blood-brain barrier, 12, 13
  drug interactions affecting transport across membrane barriers, 30
  placental barrier, 13–14
Bartonella bacilliformis, drugs affecting, 420
Bavachi, adverse effects of, 570
Bayer 205, 422
BBK8, 441
Bedsonia agents. See Chlamydiae
Belladonna alkaloids
  adverse effects of, 569, 570
  in parkinsonism, 252
  poisoning from, 134

Belladonna alkaloids (continued)
  therapeutic use of, 131–133
Bemegride, as central stimulant, 253
Benactyzine, in anxiety, 210
Benadryl hydrochloride, 386
Bendroflumethiazide, diuretic action of, 304
Benzalkonium chloride, 489
  in tinea infections, 521
Benzedrine. See Amphetamine
Benzene
  adverse effects of, 570
  chemical structure of, 22
γ-Benzene hexachloride, blood dyscrasias from, 573
Benzestriol, 372
Benzethonium chloride, 489
Benzocaine, adverse effects of, 568
Benzodiazepines
  absorption, metabolism and excretion of, 207–209
  actions of, 209
  adverse effects of, 209–210
  as anticonvulsant agents, 246
  in anxiety, 207–210
  chemistry of, 207
  therapeutic uses of, 209
Benzoic acid, 489
  substituted, adverse effects of, 570
Benzopyrine, adverse effects of, 570
Benzothiadiazides, diuretic action of, 304, 308–309
Benzoyl peroxide, adverse effects of, 568
Benztropine, in parkinsonism, 252
Bephenium hydroxynaphthoate, 518
  in helminthiasis, 513, 514
Bergamot, adverse effects of, 570
Beta receptors, blocking agents for, 135–136. See also Adrenergic receptor blocking drugs
Betahistine, 384
Betaine hydrochloride, 289
Betamethasone, 359, 361
Betazole, 384, 548
Bethanechol, 118
Bethanidine, 157
  interaction with other drugs, 567
Bezold-Jarisch reflex, 152
Bicarbonate
  renal handling of, 303
  tests for, drugs affecting, 580, 582, 584, 586
Bicarbonate sodium, 292, 293
  affecting laboratory tests, 588–589, 595, 597
  in gastric lavage, 96
  interaction with other drugs, 565
  as poison antidote, 101
Biguanides
  affecting laboratory tests, 580–581, 592
  as hypoglycemic agents, 354–355
  in malaria, 500
Bile, acids in, resins binding, 282–283, 301
  cholesterol in, chenodeoxycholic acid affecting, 290

Bile (continued)
  drugs affecting secretion of, 289
Biliary excretion of drugs, 16
Bilirubin
  affecting laboratory tests, 580–581
  enzyme inducers in hyperbilirubinemia, 31
  levels in infants, from maternal drugs, 84
  tests for, drugs affecting, 580, 582, 584, 586
Binding of drugs and receptors, 3–4
  and intrinsic activity, 4
  displacement of drugs from sites of, 29
  by plasma proteins, 14
Bioassay of drugs, 33–38
  and biologic variation, 33
    minimization of, 35
  classification of, 36
  and clinical trials, 37
  compared to chemical assays, 37
  design of, 35–36
  direct, 36
  and dose-response curves, 33–35
  indirect, 36
  of insulin, 39
  objective evaluation in, 35–36
  reference standard in, 35
Biogastrone, 294
Biotin, 557
Bisacodyl, 298
  malabsorption from, 577
Bishydroxycoumarin, 319, 321
  affecting laboratory tests, 580–581, 592, 596, 598
  crossing placental barrier, 575
  excretion in milk, 576
  interaction with phenobarbital, 30–31
Bismuth
  adverse effects of, 568, 569, 570, 571, 572
  affecting laboratory tests, 580–581, 592, 596
Bismuth subcarbonate, in diarrhea, 302
Bithionol, 422
  adverse effects of, 570
  in helminthiasis, 514
Bladder
  antimuscarinic agents affecting, 131
  responses to autonomic activity, 111
Blankophores, adverse effects of, 570
Blastomycosis, 523, 524
Bleomycin, 543
  mode of action, 417
Blood
  alcohol levels in, 77
  dyscrasias of, drug-induced, 194, 470, 573–574
  free plasma levels of drugs, 16–17
  half-life of drugs in, 17
  localization of drugs in, 13
  occult, drugs affecting tests for, 598–600

Carbon tetrachloride, in helminthiasis, 514
Carbonic anhydrase inhibitors
adverse effects of, 307
as diuretics, 304, 307
and parietal cell secretion, 291
thiazides, 308
Carbromal, 199
Carbutamide, adverse effects of,
570
Carcinoid syndrome, serotonin role
in, 393—394
Cardiovascular system
blood perfusion rate in heart, 13
drugs affecting
acetylcholine, 117
alpha receptor blocking agents,
145, 146
antianginal drugs, 276—279
antiarrhythmic drugs, 266—275
antimuscarinic agents, 130,
132—133
digitalis. See Digitalis
emetine, 503
ephedrine, 141
epinephrine, 136—137, 138—
139
ganglionic blocking agents, 154
glycosides, 258—265
histamine, 381—382
isoproterenol, 140
local anesthetics, 173—174
monoamine oxidase inhibitors,
184
norepinephrine, 139
propranolol, 148
prostaglandins, 396—397
serotonin, 391—392
vasodilator drugs, 279
xanthines, 254
localization of drugs in heart, 13
signs in poisoning, 95
treatment of hyperlipidemia,
280—284
vascular responses to autonomic
activity, 111
Cardrase. See Ethoxyzolamide
Carisoprodol, 169
affecting laboratory tests, 598
Carminatives, 288
Carrier-mediated transport of drugs,
9, 12
Carrier state, in amebiasis, 508
Cascara sagrada, 298
excretion in milk, 576
Castellani's paint, in tinea infections, 521
Castle's intrinsic factor, 316
Castor oil, 298
Catecholamines. See also Sympathomimetic drugs
adverse effects of, 568
in urine, drugs affecting tests for,
592—595
Cathartics, 296—301
adverse effects of, 297
bulk, 299
habituation to, 297
interaction with other drugs, 28
as lubricants, 299—300
saline, 299
stimulant, 297—299

Cathartics (continued)
therapeutic uses of, 300, 301
withdrawal from, 297
Caytine, 143
Cedar oil, adverse effects of, 570
Cefazolin, in renal failure, 604—605
Cellulitis, treatment of, 422
Celluloses, as cathartics, 300
Celontin. See Methsuximide
Central nervous system
drugs affecting. See also Psychotropic drugs
amphetamine, 142
anesthetic agents, 173, 211—
220
anticonvulsants, 239—247
antihistamines, 386
antiinflammatory agents, 221—
229
antimuscarinic agents, 131, 132
antiparkinson drugs, 248—252
ephedrine, 141
epinephrine, 138
imipramine, 181
lithium carbonate, 185
monoamine oxidase inhibitors,
183
narcotics, 231—238
prostaglandins, 396
serotonin, 392
stimulants, 186, 253—255
transmitter mechanisms in, 176—
180
Cephalexin, 438
in renal failure, 604—605
Cephalin flocculation test, drugs
affecting, 580, 582, 584, 586
Cephaloglycine, 439
Cehaloridine, 438
affecting laboratory tests, 580—
581, 590, 592, 596, 598
in renal failure, 604—605
Cephalosporins, 432—439
adverse effects of, 437, 571
bacterial resistance to, 436
interaction with probenecid, 32
mode of action, 412—413
preparations of, 438—439
spectrum of activity, 436
therapeutic uses of, 437
Cephalothin, 438
affecting laboratory tests, 580—
581, 590, 592, 596, 598
blood dyscrasias from, 573
interaction with other drugs, 565
in renal failure, 604—605
Cephazolin, 438
Cephradine, 439
Cerebral stimulants, 253
Cerebrospinal fluid, protein in,
drugs affecting tests for, 598—
600
Ceruloplasmin, tests for, drugs
affecting, 580, 582, 584, 586
Cestode infections, 513
Cestocide, 516
Cetrimide, adverse effects of, 568
Cetylpyridinium chloride, 489
Cetyltrimethylammonium bromide,
in tinea infections, 521
Chagas' disease, 422, 510
Chalf, precipitated, 293

Chancroid, treatment of, 420
Charcoal, activated
in diarrhea, 302
in poisonings, 96—97, 101
Chelating agents, intestinal, 301
Chemotherapy
antimicrobial, 400—467. See also
Antibiotics
in cancer, 535—544
capreomycin, 466
in helminthiasis, 512—518
in leprosy, 483—484
in mycotic diseases, 519—527
in protozoal diseases, 492—511
sulfonamides, 467—477
in tuberculosis, 478—483
in urinary tract infections, 484—
487
in viral diseases, 528—534
Chenodeoxycholic acid, 290
Chenopodium oil, adverse effects
of, 571
Childhood. See Pediatric pharmacology
Chiniofon, 506
affecting laboratory tests, 580—
581, 592, 598
Chlamydiae, 528
drugs affecting, 420, 452, 456
Chloral betaine, 200
Chloral hydrate, 200, 203
adverse effects of, 203, 568, 569,
571
affecting laboratory tests, 580—
581, 590, 592, 596, 598
crossing placental barrier, 575
excretion in milk, 576
interaction with other drugs, 566
Chlorambucil, crossing placental
barrier, 575
Chloramphenicol, 455, 456—457
adverse effects of, 456—457, 568,
570, 571, 572
affecting laboratory tests, 580—
581, 590, 592, 598
affecting protein synthesis, 414
bacterial resistance to, 456
blood dyscrasias from, 573
excretion in milk, 576
gray syndrome from, 83
preparations and dosage of, 457
in renal failure, 604—605
spectrum of activity, 456
with streptomycin, 443
sulfonamides with, 476
Chlorcyclizine, 385, 386
adverse effects of, 568
Chlordantoin, in candidiasis, 523
Chlordiazepoxide, 206, 207—210
adverse effects of, 568, 570, 571
affecting laboratory tests, 580—
581, 590, 598, 601
Chlorguanide, adverse effects of,
569
Chlorhexidine
adverse effects of, 568
mode of action, 414
Chlorhydroxyquinoline, adverse
effects of, 568
Chloride, 490
in parenteral solutions, 610
renal handling of, 304

Chloride
(continued)
tests for, drugs affecting, 580, 582, 584, 586
Chlorisondamine chloride, 155
Chlormerodrin, 304, 307
Chlorobutanol, affecting laboratory tests, 580–581, 590
Chloroform, 213, 219
affecting laboratory tests, 592
excretion in milk, 576
Chloroguanide, 497, 500–501
adverse effects of, 501
Chloromycetin succinate, interaction with other drugs, 564
Chloroquinaldol, in candidiasis, 523
Chloroquine
adverse effects of, 499, 568, 569, 570, 571, 572
affecting laboratory tests, 582–583, 592, 596
in amebiasis, 505, 506
blood dyscrasias from, 573
crossing placental barrier, 575
in helminthiasis, 514
in malaria, 496, 499
mode of action, 417
Chlorothiazide
adverse effects of, 568, 569, 571
blood dyscrasias from, 573
diuretic action of, 304, 308
in hypertension, 158
Chlorotrianisene, 371
Chloroxylenol, adverse effects of, 568
Chlorphenesin, adverse effects of, 568
Chlorpheniramine, 385, 386
interaction with other drugs, 564
Chlorphenoxamine, in parkinsonism, 252
Chlorproguanil, 501
Chlorpromazine, 187, 188, 189
adverse effects of, 568, 569, 570, 571
affecting histamine levels, 381
as antiemetic, 289
blood dyscrasias from, 573
crossing placental barrier, 575
excretion in milk, 576
interaction with other drugs, 566
localization in organs, 13
in mania, 193
as poison antidote, 101
and prolactin levels, 340
properties of, 192
Chlorpropamide, 353
adverse effects of, 570, 571
affecting laboratory tests, 582–583, 592, 596, 598
blood dyscrasias from, 573
crossing placental barrier, 575
Chlorprothixene, 190, 192
Chlortetracycline, 451, 452
adverse effects of, 569, 570, 571, 572
in amebiasis, 508
in balantidiasis, 511
interaction with other drugs, 564
in renal failure, 604–605
Chlorthalidone, affecting laboratory tests, 582–583

Chlorthalidone (continued)
diuretic action of, 304
Chlor-trimeton maleate, 386
Chlorzoxazone, affecting laboratory tests, 593, 596
Cholecalciferol, 556
Cholera. See Vibrio cholera
Cholesterol
in bile, chenodeoxycholic acid affecting, 290
drugs affecting levels of, 282–284
tests for, drugs affecting, 580, 582, 584, 586
Cholestyramine, 282, 301
adverse effects of, 301
affecting laboratory tests, 582–583, 593
malabsorption from, 577
preparations and dosage of, 301
therapeutic uses of, 301
toxicity of, 282
Choline acetylase, 113
activity in Huntington's chorea, 249
Choline dihydrogen citrate, 289
Cholinergic transmission, 113
blocking by antimuscarinic agents, 128
Cholinesterase inhibitors, 120–127
ambenonium, 123, 126
chemistry and mechanism of action, 120–121
crossing placental barrier, 575
decurarizing action of, 164
edrophonium, 124, 126
neostigmine, 123, 126
nonreversible, 122
organophosphate, 125, 126
poisoning from, 125
pharmacologic actions of, 122–123
physostigmine, 123, 126
poisoning from, treatment of, 101, 125–127
pyridostigmine bromide, 125, 126
reversible, 121–122
therapeutic use of, 124–125
Cholinesterase variants, affecting responses to succinylcholine, 62–63
Cholografin, 547
Choreoathetosis, from L-dopa, 251
Chorionic gonadotropin, human, 338–339, 373
adverse effects of, 572
in pregnancy, 367–368
therapeutic uses of, 339
Chromoblastomycosis, 524
Chrysophanic acid, 297, 299
Chylomicronemia, 281
Chymotrypsin, 550
Cimetidine, 387
and parietal cell secretion, 291
Cinchona alkaloids, 495–498
Cinchonism, 272, 498
Cinchophen
adverse effects of, 569, 570, 571
affecting laboratory tests, 582–583, 593, 598
blood dyscrasias from, 573
Circadian rhythm
of adrenocorticoids, 357

Circadian rhythm (continued)
and adverse drug reactions, 54
Citron oil, adverse effects of, 570
Clindamycin, 462–463
affecting protein synthesis, 415
in renal failure, 604–605
Clinical trials of new drugs, 41–44
Clofibrate, 283, 284
adverse effects of, 571
affecting laboratory tests, 582–583, 590
blood dyscrasias from, 573
interaction with other drugs, 566
malabsorption from, 577
toxicity of, 284
Clomiphene, affecting laboratory tests, 582–583
Clopenthixol. See Perphenazine
Clorazepate, 207, 208, 209
Clostridia, drugs affecting, 420, 427, 436, 452
Clotrimazole, 526
Clotting time determinations
drugs affecting, 580, 582, 584, 586
whole blood, 318
Cloxacillin, 434
affecting laboratory tests, 582–583, 593, 598
in renal failure, 604–605
Clozapine, 191, 192
Coagulation, 318
and anticoagulant therapy, 318–323
oral contraceptives affecting, 377
tetracycline affecting, 454
Coagulation factors, tests for, drugs affecting, 581, 583, 585, 587
Coagulation time, drugs affecting, 580, 582, 584, 586
with whole blood, 318
Coal tar, adverse effects of, 570
Cobalt poisoning, antidote in, 101
Cobefrin hydrochloride, 143
Cocaine, 71
abuse of, 72
as local anesthetic, 173
Coccidioidomycosis, 524
Codeine, 231, 232, 234, 235
adverse effects of, 570
affecting laboratory tests, 582–583
antitussive effects of, 238
in diarrhea, 301
excretion in milk, 576
poisoning from, antidote in, 103
Cogentin. See Benztropine
Colchicine, 228
affecting laboratory tests, 582–583, 598
blood dyscrasias from, 573
malabsorption from, 577
preparations and dosage of, 228
Colestipol, 282
Colistimethate, in renal failure, 604–605
Colistin, 460–461
adverse effects of, 461
affecting laboratory tests, 582–583, 593
interaction with other drugs, 566
preparations and dosage of, 461

Colitis
  in amebiasis, 508
  ulcerative, adrenocorticoids in,
    360
Collage disease, drug-induced, 571
Color
  of feces, in poisoning, 93
  of skin. See Skin, color of
  of urine
    drugs affecting, 592—595
    in poisoning, 94
  of vomitus, in poisoning, 93
Combinations of drugs, 401—402,
    405
  adverse reactions from, 50
  and benefit:risk ratio for each
    agent, 50
  in cancer, 541
Compazine. See Prochlorperazine
Conduction, cardiac, 266—267
  digitalis affecting, 259
Conjugation reactions, in metabo-
    lism of drugs, 24
  hereditary defects in, 64
Conjunctivitis, treatment of, 420
Conray, 548
Consent, informed, in clinical trials
    of drugs, 42
Constipation, 296—297
  from antipsychotic drugs, 196
  from narcotics, 233, 237
Contraception, prostaglandins in,
    397
Contraceptives, oral, 373—379
  adverse effects of, 376—377, 569,
    570, 571, 572
  affecting laboratory tests, 586—
    587, 590, 594, 599, 601
  blood dyscrasias from, 573
  contraindications to, 377
  estrogens in, 369
  excretion in milk, 576
  interaction with thyroid hor-
    mones, 331
  malabsorption from, 577
  physiologic aspects of, 373—374
  preparations of, 377—379
  progestogens crossing placental
    barrier, 575
Contraction, myocardial, digitalis
    affecting, 258—259
Contrast media, 547—548
  affecting laboratory tests, 588—
    589, 591, 595, 597, 600
Convulsions. See Seizures
Coombs test, drugs affecting, 580,
    582, 584, 586
Copper
  affecting laboratory tests, 582—
    583, 593
  excretion in milk, 576
  poisoning from, antidote in, 101
  tests for, drugs affecting, 580,
    582, 584, 586
Copper sulfate, as poison antidote,
    102
Coramine, as central stimulant, 254
Corpus luteum, 373
Corticosteroids. See Adrenocorti-
    coids
Corticosterone, 361
Corticotropin, 335

Corticotropin (continued)
  and adrenal steroidogenesis, 357
  adverse effects of, 568, 569, 571
  affecting laboratory tests, 582—
    583, 593, 598, 601
  blood dyscrasias from, 573
  chemistry of, 335
  interaction with other drugs, 564
  mechanism of action, 335
  releasing hormone, 327, 328—329
  therapeutic uses of, 335
Cortisol. See Hydrocortisone
Cortisone, 361
  crossing placental barrier, 575
  excretion in milk, 576
Corylifolia, adverse effects of, 570
Corynebacterium diphtheriae, drugs
    affecting, 420, 427, 436, 458,
    462, 467
Cosmegen, 543
Cotazym, 289
Cough reflex, narcotics affecting,
    233, 235, 238
Coumadin. See Warfarin
Coumarin anticoagulants, 319,
    321—322
  adverse effects of, 322
  antidote for, 104
  interaction with other drugs, 227,
    275, 331, 566
  resistance to, inherited, 64
  therapeutic uses of, 322
Covalent bonds, in drug-receptor
    interaction, 4
Coxiella burnetii, drugs affecting,
    420
Cranial nerves, 110
Cream of tartar, 299
Creatine in urine, drugs affecting
    tests for, 592—595
Creatinine, tests for, drugs affect-
    ing, 581, 583, 585, 587
Cresol, 490
Crigler-Najjar syndrome, and jaun-
    dice induction by drugs, 53
Crisis, hypertensive, from drug
    interactions, 185
Cromolyn sodium, 388—389
  adverse effects of, 388
  preparations and dosage of, 388—
    389
Crotamiton, adverse effects of, 568
Cryptococcosis, 524
Cryptorchidism, hormone therapy
    in, 364
Crystalluria
  from p-aminosalicylic acid, 481
  from sulfonamides, 474
Cumertilin, 304
Curare, 160—163
Cushing's syndrome, enzyme
    inducers in, 31
Cyanide
  antidotes to, 104
  poison kit, 102
Cyanocobalamin, 315, 316, 555
Cyanoketone, 379
Cyclamates, adverse effects of, 570
Cyclizine hydrochloride, 386
Cycloguanil pamoate, 501
Cyclomethycaine, adverse effects
    of, 568

Cyclopentolate, ophthalmologic use
    of, 132
Cyclophosphamide, 539, 542
  adverse effects of, 571
  crossing placental barrier, 575
  excretion in milk, 576
Cycloplegia, from antimuscarinic
    agents, 132
Cyclopropane, 213, 219—220
  crossing placental barrier, 575
  excretion in milk, 576
Cycloserine, 424—425
  affecting laboratory tests, 582—
    583
  blood dyscrasias from, 573
  excretion in milk, 576
  mode of action, 413
Cyproheptadine, 393, 395
  affecting laboratory tests, 582—
    583, 593
Cyproterone acetate, 366
Cysticercosis, 513
Cystinuria, diuretics in, 313
Cytarabine. See Cytosine
    arabinoside
Cytomel, 345
Cytosine arabinoside, 533, 539,
    541, 542
  adverse effects of, 533
  blood dyscrasias from, 573
  mode of action, 417
Cytotoxic agents, adverse effects
    of, 568
Cytoxan. See Cyclophosphamide

D

Dactinomycin. See Actinomycin D
Dalmane. See Flurazepam
Danthron, excretion in milk, 576
Dantrolene sodium, 167—168
Dapsone, 483, 484
  adverse effects of, 572
Daranide. See Dichlorphenamide
Daraprim. See Pyrimethamine
Darenthin. See Bretylium
Darvon. See Propoxyphene
DDT
  excretion in milk, 576
  exposure to, and adverse drug
    reactions, 52
Deafness, from salicylates, 225
Decamethonium, 164—165
Decholin. See Dehydrocholic acid
Decongestants, nasal, 141—142,
    143
  rebound congestion from, 142
Defecation, physiology of, 297
Deferoxamine B, as poison anti-
    dote, 102
Defibrination, from arvin, 322—323
Degradation of drugs, and adverse
    reactions, 49
Dehydrocholic acid, 289
  affecting laboratory tests, 582—
    583
Dehydroemetine, 422, 506
Dehydrogenases, and metabolism of
    drugs, 20—24

Diphenoxylate *(continued)*
  in diarrhea, 301
Diphenylhydantoin, 241–244, 247.
    See also Phenytoin
  actions and pharmacology of,
    242–243
  adverse effects of, 243–244, 274,
    569, 570, 571, 572
  affecting laboratory tests, 582–
    583, 590, 593, 596, 598, 601
  in arrhythmias, 274, 275
  blood dyscrasias from, 573
  chemical structure of, 21
  in convulsions from poisoning, 98
  crossing placental barrier, 575
  enzyme inhibitors affecting, 32
  excretion in milk, 576
  interaction with other drugs, 275,
    564
  malabsorption from, 577
  metabolism of, 243
    hereditary variations in, 63
  preparations and dosage of, 274
Diphtheria
  antitoxin, 561, 562
  treatment of, 420
Diphyllobothrium latum, 513
Diplococcus pneumoniae, drugs
    affecting, 420, 427, 436, 442
Dipyrone, blood dyscrasias from,
    573
Disinfectants. *See* Antiseptics and
    disinfectants
Displacement of drugs from plasma
    binding sites, 29
Distribution of drugs, 11–15
  in adipose tissue, 14
  blood-brain barrier affecting, 12,
    13
  drug interactions affecting, 29
  and pharmacokinetics, 16–18
  placental barrier affecting, 13–14
  plasma protein binding affecting,
    14
  volume of, 14–15
Disulfiram, 80
  adverse effects of, 569
  interaction with alcohol, 566
Dithiazanine iodide, 518
  affecting laboratory tests, 582–
    583, 593, 598
Dithizon, as poison antidote, 102
Diuresis, forced, in poisoning, 99
Diuretics, 303–313
  action of, 304
  adverse effects of, 158, 569
  and aldosterone levels, 310–311
  amiloride, 311
  in barbiturate poisoning, 313
  and calcium levels, 313
  carbonic anhydrase inhibitors,
    304, 307
  in cystinuria, 313
  ethacrynic acid, 304, 309–310
  furosemide, 304, 310
  in hypertension, 158
  interactions with other drugs, 566
  mercurial, 304, 306–307
    adverse effects of, 306–307,
      569, 570, 571, 572
    affecting laboratory tests, 584–
      585, 594, 599, 601

Diuretics *(continued)*
  potassium deficiency from, 308,
    310
  in renal tubular acidosis, 311–
    313
  in salicylate poisoning, 313
  spironolactone, 304, 310–311
  thiazide, 304, 308–309
    adverse effects of, 309, 570,
      571
    affecting laboratory tests, 588–
      589, 595, 600
    antidiuretic effect of, 308–309
    excretion in milk, 576
    in hypertension, 158
    interaction with other drugs,
      309, 567
    malabsorption from, 577
    therapeutic uses of, 308–309
  triamterene, 304, 311
  and uric acid levels, 313
Diuril. *See* Chlorothiazide
Diurnal rhythm. *See* Circadian
    rhythm
DNA synthesis, inhibition by anti-
    biotics, 416–417
Dolophine. *See* Methadone
Domiphen bromide, adverse effects
    of, 568
L-Dopa
  choreoathetosis from, 251
  in parkinsonism, 190, 251–252
Dopamine, 140–141
  and neurotransmission, 177
  phenothiazines affecting turnover
    of, 190
  striatal, in parkinsonism, 248, 249
  synthesis of, 113, 114
Dopamine β-hydroxylase, 113
  and metabolism of drugs, 20
Doriden. *See* Glutethimide
Dormison, 204
Dosage of drugs, 5
  and adverse drug reactions, 50
  and dose-response curve, 6–7,
    33–35
  effective, 7
  maximum, 6
  in pediatric pharmacology, 83–84
  and pharmacokinetics, 16–18
  relation to drug effects, 6–7
  threshold, 6
Doubling of active fraction of
    drugs, after displacement from
    binding sites, 29
Doxapran, as central stimulant, 254
Doxepin, 181
Doxycycline, 451, 452
  adverse effects of, 570
  in renal failure, 604–605
Dozoff, 199
Dracunculiasis, treatment of, 422
Dramamine. *See* Dimenhydrinate
Droperidol, interaction with other
    drugs, 275
Drug fever, from sulfonamides, 470
Drug-induced disease, 568–577
Drug-receptor binding, 3–4
DTPA, as poison antidote, 101
Dumping syndrome, serotonin role
    in, 393
Duodenal ulcer, 296

Duogastrone, 294
Dwarfism, growth hormone therapy
    in, 336
Dyrenium. *See* Triamterene
Dysentery
  amebic. *See* Amebiasis
  bacillary, treatment of, 421
  ciliate, 511
Dyskinesia, tardive, from antipsy-
    chotic drugs, 192, 195
Dysmenorrhea
  estrogen therapy in, 369
  progestational agents in, 376
  prostaglandin role in, 397
Dysphoria, from nalorphine, 233
Dystonic reactions, from antipsy-
    chotic drugs, 195

E

Ears
  salicylates affecting, 225
  signs in poisoning, 94
Echothiophate, 122, 125, 126
  in glaucoma, 125
Ecolid. *See* Chlorisondamine
Edecrin. *See* Ethacrynic acid
Edema, from oral contraceptives,
    377
Edrophonium, 124, 126
EDTA. *See* Ethylenediaminetetra-
    acetic acid
Efficacy evaluation, preclinical,
    40–41
Eggs, as poison antidote, 102
Elavil. *See* Amitriptyline
Electrocardiogram, drugs affecting,
    262, 274, 598–600
Electroencephalography, in
    seizures, 240
Electrolytes, renal handling of,
    303–304
Electrophoresis, paper, drugs affect-
    ing, 581, 583, 585, 587
Ellsworth-Howard test, 348
Emesis. *See* Vomiting
Emetine, 503–506
  affecting laboratory tests, 598,
    601
  bismuth iodide, 506
  in helminthiasis, 515
Emivan, as central stimulant, 254
Emodin cathartics, 297–299
Encephalitis
  immune globulins in, 561, 562
  vaccine for, 561
Endocarditis, bacterial, treatment
    of, 420, 421, 422
Endocrine pharmacology
  adrenocorticoids, 356–362
  androgens, 363–366
  in cancer therapy, 539, 543
  estrogens, 366–372
  glucagon, 355
  histamine and antihistamines,
    380–388
  hypoglycemic drugs, oral, 353–
    355

Excretion of drugs *(continued)*
  in childhood, 82
  drug interactions affecting, 32
  increased by dialysis, in poison-
    ing, 97—98
  renal, 15—16
Extrasystoles, from digitalis, 264
Eyes
  adrenocorticoids affecting, 361
  antimuscarinic eyedrops, 132
  antipsychotic drugs affecting, 196
  atropine affecting, 130
  chemical burns of, 100
  disorders of
    cholinesterase inhibitors in,
      124—125
    muscarinic agents in, 118—119
  ephedrine affecting, 141
  epinephrine affecting, 138
  morphine affecting, 231, 233
  muscle relaxants affecting, 166
  responses to autonomic activity,
    111
  symptoms in poisoning, 92
  treatment of conjunctivitis, 420

F

Facial signs, in poisoning, 92
Fat
  metabolism of, insulin affecting,
    351
  tests for, drugs affecting, 598—
    600
Fatty acids, in tinea infections, 521
Feces
  color of, in poisoning, 93
  defecation physiology, 297
  softeners of, 299—300
Fellypressin, with local anesthetics,
    173
Fennel oil, adverse effects of, 570
Fentanyl, 237
Fentichlor, adverse effects of, 570
Ferritin, 314
Ferroglycine sulfate complex, 315
Ferrous fumarate, 315
Ferrous gluconate, 315
Ferrous sulfate, 314, 315
Fertility control. *See* Contracep-
    tives, oral
Fetamin. *See* Metamphetamine
Fetus
  drugs affecting, 56—57, 84—85,
    470, 575—576
  masculinization of female fetus,
    57
Fever
  antipyretics in, 224, 226, 227
  drug fever, 470
  malignant hyperthermia from
    anesthesia, 64—65
Fibrillation, atrial, digitalis in,
    261—262
Fibrinogen, arvin affecting, 322—
    323
Filariasis, 513
Florantyrone, affecting laboratory
    tests, 582—583

Flowmeter, in anesthesia machine,
    214—215
Flucloxacillin, 434
Fludrocortisone, 359, 361
Fluids, intravenous, solutions for,
    609—611
Flumethiazide, diuretic action of,
    304
Fluomar. *See* Fluroxene
Fluorescein dyes, adverse effects of,
    570
Fluoride
  affecting laboratory tests, 582—
    583, 599
  poisoning from, antidote in, 101
5-Fluorocytosin, 525—526
  adverse effects of, 526
5-Fluorodeoxyuridine, 417
5-Fluorouracil, 539
  adverse effects of, 570, 571
  blood dyscrasias from, 573
  in cancer therapy, 542
  malabsorption from, 577
  mode of action, 417
Fluothane. *See* Halothane
Fluoxymesterone, 366
  adverse effects of, 571
Flupenthixol. *See* Fluphenazine
Fluphenazine, 188, 189, 190
  in Huntington's chorea, 194
  properties of, 192
Flurazepam, 200, 205—206, 209
  adverse effects of, 206
Fluroxene, 213, 219
Flutter, atrial, digitalis in, 262
Folic acid, 315, 316—317, 556—
    557
  excretion in milk, 576
Follicle-stimulating hormone, 337—
    338, 373
  and estrogen synthesis, 367
  releasing hormone, 327, 328, 329
  therapeutic uses of, 337—338
Foods. *See* Diet
Formaldehyde, adverse effects of,
    568
  antidote in poisoning from, 101
Formaldehyde sulfoxalate sodium,
    as poison antidote, 104
Formalin, adverse effects of, 569
Frangula, adverse effects of, 569
Fuadin. *See* Stibophen
Fungicidal agents, 401, 519
Fungistatic agents, 401, 519
Fungus diseases. *See* Mycotic
    diseases
Furazolidone, 486, 487
  adverse effects of, 572
  affecting laboratory tests, 582—
    583, 593, 596
  blood dyscrasias from, 573
  interaction with other drugs, 566
Furmethonol, adverse effects of,
    572
Furosemide
  adverse effects of, 570
  affecting laboratory tests, 582—
    583
  diuretic action of, 304, 310
Fusidic acid, 464
  affecting protein synthesis,
    415

Fusobacterium fusiformis, drugs
    affecting, 420, 422

G

Galactose, in urine, drugs affecting
    tests for, 592—595
Gallamine triethiodide, 164
Gallbladder, contrast media for,
    547
Gallstones, chenodeoxycholic acid
    affecting, 290
Gametocidal drugs, in malaria, 495
Gamma globulin therapy, 528,
    559—560
Ganglia, paravertebral, 109, 110
Ganglionic blocking agents, 154—
    155
  adverse effects of, 155
  crossing placental barrier, 575
  interaction with other drugs, 28
  preparations and dosage of, 155
Ganglionic stimulating agents, 154
Gantrisin. *See* Sulfisoxazole
Gas gangrene, treatment of, 420
Gastric acid secretion, 290—291
  histamine affecting, 382
  prostaglandins affecting, 397
Gastric function tests, drugs in, 548
Gastric lavage, in treatment of
    poisoning, 91—97
Gastric ulcer, 295—296
Gastrocolic reflex, 297
Gastroenteritis, treatment of, 420
Gastrografin, 547
Gastrointestinal tract
  absorption of drugs in, 9—11. *See
    also* Absorption
  cholinesterase inhibitors in dis-
    orders of, 125
  contrast media for, 547
  diarrhea, 301—302
  drugs affecting, 288—302
    p-aminosalicylic acid, 481
    antimuscarinic agents, 130—
      131, 132
    cathartics, 296—301
    chelating agents, 301
    digitalis, 264
    epinephrine, 138
    furazolidone, 487
    indomethacin, 228
    morphine, 233
    nitrofurantoin, 487
    phenylbutazone, 227
    prostaglandins, 397
    salicylates, 225
    serotonin, 392—393
    sulfonamides, 470
  muscarinic agents in disorders of,
    118
  peptic ulcer, 290—296
  responses to autonomic activity,
    111
  signs in poisonings, 93
Gefarnate, 294
Genetics
  and adverse drug reactions, 52.
    See also Pharmacogenetics

Genetics (continued)
  and resistance to antimicrobial drugs, 404
Genital infections, treatment of, 421
Gentamicin, 445, 446–447
  adverse effects of, 447, 571
  affecting laboratory tests, 582–583, 593, 599
  in renal failure, 604–605
Gentian violet
  in candidiasis, 523
  in helminthiasis, 513, 515
Geotrichosis, 524
Geriatric age group, adverse drug reactions in, 51
Germicidal agents, 488–491
Giardiasis, 487, 511
  metronidazole in, 507
Gilles de la Tourette disease, antipsychotic drugs in, 193
Glanders, treatment of, 421
Glands
  acetylcholine affecting, 117
  antimuscarinic agents affecting, 131
  epinephrine affecting, 138
  responses to autonomic activity, 111
Glauber's salt, 299
Glaucoma
  cholinesterase inhibitors in, 124–125
  muscarinic agents in, 118–119
Globulins
  corticosteroid-binding, 331–332
  gamma globulin therapy, 528, 559–560
  sex hormone binding, 332
Glomerular filtration, 303
Glucagon, 355
  in test for pheochromocytoma, 384
Glucocorticoids, 356, 360. See also Adrenocorticoids
Glucose
  hypoglycemic agents, 353–355. See also Hypoglycemic agents
  serum levels
    adrenocorticoids affecting, 360
    alcohol affecting, 78
    disease states and drugs affecting, 353
    insulin affecting, 352
    tests for, drugs affecting, 581, 585, 586, 587
    therapy with, affecting laboratory tests, 582–583, 590, 593
    tolerance test, drugs affecting, 581, 583, 585, 587
  in urine, drugs affecting tests for, 592–595
Glucose-6-phosphate dehydrogenase deficiency, and responses to drugs, 63–64, 572
Glutamic oxalacetic transaminase in serum, drugs affecting, 581, 583, 585, 587
Glutamic pyruvic transaminase in serum, drugs affecting, 581, 583, 585, 587
Glutethimide, abuse of, 70

Glutethimide (continued)
  adverse effects of, 571
  affecting laboratory tests, 582–583, 590, 593, 596, 599, 601
  blood dyscrasias from, 573
  as hypnotic, 200, 204–205
  interaction with other drugs, 32, 566
  tolerance to, 31
Glycerine suppositories, 301
Glyceryl p-aminobenzoate, adverse effects of, 570
Glyceryl guaiacolate, affecting laboratory tests, 593
Glyceryl triacetate, in tinea infections, 521
Glyceryl trinitrate, 277
Glycobiarsol, in amebiasis, 505, 507
Glycogenolysis, epinephrine affecting, 138
Glycosides, cardiac, 258–265. See also Digitalis
Glycyrrhizinic acid, 295
Gold compounds
  adverse effects of, 569, 570, 571
  affecting laboratory tests, 584–585, 593, 599
  blood dyscrasias from, 573
  poisoning from, antidote in, 102
Gonadotropin
  human chorionic, 338–339, 373
    adverse effects of, 572
    in pregnancy, 367–368
    therapeutic uses of, 339
  human menopausal, 337
  releasing factor, 327, 329
Gonorrhea, treatment of, 421
Gout
  alcohol affecting, 78
  induction by drugs, 53
Gouty arthritis
  allopurinol in, 230
  colchicine in, 228
Gramicidin, 459
  mode of action, 414
Granuloma inguinale, treatment of, 420
Granulomata, treatment of, 421
Gravity, specific, of urine, drugs affecting, 592–595
Gray syndrome, from chloramphenicol, 83
Griseofulvin
  adverse effects of, 520, 568, 569, 570, 571, 572
  affecting laboratory tests, 584–585, 593, 596
  interaction with other drugs, 566
  in tinea infections, 520–522
Growth
  adrenocorticoids affecting, 360
  parathyroid hormone affecting, 347
Growth hormone. See Somatotropin
Guanethidine, 155–157
  adverse effects of, 156–157
  affecting laboratory tests, 584–585, 593
  interaction with other drugs, 30, 182, 566, 567

Guanethidine (continued)
  preparations and dosage of, 157
Guanoxan, affecting laboratory tests, 584–585, 593
Gyancydine, 153
Gynecomastia, drug-induced, 572

H

Habituation, to cathartics, 297
Haemophilus
  ducreyi, drugs affecting, 420, 427, 442, 452, 467
  influenzae, drugs affecting, 420, 427, 436, 442, 452, 457, 458, 459, 467, 475
Half-life
  of drugs in serum, 17, 604
    and abuse of drugs, 70
    accelerated, after displacement from binding sites, 29
    adrenocorticoids, 357
    and preclinical evaluation of new agents, 41
    in twins, 61
  of hormones, 330
    parathyroid, 347
Hallocinogens, 72–73
Halogens, germicidal activity of, 490
Haloperidol, 190–191
  adverse effects of, 572
  affecting laboratory tests, 584–585
  in Gilles de la Tourette disease, 193
  in Huntington's disease, 194
  in mania, 193
  properties of, 192
Haloprogin, in tinea infections, 521
Halothane, 213, 217–218
Hamycin, 526
Harisch-Herxheimer reactions, 430
Hartmann's solution, 610
Headache. See also Migraine
  from histamine, 382
Hearing loss, from salicylates, 225
Heart. See Cardiovascular system
Heart block
  from digitalis, 264
  ephedrine in, 142
  isoproterenol in, 140
Heart failure
  digitalis in, 260–261
  xanthines in, 255
Heart rate
  digitalis affecting, 261
  nitrites affecting, 277
Heat, germicidal activity of, 488–489
Helminthiasis, 512–518
  treatment of, 422
Hemochromatosis, treatment of, 102
Hemodialysis
  antibiotic therapy during, 603, 605
  in poisoning, 97

Indanedione anticoagulants
(continued)
  therapeutic uses of, 322
Inderal. See Propranolol
Indigo carmine, 548
Indomethacin, 227–228
  absorption, excretion and meta-
    bolism of, 227–228
  adverse effects of, 228
  affecting laboratory tests, 584–
    585, 593, 599
  blood dyscrasias from, 573
  interaction with other drugs, 32,
    566
  preparations and dosage of, 228
  as prostaglandin inhibitor, 397
  therapeutic uses of, 228
Inflammation
  antiinflammatory analgesics in,
    223–229
  prostaglandin role in, 397
  targets of drug therapy in, 221–
    223
Informed consent, in clinical trials
  of drugs, 42
Insect bites, antidote for, 101
Insecticides, exposure to, and
  adverse drug reactions, 52
Insulin, 350–353
  adverse effects of, 352–353, 568,
    569, 571, 572
  affecting laboratory tests, 584–
    585
  chemistry of, 350
  circulating, 332
  dosage of, 352
  indirect bioassay of, 39
  interaction with other drugs, 352,
    564, 566
  mechanism of action, 351–352
  preparations of, 352
  synthesis and metabolism of,
    350–351
Interactions of drugs, 27–32,
  563–567
  and adverse drug reactions, 48–
    49
  before administration, 28
  from alteration in function, 28
  and alterations in mucosa, 28
  with antiarrhythmic drugs, 275
  and blood flow changes, 29–30
  in cancer therapy, 540
  classification and categories of, 27
  and displacement from plasma
    binding sites, 29
  and distribution alterations, 29–
    30
  drug-receptor interactions, 3–7
  during absorption, 28
  during excretion, 32
  with hormones, 331
  and metabolism rate, 30–32
  and properties of lumenal con-
    tents, 28
  at receptor and acceptor sites, 30
  and transport mechanisms, 29
Interferon, 534
Intestines. See Gastrointestinal
  tract
Intolerance to drugs. See Adverse
  drug reactions

Intoxications. See Poisoning
Intravenous fluid therapy, solutions
  for, 609–611
Intrinsic activity of drugs, 4
Intrinsic factor of Castle, 316
Inulin, 548
Inversine. See Mecamylamine
Iodides
  adverse effects of, 568, 570, 571,
    572
  affecting laboratory tests, 584–
    585, 590, 593, 599
  crossing placental barrier, 575
  in hyperthyroidism, 346
  interaction with other drugs, 565
Iodine, 490
  adverse effects of, 568, 569, 571
  antidotes to, 102, 104
  drugs containing, affecting labora-
    tory tests, 584–585, 590,
    593, 599
  as poison antidote, 102
  protein-bound, drugs affecting
    tests for, 598–600
  radioactive, 346
    crossing placental barrier, 575
    drugs affecting uptake of, 598–
      600
    excretion in milk, 576
  in tinea infections, 521
Iodipamide, 547
Iodized oil, 547
Iodochlorhydroxyquin, 506
  adverse effects of, 568
  affecting laboratory tests, 584–
    585, 590, 593, 599, 601
5-Iododeoxyuridine, 417
Iodophores, 490
Iodopyracet, 547
  adverse effects of, 571
Iodopyrine, affecting laboratory
  tests, 593, 599
Ion exchange resin, affecting
  laboratory tests, 584–585
Ionic bonds, in drug-receptor inter-
  action, 4
Ionization of compounds, 8
  intestinal pH affecting, 28
Ionophores, activity of, 414
Iopanoic acid, 547
  excretion in milk, 576
Iophendylate, 547
Iophenoxic acid, crossing placental
  barrier, 575
Iothalamate, 548
Iothiouracil
  affecting laboratory tests, 584–
    585, 599
  blood dyscrasias from, 573
  crossing placental barrier, 575
Ipecac
  adverse effects of, 569, 571
  emetic effects of, 90–91
Ipecacuanha alkaloids, 503
Ipodate calcium of sodium, 547
Iproniazid, 183
  adverse effects of, 571
Iron
  absorption and metabolism of,
    314
  poisoning from, antidote in, 101,
    102

Iron (continued)
  preparations of, 314–316
    adverse effects of, 316
    affecting laboratory tests, 584–
      585, 593, 596, 599, 601
    tests for, drugs affecting, 581,
      583, 585, 587
Ismelin. See Guanethidine
Isocarboxazid, 183
  affecting laboratory tests, 584–
    585
Isoflurane, 213
Isoflurophate, 126
  in glaucoma, 125
Isoniazid. See Isonicotinic acid
  hydrazide
Isonicotinic acid hydrazide, 478–
  480
  absorption, metabolism and
    excretion of, 479
  adverse effects of, 479–480, 568,
    571, 572
  affecting laboratory tests, 584–
    585, 593, 596
  bacterial resistance to, 478
  blood dyscrasias from, 573
  chemical structure of, 22
  crossing placental barrier, 575
  excretion in milk, 576
  hereditary variations in metabo-
    lism of, 63
  interaction with other drugs, 275,
    566
  preparations of, 480
  in renal failure, 604–605
  in tuberculosis, 448, 449
Isoprinosine, in virus infections,
  534
Isopropylnorepinephrine. See Isoproterenol
Isoproterenol, 140, 148
  adverse effects of, 140
  dichloro derivative of, 147
  mechanism of action, 135–136
  pharmacologic actions of, 140
  preparations and dosage of, 140
  therapeutic uses of, 140
Isosorbide dinitrate, 277
  adverse effects of, 570
Isothipendyl, adverse effects of,
  570
Isoxsuprine hydrochloride, 143
  vasodilator action of, 279
Isuprel. See Isoproterenol

J

Jadit, adverse effects of, 570
Jaundice, from antipsychotic drugs,
  194

K

Kala-azar, 509–510
Kallidin, 552
Kanamycin, 444, 446

Kanamycin *(continued)*
  adverse effects of, 446
  affecting laboratory tests, 584–585, 593, 599
  dosage of, 446
  interaction with other drugs, 564, 566
  malabsorption from, 577
  in renal failure, 604–605
  therapeutic uses of, 446
Kaolin
  affecting laboratory tests, 593, 596
  in diarrhea, 302
Kaopectate, 302
Karaya gum, adverse effects of, 569
Keflin. *See* Cephalothin
Kemadrin, in parkinsonism, 252
Kernicterus, from maternal drug use, 84, 470
Ketamine, 220
  mental effects of, 73
17-Ketosteroids, tests for, drugs affecting, 598–600
Kidney
  amphotericin B affecting, 525
  antibiotics in renal failure, 603–605
  blood perfusion rate in, 13
  dialysis of. *See* Dialysis
  digitalis affecting, 261
  drugs in function tests of, 548
  and excretion of drugs, 15–16
    in childhood, 82
  drug interactions affecting, 32
  handling of electrolytes, 303–304
  localization of drugs in, 13
  polymyxin B affecting, 460
  sulfonamides affecting, 469–470
  tetracyclines affecting, 454
Klebsiella, drugs affecting, 420, 427, 436, 442, 453, 459, 485

L

Labor, induction of, 342
Laboratory tests, drugs affecting, 579–601
β-Lactamases, production of, 427
Lactation
  and effects of maternal drugs on infants, 53, 85
  and excretion of drugs in milk, 16, 576
  prolactin secretion in, 339
Lactic dehydrogenase, tests for, drugs affecting, 581, 583, 585, 587
Lactobacillus acidophilus, affecting laboratory tests, 584–585
Lambliasis. *See* Giardiasis
Lanolin, adverse effects of, 568
Lantinin, adverse effects of, 570
Lasix. *See* Furosemide
Laudanum, in diarrhea, 301
Lavage, gastric, in treatment of poisoning, 91–97
  in childhood, 91
  fluids used in, 91, 95–96

Lavender oil, adverse effects of, 570
Laxatives, 296
LE cell test, drugs affecting, 581, 583, 585, 587
Lead poisoning, antidote in, 101, 102, 103
Lee-White clotting time, 318
Legal aspects
  informed consent in clinical trials of drugs, 42
  in prescription writing, 86–88
Leishmaniasis, 509–510
  antimony compounds in, 509
  aromatic diamidines in, 509
  mucocutaneous, 509
    treatment of, 510
  treatment of, 422
Leponex. *See* Clozapine
Leprosy, 421, 483–484
Leptospira
  canicola, drugs affecting, 420
  icterohaemorrhagiae, drugs affecting, 421, 427, 452
Leukocyte count, drugs affecting, 581, 583, 585, 587
Leukopenia, drug-induced, 573–574
Levallorphan, 232, 235
  as poison antidote, 103
Levarterenol. *See* Norepinephrine
Levorphanol, 232, 235, 236
  crossing placental barrier, 575
Leydig cells, 364
Librium. *See* Chlordiazepoxide
Lichenoid reactions, drug-induced, 571
Lidocaine, 171
  adverse effects of, 274
  in arrhythmias, 273–274, 275
  interaction with other drugs, 275
  preparations and dosage of, 274
Lime oil, adverse effects of, 570
Lincomycin, 462–463
  affecting laboratory tests, 584–585
  affecting protein synthesis, 415
  interaction with other drugs, 564
  in renal failure, 604–605
Liothyronine sodium, 345
Liothrix, 345
Lipemia, mixed, 281, 284
Lipids
  alcohol affecting levels of, 78
  hyperlipidemia. *See* Hyperlipidemia
  tests for, drugs affecting, 581, 583, 585, 587
Lipiodol, 547
Lipolysis, epinephrine affecting, 138
Lipoprotein lipase enzyme system, 280
Lipoproteins, plasma, 280
  and treatment of hyperlipidemia, 282–284
  and types of hyperlipidemia, 280–281
Liquorice compounds, 294
Listeria monocytogenes, drugs affecting, 421, 427, 436, 442, 452, 458

Lithium carbonate, 185–186
  absorption and excretion of, 185–186
  actions of, 185
  adverse effects of, 186
  affecting laboratory tests, 584–585, 593, 596, 599, 601
  in alcohol withdrawal reactions, 80
  crossing placental barrier, 575
  interaction with thiazides, 309
  in mania, 193
  preparations and dosage of, 186
  therapeutic uses of, 185, 186
Liver
  and androgen metabolism, 364
  blood perfusion rate in, 13
  and excretion of drugs, 16
  extracts of, adverse effects of 571
  insulin affecting, 351
  localization of drugs in, 13
  mixed function oxidase, 19–20
  salicylates affecting, 225
  tetracyclines affecting, 454
Loa loa, 513
Lomidine. *See* Pentamidine isethionate
Lomotil. *See* Diphenoxylate
LSD. *See* Lysergic acid diethylamide
Lucanthone, 518
  adverse effects of, 569
  in helminthiasis, 515
  mode of action, 417
Luminal. *See* Phenobarbital
Lungs
  blood perfusion rate in, 13
  and excretion of drugs, 16
  localization of drugs in, 13
Lupus erythematosus
  drug-induced, 571
  drugs affecting LE cell test in, 581, 583, 585, 587
Lupus-like syndrome
  from diphenylhydantoin, 244
  from procainamide, 273
Luteinizing hormone, 338–339, 373
  and estrogen synthesis, 367
  releasing hormone, 327, 328, 329
  therapeutic uses of, 339
Lymphogranuloma venereum, treatment of, 420
Lysergic acid diethylamide, 72–73, 146, 393, 394
  crossing placental barrier, 575

M

Macrolide antibiotics, 457–458
Macrotetralideactins, 414
Maduromycosis, 524
Mafenide, 472
Magnesium antacids, affecting laboratory tests, 584–585, 590, 593, 596
Magnesium hydroxide, 293
  adverse effects of, 569
Magnesium oxide, 293

Methadone *(continued)*
  poisoning from, antidote in, 103
Methadyl acetate, 70
Methallenestril, 372
Methaminodiazepoxide, adverse
    effects of, 568
Methamphetamine, 143, 186
  abuse of, 71
Methandrostenolone, 366
  adverse effects of, 569
  interaction with other drugs, 566
Methanol, 79
Methaqualone, 200, 205
  abuse of, 70
  adverse effects of, 205
Methdilazine
  excretion in milk, 576
  in pruritus, 194
Methedrine. *See* Methamphetamine
Methemoglobin, tests for, drugs
    affecting, 581, 583, 585, 587
Methemoglobinemia, treatment of,
    103
Methenamine
  adverse effects of, 569
  hippurate, affecting laboratory
    tests, 596
  mandelate, 484–485
    adverse effects of, 485
    affecting laboratory tests, 594,
      596, 599, 601
Methicillin, 433
  affecting laboratory tests, 584–
    585, 594, 599
  interaction with other drugs, 564
  in renal failure, 604–605
Methimazole, 346
  adverse effects of, 571
  blood dyscrasias from, 573
  crossing placental barrier, 575
  excretion in milk, 576
Methiodal sodium, 548
Methisazone, 483, 532–533
Methocarbamol
  affecting laboratory tests, 584–
    585, 594, 596
  excretion in milk, 576
  as muscle relaxant, 169
Methonium series of drugs, 164–
    165
Methophenobarbital, blood dyscra-
    sias from, 573
Methoprim, 416–417
D-Methorphan, 232, 235, 236, 238
Methosarb, in cancer therapy, 543
Methotrexate, 539, 542
  adverse effects of, 571
  affecting laboratory tests, 584–
    585, 599
  blood dyscrasias from, 573
  crossing placental barrier, 575
  displacement from plasma binding
    sites, 29
  interaction with other drugs, 28,
    32, 566
  malabsorption from, 577
  mode of action, 416–417, 536
Methotrimeprazine, 233, 235, 236
  adverse effects of, 570
Methoxamine hydrochloride, 143
Methoxsalen, adverse effects of,
    570

Methoxyflurane, 213, 218–219
Methoxypsoralen, adverse effects
    of, 570
Methsuximide, 242, 246
  adverse effects of, 571
Methylatropine, localization in
    organs, 13
α-Methyldopa, 157–158
  adverse effects of, 157, 571, 572
  affecting laboratory tests, 584–
    585, 590, 594, 596
  blood dyscrasias from, 573
  interaction with other drugs, 566
  preparations and dosage of, 157–
    158
Methylene blue
  adverse effects of, 572
  affecting laboratory tests, 584–
    585, 594, 596
  blood dyscrasias from, 573
  as poison antidote, 103
Methylergonovine, 147
Methylphenidate, 186
  interaction with other drugs, 566
Methylphenylethylhydantoin,
    adverse effects of, 570
Methylprednisolone, 361
Methylsalicylate, adverse effects of,
    571
Methyltestosterone, 366
  adverse effects of, 572
Methylthiouracil, 346
  adverse effects of, 571
Methylxanthines, 254, 255
Methyprylon, 200, 205
Methysergide, 393, 395
  affecting laboratory tests, 584–
    585, 594
Metiamide, 385, 387
  and parietal cell secretion, 291
Metopirone. *See* Metyrapone
Metrazol, as central stimulant,
    253–254
Metrecal, affecting laboratory tests,
    599, 601
Metronidazole
  adverse effects of, 507
  affecting laboratory tests, 594,
    596
  in amebiasis, 505, 507
  excretion in milk, 576
  in giardiasis, 507
  interaction with other drugs, 566
  in trichomoniasis, 507, 511
Metyrapone diagnostic test, 362,
    548
  drugs affecting, 598–600
Miconazole nitrate
  in candidiasis, 523
  in tinea infections, 521
Microflora status, and adverse drug
    reactions, 54, 55
Microsomal enzymes
  inhibition by drugs, 31–32
  and metabolism of drugs, 19
Migraine
  ergot alkaloids in, 146–147
  methysergide in, 395
  serotonin metabolism in, 394
  xanthines in, 255
Milk
  as antacid, 293

Milk *(continued)*
  in gastric lavage, 96
  human, drugs excreted in, 16, 576
  as poison antidote, 102
Milk of magnesia, 293, 299
Milontin. *See* Phensuximide
Miltown. *See* Meprobamate
Mineral oil, 300
  as poison antidote, 103
Mineralocorticoids, 356, 360
Minocycline, 451, 452
  in renal failure, 604–605
Minoxidil, 153
Mintezol, 517
Miosis, morphine-induced, 233
Miracil-D. *See* Lucanthone
Mithramycin, in cancer, 543
Mitomycin C, 417
Monichol. *See* Choline dihydrogen
    citrate
Moniliasis. *See* Candidiasis
Monoacetin, as poison antidote,
    103
Monoamine(s)
  imipramine affecting, 182
  and neurotransmission, 177
Monoamine oxidase
  inhibitors, 183–185
    actions of, 183–184
    adverse effects of, 184
    affecting laboratory tests, 586–
      587, 599
    as antihypertensive drugs, 158
    chemistry of, 183
    interaction with other drugs, 32,
      52, 183, 184–185, 566, 567
    overdosage of, 184
    preparations and dosage of, 185
    therapeutic uses of, 185
  and metabolism of drugs, 20
Monoglycerol p-aminobenzoate,
    adverse effects of, 570
Morphine, 231, 232, 234, 235
  affecting laboratory tests, 586–
    587, 594, 596, 599, 601
  antitussive effects of, 238
  conversion to heroin, 68–69
  crossing placental barrier, 575
  excretion in milk, 576
  interaction with other drugs, 564
  with oxygen, as anesthetic, 220
  poisoning from, antidote in, 103
Motion sickness, antihistamines in,
    388
Mouth. *See* Oral conditions
Mucin, gastric, 291, 293
Multiple drugs. *See* Combinations
    of drugs
Muscarine poisoning, antimusca-
    rinic agents in, 133
Muscarinic agents, 116–119
  acetylcholine, 116–117
  adverse effects of, 119
  bethanechol, 118
  carbamylcholine, 118
  contraindications to, 119
  methacholine, 118
  pilocarpine, 118–119
  therapeutic use of, 118–119
Muscarinic receptors, 114
  antagonism by antimuscarinic
    agents, 128–134

Muscle
  acetylcholine affecting, 117
  blood perfusion rate in, 12
  localization of drugs in, 13
Muscle relaxants, 160—169
  adverse effects of, 167
  anesthetic agents affecting, 166
  antagonists of, 164, 167
  antodyne, 168—169
  carisoprodol, 169
  centrally acting, 168—169
  dantrolene sodium, 167—168
  decamethonium, 164—165
  depolarizing, 164—165
  diazepam, 169
  directly acting, 167—168
  dosage of, 166
  gallamine triethiodide, 164
  interaction with other drugs, 566
  mephenesin, 169
  meprobamate, 169
  methocarbamol, 169
  nondepolarizing, 162—164
  pancuronium bromide, 163—164
  peripherally acting, 160—168
  selection of, 166
  succinylcholine, 164—165
  therapeutic uses of, 165—166
  d-tubocurarine, 162—163
  ventilatory effects of, 162—163,
    167
Mushroom poisoning, antimuscarinic agents in, 133
Mustards, adverse effects of, 570
Mustargen, 542
Mutations, bacterial, and resistance
  to antimicrobial drugs, 403
Myasthenia gravis
  cholinesterase inhibitors in, 124
  and sensitivity to muscle
    relaxants, 166
Mycobacterial infections
  atypical, drugs affecting, 421, 449
  tuberculosis. See Tuberculosis
Mycobacterium
  leprae, drugs affecting, 421,
    483—484
  tuberculosis, drugs affecting, 442,
    464—465
Mycoplasma pneumoniae, drugs
  affecting 421, 458
Mycostatin, in candidiasis, 522
Mycotic diseases, 519—527
  actinomycosis, 523
  amphotericin B in, 524—525
  blastomycosis, 523
  candidiasis, 522—523, 525
  clotrimazole in, 526
  deep, 523—527
  5-fluorocytosine in, 525—526
  griseofulvin in, 520—522
  hamycin in, 526
  natamycin in, 526
  nocardiosis, 523
  mystatin in, 522
  penicillin in, 523
  potassium iodide in, 523—524
  sulfonamides in, 475, 523
  superficial, 519—523
  tinea infections, 520—522
  X-5079C in, 526—527

Mydriasis
  from antimuscarinic agents, 132
  from ephedrine, 141, 142
Myleran. See Busulfan
Myocardial contraction, digitalis
  affecting, 258—259
Mysoline. See Primidone
Mytelase chloride. See Ambenonium

N

Nafcillin, 434
  affecting laboratory tests, 586—
    587, 594, 599
  in renal failure, 604—605
Nalidixic acid, 385—386
  adverse effects of, 485, 570, 572
  affecting laboratory tests, 586—
    587, 594, 599
  mode of action, 417
Nalorphine, 231, 232, 233, 235
  as poison antidote, 103
Naloxone, 231, 232, 235, 237
  as poison antidote, 103
Naphthalene, adverse effects of,
  570, 572
Narcolepsy, monoamine oxidase
  inhibitors in, 184, 185
Narcotics, 231—238
  abuse of, 68—70
  adverse effects of, 237
  antagonists of, 231, 235, 237—
    238
  as antitussive agents, 233, 235,
    238
  choice of drugs, 234—237
  excretion in milk, 576
  interaction with other drugs, 565
  overdosage of, 237
  pharmacologic action of, 231—
    233
  for preanesthetic medication, 234
  therapeutic uses of, 233—234
Nardil. See Phenelzine
Nasal decongestants, 141—142, 143
  rebound congestion from, 142
Natamycin, 526
Naturetin. See Bendroflumethiazide
Necator americanus, 513
Necrolysis, epidermal, drug-
  induced, 571
Neisseria
  gonorrhoeae, drugs affecting, 421,
    427, 436, 442, 452, 458, 464
  meningitidis, drugs affecting, 421,
    427, 436, 452, 475
Nematode infections, 513
Nembutal. See Pentobarbital
Neoarsphenamine, adverse effects
  of, 569, 572
Neohydrin. See Chlormerodrin
Neomycin, 443, 444, 446
  affecting laboratory tests, 586—
    587, 594, 599
  in amebiasis, 508
  blood dyscrasias from, 573
  excretion in milk, 576
  interaction with other drugs, 566

Neomycin (continued)
  malabsorption from, 577
  therapeutic uses of, 446
Neostam, 509
Neostibosan, 509
Neostigmine, 123, 126
  as antagonist to muscle relaxants,
    167
Neo-synephrine. See Phenylephrine
Nervous system. See also Central
    nervous system; Peripheral
    nervous system
  signs in poisonings, 92—93
Nethalide, 147
Neuroeffector junction, 108
Neurohumoral transmission, 110—
    114, 161—162. See also Trans-
    mission
Neurohypophysis, 327, 340
Neuroleptanalgesia, 234
Neuromuscular blocking agents
    160—169. See also Muscle
    relaxants
Neuromuscular junction, 108
  physiology of, 160—161
  transmission at, 161—162
Neurophysin, 340
Neuroses, amphetamine in, 142
Neurotransmitters, 176—180
  biosynthesis of, 178
  false, 20, 157
  in parkinsonism, 248—249
  receptor interaction with, 179
  release of, 179
  storage of, 179
  termination of action of, 179
Neutral red, 417
New drugs, development of, 39—45
Newborn
  development affected by maternal
    use of drugs, 57
  and drugs excreted in human
    milk, 16, 576
  sulfonamides affecting, 470
Niacin, 554—555
  excretion in milk, 576
Nialamide, 183
Niamid, 183
Nickel poisoning, antidote in, 101
Niclosamide, 422, 518, 561
  in helminthiasis, 513, 516
Nicotine
  crossing placental barrier, 575
  and effects of smoking, 66
  excretion in milk, 576
  as ganglionic stimulating agent,
    154
  poisoning from, antidote in, 103
Nicotinic acid, 554—555
  adverse effects of, 283
  affecting laboratory tests, 586—
    587, 594, 596
  in hyperlipidemia, 283
Nicotinic receptors, 114
Nifuroxime, 486
Nikethamide, as central stimulant,
    254
Niridazole, 422, 518
  adverse effects of, 572
  in helminthiasis, 513, 516
Nirvanol, adverse effects of, 571
Nitrites, 276—278

Nitrites *(continued)*
  actions of, 276—277
  adverse effects of, 278
  contraindications to, 278
  preparations and dosage of, 277
  therapeutic uses of, 277—278
  tolerance to, 278
Nitrofurantoin, 486—487
  adverse effects of, 487, 569, 571, 572
  affecting laboratory tests, 586—587, 594, 596, 599
  blood dyscrasias from, 573
  crossing placental barrier, 575
  excretion in milk, 576
  interaction with other drugs, 565
  in renal failure, 604—605
  with streptomycin, 443
Nitrofurazone, 486
  adverse effects of, 568, 572
  blood dyscrasias from, 573
Nitrogen mustard, 542
  mode of action, 417
Nitroglycerin, 277
  adverse effects of, 570
  interaction with other drugs, 566
Nitroprusside sodium, in hypertensive crises, 158
Nitrosoureas, 537
Nitrous oxide, 213, 217
  crossing placental barrier, 575
Nocardiosis, 524
  sulfonamides in, 467, 523
Noncompliance of patients, and adverse drug reactions, 53—54
Nordefrin hydrochloride, 143
Norepinephrine, 139—140
  adverse effects of, 140
  interaction with other drugs, 564
  with local anesthetics, 173
  mechanism of action, 135—136
  and neurotransmission, 177
  pharmacologic actions of, 139
  preparations and dosage of, 139—140
  synthesis of, 113, 114
  therapeutic uses of, 139
Norethandrolone, 366
Norethindrone, 377
  adverse effects of, 571
Norethynodrel, 374, 377
Norgestrel, 378
Norpramin, 181
Nortriptyline, 181
  adverse effects of, 570
Noscapine, 231
Nose drops, 141—142
Novobiocin
  adverse effects of, 569, 571
  affecting laboratory tests, 586—587, 590, 594
  blood dyscrasias from, 573
  crossing placental barrier, 575
  excretion in milk, 576
  interaction with other drugs, 565
  mode of action, 413
  in renal failure, 604—605
Novocain. *See* Procaine hydrochloride
Nucleic acid metabolism, inhibition by antibiotics, 416—417
Numorphan. *See* Oxymorphone

Nylidrin hydrochloride, 143
  vasodilator action of, 279
Nyquil, 199
Nystatin, in candidiasis, 522

O

Obesity, appetite suppressants in, 142, 288
Oblivon, 204
Octylphenoxyethoxyethyl ether sulfonate, 489
Ocular conditions. *See* Eyes
Oleandomycin, 455, 458
Oleum ricini, 298
Onchocerca volvulus, 513
Onchocerciasis, 513
Oncovin, 543
Ophthalmological disorders. *See* Eyes
Opiates
  addiction to, 68—70
  adverse effects of, 569, 571
  in diarrhea, 301
  interaction with other drugs, 28
Opium, 231
  adverse effects of, 569
Opportunistic infections, 408
  treatment of, 421
Oragrafin, 547
Oral administration of drugs, 11, 12
  interactions in, 28—29
Oral contraceptives. *See* Contraceptives, oral
Oral infections, treatment of, 422
Oral signs in poisoning, 94
Oretic. *See* Hydrochlorothiazide
Organic brain syndromes, antipsychotic drugs in, 193
Organic compounds
  adverse effects of, 568
  ionization of, 8
Organophosphates
  cholinesterase inhibitors, 122, 125, 126
  poisoning from, antidote for, 101, 103
Oriental sore, 509
  treatment of, 510
Orinase. *See* Tolbutamide
Ornithosis, treatment of, 420
Oroya fever, treatment of, 420
Orphenadrine
  interaction with other drugs, 566
  as muscle relaxant, 169
Orthostatic hypotension, 151
Osmotic cathartics, 299
Osteomyelitis, treatment of, 420, 421
Osteoporosis, from adreno-corticoids, 360
Otitis media, treatment of, 420, 422
Ouabain, 262, 263
Overdose
  of barbiturates, 202
  of monoamine oxidase inhibitors, 184
  of narcotics, 237

Ovulation prevention, with oral contraceptives, 373—379
Oxacillin, 434
  affecting laboratory tests, 586—587, 594, 599
  excretion in milk, 576
  in renal failure, 604—605
Oxalate poisoning, antidote in, 101
Oxandrolone, 366
Oxazepam, 207, 208, 209
Oxazolidinediones, as anticonvulsant agents, 246
Oxidation, 19—24
Oxidizing agents, germicidal activity of, 490
Oxophenarsine, adverse effects of, 569
Oxphenisatin, 298
Oxycodone, 232, 234, 235
Oxygen
  consumption of, epinephrine affecting, 138
  hyperbaric, 551
  morphine with, as anesthetic, 220
Oxymorphone, 232, 234, 235
Oxyphenbutazone, 227
  blood dyscrasias from, 573
  excretion in milk, 576
  interaction with other drugs, 566, 567
Ocyphenisatin, adverse effects of, 571
Oxytetracycline, 451, 452
  adverse effects of, 569, 570
  in amebiasis, 508
  in balantidiasis, 511
  in helminthiasis, 513
  interaction with other drugs, 565
Oxytocic action, of ergot alkaloids, 147
Oxytocin, 341—342
  secretion affected by alcohol, 78
  therapeutic uses of, 342

P

Pain, analgesics in. *See* Analgesics
Pamaquine
  adverse effects of, 572
  blood dyscrasias from, 573
Pancreas, insulin secretion in, 350
Pancreatic extracts, 289
Pancreatin, 289
Pancreatitis, antacids in, 296
Pancrelipase, 289
Pancreomyzin, affecting laboratory tests, 586—587
Pancuronium bromide, 163—164
Pantopaque, 547
Pantopon, poisoning from, antidote in, 103
Pantothenic acid, 557—558
  excretion in milk, 576
Papaverine, 231
  excretion in milk, 576
  vasodilator action of, 279
Para-aminobenzoic acid. *See* Aminobenzoic acid

Pimafucin, 526
Pimaricin, 526
Piperazine, 518
  affecting laboratory tests, 586–587
  in helminthiasis, 513, 516
Piperazine estrone sulfate, 372
Pipradrol, 186
Pitocin, 342
Pitressin
  affecting laboratory tests, 586–587, 594
  in diabetes insipidus, 340
Pituitary gland
  anterior hormones, 333–340
    corticotropin, 335
    follicle-stimulating hormone, 337–338
    interactions with target organs, 333–335
    prolactin, 339–340
    somatotropin, 335–336
    thyrotropin, 337
  posterior hormones, 340–342
    antidiuretic hormone, 340–341
    oxytocin, 341–342
  relation to hypothalamus, 327
Placebos
  adverse reactions to, 57
  in clinical trials of drugs, 43
Placental barrier
  and distribution of drugs, 13–14
  drugs crossing, 575–576
Placidyl. See Ethclorvynol
Plague, treatment of, 421
Plantago seed, 300
Plaquenil. See Hydroxychloroquine
Plasma. See Blood
Plasmids, and resistance to antimicrobial drugs, 404
Plasmodia. See Malaria
Platelets
  drugs affecting count of, 581, 583, 585, 587
  prostaglandins affecting aggregation of, 397
  salicylates affecting, 224
  serotonin in, 393
    in carcinoid syndrome, 394
  thrombocytopenia from drugs, 573–574
Pneumococci, drugs affecting, 458, 462, 467
Pneumocystis carinii pneumonia, treatment of, 422, 509
Pneumonia, treatment of, 420, 421, 422
Podophyllum, crossing placental barrier, 575
Poisoning, 90–104
  from absorbed dermal poisons, 100
  activated charcoal in, 96–97, 101
  antibiotics in, 97
  anticholinesterase, antimuscarinic agents in, 133
  antidotes in, 97, 101–104
  barbiturate, 99
  by belladonna alkaloids, 134
  and chemical eye burns, 100
  convulsions in, 98
  dialysis in, 97–98

Poisoning (continued)
  exchange transfusions in, 99
  gastric lavage in, 91–97
  general therapeutic measures in, 99–100
  from inhaled poisons, 100
  from injected poisons, 100
  muscarine, antimuscarinic agents in, 133
  from organophosphate cholinesterase inhibitors, 122, 125
  from overdosage. See Overdose and preclinical evaluation of toxicity, 41
  from salicylates, 225–226
  symptoms of, 92–95
  vomiting induction in, 90–91
Polarity, 8
  and adverse drug reactions, 48
Polio vaccine, adverse effects of, 571
Poloxalkol, 300
Polycarbophil, in diarrhea, 302
Polyestradiol phosphate, 372
Polymyxin B, 459–460
  absorption, metabolism and excretion of, 460
  adverse effects of, 460
  affecting laboratory tests, 586–587, 594, 600
  bacterial resistance to, 460
  interaction with other drugs, 566
  malabsorption from, 577
  preparations and dosage of, 460
  in renal failure, 604–605
  spectrum of activity, 459–460
  therapeutic uses of, 460
Polypeptides, vasoactive, 552
Polythiazide, diuretic action of, 304
Porphyria, drug-induced, 53, 571
Porphyrins in urine, drugs affecting tests for, 592–595
Postural hypotension, 151
Potassium
  affecting cardiac rhythm, 267
  deficiency from diuretics, 308, 310
  tests for, drugs affecting, 581, 583, 585, 587
Potassium bitartrate, 299
Potassium chlorate, adverse effects of, 569
Potassium chloride
  affecting laboratory tests, 586–587, 600, 601
  malabsorption from, 577
Potassium hydroxyquinoline sulfate, adverse effects of, 568
Potassium iodide
  adverse effects of, 568
  crossing placental barrier, 575
  excretion in milk, 576
  in mycoses, 523–524
Potassium perchlorate, and thyroid gland function, 346
Potassium permanganate, 490
  in gastric lavage, 95
  as poison antidote, 103
  poisoning from, antidote in, 102
Potassium sodium tartrate, 299
Potency of drugs, 5–6

Povan, 516
Practolol, 148
Pralidoxime, as poison antidote, 103, 125–127
Prednisolone, 359, 361
  interaction with other drugs, 565
Prednisone, 359, 361
  in cancer, 539, 541, 543
Pregnancy
  and adverse drug reactions, 53, 56–57
  diagnosis of, 376
  drugs affecting tests for, 598–600
  and effects of drugs on fetus, 84–85
  estrogen secretion in, 367
  and labor induction, 342
  placental barrier in, 13–14
    drugs crossing, 575–576
  prevention with oral contraceptives, 373–379
  progesterone secretion in, 373
Prescription writing, 86–89
  components in, 88–89
  Latin words and phrases in, 87
  legal aspects of, 86–88
Prilocaine, affecting laboratory tests, 586–587
Primamycin, 526
Primaquine, 497, 500
  adverse effects of, 572
  affecting laboratory tests, 586–587, 594, 597
  blood dyscrasias from, 574
Primidone, 242, 245
  adverse effects of, 568, 571
  affecting laboratory tests, 586–587
  blood dyscrasias from, 574
  interaction with other drugs, 566
Priscoline. See Tolazoline
Probenecid
  affecting laboratory tests, 586–587, 594, 600
  with p-aminosalicylic acid, 481
  blood dyscrasias from, 574
  interaction with other drugs, 32, 566, 567
  with penicillin, 32, 431–432
  uricosuric effect of, 229
Procainamide, 273, 275
  adverse effects of, 273, 571, 572
  affecting laboratory tests, 586–587
  blood dyscrasias from, 574
  hydrolysis of, 25
  interaction with other drugs, 275
  preparations and dosage of, 273
Procaine hydrochloride, 171
  adverse effects of, 568
  affecting laboratory tests, 586–587, 594, 597
  hydrolysis of, 25
  interaction with other drugs, 565
Procarbazine, in cancer, 537
Prochlorperazine
  adverse effects of, 570
  as antiemetic, 289
  blood dyscrasias from, 574
  excretion in milk, 576
  interaction with other drugs, 565
  in vomiting, 194

Procyclidine, in parkinsonism, 252
Proflavine, 417
Progesterone, 373
  affecting laboratory tests, 586–587, 600, 601
  mechanism of action, 375
  receptors for, 375
  synthesis, metabolism and excretion of, 374–375
Progestogens, oral. See Contraceptives, oral
Proguanil. See Chloroguanide
Prolactin, 339–340
  drugs affecting levels of, 340
  inhibitory hormone, 328, 330
  releasing hormone, 328, 330
Prolidoxime, 133
Prolixin. See Fluphenazine
Prolonging drug action, methods for, 607–608
Promazine
  adverse effects of, 570
  as antiemetic, 289
  blood dyscrasias from, 574
  interaction with other drugs, 565
Promethazine hydrochloride, 386
  adverse effects of, 568, 570
  interaction with other drugs, 565, 566
Promethazone, 385
Pronestyl. See Procainamide
Pronethalol, 147
Prontosil, and sulfanilamide formation, 24
Propadrine, 143
Propamidine, adverse effects of, 568
Propanediols, in anxiety, 207
Propoxyphene, 68, 235, 236
  adverse effects of, 571
  affecting laboratory tests, 588–589, 600
  excretion in milk, 576
Propranolol, 147–148, 158
  adverse effects of, 148–149, 571
  affecting laboratory tests, 588–589, 590
  in alcohol withdrawal reactions, 80
  in angina pectoris, 278–279
  in arrhythmias, 273, 275
  dosage of, 279
  interaction with other drugs, 275
  therapeutic uses of, 148
Propyliodone, 547
Propylthiouracil, 346
  adverse effects of, 571
  affecting laboratory tests, 600
  blood dyscrasias from, 574
  crossing placental barrier, 575
  excretion in milk, 576
  interaction with thyroid hormones, 331
Proquil, 199
Prostaglandins, 396–398
  chemistry of, 396
  inhibitors of, 397–398
  salicylates affecting synthesis of, 224
  therapeutic uses of, 397
Prostatic cancer, estrogen therapy in, 369, 370

Prostigmine. See Neostigmine
Protamine sulfate
  as anticoagulant antagonist, 320–321
  as poison antidote, 104
Protein
  antibiotics affecting synthesis of, 414–415, 441–458
  binding to adrenocorticoids, 331, 357
  binding to steroid hormones, 330–331
  binding to sulfonamides, 469
  binding to thyroid hormones, 330
  in cerebrospinal fluid, drugs affecting tests for, 598–600
  displacement of drugs from binding sites, 29
  metabolism of, insulin affecting, 351
  plasma proteins binding to drugs, 14
  tests for, drugs affecting, 581, 583, 585, 587
  in urine, drugs affecting tests for, 592–595
Proteus, drugs affecting, 421, 427, 436, 442, 460, 485, 487
Prothrombin time determination, 318–319
  drugs affecting, 581, 583, 585, 587
Protokylol hydrochloride, 143
Protozoal diseases, 492–511
  amebiasis, 502–509
  belantidiasis, 511
  furazolidone in, 487
  giardiasis, 511
  leishmaniasis, 509–510
  malaria, 492–502
  sulfonamides in, 475
  toxoplasmosis, 511
  trichomoniasis, 511
  trypanosomiasis, 510–511
Protriptyline, 181
  adverse effects of, 570
Provera. See Medroxyprogesterone acetate
Providencia, drugs affecting, 421
Pruritus, treatment of, 194, 387
Pseudocholinesterase, 24–25, 120
Pseudoephedrine, excretion in milk, 576
Pseudolymphoma, drugs affecting tests for, 598–600
Pseudomonas
  aeruginosa, drugs affecting, 421, 442, 460
  pseudomalleii, drugs affecting, 452
Pseudotumor cerebri, from tetracyclines, 454
Psilocine, 393
Psilocybin, 72–73, 393
Psittacosis, treatment of, 420
Psoralens, adverse effects of, 570
Psychoses
  from adrenocorticoids, 361
  amphetamine in, 142
  amphetamine-induced, 144, 190
  antipsychotic drugs in, 187–196
  serotonin metabolism in, 392

Psychotropic drugs
  antianxiety agents, 206–210
  antidepressants, tricyclic, 181–183
  antipsychotic agents, 187–196
  classification of, 179–180
  lithium carbonate, 185–186
  monoamine oxidase inhibitors, 183–185
  sedative-hypnotics, 197–206
  stimulants, 186
Psyllium, in diarrhea, 301
Pteroylglutamic acid, 317
Pteroylmonoglutamic acid, 556
Pulse, in poisoning, 95
Purgatives, 296
Purine metabolism, 230
Purity of drugs, and adverse reactions, 49–50
Puromycin, affecting protein synthesis, 414
Purpura, drug-induced, 571
Pyelography, contrast media for, 547–548
Pyramidone, adverse effects of, 572
Pyrantel, in helminthiasis, 513, 516
Pyrathiazine hydrochloride, adverse effects of, 570
Pyrazinamide
  adverse effects of, 482
  affecting laboratory tests, 588–589, 600
  in tuberculosis, 480, 482
Pyribenzamine. See Tripelennamine
Pyridine, adverse effects of, 570
Pyridium, adverse effects of, 572
Pyridostigmine, 123, 126
  as antagonist to muscle relaxants, 167
Pyridoxine, 555
Pyrilamine, 385, 386
  adverse effects of, 568
Pyrimethamine, 497, 501
  affecting laboratory tests, 588–589
  blood dyscrasias from, 574
  excretion in milk, 576
  mode of action, 416–417
  sulfonamides with, 418
  in toxoplasmosis, 511
Pyrimidine, adverse effects of, 569
Pyromen, adverse effects of, 571
Pyrvinium pamoate, 518
  in helminthiasis, 513, 516

Q

Q fever, treatment of, 420, 421
Quaalude. See Methaqualone
Questran. See Cholestyramine
Quick's prothrombin time determination, 318–319
Quinacrine, 496, 498
  adverse effects of, 498, 568, 569, 570, 571, 572
  affecting laboratory tests, 588–589, 595, 597
  blood dyscrasias from, 574
  in giardiasis, 511

Quinacrine *(continued)*
  in helminthiasis, 513, 517
  mode of action, 417
  in virus infections, 534
Quinestrol, 372, 378
Quinethazone
  adverse effects of, 570
  affecting laboratory tests, 588–
    589
Quinidine, 271–272, 274–275
  adverse effects of, 272, 568, 569,
    570, 571, 572
  affecting laboratory tests, 588–
    589, 590, 595, 597, 600, 601
  blood dyscrasias from, 574
  cardiac effects of, 272
  excretion in milk, 576
  extracardiac effects of, 272
  interaction with other drugs, 275,
    566
  preparations and dosage of, 272
Quinine, 495–498
  adverse effects of, 498, 568, 569,
    570, 571, 572
  affecting laboratory tests, 588–
    589, 590, 595, 597, 600, 601
  antidote to, 103
  blood dyscrasias from, 574
  crossing placental barrier, 575
  excretion in milk, 576
  mode of action, 417
Quinocide, adverse effects of, 572

R

R factors, and resistance to anti-
    microbial drugs, 404
Radiation therapy, in peptic ulcer,
    295
Radioactive drugs
  adverse reactions to, 55
  blood dyscrasias from, 573
  iodine, 346
    crossing placental barrier, 575
    drugs affecting uptake of, 598–
      600
    excretion in milk, 576
Rash, drug-induced, 428–429, 568
Rat-bite fever, treatment of, 421,
    422
Rauwolfia alkaloids, 152, 191
Receptors
  adrenergic, blocking of. *See*
    Adrenergic receptor blocking
    drugs
  for adrenocorticoids, 357
  binding with drugs, 3–4
    covalent bonds in, 4
    hydrogen bonds in, 4
    and intrinsic activity, 4
    ionic bonds in, 4
    van der Waals forces in, 3
  compared to acceptors, 4
  for dopamine, 140
  drug interactions at sites of, 30
  for estrogen, 368
  for histamine, 382–383
  interaction with neurotrans-
    mitters, 179

Receptors *(continued)*
  muscarinic, 114
  in neurohumoral transmission,
    113
  nicotinic, 114
  for progesterone, 375
  for serotonin, 392
Reduction reaction, in metabolism
    of drugs, 24
Reentry phenomenon, in conduc-
    tion defects, 267
Regitine. *See* Phentolamine
Relapsing fever, treatment of, 420,
    422
Renin, and aldosterone release, 357
Renografin, 548
Reserpine, 152–153, 191
  adverse effects of, 152–153, 568,
    569, 570, 571, 572
  affecting laboratory tests, 588–
    589, 595, 600, 601
  crossing placental barrier, 575
  excretion in milk, 576
  interaction with other drugs, 566
  preparations and dosage of, 153
  and prolactin levels, 340
  and serotonin uptake, 391
Resins
  anion exchange, 293
  binding bile acids, 282–283, 301
  ion exchange, affecting laboratory
    tests, 584–585
Resistance
  bacterial, 403–405
    to aminoglycosides, 441
    to antitubercular drugs, 448
    to cephalosporins, 436
    to chloramphenicol, 456
    to erythromycin, 458
    to isoniazid, 478
    to penicillins, 427
    to polymyxin B, 460
    to streptomycin, 442
    to sulfonamides, 468
    to tetracyclines, 450
  of cells, to cancer therapy, 540–
    541
Resorcinol
  adverse effects of, 568
  affecting laboratory tests, 600
Respiration
  morphine affecting, 231, 232,
    237
  muscle relaxants affecting, 162–
    163, 167
Respiratory system
  antimuscarinic agents affecting,
    131
  prostaglandins affecting, 397
  signs in poisoning, 94–95
  treatment of infections, 421
Retinol, 553
Rh antibodies, excretion in milk,
    576
Rheumatic fever, salicylates in, 224
Rhinosporidiosis, 524
Rhubarb, 298
  excretion in milk, 576
Riboflavin, 554
  affecting laboratory tests, 595,
    597
  excretion in milk, 576

Rickettsiae, drugs affecting, 421,
    452, 457, 458
Rifampin, 464–465
  adverse effects of, 465
  blood dyscrasias from, 574
  mode of action, 417
  in renal failure, 604–605
  in tuberculosis, 448
  in virus infections, 534
Ringer's solution, 611
  lactated, 610
Ristocetin, 413
Ritalin. *See* Methylphenidate
RNA synthesis, inhibition by anti-
    biotics, 416–417
Ro-2-7758, in mycoses, 526–527
Rochelle salt, 299
Rocky Mountain spotted fever,
    treatment of, 421
Rolitetracycline, 451, 542
Rose bengal perfume, adverse
    effects of, 570
Rose bengal sodium, 548
Routes of administration, 12
  and absorption of drugs, 10–11
  and adverse drug reactions, 50
  for digitalis, 263
  for diphenylhydantoin, 243
  and drug interactions, 28–29
  intraarterial, 11
  for local anesthesia, 174
  oral, 11, 12
  parenteral, 11
  in pediatric pharmacology, 81
  subcutaneous, 11
  topical, 12
Rue, adverse effects of, 570

S

Saccharin, adverse effects of, 569
Salicylanilide
  adverse effects of, 570
  in tinea infections, 521
Salicylates, 223–226. *See also*
    Acetylsalicylic acid
  absorption and metabolism of,
    225
  adverse effects of, 225, 568, 569,
    570, 571, 572
  affecting laboratory tests, 588–
    589, 590, 595, 597, 600, 601
  blood dyscrasias from, 574
  chemistry of, 223
  crossing placental barrier, 575
  excretion in milk, 576
  interaction with other drugs, 225,
    566, 567
  interaction with thyroid hor-
    mones, 331
  pharmacologic effects of, 223–
    224
  poisoning from, 225–226
    diuretics in, 313
  preparations and dosage of, 226
  as prostaglandin inhibitors, 397
Salicylazosulfapyridine, 473
  adverse effects of, 572
Salicylic acid, 489

Salicylic acid *(continued)*
  chemical structure of, 22
Saline cathartics, 299
Saline solution, 611
  in gastric lavage, 96
Salmonellae, drugs affecting, 421,
    427, 436, 442, 452, 457, 460,
    487
Saluretics, 303
Saluron. *See* Hydroflumethiazide
Salyrgan. *See* Mersalyl sodium
Sandalwood oil, adverse effects of,
    570
Santonin, adverse effects of, 569
Saramycetin, in mycoses, 526–527
Sarcoidosis, drugs affecting tests
    for, 598–600
Sarin, 126
Scalp signs, in poisonings, 92
Scarlet fever, treatment of, 422
Schilling test, drugs affecting,
    598–600
Schistosomiasis, treatment of, 422
Schizophrenia. *See* Psychoses
Scopolamine, 128–134
  absorption, excretion and meta-
    bolism of, 131
  adverse effects of, 569
  chemistry of, 128–129
  excretion in milk, 576
  mechanism of action, 129
  pharmacologic effects of, 130–
    131
  poisoning from, 134
  preanesthetic medication with,
    220
  therapeutic uses of, 131–133
Secobarbital, 201
  abuse of, 70
  interaction with other drugs, 565
Seconal. *See* Secobarbital
Sedative-hypnotics, 197–206
  abuse of, 70–71
  antihistamines, 387
  barbiturates, 201–203
  bromides, 199
  chloral hydrate, 200, 203
  classification of, 199
  in diarrhea, 301
  effect on sleep, 198–199
  ethclorvynol, 200, 204
  ethinamate, 200, 204
  flurazepam, 200, 205–206, 209
  glutethimide, 200, 204–205
  mechanism of action, 198
  meparfynol, 204
  methaqualone, 200, 205
  methyprylon, 200, 205
  nonprescription, 199–201
  paraldehyde, 200, 203–204
  in peptic ulcer, 295
Sedimentation rate, drugs affecting,
    581, 583, 585, 587
Seizures
  from alcohol withdrawal, 80
  anticonvulsant agents in, 241–
    247
  and education of patient and
    family, 240
  electroencephalogram in, 240
  focal, 240
  grand mal, 239

Seizures *(continued)*
  petit mal, 239–240
  in poisoning, treatment of, 98
  principles of drug therapy in, 241
  psychomotor, 240
  status epilepticus, 240
    treatment of, 247
  temporal lobe, 240
Selective activity of drugs, 3
  and accessibility, 6
Selenium
  poisoning from, antidote for, 101
  in tinea infections, 521
Selenium sulfide, adverse effects of,
    568, 571
Self-medication, and adverse drug
    reactions, 54
Senna, 298
  excretion in milk, 576
Serax. *See* Oxazepam
Sernylan, 73
Serotonin, 390–394
  antagonists of, 394–395
  and carcinoid syndrome, 393–
    394
  and dumping syndrome, 393
  metabolism of, 391
  and migraine attacks, 394
  and neurotransmission, 177
  pharmacologic actions of, 391–
    392
  receptors for, 392
  striatal, in parkinsonism, 249
  synthesis, distribution and storage
    of, 390–391
  tests for, drugs affecting, 581,
    583, 585, 587
Serratia marcessens, drugs affecting,
    421
Sertoli cells, 364
Serums, adverse effects of, 568,
    571, 572
Serutan, 302
Sex chromatin, drugs affecting tests
    for, 598–600
Sex factors, in adverse drug reac-
    tions, 51–52
Sex hormones
  binding globulins, 332
  female, 366
  male, 363
Sex organ responses, to autonomic
    activity, 111
Shigellae, drugs affecting, 421, 427,
    436, 442, 452, 460, 487
Shigellosis, sulfonamides in, 475
Shock
  anaphylactic, 383
  norepinephrine in, 139
Side effects of drugs. *See* Adverse
    drug reactions
Silver nitrate, 491
  antidote for, 104
Silver salts, adverse effects of, 568,
    570
Sinequan, 181
Sinus node, digitalis affecting, 259
Sisomycin, 441
Skin
  blood perfusion rate in, 12
  color of
    and adverse drug reactions, 52

Skin
  color of *(continued)*
    drug-induced pigmentation, 568
    in poisonings, 92
  poisons absorbed through, 100
  rash from drugs, 428–429, 568
  responses to autonomic activity,
    111
Skin tests
  antigens in, 561
  drugs affecting, 598–600
Skiodan, 548
Sleep
  monoamine oxidase inhibitors
    affecting, 184
  morphine-induced, 231, 232
  nonrapid-eye-movement in, 198
  rapid-eye-movement in, 198–199
  sedative-hypnotics affecting,
    198–199, 202
Sleep Eze, 199
Sleeping sickness, 422, 510
Smallpox, 559
  methisazone prophylaxis in, 532
Smallpox vaccine, 559
  adverse effects of, 570
  crossing placental barrier, 576
Smoking. *See also* Nicotine
  and adverse drug reactions, 52
  and effects of nicotine, 66
  and peptic ulcer disease, 295
Snake bite, antivenins in, 561, 562
Soaps, 489
Sodium
  renal handling of, 303
  tests for, drugs affecting, 581,
    583, 585, 587
Sodium chloride
  affecting laboratory tests, 588–
    589
  in parenteral solutions, 611
  as poison antidote, 104
Sodium phosphate, 299
Sodium sulfate, 299
  as poison antidote, 103
Soluthricin, 459
Somatostatin, 330
Somatotropin, 335–336
  agents affecting plasma levels of,
    336
  chemistry of, 336
  inhibitory hormone, 328, 329–
    330
  releasing hormone, 327, 328,
    329–330
  therapeutic uses of, 336
Sominex, 199
Sorboquel, in diarrhea, 302
Sparteine, 342
Spectinomycin, 463–464
Spermatozoa, postcoital tests of,
    drugs affecting, 598–600
Spider bites, antidote for, 101
Spinal cord stimulants, 254
Spiramycin, 455, 458
  adverse effects of, 568
Spirillum minus, drugs affecting,
    421, 427
Spirochetes, drugs affecting, 458
Spironolactone
  adverse effects of, 572

Ultraviolet light
  absorption by drugs, 48, 56
  germicidal activity of, 489
Undecylenic acid, in tinea infec-
    tions, 521
Uracil mustard, adverse effects of,
    571
Urea nitrogen, tests for, drugs
    affecting, 580, 582, 584, 586
Urecholine. See Bethanechol
Uremia, antibiotic therapy in,
    603–605
Urethanes, 204
Uric acid levels
  allopurinol affecting, 229–230
  diuretics affecting, 313
  probenecid affecting, 229
  salicylates affecting, 224
  sulfinpyrazone affecting, 229
  in urine, drugs affecting tests for,
    592–595
Urinary tract
  epinephrine affecting, 138
  infections of, 484–487
    antimicrobial drugs in, 420,
      421, 422
    cholinesterase inhibitors in, 125
    methenamine mandelate in,
      484–485
    muscarinic agents in, 118
    nalidixic acid in, 485–486
    5-nitrofurans in, 486–487
Urine
  androgen metabolites in, 364
  color of, in poisoning, 94
  estrogens in, 368
  formation of, 303
  progesterone metabolites in, 374
  tests of, drugs affecting, 592–597
Urobilinogen
  drugs affecting tests for, 598–600
  in urine, drugs affecting tests for,
    592–595
Urticaria
  antihistamines in, 387
  drug-induced, 571
Uterus
  epinephrine affecting, 138
  ergot alkaloids affecting, 147
  estrogens affecting, 368, 373
  histamine affecting, 382
  oxytocin affecting, 341, 342
  progestational agents in func-
    tional bleeding of, 370, 376
  progesterone affecting, 373
  prostaglandins affecting, 396, 397
  signs in poisoning, 94

V

Vaccination, 528, 559–562
Vaccines, 561
  adverse effects of, 569, 572
  measles, adverse effects of, 570
  polio, adverse effects of, 571
  smallpox, 559
    adverse effects of, 570
    crossing placental barrier, 575
Vaccinia, immune globulin, 561, 562

Vagina, estrogens affecting, 368
Valium. See Diazepam
Vancomycin, 425
  affecting laboratory tests, 588–
    589
  interaction with other drugs, 565,
    566
  mode of action, 413
  in renal failure, 604–605
Van der Waals forces, 3
Vanillin oils, adverse effects of, 570
Vanillylmandelic acid, in urine,
    drugs affecting tests for,
    592–595
Vaporizer, in anesthesia machine,
    215
Vascular conditions. See Cardio-
    vascular system
Vasoactive polypeptides, 552
Vasodilan hydrochloride. See
    Isoxsuprine hydrochloride
Vasodilator drugs, 279
  isoproterenol, 140
Vasopressin. See Antidiuretic hor-
    mone
Vasotonin, 390
Vasoxyl hydrochloride, 143
Velban, 543
Venoconstriction, from digitalis,
    261
Ventilation. See Respiration
Ventricular conduction system,
    digitalis affecting, 259
Veratrum alkaloids, 151–152
  adverse effects of, 152
Vermox, 515
Veronal. See Barbital
Vesicles, in neurohumoral trans-
    mission, 112–113
Vesprin. See Triflupromazine
Vestibular disorders, antimuscarinic
    agents in, 132
Vibrio cholerae, drugs affecting,
    422, 452, 467, 487
Vidarabine, 534
Vinblastine, 538, 539, 543
  adverse effects of, 571
Vinca alkaloids, 538, 539, 543
  mechanism of action, 537
Vincent's angina, treatment of,
    420, 422
Vincristine, 538, 539, 543
  adverse effects of, 571, 572
Vinegar, in alkali poisoning, 101
Viomycin, 445, 447
  affecting laboratory tests, 588–
    589, 595
Virilization, from androgen
    therapy, 57, 365
Virus diseases, 528–534
  amantadine in, 530–531
  cytosine arabinoside in, 533
  erythromycin in, 458
  idoxuridine in, 531–532
  interferon in, 534
  methisazone in, 532–533
  and photodynamic inactivation of
    herpesviruses, 533–534
Viruses
  drugs affecting, 467, 530–534
  large, 528
    drugs affecting, 467, 475

Viruses (continued)
  reproduction of, 529–530
  small, 528
  specificity of, 528–529
  structure of, 528
Visceral fibers, afferent and
    efferent, 108
Vitamin(s), 553–558
  biotin, 557
  folic acid, 556–557. See also
    Folic acid
  increased requirements for, 64
  niacin, 554–555
    excretion in milk, 576
  pantothenic acid, 557–558
    excretion in milk, 576
Vitamin A, 553
  adverse effects of, 570, 571
  affecting laboratory tests, 588–
    589, 600
  crossing placental barrier, 576
  excretion in milk, 576
Vitamin B_1, 553–554. See also
    Thiamine
Vitamin B_2, 554. See also Ribo-
    flavine
Vitamin B_6, 555
Vitamin B_{12}, 316–317, 555–556
  adverse effects of, 569
  affecting laboratory tests, 588–
    589, 595, 600
  excretion in milk, 576
  interaction with other drugs, 565
Vitamin B complex
  affecting laboratory tests, 595
  excretion in milk, 576
  with vitamin C, interaction with
    other drugs, 565
Vitamin C, 556
  affecting laboratory tests, 588–
    589, 595, 597, 600, 601
  excretion in milk, 576
Vitamin D, 556
  adverse effects of, 572
  affecting laboratory tests, 588–
    589, 595, 600
  and calcium absorption, 348
  crossing placental barrier, 576
  excretion in milk, 576
Vitamin E, 558
  affecting laboratory tests, 588–
    589, 595
  excretion in milk, 576
Vitamin K, 558
  adverse effects of, 572
  affecting laboratory tests, 588–
    589, 591
  blood dyscrasias from, 574
  crossing placental barrier, 576
  excretion in milk, 576
Vitamin K_1, 321
  as poison antidote, 104
Vitamin K_3, 321, 558
Vivactil. See Protriptyline
Vomiting
  antiemetics in, 289
  antihistamines in, 388
  antipsychotic drugs in, 194
  induction of, 90–91, 288
  from morphine, 231, 232
Vomitus, in poisoning, 93

W

Warfarin, 319
    adverse effects of, 571
    crossing placental barrier, 576
    displacement from plasma binding sites, 29
    interaction with other drugs, 275, 565
    resistance to, in rats, 64
Water ash, adverse effects of, 570
Weight
    and adverse drug reactions, 51
    gain from antipsychotic drugs, 196
Weil's disease, treatment of, 421
Wheat germ extracts, affecting laboratory tests, 595
Whitfield's ointment, in tinea infections, 521
Whooping cough, treatment of, 420
Withdrawal reactions
    after alcohol, 80
    after barbiturates, 70
    after cathartics, 297

Withdrawal reactions (continued)
    symptoms in, 68
Worm infections. See Helminthiasis
Wound infections, antimicrobial drugs in, 420, 421, 422
Wuchereria bancrofti, 513
Wyamin sulfate, 143

X

X-5079C, in mycoses, 526–527
Xanthine(s), 254–255
    adverse effects of, 255
    preparation and dosage of, 255
    synthesis of, 229
    therapeutic uses of, 255
Xanthine oxidase inhibitors, interaction with other drugs, 32
Xenalamine, in virus infections, 534
Xerostomia
    from atropine, 131
    from ganglionic blocking agents, 155

Xylene, adverse effects of, 570
Xylocaine. See Lidocaine

Y

Yarrow, adverse effects of, 570
Yomesan, 516, 561

Z

Zarotin. See Ethosuximide
Zephiran. See Benzalkonium chloride
Zinc, tests for, drugs affecting, 581, 583, 585, 587
Zinc oxide, adverse effects of, 568
Zinc undecylenate, in tinea infections, 521
Zoster immune globulin, 561, 562